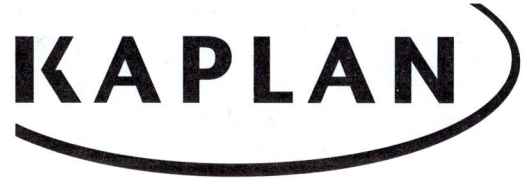

NBDE

Part I Lecture Notes

© 2017 by Kaplan, Inc.

Published by Kaplan Publishing, a division of Kaplan, Inc.
750 Third Avenue
New York, NY 10017

10 9 8 7 6 5 4 3 2 1

Retail ISBN-13: 978-1-5062-0783-4

Course ISBN-13: 978-1-5062-0784-1

Kaplan Publishing print books are available at special quantity discounts to use for sales promotions, employee premiums, or educational purposes. For more information or to purchase books, please call the Simon & Schuster special sales department at 866-506-1949.

Microbiology/Immunology

Tiffany L. Alley, Ph.D.
Lincoln Memorial University
DeBusk College of Osteopathic Medicine

Kim Moscatello, Ph.D.
Lake Erie College of Osteopathic Medicine

Pathology

John Barone, M.D.
Anatomic and Clinical Pathologist

Manuel A. Castro, M.D., AAHIVS
Wilton Health Center (Private Practice)
Nova Southeastern University
LECOM College of Osteopathy

Contents

BIOCHEMISTRY

Section I: Molecular Biology and Biochemistry

Section II: Medical Genetics

PHYSIOLOGY

Section IX: Acid–Base Disturbances

Section X: Endocrinology

Section XI: Gastrointestinal Physiology

ANATOMY

Section I: Early Embryology and Histology: Epithelia

Section II: Gross Anatomy

Section III: Neuroscience

MICROBIOLOGY

IMMUNOLOGY

PATHOLOGY

DENTAL ANATOMY

Biochemistry

Nucleic Acid Structure and Organization

1

Learning Objectives

❏ Explain information related to nucleotide structure and nomenclature

❏ Answer questions about nucleic acids

❏ Use knowledge of organization of DNA

OVERVIEW: CENTRAL DOGMA OF MOLECULAR BIOLOGY

An organism must be able to store and preserve its genetic information, pass that information along to future generations, and express that information as it carries out all the processes of life. The major steps involved in handling genetic information are illustrated by the central dogma of molecular biology. Genetic information is stored in the base sequence of DNA molecules. Ultimately, during the process of gene expression, this information is used to synthesize all the proteins made by an organism. Classically, a gene is a unit of the DNA that encodes a particular protein or RNA molecule. Although this definition is now complicated by our increased appreciation of the ways in which genes may be expressed, it is still useful as a general, working definition.

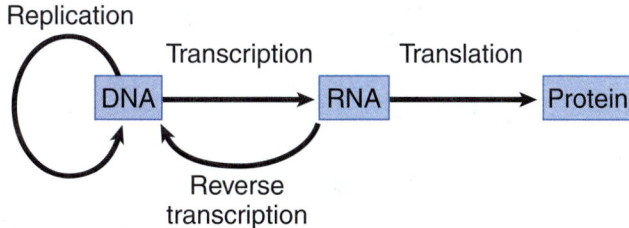

Figure 1-1. Central Dogma of Molecular Biology

Gene Expression and DNA Replication

Gene expression and DNA replication are compared in Table 1-1. Transcription, the first stage in gene expression, involves transfer of information found in a double-stranded DNA molecule to the base sequence of a single-stranded RNA molecule. If the RNA molecule is a messenger RNA, then the process known as translation converts the information in the RNA base sequence to the amino acid sequence of a protein.

When cells divide, each daughter cell must receive an accurate copy of the genetic information. DNA replication is the process in which each chromosome is duplicated before cell division.

Table 1-1. Comparison of Gene Expression and DNA Replication

Gene Expression	DNA Replication
Produces all the proteins an organism requires	Duplicates the chromosomes before cell division
Transcription of DNA: RNA copy of a small section of a chromosome (average size of human gene, 10^4–10^5 nucleotide pairs)	DNA copy of entire chromosome (average size of human chromosome, 10^8 nucleotide pairs)
Transcription occurs in the nucleus throughout interphase	Occurs during S phase
Translation of RNA (protein synthesis) occurs in the cytoplasm throughout the cell cycle.	Replication in nucleus

The concept of the cell cycle can be used to describe the timing of some of these events in a eukaryotic cell. The M phase (mitosis) is the time in which the cell divides to form two daughter cells. Interphase is the term used to describe the time between two cell divisions or mitoses. Gene expression occurs throughout all stages of interphase. Interphase is subdivided as follows:

- G_1 phase (gap 1) is a period of cellular growth preceding DNA synthesis. Cells that have stopped cycling, such as muscle and nerve cells, are said to be in a special state called G_0.

- S phase (DNA synthesis) is the period of time during which DNA replication occurs. At the end of S phase, each chromosome has doubled its DNA content and is composed of two identical sister chromatids linked at the centromere.

- G_2 phase (gap 2) is a period of cellular growth after DNA synthesis but preceding mitosis. Replicated DNA is checked for any errors before cell division.

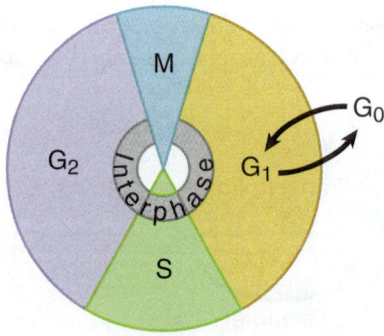

Figure 1-2. The Eukaryotic Cell Cycle

Control of the cell cycle is accomplished at checkpoints between the various phases by strategic proteins such as cyclins and cyclin-dependent kinases. These checkpoints ensure that cells will not enter the next phase of the cycle until the molecular events in the previous cell cycle phase are concluded.

Reverse transcription, which produces DNA copies of an RNA, is more commonly associated with life cycles of retroviruses, which replicate and express their genome through a DNA intermediate (an integrated provirus). Reverse transcription also occurs to a limited extent in human cells, where it plays a role in amplifying certain highly repetitive sequences in the DNA (Chapter 7).

NUCLEOTIDE STRUCTURE AND NOMENCLATURE

Nucleic acids (DNA and RNA) are assembled from nucleotides, which consist of three components: a nitrogenous base, a five-carbon sugar (pentose), and phosphate.

Five-Carbon Sugars

Nucleic acids (as well as nucleosides and nucleotides) are classified according to the pentose they contain. If the pentose is ribose, the nucleic acid is RNA (ribonucleic acid); if the pentose is deoxyribose, the nucleic acid is DNA (deoxyribonucleic acid).

Bases

There are two types of nitrogen-containing bases commonly found in nucleotides: purines and pyrimidines:

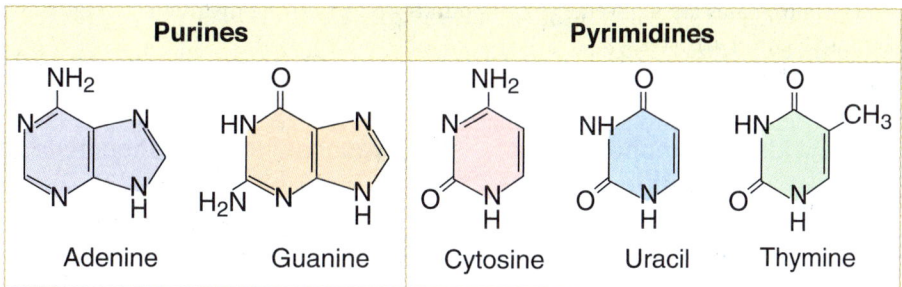

Figure 1-3. Bases Commonly Found in Nucleic Acids

- Purines contain two rings in their structure. The two purines commonly found in nucleic acids are adenine (A) and guanine (G); both are found in DNA and RNA. Other purine metabolites, not usually found in nucleic acids, include xanthine, hypoxanthine, and uric acid.
- Pyrimidines have only one ring. Cytosine (C) is present in both DNA and RNA. Thymine (T) is usually found only in DNA, whereas uracil (U) is found only in RNA.

Nucleosides and Nucleotides

Nucleosides are formed by covalently linking a base to the number 1 carbon of a sugar. The numbers identifying the carbons of the sugar are labeled with "primes" in nucleosides and nucleotides to distinguish them from the carbons of the purine or pyrimidine base.

Adenosine	Deoxythymidine

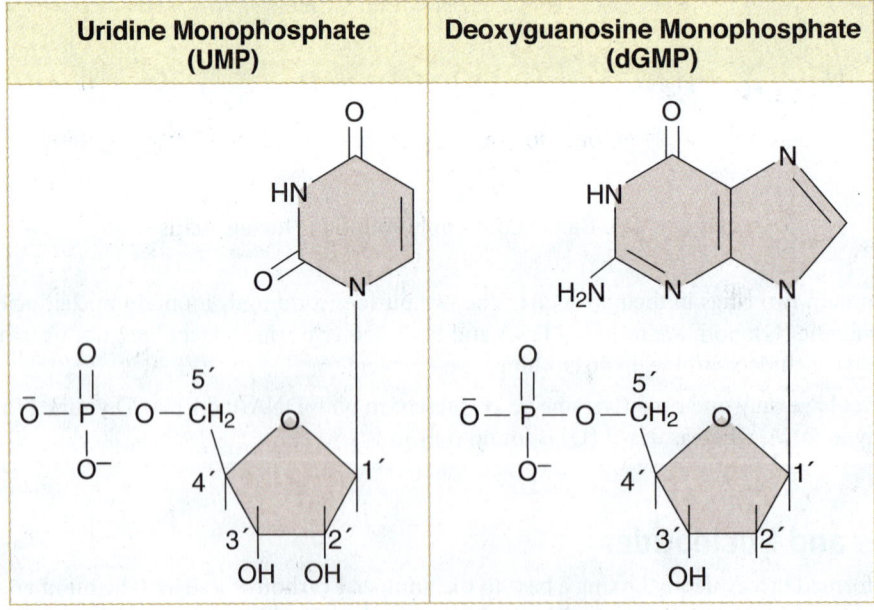

Figure 1-4. Examples of Nucleosides

Nucleotides are formed when one or more phosphate groups is attached to the 5′ carbon of a nucleoside (Figure 1-5). Nucleoside di- and triphosphates are high-energy compounds because of the hydrolytic energy associated with the acid anhydride bonds (Figure 1-6).

Uridine Monophosphate (UMP)	Deoxyguanosine Monophosphate (dGMP)

Figure 1-5. Examples of Nucleotides

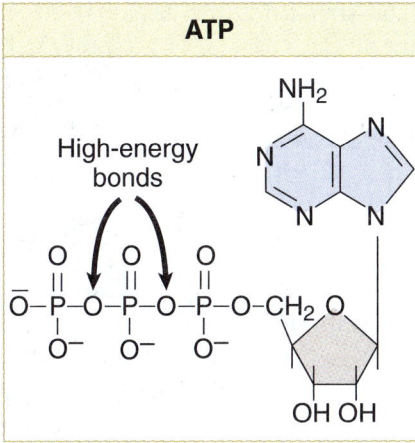

Figure 1-6. High-Energy Bonds in a Nucleoside Triphosphate

The nomenclature for the commonly found bases, nucleosides, and nucleotides is shown in Table 1-2. Note that the "deoxy" part of the names deoxythymidine, dTMP, etc., is sometimes understood, and not expressly stated, because thymine is almost always found attached to deoxyribose.

Table 1-2. Nomenclature of Important Bases, Nucleosides, and Nucleotides

Base	Nucleoside	Nucleotides		
Adenine	Adenosine (Deoxyadenosine)	AMP (dAMP)	ADP (dADP)	ATP (dATP)
Guanine	Guanosine (Deoxyguanosine)	GMP (dGMP)	GDP (dGDP)	GTP (dGTP)
Cytosine	Cytidine (Deoxycytidine)	CMP (dCMP)	CDP (dCDP)	CTP (dCTP)
Uracil	Uridine (Deoxyuridine)	UMP (dUMP)	UDP (dUDP)	UTP (dUTP)
Thymine	(Deoxythymidine)	(dTMP)	(dTDP)	(dTTP)

Names of nucleosides and nucleotides attached to deoxyribose are shown in parentheses.

NUCLEIC ACIDS

Nucleic acids are polymers of nucleotides joined by 3′, 5′-phosphodiester bonds; that is, a phosphate group links the 3′ carbon of a sugar to the 5′ carbon of the next sugar in the chain. Each strand has a distinct 5′ end and 3′ end, and thus has polarity. A phosphate group is often found at the 5′ end, and a hydroxyl group is often found at the 3′ end.

The base sequence of a nucleic acid strand is written by convention, in the 5′→3′ direction (left to right). According to this convention, the sequence of the strand on the left in Figure 1-7 must be written

5′-TCAG-3′ or TCAG:

- If written backward, the ends must be labeled: 3′-GACT-5′
- The positions of phosphates may be shown: pTpCpApG
- In DNA, a "d" (deoxy) may be included: dTdCdAdG

In eukaryotes, DNA is generally double-stranded (dsDNA) and RNA is generally single-stranded (ssRNA). Exceptions occur in certain viruses, some of which have ssDNA genomes and some of which have dsRNA genomes.

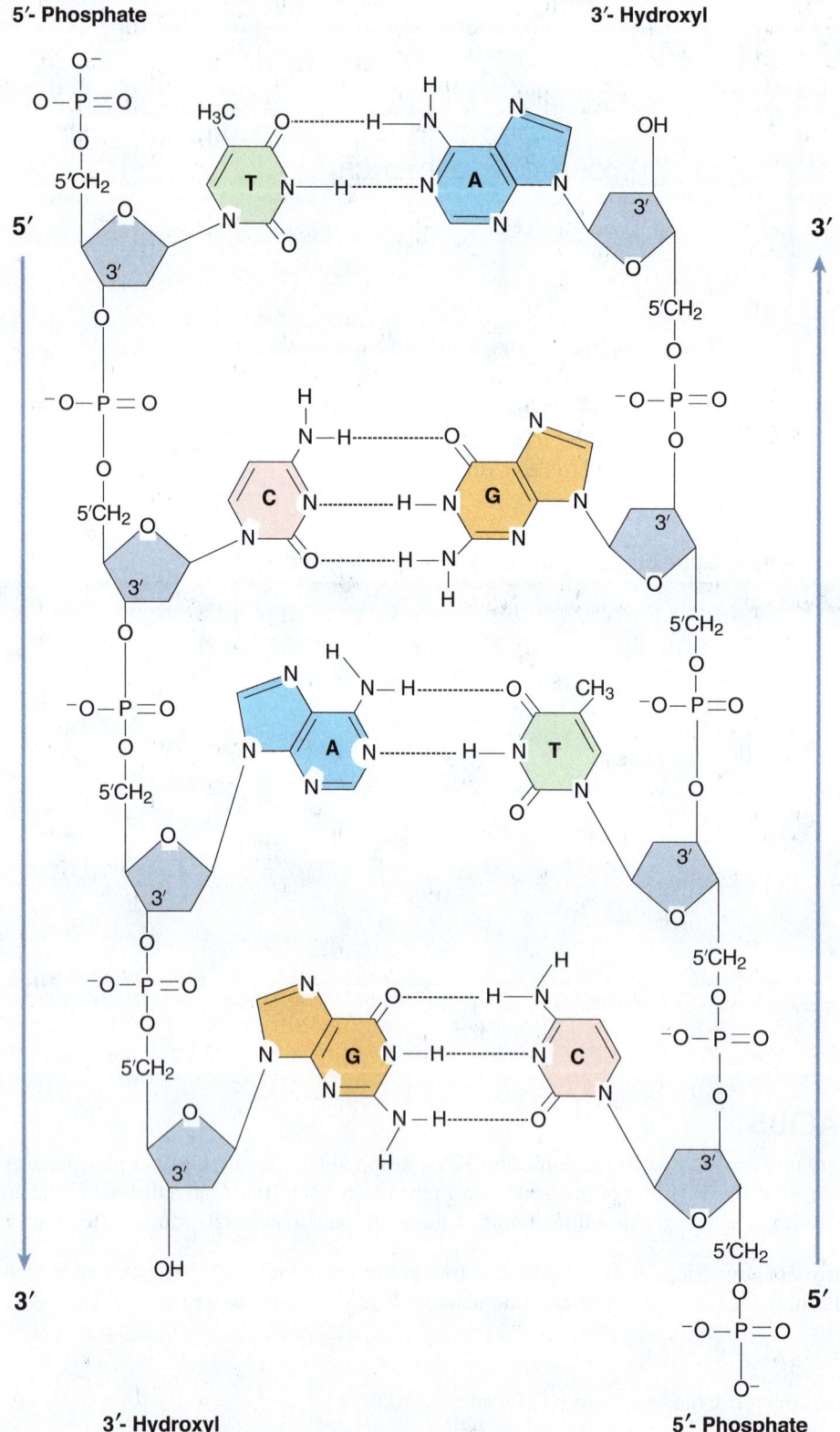

Figure 1-7. Hydrogen-Bonded Base Pairs in DNA

DNA Structure

Figure 1-8 shows an example of a double-stranded DNA molecule. Some of the features of double-stranded DNA include:

- The two strands are antiparallel (opposite in direction).
- The two strands are complementary. A always pairs with T (two hydrogen bonds), and G always pairs with C (three hydrogen bonds). Thus, the base sequence on one strand defines the base sequence on the other strand.
- Because of the specific base pairing, the amount of A equals the amount of T, and the amount of G equals the amount of C. Thus, total purines equals total pyrimidines. These properties are known as Chargaff's rules.

Note

Using Chargaff's Rules

In dsDNA (or dsRNA) (ds = double-stranded)

% A = % T (% U)

% G = % C

% purines = % pyrimidines

A sample of DNA has 10% G; what is the % T?

10% G + 10% C = 20%

therefore, % A + % T must total 80%

40% A and 40% T

Ans: 40% T

With minor modification (substitution of U for T) these rules also apply to dsRNA.

Most DNA occurs in nature as a right-handed double-helical molecule known as Watson-Crick DNA or B-DNA. The hydrophilic sugar-phosphate backbone of each strand is on the outside of the double helix. The hydrogen-bonded base pairs are stacked in the center of the molecule. There are about 10 base pairs per complete turn of the helix. A rare left-handed double-helical form of DNA that occurs in G-C–rich sequences is known as Z-DNA. The biologic function of Z-DNA is unknown, but may be related to gene regulation.

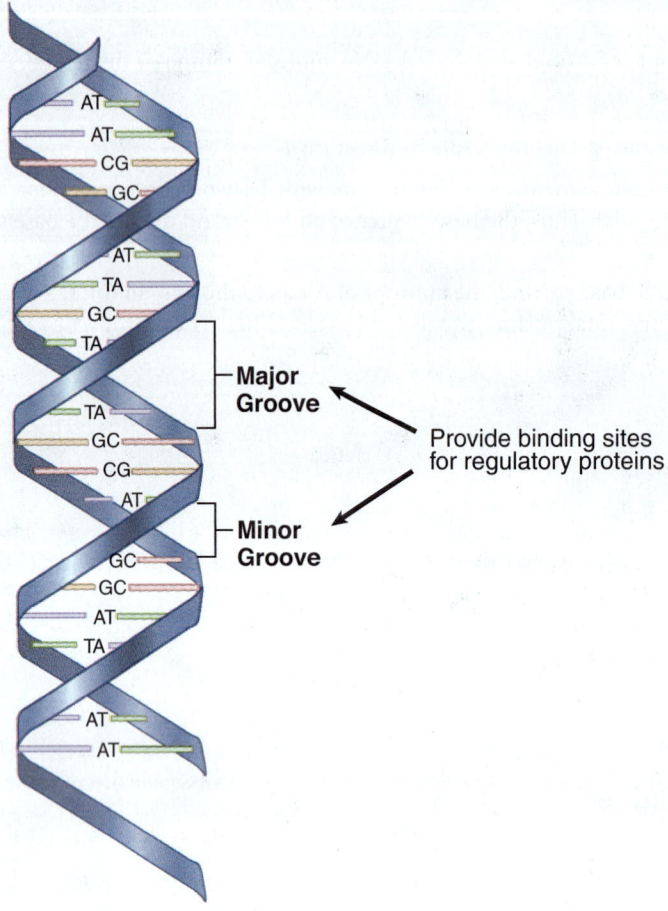

Figure 1-8. The B-DNA Double Helix

Denaturation and Renaturation of DNA

Double-helical DNA can be denatured by conditions that disrupt hydrogen bonding and base stacking, resulting in the "melting" of the double helix into two single strands that separate from each other. No covalent bonds are broken in this process. Heat, alkaline pH, and chemicals such as formamide and urea are commonly used to denature DNA.

Denatured single-stranded DNA can be renatured (annealed) if the denaturing condition is slowly removed. For example, if a solution containing heat-denatured DNA is slowly cooled, the two complementary strands can become base-paired again.

Such renaturation or annealing of complementary DNA strands is an important step in probing a Southern blot and in performing the polymerase chain reaction (reviewed in Chapter 7). In these techniques, a well-characterized probe DNA is added to a mixture of target DNA molecules. The mixed sample is denatured and then renatured. When probe DNA binds to target DNA sequences of sufficient complementarity, the process is called hybridization.

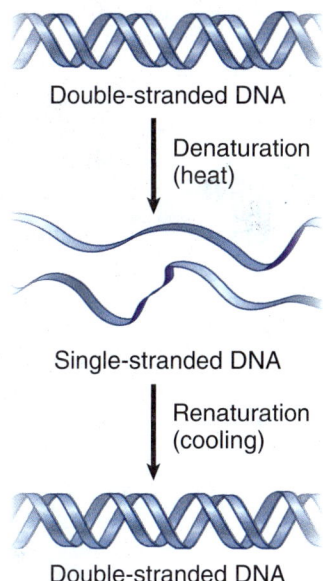

Double-stranded DNA

Denaturation
(heat)

Single-stranded DNA

Renaturation
(cooling)

Double-stranded DNA

Figure 1-9. Denaturation and Renaturation of DNA

ORGANIZATION OF DNA

Large DNA molecules must be packaged in such a way that they can fit inside the cell and still be functional.

Supercoiling

Mitochondrial DNA and the DNA of most prokaryotes are closed circular structures. These molecules may exist as relaxed circles or as supercoiled structures in which the helix is twisted around itself in three-dimensional space. Supercoiling results from strain on the molecule caused by under- or overwinding the double helix:

- Negatively supercoiled DNA is formed if the DNA is wound more loosely than in Watson-Crick DNA. This form is required for most biologic reactions.
- Positively supercoiled DNA is formed if the DNA is wound more tightly than in Watson-Crick DNA.
- Topoisomerases are enzymes that can change the amount of supercoiling in DNA molecules. They make transient breaks in DNA strands by alternately breaking and resealing the sugar-phosphate backbone. For example, in Escherichia coli, DNA gyrase (DNA topoisomerase II) can introduce negative supercoiling into DNA.

Nucleosomes and Chromatin

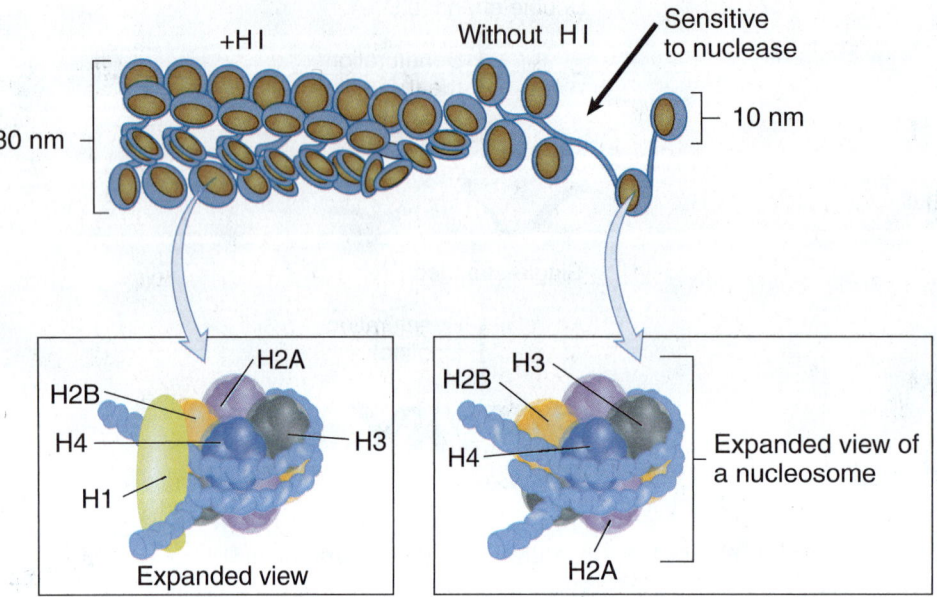

Figure 1-10. Nucleosome and Nucleofilament Structure in Eukaryotic DNA

Nuclear DNA in eukaryotes is found in chromatin associated with histones and nonhistone proteins. The basic packaging unit of chromatin is the nucleosome:

- Histones are rich in lysine and arginine, which confer a positive charge on the proteins.
- Two copies each of histones H2A, H2B, H3, and H4 aggregate to form the histone octamer.
- DNA is wound around the outside of this octamer to form a nucleosome (a series of nucleosomes is sometimes called "beads on a string", but is more properly referred to as a 10nm chromatin fiber).
- Histone H1 is associated with the linker DNA found between nucleosomes to help package them into a solenoid-like structure, which is a thick 30-nm fiber.
- Further condensation occurs to eventually form the chromosome. Each eukaryotic chromosome in Go or G1 contains one linear molecule of double-stranded DNA.

Cells in interphase contain two types of chromatin: euchromatin (more opened and available for gene expression) and heterochromatin (much more highly condensed and associated with areas of the chromosomes that are not expressed).

Euchromatin generally corresponds to the nucleosomes (10-nm fibers) loosely associated with each other (looped 30-nm fibers). Heterochromatin is more highly condensed, producing interphase heterochromatin as well as chromatin characteristic of mitotic chromosomes. Figure 1-11 shows an electron micrograph of an interphase nucleus containing euchromatin, heterochromatin, and a nucleolus. The nucleolus is a nuclear region specialized for ribosome assembly (discussed in Chapter 3).

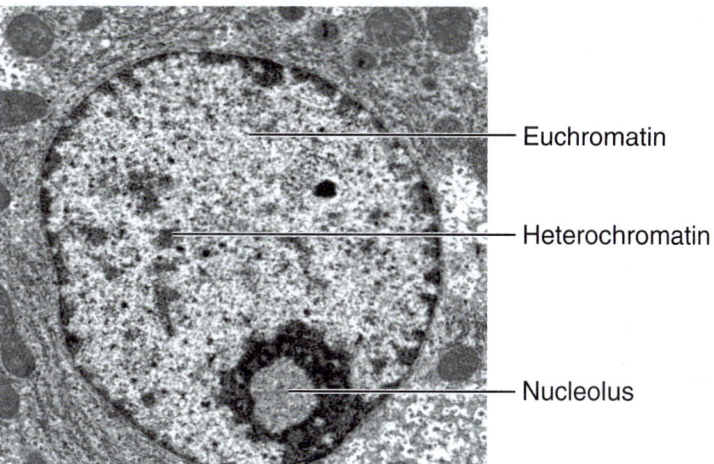

Euchromatin

Heterochromatin

Nucleolus

Figure 1-11. An Interphase Nucleus

During mitosis, all the DNA is highly condensed to allow separation of the sister chromatids. This is the only time in the cell cycle when the chromosome structure is visible. Chromosome abnormalities may be assessed on mitotic chromosomes by karyotype analysis (metaphase chromosomes) and by banding techniques (prophase or prometaphase), which identify aneuploidy, translocations, deletions, inversions, and duplications.

DNA Replication and Repair

Learning Objectives

❏ Explain information related to comparison of DNA and RNA synthesis

❏ Answer questions about steps of DNA replication

❏ Solve problems concerning DNA repair

OVERVIEW OF DNA REPLICATION

Genetic information is transmitted from parent to progeny by replication of parental DNA, a process in which two daughter DNA molecules are produced that are each identical to the parental DNA molecule. During DNA replication, the two complementary strands of parental DNA are pulled apart. Each of these parental strands is then used as a template for the synthesis of a new complementary strand (semiconservative replication). During cell division, each daughter cell receives one of the two identical DNA molecules.

Replication of Prokaryotic and Eukaryotic Chromosomes

The overall process of DNA replication in prokaryotes and eukaryotes is compared here:

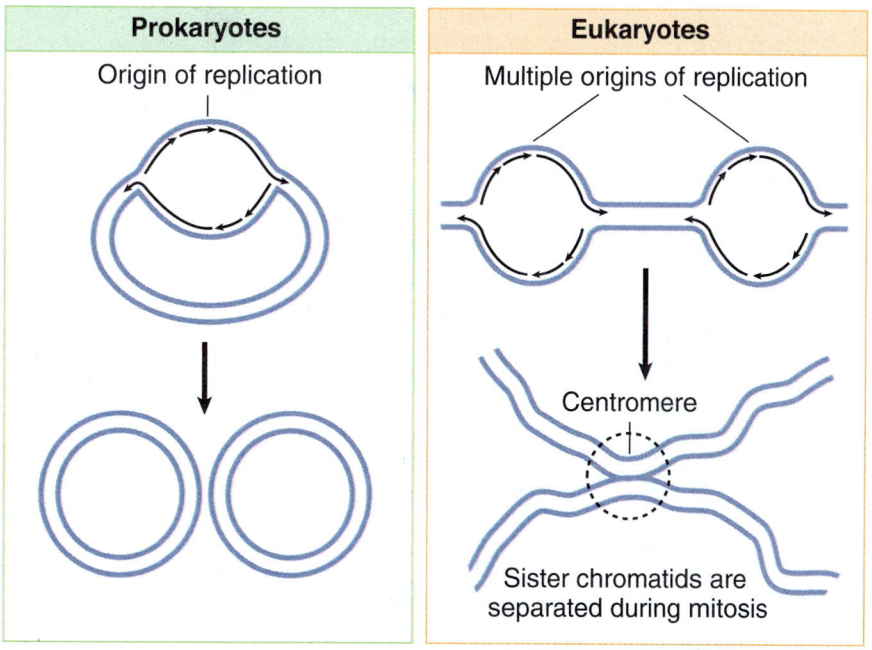

Figure 2-1. DNA Replication by a Semi-Conservative, Bidirectional Mechanism

The bacterial chromosome is a closed, double-stranded circular DNA molecule having a single origin of replication. Separation of the two parental strands of DNA creates two replication forks that move away from each other in opposite directions around the circle. Replication is, thus, a bidirectional process. The two replication forks eventually meet, resulting in the production of two identical circular molecules of DNA.

Each eukaryotic chromosome contains one linear molecule of dsDNA having multiple origins of replication. Bidirectional replication occurs by means of a pair of replication forks produced at each origin. Completion of the process results in the production of two identical linear molecules of dsDNA (sister chromatids). DNA replication occurs in the nucleus during the S phase of the eukaryotic cell cycle. The two identical sister chromatids are separated from each other when the cell divides during mitosis.

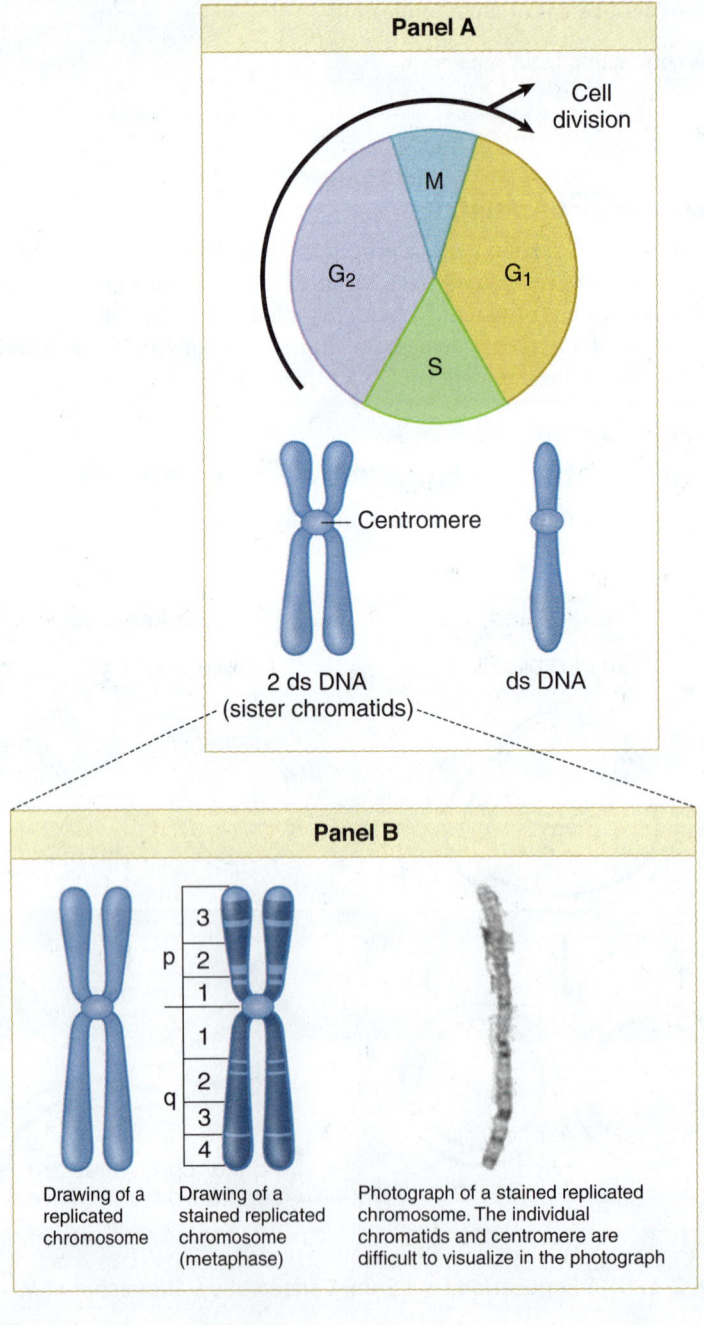

Figure 2-2. Panel A: Eukaryotic Chromosome Replication During S-Phase
Panel B: Different Representations of a Replicated Eukaryotic Chromosome

COMPARISON OF DNA AND RNA SYNTHESIS

The overall process of DNA replication requires the synthesis of both DNA and RNA. These two types of nucleic acids are synthesized by DNA polymerases and RNA polymerases, respectively. DNA synthesis and RNA synthesis are compared in the following figure and table.

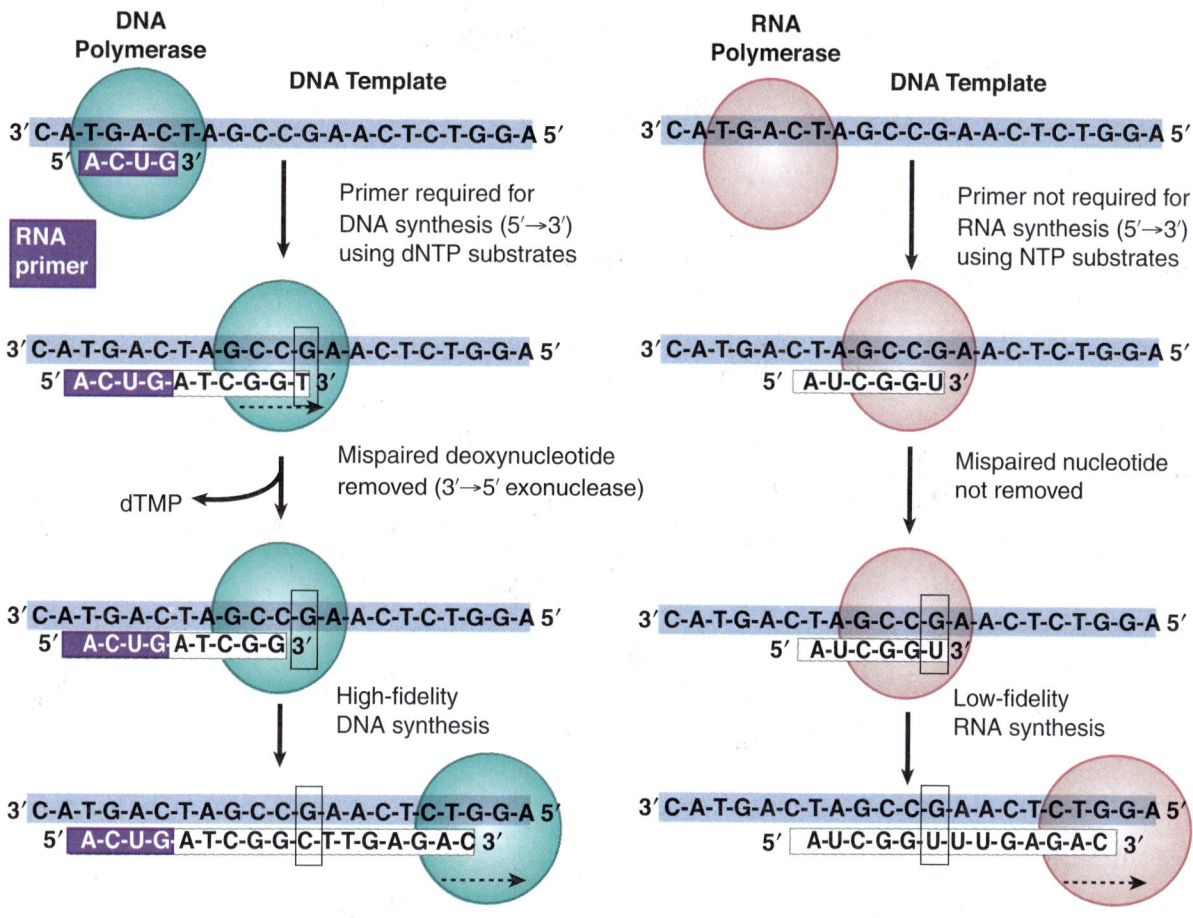

Figure 2-3. Polymerase Enzymes Synthesize DNA and RNA

Table 2-1. Comparison of DNA and RNA Polymerases

	DNA Polymerase	RNA Polymerase
Nucleic acid synthesized (5′ → 3′)	DNA	RNA
Required template (copied 3′ → 5′)	DNA*	DNA*
Required substrates	dATP, dGTP, dCTP, dTTP	ATP, GTP, CTP, UTP
Required primer	RNA (or DNA)	None
Proofreading activity (3′ → 5′ exonuclease)	Yes	No

* Certain DNA and RNA polymerases require RNA templates. These enzymes are most commonly associated with viruses.

Similarities include:

- The newly synthesized strand is made in the $5' \rightarrow 3'$ direction.
- The template strand is scanned in the $3' \rightarrow 5'$ direction.
- The newly synthesized strand is complementary and antiparallel to the template strand.
- Each new nucleotide is added when the $3'$ hydroxyl group of the growing strand reacts with a nucleoside triphosphate, which is base-paired with the template strand. Pyrophosphate (PPi, the last two phosphates) is released during this reaction.

Differences include:

- The substrates for DNA synthesis are the dNTPs, whereas the substrates for RNA synthesis are the NTPs.
- DNA contains thymine, whereas RNA contains uracil.
- DNA polymerases require a primer, whereas RNA polymerases do not. That is, DNA polymerases cannot initiate strand synthesis, whereas RNA polymerases can.
- DNA polymerases can correct mistakes ("proofreading"), whereas RNA polymerases cannot. DNA polymerases have $3' \rightarrow 5'$ exonuclease activity for proofreading.

STEPS OF DNA REPLICATION

The molecular mechanism of DNA replication is shown in Figure 2-4. The sequence of events is as follows:

1. The base sequence at the origin of replication is recognized.
2. Helicase breaks the hydrogen bonds holding the base pairs together. This allows the two parental strands of DNA to begin unwinding and forms two replication forks.
3. Single-stranded DNA binding protein (SSB) binds to the single-stranded portion of each DNA strand, preventing them from reassociating and protecting them from degradation by nucleases.
4. Primase synthesizes a short (about 10 nucleotides) RNA primer in the $5' \rightarrow 3'$ direction, beginning at the origin on each parental strand. The parental strand is used as a template for this process. RNA primers are required because DNA polymerases are unable to initiate synthesis of DNA, and can only extend a strand from the $3'$ end of a preformed "primer."
5. DNA polymerase III begins synthesizing DNA in the $5' \rightarrow 3'$ direction, beginning at the $3'$ end of each RNA primer. The newly synthesized strand is complementary and antiparallel to the parental strand used as a template. This strand can be made continuously in one long piece and is known as the "leading strand."
   - The "lagging strand" is synthesized discontinuously as a series of small fragments (about 1,000 nucleotides long) known as Okazaki fragments. Each Okazaki fragment is initiated by the synthesis of an RNA primer by primase, and then completed by the synthesis of DNA using DNA polymerase III. Each fragment is made in the $5' \rightarrow 3'$ direction.
   - There is a leading and a lagging strand for each of the two replication forks on the chromosome.
6. RNA primers are removed by RNAase H in eukaryotes and an uncharacterized DNA polymerase fills in the gap with DNA. In prokaryotes DNA polymerase I both removes the primer ($5'$ exonuclease) and synthesizes new DNA, beginning at the $3'$ end of the neighboring Okazaki fragment.
7. Both eukaryotic and prokaryotic DNA polymerases have the ability to "proofread" their work by means of a $3' \rightarrow 5'$ exonuclease activity. If DNA polymerase makes a mistake during DNA synthesis, the resulting unpaired base at the $3'$ end of the growing strand is removed before synthesis continues.
8. DNA ligase seals the "nicks" between Okazaki fragments, converting them to a continuous strand of DNA.

9. DNA gyrase (DNA topoisomerase II) provides a "swivel" in front of each replication fork. As helicase unwinds the DNA at the replication forks, the DNA ahead of it becomes overwound and positive supercoils form. DNA gyrase inserts negative supercoils by nicking both strands of DNA, passing the DNA strands through the nick, and then resealing both strands. Quinolones are a family of drugs that block the action of topoisomerases. Nalidixic acid kills bacteria by inhibiting DNA gyrase. Inhibitors of eukaryotic topoisomerase II (etoposide, teniposide) are becoming useful as anticancer agents.

The mechanism of replication in eukaryotes is believed to be very similar to this. However, the details have not yet been completely worked out. The steps and proteins involved in DNA replication in prokaryotes are compared with those used in eukaryotes in Table 2-2.

Eukaryotic DNA Polymerases

- DNA α and δ work together to synthesize both the leading and lagging strands.
- DNA polymerase γ replicates mitochondrial DNA.
- DNA polymerases β and ε are thought to participate primarily in DNA repair. DNA polymerase ε may substitute for DNA polymerase δ in certain cases.

Telomerase

Telomeres are repetitive sequences at the ends of linear DNA molecules in eukaryotic chromosomes. With each round of replication in most normal cells, the telomeres are shortened because DNA polymerase cannot complete synthesis of the 5′ end of each strand. This contributes to the aging of cells, because eventually the telomeres become so short that the chromosomes cannot function properly and the cells die.

Telomerase is an enzyme in eukaryotes used to maintain the telomeres. It contains a short RNA template complementary to the DNA telomere sequence, as well as telomerase reverse transcriptase activity (hTRT). Telomerase is thus able to replace telomere sequences that would otherwise be lost during replication. Normally telomerase activity is present only in embryonic cells, germ (reproductive) cells, and stem cells, but not in somatic cells.

Cancer cells often have relatively high levels of telomerase, preventing the telomeres from becoming shortened and contributing to the immortality of malignant cells.

Table 2-2. Steps and Proteins Involved in DNA Replication

Step in Replication	Prokaryotic Cells	Eukaryotic Cells (Nuclei)
Origin of replication (ori)	One ori site per chromosome	Multiple ori sites per chromosome
Unwinding of DNA double helix	Helicase	Helicase
Stabilization of unwound template strands	Single-stranded DNA-binding protein (SSB)	Single-stranded DNA-binding protein (SSB)
Synthesis of RNA primers	Primase	Primase

Synthesis of DNA
  Leading strand
  Lagging strand
    (Okazaki fragments)
	DNA polymerase III
	DNA polymerase III
		DNA polymerases $\alpha + \delta$
		DNA polymerases $\alpha + \delta$

(Continue)

Step in Replication	Prokaryotic Cells	Eukaryotic Cells (Nuclei)
Removal of RNA primers	DNA polymerase I (5′ → 3′ exonuclease)	RNase H (5′ → 3′ exonuclease)
Replacement of RNA with DNA	DNA polymerase I	DNA polymerase δ
Joining of Okazaki fragments	DNA ligase	DNA ligase
Removal of positive supercoils ahead of advancing replication forks	DNA topoisomerase II (DNA gyrase)	DNA topoisomerase II
Synthesis of telomeres	Not required	Telomerase

Reverse Transcriptase

Reverse transcriptase is an RNA-dependent DNA polymerase that requires an RNA template to direct the synthesis of new DNA. Retroviruses, most notably HIV, use this enzyme to replicate their RNA genomes. DNA synthesis by reverse transcriptase in retroviruses can be inhibited by AZT, ddC, and ddI. These are first generation antiretrovirals.

Eukaryotic cells also contain reverse transcriptase activity:

- Associated with telomerase (hTRT).
- Encoded by retrotransposons (residual viral genomes permanently maintained in human DNA) that play a role in amplifying certain repetitive sequences in DNA (see Chapter 7).

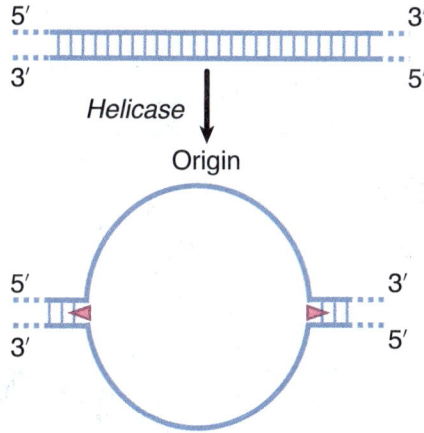

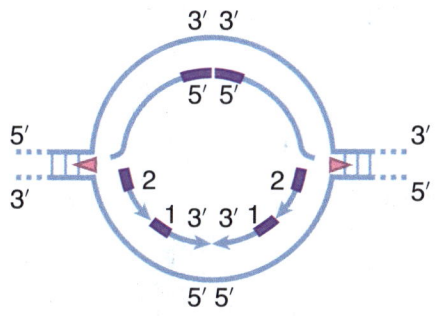

Leading Strand Synthesis (Continuous)

1. *Primase* synthesizes the primer (▬) 5′ to 3′.

2. *DNA polymerases* α and δ extend the primer, moving **into** the replication fork (Leading strand synthesis).

3. *Helicase* (◄) continues to unwind the DNA.

Lagging Strand Synthesis (Discontinuous)

1. *Primase* synthesizes the primer (▬) 5′ to 3′.

2. *DNA polymerases* α and δ extend the primer, moving **away from** the replication fork (Lagging strand synthesis).

3. Synthesis stops when *DNA polymerase* encounters the primer of the leading strand on the other side of the diagram (not shown), or the primer of the previous (Okasaki) fragment.

4. As *helicase* opens more of the replication fork, a third Okasaki fragment will be added.

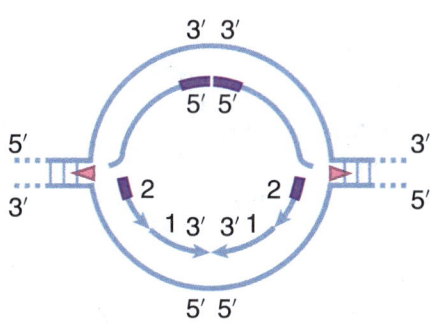

RNase H (5′ exoribonuclease activity) digests the RNA primer from fragment 1. In the eukaryotic cell, *DNA polymerase* extends the next fragment (2), to fill in the gap.

In prokaryotic cells *DNA polymerase 1* has both the 5′ exonuclease activity to remove primers, and the *DNA polymerase* activity to extend the next fragment (2) to fill in the gap.

In both types of cells *DNA ligase* connects fragments 1 and 2 by making a phosphodiester bond.

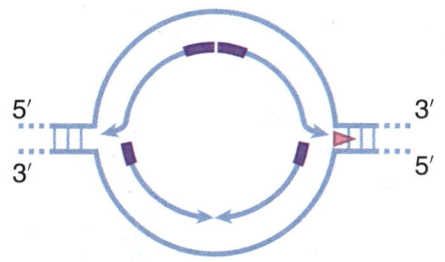

This whole process repeats to remove all RNA primers from both the leading and lagging strands.

Figure 2-4. DNA Replication

DNA REPAIR

The structure of DNA can be damaged in a number of ways through exposure to chemicals or radiation. Incorrect bases can also be incorporated during replication. Multiple repair systems have evolved, allowing cells to maintain the sequence stability of their genomes. If cells are allowed to replicate their DNA using a damaged template, there is a high risk of introducing stable mutations into the new DNA. Thus any defect in DNA repair carries an increased risk of cancer. Most DNA repair occurs in the G1 phase of the eukaryotic cell cycle. Mismatch repair occurs in the G2 phase to correct replication errors.

Table 2-3. DNA Repair

Damage	Cause	Recognition/Excision Enzyme	Repair Enzymes
Thymine dimers (G_1)	UV radiation	Excision endonuclease (deficient in Xeroderma pigmentosum)	DNA polymerase DNA ligase
Mismatched base (G_2)	DNA replication errors	A mutation on one of two genes, hMSH2 or hMLH1, initiates defective repair of DNA mismatches, resulting in a condition known as hereditary nonpolyposis colorectal cancer—HNPCC.	DNA polymerase DNA ligase
Cytosine deamination G_1	Spontaneous/heat	Uracil glycosylase AP endonuclease	DNA polymerase DNA ligase

Repair of Thymine Dimers

Ultraviolet light induces the formation of dimers between adjacent thymines in DNA (also occasionally between other adjacent pyrimidines). The formation of thymine dimers interferes with DNA replication and normal gene expression. Thymine dimers are eliminated from DNA by a nucleotide excision-repair mechanism.

Transcription and RNA Processing 3

Learning Objectives

❏ Interpret scenarios about production of other classes of RNA

❏ Demonstrate understanding of transcription terminology

❏ Answer questions about production of messenger RNA

❏ Demonstrate understanding of how ribosomal RNA (rRNA) is used to construct ribosomes

❏ Explain information related to how transfer RNA (tRNA) carries activated amino acids for translation

OVERVIEW OF TRANSCRIPTION

The first stage in the expression of genetic information is transcription of the information in the base sequence of a double-stranded DNA molecule to form the base sequence of a single-stranded molecule of RNA. For any particular gene, only one strand of the DNA molecule, called the template strand, is copied by RNA polymerase as it synthesizes RNA in the 5′ to 3′ direction. Because RNA polymerase moves in the 3′ to 5′ direction along the template strand of DNA, the RNA product is antiparallel and complementary to the template. RNA polymerase recognizes start signals (promoters) and stop signals (terminators) for each of the thousands of transcription units in the genome of an organism. The following figure illustrates the arrangement and direction of transcription for several genes on a DNA molecule.

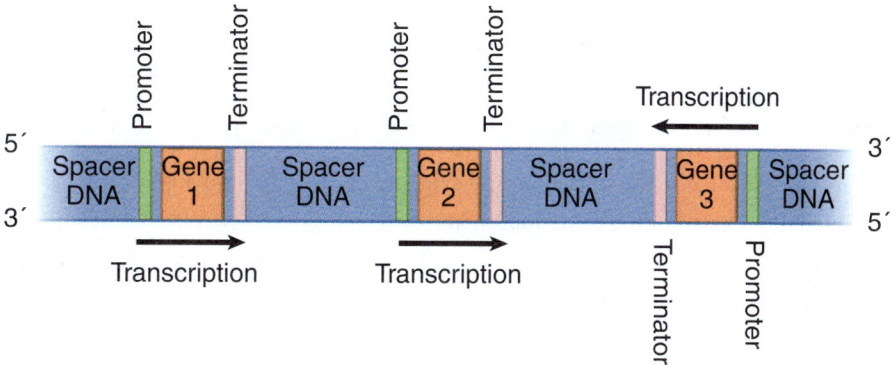

Figure 3-1. Transcription of Several Genes on a Chromosome

TYPES OF RNA

RNA molecules play a variety of roles in the cell. The major types of RNA are:

- Ribosomal RNA (rRNA), which is the most abundant type of RNA in the cell. It is used as a structural component of the ribosome. Ribosomal RNA associates with ribosomal proteins to form the complete, functional ribosome.

- Transfer RNA (tRNA), which is the second most abundant type of RNA. Its function is to carry amino acids to the ribosome, where they will be linked together during protein synthesis.

- Messenger RNA (mRNA), which carries the information specifying the amino acid sequence of a protein to the ribosome. Messenger RNA is the only type of RNA that is translated. The mRNA population in a cell is very heterogeneous in size and base sequence, as the cell has essentially a different mRNA molecule for each of the thousands of different proteins made by that cell.

- Heterogeneous nuclear RNA (hnRNA or pre-mRNA), which is found only in the nucleus of eukaryotic cells. It represents precursors of mRNA, formed during its posttranscriptional processing.

- Small nuclear RNA (snRNA), which is also only found in the nucleus of eukaryotes. One of its major functions is to participate in splicing (removal of introns) mRNA.

- Ribozymes, which are RNA molecules with enzymatic activity. They are found in both prokaryotes and eukaryotes.

PRODUCTION OF OTHER CLASSES OF RNA

Genes encoding other classes of RNA are also expressed. The RNA products are not translated to produce proteins, but rather serve different roles in the process of translation.

RNA POLYMERASES

There is a single prokaryotic RNA polymerase that synthesizes all types of RNA in the cell. The core polymerase responsible for making the RNA molecule has the subunit structure $\alpha2\beta\beta'$. A protein factor called sigma (σ) is required for the initiation of transcription at a promoter. Sigma factor is released immediately after initiation of transcription. Termination of transcription sometimes requires a protein called rho (ρ) factor. The prokaryotic RNA polymerase is inhibited by rifampin. Actinomycin D binds to the DNA, preventing transcription.

There are three eukaryotic RNA polymerases, distinguished by the particular types of RNA they produce.

- RNA polymerase I is located in the nucleolus and synthesizes 28S, 18S, and 5.8S rRNAs.
- RNA polymerase II is located in the nucleoplasm and synthesizes hnRNA/mRNA and some snRNA.
- RNA polymerase III is located in the nucleoplasm and synthesizes tRNA, some snRNA, and 5S rRNA.

Transcription factors (such as TFIID for RNA polymerase II) help to initiate transcription. The requirements for termination of transcription in eukaryotes are not well understood. All transcription can be inhibited by actinomycin D. In addition, RNA polymerase II is inhibited by α-amanitin (a toxin from certain mushrooms).

Table 3-1. Comparison of RNA Polymerases

Prokaryotic	Eukaryotic
Single RNA	RNAP 1: rRNA (nucleolus) Except 5S rRNA
polymerase	RNAP 2: hnRNA/mRNA and some snRNA
($\alpha^2\beta\beta'$)	RNAP 3: tRNA, 5S rRNA

(Continue)

Prokaryotic	Eukaryotic
Requires sigma (σ) to initiate at a promoter	No sigma, but transcription factors (TFIID) bind before RNA polymerase
Sometimes requires rho (ρ) to terminate	No rho required
Inhibited by rifampin Actinomycin D	RNAP 2 inhibited by α-amanitin (mushrooms) Actinomycin D

TRANSCRIPTION: IMPORTANT CONCEPTS AND TERMINOLOGY

RNA is synthesized by a DNA-dependent RNA polymerase (uses DNA as a template for the synthesis of RNA). Important terminology used when discussing transcription is illustrated in Figure 3-2.

- RNA polymerase locates genes in DNA by searching for promoter regions. The promoter is the binding site for RNA polymerase. Binding establishes where transcription begins, which strand of DNA is used as the template, and in which direction transcription proceeds. No primer is required.

- RNA polymerase moves along the template strand in the 3′ to 5′ direction as it synthesizes the RNA product in the 5′ to 3′ direction using NTPs (ATP, GTP, CTP, UTP) as substrates. RNA polymerase does not proof-read its work. The RNA product is complementary and antiparallel to the template strand.

- The coding (antitemplate) strand is not used during transcription. It is identical in sequence to the RNA molecule, except that RNA contains uracil instead of the thymine found in DNA.

- By convention, the base sequence of a gene is given from the coding strand (5′ → 3′).

- In the vicinity of a gene, a numbering system is used to identify the location of important bases. The first base transcribed as RNA is defined as the +1 base of that gene region.

  – To the left (5′, or upstream) of this starting point for transcription, bases are −1, −2, −3, etc.

  – To the right (3′, or downstream) of this point, bases are +2, +3, etc.

- Transcription ends when RNA polymerase reaches a termination signal.

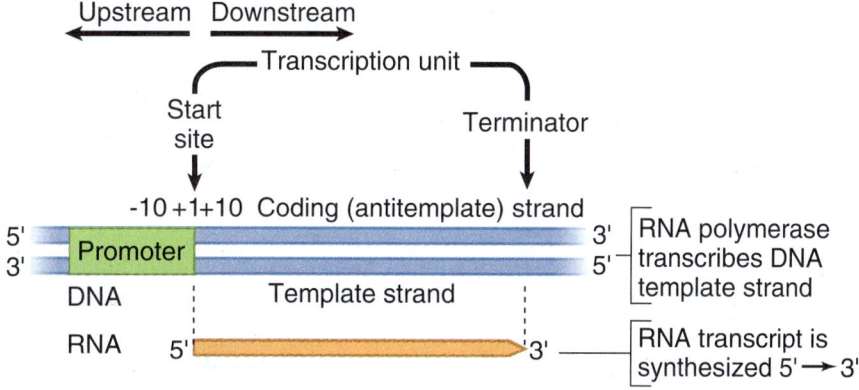

Figure 3-2. Transcription of DNA

Flow of Genetic Information From DNA to Protein

For the case of a gene coding for a protein, the relationship among the sequences found in double-stranded DNA, single-stranded mRNA, and protein is illustrated in Figure 3-3. Messenger RNA is synthesized in the 5′ to 3′ direction. It is complementary and antiparallel to the template strand of DNA. The ribosome translates the mRNA in the 5′ to 3′ direction, as it synthesizes the protein from the amino to the carboxyl terminus.

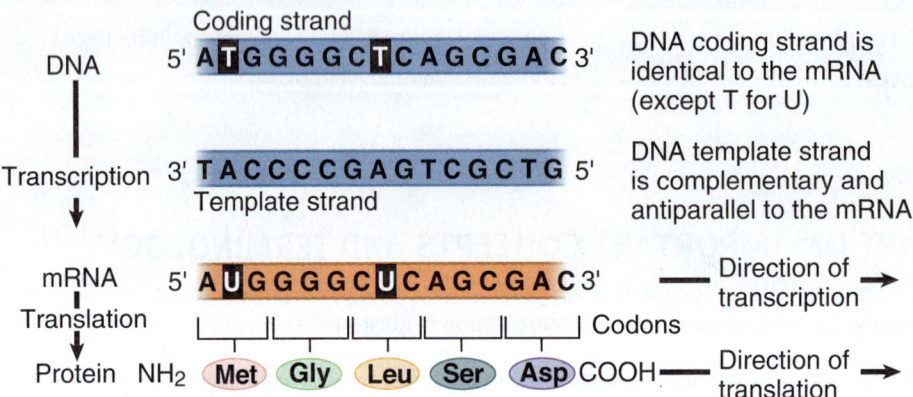

Figure 3-3. Flow of Genetic Information from DNA to Protein

PRODUCTION OF PROKARYOTIC MESSENGER RNA

The structure and expression of a typical prokaryotic gene coding for a protein are illustrated in Figure 3-4. The following events occur during the expression of this gene:

1. With the help of sigma factor, RNA polymerase recognizes and binds to the promoter region. The bacterial promoter contains two "consensus" sequences, called the Pribnow box (or TATA box) and the –35 sequence. The promoter identifies the start site for transcription and orients the enzyme on the template strand. The RNA polymerase separates the two strands of DNA as it reads the base sequence of the template strand.

2. Transcription begins at the +1 base pair. Sigma factor is released as soon as transcription is initiated.

3. The core polymerase continues moving along the template strand in the 3′ to 5′ direction, synthesizing the mRNA in the 5′ to 3′ direction.

4. RNA polymerase eventually reaches a transcription termination signal, at which point it will stop transcription and release the completed mRNA molecule. There are two kinds of transcription terminators commonly found in prokaryotic genes:

   • Rho-independent termination occurs when the newly formed RNA folds back on itself to form a GC-rich hairpin loop closely followed by 6–8 U residues. These two structural features of the newly synthesized RNA promote dissociation of the RNA from the DNA template. This is the type of terminator shown in Figure 3-4.

   • Rho-dependent termination requires participation of rho factor. This protein binds to the newly formed RNA and moves toward the RNA polymerase that has paused at a termination site. Rho then displaces RNA polymerase from the 3′ end of the RNA.

5. Transcription and translation can occur simultaneously in bacteria. Because there is no processing of prokaryotic mRNA (no introns), ribosomes can begin translating the message even before transcription is complete. Ribosomes bind to a sequence called the Shine-Dalgarno sequence in the 5′ untranslated region (UTR) of the message. Protein synthesis begins at an AUG codon at the beginning of the coding region and continues until the ribosome reaches a stop codon at the end of the coding region.

6. The ribosome translates the message in the 5′ to 3′ direction, synthesizing the protein from amino terminus to carboxyl terminus.

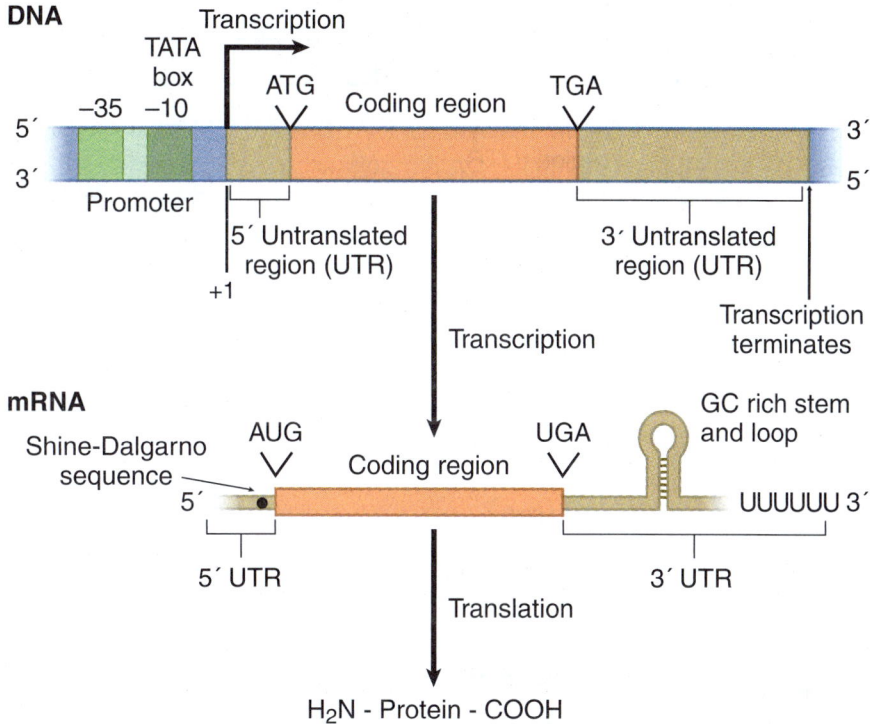

Figure 3-4. Expression of a Prokaryotic Protein Coding Gene

The mRNA produced by the gene shown is a monocistronic message. That is, it is transcribed from a single gene and codes for only a single protein. The word cistron is another name for a gene. Some bacterial operons (for example, the lactose operon) produce polycistronic messages. In these cases, related genes grouped together in the DNA are transcribed as one unit. The mRNA in this case contains information from several genes and codes for several different proteins.

PRODUCTION OF EUKARYOTIC MESSENGER RNA

In eukaryotes, most genes are composed of coding segments (exons) interrupted by noncoding segments (introns). Both exons and introns are transcribed in the nucleus. Introns are removed during processing of the RNA molecule in the nucleus. In eukaryotes, all mRNA is monocistronic. The mature mRNA is translated in the cytoplasm. The structure and transcription of a typical eukaryotic gene coding for a protein is illustrated in Figure 3-5. Transcription of this gene occurs as follows:

1. With the help of proteins called transcription factors, RNA polymerase II recognizes and binds to the promoter region. The basal promoter region of eukaryotic genes usually has two consensus sequences called the TATA box (also called Hogness box) and the CAAT box.

2. RNA polymerase II separates the strands of the DNA over a short region to initiate transcription and read the DNA sequence. The template strand is read in the 3′ to 5′ direction as the RNA product (the primary transcript) is synthesized in the 5′ to 3′ direction. Both exons and introns are transcribed.

3. RNA polymerase II ends transcription when it reaches a termination signal. These signals are not well understood in eukaryotes.

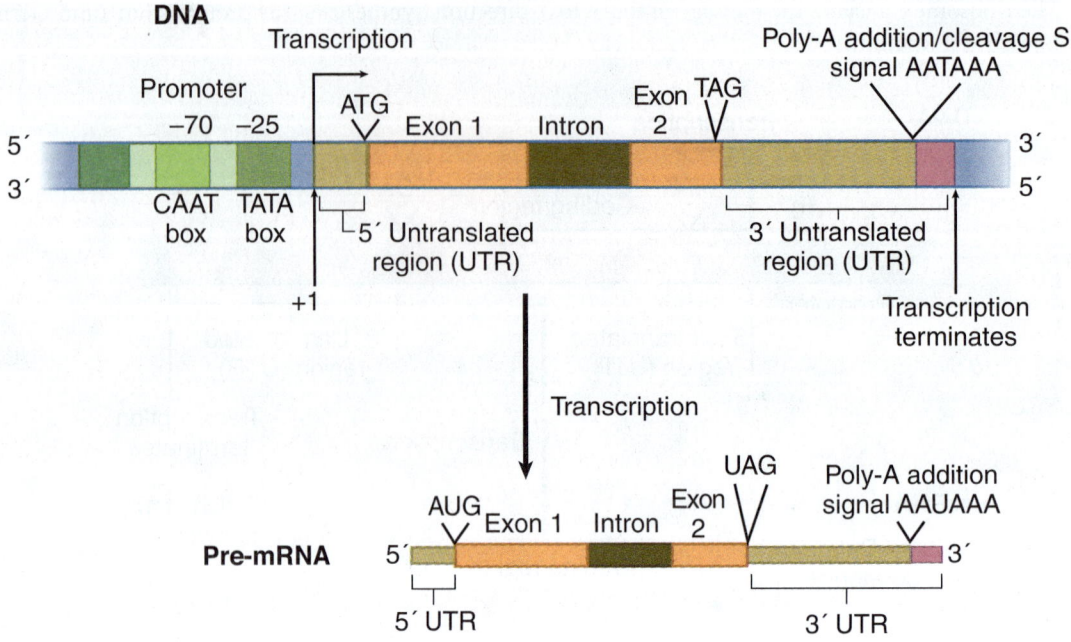

Figure 3-5. A Eukaryotic Transcription Unit

Processing of Eukaryotic Pre-Messenger RNA

The primary transcript must undergo extensive posttranscriptional processing inside the nucleus to form the mature mRNA molecule. These processing steps include the following:

1. A 7-methylguanosine cap is added to the 5′ end while the RNA molecule is still being synthesized. The cap structure serves as a ribosome-binding site and also helps to protect the mRNA chain from degradation.

2. A poly-A tail is attached to the 3′ end. In this process, an endonuclease cuts the molecule on the 3′ side of the sequence AAUAAA (poly-A addition signal), then poly-A polymerase adds the poly-A tail (about 200 As) to the new 3′ end. The poly-A tail protects the message against rapid degradation and aids in its transport to the cytoplasm. A few mRNAs (for example, histone mRNAs) have no poly-A tails.

3. Introns are removed from hnRNA by splicing, accomplished by spliceosomes (also known as an snRNP, or snurp), which are complexes of snRNA and protein. The hnRNA molecule is cut at splice sites at the 5′ (donor) and 3′ (acceptor) ends of the intron. The intron is excised in the form of a lariat structure and degraded. Neighboring exons are joined together to assemble the coding region of the mature mRNA.

4. All of the intermediates in this processing pathway are collectively known as hnRNA.

5. The mature mRNA molecule is transported to the cytoplasm, where it is translated to form a protein.

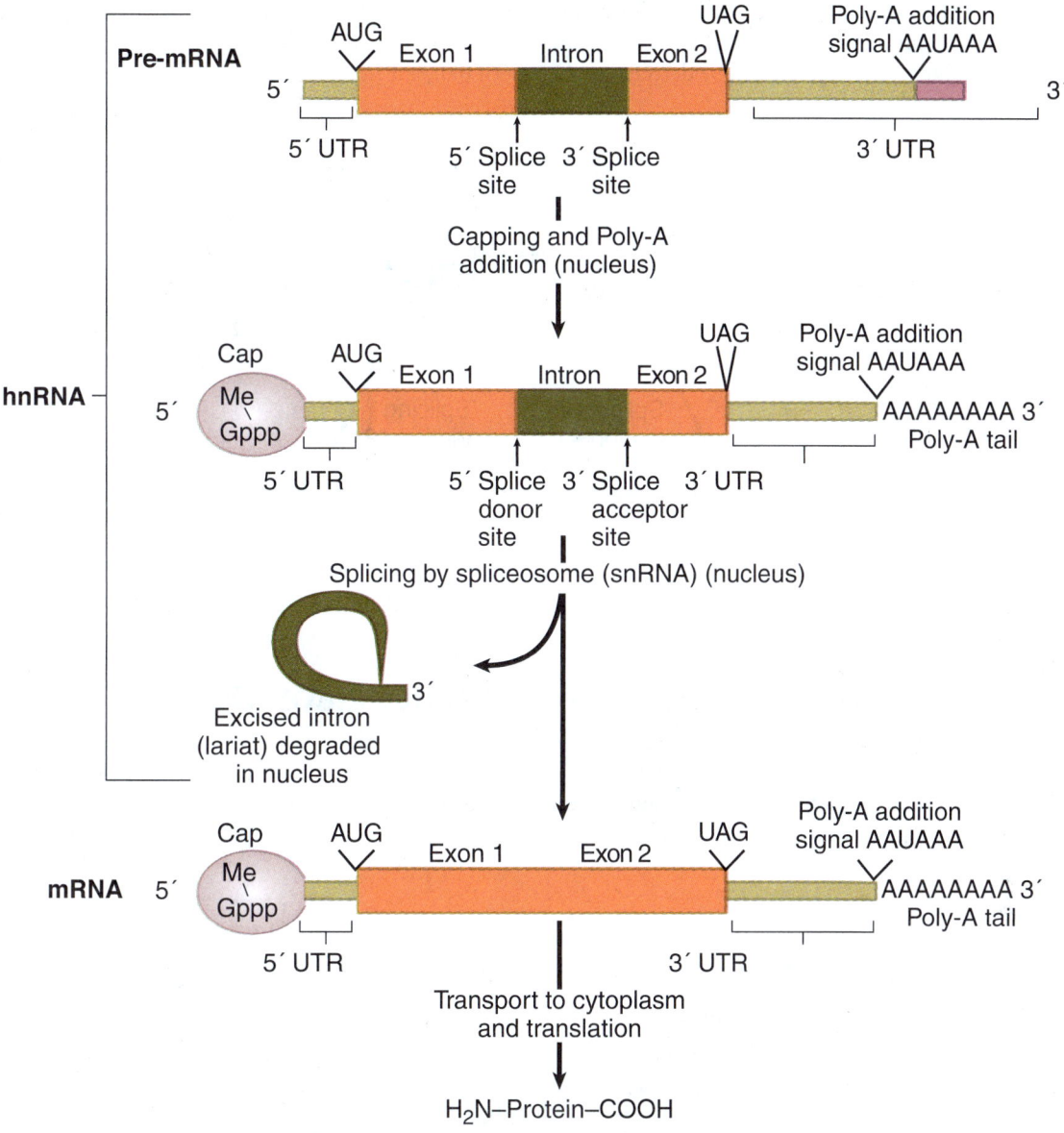

Figure 3-6. Processing Eukaryotic Pre-mRNA

ALTERNATIVE SPLICING OF EUKARYOTIC PRIMARY PRE-mRNA TRANSCRIPTS

For some genes, the primary transcript is spliced differently to produce two or more variants of a protein from the same gene. This process is known as alternative splicing and is illustrated in Figure 3-7. Variants of the muscle proteins tropomyosin and troponin T are produced in this way. The synthesis of membrane-bound immunoglobulins by unstimulated B lymphocytes, as opposed to secreted immunoglobulins by antigen-stimulated B lymphocytes, also involves alternative splicing.

The primary transcripts from a large percentage of genes undergo alternative splicing. This may occur within the same cell, or the primary transcript of a gene may be alternatively spliced in different tissues, giving rise to tissue-specific protein products. By alternative splicing, an organism can make many more different proteins than it has genes to encode. A current estimate of the number of human proteins is at least 100,000, whereas the current estimate of human genes is about only 20,000 to 25,000. These figures should not be memorized because they may change upon more research. Alternative splicing can be detected by Northern blot, a technique discussed in chapter 7.

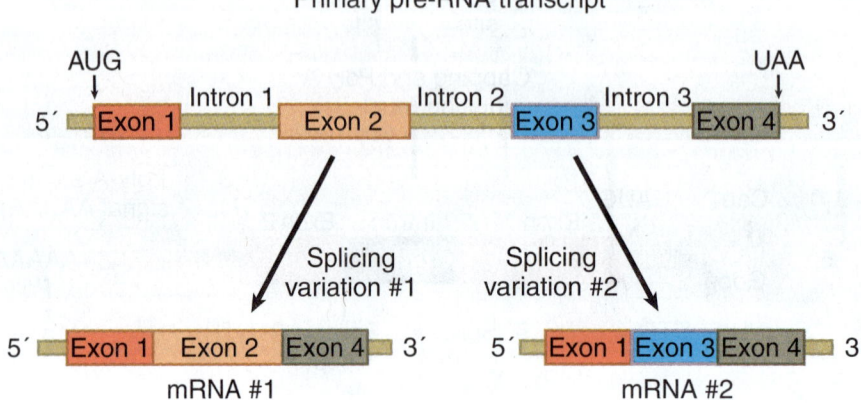

Figure 3-7. Alternative Splicing of Eukaryotic hnRNA (pre-mRNA) to Produce Different Proteins

RIBOSOMAL RNA (rRNA) IS USED TO CONSTRUCT RIBOSOMES

Eukaryotic ribosomal RNA is transcribed in the nucleolus by RNA polymerase I as a single piece of 45S RNA, which is subsequently cleaved to yield 28S rRNA, 18S rRNA, and 5.8S rRNA. RNA polymerase III transcribes the 5S rRNA unit from a separate gene. The ribosomal subunits assemble in the nucleolus as the rRNA pieces combine with ribosomal proteins. Eukaryotic ribosomal subunits are 60S and 40S. They join during protein synthesis to form the whole 80S ribosome.

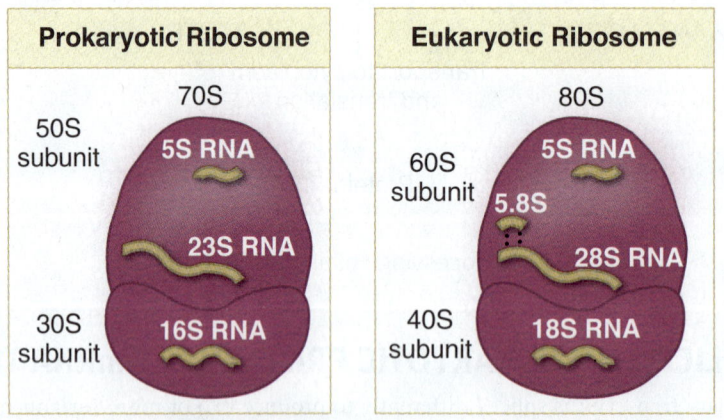

Figure 3-8. The Composition of Prokaryotic and Eukaryotic Ribosomes

The large and small prokaryotic ribosomal subunits are 50S and 30S, respectively. The complete prokaryotic ribosome is a 70S particle. (Note: The S values are determined by behavior of the particles in an ultracentrifuge. They are a function of both size and shape, and therefore the numbers are not additive.) Note also that the differences in the prokaryotic and eukaryotic ribosome contribute to selective toxicity-the ability of antibiotics to kill a bacterial cell while not harming a human cell.

TRANSFER RNA (tRNA) CARRIES ACTIVATED AMINO ACIDS FOR TRANSLATION

There are many different specific tRNAs. Each tRNA carries only one type of activated amino acid for making proteins during translation. The genes encoding these tRNAs in eukaryotic cells are transcribed by RNA polymerase III. The tRNAs enter the cytoplasm where they combine with their appropriate amino acids. Although all tRNAs have the same general shape shown in Figure 3-9, small structural features distinguish among them.

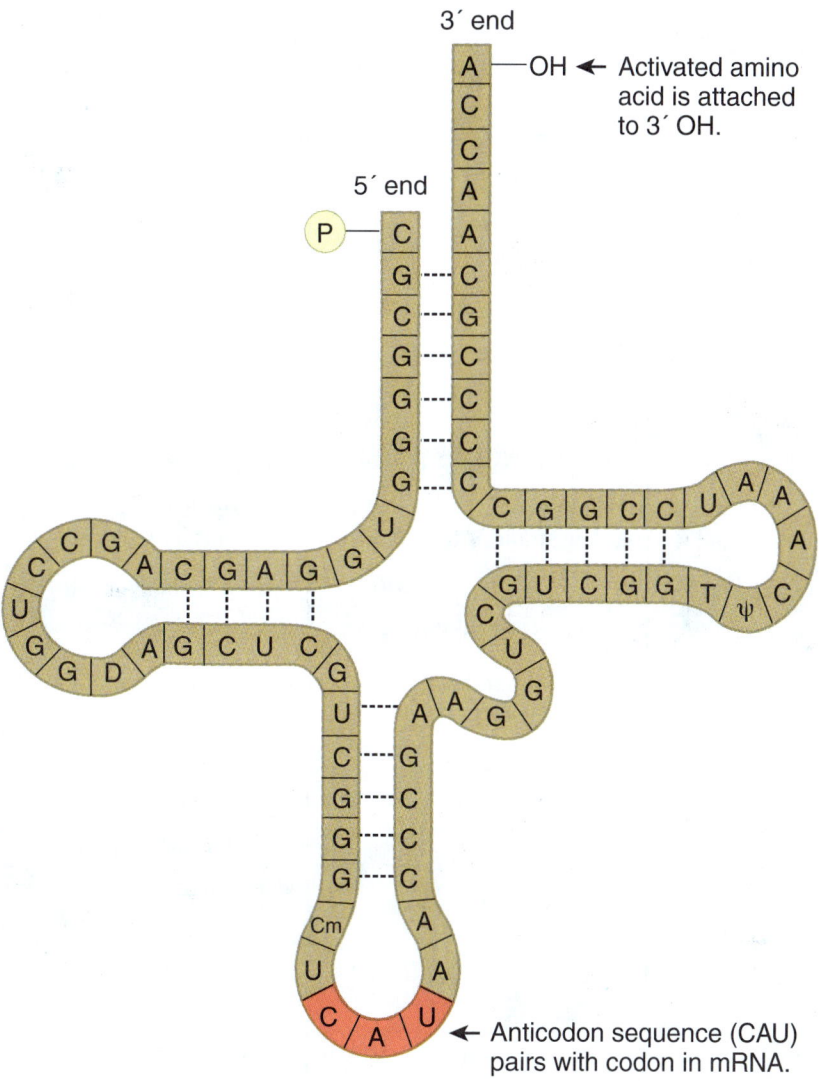

Figure 3-9. Transfer RNA (tRNA)

RNA Editing

RNA editing is a process by which some cells make discrete changes to specific nucleotide sequences within a RNA molecule after its gene has been transcribed by RNA polymerase. Posttranscription editing events may include insertion, deletion, and base alterations of nucleotides (such as adenine deamination) within the edited RNA molecule. RNA editing has been observed in some mRNA, rRNA, mRNA, or tRNA molecules in humans. An important example is cytosine-to-uracil deamination in the apoprotein B gene. Apoprotein B100 is expressed in the liver, and apoprotein B48 is expressed in the intestines. In the intestines, the mRNA is edited from a CAA sequence to be UAA, a stop codon, thus producing the shorter apoprotein B48 form.

Table 3-2. Summary of Important Points About Transcription and RNA Processing

	Prokaryotic	Eukaryotic
Gene regions	May be polycistronic	Always monocistronic
	Genes are continuous coding regions	Genes have exons and introns
	Very little spacer (noncoding) DNA between genes	Large spacer (noncoding) DNA between genes
RNA polymerase	Core enzyme: $\alpha_2\beta\beta'$	RNA polymerase I: rRNA
		RNA polymerase II: mRNA; snRNA
		RNA polymerase III: tRNA, 5S RNA
Initiation of transcription	Promoter (−10) TATAAT and (−35) sequence	Promoter (−25) TATA and (−70) CAAT
	Sigma initiation subunit required to recognize promoter	Transcription factors (TFIID) bind promoter
mRNA synthesis	Template read 3′ to 5′; mRNA synthesized 5′ to 3′; gene sequence specified from coding strand 5′ to 3′; transcription begins at +1 base	
Termination of transcription	Stem and loop + UUUUU	Not well characterized
	Stem and loop + rho factor	
Relationship of RNA transcript to DNA	RNA is antiparallel and complementary to DNA template strand; RNA is identical (except U substitutes for T) to DNA coding strand	
Posttranscriptional processing of hnRNA (pre-mRNA)	None	In nucleus:
		5′ cap (7-MeG)
		3′ tail (poly-A sequence)
		Removal of introns from pre-RNA
		• Alternative splicing yields variants of protein product
Ribosomes	70S (30S and 50S)	80S (40S and 60S)
	rRNA and protein	rRNA and protein
tRNA	Cloverleaf secondary structure	
	• Acceptor arm (CCA) carries amino acid	
	• Anticodon arm; anticodon complementary and antiparallel to codon in mRNA	

The Genetic Code, Mutations, and Translation

4

Learning Objectives

❏ Demonstrate understanding of the Genetic Code

❏ Demonstrate understanding of translation (protein synthesis)

❏ Interpret scenarios about protein synthesis and protein folding

❏ Demonstrate understanding of co- and posttranslational covalent modifications

❏ Solve problems concerning posttranslational modifications of collagen

OVERVIEW OF TRANSLATION

The second stage in gene expression is translating the nucleotide sequence of a messenger RNA molecule into the amino acid sequence of a protein. The genetic code is defined as the relationship between the sequence of nucleotides in DNA (or its RNA transcripts) and the sequence of amino acids in a protein. Each amino acid is specified by one or more nucleotide triplets (codons) in the DNA.

During translation, mRNA acts as a working copy of the gene in which the codons for each amino acid in the protein have been transcribed from DNA to mRNA. tRNAs serve as adapter molecules that couple the codons in mRNA with the amino acids they each specify, thus aligning them in the appropriate sequence before peptide bond formation. Translation takes place on ribosomes, complexes of protein and rRNA that serve as the molecular machines coordinating the interactions between mRNA, tRNA, the enzymes, and the protein factors required for protein synthesis. Many proteins undergo posttranslational modifications as they prepare to assume their ultimate roles in the cell.

THE GENETIC CODE

Most genetic code tables designate the codons for amino acids as mRNA sequences. Important features of the genetic code include:

- Each codon consists of three bases (triplet). There are 64 codons. They are all written in the 5′ to 3′ direction.
- 61 codons code for amino acids. The other three (UAA, UGA, UAG) are stop codons (or nonsense codons) that terminate translation.
- There is one start codon (initiation codon), AUG, coding for methionine. Protein synthesis begins with methionine (Met) in eukaryotes, and formylmethionine (fmet) in prokaryotes.
- The code is unambiguous. Each codon specifies no more than one amino acid.
- The code is degenerate. More than one codon can specify a single amino acid. All amino acids, except Met and tryptophan (Trp), have more than one codon.
- For those amino acids having more than one codon, the first two bases in the codon are usually the same. The base in the third position often varies.
- The code is universal (the same in all organisms). Some minor exceptions to this occur in mitochondria.
- The code is commaless (contiguous). There are no spacers or "commas" between codons on an mRNA.
- Neighboring codons on a message are nonoverlapping.

First Position (5' End)	Second Position				Third Position (3' End)
	U	**C**	**A**	**G**	
U	UUU }Phe UUC UUA }Leu UUG	UCU UCC }Ser UCA UCG	UAU }Tyr UAC UAA }Stop UAG	UGU }Cys UGC UGA Stop UGG Trp	U C A G
C	CUU CUC }Leu CUA CUG	CCU CCC }Pro CCA CCG	CAU }His CAC CAA }Gln CAG	CGU CGC }Arg CGA CGG	U C A G
A	AUU }Ile AUC AUA AUG Met	ACU ACC }Thr ACA ACG	AAU }Asn AAC AAA }Lys AAG	AGU }Ser AGC AGA }Arg AGG	U C A G
G	GUU GUC }Val GUA GUG	GCU GCC }Ala GCA GCG	GAU }Asp GAC GAA }Glu GAG	GGU GGC }Gly GGA GGG	U C A G

Figure 4-1. The Genetic Code

MUTATIONS

A mutation is any permanent, heritable change in the DNA base sequence of an organism. This altered DNA sequence can be reflected by changes in the base sequence of mRNA, and, sometimes, by changes in the amino acid sequence of a protein. Mutations can cause genetic diseases. They can also cause changes in enzyme activity, nutritional requirements, antibiotic susceptibility, morphology, antigenicity, and many other properties of cells.

A very common type of mutation is a single base alteration or point mutation.

- A transition is a point mutation that replaces a purine-pyrimidine base pair with a different purine-pyrimidine base pair. For example, an A-T base pair becomes a G-C base pair.
- A transversion is a point mutation that replaces a purine-pyrimidine base pair with a pyrimidine-purine base pair. For example, an A-T base pair becomes a T-A or a C-G base pair.

Mutations are often classified according to the effect they have on the structure of the gene's protein product. This change in protein structure can be predicted using the genetic code table in conjunction with the base sequence of DNA or mRNA. A variety of such mutations is listed in the following table. Point mutations and frameshifts are illustrated in more detail in Figure 4-2.

Table 4-1. Effects of Some Common Types of Mutations on Protein Structure

Type of Mutation	Effect on Protein
Silent: new codon specifies same amino acid	None
Missense: new codon specifies different amino acid	Possible decrease in function; variable effects
Nonsense: new codon is stop codon	Shorter than normal; usually nonfunctional
Frameshift/in-frame: addition or deletion of base(s)	Usually nonfunctional; often shorter than normal
Large segment deletion (unequal crossover in meiosis)	Loss of function; shorter than normal or entirely missing
5′ splice site (donor) or 3′ splice site (acceptor)	Variable effects ranging from addition or deletion of a few amino acids to deletion of an entire exon
Trinucleotide repeat expansion	Expansions in coding regions cause protein product to be longer than normal and unstable. Disease often shows anticipation in pedigree.

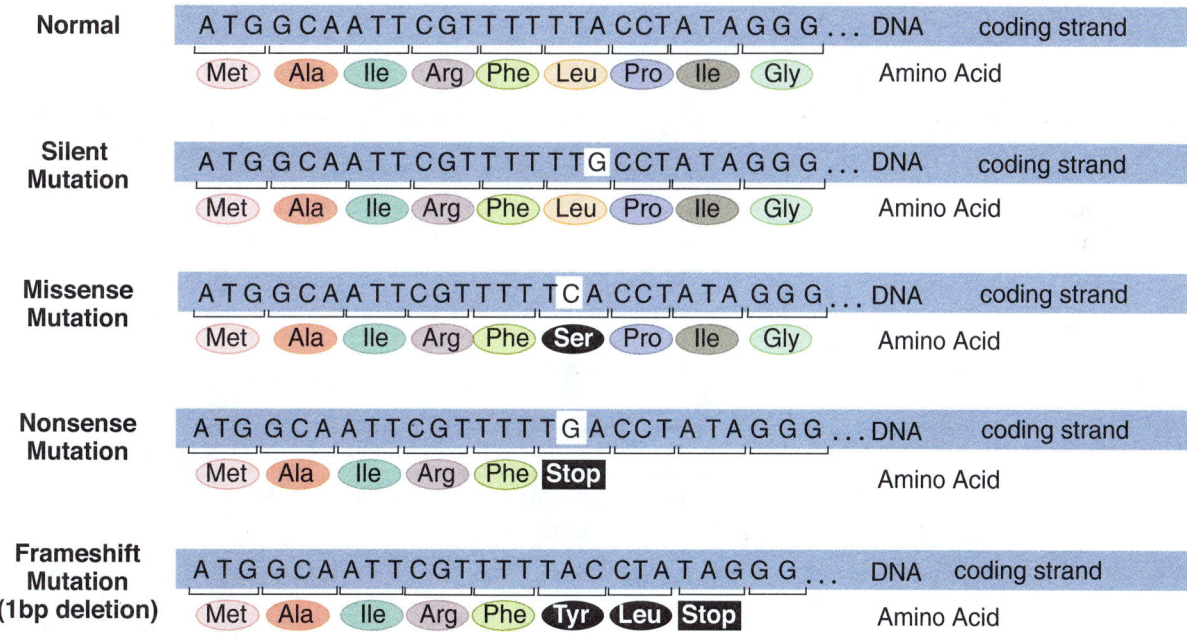

Figure 4-2. Some Common Types of Mutations in DNA

Large Segment Deletions

Large segments of DNA can be deleted from a chromosome during an unequal crossover in meiosis. Crossover or recombination between homologous chromosomes is a normal part of meiosis I that generates genetic diversity in reproductive cells (egg and sperm), a largely beneficial result. In a normal crossover event, the homologous maternal and paternal chromosomes exchange equivalent segments, and although the resultant chromosomes are mosaics of maternal and paternal alleles, no genetic information has been lost from either one. On rare occasions, a crossover can be unequal and one of the two homologs loses some of its genetic information.

α-thalassemia is a well-known example of a genetic disease in which unequal crossover has deleted one or more α-globin genes from chromosome 16. Cri-du-chat (mental retardation, microcephaly, wide-set eyes, and a characteristic kittenlike cry) results from a terminal deletion of the short arm of chromosome 5.

Mutations in Splice Sites

Mutations in splice sites affect the accuracy of intron removal from hnRNA during posttranscriptional processing. If a splice site is lost through mutation, spliceosomes may:

- Delete nucleotides from the adjacent exon.
- Leave nucleotides of the intron in the processed mRNA.
- Use the next normal upstream or downstream splice site, deleting an exon from the processed mRNA.

Mutations in splice sites have now been documented in many different diseases, including β-thalassemia, Gaucher disease, and Tay-Sachs.

AMINO ACID ACTIVATION AND CODON TRANSLATION BY tRNAS

Inasmuch as amino acids have no direct affinity for mRNA, an adapter molecule, which recognizes an amino acid on one end and its corresponding codon on the other, is required for translation. This adapter molecule is tRNA.

Amino Acid Activation

As tRNAs enter the cytoplasm, each combines with its cognate amino acid in a process called amino acid activation.

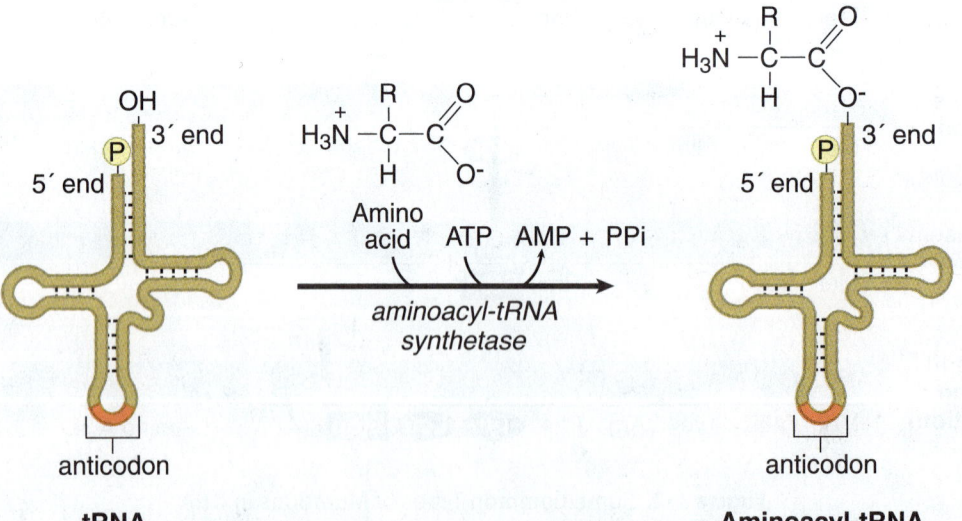

Figure 4-3. Activation of Amino Acid for Protein Synthesis

- Each type of amino acid is activated by a different aminoacyl tRNA synthetase.
- Two high-energy bonds from an ATP are required.
- The aminoacyl tRNA synthetase transfers the activated amino acid to the 3´ end of the correct tRNA.
- The amino acid is linked to its cognate tRNA with an energy-rich bond.
- This bond will later supply energy to make a peptide bond linking the amino acid into a protein.

Aminoacyl tRNA synthetases have self-checking functions to prevent incorrectly paired aminoacyl tRNAs from forming. If, however, an aminoacyl tRNA synthetase does release an incorrectly paired product (ala-tRNA^{ser}), there is no mechanism during translation to detect the error and an incorrect amino acid will be introduced into some protein.

Each tRNA has an anticodon sequence that allows it to pair with the codon for its cognate amino acid in the mRNA. Because base pairing is involved, the orientation of this interaction will be complementary and antiparallel. For example, the amino acyl tRNA arg-tRNA^{arg} has an anticodon sequence, UCG, allowing it to pair with the arginine codon CGA.

TRANSLATION (PROTEIN SYNTHESIS)

Protein synthesis occurs by peptide bond formation between successive amino acids whose order is specified by a gene and thus by an mRNA. The formation of a peptide bond between the carboxyl group on one amino acid and the amino group of another is illustrated in the following figure.

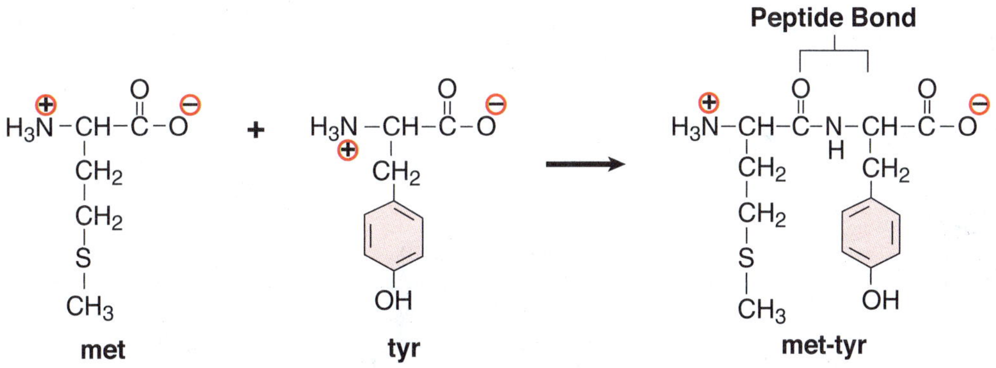

Figure 4-4. Peptide Bond Formation

During translation, the amino acids are attached to the 3′ ends of their respective tRNAs. The aminoacyl–tRNAs are situated in the P and A sites of the ribosome as shown in Figure 4-5. Notice that the peptide bond forms between the carboxyl group of the amino acid (or growing peptide) in the P site and the amino group of the next amino acid in the A site. Proteins are synthesized from the amino to the carboxyl terminus.

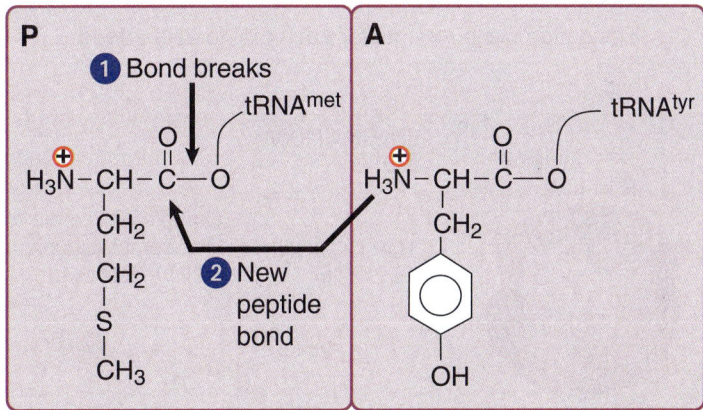

Figure 4-5. Formation of a Peptide Bond by a Ribosome During Translation

Steps of Translation

Translation occurs in the cytoplasm of both prokaryotic (Pr) and eukaryotic (Eu) cells. In prokaryotes, ribosomes can begin translating the mRNA even before RNA polymerase completes its transcription. In eukaryotes, translation and transcription are completely separated in time and space with transcription in the nucleus and translation in the cytoplasm. The process of protein synthesis occurs in 3 stages: initiation, elongation, and termination. Special protein factors for initiation (IF), elongation (EF), and termination (release factors), as well as GTP, are required for each of these stages.

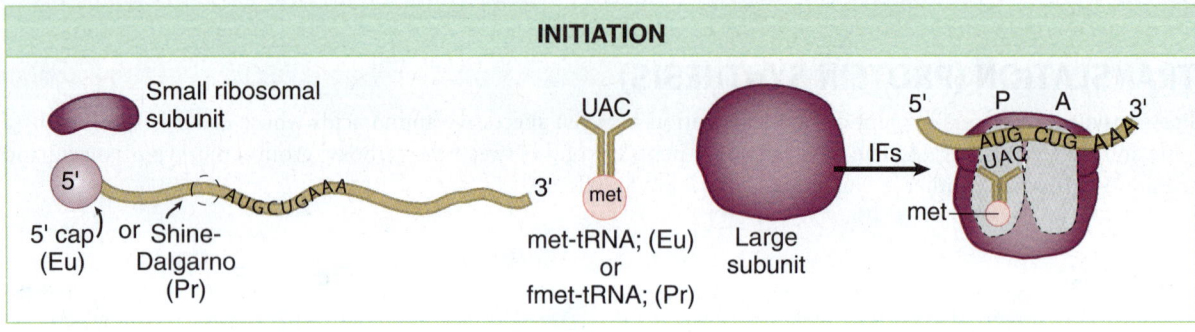

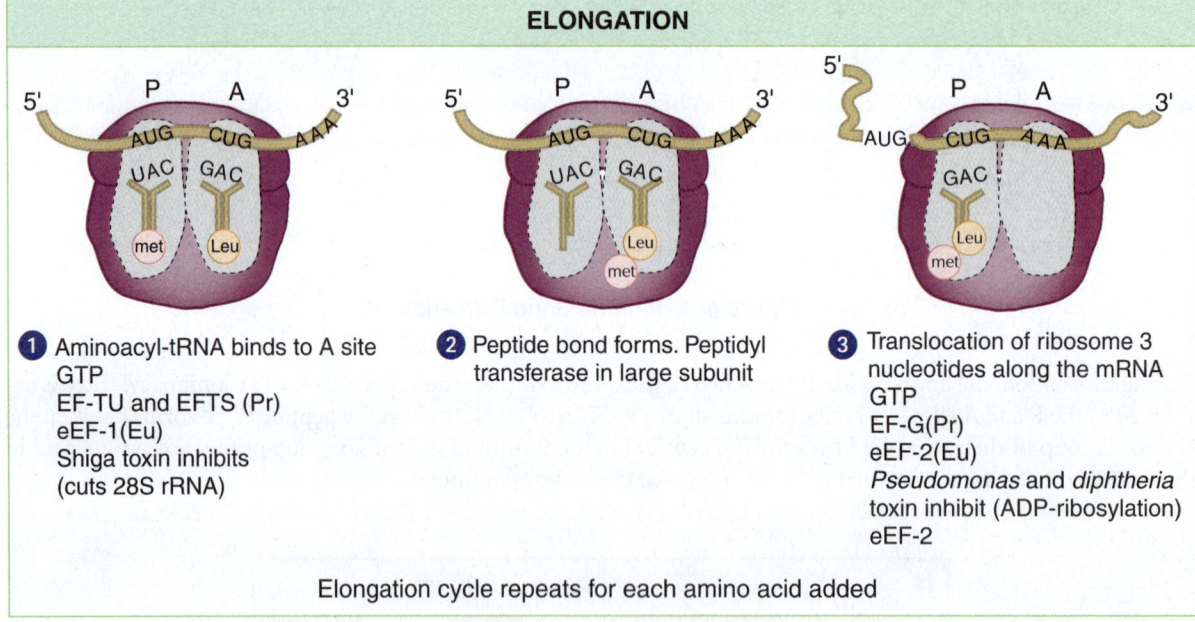

① Aminoacyl-tRNA binds to A site
GTP
EF-TU and EFTS (Pr)
eEF-1(Eu)
Shiga toxin inhibits
(cuts 28S rRNA)

② Peptide bond forms. Peptidyl transferase in large subunit

③ Translocation of ribosome 3 nucleotides along the mRNA
GTP
EF-G(Pr)
eEF-2(Eu)
Pseudomonas and *diphtheria* toxin inhibit (ADP-ribosylation) eEF-2

Elongation cycle repeats for each amino acid added

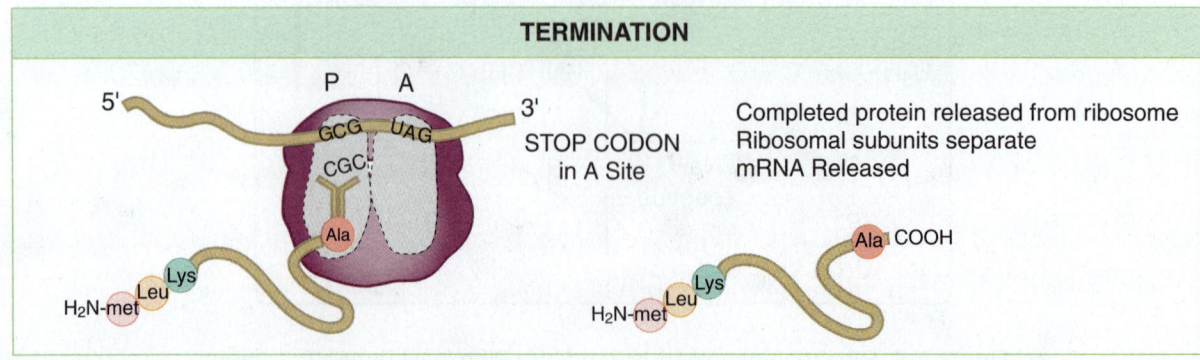

Figure 4-6. Steps in Translation

Initiation

The small ribosomal subunit binds to the mRNA. In prokaryotes, the 16S rRNA of the small subunit binds to the Shine-Dalgarno sequence in the 5′ untranslated region of the mRNA. In eukaryotes, the small subunit binds to the 5′ cap structure and slides down the message to the first AUG.

The charged initiator tRNA becomes bound to the AUG start codon on the message through base pairing with its anticodon. The initiator tRNA in prokaryotes carries fmet, whereas the initiator tRNA in eukaryotes carries Met.

The large subunit binds to the small subunit, forming the completed initiation complex.

There are two important binding sites on the ribosome called the P site and the A site.

- The peptidyl site (P site) is the site on the ribosome where (f)met–tRNA$_i$ initially binds. After formation of the first peptide bond, the P site is a binding site for the growing peptide chain.
- The aminoacyl site (A site) binds each new incoming tRNA molecule carrying an activated amino acid.

Elongation

Elongation is a 3-step cycle that is repeated for each amino acid added to the protein after the initiator methionine. Each cycle uses 4 high-energy bonds (2 from the ATP used in amino acid activation to charge the tRNA, and 2 from GTP). During elongation, the ribosome moves in the 5′ to 3′ direction along the mRNA, synthesizing the protein from amino to carboxyl terminus. The three steps are:

- A charged tRNA binds in the A site. The particular aminoacyl–tRNA is determined by the mRNA codon aligned with the A site.
- Peptidyl transferase, an enzyme that is part of the large subunit, forms the peptide bond between the new amino acid and the carboxyl end of the growing polypeptide chain. The bond linking the growing peptide to the tRNA in the P site is broken, and the growing peptide attaches to the tRNA located in the A site.
- In the translocation step, the ribosome moves exactly three nucleotides (one codon) along the message. This moves the growing peptidyl–tRNA into the P site and aligns the next codon to be translated with the empty A site.

In eukaryotic cells, elongation factor-2 (eEF-2) used in translocation is inactivated through ADP-ribosylation by *Pseudomonas* and *Diphtheria* toxins.

Shiga and Shiga-like toxins clip an adenine residue from the 28S rRNA in the 60S subunit stopping protein synthesis in eukaryotic cells.

Termination

When any of the 3 stop (termination or nonsense) codons moves into the A site, peptidyl transferase (with the help of release factor) hydrolyzes the completed protein from the final tRNA in the P site. The mRNA, ribosome, tRNA, and factors can all be reused for additional protein synthesis.

POLYSOMES

Messenger RNA molecules are very long compared with the size of a ribosome, allowing room for several ribosomes to translate a message at the same time. Because ribosomes translate mRNA in the 5′ to 3′ direction, the ribosome closest to the 3′ end has the longest nascent peptide. Polysomes are found free in the cytoplasm or attached to the rough endoplasmic reticulum (RER), depending on the protein being translated.

INHIBITORS OF PROTEIN SYNTHESIS

Some well-known inhibitors of prokaryotic translation include streptomycin, erythromycin, clindamycin, tetracycline, and chloramphenicol. Inhibitors of eukaryotic translation include cycloheximide and *Diphtheria* and *Pseudomonas* toxins.

Clinical Correlate

Gray Baby Syndrome

Gray syndrome is a dangerous condition that occurs in newborns (especially premature babies) who are given the drug chloramphenicol. Chloramphenicol is a drug used to fight bacterial infections, including meningitis. If given to a newborn, however, this drug can trigger a potentially deadly reaction. Babies do not have sufficient UDP-glucuronyl transferase activity needed to allow excretion of this drug. The drug builds up in the baby's bloodstream and can lead to:

- Blue lips, nail beds, and skin (cyanosis)
- Death
- Low blood pressure

Certain antibiotics (for example, chloramphenicol) inhibit mitochondrial protein synthesis, but not cytoplasmic protein synthesis, because mitochondrial ribosomes are similar to prokaryotic ribosomes.

PROTEIN FOLDING AND SUBUNIT ASSEMBLY

As proteins emerge from ribosomes, they fold into three-dimensional conformations that are essential for their subsequent biologic activity. Generally, four levels of protein shape are distinguished:

Primary—sequence of amino acids specified in the gene.

Secondary—folding of the amino acid chain into an energetically stable structure. Two common examples are the α-helix and the β-pleated sheet. These shapes are reinforced by hydrogen bonds. An individual protein may contain both types of secondary structures. Some proteins, like collagen, contain neither but have their own more characteristic secondary structures.

Tertiary—positioning of the secondary structures in relation to each other to generate higher-order three-dimensional shapes (the domains of the IgG molecule are examples). Tertiary structure also includes the shape of the protein as a whole (globular, fibrous). Tertiary structures are stabilized by weak bonds (hydrogen, hydrophobic, ionic) and, in some proteins, strong, covalent disulfide bonds. Agents such as heat or urea disrupt tertiary structure to denature proteins, causing loss of function.

Quaternary—in proteins such as hemoglobin that have multiple subunits, quaternary structure describes the interactions among subunits.

TRANSLATION OCCURS ON FREE RIBOSOMES AND ON THE ROUGH ENDOPLASMIC RETICULUM

Although all translation of eukaryotic nuclear genes begins on ribosomes free in the cytoplasm, the proteins being translated may belong in other locations. For example, certain proteins are translated on ribosomes associated with the rough endoplasmic reticulum (RER), including:

- Secreted proteins
- Proteins inserted into the cell membrane
- Lysosomal enzymes

Proteins translated on free cytoplasmic ribosomes include:

- Cytoplasmic proteins
- Mitochondrial proteins (encoded by nuclear genes)

Molecular Chaperones and Proteasomes

Protein folding is an essential step in the final synthesis of any protein. There is a class of specialized proteins, **chaperones**, whose function is to assist in this process. Molecular chaperones function in many cell compartments, including the endoplasmic reticulum, where extensive protein synthesis occurs. Failure to fold correctly usually results in eventual destruction of the protein.

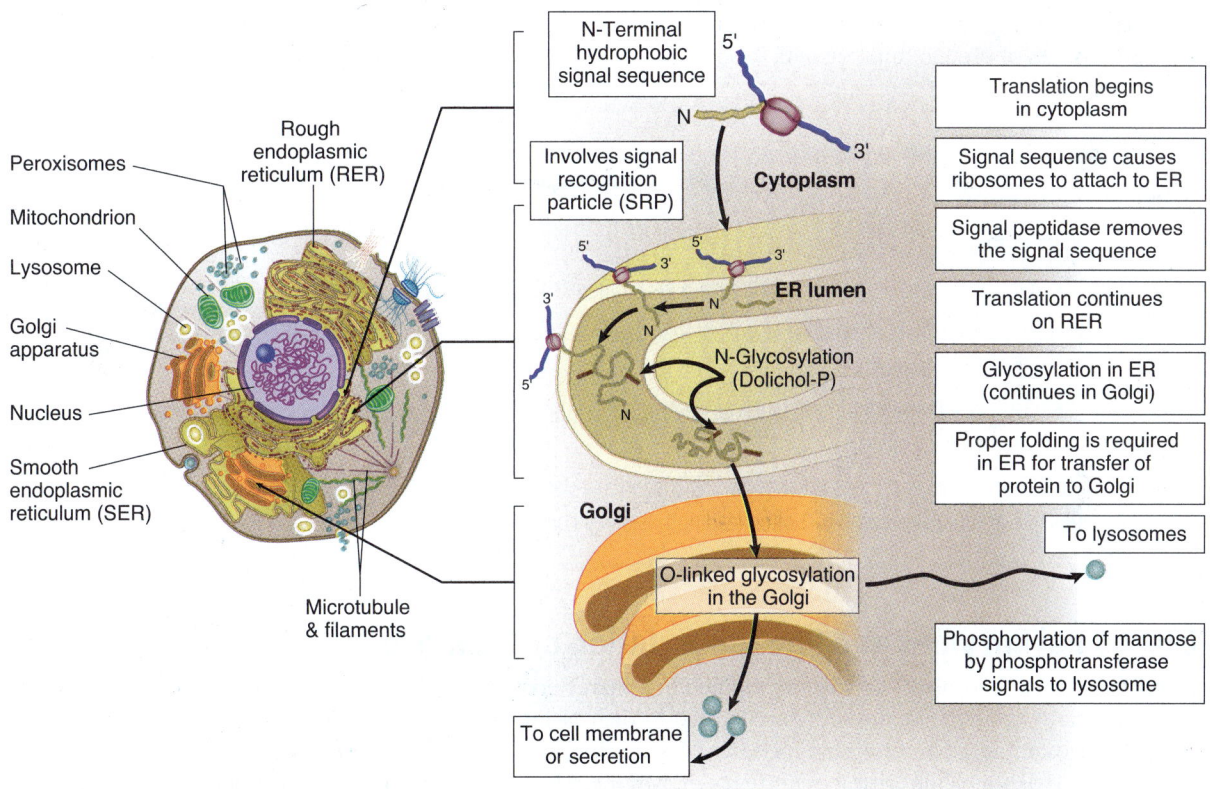

Figure 4-7. Synthesis of Secretory, Membrane, and Lysosomal Proteins

N-Terminal Hydrophobic Signal Sequence

This sequence is found on proteins destined to be secreted (insulin), placed in the cell membrane (Na^+-K^+ ATPase), or ultimately directed to the lysosome (sphingomyelinase). These proteins all require N-terminal hydrophobic signal sequences as part of their primary structure. Translation begins on free cytoplasmic ribosomes, but after translation of the signal sequence, the ribosome is positioned on the ER (now RER) with the help of a signal recognition particle. During translation, the nascent protein is fed through the membrane of the RER and captured in the lumen. The signal sequence is cleaved off in the ER, and then the protein passes into the Golgi for further modification and sorting.

In transit through the ER and Golgi, most proteins acquire oligosaccharide side chains, becoming glycoproteins. N-glycosylation refers to the addition of sugar chains to the nitrogen of asparagine residues (N-linked). The attachment of sugars in N-glycosylation begins in the ER (cotranslational modification) and requires the participation of a special lipid called dolichol phosphate. The N-linked sugar chain can further be modified upon entry in the Golgi (posttranslational modification). O-glycosylation refers to the addition of sugar chains to the hydroxyl group of either serine or threonine residues of the protein, and it occurs exclusively in the Golgi (posttranslational modification). Depending of the particular glycoprotein, some proteins are solely N-glycosylated (for example, transferrin); some are solely O-glycosylated (for example, heparin); and some are both N- and O-glycosylated (for example, LDL receptor). Significantly, the structure and sequence of the oligosaccharide chains on proteins and lipids (glycolipids) are the basis of the A, B, O blood groups.

Accumulation or ineffective targeting of misfolded proteins

Proteins synthesized in the endoplasmic reticulum must fold correctly for transport to the Golgi and then to their final destinations. In certain genetic diseases, the mutation may cause all copies of the protein to fold incorrectly. The result is loss of protein function and, in some cases, accumulation of the misfolded protein in the endoplasmic reticulum.

Bridge to Anatomy

Lysosomes

- Organelles whose major function is to digest materials that the cell has ingested by endocytosis.

- Contain multiple enzymes that, collectively, digest carbohydrates (glycosylases), lipids (lipases), and proteins (proteases).

- Especially prominent in cells such as neutrophils and macrophages, though they serve this essential role in almost all cells.

When a lysosomal enzyme is missing (for instance in a genetic disease such as Tay-Sachs), the undigested substrate accumulates in the cell, often leading to serious consequences.

Lysosomal Enzymes and Phosphorylation of Mannose

Lysosomal enzymes are glycosylated and modified in a characteristic way. Most importantly, when they arrive in the Golgi apparatus, specific mannose residues located in their N-linked oligosaccharide chains are phosphorylated by N-acetylglucosamine-1 phosphotransferase, forming a critical mannose-6-phosphate in the oligosaccharide chain. This phosphorylation is the critical event that removes them from the secretion pathway and directs them to lysosomes. Genetic defects affecting this phosphorylation produce I-cell disease in which lysosomal enzymes are released into the extracellular space, and inclusion bodies accumulate in the cell, compromising its function.

CO- AND POSTTRANSLATIONAL COVALENT MODIFICATIONS

In addition to disulfide bond formation while proteins are folding, other covalent modifications include:

- Glycosylation: addition of oligosaccharide as proteins pass through the ER and Golgi apparatus
- Proteolysis: cleavage of peptide bonds to remodel proteins and activate them (proinsulin, trypsinogen, prothrombin)
- Phosphorylation: addition of phosphate by protein kinases
- γ-Carboxylation: produces Ca^{2+} binding sites
- Prenylation: addition of farnesyl or geranylgeranyl lipid groups to certain membrane-associated proteins

POSTTRANSLATIONAL MODIFICATIONS OF COLLAGEN

Collagen is an example of a protein that undergoes several important co- and posttranslational modifications. It has a somewhat unique primary structure in that much of its length is composed of a repeating tripeptide Gly-X-Y-Gly-X-Y-etc. Hydroxyproline is an amino acid unique to collagen. The hydroxyproline is produced by hydroxylation of prolyl residues at the Y positions in procollagen chains as they pass through the RER. Important points about collagen synthesis are summarized here:

1. Prepro-α chains containing a hydrophobic signal sequence are synthesized by ribosomes attached to the RER.

2. The hydrophobic signal sequence is removed by signal peptidase in the RER to form pro-α chains.

3. Selected prolines and lysines are hydroxylated by prolyl and lysyl hydroxylases. These enzymes, located in the RER, require ascorbate (vitamin C), deficiency of which produces scurvy.

4. Selected hydroxylysines are glycosylated.

5. Three pro-α chains assemble to form a triple helical structure (procollagen), which can now be transferred to the Golgi. Modification of oligosaccharide continues in the Golgi.

6. Procollagen is secreted from the cell.

7. The propeptides are cleaved from the ends of procollagen by proteases to form collagen molecules (also called tropocollagen).

8. Collagen molecules assemble into fibrils. Cross-linking involves lysyl oxidase, an enzyme that requires O_2 and copper.

9. Fibrils aggregate and cross-link to form collagen fibers.

Table 4-2. Collagen

Collagen Type	Characteristics	Tissue Distribution	Associated Diseases
I	Bundles of fibers High tensile strength	Bone, skin, tendons	Osteogenesis imperfecta Ehlers-Danlos (various)
II	Thin fibrils Structural	Cartilage Vitreous humor	----------
III	Thin fibrils Pliable	Blood vessels Granulation tissue	Ehlers-Danlos Type IV Keloid formation
IV	Amorphous	Basement membranes	Goodpasture syndrome Alport disease Epidermolysis bullosa

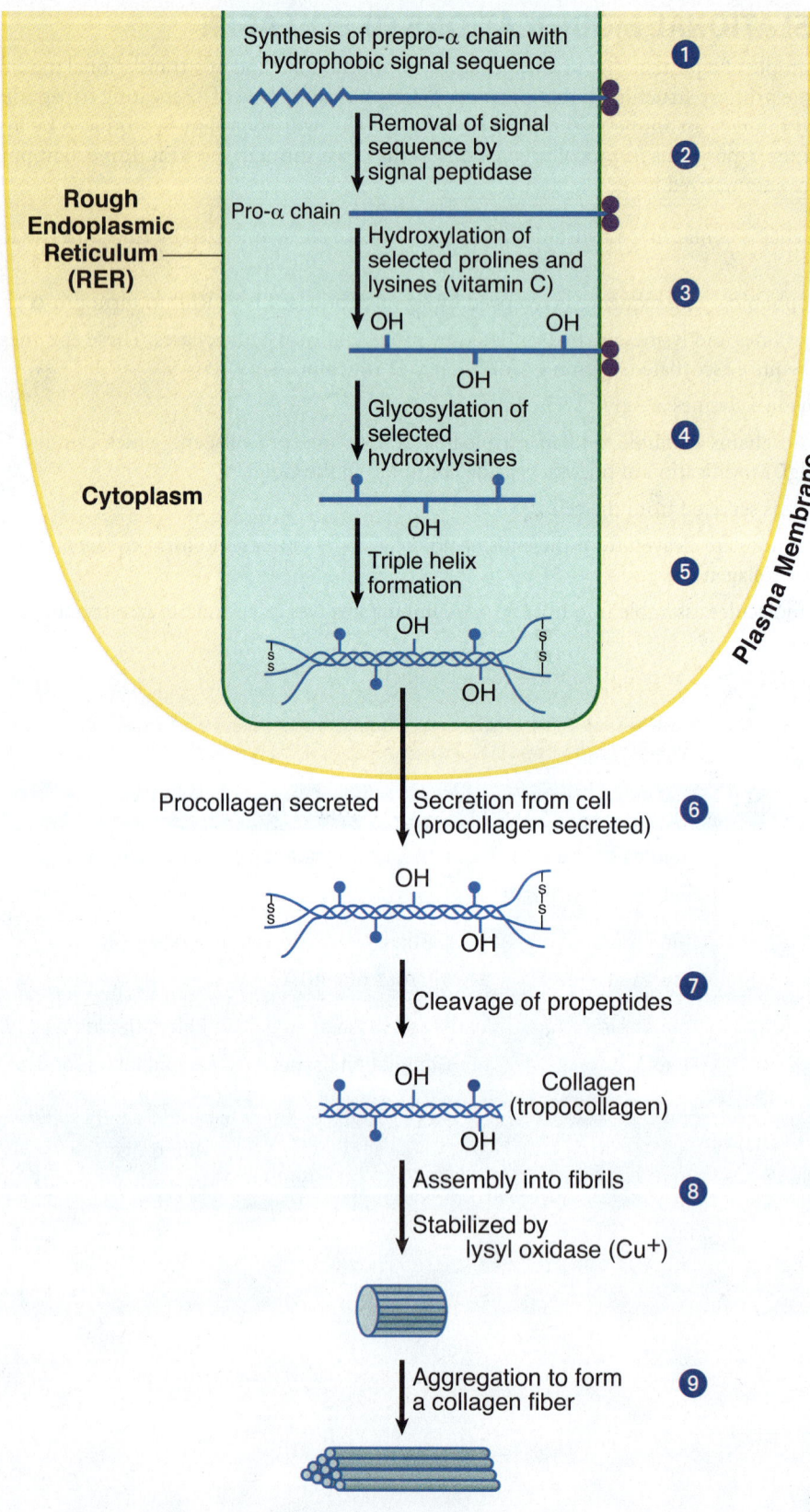

Figure 4-8. Synthesis of Collagen

Table 4-3. Important Points About the Genetic Code, Mutations, and Translation

	Prokaryotic	Eukaryotic
Genetic code	Start: AUG (also codes for Met) Stop: UAG, UGA, UAA Unambiguous (1 codon = 1 amino acid) Redundant (1 amino acid >1 codon); often differ at base 3	
Mutations	Point mutations: silent, missense, nonsense Frameshift (delete 1 or 2 nucleotides; not multiple of 3) Large segment deletion	
		Mutation in splice site Trinucleotide repeat expansion
Amino acid activation	Aminoacyl-tRNA synthetase: two high-energy bonds (ATP) to link amino acid to tRNA	
Translation: Initiation	30S subunit binds to Shine-Dalgarno sequence on mRNA	40S subunit associates with 5′ cap on mRNA
	fMet–tRNA$_i$ binds to P site	Met–tRNA$_i$ binds to P site
	GTP required	GTP required
Translation: Elongation	Charged aminoacyl–tRNA binds to A site (GTP)	Charged aminoacyl–tRNA binds to A site (GTP)
	Peptide bond forms (two high-energy bonds from amino acid activation)	28S rRNA is cut by Shiga and Shiga-like toxins removing an adenine residue. Prevents protein synthesis.
		Peptide bond forms (two high-energy bonds from amino acid activation)
	Peptidyl synthase (50S sub-unit)	Peptidyl synthase (60S subunit)
	Translocation: GTP required	Translocation: GTP required
		eEF-2 inhibited by *Diphtheria* and *Pseudomonas* toxins
Termination	Release of protein; protein synthesized N to C	
Protein targeting		Secreted or membrane proteins: N-terminal hydrophobic signal sequence
		Lysosomal enzymes: phosphorylation of mannose by phosphotransferase in Golgi
		I-cell disease
Other important disease associations		Scurvy (prolyl hydroxylase, Vit C)
		Menke Disease (Cu deficiency, lysyl oxidase)

Regulation of Eukaryotic Gene Expression

5

Learning Objectives

❏ Demonstrate understanding of regulation of eukaryotic gene expression

OVERVIEW OF GENETIC REGULATION

Regulation of gene expression is an essential feature in maintaining the functional integrity of a cell. Increasing or decreasing the expression of a gene can occur through a variety of mechanisms, but many of the important ones involve regulating the rate of transcription. In addition to the basic transcription proteins, RNA polymerase and TFIID in eukaryotes activator and repressor proteins help control the rate of the process. These regulatory proteins bind to specific DNA sequences (enhancer or silencer elements) associated with eukaryotic gene regions.

Other mechanisms are important, and gene expression is controlled at multiple levels.

REGULATION OF EUKARYOTIC GENE EXPRESSION

In eukaryotic cells, DNA is packaged in chromatin structures, and gene expression typically requires chromatin remodeling in order to make the desired gene region accessible to RNA polymerase and other proteins (transcription factors) required for gene expression. Important aspects of chromatin remodeling include:

- Transcription factors that bind to the DNA and recruit other coactivators such as histone acetylases
- Histone acetylases (favor gene expression) and deacetylases (favor inactive chromatin)
- Certain lysyl residues in the histones are acetylated decreasing the positive charge and weakening the interaction with DNA.
- A chromatin remodeling engine that binds to acetylated lysyl residues and reconfigures the DNA to expose the promoter region.
- Additional transcription factors bind in the promoter region and recruit RNA polymerase.

Once the transcription complex is formed, basal (low level) transcription occurs, maintaining moderate, but adequete, levels of the protein encoded by this gene in the cell. The transcription factors assembled in this complex are referred to as general transcription factors.

There are times when the expression of the gene should be increased in response to specific signals such as hormones, growth factors, intracellular conditions. In this case there are DNA sequences referred to as response elements that bind specific transcription factors. Several of these response elements may be grouped together to form an enhancer that allows control of gene expression by multiple signals.

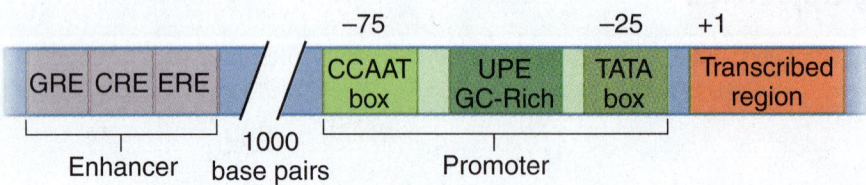

Figure 5-1. Enhancers and Upstream Promoter Elements

Upstream Promoter Elements

Only the proximity of the upstream promoter element to the –25 sequence distinguishes it from an enhancer. Upstream promoter elements include:

- A CCAAT box (around –75) that binds a transcription factor NF-1
- A GC-rich sequence that binds a general transcription factor SP-1

Enhancers

Enhancers in the DNA are binding sites for activator proteins. Enhancers have the following characteristics:

- They may be up to 1,000 base pairs away from the gene.
- They may be located upstream, downstream, or within an intron of the gene they control.
- The orientation of the enhancer sequence with respect to the gene is not important.
- Enhancers can appear to act in a tissue-specific manner if the DNA-binding proteins that interact with them are present only in certain tissues.
- Enhancers may be brought close to the basal promoter region in space by bending of the DNA molecule (Figure 5-2).

Similar sequences that bind repressor proteins in eukaryotes are called silencers. There are fewer examples of these sequences known.

Note

Cis and *Trans* Regulatory Elements

The DNA regulatory base sequences (e.g., promoters, enhancers, response elements, and UPEs) in the vicinity of genes that serve as binding sites for proteins are often called "*cis*" regulators.

Transcription factors (and the genes that code for them) are called "*trans*" regulators. *Trans* regulatory proteins can diffuse through the cell to their point of action.

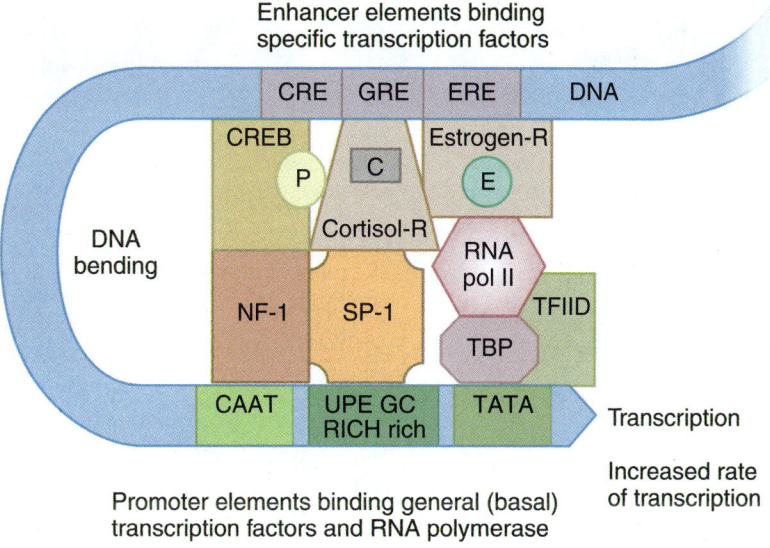

Figure 5-2. Stimulation of Transcription by an Enhancer and Its Associated Transcription Factors

Transcription Factors

The activator proteins that bind response elements are often referred to as transcription factors. Typically, transcription factors contain at least two recognizable domains, a DNA-binding domain and an activation domain.

1. The DNA-binding domain binds to a specific nucleotide sequence in the promoter or response element. Several types of DNA-binding domain motifs have been characterized and have been used to define certain families of transcription factors. Some common DNA-binding domains include:
   - Zinc fingers (steroid hormone receptors)
   - Leucine zippers (cAMP-dependent transcription factor)
   - Helix-loop-helix
   - Helix-turn-helix (homeodomain proteins encoded by homeotic/homeobox genes)

2. The activation domain allows the transcription factor to:
   - Bind to other transcription factors and coregulators
   - Interact with RNA polymerase II to stabilize the formation of the initiation complex
   - Recruit chromatin-modifying proteins such as histone acetylases or deacetylases

Two types can be distinguished: general transcription factors and specific transcription factors.

Table 5-1. Properties of Important Specific Transcription Factors

Transcription Factor (DNA-Binding Protein)	Response Element (Binding Site)	Function	Protein Class
Steroid receptors	HRE	Steroid response	Zinc finger
cAMP response element binding (CREB) protein	CRE	Response to cAMP	Leucine zipper
Peroxisome proliferator-activated receptors (PPARs)	PPREs	Regulate multiple aspects of lipid metabolism Activated by fibrates and thiazolidinediones	Zinc finger
NFkB (nuclear factor kappa-B)	kB elements	Regulates expression of many genes in immune system	Rel domains
Homeodomain proteins	——	Regulate gene expression during development	Helix-turn-helix

General Transcription Factors

In eukaryotes, general transcription factors must bind to the promoter to allow RNA polymerase II to bind and form the initiation complex at the start site for transcription. General transcription factors are common to most genes. The general transcription factor TFIID with its TATA box-binding protein subunit (TBP) must bind to the TATA box before RNA polymerase II can bind. Other examples include SP-1 and NF-1 that modulate basal transcription of many genes.

Specific Transcription Factors

Specific transcription factors bind to enhancer regions or, in a few cases, to silencers and modulate the formation of the initiation complex, thus regulating the rate of initiation of transcription. Each gene contains a variety of enhancer or silencer sequences in its regulatory region. The exact combination of specific transcription factors available (and active) in a particular cell at a particular time determines which genes will be transcribed at what rates. Because specific transcription factors are proteins, their expression can be cell-type specific. Additionally, hormones may regulate the activity of some specific transcription factors. Examples include steroid receptors and the CREB protein.

Peroxisome proliferator-activated receptors (PPARs) are transcription factors that bind to DNA response elements (PPREs) and control multiple aspects of lipid metabolism. Individual members of this family of zinc-finger proteins are activated by a variety of natural and xenobiotic ligands, including:

- Fatty acids
- Prostaglandin derivatives
- Fibrates
- Thiazolidinediones

The improvement in insulin resistance seen with thiazolidinediones is thought to be mediated through their interaction with PPARγ. Clofibrate binds PPARα, affecting different aspects of lipid metabolism than the thiazolidinediones.

Co-Expression of Genes

Most eukaryotic cells are diploid, each chromosome being present in two homologous copies. The alleles of a gene on the two homologous chromosomes are usually co-expressed. In a person heterozygous for the alleles of a particular gene, for example a carrier of sickle cell trait, two different versions of the protein will be present in cells that express the gene. In the person heterozygous for the normal and sickle alleles, about 50% of the β-globin chains will contain glutamate and 50% valine at the variable position (specified by codon 6).

Major exceptions to this rule of codominant expression include genes:

- On the Barr body (inactivated X chromosome) in women
- In the immunoglobulin heavy and light chain loci (ensuring that one B cell makes only one specificity of antibody)
- In the T-cell receptor loci

Other Mechanisms for Controlling Gene Expression in Eukaryotes

The following table summarizes some of the mechanisms that control gene expression in eukaryotic cells.

Table 5-2. Control of Eukaryotic Gene Expression and Protein Levels

Control Point	Example
Inactivation of specific chromo somes or chromosomal regions during development	One X chromosome in each cell of a woman is inactivated by condensation to heterochromatin (Barr bodies)
Local chromatin-modifying activities	Acetylation of histones increases gene expression (many genes) Methylation of DNA silences genes in genetic imprinting (Prader-Willi and Angelman syndromes)
Gene amplification	Many oncogenes are present in multiple copies: *erbB* amplified in certain breast cancers Dihydrofolate reductase genes are amplified in some tumors, leading to drug resistance
Specific transcription factors	Steroid hormone receptors, CREB, and homeodomain proteins
Processing mRNA	Alternative splicing of mRNA in the production of membrane-bound vs. secreted antibodies
Rate of translation	Heme increases the initiation of β-globin translation
Protein modification	Proinsulin is cleaved to form active insulin
Protein degradation rate	ALA synthase has a half-life of 1 hour in the hepatocyte

Genetic Strategies in Therapeutics 6

Learning Objectives

❏ Demonstrate understanding of the Human Genome Project

❏ Solve problems concerning cloning genes as cDNA produced by reverse transcription of cellular mRNA

❏ Answer questions about medical applications of recombinant DNA

OVERVIEW OF RECOMBINANT DNA TECHNOLOGY

Recombinant DNA technology allows a DNA fragment from any source to be joined *in vitro* with a nucleic acid vector that can replicate autonomously in microorganisms. This provides a means of analyzing and altering genes and proteins. It also provides the reagents necessary for genetic testing for carrier detection and prenatal diagnosis of genetic diseases and for gene therapy. Additionally, this technology can provide a source of a specific protein, such as recombinant human insulin, in almost unlimited quantities.

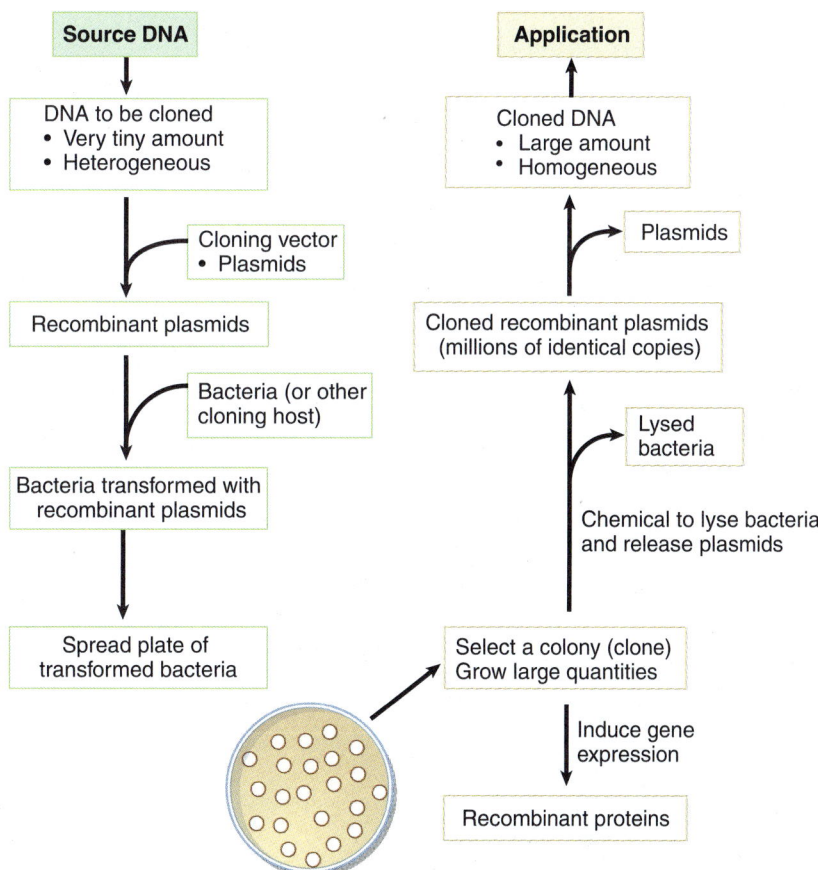

Figure 6-1. Cloning Recombinant DNA

The DNA to be cloned is usually present in a small quantity and is part of a heterogeneous mixture containing other DNA sequences. The goal is to produce a large quantity of homogeneous DNA for one of the above applications. The general strategy for cloning DNA and isolating the cloned material is shown in Figure 6-1. The steps include:

- Ligate the DNA into a piece of nucleic acid (the vector) that can be autonomously replicated in a living organism. The vector containing the new DNA is referred to as a recombinant vector.
- Transfer the recombinant vectors into host cells.
- Grow the host cells in isolated colonies so that each colony contains only one recombinant vector.
- Each cultured colony is a clone; all members are genetically identical.
- Select a colony for study.
- Grow a large quantity of that colony.
- Lyse the host cells and re-isolate the replicated recombinant vectors.
- Remove (by restriction enzyme cutting) the cloned DNA from the vector.

Techniques of Genetic Analysis 7

Learning Objectives

❏ Interpret scenarios about blotting technique

❏ Explain the use of DNA probes in blotting technique

Techniques of genetic analysis are assuming an increasingly larger role in medical diagnosis. These techniques, which once were a specialized part of medical genetics, are now becoming essential tools for every physician to understand. Blotting techniques allow testing for genetic diseases, gene expression profiling, and routine testing for antigens and antibodies. DNA probes can be useful in the analysis of blots.

BLOTTING TECHNIQUES

Blotting techniques have been developed to detect and visualize specific DNA, RNA, and protein among complex mixtures of contaminating molecules. These techniques have allowed the identification and characterization of the genes involved in numerous inherited diseases. The general method for performing a blotting technique is illustrated in Figure 7-1.

The fragments in the material to be analyzed (DNA, RNA, or protein) are separated by gel electrophoresis. The smaller molecules travel faster and appear nearer the bottom of the gel. The bands of material in the gel are transferred, or blotted, to the surface of a membrane. The membrane is incubated with a (usually radioactive) labeled probe that will specifically bind to the molecules of interest. Visualization of the labeled probe (usually by autoradiography) will reveal which band(s) interacted with the probe. The most common types of blots are compared in Table 7-1. Most typically, DNA restriction fragments are analyzed on a Southern blot.

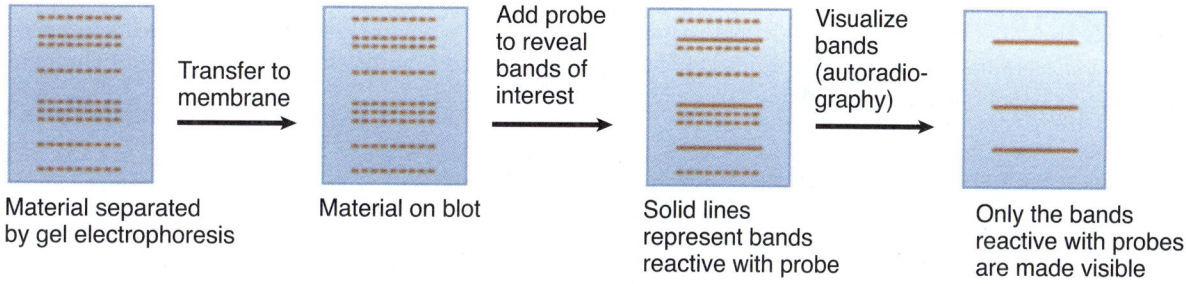

Material separated by gel electrophoresis → Transfer to membrane → Material on blot → Add probe to reveal bands of interest → Solid lines represent bands reactive with probe → Visualize bands (autoradiography) → Only the bands reactive with probes are made visible

Figure 7-1. Blotting Technique

Table 7-1. Types of Blots

Blot Type	Material Analyzed	Electro-phoresis Required	Probe Used	Purpose
Southern	DNA	Yes	^{32}P-DNA	To determine which restriction fragments of DNA are associated with a particular gene
Northern	RNA	Yes	^{32}P-DNA	To measure sizes and amounts of specific mRNA molecules to answer questions about gene expression
Western	Protein	Yes	^{125}I- or enzyme-linked antibody	To measure amount of antigen (proteins) or antibody
Dot (slot) (Figure 7-1)	RNA, DNA, or protein	No	Same as for blots above	To detect specific DNA, RNA, protein, or antibody

Probes

DNA probes are radioactively labeled single-stranded DNA molecules that are able to specifically hybridize (anneal) to particular denatured DNA sequences. Examples include:

- Probes that bind to part of a specific gene region. These are often produced by cloning cDNA transcribed from the gene and labeling it with ^{32}P, a radioactive isotope of phosphorus.
- Probes that bind to markers known to be in close proximity (closely linked) to a gene
- Probes that bind specifically to a single allele of a gene—allele-specific oligonucleotide (ASO) probes

When protein is separated and analyzed on a Western blot, ^{125}I-labeled antibody specific for the protein of interest is used as a probe.

The probe is an important part of analyzing any blot because the only bands that will appear on the final autoradiogram are those to which the probe has hybridized.

DNA probes are used to selectively detect DNA fragments. Staining with ethidium bromide can be used to visualize and detect *all* DNA fragments in a gel, provided the fragments are present in sufficient quantities. Ethidium bromide intercalates between stacked bases and fluoresces when exposed to UV light.

Amino Acids, Proteins, and Enzymes 8

Learning Objectives

❏ Explain information related to amino acids

❏ Answer questions about protein turnover and amino acid nutrition

❏ Answer questions about biochemical reactions

AMINO ACIDS

General Structure

All amino acids have a central carbon atom attached to a carboxyl group, an amino group, and a hydrogen atom, as shown in Figure 8-1. The amino acids differ from one another only in the chemical nature of the side chain (R). There are hundreds of amino acids in nature, but only 20 are used as building blocks of proteins in humans.

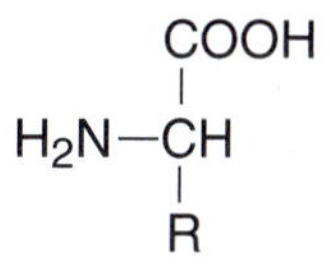

$$
\begin{array}{c}
\text{COOH} \\
| \\
\text{H}_2\text{N}-\text{CH} \\
| \\
\text{R}
\end{array}
$$

Figure 8-1. Generalized Structure of Amino Acids

Classification

The amino acids can be classified as either hydrophobic or hydrophilic, depending on the ease with which their side chains interact with water. In general, proteins fold so that amino acids with hydrophobic side chains are in the interior of the molecule where they are protected from water and those with hydrophilic side chains are on the surface.

Hydrophobic amino acids are shown in Figure 8-2. Additional points about some of these amino acids include:

- Phenylalanine and tyrosine are precursors for catecholamines.
- Tryptophan can form serotonin and niacin.
- Valine, leucine, and isoleucine are branched-chain amino acids whose metabolism is abnormal in maple syrup urine disease (discussed in chapter 17).
- Proline is a secondary amine whose presence in a protein disrupts normal secondary structure.

Hydrophilic amino acids have side chains that contain O or N atoms. Some of the hydrophilic side chains are charged at physiologic pH. The acidic amino acids (aspartic and glutamic acids) have carboxyl groups that are negatively charged, whereas the basic amino acids (lysine, arginine, and histidine) have nitrogen atoms that are positively charged. The structures of the hydrophilic amino acids are shown in Figure 8-3. Additional points about some of these amino acids include:

- Serine and threonine are sites for O-linked glycosylation of proteins, a posttranslational modification that should be associated with the Golgi apparatus.

- Asparagine is a site for N-linked glycosylation of proteins, a posttranslational modification that should be associated with the endoplasmic reticulum.

- Cysteine contains sulfur and can form disulfide bonds to stabilize the shape (tertiary structure) of proteins. Destroying disulfide bonds denatures proteins.

- Methionine, another sulfur-containing amino acid, is part of S-adenosylmethionine (SAM), a methyl donor in biochemical pathways.

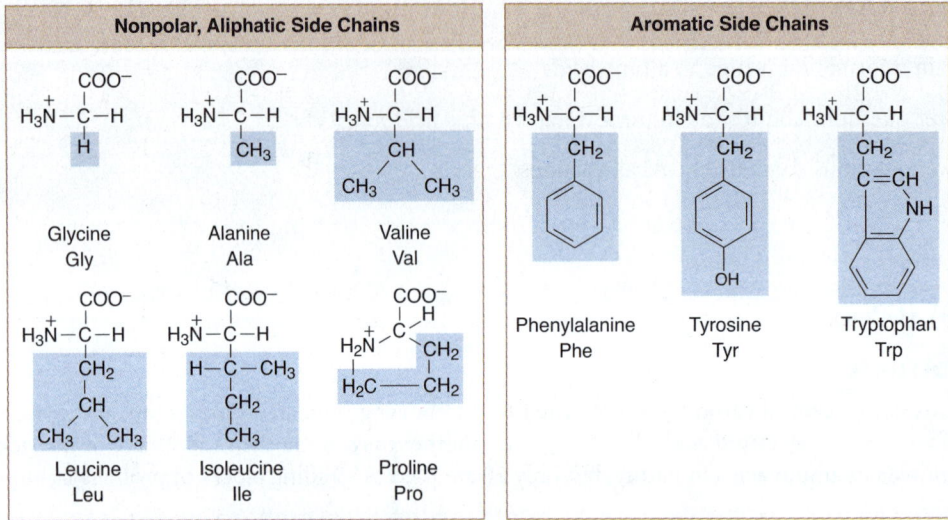

Figure 8-2. The Hydrophobic Amino Acids

Note: Tyrosine can be considered either nonpolar or polar because of the ability of the -OH group to form a hydrogen bond.

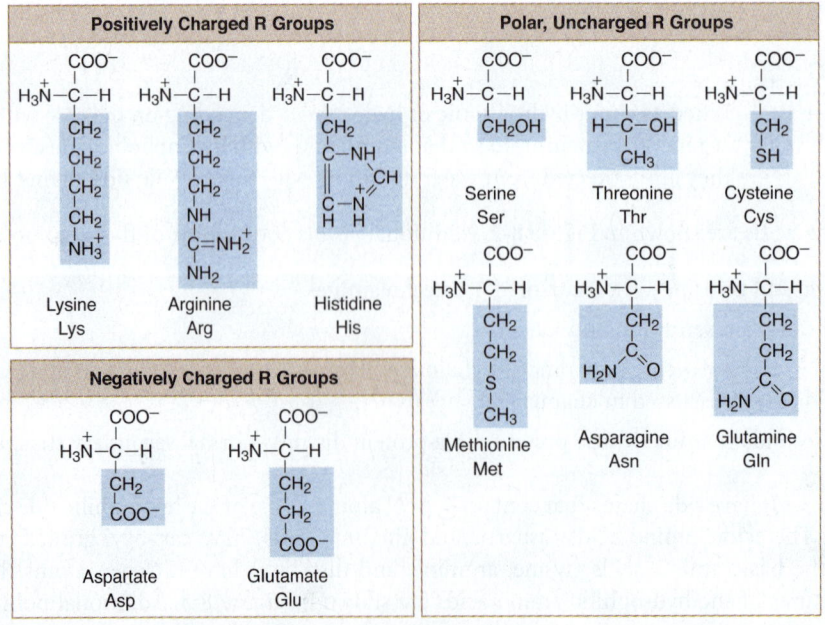

Figure 8-3. The Hydrophilic Amino Acids

Note: Methionine can be considered nonpolar or polar because it has a sulfur in it.

PROTEIN TURNOVER AND AMINO ACID NUTRITION

When older proteins are broken down in the body, they must be replaced. This concept is called protein turnover, and different types of proteins have very different turnover rates. Protein synthesis occurs during the process of translation on ribosomes. Protein breakdown occurs generally in two cellular locations:

- Lysosomal proteases digest endocytosed proteins.
- Large cytoplasmic complexes, called proteasomes, digest older or abnormal proteins that have been covalently tagged with a protein (called ubiquitin) for destruction.

Essential Amino Acids

All 20 types of amino acids are required for protein synthesis. These amino acids can be derived from digesting dietary protein and absorbing their constituent amino acids or, alternatively, by synthesizing them *de novo*.

The 10 amino acids listed in the following table cannot be synthesized in humans and therefore must be provided from dietary sources. These are called the essential amino acids. Arginine is required only during periods of growth, or positive nitrogen balance.

Table 8-1. Essential Amino Acids

Arginine*	Methionine
Histidine	Phenylalanine
Isoleucine	Threonine
Leucine	Tryptophan
Lysine	Valine

*Essential only during periods of positive nitrogen balance.

Nitrogen Balance

Nitrogen balance is the (normal) condition in which the amount of nitrogen incorporated into the body each day exactly equals the amount excreted.

Negative nitrogen balance occurs when nitrogen loss exceeds incorporation and is associated with:

- Protein malnutrition (kwashiorkor)
- A dietary deficiency of even one essential amino acid
- Starvation
- Uncontrolled diabetes
- Infection

Note

Do not confuse kwashiorkor with marasmus, which is a chronic deficiency of calories. Patients with marasmus do not present with edema as patients do with kwashiorkor.

Positive nitrogen balance occurs when the amount of nitrogen incorporated exceeds the amount excreted and is associated with:

- Growth
- Pregnancy
- Convalescence (recovery phase of injury or surgery)
- Recovery from condition associated with negative nitrogen balance

BIOCHEMICAL REACTIONS

Chemical reactions have two independent properties, their energy and their rate. ΔG represents the amount of energy released or required per mole of reactant. The amount or sign of ΔG indicates nothing about the rate of the reaction.

Table 8-2. Comparison of Energy and Rate

Energy (ΔG)	Rate (v)
Not affected by enzymes	Increased by enzymes
$\Delta G < 0$, thermodynamically spontaneous (energy released, often irreversible)	Decrease energy of activation, $\Delta G^{\ddagger}$
$\Delta G > 0$, thermodynamically nonspontaneous (energy required)	
$\Delta G = 0$, reaction at equilibrium (freely reversible)	
ΔG^0 = energy involved under standardized conditions	

The rate of the reaction is determined by the energy of activation ($\Delta G^{\ddagger}$), which is the energy required to initiate the reaction. ΔG and $\Delta G^{\ddagger}$ are represented in Figure 8-4. Enzymes lower the energy of activation for a reaction; they do not affect the value of ΔG or the equilibrium constant for the reaction, K_{eq}.

Note
Hydrolysis of high-energy bonds in ATP or GTP provide energy to drive reactions in which $\Delta G > 0$.

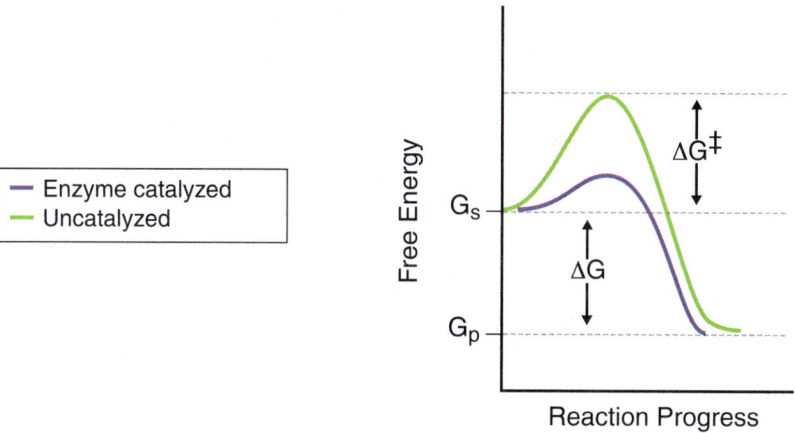

Figure 8-4. Energy Profile for a Catalyzed and Uncatalyzed Reaction

Michaelis-Menten Equation

The Michaelis-Menten equation describes how the rate of the reaction, V, depends on the concentration of both the enzyme [E] and the substrate [S], which forms product [P].

$$E + S \leftrightharpoons E - S \rightarrow E + P$$

$$V = \frac{k_2[E][S]}{K_m + [S]} \quad \text{or, with [E] held constant,} \quad V = \frac{V_{max}[S]}{K_m + [S]}$$

Note: $V_{max} = k_2[E]$

V_{max} is the maximum rate possible to achieve with a given amount of enzyme. The only way to increase V_{max} is by increasing the [E]. In the cell, this can be accomplished by inducing the expression of the gene encoding the enzyme.

The other constant in the equation, K_m is often used to compare enzymes. K_m is the substrate concentration required to produce half the maximum velocity. Under certain conditions, K_m is a measure of the affinity of the enzyme for its substrate. When comparing two enzymes, the one with the higher K_m has a lower affinity for its substrate. The K_m value is an intrinsic property of the enzyme-substrate system and cannot be altered by changing [S] or [E].

Bridge to Medical Genetics

A missense mutation in the coding region of a gene may yield an enzyme with a different K_m.

When the relationship between [S] and V is determined in the presence of constant enzyme, many enzymes yield the graph shown in Figure 8-5, a hyperbola.

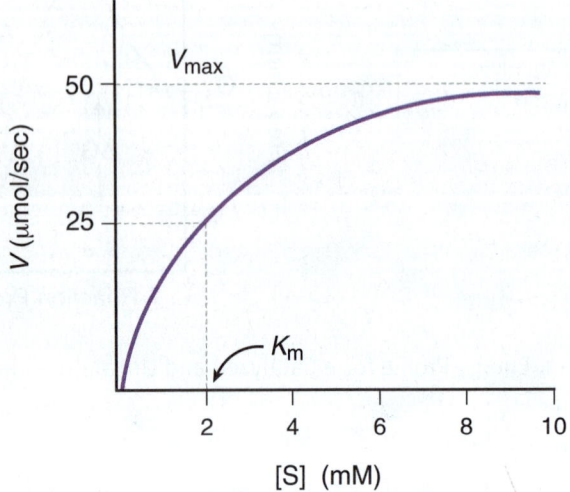

Figure 8-5. Michaelis-Menten Plot

Lineweaver-Burk Equation

The Lineweaver-Burk equation is a reciprocal form of the Michaelis-Menten equation. The same data graphed in this way yield a straight line as shown in Figure 8-6. The actual data are represented by the portion of the graph to the right of the y-axis, but the line is extrapolated into the left quadrant to determine its intercept with the x-axis. The intercept of the line with the x-axis gives the value of $-1/K_m$. The intercept of the line with the y-axis gives the value of $1/V_{max}$.

$$\frac{1}{V} = \frac{K_m}{V_{max}} \frac{1}{[S]} + \frac{1}{V_{max}}$$

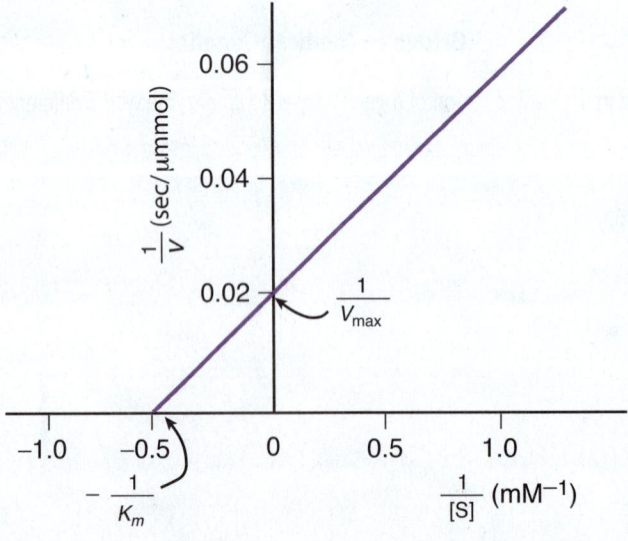

Figure 8-6. Lineweaver-Burk Plot

Inhibitors and Activators

Two important classes of inhibitors are shown in the following table. Competitive inhibitors resemble the substrate and compete for binding to the active site of the enzyme. Noncompetitive inhibitors do not bind at the active site. They bind to regulatory sites on the enzyme.

Table 8-3. Important Classes of Enzyme Inhibitors

Class of Inhibitor	K_m	V_{max}
Competitive	Increase	No effect
Noncompetitive	No effect	Decrease

The effects of these classes of inhibitors on Lineweaver-Burk kinetics are shown in the two figures that follow. Notice that on a Lineweaver-Burk graph, inhibitors always lie above the control on the right side of the *y*-axis.

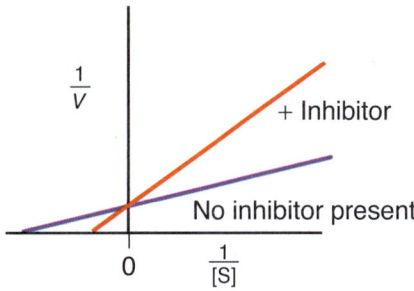

Figure 8-7. Lineweaver-Burk Plot of Competitive Inhibition

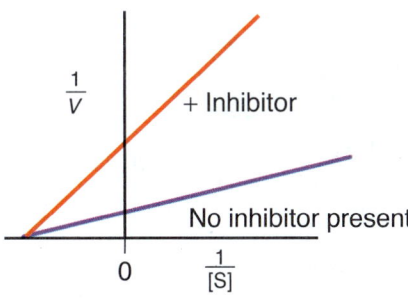

Figure 8-8. Lineweaver-Burk Plot of Noncompetitive Inhibition

Note

Drugs That Noncompetitively Inhibit Enzymes

An example of a noncompetitive inhibitor is allopurinol, which noncompetitively inhibits xanthine oxidase.

Figure 8-9 shows the effect on a Lineweaver-Burk plot of adding more enzyme. It might also represent adding an activator to the existing enzyme or a covalent modification of the enzyme. An enzyme activator is a molecule that binds to an enzyme and increases its activity. In these latter two cases the K_m might decrease and/or the V_{max} might increase but the curve would always be below the control curve in the right-hand quadrant of the graph.

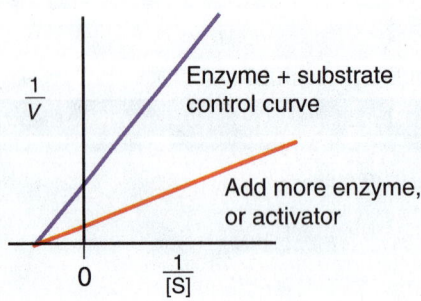

Figure 8-9. Lineweaver-Burk Plot Showing the Addition of More Enzyme or the Addition of an Activator

Cooperative Enzyme Kinetics

Certain enzymes do not show the normal hyperbola when graphed on a Michaelis-Menten plot ([S] versus V), but rather show sigmoid kinetics owing to cooperativity among substrate binding sites. Cooperative enzymes have multiple subunits and multiple active sites. Enzymes showing cooperative kinetics are often regulatory enzymes in pathways (for example, phosphofructokinase-1 [PFK-1] in glycolysis).

In addition to their active sites, these enzymes often have multiple sites for a variety of activators and inhibitors (e.g., AMP, ATP, citrate, fructose-2,6-bisphosphate [F2,6-BP]). Cooperative enzymes are sometimes referred to as allosteric enzymes because of the shape changes that are induced or stabilized by binding substrates, inhibitors, and activators.

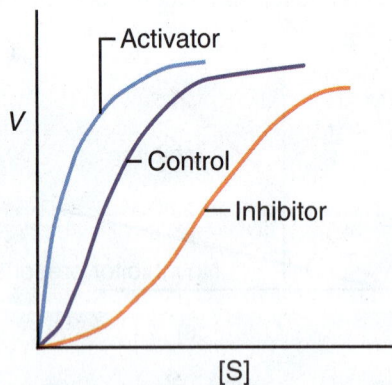

Figure 8-10. Cooperative Kinetics

Transport Kinetics

The K_m and V_{max} parameters that apply to enzymes are also applicable to transporters in membranes. The kinetics of transport can be derived from the Michaelis-Menten and Lineweaver-Burk equations, where K_m refers to the solute concentration at which the transporter is functioning at half its maximum activity. The importance of K_m values for membrane transporters is exemplified with the variety of glucose transporters (GLUT) and their respective physiologic roles (see chapter 12).

Learning Objectives

❏ Solve problems concerning hormones and signal transduction

❏ Interpret scenarios about mechanism of water-soluble hormones

❏ Answer questions about G-proteins in signal transduction

❏ Answer questions about lipid-soluble hormones

HORMONES AND SIGNAL TRANSDUCTION

Broadly speaking, a hormone is any compound produced by a cell, which by binding to its cognate receptor alters the metabolism of the cell bearing the hormone–receptor complex. Although a few hormones bind to receptors on the cell that produces them (autoregulation or autocrine function), hormones are more commonly thought of as acting on some other cell, either close by (paracrine) or at a distant site (telecrine). Paracrine hormones are secreted into the interstitial space and generally have a very short half-life. These include the prostaglandins and the neurotransmitters. The paracrine hormones are discussed in the various Lecture Notes, as relevant to the specific topic under consideration. Telecrine hormones are secreted into the bloodstream, generally have a longer half-life, and include the endocrine and gastrointestinal (GI) hormones. The endocrine hormones are the classic ones, and it is sometimes implied that reference is being made to endocrine hormones when the word hormones is used in a general sense. The GI and endocrine hormones are discussed in detail in the GI and endocrinology chapters in the Physiology Lecture Notes. Although there is some overlap, this chapter presents basic mechanistic concepts applicable to all hormones, whereas coverage in the Physiology notes emphasizes the physiologic consequences of hormonal action.

Hormones are divided into two major categories, those that are water soluble (hydrophilic) and those that are lipid soluble (lipophilic, also known as hydrophobic). Important properties of these two classes are shown in Table 9-1.

Table 9-1. Two Classes of Hormones

Water Soluble	Lipid Soluble
Receptor in cell membrane	Receptor inside cell
Second messengers often involved Protein kinases activated	Hormone–receptor complex binds hormone response elements (HRE) of enhancer regions in DNA
Protein phosphorylation to modify activity of enzymes (requires minutes)	——
Control of gene expression through proteins such as cAMP response element binding (CREB) protein (requires hours)	Control of gene expression (requires hours)
Examples: • Insulin • Glucagon • Catecholamines	Examples: • Steroids • Calcitriol • Thyroxines • Retinoic acid

MECHANISM OF WATER-SOLUBLE HORMONES

Water-soluble hormones must transmit signals to affect metabolism and gene expression without themselves entering the cytoplasm. They often do so via second messenger systems that activate protein kinases.

Protein Kinases

A protein kinase is an enzyme that phosphorylates other proteins, changing their activity (e.g., phosphorylation of acetyl CoA carboxylase inhibits it). Examples of protein kinases are listed in the following table along with the second messengers that activate them.

Table 9-2. Summary of Signal Transduction by Water-Soluble Hormones

Pathway	G Protein	Enzyme	Second Messenger(s)	Protein Kinase	Examples
cAMP	G_s (G_i)	Adenyl cyclase	cAMP	Protein kinase A	Glucagon Epinephrine (β, α-2) Vasopressin (V2, ADH) kidney
PIP_2	G_q	Phospholipase C	DAG, IP_3, Ca^{2+}	Protein kinase C	Vasopressin (V1, V3) vascular smooth muscle Epinephrine (α_1)
cGMP	None	Guanyl cyclase	cGMP	Protein kinase G	Atrial natriuretic factor (ANF) Nitric oxide (NO)
Insulin, growth factors	Monomeric p21^{ras}	——	——	Tyrosine kinase activity of receptor	Insulin Insulin-like growth factor (IGF) Platelet-derived growth factor (PDGF) Epidermal growth factor (EGF)

Some water-soluble hormones bind to receptors with intrinsic protein kinase activity (often tyrosine kinases). In this case, no second messenger is required for protein kinase activation. The insulin receptor is an example of a tyrosine kinase receptor.

Activation of a protein kinase causes:

- Phosphorylation of enzymes to rapidly increase or decrease their activity.
- Phosphorylation of gene regulatory proteins such as CREB to control gene expression, usually over several hours. The typical result is to add more enzyme to the cell. CREB induces the phosphoenolpyruvate carboxykinase (PEPCK) gene. Kinetically, an increase in the number of enzymes means an increase in V_{max} for that reaction.

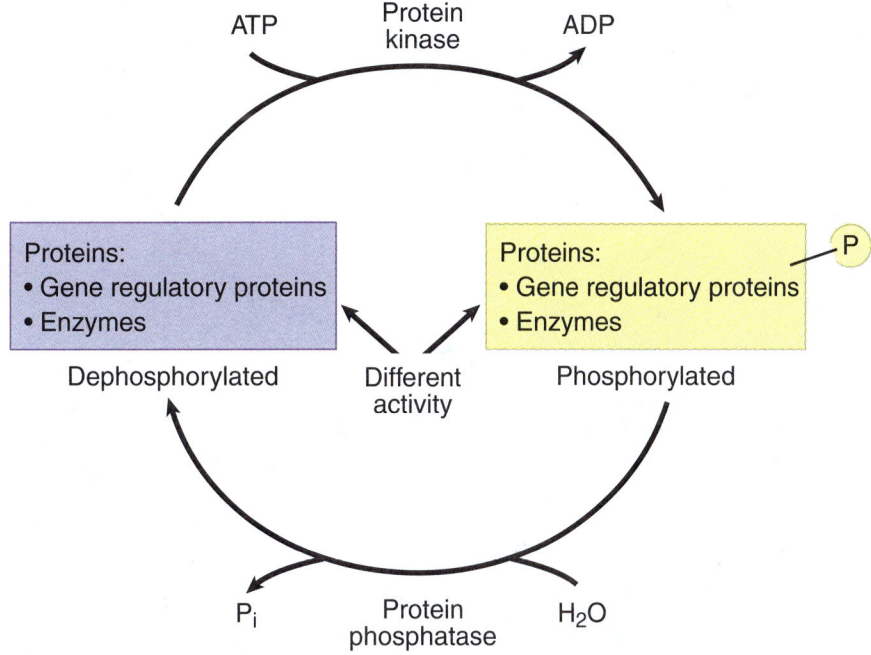

Figure 9-1. Protein Kinases and Phosphatases

Both represent strategies to control metabolism. The action of protein kinases is reversed by protein phosphatases.

Sequence of Events From Receptor to Protein Kinase

G Protein

Receptors in these pathways are coupled through trimetric G proteins in the membrane. The 3 subunits in this type of G protein are α, β, and γ. In its inactive form, the α subunit binds GDP and is in complex with the β and γ subunits. When a hormone binds to its receptor, the receptor becomes activated and, in turn, engages the corresponding G protein (step 1 in Figure 9-2). The GDP is replaced with GTP, enabling the α subunit to dissociate from the β and γ subunits (step 2). The activated α subunit alters the activity of adenylate cyclase. If the α subunit is α_s, then the enzyme is activated; if the α subunit is α_i, then the enzyme is inhibited. The GTP in the activated α subunit will be dephosphorylated to GDP (step 3) and will rebind to the β and γ subunits (step 4), rendering the G protein inactive.

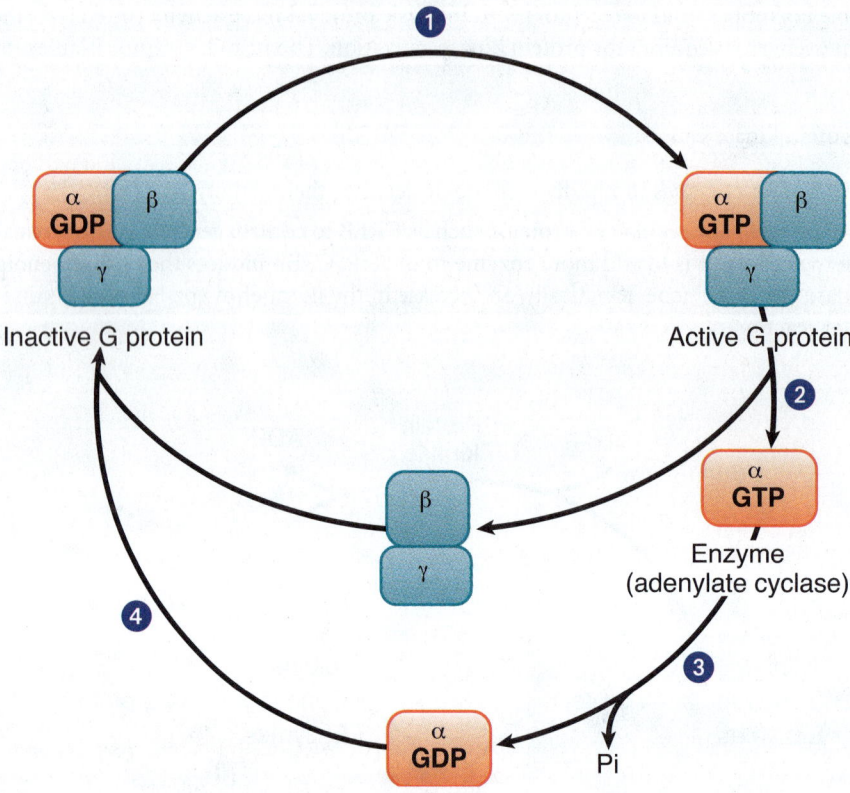

Figure 9-2. Trimeric G Protein Cycle

Cyclic AMP (cAMP) and phosphatidylinositol bisphosphate (PIP$_2$)

The receptors all have characteristic 7-helix membrane-spanning domains.

The sequence of events (illustrated in Figure 9-3) leading from receptor to activation of the protein kinase via the cAMP and PIP$_2$ second messenger systems is as follows:

- Hormone binds receptor
- Trimeric G protein in membrane is engaged
- Enzyme (adenylate cyclase or phospholipase) activated
- Second messenger generated
- Protein kinase activated
- Protein phosphorylation (minutes) and gene expression (hours)

An example of inhibition of adenylate cyclase via G$_i$ is epinephrine inhibition (through its binding to α_2 adrenergic receptor) of insulin release from β cells of the pancreas.

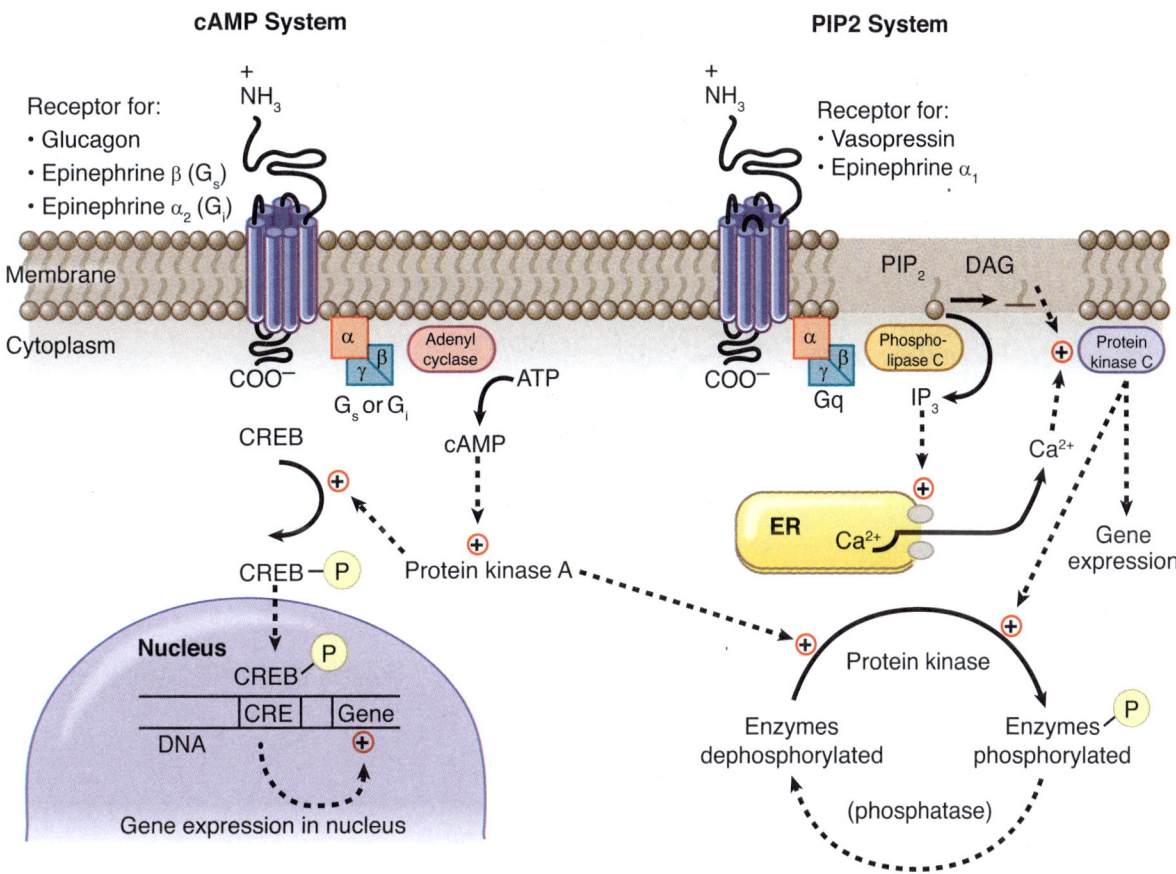

Figure 9-3. Cyclic AMP and Phosphatidylinositol Bisphosphate (PIP$_2$)

cGMP

Atrial natriuretic factor (ANF), produced by cells in the atrium of the heart in response to distension, binds the ANF receptor in vascular smooth muscle and in the kidney. The ANF receptor spans the membrane and has guanylate cyclase activity associated with the cytoplasmic domain. It causes relaxation of vascular smooth muscle, resulting in vasodilation, and in the kidney it promotes sodium and water excretion.

Nitric oxide (NO) is synthesized by vascular endothelium in response to vasodilators. It diffuses into the surrounding vascular smooth muscle, where it directly binds the heme group of soluble guanylate cyclase, activating the enzyme.

Note
Once generated, the second messengers cAMP and cGMP are slowly degraded by a class of enzymes called phosphodiesterases (PDEs).

Both the ANF receptor and the soluble guanylate cyclase are associated with the same vascular smooth muscle cells. These cGMP systems are shown in the following figure.

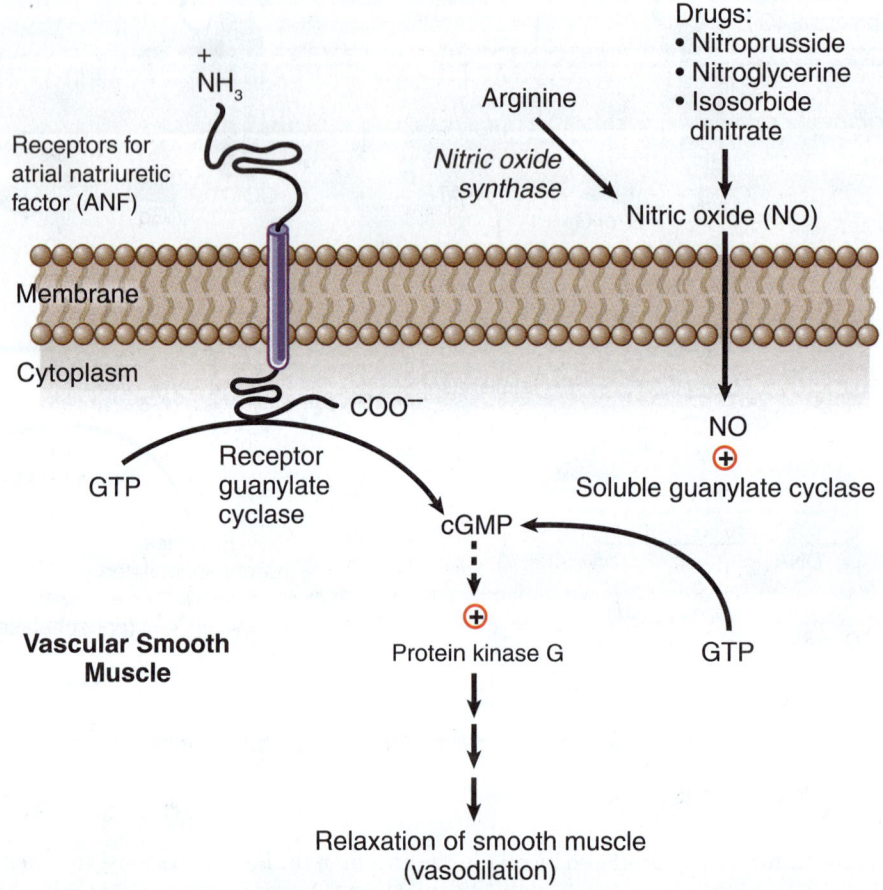

Figure 9-4. Cyclic GMP

The sequence from receptor to protein kinase is quite similar to the one above for cAMP with two important variations:

- The ANF receptor has intrinsic guanylate cyclase activity. Because no G protein is required in the membrane, the receptor lacks the 7-helix membrane-spanning domain.
- Nitric oxide diffuses into the cell and directly activates a soluble, cytoplasmic guanylate cyclase, so no receptor or G protein is required.

The Insulin Receptor: A Tyrosine Kinase

Insulin binding activates the tyrosine kinase activity associated with the cytoplasmic domain of its receptor as shown in Figure 9-5. There is no trimeric G protein, enzyme, or second messenger required to activate this protein tyrosine kinase activity:

- Hormone binds receptor
- Receptor tyrosine kinase (protein kinase) is activated
- Protein phosphorylation (autophosphorylation and activation of other proteins)

Once autophosphorylation begins, a complex of other events ensues. An insulin receptor substrate (IRS-1) binds the receptor and is phosphorylated on tyrosine residues, allowing proteins with SH2 (*src* homology) domains to bind to the phosphotyrosine residues on IRS-1 and become active. In this way, the receptor activates several enzyme cascades, which involve:

- Activation of phosphatidylinositol-3 kinase (PI-3 kinase), one of whose effects in adipose and muscle tissues is to increase GLUT-4 in the membrane
- Activation of protein phosphatases. Paradoxically, insulin stimulation via its tyrosine kinase receptor ultimately may lead to dephosphorylating enzymes
- Stimulation of the monomeric G protein (p21^{ras}) encoded by the normal *ras* gene

All these mechanisms can be involved in controlling gene expression, although the pathways by which this occurs have not yet been completely characterized.

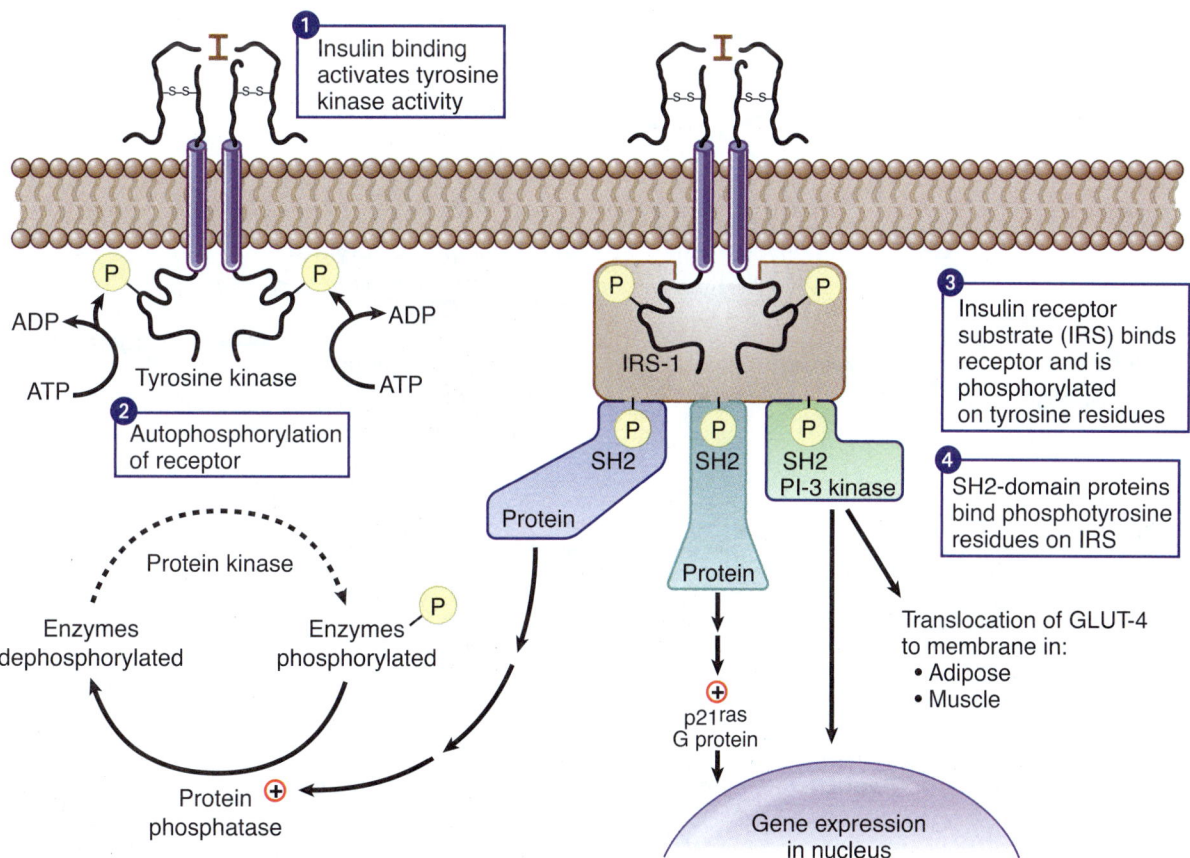

Figure 9-5. Insulin Receptor

Tyrosine kinase receptors are also involved in signaling by several growth factors, including platelet-derived growth factor (PDGF) and epidermal growth factor (EGF).

Functional Relationship of Glucagon and Insulin

Insulin, associated with well-fed, absorptive metabolism, and glucagon, associated with fasting and postabsorptive metabolism, usually oppose each other with respect to pathways of energy metabolism. Glucagon works through the cAMP system to activate protein kinase A favoring phosphorylation of rate-limiting enzymes, whereas insulin often activates protein phosphatases that dephosphorylate many of the same enzymes. An example of this opposition in glycogen metabolism is shown in Figure 9-6. Glucagon promotes phosphorylation of both rate-limiting enzymes (glycogen phosphorylase for glycogenolysis and glycogen synthase for glycogen synthesis). The result is twofold in that synthesis slows and degradation increases, but both effects contribute to the same physiologic outcome, release of glucose from the liver during hypoglycemia. Insulin reverses this pattern, promoting glucose storage after a meal. The reciprocal relationship between glucagon and insulin is manifested in other metabolic pathways, such as triglyceride synthesis and degradation.

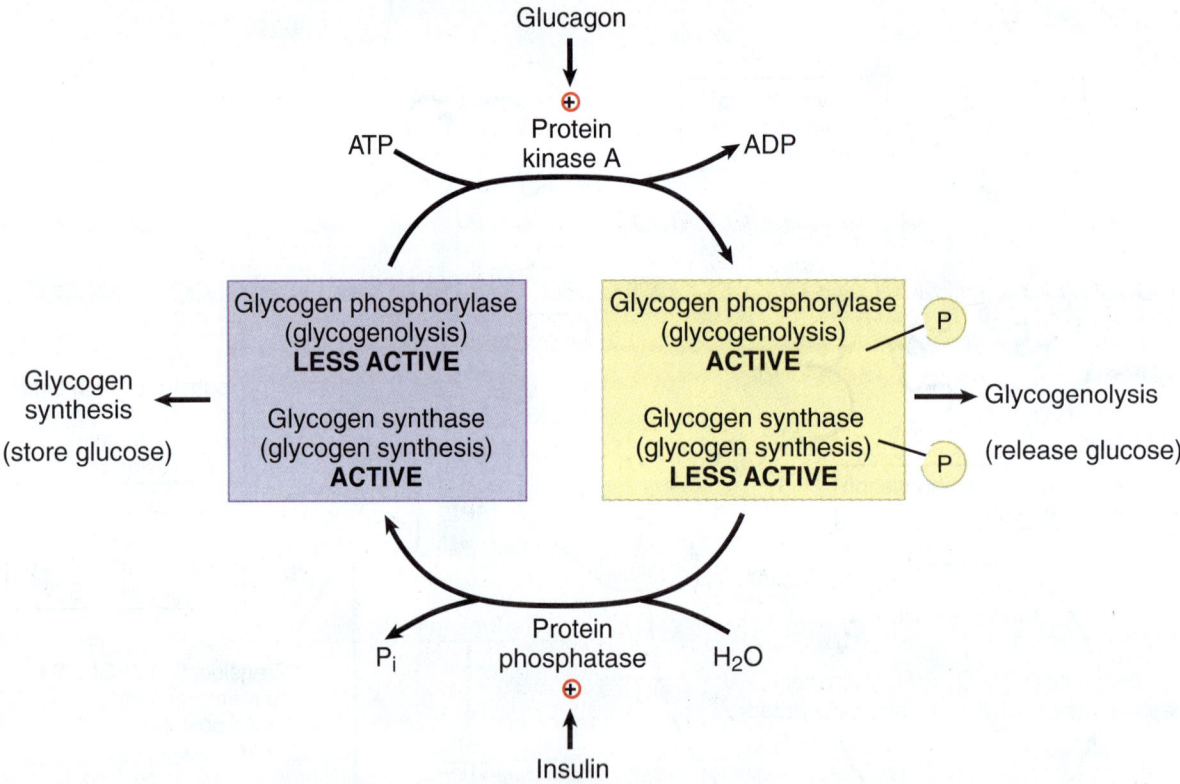

Figure 9-6. Opposing Activities of Insulin and Glucagon

Learning Objectives

❏ Answer questions about vitamin D and calcium homeostasis

❏ Interpret scenarios about vitamin A

❏ Answer questions about vitamin K

❏ Explain information related to vitamin E

OVERVIEW OF VITAMINS

Vitamins have historically been classified as either water soluble or lipid soluble. Water-soluble vitamins are precursors for coenzymes and are reviewed in the context of the reactions for which they are important. A summary of these vitamins is shown in the following table.

Table 10-1. Water-Soluble Vitamins

Vitamin or Coenzyme	Enzyme	Pathway	Deficiency
Biotin	Pyruvate carboxylase	Gluconeogenesis	MCC* (rare): excessive consumption of raw eggs (contain avidin, a biotin-binding protein); also caused by biotinidase deficiency
	Acetyl CoA carboxylase	Fatty acid synthesis	
	Propionyl CoA carboxylase	Odd-carbon fatty acids, Val, Met, Ile, Thr	Alopecia (hair loss), bowel inflammation, muscle pain
Thiamine (B$_1$)	Pyruvate dehydrogenase	PDH	MCC: alcoholism (alcohol interferes with absorption)
	α-Ketoglutarate dehydrogenase	TCA cycle	Wernicke (ataxia, nystagmus, ophthal-moplegia)
			Korsakoff (confabulation, psychosis)
	Transketolase	HMP shunt	Wet beri-beri (high-output cardiac failure, fluid retention, vascular leak) and dry beri-beri (peripheral neuropathy)
	Branched chain keto-acid dehydrogenase	Metabolism of valine isoleucine and leucine	
Niacin (B$_3$)	Dehydrogenases	Many	Pellagra: diarrhea, dementia, dermatitis, and, if not treated, death
NAD(H) NADP(H)			Pellagra may also be related to deficiency of tryptophan (corn is low in triptophan), which supplies a portion of the niacin requirement.

(Continued)

Vitamin or Coenzyme	Enzyme	Pathway	Deficiency
Folic acid THF	Thymidylate synthase Enzymes in purine synthesis need not be memorized	Thymidine (pyrimidine) synthesis Purine synthesis	MCC: alcoholism and pregnancy (body stores depleted in 3 months), hemodialysis Homocystinemia with risk of deep vein thrombosis and atherosclerosis Megaloblastic (macrocytic) anemia Deficiency in early pregnancy causes neural tube defects in fetus
Cyanocobalamin (B_{12})	Homocysteine methyltransferase Methylmalonyl CoA mutase	Methionine, SAM Odd-carbon fatty acids, Val, Met, Ile, Thr	MCC: pernicious anemia. Also in aging, especially with poor nutrition, bacterial overgrowth of terminal ileum, resection of the terminal ileum secondary to Crohn disease, chronic pancreatitis, and, rarely, vegans, or infection with *D. latum* Megaloblastic (macrocytic) anemia Progressive peripheral neuropathy
Pyridoxine (B_6) Pyridoxal-P (PLP)	Aminotransferases (transaminase): AST (GOT), ALT (GPT) δ-Aminolevulinate synthase	Protein catabolism Heme synthesis	MCC: isoniazid therapy Sideroblastic anemia Cheilosis or stomatitis (cracking or scaling of lip borders and corners of the mouth) Convulsions
Riboflavin (B_2) FAD(H_2)	Dehydrogenases	Many	Corneal neovascularization Cheilosis or stomatitis (cracking or scaling of lip borders and corners of the mouth) Magenta-colored tongue
Ascorbate (C)	Prolyl and lysyl hydroxylases Dopamine hydroxylase Dopamine hydroxylase	Collagen synthesis Catecholamine synthesis Absorption of iron in GI tract	MCC: diet deficient in citrus fruits and green vegetables Scurvy: poor wound healing, easy bruising (perifollicular hemorrhage), bleeding gums, increased bleeding time, painful glossitis, anemia
Pantothenic acid CoA	Fatty acid synthase Fatty acyl CoA synthetase Pyruvate dehydrogenase α-Ketoglutarate dehydrogenase	Fatty acid metabolism PDH TCA cycle	Rare

*MCC, most common cause

There are four important lipid-soluble vitamins, D, A, K, and E. Two of these vitamins, A and D, work through enhancer mechanisms similar to those for lipid-soluble hormones. In addition, all four lipid-soluble vitamins have more specialized mechanisms through which they act. The following table lists their major functions.

Table 10-2. Lipid-Soluble Vitamins

Vitamin	Important Functions
D (cholecalciferol)	In response to hypocalcemia, helps normalize serum calcium levels
A (carotene)	Retinoic acid and retinol act as growth regulators, especially in epithelium
	Retinal is important in rod and cone cells for vision
K (menaquinone, bacteria; phytoquinone, plants)	Carboxylation of glutamic acid residues in many Ca^{2+}-binding proteins, importantly coagulation factors II, VII, IX, and X, as well as protein C and protein S
E (α-tocopherol)	Antioxidant in the lipid phase. Protects membrane lipids from peroxidation

VITAMIN D AND CALCIUM HOMEOSTASIS

Hypocalcemia (below-normal blood calcium) stimulates release of parathyroid hormone (PTH), which in turn binds to receptors on cells of the renal proximal tubules. The receptors are coupled through cAMP to activation of a 1α-hydroxylase important for the final, rate-limiting step in the conversion of vitamin D to 1,25-DHCC (dihydroxycholecalciferol or calcitriol).

Once formed, 1,25-DHCC acts on duodenal epithelial cells as a lipid-soluble hormone. Its intracellular receptor (a Zn-finger protein) binds to response elements in enhancer regions of DNA to induce the synthesis of calcium-binding proteins thought to play a role in stimulating calcium uptake from the GI tract.

1,25-DHCC also facilitates calcium reabsorption in the kidney and mobilizes calcium from bone when PTH is also present. All these actions help bring blood calcium levels back within the normal range.

The relation of vitamin D to calcium homeostasis and its *in vivo* activation are shown in the following figure.

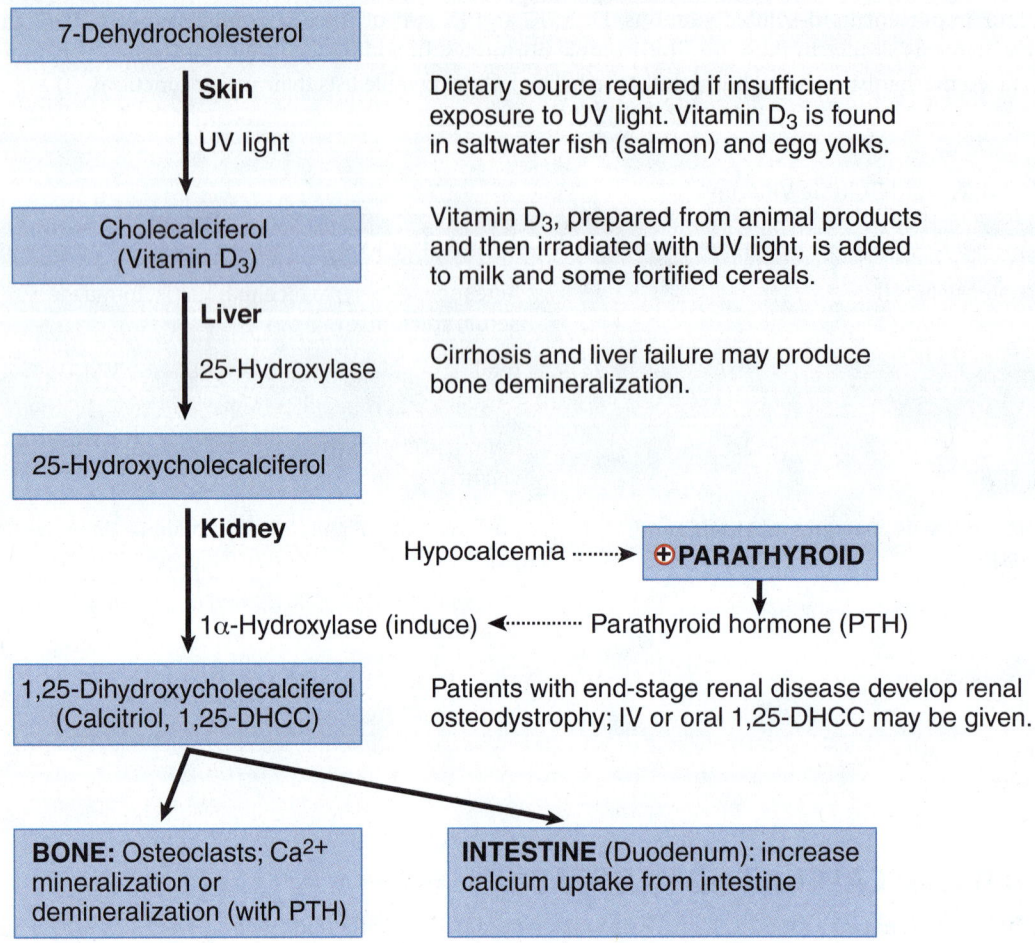

Figure 10-1. Synthesis and Activation of Vitamin D

Synthesis of 1, 25-Dihydroxycholecalciferol (Calcitriol)

Humans can synthesize calcitriol from 7-dehydrocholesterol derived from cholesterol in the liver. Three steps are involved, each occurring in a different tissue:

1. Activation of 7-dehydrocholesterol by UV light in the skin produces cholecalciferol (vitamin D_3) This step is insufficient in many people in cold, cloudy climates, and vitamin D_3 supplementation is necessary.

2. 25-Hydroxylation in the liver (patients with severe liver disease may need to be given 25-DHCC or 1,25-DHCC).

3. 1α-Hydroxylation in the proximal renal tubule cells in response to PTH. Genetic deficiencies or patients with end-stage renal disease develop renal osteodystrophy because of insufficiency of 1,25-DHCC and must be given 1,25-DHCC or a drug analog that does not require metabolism in the kidney. Such patients include those with:
    *   End-stage renal disease secondary to diabetes mellitus
    *   Fanconi renal syndrome (renal proximal tubule defect)
    *   Genetic deficiency of the 1α-hydroxylase (vitamin D-resistant rickets)

Vitamin D Deficiency

Deficiency of vitamin D in childhood produces rickets, a constellation of skeletal abnormalities most strikingly seen as deformities of the legs, but many other developing bones are affected. Muscle weakness is common.

Vitamin D deficiency after epiphyseal fusion causes osteomalacia, which produces less deformity than rickets. Osteomalacia may present as bone pain and muscle weakness.

VITAMIN A

Vitamin A (carotene) is converted to several active forms in the body associated with two important functions, maintenance of healthy epithelium and vision. Biochemically, there are three vitamin A structures that differ on the basis of the functional group on C-1: hydroxyl (retinol), carboxyl (retinoic acid), and aldehyde (retinal).

Maintenance of Epithelium

Retinol and retinoic acid are required for the growth, differentiation, and maintenance of epithelial cells. In this capacity they bind intracellular receptors, which are in the family of Zn-finger proteins, and they regulate transcription through specific response elements.

Vision

When first formed, all the double bonds in the conjugated double bond system in retinal are in the *trans* configuration. This form, all-*trans* retinal is not active. The conversion of all-*trans* retinal to the active form *cis*-retinal takes place in the pigmented epithelial cells. *Cis*-retinal is then transferred to opsin in the rod cells forming the light receptor rhodopsin. It functions similarly in rod and cone cells. When exposed to light, *cis*-retinal is converted all-*trans* retinal. A diagram of the signal transduction pathway for light-activated rhodopsin in the rod cell is shown in Figure 10-2, along with the relationship of this pathway to rod cell anatomy and changes in the membrane potential. Note the following points:

- Rhodopsin is a 7-pass receptor coupled to the trimeric G protein transducin (G_t).
- When light is present, the pathway activates cGMP phosphodiesterase, which lowers cGMP.
- Rhodopsin and transducin are embedded in the disk membranes in the outer rod segment.
- cGMP-gated Na^+ channels in the cell membrane of the outer rod segment respond to the decrease in cGMP by closing and hyperpolarizing the membrane.
- The rod cell is unusual for an excitable cell in that the membrane is partially depolarized (~ -30 mV) at rest (in darkness) and hyperpolarizes on stimulation.

Because the membrane is partially depolarized in the dark, its neurotransmitter glutamate is continuously released. Glutamate inhibits the optic nerve bipolar cells with which the rod cells synapse. By hyperpolarizing the rod cell membrane, light stops the release of glutamate, relieving inhibition of the optic nerve bipolar cell and thus initiating a signal into the brain.

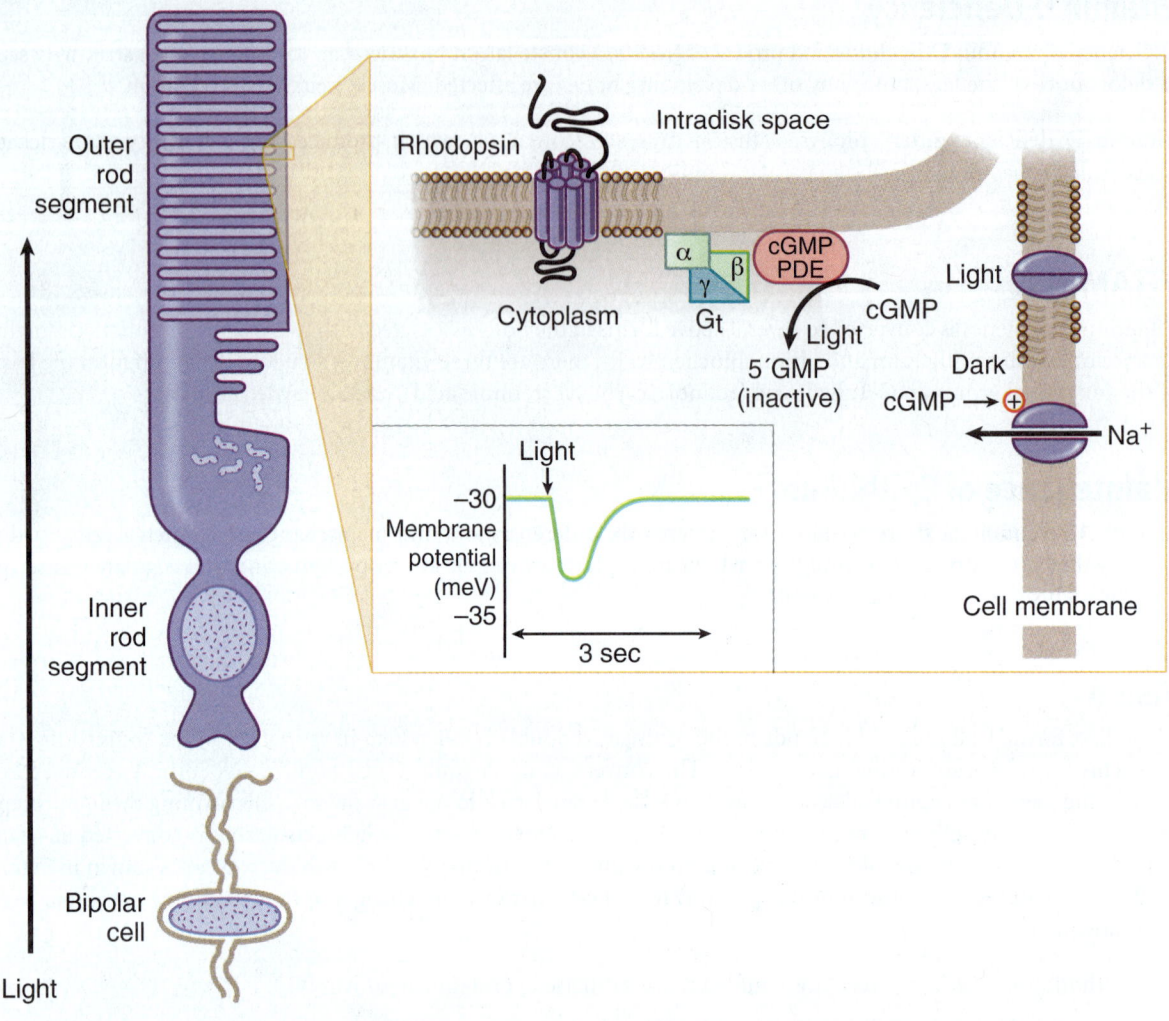

Figure 10-2. Light-Activated Signal Transduction in the Retinal Rod Cell

VITAMIN K

Vitamin K is required to introduce Ca^{2+} binding sites on several calcium-dependent proteins. The modification that introduces the Ca^{2+} binding site is a γ-carboxylation of glutamyl residue(s) in these proteins, often identified simply as the γ-carboxylation of glutamic acid. Nevertheless, this vitamin K-dependent carboxylation is a cotranslational modification occurring as the proteins are synthesized on ribosomes associated with the rough endoplasmic reticulum (RER) during translation.

Examples of proteins undergoing this vitamin K–dependent carboxylation include the coagulation factors II (prothrombin), VII, IX, and X, as well as the anticoagulant proteins C and S. All these proteins require Ca^{2+} for their function. Vitamin K deficiencies produce prolonged bleeding, easy bruising, and potentially fatal hemorrhagic disease. Conditions predisposing to a vitamin K deficiency include:

- Fat malabsorption (bile duct occlusion)
- Prolonged treatment with broad-spectrum antibiotics (eliminate intestinal bacteria that supply vitamin K)
- Breast-fed newborns (little intestinal flora, breast milk very low in vitamin K), especially in a home-birth where a postnatal injection of vitamin K may not be given
- Infants whose mothers have been treated with certain anticonvulsants during pregnancy such as phenytoin (Dilantin)

Poor nutrition and malnourishment, lack of medications, occult blood in the stool specimen, prolonged PT, and normal LFTs are all consistent with vitamin K deficiency. Without vitamin K, several blood clotting factors (prothrombin, X, IX, VII) are not γ-carboxylated on glutamate residues by the γ-glutamyl carboxylase during their synthesis (cotranslational modification) in hepatocytes.

Vitamin K deficiency should be distinguished from vitamin C deficiency.

Table 10-3. Comparison of Vitamin K and Vitamin C Deficiencies

Vitamin K Deficiency	Vitamin C Deficiency
Easy bruising, bleeding	Easy bruising, bleeding
Normal bleeding time	Increased bleeding time
Increased PT	Normal PT
Hemorrhagic disease with no connective tissue problems	• Gum hyperplasia, inflammation, loss of teeth • Skeletal deformity in children • Poor wound healing • Anemia
Associated with: • Fat malabsorption • Long-term antibiotic therapy • Breast-fed newborns • Infant whose mother was taking anticonvulsant therapy during pregnancy	Associated with: • Diet deficient in citrus fruit, green vegetables

VITAMIN E

Vitamin E (α-tocopherol) is an antioxidant. As a lipid-soluble compound, it is especially important for protecting other lipids from oxidative damage.

It prevents peroxidation of fatty acids in cell membranes, helping to maintain their normal fluidity. Deficiency can lead to hemolysis, neurologic problems, and retinitis pigmentosa.

High blood levels of Vitamin E can cause hemorrhage in patients given warfarin.

Learning Objectives

❏ Explain information related to metabolic sources of energy

❏ Interpret scenarios about metabolic energy storage

❏ Interpret scenarios about regulation of fuel metabolism

❏ Answer questions about patterns of fuel metabolism in tissues

METABOLIC SOURCES OF ENERGY

Energy is extracted from food via oxidation, resulting in the end products carbon dioxide and water. This process occurs in four stages, shown in Figure 11-1.

In stage 1, metabolic fuels are hydrolyzed in the gastrointestinal tract to a diverse set of monomeric building blocks (glucose, amino acids, and fatty acids) and absorbed.

In stage 2, the building blocks are degraded by various pathways in tissues to a common metabolic intermediate, acetyl-CoA. Most of the energy contained in metabolic fuels is conserved in the chemical bonds (electrons) of acetyl-CoA. A smaller portion is conserved in reducing nicotinamide adenine dinucleotide (NAD) to NADH or flavin adenine dinucleotide (FAD) to $FADH_2$. Reduction indicates the addition of electrons that may be free, part of a hydrogen atom (H), or a hydride ion (H^-).

In stage 3, the citric acid (Krebs, or tricarboxylic acid [TCA]) cycle oxidizes acetyl-CoA to CO_2. The energy released in this process is primarily conserved by reducing NAD to NADH or FAD to $FADH_2$.

The final stage is oxidative phosphorylation, in which the energy of NADH and $FADH_2$ is released via the electron transport chain (ETC) and used by an ATP synthase to produce ATP. This process requires O_2.

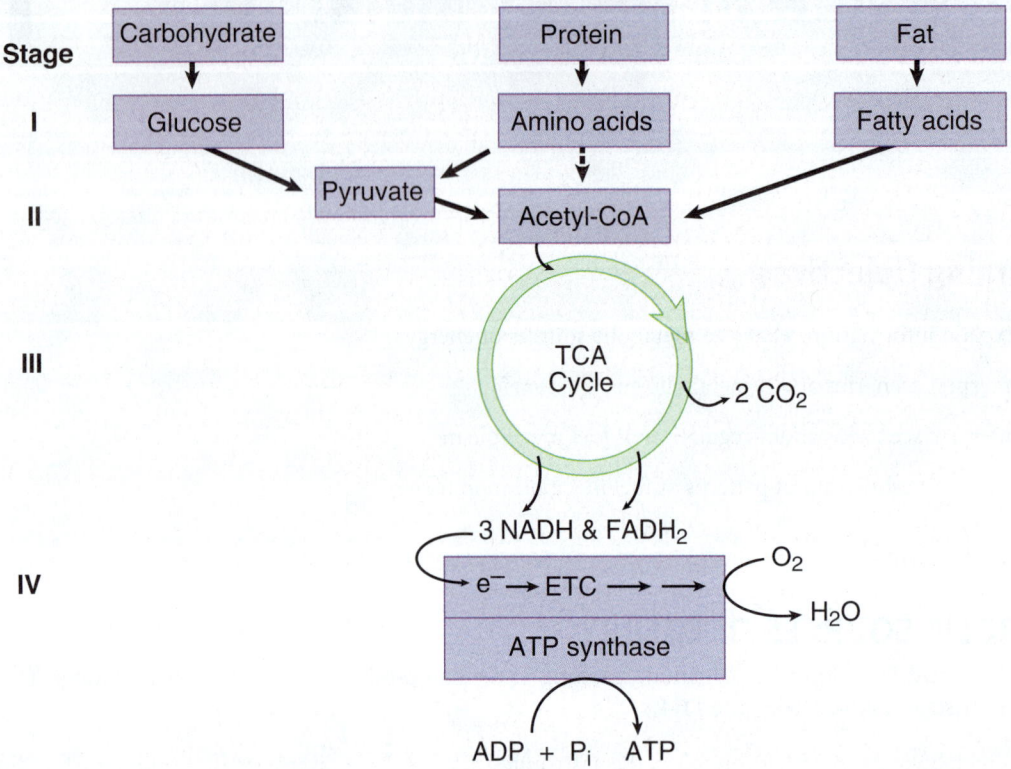

Figure 11-1. Energy from Metabolic Fuels

METABOLIC ENERGY STORAGE

ATP is a form of circulating energy currency in cells. It is formed in catabolic pathways by phosphorylation of ADP and may provide energy for biosynthesis (anabolic pathways). There is a limited amount of ATP in circulation. Most of the excess energy from the diet is stored as fatty acids (a reduced polymer of acetyl CoA) and glycogen (a polymer of glucose). Although proteins can be mobilized for energy in a prolonged fast, they are normally more important for other functions (contractile elements in muscle, enzymes, intracellular matrix, etc.).

In addition to energy reserves, many other types of biochemicals are required to maintain an organism. Cholesterol is required for cell membrane structure, proteins for muscle contraction, and polysaccharides for the intracellular matrix, to name just a few examples. These substances may be produced from transformed dietary components.

REGULATION OF FUEL METABOLISM

The pathways that are operational in fuel metabolism depend on the nutritional status of the organism. Shifts between storage and mobilization of a particular fuel, as well as shifts among the types of fuel being used, are very pronounced in going from the well-fed state to an overnight fast, and finally to a prolonged state of starvation. The shifting metabolic patterns are regulated mainly by the insulin/glucagon ratio. Insulin is an anabolic hormone that promotes fuel storage. Its action is opposed by a number of hormones, including glucagon, epinephrine, cortisol, and growth hormone. The major function of glucagon is to respond rapidly to decreased blood glucose levels by promoting the synthesis and release of glucose into the circulation. Anabolic and catabolic pathways are controlled at three important levels:

- Allosteric inhibitors and activators of rate-limiting enzymes
- Control of gene expression by insulin and glucagon
- Phosphorylation (glucagon) and dephosphorylation (insulin) of rate-limiting enzymes

Well-Fed (Absorptive) State

Immediately after a meal, the blood glucose level rises and stimulates the release of insulin. The three major target tissues for insulin are liver, muscle, and adipose tissue. Insulin promotes glycogen synthesis in liver and muscle. After the glycogen stores are filled, the liver converts excess glucose to fatty acids and triglycerides. Insulin promotes triglyceride synthesis in adipose tissue and protein synthesis in muscle, as well as glucose entry into both tissues. After a meal, most of the energy needs of the liver are met by the oxidation of excess amino acids.

Two tissues, brain and red blood cells, are insensitive to insulin (are insulin independent). The brain and other nerves derive energy from oxidizing glucose to CO_2 and water in both the well-fed and normal fasting states. Only in prolonged fasting does this situation change. Under all conditions, red blood cells use glucose anaerobically for all their energy needs.

Postabsorptive State

Glucagon and epinephrine levels rise during an overnight fast. These hormones exert their effects on skeletal muscle, adipose tissue, and liver. In liver, glycogen degradation and the release of glucose into the blood are stimulated. Hepatic gluconeogenesis is also stimulated by glucagon, but the response is slower than that of glycogenolysis. The release of amino acids from skeletal muscle and fatty acids from adipose tissue are both stimulated by the decrease in insulin and by an increase in epinephrine. The amino acids and fatty acids are taken up by the liver, where the amino acids provide the carbon skeletons and the oxidation of fatty acids provides the ATP necessary for gluconeogenesis.

Prolonged Fast (Starvation)

Levels of glucagon and epinephrine are markedly elevated during starvation. Lipolysis is rapid, resulting in excess acetyl-CoA that is used for ketone synthesis. Levels of both lipids and ketones are therefore increased in the blood. Muscle uses fatty acids as the major fuel, and the brain adapts to using ketones for some of its energy. After several weeks of fasting, the brain derives approximately two thirds of its energy from ketones and one third from glucose. The shift from glucose to ketones as the major fuel diminishes the amount of protein that must be degraded to support gluconeogenesis. There is no "energy-storage form" for protein because each protein has a specific function in the cell. Therefore, the shift from using glucose to ketones during starvation spares protein, which is essential for these other functions. Red blood cells (and renal medullary cells) that have few, if any, mitochondria continue to be dependent on glucose for their energy.

PATTERNS OF FUEL METABOLISM IN TISSUES

Fats are much more energy-rich than carbohydrates, proteins, or ketones. Complete combustion of fat results in 9 kcal/g compared with 4 kcal/g derived from carbohydrate, protein, and ketones. The storage capacity and pathways for utilization of fuels varies with different organs and with the nutritional status of the organism as a whole.

The organ-specific patterns of fuel utilization in the well-fed and fasting states are summarized in the following table.

Table 11-1. Preferred Fuels in the Well-Fed and Fasting States

Organ	Well-Fed	Fasting
Liver	Glucose and amino acids	Fatty acids
Resting skeletal muscle	Glucose	Fatty acids, ketones
Cardiac muscle	Fatty acids	Fatty acids, ketones
Adipose tissue	Glucose	Fatty acids
Brain	Glucose	Glucose (ketones in prolonged fast)
Red blood cells	Glucose	Glucose

Liver

Two major roles of liver in fuel metabolism are to maintain a constant level of blood glucose under a wide range of conditions and to synthesize ketones when excess fatty acids are being oxidized. After a meal, the glucose concentration in the portal blood is elevated. The liver extracts excess glucose and uses it to replenish its glycogen stores. Any glucose remaining in the liver is then converted to acetyl CoA and used for fatty acid synthesis. The increase in insulin after a meal stimulates both glycogen synthesis and fatty acid synthesis in liver. The fatty acids are converted to triglycerides and released into the blood as very low-density lipoproteins (VLDLs). In the well-fed state, the liver derives most of its energy from the oxidation of excess amino acids.

Between meals and during prolonged fasts, the liver releases glucose into the blood. The increase in glucagon during fasting promotes both glycogen degradation and gluconeogenesis. Lactate, glycerol, and amino acids provide carbon skeletons for glucose synthesis.

Adipose Tissue

After a meal, the elevated insulin stimulates glucose uptake by adipose tissue. Insulin also stimulates fatty acid release from VLDL and chylomicron triglyceride (triglyceride is also known as triacylglycerol). Lipoprotein lipase, an enzyme found in the capillary bed of adipose tissue, is induced by insulin. The fatty acids that are released from lipoproteins are taken up by adipose tissue and re-esterified to triglyceride for storage. The glycerol phosphate required for triglyceride synthesis comes from glucose metabolized in the adipocyte. Insulin is also very effective in suppressing the release of fatty acids from adipose tissue.

During the fasting state, the decrease in insulin and the increase in epinephrine activate hormone-sensitive lipase in fat cells, allowing fatty acids to be released into the circulation.

Skeletal Muscle

Resting muscle

The major fuels of skeletal muscle are glucose and fatty acids. Because of the enormous bulk, skeletal muscle is the body's major consumer of fuel. After a meal, under the influence of insulin, skeletal muscle takes up glucose to replenish glycogen stores and amino acids that are used for protein synthesis. Both excess glucose and amino acids can also be oxidized for energy.

In the fasting state, resting muscle uses fatty acids derived from free fatty acids in the blood. Ketones may be used if the fasting state is prolonged. In exercise, skeletal muscle may convert some pyruvate to lactate, which is transported by blood to be converted to glucose in the liver.

Clinical Correlate
Because insulin is necessary for adipose cells to take up fatty acids from triglycerides, high triglyceride levels in the blood may be an indicator of untreated diabetes.

Active muscle

The primary fuel used to support muscle contraction depends on the magnitude and duration of exercise as well as the major fibers involved. Skeletal muscle has stores of both glycogen and some triglycerides. Blood glucose and free fatty acids also may be used.

Fast-twitch muscle fibers have a high capacity for anaerobic glycolysis but are quick to fatigue. They are involved primarily in short-term, high-intensity exercise. Slow-twitch muscle fibers in arm and leg muscles are well vascularized and primarily oxidative. They are used during prolonged, low-to-moderate intensity exercise and resist fatigue. Slow-twitch fibers and the number of their mitochondria increase dramatically in trained endurance athletes.

Short bursts of high-intensity exercise are supported by anaerobic glycolysis drawing on stored muscle glycogen.

During moderately high, continuous exercise, oxidation of glucose and fatty acids are both important, but after 1 to 3 hours of continuous exercise at this level, muscle glycogen stores become depleted, and the intensity of exercise declines to a rate that can be supported by oxidation of fatty acids.

Cardiac Muscle

During fetal life cardiac muscle primarily uses glucose as an energy source, but in the postnatal period there is a major switch to β-oxidation of fatty acids. Thus, in humans fatty acids serve as the major fuel for cardiac myocytes. When ketones are present during prolonged fasting, they are also used. Thus, not surprisingly, cardiac myocytes most closely parallel the skeletal muscle during extended periods of exercise.

In patients with cardiac hypertrophy, this situation reverses to some extent. In the failing heart, glucose oxidation increases, and β-oxidation falls.

Brain

Although the brain represents 2% of total body weight, it obtains 15% of the cardiac output, uses 20% of total O_2, and consumes 25% of the total glucose. Therefore, glucose is the primary fuel for the brain. Blood glucose levels are tightly regulated to maintain the concentration levels that enable sufficient glucose uptake into the brain via GLUT 1 and GLUT 3 transporters. Because glycogen levels in the brain are minor, normal function depends upon continuous glucose supply from the bloodstream. In hypoglycemic conditions (<70 mg/dL), centers in the hypothalamus sense a fall in blood glucose level, and the release of glucagon and epinephrine is triggered. Fatty acids cannot cross the blood–brain barrier and are therefore not used at all. Between meals, the brain relies on blood glucose supplied by either hepatic glycogenolysis or gluconeogenesis. Only in prolonged fasts does the brain gain the capacity to use ketones for energy, and even then ketones supply only approximately two thirds of the fuel; the remainder is glucose.

Glycolysis and Pyruvate Dehydrogenase 12

Learning Objectives

❏ Answer questions about carbohydrate digestion

❏ Demonstrate understanding of glucose transport

❏ Solve problems concerning glycolysis

❏ Interpret scenarios about galactose and fructose metabolism

❏ Answer questions about pyruvate dehydrogenase

OVERVIEW

All cells can carry out glycolysis. In a few tissues, most importantly red blood cells, glycolysis represents the only energy-yielding pathway available. Glucose is the major monosaccharide that enters the pathway, but others such as galactose and fructose can also be used. The first steps in glucose metabolism in any cell are transport across the membrane and phosphorylation by kinase enzymes inside the cell to prevent it from leaving via the transporter.

CARBOHYDRATE DIGESTION

Only a very small amount of the total carbohydrates ingested are monosaccharides. Most of the carbohydrates in foods are in complex forms, such as starch (amylose and amylopectin) and the disaccharides sucrose and lactose. In the mouth, secreted salivary amylase randomly hydrolyzes the starch polymers to dextrins (< 8–10 glucoses). Upon entry of food into the stomach, the acid pH destroys the salivary amylase. In the intestine, the dextrins are hydrolyzed to the disaccharides maltose and isomaltose. Disaccharides in the intestinal brush border complete the digestion process:

- Maltase cleaves maltose to 2 glucoses
- Isomaltase cleaves isomaltose to 2 glucoses
- Lactase cleaves lactose to glucose and galactose
- Sucrase cleaves sucrose to glucose and fructose

Uptake of glucose into the mucosal cells is performed by the sodium/glucose transporter, an active transport system.

GLUCOSE TRANSPORT

Glucose entry into most cells is concentration driven and independent of sodium. Four glucose transporters (GLUT) are listed in Table 12-1. They have different affinities for glucose coinciding with their respective physiologic roles. Normal glucose concentration in peripheral blood is 4–6 mM (70–110 mg/dL).

- GLUT 1 and GLUT 3 mediate basal glucose uptake in most tissues, including brain, nerves, and red blood cells. Their high affinities for glucose ensure glucose entry even during periods of relative hypoglycemia. At normal glucose concentration, GLUT 1 and GLUT 3 are at V_{max}.

- GLUT 2, a low-affinity transporter, is in hepatocytes. After a meal, portal blood from the intestine is rich in glucose. GLUT 2 captures the excess glucose primarily for storage. When the glucose concentration drops below the *Km* for the transporter, much of the remainder leaves the liver and enters the peripheral circulation. In the β-islet cells of the pancreas. GLUT-2, along with glucokinase, serves as the glucose sensor for insulin release.

- GLUT 4 is in adipose tissue and muscle and responds to the glucose concentration in peripheral blood. The rate of glucose transport in these two tissues is increased by insulin, which stimulates the movement of additional GLUT 4 transporters to the membrane by a mechanism involving exocytosis.

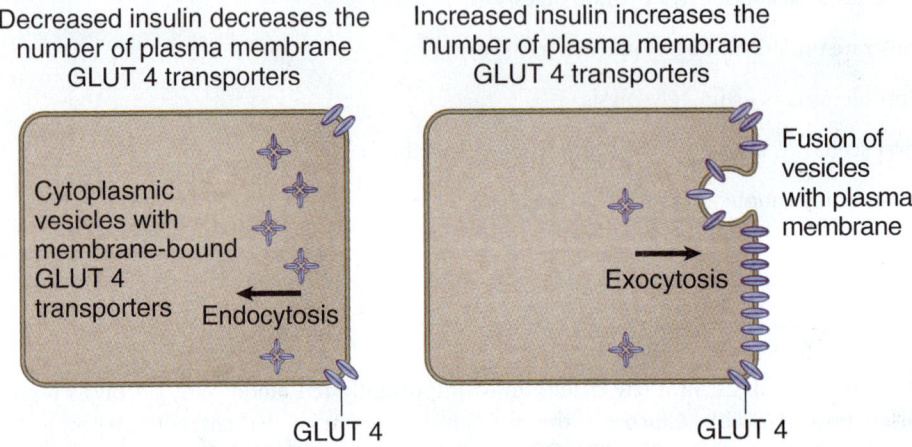

Figure 12-1. Insulin Regulation of Glucose Transport in Muscle and Adipose Cells

Although basal transport occurs in all cells independently of insulin, the transport rate increases in adipose tissue and muscle when insulin levels rise. Muscle stores excess glucose as glycogen, and adipose tissue requires glucose to form dihydroxyacetone phosphate (DHAP), which is converted to glycerol phosphate used to store incoming fatty acids as triglyceride (TGL, three fatty acids attached to glycerol).

Table 12-1. Major Glucose Transporters in Human Cells

Name	Tissues	K_m, Glucose	Functions
GLUT 1	Most tissues (brain, red cells)	~1 mM	Basal uptake of glucose
GLUT 2	Liver Pancreatic β-cells	~15 mM	Uptake and release of glucose by the liver β-cell glucose sensor
GLUT 3	Most tissues	~1 mM	Basal uptake
GLUT 4	Skeletal muscle Adipose tissue	~5 mM	Insulin-stimulated glucose uptake; stimulated by exercise in skeletal muscle

Normal blood glucose concentration is 4–6 mM (72–110 mg/dL).

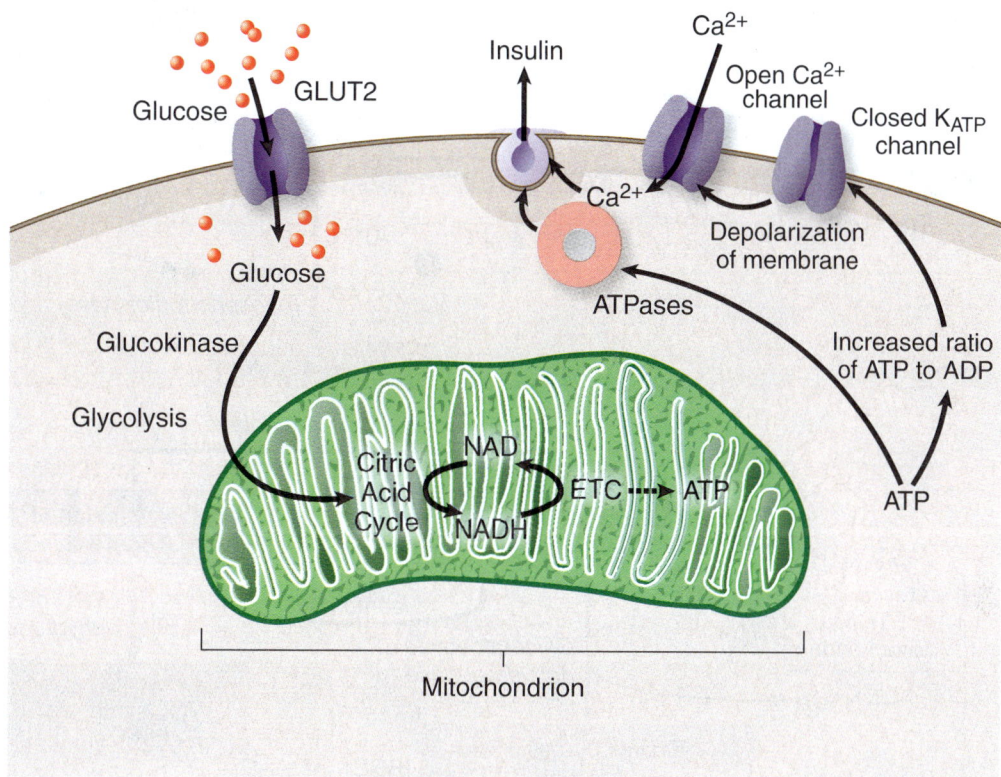

Figure 12-2. GLUT2 and Glucokinase Together Function as the Glucose Sensor in Pancreatic β-Islet Cells

GLYCOLYSIS

Glycolysis is a cytoplasmic pathway that converts glucose into two pyruvates, releasing a modest amount of energy captured in two substrate-level phosphorylations and one oxidation reaction. If a cell has mitochondria and oxygen, glycolysis is aerobic. If either mitochondria or oxygen is lacking, glycolysis may occur anaerobically (erythrocytes, exercising skeletal muscle), although some of the available energy is lost.

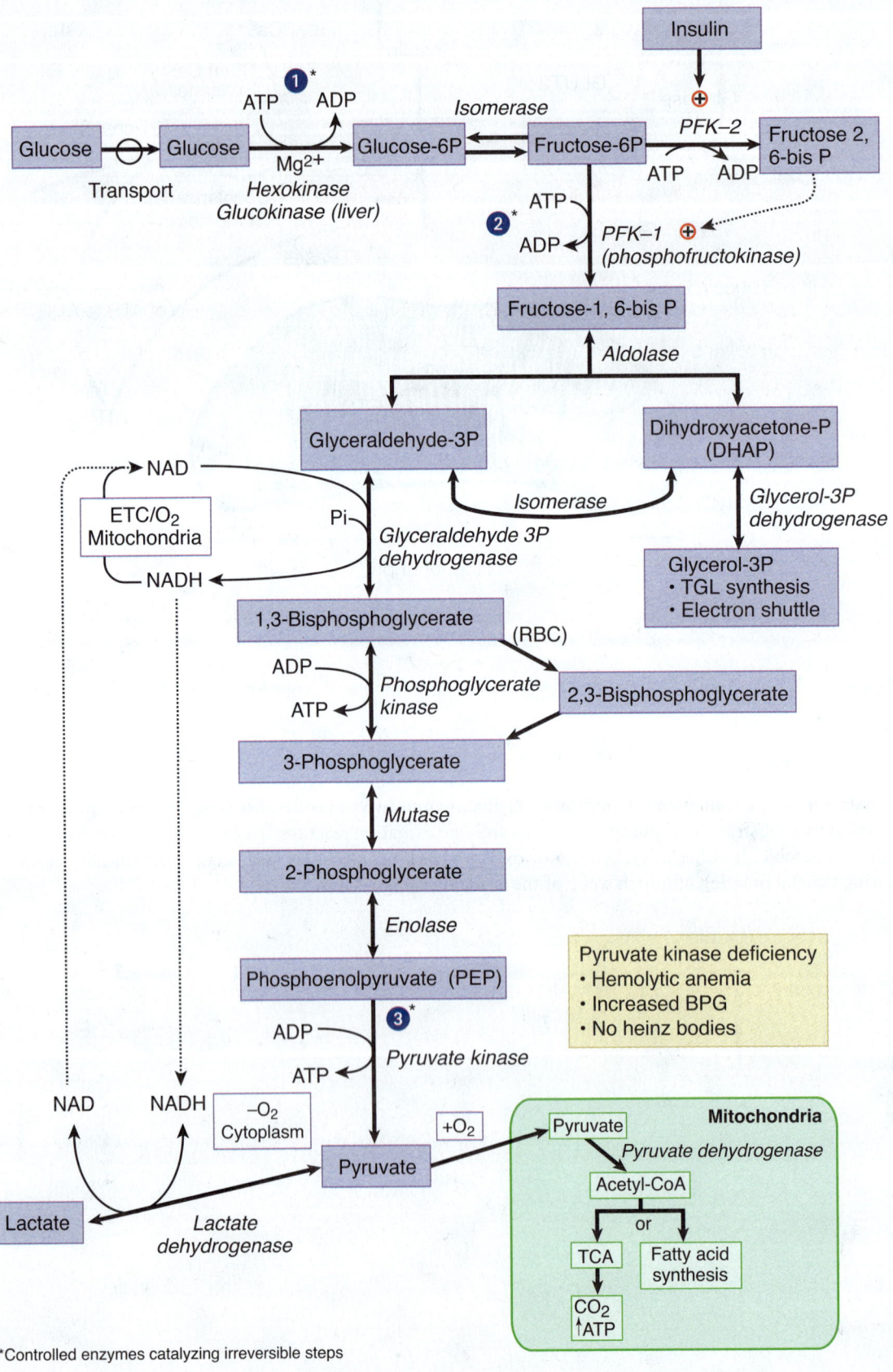

Figure 12-3. Glycolysis

Glycolysis also provides intermediates for other pathways. In the liver, glycolysis is part of the process by which excess glucose is converted to fatty acids for storage. Important enzymes in glycolysis include:

1. **Hexokinase/glucokinase:** glucose entering the cell is trapped by phosphorylation using ATP. Hexokinase is widely distributed in tissues, whereas glucokinase is found only in hepatocytes and pancreatic β-islet cells. The following table identifies the differences in their respective K_m and V_{max} values. These coincide with the differences in K_m values for the glucose transporters in these tissues.

Table 12-2. Comparison of Hexokinase and Glucokinase

Hexokinase	Glucokinase
Most tissues	Hepatocytes and pancreatic β-islet cells (along with GLUT-2, acts as the glucose sensor)
Low K_m (0.05 mM in erythrocytes)	High K_m (10 mM)
Inhibited by glucose 6-phosphate	Induced by insulin in hepatocytes

2. **Phosphofructokinases** (PFK-1 and PFK-2): PFK-1 is the rate-limiting enzyme and main control point in glycolysis. In this reaction, fructose 6-phosphate is phosphorylated to fructose 1,6-bisphosphate using ATP.

   • PFK-1 is inhibited by ATP and citrate, and activated by AMP.

   • Insulin stimulates and glucagon inhibits PFK-1 in hepatocytes by an indirect mechanism involving PFK-2 and fructose 2,6-bisphosphate (Figure 12-3).

Note

C-peptide is a short polypeptide that connects the A-chain to the B-chain in the proinsulin molecule. It is removed after proinsulin is packaged into vesicles in the Golgi apparatus.

Insulin activates PFK-2 (via the tyrosine kinase receptor and activation of protein phosphatases), which converts a tiny amount of fructose 6-phosphate to fructose 2,6-bisphosphate (F2,6-BP). F2,6-BP activates PFK-1. Glucagon inhibits PFK-2 (via cAMP-dependent protein kinase A), lowering F2,6-BP and thereby inhibiting PFK-1. PFK-1 is a multi-subunit enzyme that demonstrates cooperative kinetics (discussed in Chapter 8).

3. **Glyceraldehyde 3-phosphate dehydrogenase** : catalyzes an oxidation and addition of inorganic phosphate (P_i) to its substrate. This results in the production of a high-energy intermediate 1,3-bisphosphoglycerate and the reduction of NAD to NADH. If glycolysis is aerobic, the NADH can be reoxidized (indirectly) by the mitochondrial electron transport chain, providing energy for ATP synthesis by oxidative phosphorylation.

4. **3-Phosphoglycerate kinase:** transfers the high-energy phosphate from 1,3-bisphosphoglycerate to ADP, forming ATP and 3-phosphoglycerate. This type of reaction in which ADP is directly phosphorylated to ATP using a high-energy intermediate is referred to as a substrate-level phosphorylation. In contrast to oxidative phosphorylation in mitochondria, substrate-level phosphorylations are not dependent on oxygen, and are the only means of ATP generation in an anaerobic tissue.

5. **Pyruvate kinase:** the last enzyme in aerobic glycolysis, it catalyzes a substrate-level phosphorylation of ADP using the high-energy substrate phosphoenolpyruvate (PEP). Pyruvate kinase is activated by fructose 1,6-bisphosphate from the PFK-1 reaction (feed-forward activation).

6. **Lactate dehydrogenase**: is used only in anaerobic glycolysis. It reoxidizes NADH to NAD, replenishing the oxidized coenzyme for glyceraldehyde 3-phosphate dehydrogenase. Without mitochondria and oxygen, glycolysis would stop when all the available NAD had been reduced to NADH. By reducing pyruvate to lactate and oxidizing NADH to NAD, lactate dehydrogenase prevents this potential problem from developing. In aerobic tissues, lactate does not normally form in significant amounts. However, when oxygenation is poor (skeletal muscle during strenuous exercise, myocardial infarction), most cellular ATP is generated by anaerobic glycolysis, and lactate production increases.

Important Intermediates of Glycolysis

- Dihydroxyacetone phosphate (DHAP) is used in liver and adipose tissue for triglyceride synthesis.
- 1,3-Bisphosphoglycerate and phosphoenolpyruvate (PEP) are high-energy intermediates used to generate ATP by substrate-level phosphorylation.

Glycolysis Is Irreversible

Three enzymes in the pathway catalyze reactions that are irreversible. When the liver produces glucose, different reactions and therefore different enzymes must be used at these three points:

- Glucokinase/hexokinase
- PFK-1
- Pyruvate kinase

ATP Production and Electron Shuttles

Anaerobic glycolysis yields 2 ATP/glucose by substrate-level phosphorylation. Aerobic glycolysis yields these 2 ATP/glucose plus 2 NADH/glucose that can be utilized for ATP production in the mitochondria; however, the inner membrane is impermeable to NADH. Cytoplasmic NADH is reoxidized to NAD and delivers its electrons to one of two electron shuttles in the inner membrane. In the malate shuttle, electrons are passed to mitochondrial NADH and then to the electron transport chain. In the glycerol phosphate shuttle, electrons are passed to mitochondrial $FADH_2$. The two shuttles are diagrammed in Figure 12-3; important points include:

- Cytoplasmic NADH oxidized using the malate shuttle produces a mitochondrial NADH and yields approximately 3 ATP by oxidative phosphorylation.
- Cytoplasmic NADH oxidized by the glycerol phosphate shuttle produces a mitochondrial $FADH_2$ and yields approximately 2 ATP by oxidative phosphorylation.

Glycolysis in the Erythrocyte

In red blood cells, anaerobic glycolysis represents the only pathway for ATP production, yielding a net 2 ATP/glucose.

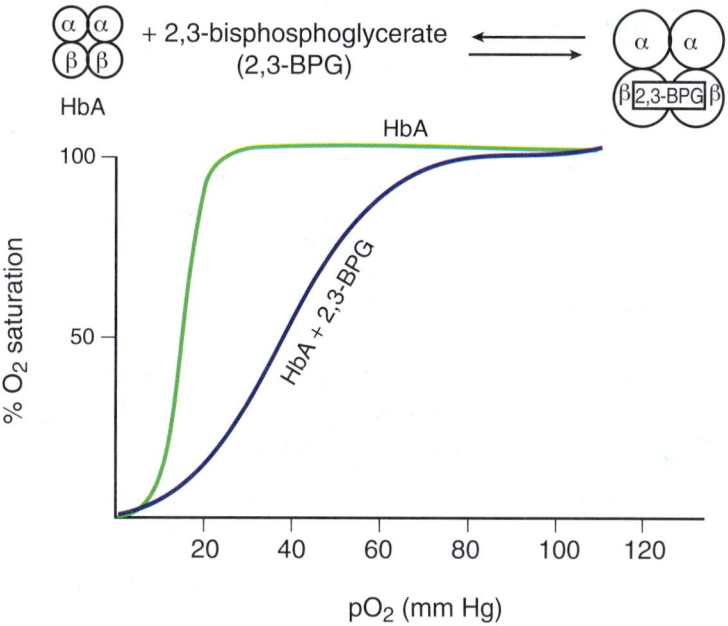

Figure 12-4. Effect of 2,3-Bisphosphoglycerate on Hemoglobin A

Erythrocytes have bisphosphoglycerate mutase, which produces 2,3-bisphosphoglycerate (BPG) from 1,3-BPG in glycolysis. 2,3-BPG binds to the β-chains of hemoglobin A (HbA) and decreases its affinity for oxygen. This effect of 2,3-BPG is seen in the oxygen dissociation curve for HbA, shown in Figure I-12-4. The rightward shift in the curve is sufficient to allow unloading of oxygen in tissues, but still allows 100% saturation in the lungs. An abnormal increase in erythrocyte 2,3-BPG might shift the curve far enough so HbA is not fully saturated in the lungs.

Although 2,3-BPG binds to HbA, it does not bind well to HbF ($\alpha_2\gamma_2$), with the result that HbF has a higher affinity for oxygen than maternal HbA, allowing transplacental passage of oxygen from mother to fetus.

Clinical Correlate

Transfused blood has lower than the expected 2,3-BPG levels, making it less efficient at delivering oxygen to peripheral tissues.

Pyruvate kinase deficiency

Pyruvate kinase deficiency is the second most common genetic deficiency that causes a hemolytic anemia (glucose 6-phosphate dehydrogenase, G6PDH, is the most common). Characteristics include:

- Chronic hemolysis
- Increased 2,3-BPG and therefore a lower-than-normal oxygen affinity of HbA
- Absence of Heinz bodies (Heinz bodies are more characteristic of G6PDH deficiency)

The red blood cell has no mitochondria and is totally dependent on anaerobic glycolysis for ATP. In pyruvate kinase deficiency, the decrease in ATP causes the erythrocyte to lose its characteristic biconcave shape and signals its destruction in the spleen. In addition, decreased ion pumping by Na^+/K^+-ATPase results in loss of ion balance and causes osmotic fragility, leading to swelling and lysis.

GALACTOSE METABOLISM

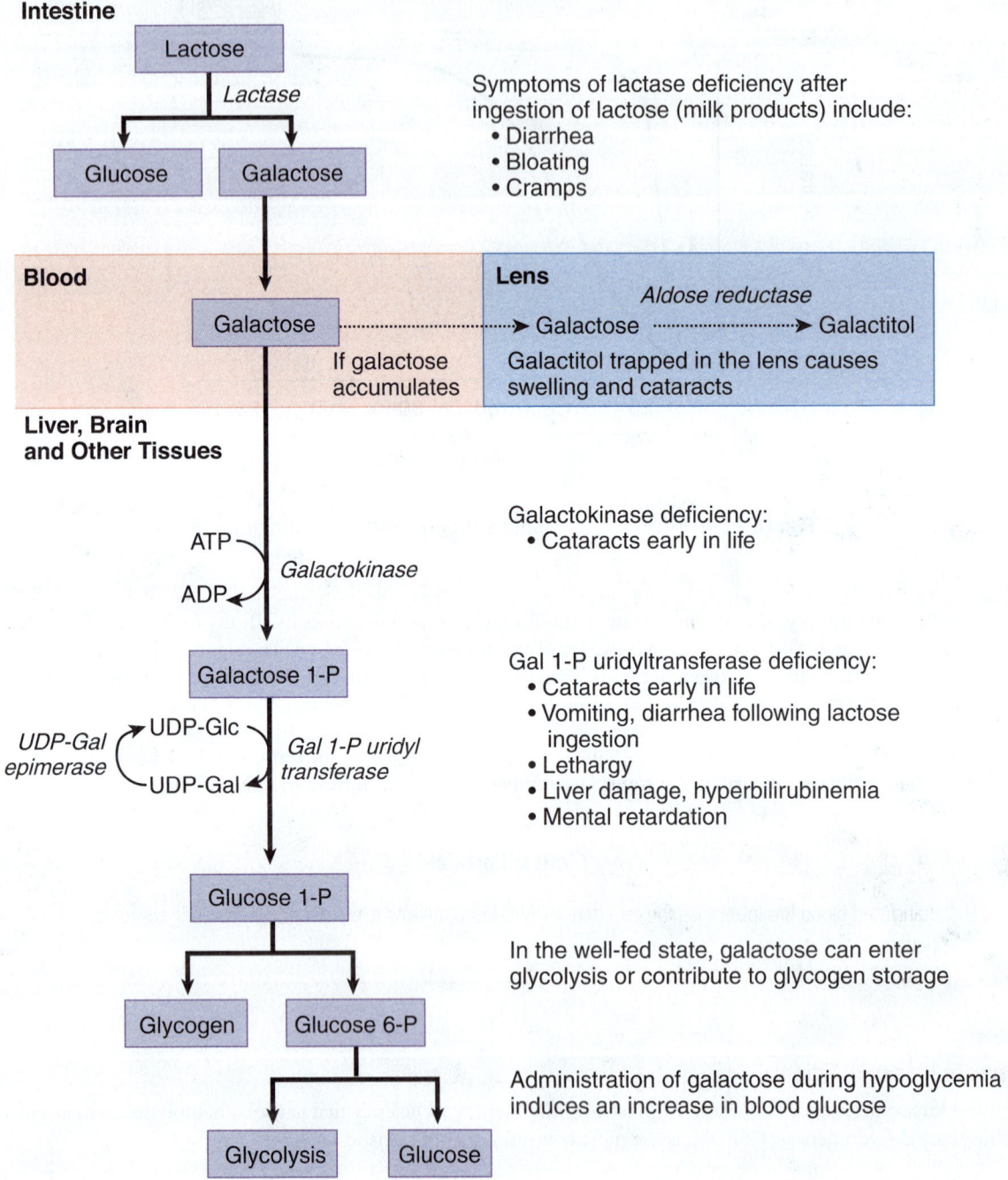

Figure 12-5. Galactose Metabolism

An important source of galactose in the diet is the disaccharide lactose present in milk. Lactose is hydrolyzed to galactose and glucose by lactase associated with the brush border membrane of the small intestine. Along with other monosaccharides, galactose reaches the liver through the portal blood.

Once transported into tissues, galactose is phosphorylated (galactokinase), trapping it in the cell. Galactose 1-phosphate is converted to glucose 1-phosphate by galactose 1-P uridyltransferase and an epimerase. The pathway is shown in Figure 12-5; important enzymes to remember are:

- Galactokinase
- Galactose 1-phosphate uridyltransferase

Genetic deficiencies of these enzymes produce galactosemia. Cataracts, a characteristic finding in patients with galactosemia, result from conversion of the excess galactose in peripheral blood to galactitol in the lens of the eye, which has aldose reductase. Accumulation of galactitol in the lens causes osmotic damage and cataracts.

The same mechanism accounts for the cataracts in diabetics because aldose reductase also converts glucose to sorbitol, which causes osmotic damage.

Deficiency of galactose 1-phosphate uridyltransferase produces a more severe disease because, in addition to galactosemia, galactose 1-P accumulates in the liver, brain, and other tissues.

Clinical Correlate

Lactose Intolerance Primary lactose intolerance is caused by a hereditary deficiency of lactase, most commonly found in persons of Asian and African descent. Secondary lactose intolerance can be precipitated at any age by gastrointestinal disturbances such as celiac sprue, colitis, or viral-induced damage to intestinal mucosa, which is why kids with diarrhea should drink clear liquids, and not milk.

Common symptoms of lactose intolerance include vomiting, bloating, explosive and watery diarrhea, cramps, and dehydration. The symptoms can be attributed to bacterial fermentation of lactose to a mixture of CH_4, H_2, and small organic acids. The acids are osmotically active and result in the movement of water into the intestinal lumen.

Diagnosis is based on a positive hydrogen breath test after an oral lactose load. Treatment is by dietary restriction of milk and milk products (except unpasteurized yogurt, which contains active *Lactobacillus*) or by lactase pills.

FRUCTOSE METABOLISM

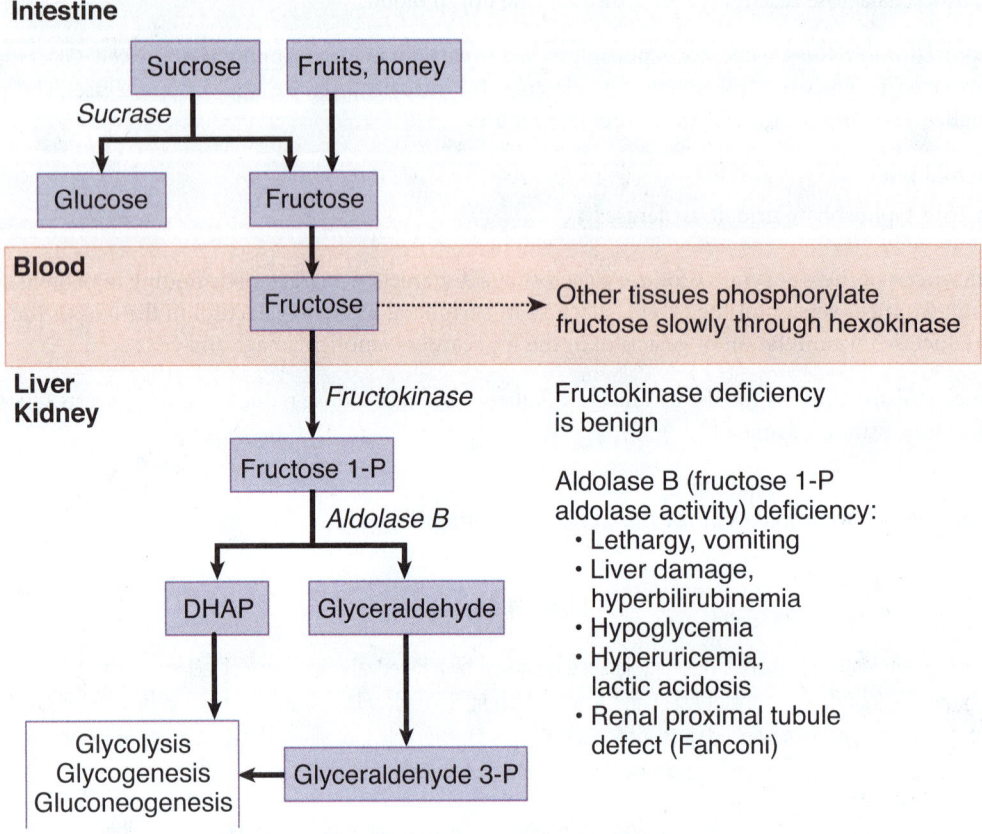

Figure 12-6. Fructose Metabolism

Fructose is found in honey and fruit and as part of the disaccharide sucrose (common table sugar). Sucrose is hydrolyzed by intestinal brush border sucrase, and the resulting monosaccharides, glucose and fructose, are absorbed into the portal blood. The liver phosphorylates fructose and cleaves it into glyceraldehyde and DHAP. Smaller amounts are metabolized in renal proximal tubules. The pathway is shown in Figure 12-6; important enzymes to remember are:

- Fructokinase
- Fructose 1-P aldolase (aldolase B)

Genetic deficiency of fructokinase is benign and often detected incidentally when the urine is checked for glucose with a dipstick. Fructose 1-phosphate aldolase deficiency is a severe disease because of accumulation of fructose 1-phosphate in the liver and renal proximal tubules. Symptoms are reversed after removing fructose and sucrose from the diet.

Cataracts are not a feature of this disease because fructose is not an aldose sugar and therefore not a substrate for aldose reductase in the lens.

PYRUVATE DEHYDROGENASE

Pyruvate from aerobic glycolysis enters mitochondria, where it may be converted to acetyl-CoA for entry into the citric acid cycle if ATP is needed, or for fatty acid synthesis if sufficient ATP is present. The pyruvate dehydrogenase (PDH) reaction is irreversible and cannot be used to convert acetyl-CoA to pyruvate or to glucose. Pyruvate dehydrogenase in the liver is activated by insulin, whereas in the brain and nerves the enzyme (actually a complex of five different enzymatic activities) is not responsive to hormones.

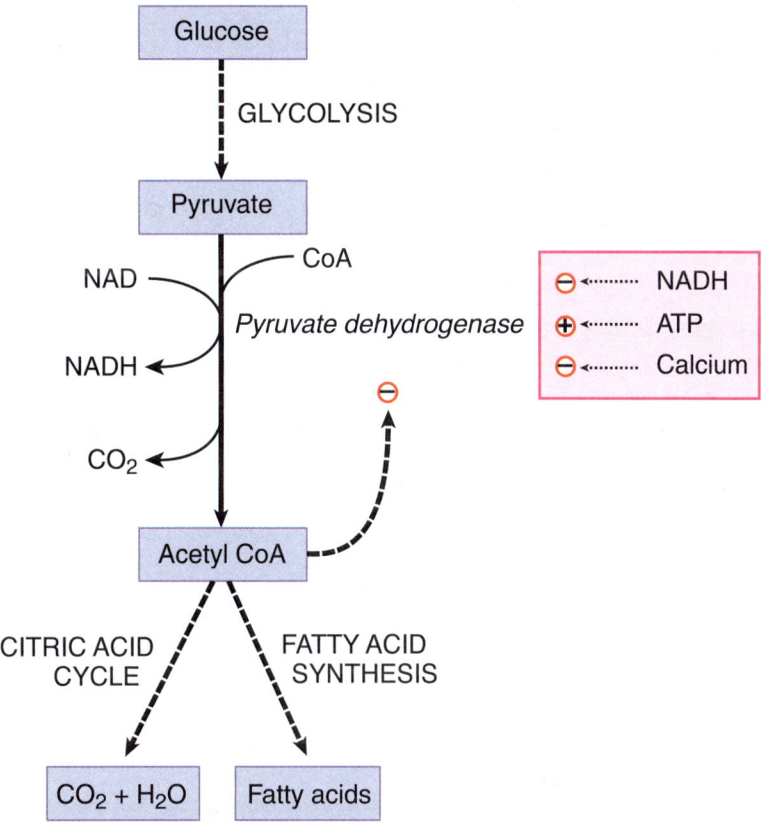

Figure 12-7. Pyruvate Dehydrogenase

Cofactors and coenzymes used by pyruvate dehydrogenase include:

- Thiamine pyrophosphate (TPP) from the vitamin thiamine
- Lipoic acid
- Coenzyme A (CoA) from pantothenate
- $FAD(H_2)$ from riboflavin
- NAD(H) from niacin (some may be synthesized from tryptophan)

Pyruvate dehydrogenase is inhibited by its product acetyl-CoA. This control is important in several contexts and should be considered along with pyruvate carboxylase, the other mitochondrial enzyme that uses pyruvate (introduced in chapter 14, Gluconeogenesis, Figure 14-5).

Thiamine Deficiency

Thiamine deficiency is commonly seen in alcoholics, who may develop a complex of symptoms associated with Wernicke peripheral neuropathy and Korsakoff psychosis. Alcohol interferes with thiamine absorption from the intestine. Symptoms include:

- Ataxia
- Ophthalmoplegia, nystagmus
- Memory loss and confabulation
- Cerebral hemorrhage

Congestive heart failure may be a complication (wet beri-beri) owing to inadequate ATP and accumulation of ketoacids in the cardiac muscle.

Clinical Correlate
If thiamine deficiency is suspected, patients should be given IV thiamine in the emergency department to prevent lactic acidosis when glucose (dextrose) is administered.

Two other enzyme complexes similar to pyruvate dehydrogenase that use thiamine are:

- α-Ketoglutarate dehydrogenase (citric acid cycle)
- Branched-chain ketoacid dehydrogenase (metabolism of branched-chain amino acids)

Insufficient thiamine significantly impairs glucose oxidation, causing highly aerobic tissues, such as brain and cardiac muscle, to fail first. In addition, branched-chain amino acids are sources of energy in brain and muscle.

Citric Acid Cycle and Oxidative Phosphorylation

13

Learning Objectives

❑ Solve problems concerning citric acid cycle

❑ Explain information related to electron transport chain

❑ Use knowledge of ATP and oxidative phosphorylation

CITRIC ACID CYCLE

The citric acid cycle, also called the Krebs cycle or the tricarboxylic acid (TCA) cycle, is in the mitochondria. Although oxygen is not directly required in the cycle, the pathway will not occur anaerobically because NADH and $FADH_2$ will accumulate if oxygen is not available for the electron transport chain.

The primary function of the citric acid cycle is oxidation of acetyl-CoA to carbon dioxide. The energy released from this oxidation is saved as NADH, $FADH_2$, and guanosine triphosphate (GTP). The overall result of the cycle is represented by the following reaction:

$$\text{Acetyl-CoA} \longrightarrow 2\ CO_2$$
$$3\ NAD + FAD + GDP + P_i \qquad\qquad 3\ NADH + FADH_2 + GTP$$

Notice that none of the intermediates of the citric acid cycle appear in this reaction, not as reactants or as products. This emphasizes an important (and frequently misunderstood) point about the cycle. It does not represent a pathway for the net conversion of acetyl-CoA to citrate, to malate, or to any other intermediate of the cycle. The only fate of acetyl-CoA in this pathway is its oxidation to CO_2. Therefore, the citric acid cycle does not represent a pathway by which there can be net synthesis of glucose from acetyl-CoA.

The cycle is central to the oxidation of any fuel that yields acetyl-CoA, including glucose, fatty acids, ketone bodies, ketogenic amino acids, and alcohol. There is no hormonal control of the cycle, as activity is necessary irrespective of the fed or fasting state. Control is exerted by the energy status of the cell through allosteric activation or deactivation. Many enzymes are subject to negative feedback.

The citric acid cycle is shown in Figure 13-1. All the enzymes are in the matrix of the mitochondria except succinate dehydrogenase, which is in the inner membrane.

Key points:

1. Isocitrate dehydrogenase, the major control enzyme, is inhibited by NADH and ATP and activated by ADP.
2. α-Ketoglutarate dehydrogenase, like pyruvate dehydrogenase, is a multienzyme complex. It requires thiamine, lipoic acid, CoA, FAD, and NAD. Lack of thiamine slows oxidation of acetyl-CoA in the citric acid cycle.
3. Succinyl-CoA synthetase (succinate thiokinase) catalyzes a substrate-level phosphorylation of GDP to GTP.
4. Succinate dehydrogenase is on the inner mitochondrial membrane, where it also functions as complex II of the electron transport chain.
5. Citrate synthase condenses the incoming acetyl group with oxaloacetate to form citrate.

Note

GTP is energetically equivalent to ATP:

GTP + ADP <---> GDP + ATP

catalyzed by nucleoside diphosphate kinase

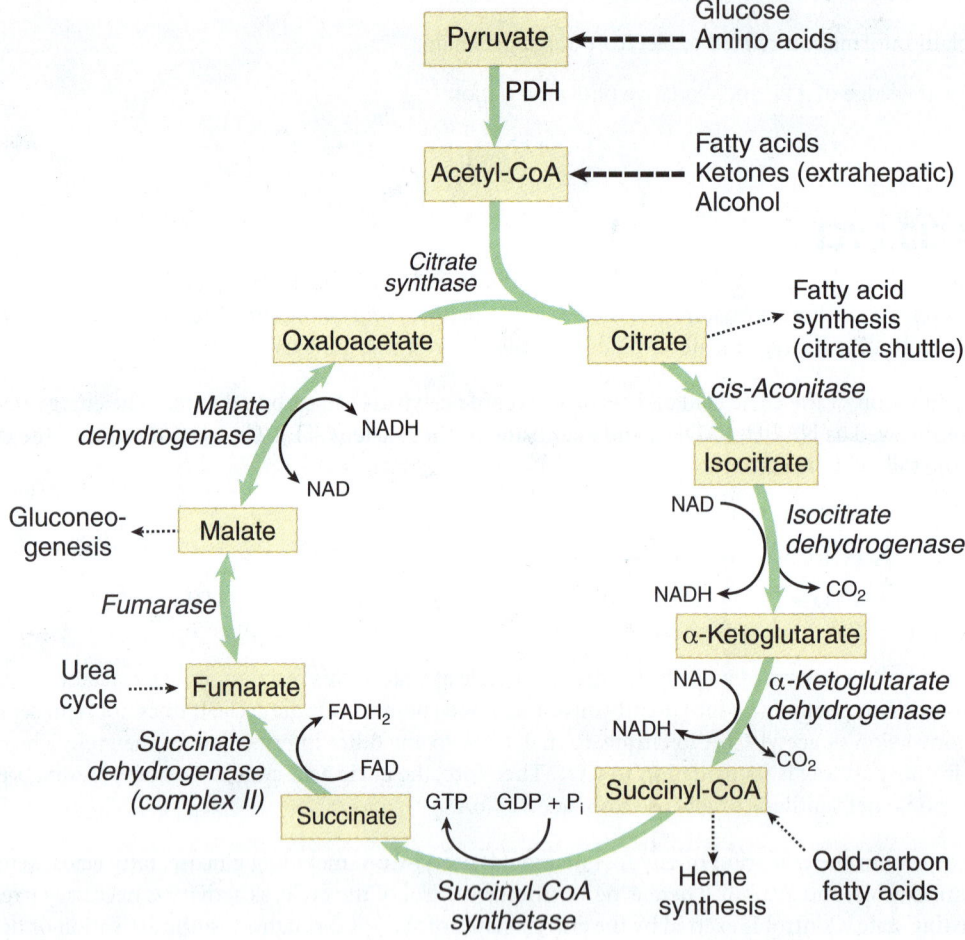

Figure 13-1. Citric Acid Cycle

Several intermediates of the cycle may serve other functions:

- Citrate may leave the mitochondria (citrate shuttle) to deliver acetyl-CoA into the cytoplasm for fatty acid synthesis.
- Succinyl-CoA is a high-energy intermediate that can be used for heme synthesis and to activate ketone bodies in extrahepatic tissues.
- Malate can leave the mitochondria (malate shuttle) for gluconeogenesis.

When intermediates are drawn out of the citric acid cycle, the cycle slows. Therefore when intermediates leave the cycle they must be replaced to ensure sufficient energy for the cell.

ELECTRON TRANSPORT CHAIN AND OXIDATIVE PHOSPHORYLATION

The mitochondrial electron transport chain (ETC) carries out the following two reactions:

$$NADH + O_2 \longrightarrow NAD + H_2O \qquad \Delta G = -56 \text{ kcal/mol}$$

$$FADH_2 + O_2 \longrightarrow FAD + H_2O \qquad \Delta G = -42 \text{ kcal/mol}$$

Although the value of ΔG should not be memorized, it does indicate the large amount of energy released by both reactions. The electron transport chain is a device to capture this energy in a form useful for doing work.

Sources of NADH, FADH$_2$, and O$_2$

Many enzymes in the mitochondria, including those of the citric acid cycle and pyruvate dehydrogenase, produce NADH, all of which can be oxidized in the electron transport chain and in the process, capture energy for ATP synthesis by oxidative phosphorylation. If NADH is produced in the cytoplasm, either the malate shuttle or the α-glycerol phosphate shuttle can transfer the electrons into the mitochondria for delivery to the ETC. Once NADH has been oxidized, the NAD can again be used by enzymes that require it.

FADH$_2$ is produced by succinate dehydrogenase in the citric acid cycle and by the α-glycerol phosphate shuttle. Both enzymes are located in the inner membrane and can reoxidize FADH$_2$ directly by transferring electrons into the ETC. Once FADH$_2$ has been oxidized, the FAD can be made available once again for use by the enzyme.

O$_2$ is delivered to tissues by hemoglobin. The majority of oxygen required in a tissue is consumed in the ETC. Its function is to accept electrons at the end of the chain, and the water formed is added to the cellular water. This scheme is shown in the following figure.

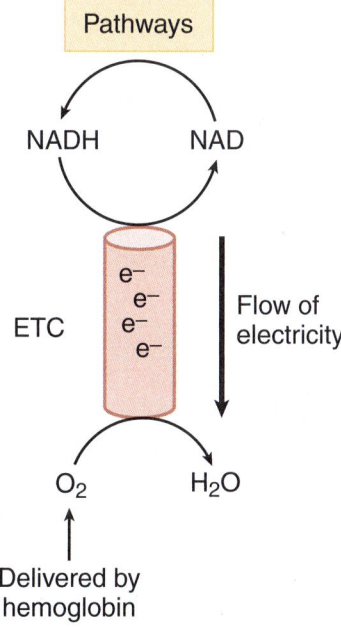

Figure 13-2. Overview of the Electron Transport Chain

Capturing Chemical Energy as Electricity

The mitochondrial electron transport chain works like a chemical battery. In one location, an oxidation reaction is poised to release electrons at very high energy; in another location, a potential electron acceptor waits to be reduced. Because the two components are physically separated, nothing happens. Once the two terminals of the battery are connected by a wire, electrons flow from one compartment to the other through the wire, producing an electrical current or electricity. A light bulb or an electrical pump inserted into the circuit will run on the electricity generated. If no electrical device is in the circuit, all the energy is released as heat. The mitochondrial electron transport chain operates according to the same principle.

Electron Transport Chain

NADH is oxidized by NADH dehydrogenase (complex I), delivering its electrons into the chain and returning as NAD to enzymes that require it. The electrons are passed along a series of protein and lipid carriers that serve as the wire. These include, in order:

- NADH dehydrogenase (complex I) accepts electrons from NADH
- Coenzyme Q (a lipid)
- Cytochrome b/c_1 (an Fe/heme protein; complex III)
- Cytochrome c (an Fe/heme protein)
- Cytochrome a/a_3 (a Cu/heme protein; cytochrome oxidase, complex IV) transfers electrons to oxygen

All these components are in the inner membrane of the mitochondria as shown in the following figure. Succinate dehydrogenase and the α-glycerol phosphate shuttle enzymes reoxidize their $FADH_2$ and pass electrons directly to CoQ.

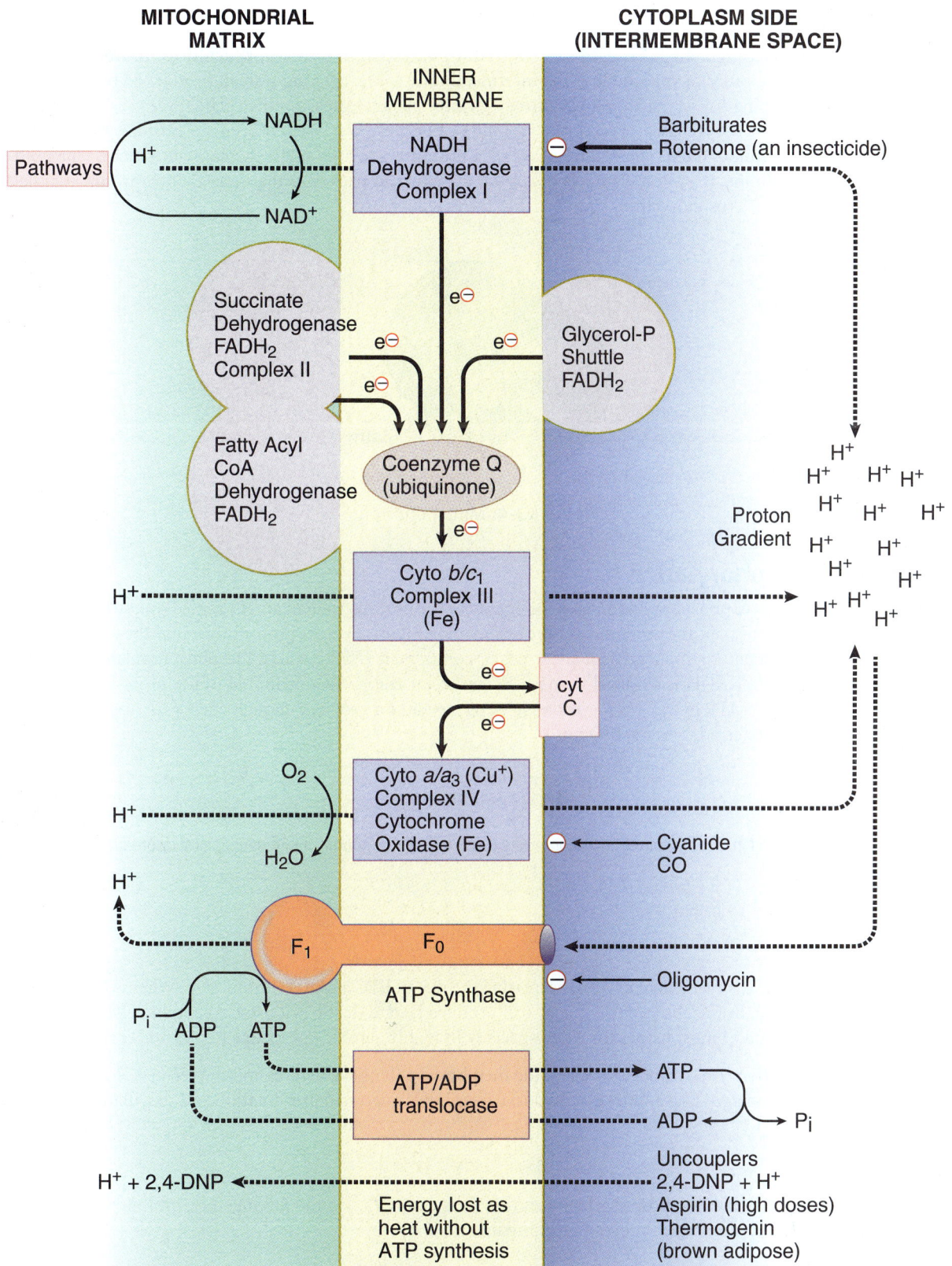

Figure 13-3. Oxidative Phosphorylation

Proton Gradient

The electricity generated by the ETC is used to run proton pumps (translocators), which drive protons from the matrix space across the inner membrane into the intermembrane space, creating a small proton (or pH) gradient. This is similar to pumping any ion, such as Na^+, across a membrane to create a gradient. The three major complexes I, III, and IV (NADH dehydrogenase, cytochrome b/c_1, and cytochrome a/a_3) each translocate protons in this way as the electricity passes through them. The end result is that a proton gradient is normally maintained across the mitochondrial inner membrane. If proton channels open, the protons run back into the matrix. Such proton channels are part of the oxidative phosphorylation complex.

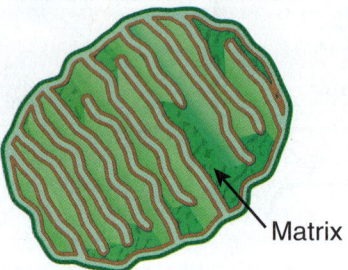

—Matrix

Figure 13-4. Mitochondrion

Oxidative Phosphorylation

ATP synthesis by oxidative phosphorylation uses the energy of the proton gradient and is carried out by the F_0F_1 ATP synthase complex, which spans the inner membrane as shown in Figure 13-3. As protons flow into the mitochondria through the F_0 component, their energy is used by the F_1 component (ATP synthase) to phosphorylate ADP using P_i. On average, when an NADH is oxidized in the ETC, sufficient energy is contributed to the proton gradient for the phosphorylation of 3 ATP by F_0F_1 ATP synthase. $FADH_2$ oxidation provides enough energy for approximately 2 ATP. These figures are referred to as the P/O ratios.

Bridge to Pathology

A genetic defect in oxidative phosphorylation is one cause of Leigh syndrome, a rare neurological disorder.

Tissue Hypoxia

Hypoxia deprives the ETC of sufficient oxygen, decreasing the rate of ETC and ATP production. When ATP levels fall, glycolysis increases and, in the absence of oxygen, will produce lactate (lactic acidosis). Anaerobic glycolysis is not able to meet the demand of most tissues for ATP, especially in highly aerobic tissues like nerves and cardiac muscle.

In a myocardial infarction (MI), myocytes swell as the membrane potential collapses and the cell gets leaky. Enzymes are released from the damaged tissue, and lactic acidosis contributes to protein precipitation and coagulation necrosis.

Inhibitors

The ETC is coupled to oxidative phosphorylation so that their activities rise and fall together. Inhibitors of any step effectively inhibit the whole coupled process, resulting in:

- Decreased oxygen consumption
- Increased intracellular NADH/NAD and $FADH_2$/FAD ratios
- Decreased ATP

Important inhibitors include cyanide and carbon monoxide.

Cyanide

Cyanide is a deadly poison because it binds irreversibly to cytochrome a/a_3, preventing electron transfer to oxygen, and producing many of the same changes seen in tissue hypoxia. Sources of cyanide include:

- Burning polyurethane (foam stuffing in furniture and mattresses)
- Byproduct of nitroprusside (released slowly; thiosulfate can be used to destroy the cyanide)

Nitrites may be used as an antidote for cyanide poisoning if given rapidly. They convert hemoglobin to methemoglobin, which binds cyanide in the blood before reaching the tissues. Oxygen is also given, if possible.

Carbon monoxide

Carbon monoxide binds to cytochrome a/a_3 but less tightly than cyanide. It also binds to hemoglobin, displacing oxygen. Symptoms include headache, nausea, tachycardia, and tachypnea. Lips and cheeks turn a cherry-red color. Respiratory depression and coma result in death if not treated by giving oxygen. Sources of carbon monoxide include:

- Propane heaters and gas grills
- Vehicle exhaust
- Tobacco smoke
- House fires
- Methylene chloride–based paint strippers

Other inhibitors include antimycin (cytochrome b/c_1), doxorubicin (CoQ), and oligomycin (F_0).

Uncouplers

Uncouplers are chemicals that decrease the proton gradient, causing:

- Decreased ATP synthesis
- Increased oxygen consumption
- Increased oxidation of NADH

Because the rate of the ETC increases, with no ATP synthesis, energy is released as heat. Important uncouplers include 2,4-dinitrophenol (2,4-DNP) and aspirin (and other salicylates). Brown adipose tissue contains a natural uncoupling protein (UCP, formerly called thermogenin), which allows energy loss as heat to maintain a basal temperature around the kidneys, neck, breastplate, and scapulae in newborns.

Reactive Oxygen Species

When molecular oxygen (O_2) is partially reduced, unstable products called reactive oxygen species (ROS) are formed. These react rapidly with lipids to cause peroxidation, with proteins, and with other substrates, resulting in denaturation and precipitation in tissues. Reactive oxygen species include:

- Superoxide $\left(O_2^- \right)$
- Hydrogen peroxide (H_2O_2)
- Hydroxyl radical ($OH\cdot$)

The polymorphonuclear neutrophil produces these substances to kill bacteria in the protective space of the phagolysosome during the oxidative burst accompanying phagocytosis. Production of these same ROS can occur at a slower rate wherever there is oxygen in high concentration. Small quantities of ROS are inevitable by-products of the electron transport chain in mitochondria. These small quantities are normally destroyed by protective enzymes such as catalase. The rate of ROS production can increase dramatically under certain conditions, such as reperfusion injury in a tissue that has been temporarily deprived of oxygen. ATP levels will be low and NADH levels high in a tissue deprived of oxygen (as in an MI). When oxygen is suddenly introduced, there is a burst of activity in the ETC, generating incompletely reduced ROS.

Defenses against ROS accumulation are particularly important in highly aerobic tissues and include superoxide dismutase and catalase. In the special case of erythrocytes, large amounts of superoxide are generated by the spontaneous dissociation of the oxygen from hemoglobin (occurrence is 0.5–3% of the total hemoglobin per day). The products are methemoglobin and superoxide. The processes that adequately detoxify the superoxide require a variety of enzymes and compounds, including superoxide dismutase, catalase, as well as glutathione peroxidase, vitamin E in membranes, and vitamin C in the cytoplasm. Low levels of any of these detoxifying substances result in hemolysis. For example, inadequate production of NADPH in glucose 6-phosphate dehydrogenase deficiency results in accumulation of the destructive hydrogen peroxide (chapter 14).

Glycogen, Gluconeogenesis, and the Hexose Monophosphate Shunt

14

Learning Objectives

❏ Interpret scenarios about glycogenesis and glycogenolysis

❏ Demonstrate understanding of glycogenolysis and glycogen synthesis

❏ Interpret scenarios about genetic deficiencies of enzymes in glycogen metabolism

❏ Solve problems concerning gluconeogenesis

❏ Use knowledge of hexose monophosphate shunt

GLYCOGENESIS AND GLYCOGENOLYSIS

Glycogen, a branched polymer of glucose, represents a storage form of glucose. Glycogen synthesis and degradation occur primarily in liver and skeletal muscle, although other tissues, including cardiac muscle and the kidney, store smaller quantities.

Glycogen is stored in the cytoplasm as either single granules (skeletal muscle) or as clusters of granules (liver). The granule has a central protein core with polyglucose chains radiating outward to form a sphere. Glycogen granules composed entirely of linear chains have the highest *density* of glucose near the core. If the chains are branched, the glucose *density* is highest at the periphery of the granule, allowing more rapid release of glucose on demand.

Glycogen stored in the liver is a source of glucose mobilized during hypoglycemia. Muscle glycogen is stored as an energy reserve for muscle contraction. In white (fast-twitch) muscle fibers, the glucose is converted primarily to lactate, whereas in red (slow-twitch) muscle fibers, the glucose is completely oxidized.

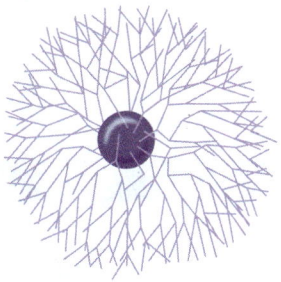

Figure 14-1. A glycogen granule

GLYCOGEN SYNTHESIS

Synthesis of glycogen granules begins with a core protein glycogenin. Glucose addition to a granule, shown in the following figure, begins with glucose 6-phosphate, which is converted to glucose 1-phosphate and activated to UDP-glucose for addition to the glycogen chain by glycogen synthase. Glycogen synthase is the rate-limiting enzyme of glycogen synthesis.

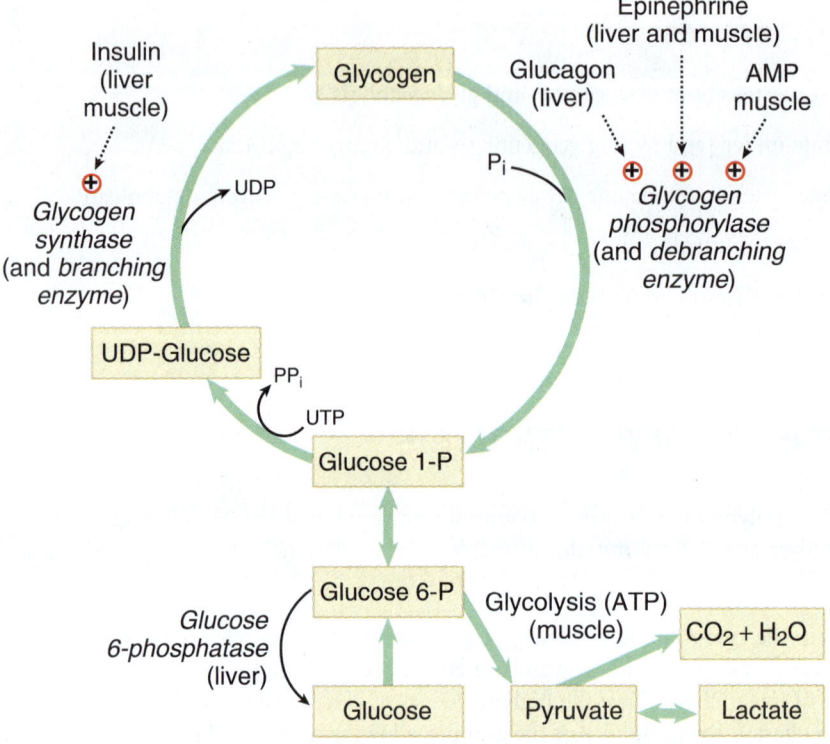

Figure 14-2. Glycogen Metabolism

Glycogen Synthase

Glycogen synthase forms the α1,4 glycosidic bond found in the linear glucose chains of the granule. The following table shows the control of glycogen synthase in liver and skeletal muscle.

Table 14-1. Comparison of Glycogen Synthase in Liver and Muscle

Glycogen Synthase	Liver	Skeletal Muscle
Activated by	Insulin	Insulin
Inhibited by	Glucagon Epinephrine	Epinephrine

Branching Enzyme (Glycosyl α 1,4: α 1,6 Transferase)

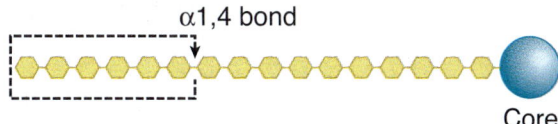

1. Glycogen synthase makes a linear α1,4-linked polyglucose chain (◦–◦–◦–◦).

2. Branching enzyme hydrolyzes an α1,4 bond.

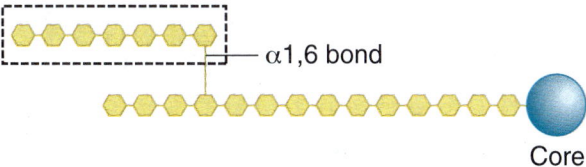

3. Transfers the oligoglucose unit and attaches it with an α1,6 bond to create a branch.

4. Glycogen synthase extends both branches.

Figure 14-3. Branching Enzyme

Branching enzyme is responsible for introducing α1,6-linked branches into the granule as it grows. The process by which the branch is introduced is shown schematically in Figure 14-3. Branching enzyme:

- Hydrolyzes one of the α1,4 bonds to release a block of oligoglucose, which is then moved and added in a slightly different location
- Forms an α1,6 bond to create a branch

GLYCOGENOLYSIS

The rate-limiting enzyme of glycogenolysis is glycogen phosphorylase (in contrast to a hydrolase, a phosphorylase breaks bonds using P_i rather than H_2O). The glucose 1-phosphate formed is converted to glucose 6-phosphate by the same mutase used in glycogen synthesis (Figure 14-2).

Glycogen Phosphorylase

Glycogen phosphorylase breaks α1,4 glycosidic bonds, releasing glucose 1-phosphate from the periphery of the granule. Control of the enzyme in liver and muscle is compared in the following table.

Table 14-2. Comparison of Glycogen Phosphorylase in Liver and Muscle

Glycogen Phosphorylase	Liver	Skeletal Muscle
Activated by	Epinephrine Glucagon	Epinephrine AMP Ca^{2+} (through calmodulin)
Inhibited by	Insulin	Insulin ATP

Glycogen phosphorylase cannot break α1,6 bonds and therefore stops when it nears the outermost branch points.

α1,4 bond nearest the branch point

to core

1. Glycogen phosphorylase releases glucose 1-P from the periphery of the granule until it encounters the first branch points.

2. Debranching enzyme hydrolyzes the α1,4 bond nearest the branch point, as shown.

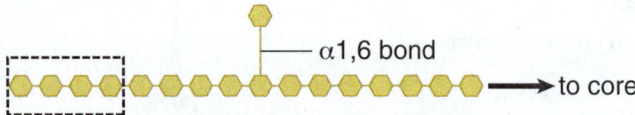

α1,6 bond

to core

3. Transfers the oligoglucose unit to the end of another chain, then

4. Hydrolyzes the α1,6 bond releasing the single glucose from the former branch.

Figure 14-4. Debranching Enzyme

Debranching Enzyme (Glucosyl α1,4: α1,4 Transferase and α1,6 Glucosidase)

Debranching enzyme deconstructs the branches in glycogen that have been exposed by glycogen phosphorylase. The two-step process by which this occurs is diagrammed in Figure 14-4. Debranching enzyme:

- Breaks an α1,4 bond adjacent to the branch point and moves the small oligoglucose chain released to the exposed end of the other chain

- Forms a new α1,4 bond

- Hydrolyzes the α1,6 bond, releasing the single residue at the branch point as free glucose. This represents the only free glucose produced directly in glycogenolysis.

GENETIC DEFICIENCIES OF ENZYMES IN GLYCOGEN METABOLISM

Important genetic deficiencies, listed in the following table, are classed as glycogen storage diseases because all are characterized by accumulation of glycogen in one or more tissues.

Table 14-3. Glycogen Storage Diseases

Type	Deficient Enzyme	Cardinal Clinical Features	Glycogen Structure
I: von Gierke	Glucose-6-phosphatase	Severe hypoglycemia, lactic acidosis, hepatomegaly, hyperlipidemia, hyperuricemia, short stature, doll-like facies, protruding abdomen emaciated extremities	Normal
II: Pompe	Lysosomal α1,4-glucosidase	Cardiomegaly, muscle weakness, death by 2 years	Glycogen-like material in inclusion bodies
III: Cori	Glycogen debranching enzyme	Mild hypoglycemia, liver enlargement	Short outer branches Single glucose residue at outer branch
IV: Andersen	Branching enzyme	Infantile hypotonia, cirrhosis, death by 2 years	Very few branches, especially toward periphery
V: McArdle	Muscle glycogen phosphorylase	Muscle cramps and weakness on exercise, myoglobinuria	Normal
VI: Hers	Hepatic glycogen phosphorylase	Mild fasting hypoglycemia, hepatomegaly, cirrhosis	Normal

GLUCONEOGENESIS

The liver maintains glucose levels in blood during fasting through either glycogenolysis or gluconeogenesis. These pathways are promoted by glucagon and epinephrine and inhibited by insulin. In fasting, glycogen reserves drop dramatically in the first 12 hours, during which time gluconeogenesis increases. After 24 hours, it represents the sole source of glucose. Important substrates for gluconeogenesis are:

- Glycerol 3-phosphate (from triacylglycerol in adipose)
- Lactate (from anaerobic glycolysis)
- Gluconeogenic amino acids (protein from muscle)

Table 14-4. Glucogenic and Ketogenic Amino Acids

Ketogenic	Ketogenic and Glucogenic	Glucogenic
Leucine Lysine	Phenylalanine Tyrosine Tryptophan Isoleucine Threonine	All others

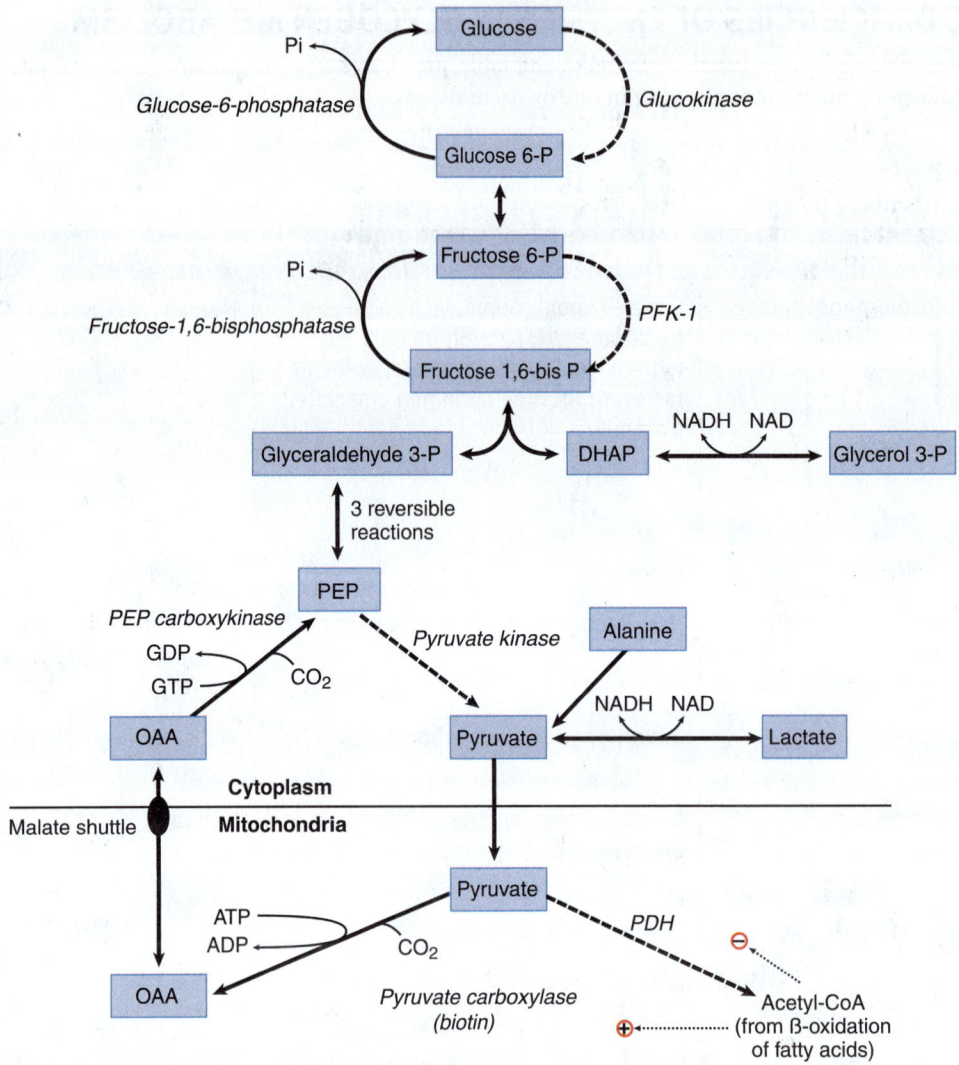

Figure 14-5. Gluconeogenesis

Dietary fructose and galactose can also be converted to glucose in the liver.

In humans, it is not possible to convert acetyl-CoA to glucose. Inasmuch as most fatty acids are metabolized solely to acetyl-CoA, they are not a major source of glucose either. One minor exception is odd-number carbon fatty acids (e.g., C17), which yield a small amount of propionyl-CoA that is gluconeogenic.

The pathway of gluconeogenesis is diagrammed in Figure 14-5. Lactate is oxidized to pyruvate by lactate dehydrogenase. The important gluconeogenic amino acid alanine is converted to pyruvate by alanine aminotransferase (ALT or GPT). Glycerol 3-phosphate is oxidized to dihydroxyacetone phosphate (DHAP) by glycerol 3-phosphate dehydrogenase. Most steps represent a reversal of glycolysis, and several of these have been omitted from the diagram. The four important enzymes are those required to catalyze reactions that circumvent the irreversible steps:

1. **Pyruvate carboxylase** is a mitochondrial enzyme requiring biotin. It is activated by acetyl-CoA (from β-oxidation). The product oxaloacetate (OAA), a citric acid cycle intermediate, cannot leave the mitochondria but is reduced to malate that can leave via the **malate shuttle**. In the cytoplasm, malate is reoxidized to OAA.

2. **Phosphoenolpyruvate carboxykinase** (PEPCK) in the cytoplasm is induced by glucagon and cortisol. It converts OAA to phosphoenolpyruvate (PEP) in a reaction that requires GTP. PEP continues in the pathway to fructose 1,6-bisphosphate.

3. **Fructose-1,6-bisphosphatase** in the cytoplasm is a key control point of gluconeogenesis. It hydrolyzes phosphate from fructose 1,6-bisphosphate rather than using it to generate ATP from ADP. A common pattern to note is that phosphatases oppose kinases. Fructose-1,6-bisphosphatase is activated by ATP and inhibited by AMP and fructose 2,6-bisphosphate. Fructose 2,6-bisphosphate, produced by PFK-2, controls both gluconeogenesis and glycolysis (in the liver). Recall from the earlier discussion of this enzyme (see Chapter 12, Figure 12-3) that PFK-2 is activated by insulin and inhibited by glucagon. Thus, glucagon will lower F 2,6-BP and stimulate gluconeogenesis, whereas insulin will increase F 2,6-BP and inhibit gluconeogenesis.

4. **Glucose-6-phosphatase** is in the lumen of the endoplasmic reticulum. Glucose 6-phosphate is transported into the ER, and free glucose is transported back into the cytoplasm from which it leaves the cell. Glucose-6-phosphatase is only in the liver. The absence of glucose-6-phosphatase in skeletal muscle accounts for the fact that muscle glycogen cannot serve as a source of blood glucose (see chapter 17, Figure 17-3).

Although alanine is the major gluconeogenic amino acid, 18 of the 20 (all but leucine and lysine) are also gluconeogenic. Most of these are converted by individual pathways to citric acid cycle intermediates, then to malate, following the same path from there to glucose.

It is important to note that glucose produced by hepatic gluconeogenesis does not represent an energy source for the liver. Gluconeogenesis requires expenditure of ATP that is provided by β-oxidation of fatty acids. Therefore, hepatic gluconeogenesis is always dependent on β-oxidation of fatty acids in the liver. During hypoglycemia, adipose tissue releases these fatty acids by breaking down triglyceride.

Although the acetyl-CoA from fatty acids cannot be converted to glucose, it can be converted to ketone bodies as an alternative fuel for cells, including the brain. Chronic hypoglycemia is thus often accompanied physiologically by an increase in ketone bodies.

Coordinate Regulation of Pyruvate Carboxylase and Pyruvate Dehydrogenase by Acetyl-CoA

The two major mitochondrial enzymes that use pyruvate, pyruvate carboxylase and pyruvate dehydrogenase, are both regulated by acetyl-CoA. This control is important in these contexts:

- Between meals, when fatty acids are oxidized in the liver for energy, accumulating acetyl-CoA activates pyruvate carboxylase and gluconeogenesis and inhibits PDH, thus preventing conversion of lactate and alanine to acetyl-CoA.

- In the well-fed, absorptive state (insulin), accumulating acetyl-CoA is shuttled into the cytoplasm for fatty acid synthesis. OAA is necessary for this transport, and acetyl-CoA can stimulate its formation from pyruvate (see chapter 15, Figure 15-1).

Cori Cycle and Alanine Cycle

During fasting, lactate from red blood cells (and possibly exercising skeletal muscle) is converted in the liver to glucose that can be returned to the red blood cell or muscle. This is called the Cori cycle. The alanine cycle is a slightly different version of the Cori cycle, in which muscle releases alanine, delivering both a gluconeogenic substrate (pyruvate) and an amino group for urea synthesis.

HEXOSE MONOPHOSPHATE SHUNT

The hexose monophosphate (HMP) shunt (pentose phosphate pathway) occurs in the cytoplasm of all cells, where it serves two major functions:

- NADPH production
- Source of ribose 5-phosphate for nucleotide synthesis

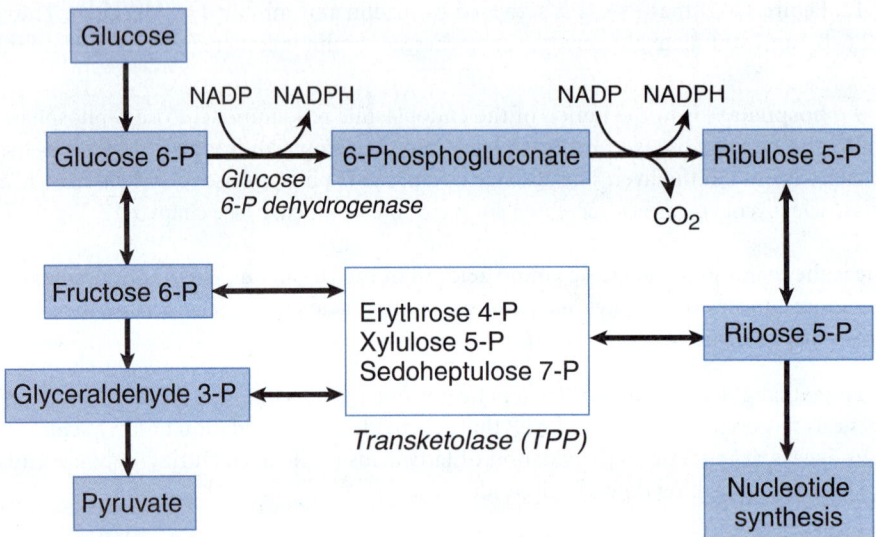

Figure 14-6. The Hexose Monophosphate Shunt

An abbreviated diagram of the pathway is shown in Figure 14-7. The first part of the HMP shunt begins with glucose 6-phosphate and ends with ribulose 5-phosphate and is irreversible. This part produces NADPH and involves the important rate-limiting enzyme glucose 6-phosphate dehydrogenase (G6PDH). G6PDH is induced by insulin, inhibited by NADPH, and activated by NADP.

The second part of the pathway, beginning with ribulose 5-phosphate, represents a series of reversible reactions that produce an equilibrated pool of sugars for biosynthesis, including ribose 5-phosphate for nucleotide synthesis. Because fructose 6-phosphate and glyceraldehyde 3-phosphate are among the sugars produced, intermediates can feed back into glycolysis; conversely, pentoses can be made from glycolytic intermediates without going through the G6PDH reaction. Transketolase, a thiamine-requiring enzyme, is important for these interconversions. Transketolase is the only thiamine enzyme in red blood cells.

Functions of NADPH

Cells require NADPH for a variety of functions, including:

- Biosynthesis
- Maintenance of a supply of reduced glutathione to protect against reactive oxygen species (ROS)
- Bactericidal activity in polymorphonuclear leukocytes (PMN)

These important roles are cell specific and shown in the following figure.

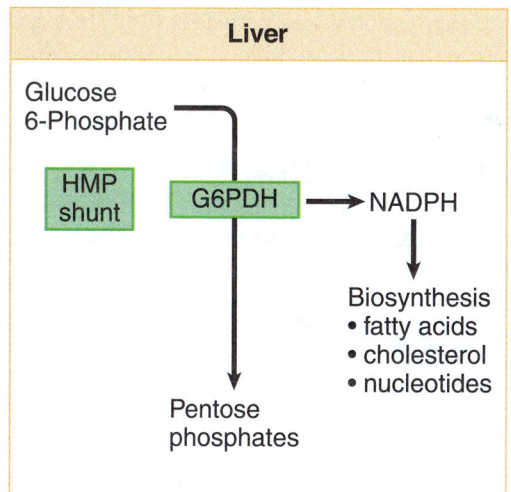

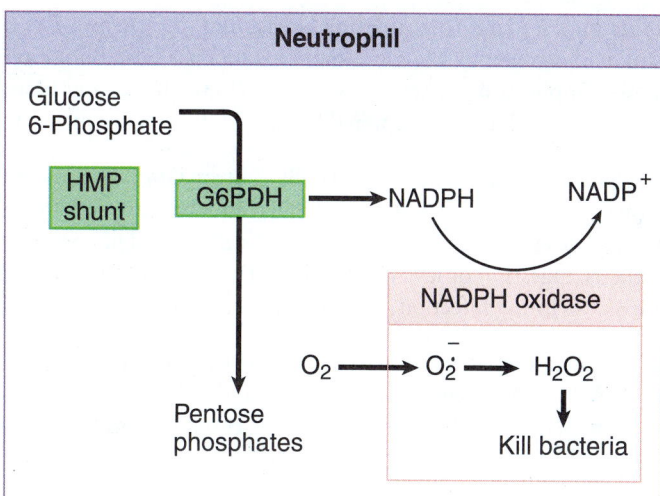

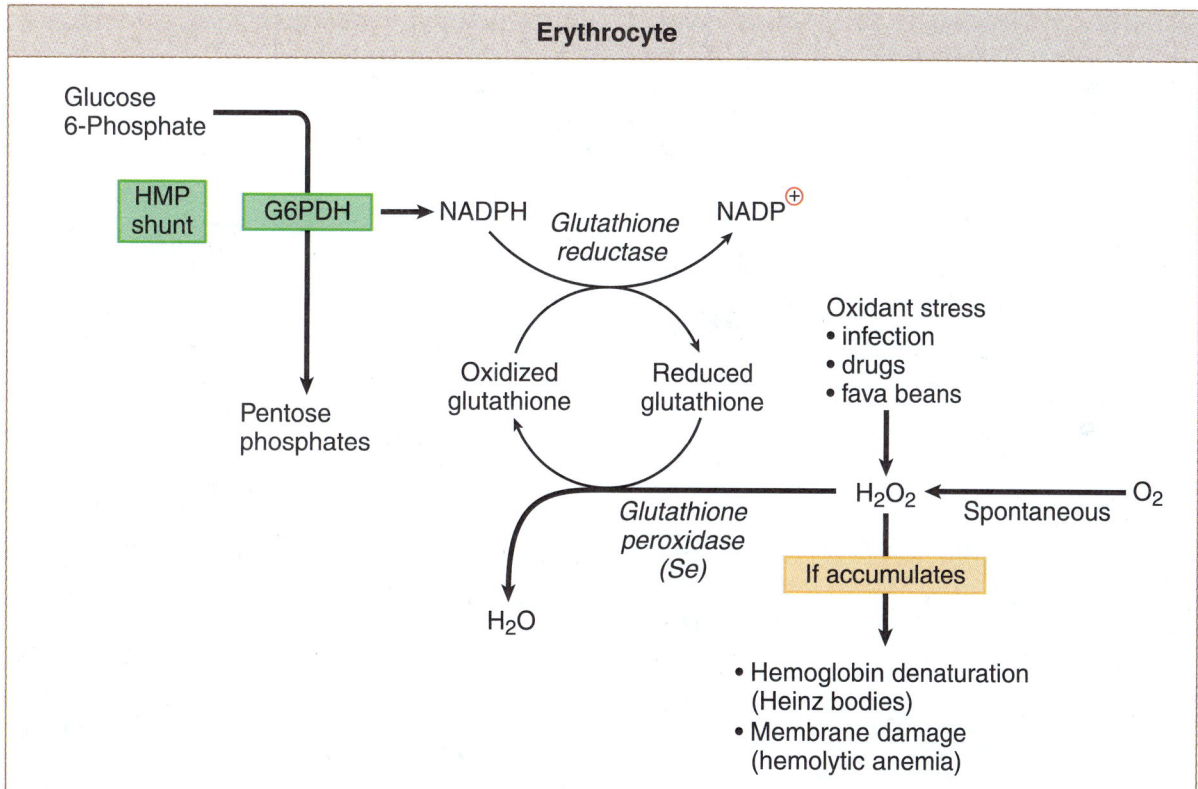

Figure 14-7. Role of the HMP Shunt in Hepatocytes, Phagocytes, and Erythrocytes

Glucose 6-Phosphate Dehydrogenase Deficiency

Deficiency of G6PDH may result in hemolytic anemia and, in rare cases, symptoms resembling chronic granuloma-tous disease (CGD). The disease shows significant allelic heterogeneity (over 400 different mutations in the G6PDH gene are known). The major symptom is either an acute episodic or (rarely) a chronic hemolysis. The disease is X-linked recessive. Females heterozygous for G6PDH deficiency have increased resistance to malaria. Consequently, the deficiency is seen more commonly in families from regions where malaria is endemic.

Because red blood cells contain a large amount of oxygen, they are prone to spontaneously generate ROS that dam-age protein and lipid in the cell. In the presence of ROS, hemoglobin may precipitate (Heinz bodies) and membrane lipids may undergo peroxidation, weakening the membrane and causing hemolysis. As peroxides form, they are rapidly destroyed by the glutathione peroxidase/glutathione reductase system in the red blood cell, thus avoiding these complications. These enzymes are shown in the red blood cell diagram in Figure 14-8. NADPH required by glutathione reductase is supplied by the HMP shunt in the erythrocyte.

Persons with mutations that partially destroy G6PDH activity may develop an acute, episodic hemolysis. Certain mutations affect the stability of G6PDH, and, because erythrocytes cannot synthesize proteins, the enzyme is gradually lost over time and older red blood cells lyse. This process is accelerated by certain drugs and, in a subset of patients, ingestion of fava beans. In the United States, the most likely cause of a hemolytic episode in these patients is overwhelming infection, often pneumonia (viral and bacterial) or infectious hepatitis.

In rare instances, a mutation may decrease the activity of G6PDH sufficiently to cause chronic nonspherocytic hemolytic anemia. Symptoms of CGD may also develop if there is insufficient activity of G6PDH (<5% of normal) in the PMN to generate NADPH for the NADPH oxidase bactericidal system.

Lipid Synthesis and Storage   15

Learning Objectives

❑ Answer questions about fatty acid nomenclature, lipid digestion, and fatty acid biosynthesis

❑ Demonstrate understanding of triglyceride (triacylglycerol) synthesis

❑ Demonstrate understanding of lipoprotein metabolism

❑ Explain information related to hyperlipidemias

❑ Use knowledge of cholesterol metabolism

FATTY ACID NOMENCLATURE

Fatty acids are long-chain carboxylic acids. The carboxyl carbon is number 1, and carbon number 2 is referred to as the α carbon. When designating a fatty acid, the number of carbons is given along with the number of double bonds (carbons:double bonds). Saturated fatty acids have no double bonds. Palmitic acid (palmitate) is the primary end product of fatty acid synthesis.

$$CH_3CH_2CH_2CH_2CH_2CH_2CH_2CH_2CH_2CH_2CH_2CH_2CH_2CH_2CH_2COO^-$$

Palmitate C16:0 or 16:0

Clinical Correlate

Cardioprotective Effects of Omega-3 Fatty Acids

Omega-3 fatty acids in the diet are correlated with a decreased risk of cardiovascular disease. These appear to replace some of the arachidonic acid (an omega-6 fatty acid) in platelet membranes and may lower the production of thromboxane and the tendency of the platelets to aggregate. A diet high in omega-3 fatty acids has also been associated with a decrease in serum triglycerides. Omega-3 fatty acids are found in cold-water fish, such as salmon, tuna, and herring, as well as in some nuts (walnuts) and seeds (flax seed).

Unsaturated fatty acids

Unsaturated fatty acids have one or more double bonds. Humans can synthesize only a few of the unsaturated fatty acids; the rest come from essential fatty acids in the diet that are transported as triglycerides from the intestine in chylomicrons. Two important essential fatty acids are linolenic acid and linoleic acid. These polyunsaturated fatty acids, as well as other acids formed from them, are important in membrane phospholipids to maintain normal fluidity of cell membranes essential for many functions.

The omega (ω) numbering system is also used for unsaturated fatty acids. The ω-family describes the position of the last double bond relative to the end of the chain. The omega designation identifies the major precursor fatty acid, e.g., arachidonic acid is formed from linoleic acid (ω-6 family). Arachidonic acid is itself an important precursor for prostaglandins, thromboxanes, and leukotrienes.

Linoleic	C18:2 (9,12) or $18^{\Delta 9,12}$	ω-6 family (18 − 12 = 6)
Linolenic	C18:3 (9,12,15) or $18^{\Delta 9,12,15}$	ω-3 family
Arachidonic	C20:4 (5,8,11,14) or $20^{\Delta 5,8,11,14}$	ω-6 family

Double bonds in fatty acids are in the *cis-* configuration. *Trans*-double bonds are unnatural and predominate in fatty acids found in margarine and other foods where partial hydrogenation of vegetable oils is used in their preparation. Compared with liquid oils, these partial hydrogenated fatty acids are conveniently solid at cool temperatures. When incorporated into phospholipids that constitute membranes, *trans*-fatty acids decrease membrane fluidity, similar to saturated fatty acids that are found in butter fat and other foods. *Trans*-fatty acids, as well as saturated fatty acids, are associated with increased risk of atherosclerosis.

Activation of Fatty Acids

When fatty acids are used in metabolism, they are first activated by attaching coenzyme A (CoA); fatty acyl CoA synthetase catalyzes this activation step. The product is generically referred to as a fatty acyl CoA or sometimes just acyl CoA. Specific examples would be acetyl CoA with a 2-carbon acyl group, or palmitoyl CoA with a 16-carbon acyl group.

Fatty acid + CoA + ATP $\rightarrow$ Fatty acyl CoA + AMP + PP$_i$

LIPID DIGESTION

Typical high-fat meals contain gram-level amounts of triglycerides and milligram-level amounts of cholesterol and cholesterol esters. Upon entry into the intestinal lumen, bile is secreted by the liver to emulsify the lipid contents. The pancreas secretes pancreatic lipase, colipase, and cholesterol esterase that degrade the lipids to 2-monoglyceride, fatty acids, and cholesterol. These lipids are absorbed and re-esterified to tryglycerides and cholesterol esters and packaged, along with apoprotein B-48 and other lipids (e.g., fat-soluble vitamins), into chylomicrons. Normally, there is very little lipid loss in stools. Defects in lipid digestion result in steatorrhea, in which there is an excessive amount of lipids in stool (fatty stools).

FATTY ACID BIOSYNTHESIS

Excess dietary glucose can be converted to fatty acids in the liver and subsequently sent to the adipose tissue for storage. Adipose tissue synthesizes smaller quantities of fatty acids. The pathway is shown in Figure 15-1. Insulin promotes many steps in the conversion of glucose to acetyl CoA in the liver:

- Glucokinase (induced)
- PFK-2/PFK-1 (PFK-2 dephosphorylated)
- Pyruvate dehydrogenase (dephosphorylated)

Both of the major enzymes of fatty acid synthesis are also affected by insulin:

- Acetyl CoA carboxylase (dephosphorylated, activated)
- Fatty acid synthase (induced)

Citrate Shuttle and Malic Enzyme

The citrate shuttle transports acetyl CoA groups from the mitochondria to the cytoplasm for fatty acid synthesis. Acetyl CoA combines with oxaloacetate in the mitochondria to form citrate, but rather than continuing in the citric acid cycle, citrate is transported into the cytoplasm. Factors that indirectly promote this process include insulin and high-energy status.

In the cytoplasm, citrate lyase splits citrate back into acetyl CoA and oxaloacetate. The oxaloacetate returns to the mitochondria to transport additional acetyl CoA. This process is shown in Figure 15-1 and includes the important malic enzyme. This reaction represents an additional source of cytoplasmic NADPH in liver and adipose tissue, supplementing that from the HMP shunt.

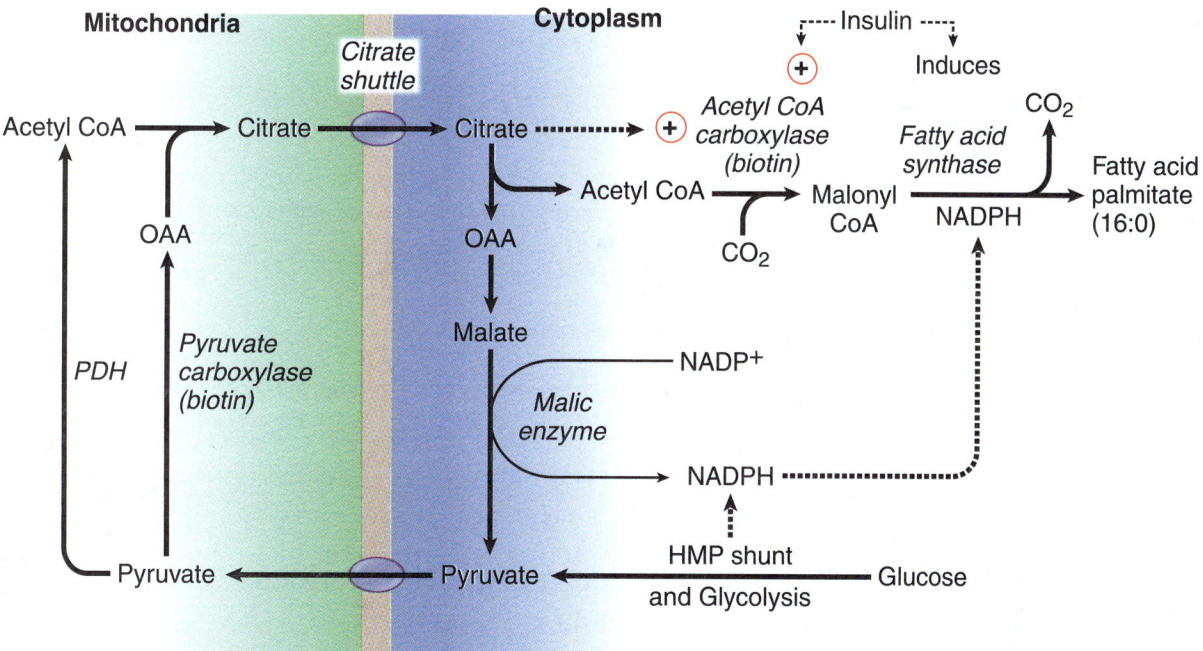

Figure 15-1. Synthesis of Palmitate From Glucose

Acetyl CoA Carboxylase

Acetyl CoA is activated in the cytoplasm for incorporation into fatty acids by acetyl CoA carboxylase, the rate-limiting enzyme of fatty acid biosynthesis. Acetyl CoA carboxylase requires biotin, ATP, and CO_2. Controls include:

- Activation by insulin (dephosphorylated)
- Activation by citrate

The CO_2 added to form malonyl CoA is never incorporated into the fatty acid because it is removed by fatty acid synthase during the addition of the acetyl group to the fatty acid.

Fatty Acid Synthase

Fatty acid synthase is more appropriately called palmitate synthase because palmitate is the only fatty acid that humans can synthesize *de novo*. This enzyme is a large, multienzyme complex in the cytoplasm that is rapidly induced in the liver after a meal by high carbohydrate and concomitantly rising insulin levels. It contains an acyl carrier protein (ACP) that requires the vitamin pantothenic acid. Although malonyl CoA is the substrate used by fatty acid synthase, only the carbons from the acetyl CoA portion are actually incorporated into the fatty acid produced. Therefore, the fatty acid is derived entirely from acetyl CoA.

NADPH is required to reduce the acetyl groups added to the fatty acid. Eight acetyl CoA groups are required to produce palmitate (16:0).

Fatty acyl CoA may be elongated and desaturated (to a limited extent in humans) using enzymes associated with the smooth endoplasmic reticulum (SER). Cytochrome b_5 is involved in the desaturation reactions. These enzymes cannot introduce double bonds past position 9 in the fatty acid.

TRIGLYCERIDE (TRIACYLGLYCEROL) SYNTHESIS

Triglycerides

Triglycerides, the storage form of fatty acids, are formed by attaching three fatty acids (as fatty acyl CoA) to glycerol. Triglyceride formation from fatty acids and glycerol 3-phosphate occurs primarily in liver and adipose tissue.

Liver sends triglycerides to adipose tissue packaged as very low-density lipoproteins (VLDL; reviewed later in this chapter). A small amount of triglyceride may be stored in the liver. Accumulation of significant triglyceride in tissues other than adipose tissue usually indicates a pathologic state.

Bridge to Pathology

Chronic alcohol use can interfere with lipid metabolism in the liver, leading to steatosis, or fatty degeneration of the liver parenchyma.

Sources of Glycerol 3-Phosphate for Synthesis of Triglycerides

There are two sources of glycerol 3-P for triglyceride synthesis:

- Reduction of dihydroxyacetone phosphate (DHAP) from glycolysis by glycerol 3-P dehydrogenase, an enzyme in both adipose tissue and liver
- Phosphorylation of free glycerol by glycerol kinase, an enzyme found in liver but not in adipose tissue

Glycerol kinase allows the liver to recycle the glycerol released during VLDL metabolism (insulin) back into new triglyceride synthesis. During fasting (glucagon), this same enzyme allows the liver to trap glycerol released into the blood from lipolysis in adipose tissue for subsequent conversion to glucose.

Adipose tissue lacks glycerol kinase and is strictly dependent on glucose uptake to produce DHAP for triglyceride synthesis. In adipose tissue, the GLUT 4 transporter is stimulated by insulin, ensuring a good supply of DHAP for triglyceride synthesis.

The roles of glycerol kinase and glycerol 3-P dehydrogenase during triglyceride synthesis and storage are shown in the following figure.

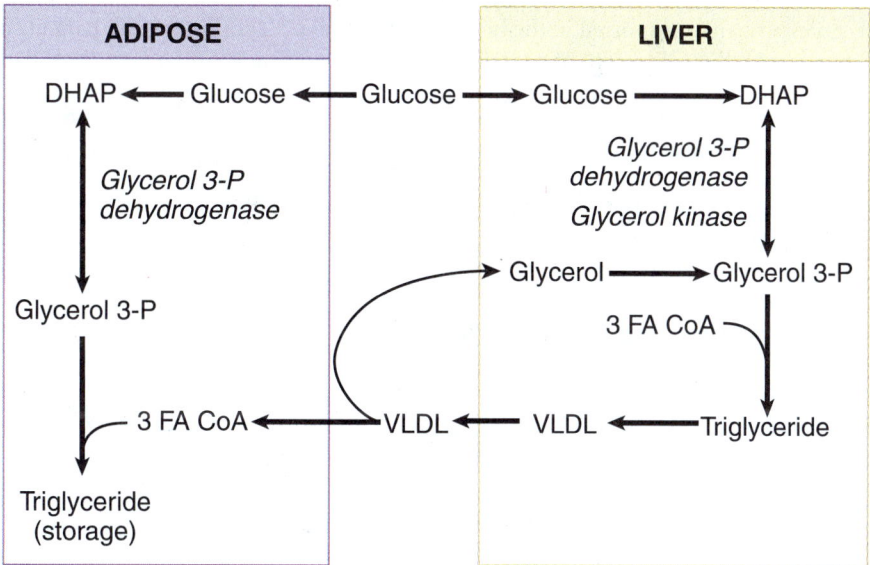

Figure 15-2. Glycerol 3-P Dehydrogenase and Glycerol Kinase in Triglyceride Synthesis and Storage

Glycerophospholipids

Glycerophospholipids are used for membrane synthesis and for producing a hydrophilic surface layer on lipoproteins such as VLDL. In cell membranes, they also serve as a reservoir of second messengers such as diacylglycerol, inositol 1,4,5-triphosphate, and arachidonic acid. Their structure is similar to triglycerides, except that the last fatty acid is replaced by phosphate and a water-soluble group such as choline (phosphatidylcholine, lecithin) or inositol (phosphatidylinositol).

A comparison of the structures is diagrammed here:

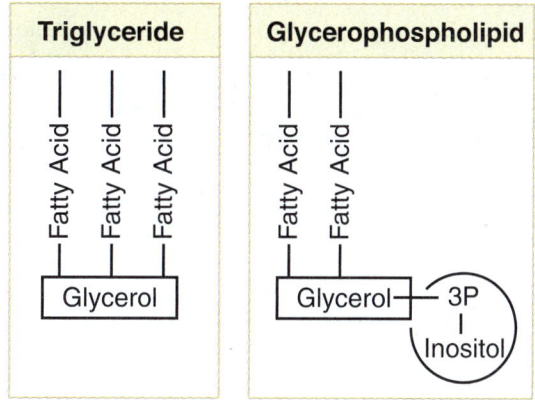

Figure 15-3. Triglycerides and Glycerophospholipids

LIPOPROTEIN METABOLISM

General Concepts: Cholesterol Digestion

Triglycerides and cholesterol are transported in the blood as lipoproteins. Lipoproteins are named according to their density, which increases with the percentage of protein in the particle. From least dense to most dense:

chylomicrons < VLDL < IDL (intermediate-density lipoproteins) < LDL (low-density lipoproteins) < HDL (high-density lipoproteins). An example of a lipoprotein is shown in Figure 15-4.

The classes of lipoproteins and the important apoproteins associated with their functions are summarized in Table 15-1 and Figure 15-4.

Classes of Lipoproteins and Important Apoproteins

Table 15-1. Classes of Lipoproteins and Important Apoproteins

Lipoprotein	Functions	Apoproteins	Functions
Chylomicrons	Transport dietary triglyceride and cholesterol from intestine to tissues	apoB-48 apoC-II apoE	Secreted by intestine Activates lipoprotein lipase Uptake of remnants by the liver
VLDL	Transports triglyceride from liver to tissues	apoB-100 apoC-II apoE	Secreted by liver Activates lipoprotein lipase Uptake of remnants (IDL) by liver
IDL (VLDL remnants)	Picks up cholesterol from HDL to become LDL Picked up by liver	apoE apoB-100	Uptake by liver
LDL	Delivers cholesterol into cells	apoB-100	Uptake by liver and other tissues via LDL receptor (apoB-100 receptor)
HDL	Picks up cholesterol accumulating in blood vessels Delivers cholesterol to liver and steroidogenic tissues via scavenger receptor (SR-B1) Shuttles apoC-II and apoE in blood	apoA-1	Activates lecithin cholesterol acyltransferase (LCAT) to produce cholesterol esters

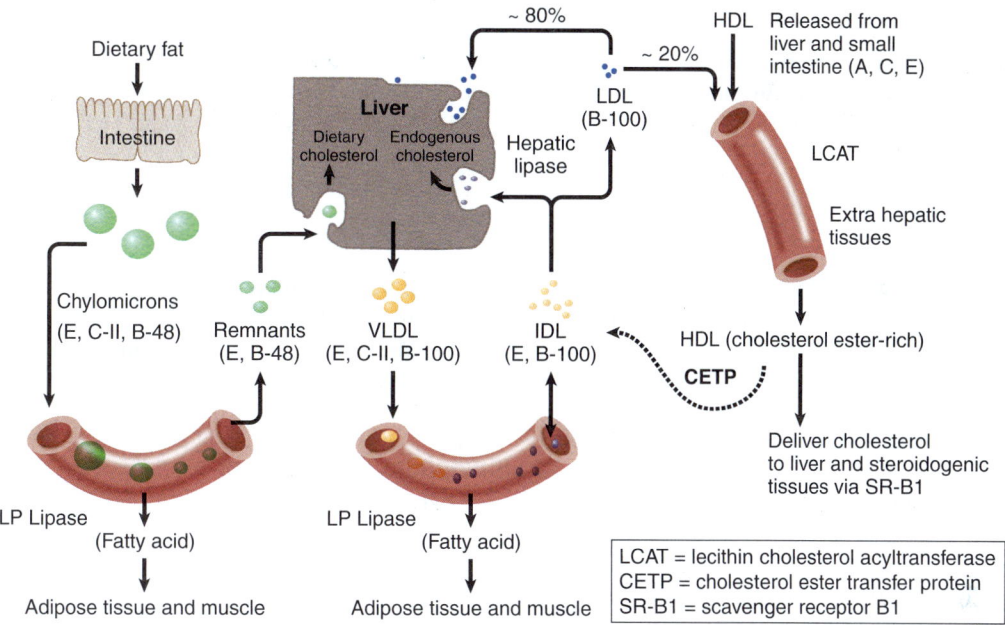

Figure 15-4. Overview of Lipoprotein Metabolism

Chylomicrons, VLDL, and IDL (VLDL Remnants)

Chylomicrons and VLDL are primarily triglyceride particles, although they each have small quantities of cholesterol esters. Chylomicrons transport dietary triglyceride to adipose tissue and muscle, whereas VLDL transport triglyceride synthesized in the liver to these same tissues. Both chylomicrons and VLDL have apoC-II, apoE, and apoB (apoB-48 on chylomicrons and apoB-100 on VLDL). The metabolism of these particles is shown in the following figure.

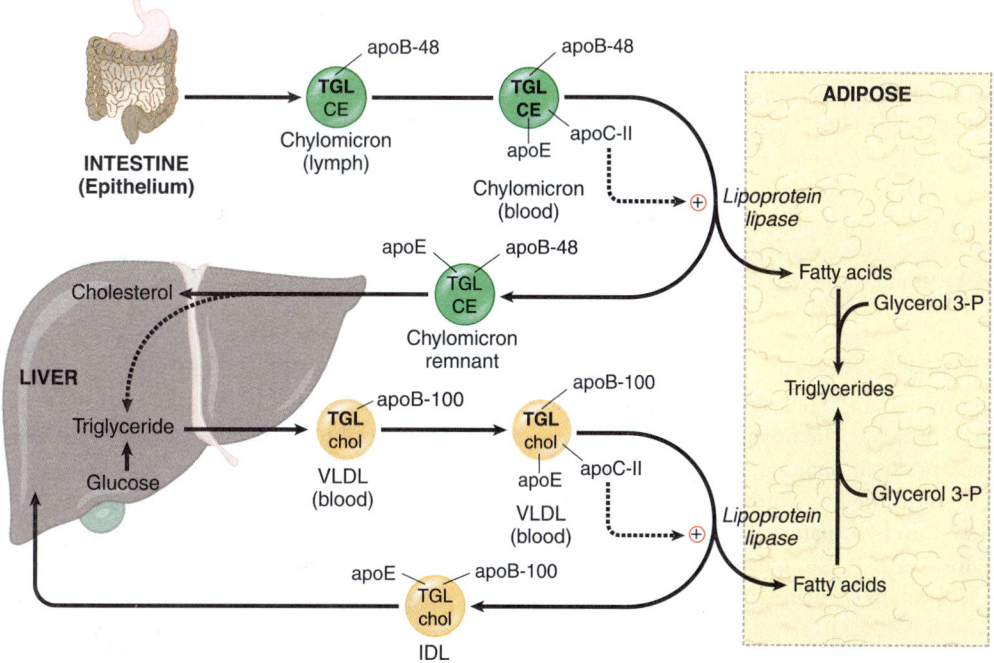

Figure 15-5. Chylomicron and VLDL Metabolism

Lipoprotein Lipase

Lipoprotein (LPLase) is required for the metabolism of both chylomicrons and VLDL. This enzyme is induced by insulin and transported to the luminal surface of capillary endothelium, where it is in direct contact with the blood. Lipoprotein lipase hydrolyzes the fatty acids from triglycerides carried by chylomicrons and VLDL and is activated by apoC-II.

Chylomicrons

Chylomicrons are assembled from dietary triglycerides (containing predominantly the longer chain fatty acids, including the essential fatty acids), cholesterol esters, and the four lipid-soluble vitamins. The core lipid is surrounded by phospholipids similar to those found in cell membranes, which increase the solubility of chylomicrons in lymph and blood. ApoB-48 is attached and required for release from the epithelial cells into the lymphatics.

Chylomicrons leave the lymph and enter the peripheral blood, where the thoracic duct joins the left subclavian vein, thus initially bypassing the liver. After a high-fat meal, chylomicrons cause serum to become turbid or milky. While in the blood, chylomicrons acquire apoC-II and apoE from HDL particles.

In capillaries of adipose tissue (and muscle), apoC-II activates lipoprotein lipase , the fatty acids released enter the tissue for storage, and the glycerol is retrieved by the liver, which has glycerol kinase. The chylomicron remnant is picked up by hepatocytes through the apoE receptor; thus, dietary cholesterol, as well as any remaining triglyceride, is released in the hepatocyte.

VLDL (very low-density lipoprotein)

The metabolism of VLDL is very similar to that of chylomicrons, the major difference being that VLDL are assembled in hepatocytes to transport triglyceride containing fatty acids newly synthesized from excess glucose, or retrieved from the chylomicron remnants, to adipose tissue and muscle. ApoB-100 is added in the hepatocytes to mediate release into the blood. Like chylomicrons, VLDL acquire apoC-II and apoE from HDL in the blood and are metabolized by lipoprotein lipase in adipose tissue and muscle.

VLDL remnants (IDL, intermediate-density lipoprotein)

After triglyceride is removed from the VLDL, the resulting particle is referred to as either a VLDL remnant or as an IDL. A portion of the IDLs is picked up by hepatocytes through their apoE receptor, but some of the IDLs remain in the blood, where they are further metabolized. These IDLs are transition particles between triglyceride and cholesterol transport. In the blood, they can acquire cholesterol esters transferred from HDL particles and thus become converted into LDLs, as shown in Figures 15-4 and 15-5.

LDL and HDL

LDL (low-density lipoprotein)

Although both LDL and HDL are primarily cholesterol particles, most of the cholesterol measured in the blood is associated with LDL. The normal role of LDL is to deliver cholesterol to tissues for biosynthesis. When a cell is repairing membrane or dividing, the cholesterol is required for membrane synthesis. Bile acids and salts are made from cholesterol in the liver, and many other tissues require some cholesterol for steroid synthesis. About 80% of LDL are picked up by hepatocytes, the remainder by peripheral tissues. ApoB-100 is the only apoprotein on LDL, and endocytosis of LDL is mediated by apoB-100 receptors (LDL receptors) clustered in areas of cell membranes lined with the protein clathrin.

Regulation of the Cholesterol Level in Hepatocytes

The liver has multiple pathways for acquiring cholesterol, including:

- *De novo* synthesis
- Endocytosis of LDL
- Transfer of cholesterol from HDL via the SR-B1 receptor
- Endocytosis of chylomicron remnants with residual dietary cholesterol

Increased cholesterol in the hepatocytes inhibits further accumulation by repressing the expression of the genes for HMG-CoA reductase, the LDL receptor, and the SR-B1 receptor.

Endocytosis involves:

- Formation of a coated pit, which further invaginates to become an endosome
- Fusion of the endosome with a lysosome, accompanied by acidification and activation of lysosomal enzymes
- Release of LDL from the LDL receptor

The receptor may recycle to the surface, the LDL is degraded, and cholesterol is released into the cell. Expression of the gene for LDL receptors (apoB-100 receptor) is regulated by the cholesterol level within the cell. High cholesterol decreases expression of this gene as well as the gene for HMG-CoA reductase, the rate limiting enzyme of *de novo* cholesterol synthesis.

HDL (high-density lipoprotein)

HDL is synthesized in the liver and intestines and released as dense, protein-rich particles into the blood. They contain apoA-1 used for cholesterol recovery from fatty streaks in the blood vessels. HDL also carry apoE and apoC-II, but those apoproteins are primarily to donate temporarily to chylomicrons and VLDL.

Lecithin–cholesterol acyltransferase (LCAT)

LCAT (or PCAT, phosphatidylcholine–cholesterol acyltransferase) is an enzyme in the blood that is activated by apoA-1 on HDL. LCAT adds a fatty acid to cholesterol, producing cholesterol esters, which dissolve in the core of the HDL, allowing HDL to transport cholesterol from the periphery to the liver. This process of reverse cholesterol transport is shown in Figure 15-8.

Cholesterol ester transfer protein (CETP)

HDL cholesterol esters picked up in the periphery can be distributed to other lipoprotein particles such as VLDL remnants (IDL), converting them to LDL. The cholesterol ester transfer protein facilitates this transfer.

Scavenger receptors (SR-B1)

HDL cholesterol picked up in the periphery can also enter cells through a scavenger receptor, SR-B1. This receptor is expressed at high levels in hepatocytes and the steroidogenic tissues, including ovaries, testes, and areas of the adrenal glands. This receptor does not mediate endocytosis of the HDL, but rather transfer of cholesterol into the cell by a mechanism not yet clearly defined.

CHOLESTEROL METABOLISM

Cholesterol is required for membrane synthesis, steroid and vitamin D synthesis, and in the liver, bile acid synthesis. Most cells derive their cholesterol from LDL or HDL, but some cholesterol may be synthesized *de novo*. Most *de novo* synthesis occurs in the liver, where cholesterol is synthesized from acetyl-CoA in the cytoplasm. The citrate shuttle carries mitochondrial acetyl-CoA into the cytoplasm, and NADPH is provided by the HMP shunt and malic enzyme. Important points are noted in the following figure.

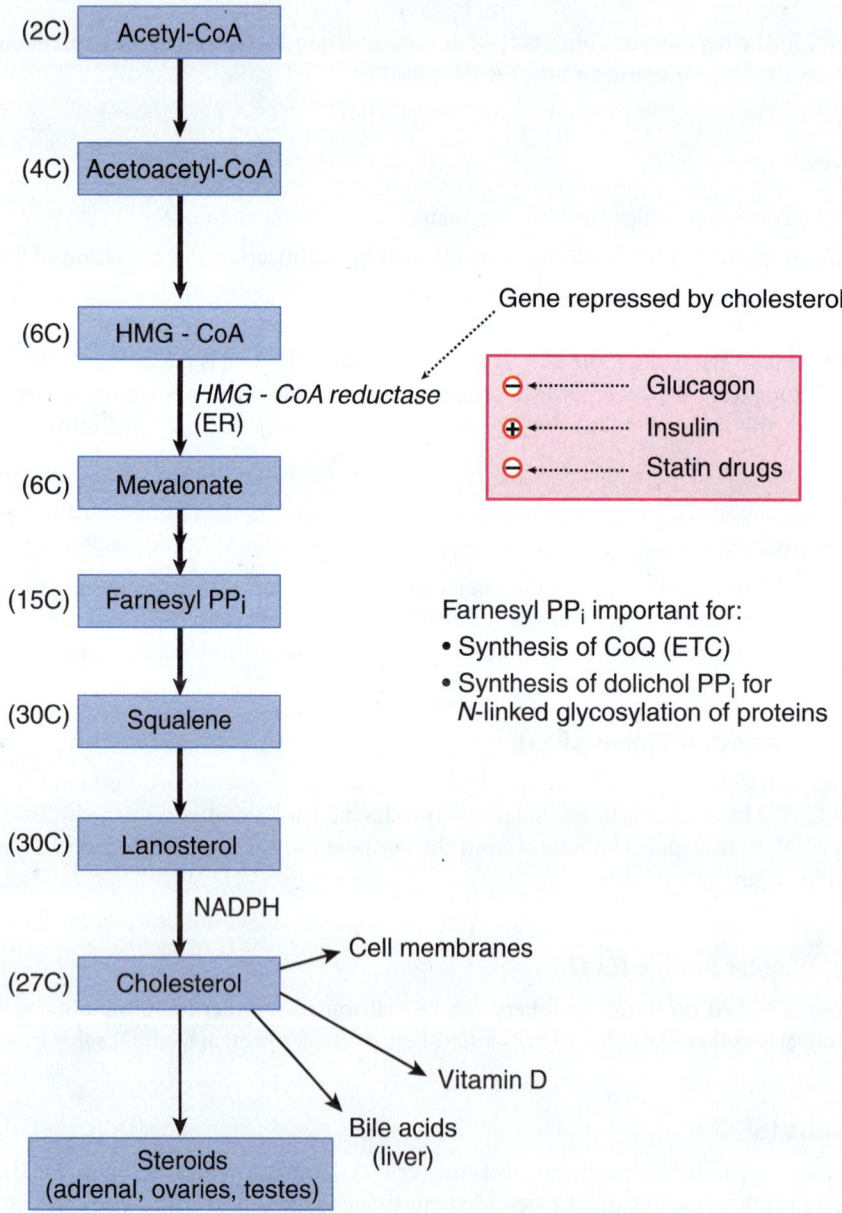

Figure 15-6. Synthesis of Cholesterol

3-Hydroxy-3-methylglutaryl (HMG)-CoA reductase on the smooth endoplasmic reticulum (SER) is the rate-limiting enzyme. Insulin activates the enzyme (dephosphorylation), and glucagon inhibits it. Mevalonate is the product, and the statin drugs competitively inhibit the enzyme. Cholesterol represses the expression of the HMG-CoA reductase gene and also increases degradation of the enzyme.

Farnesyl pyrophosphate, an intermediate in the pathway, may also be used for:

- Synthesis of CoQ for the mitochondrial electron transport chain
- Synthesis of dolichol pyrophosphate, a required cofactor in *N*-linked glycosylation of proteins in the endoplasmic reticulum
- Prenylation of proteins (a posttranslational modification) that need to be held in the cell membrane by a lipid tail. An example is the p21^{ras} G protein in the insulin and growth factor pathways.

Lipid Mobilization and Catabolism 16

Learning Objectives

❏ Solve problems concerning lipid mobilization

❏ Interpret scenarios about fatty acid oxidation

❏ Demonstrate understanding of ketone body metabolism

❏ Use knowledge of sphingolipids

LIPID MOBILIZATION

In the postabsorptive state, fatty acids can be released from adipose tissue to be used for energy. Although human adipose tissue does not respond directly to glucagon, the fall in insulin activates a hormone-sensitive triacylglycerol lipase (HSL) that hydrolyzes triglycerides, yielding fatty acids and glycerol. Epinephrine and cortisol also activate HSL. These steps are shown in Figure 16-1.

Glycerol may be picked up by liver and converted to dihydroxyacetone phosphate (DHAP) for gluconeogenesis, and the fatty acids are distributed to tissues that can use them. Free fatty acids are transported through the blood in association with serum albumin.

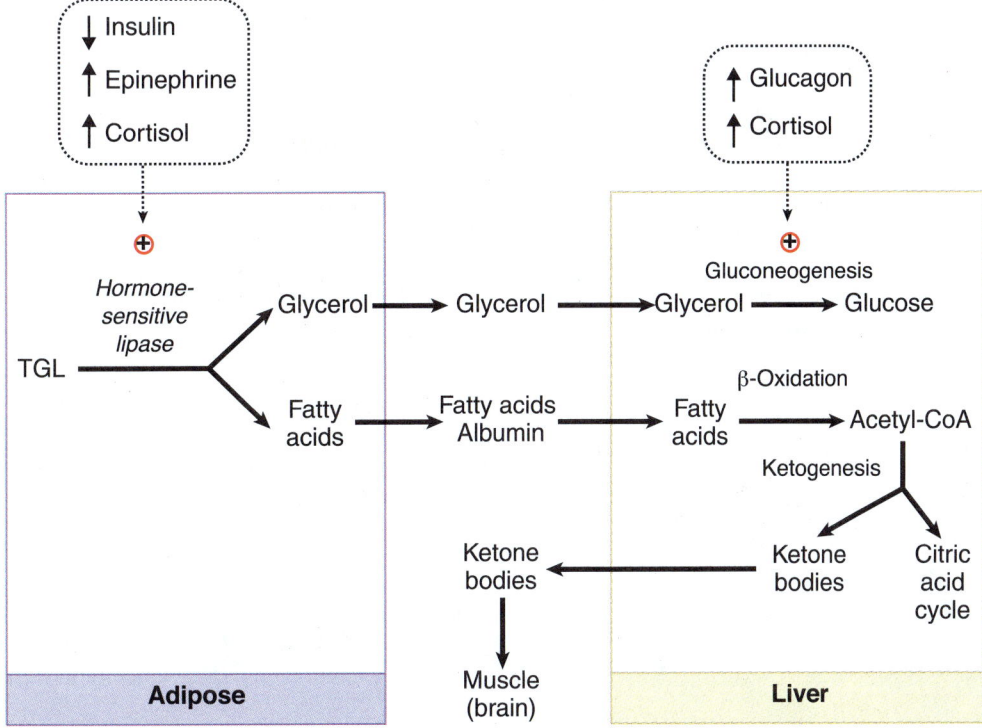

Figure 16-1. Lipolysis of Triglyceride in Response to Hypoglycemia and Stress

FATTY ACID OXIDATION

Fatty acids are oxidized in several tissues, including liver, muscle, and adipose tissue, by the pathway of β-oxidation. Neither erythrocytes nor brain can use fatty acids and so continue to rely on glucose during normal periods of fasting. Erythrocytes lack mitochondria, and fatty acids do not cross the blood–brain barrier efficiently.

Short-chain fatty acids (2–4 carbons) and medium-chain fatty acids (6–12 carbons) diffuse freely into mitochondria to be oxidized. Long-chain fatty acids (14–20 carbons) are transported into the mitochondrion by a carnitine shuttle (Figure 16-2) to be oxidized. Very long-chain fatty acids (>20 carbons) enter peroxisomes via an unknown mechanism for oxidation.

Fatty Acid Entry Into Mitochondria

Long-chain fatty acids must be activated and transported into the mitochondria. Fatty acyl-CoA synthetase, on the outer mitochondrial membrane, activates the fatty acids by attaching CoA. The fatty acyl portion is then transferred onto carnitine by carnitine acyltransferase-1 for transport into the mitochondria. The sequence of events is shown in Figure 16-2 and includes the following steps:

- Fatty acyl synthetase activates the fatty acid (outer mitochondrial membrane).
- Carnitine acyltransferase-1 transfers the fatty acyl group to carnitine (outer mitochondrial membrane).
- Fatty acylcarnitine is shuttled across the inner membrane.
- Carnitine acyltransferase-2 transfers the fatty acyl group back to a CoA (mitochondrial matrix).

Carnitine acyltransferase-1 is inhibited by malonyl-CoA from fatty acid synthesis and thereby prevents newly synthesized fatty acids from entering the mitochondria. Insulin indirectly inhibits β-oxidation by activating acetyl-CoA carboxylase (fatty acid synthesis) and increasing the malonyl-CoA concentration in the cytoplasm. Glucagon reverses this process.

β-Oxidation in Mitochondria

β-oxidation reverses the process of fatty acid synthesis by oxidizing (rather than reducing) and releasing (rather than linking) units of acetyl-CoA. The pathway is a repetition of four steps and is shown in Figure 16-2. Each four-step cycle releases one acetyl-CoA and reduces NAD and FAD (producing NADH and $FADH_2$).

The $FADH_2$ and NADH are oxidized in the electron transport chain, providing ATP. In muscle and adipose tissue, the acetyl-CoA enters the citric acid cycle. In liver, the ATP may be used for gluconeogenesis, and the acetyl-CoA (which cannot be converted to glucose) stimulates gluconeogenesis by activating pyruvate carboxylase.

In a fasting state, the liver produces more acetyl-CoA from β-oxidation than is used in the citric acid cycle. Much of the acetyl-CoA is used to synthesize ketone bodies (essentially two acetyl-CoA groups linked together) that are released into the blood for other tissues.

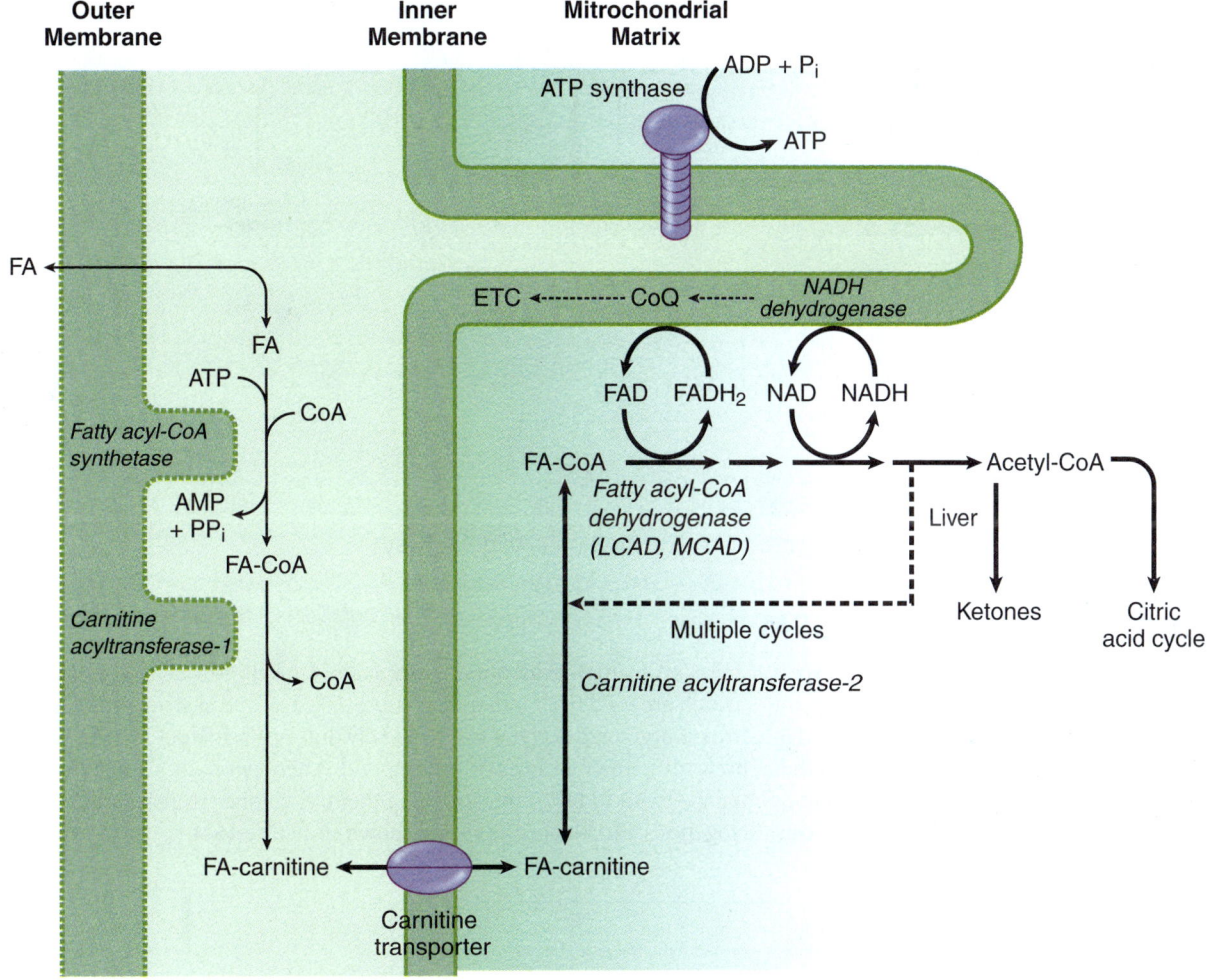

Figure 16-2. Fatty Acid Activation, Transport, and β-Oxidation

Propionic Acid Pathway

Fatty acids with an odd number of carbon atoms are oxidized by β-oxidation identically to even-carbon fatty acids. The difference results only from the final cycle, in which even-carbon fatty acids yield two acetyl-CoA (from the 4-carbon fragment remaining) but odd-carbon fatty acids yield one acetyl-CoA and one propionyl-CoA (from the 5-carbon fragment remaining).

Propionyl-CoA is converted to succinyl-CoA, a citric acid cycle intermediate, in the two-step propionic acid pathway. Because this extra succinyl-CoA can form malate and enter the cytoplasm and gluconeogenesis, odd-carbon fatty acids represent an exception to the rule that fatty acids cannot be converted to glucose in humans. The propionic acid pathway is shown in Figure 16-3 and includes two important enzymes, both in the mitochondria:

- Propionyl-CoA carboxylase requires biotin.
- Methylmalonyl-CoA mutase requires vitamin B_{12}, cobalamin.

Vitamin B_{12} deficiency can cause a megaloblastic anemia of the same type seen in folate deficiency (discussed in chapter 17). In a patient with megaloblastic anemia, it is important to determine the underlying cause because B_{12} deficiency, if not corrected, produces a peripheral neuropathy owing to aberrant fatty acid incorporation into the myelin sheath associated with inadequate methylmalonyl-CoA mutase activity. Excretion of methylmalonic acid indicates a vitamin B_{12} deficiency rather than folate.

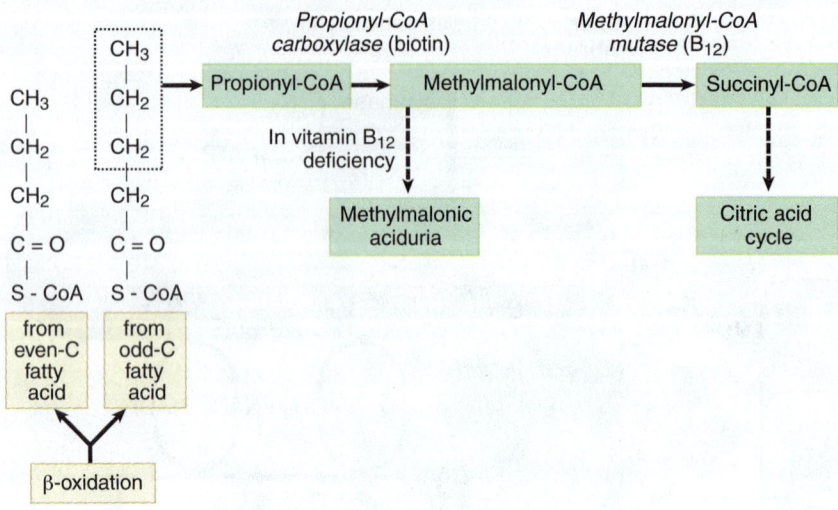

Figure 16-3. The Propionic Acid Pathway

KETONE BODY METABOLISM

In the fasting state, the liver converts excess acetyl-CoA from β-oxidation of fatty acids into ketone bodies, acetoacetate and 3-hydroxybutyrate (β-hydroxybutyrate), which are used by extrahepatic tissues. Cardiac and skeletal muscles and renal cortex metabolize acetoacetate and 3-hydroxybutyrate to acetyl-CoA. Normally during a fast, muscle metabolizes ketones as rapidly as the liver releases them, preventing their accumulation in blood. After a week of fasting, ketones reach a concentration in blood high enough for the brain to begin metabolizing them. If ketones increase sufficiently in the blood, they can lead to ketoacidosis. Ketogenesis and ketogenolysis are shown in Figure 16-4.

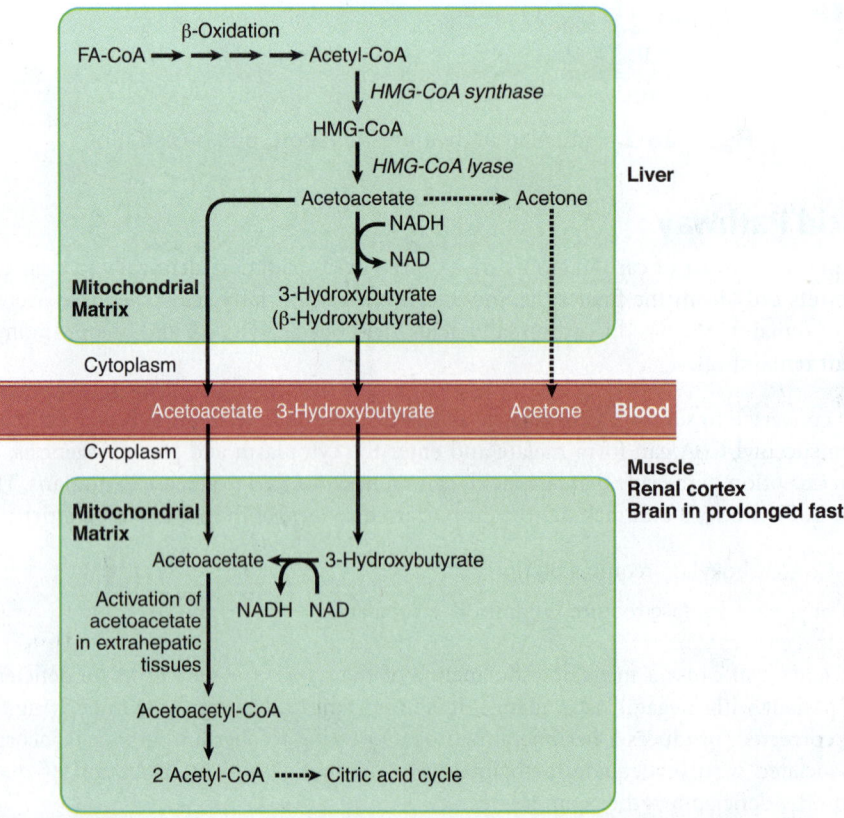

Figure 16-4. Ketogenesis (Liver) and Ketogenolysis (Extrahepatic)

Ketogenesis

Ketogenesis occurs in mitochondria of hepatocytes when excess acetyl-CoA accumulates in the fasting state. HMG-CoA synthase forms HMG-CoA, and HMG-CoA lyase breaks HMG-CoA into acetoacetate, which can subsequently be reduced to 3-hydroxybutyrate. Acetone is a minor side product formed nonenzymatically but is not used as a fuel in tissues. It does, however, impart a strong odor (sweet or fruity) to the breath, which is almost diagnostic for ketoacidosis.

> ### Clinical Correlate
>
> In untreated type 1 diabetes mellitus, there is no insulin. Although glucose may be high, no insulin is released, HSL is active, β-oxidation is not inhibited, and ketone bodies are generated.

Ketogenolysis

Acetoacetate picked up from the blood is activated in the mitochondria by succinyl-CoA acetoacetyl-CoA transferase (common name thiophorase), an enzyme present only in extrahepatic tissues; 3-hydroxybutyrate is first oxidized to acetoacetate. Because the liver lacks this enzyme, it cannot metabolize the ketone bodies.

Ketogenolysis in brain

Figure 16-5 shows the major pathways producing fuel for the brain. Note the important times at which the brain switches from:

- Glucose derived from liver glycogenolysis to glucose derived from gluconeogenesis (~12 hours)
- Glucose derived from gluconeogenesis to ketones derived from fatty acids (~1 week)

In the brain, when ketones are metabolized to acetyl-CoA, pyruvate dehydrogenase is inhibited. Glycolysis and subsequently glucose uptake in brain decreases. This important switch spares body protein (which otherwise would be catabolized to form glucose by gluconeogenesis in the liver) by allowing the brain to indirectly metabolize fatty acids as ketone bodies.

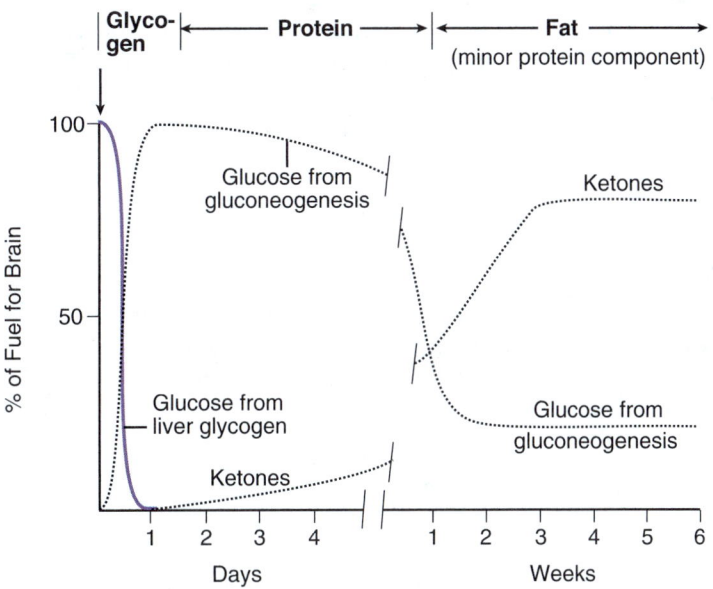

Figure 16-5. Fuel Use in the Brain During Fasting and Starvation

Ketoacidosis

In patients with type 1 insulin-dependent diabetes mellitus not adequately treated with insulin, fatty acid release from adipose tissue and ketone synthesis in the liver exceed the ability of other tissues to metabolize them, and a profound, life-threatening ketoacidosis may occur. An infection or trauma (causing an increase in cortisol and epinephrine) may precipitate an episode of ketoacidosis by activating HSL. Patients with type 2 non–insulin-dependent diabetes mellitus (NIDDM) are much less likely to show ketoacidosis. The basis for this observation is not completely understood, although type 2 disease has a much slower, insidious onset, and insulin resistance in the periphery is usually not complete. Type 2 diabetics can develop ketoacidosis after an infection or trauma. In certain populations with NIDDM, ketoacidosis is much more common than previously appreciated.

Clinical Correlate

Insulin facilitates uptake of potassium by cells, so K⁺ levels may be normal before DKA is treated with insulin. Once insulin is administered, however, blood potassium levels need to be monitored.

Alcoholics can also develop ketoacidosis. Chronic hypoglycemia, which is often present in chronic alcoholism, favors fat release from adipose. Ketone production increases in the liver, but utilization in muscle may be slower than normal because alcohol is converted to acetate in the liver, diffuses into the blood, and oxidized by muscle as an alternative source of acetyl-CoA.

Associated with ketoacidosis:

- Polyuria, dehydration, and thirst (exacerbated by hyperglycemia and osmotic diuresis)
- CNS depression and coma
- Potential depletion of K⁺ (although loss may be masked by a mild hyperkalemia)
- Decreased plasma bicarbonate
- Breath with a sweet or fruity odor, acetone

Laboratory measurement of ketones

In normal ketosis (that accompanies fasting and does not produce an acidosis), acetoacetate and β-hydroxybutyrate are formed in approximately equal quantities. In pathologic conditions, such as diabetes and alcoholism, ketoacidosis may develop with life-threatening consequences. In diabetic and alcoholic ketoacidosis, the ratio between acetoacetate and β-hydroxybutyrate shifts and β-hydroxybutyrate predominates. The urinary nitroprusside test detects only acetoacetate and can dramatically underestimate the extent of ketoacidosis and its resolution during treatment. β-hydroxybutyrate should be measured in these patients. Home monitors of both blood glucose and β-hydroxybutyrate are available for diabetic patients.

SPHINGOLIPIDS

Sphingolipids are important constituents of cell membranes, as shown in Figure 16-6. Although sphingolipids contain no glycerol, they are similar in structure to the glycerophospholipids in that they have a hydrophilic region and two fatty acid–derived hydrophobic tails. The various classes of sphingolipids shown in Figure 16-7 differ primarily in the nature of the hydrophilic region.

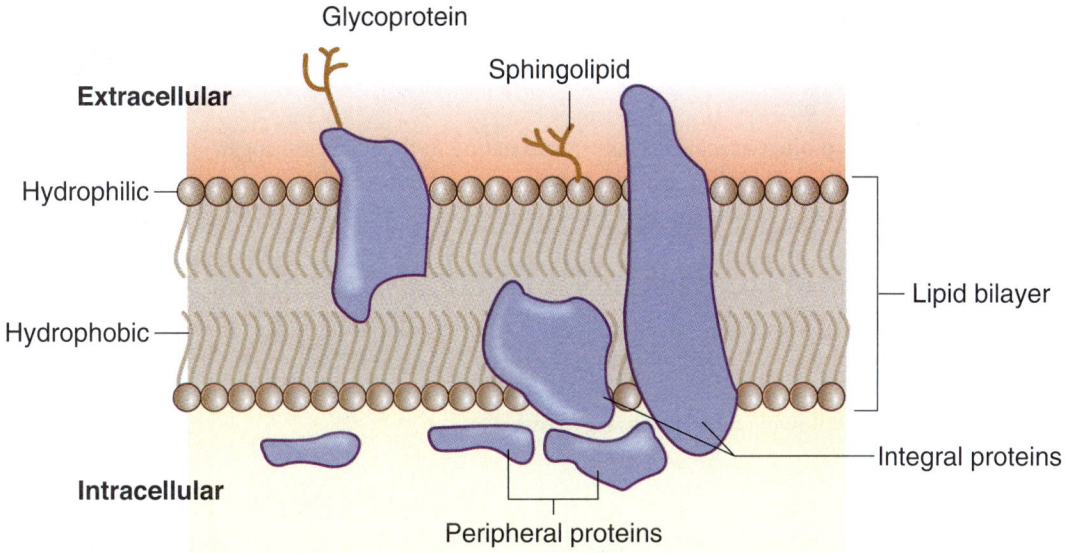

Figure 16-6. Plasma Membrane

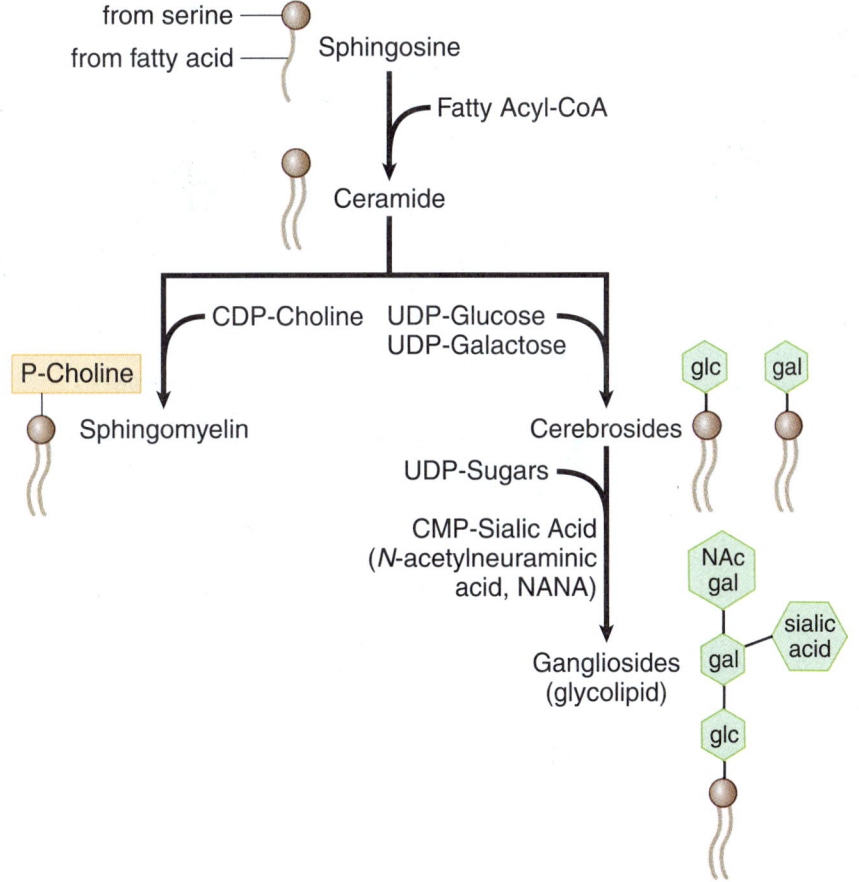

Figure 16-7. Synthesis of Sphingolipids

Classes of sphingolipids and their hydrophilic groups include:

- Sphingomyelin: phosphorylcholine
- Cerebrosides: galactose or glucose
- Gangliosides: branched oligosaccharide chains terminating in the 9-carbon sugar, sialic acid (*N*-acetylneuraminic acid, NANA)

Genetic Deficiencies of Enzymes in Sphingolipid Catabolism

Sphingolipids released when membrane is degraded are digested in endosomes after fusion with lysosomes. Lysosomes contain many enzymes, each of which removes specific groups from individual sphingolipids. Genetic deficiencies of many of these enzymes are known, and the diseases share some of the characteristics of I-cell disease discussed in chapter 4. The following table summarizes these.

Table 16-1. Genetic Deficiencies of Sphingolipid Catabolism

Disease	Lysosomal Enzyme Missing	Substrate Accumulating in Inclusion Body	Symptoms
Tay-Sachs	Hexosaminidase A	Ganglioside GM 2	Cherry red spots in macula Blindness Psychomotor retardation Death usually < 2 years Startle reflex
Gaucher	Glucocerebrosidase	Glucocerebroside	Type 1 (99%): Adult hepatosplenomegaly Erosion of bones, fractures Pancytopenia or thrombocytopenia Characteristic macrophages (crumpled paper inclusions)
Niemann-Pick	Sphingomyelinase	Sphingomyelin	May see cherry red spot in macula Hepatosplenomegaly Microcephaly, severe mental retardation Foamy macrophages with zebra bodies Early death

Amino Acid Metabolism 17

Learning Objectives

❏ Explain information related to removal and excretion of amino groups

❏ Answer questions about disorders of amino acid metabolism

❏ Use knowledge of s-adenosylmethionine, folate, and cobalamin

❏ Solve problems concerning heme synthesis and bilirubin metabolism

❏ Use knowledge of iron transport and storage

OVERVIEW

Protein obtained from the diet or from body protein during prolonged fasting or starvation may be used as an energy source. Body protein is catabolized primarily in muscle and in liver. Amino acids released from proteins usually lose their amino group through transamination or deamination. The carbon skeletons can be converted in the liver to glucose (glucogenic amino acids), acetyl CoA, and ketone bodies (ketogenic), or in a few cases both may be produced (glucogenic and ketogenic).

REMOVAL AND EXCRETION OF AMINO GROUPS

Excess nitrogen is eliminated from the body in the urine. The kidney adds small quantities of ammonium ion to the urine in part to regulate acid-base balance, but nitrogen is also eliminated in this process. Most excess nitrogen is converted to urea in the liver and goes through the blood to the kidney, where it is eliminated in urine.

Amino groups released by deamination reactions form ammonium ion (NH_4^+), which must not escape into the peripheral blood. An elevated concentration of ammonium ion in the blood, hyperammonemia, has toxic effects in the brain (cerebral edema, convulsions, coma, and death). Most tissues add excess nitrogen to the blood as glutamine by attaching ammonia to the γ-carboxyl group of glutamate. Muscle sends nitrogen to the liver as alanine and smaller quantities of other amino acids, in addition to glutamine. The following figure summarizes the flow of nitrogen from tissues to either the liver or kidney for excretion.

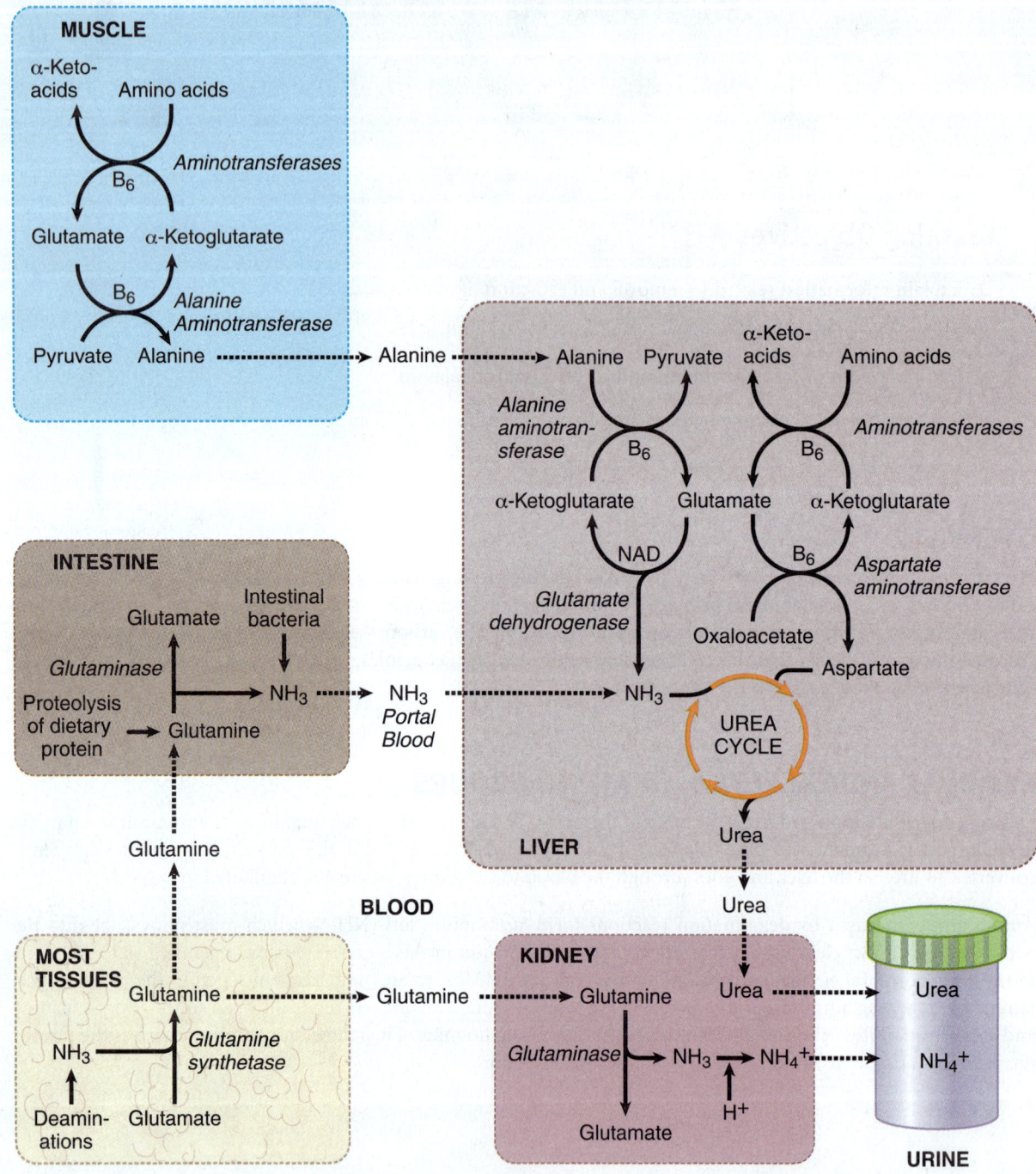

Figure 17-1. Amino Group Removal for Elimination as Urea and Ammonia

Glutamine Synthetase

Most tissues, including muscle, have glutamine synthetase, which captures excess nitrogen by aminating glutamate to form glutamine. The reaction is irreversible. Glutamine, a relatively nontoxic substance, is the major carrier of excess nitrogen from tissues.

Glutaminase

The kidney contains glutaminase, allowing it to deaminate glutamine arriving in the blood and to eliminate the amino group as ammonium ion in urine. The reaction is irreversible. Kidney glutaminase is induced by chronic acidosis, in which excretion of ammonium may become the major defense mechanism. The liver has only small quantities of glutaminase; however, levels of the enzyme are high in the intestine where the ammonium ion from deamination can be sent directly to the liver via the portal blood and used for urea synthesis. The intestinal bacteria and glutamine from dietary protein contribute to the intestinal ammonia entering the portal blood.

Aminotransferases (Transaminases)

Both muscle and liver have aminotransferases, which, unlike deaminases, do not release the amino groups as free ammonium ion. This class of enzymes transfers the amino group from one carbon skeleton (an amino acid) to another (usually α-ketoglutarate, a citric acid cycle intermediate). Pyridoxal phosphate (PLP) derived from vitamin B_6 is required to mediate the transfer.

Aminotransferases are named according to the amino acid donating the amino group to α-ketoglutarate. Two important examples are alanine aminotransferase (ALT, formerly GPT) and aspartate aminotransferase (AST, formerly GOT). Although the aminotransferases are in liver and muscle, in pathologic conditions these enzymes may leak into the blood, where they are useful clinical indicators of damage to liver or muscle.

The reactions catalyzed by aminotransferases are reversible and play several roles in metabolism:

- During protein catabolism in muscle, they move the amino groups from many of the different amino acids onto glutamate, thus pooling it for transport. A portion of the glutamate may be aminated by glutamine synthetase (as in other tissues) or may transfer the amino group to pyruvate, forming alanine using the aminotransferase ALT.

- In liver, aminotransferases ALT and AST can move the amino group from alanine arriving from muscle into aspartate, a direct donor of nitrogen into the urea cycle.

Glutamate Dehydrogenase

This enzyme is found in many tissues, where it catalyzes the reversible oxidative deamination of the amino acid glutamate. It produces the citric acid cycle intermediate α-ketoglutarate, which serves as an entry point to the cycle for a group of glucogenic amino acids. Its role in urea synthesis and nitrogen removal is still controversial, but has been included in Figure 17-1.

UREA CYCLE

Urea, which contains two nitrogens, is synthesized in the liver from aspartate and carbamoyl phosphate, which in turn is produced from ammonium ion and carbon dioxide by mitochondrial carbamoyl phosphate synthetase. This enzyme requires N-acetylglutamate as an activator. N-acetylglutamate is produced only when free amino acids are present.

The urea cycle and the carbamoyl phosphate synthetase reaction are shown in the following figure.

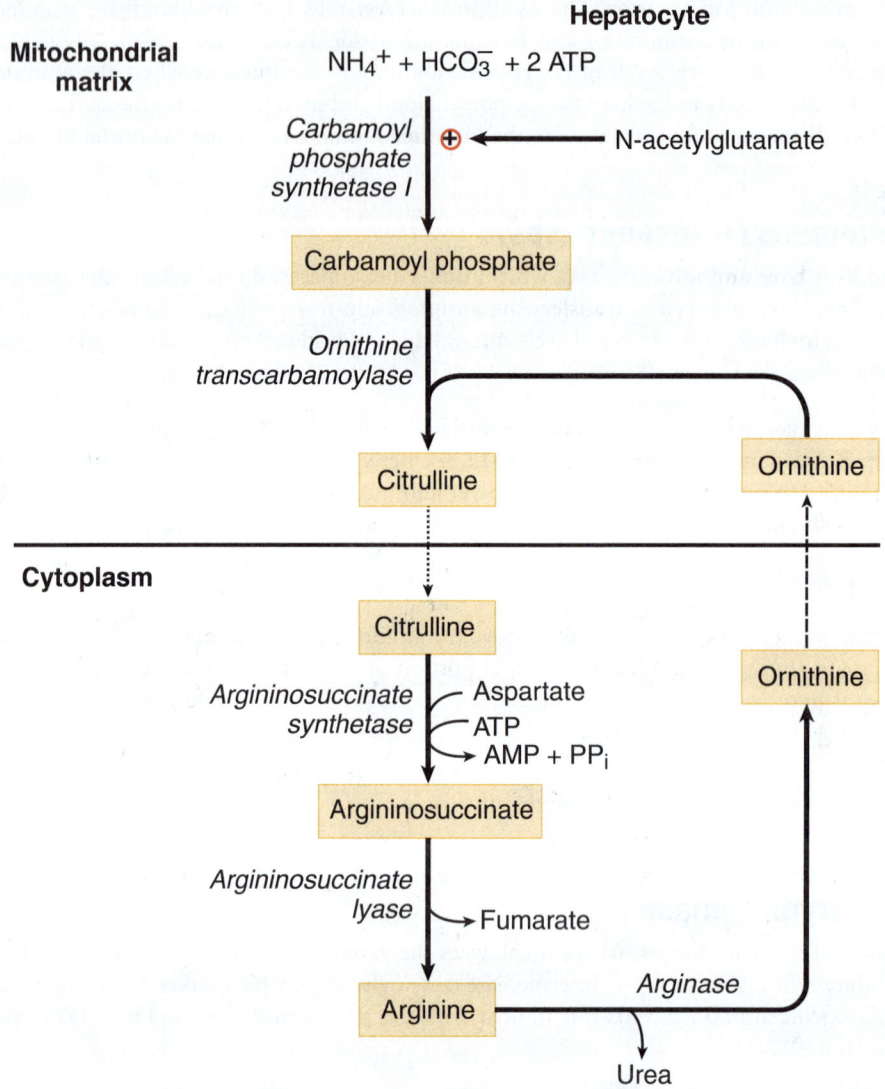

Figure 17-2. The Urea Cycle in the Liver

The urea cycle, like the citric acid cycle, acts catalytically. Small quantities of the intermediates are sufficient to synthesize large amounts of urea from aspartate and carbamoyl phosphate. The cycle occurs partially in the mitochondria and partially in the cytoplasm.

- Citrulline enters the cytoplasm, and ornithine returns to the mitochondria.
- Carbamoyl phosphate synthetase and ornithine transcarbamoylase are mitochondrial enzymes.
- Aspartate enters the cycle in the cytoplasm and leaves the cycle (minus its amino group) as fumarate. If gluconeogenesis is active, fumarate can be converted to glucose.
- The product urea is formed in the cytoplasm and enters the blood for delivery to the kidney.

DISORDERS OF AMINO ACID METABOLISM

The following figure presents a diagram of pathways in which selected amino acids are converted to citric acid cycle intermediates (and glucose) or to acetyl-CoA (and ketones). Important genetic deficiencies are identified on the diagram.

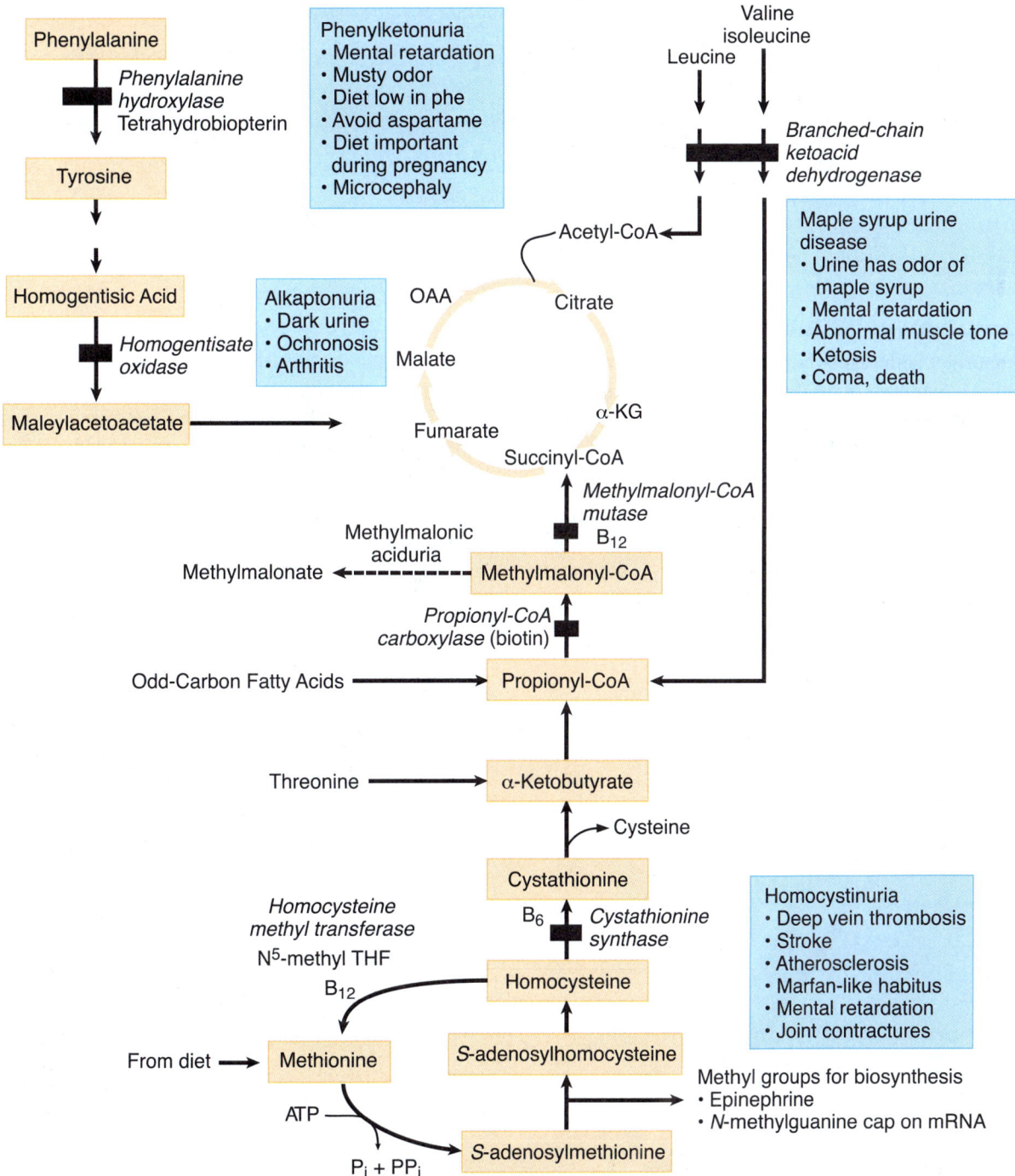

Figure 17-3. Genetic Deficiencies of Amino Acid Metabolism

S-ADENOSYLMETHIONINE, FOLATE, AND COBALAMIN

One-Carbon Units in Biochemical Reactions

One-carbon units in different oxidation states are required in the pathways producing purines, thymidine, and many other compounds. When a biochemical reaction requires a methyl group (methylation), *S*-adenosylmethionine (SAM) is generally the methyl donor. If a 1-carbon unit in another oxidation state is required (methylene, methenyl, formyl), tetrahydrofolate (THF) typically serves as its donor.

Note
THB (BH4) is necessary for tyrosine hydroxylase, phenylalanine hydroxylase, and tryptophan hydroxylase (serotonin synthesis) and is regenerated by dihydropteridine reductase.

S-Adenosylmethionine

Important pathways requiring SAM include synthesis of epinephrine and of the 7-methylguanine cap on eukaryotic mRNA. Synthesis of SAM from methionine is shown in Figure 17-3. After donating the methyl group, SAM is converted to homocysteine and remethylated in a reaction catalyzed by *N*-methyl THF–homocysteine methyltransferase requiring both vitamin B_{12} and *N*-methyl-THF. The methionine produced is once again used to make SAM.

Clinical Correlate
Parkinson's disease is caused by loss of dopaminergic neurons in the substantia nigra. It is treated with levodopa (L-dopa).

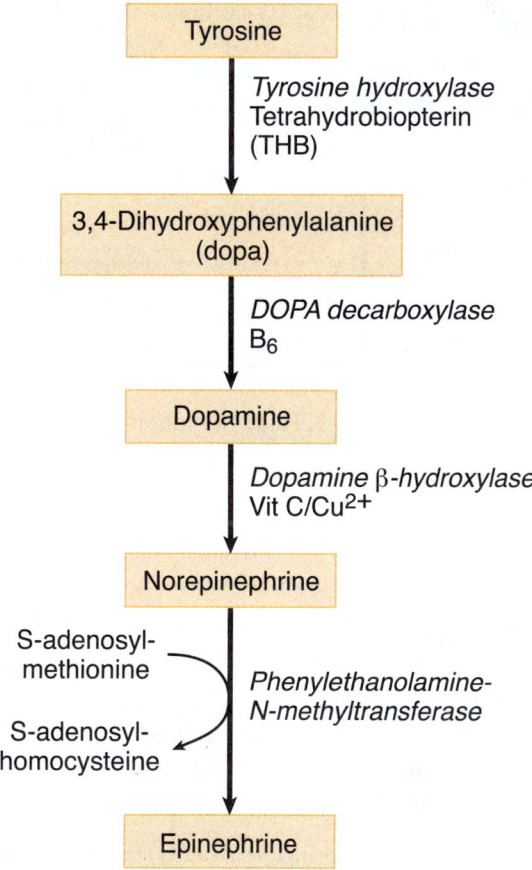

Figure 17-4. Catecholamine Synthesis

Tetrahydrofolate

THF is formed from the vitamin folate through two reductions involving NADPH and catalyzed by dihydrofolate reductase shown in Figure 17-5. It picks up a 1-carbon unit from a variety of donors and enters the active 1-carbon pool. Important pathways requiring forms of THF from this pool include the synthesis of all purines and thymidine, which in turn are used for DNA and RNA synthesis during cell growth and division.

Megaloblastic anemia results from insufficient active THF to support cell division in the bone marrow. Methotrexate inhibits DHF reductase, making it a useful antineoplastic drug. Folate deficiencies may be seen during pregnancy and in alcoholism.

Additional folate may be stored as the highly reduced N^5-methyl-THF. This form is referred to as the storage pool as there is only one known enzyme that uses it, and in turn moves it back into the active pool. This enzyme is N-methyl THF-homocysteine methyltransferase, discussed above, which also requires vitamin B_{12} and is involved in regenerating SAM as a methyl donor for reactions.

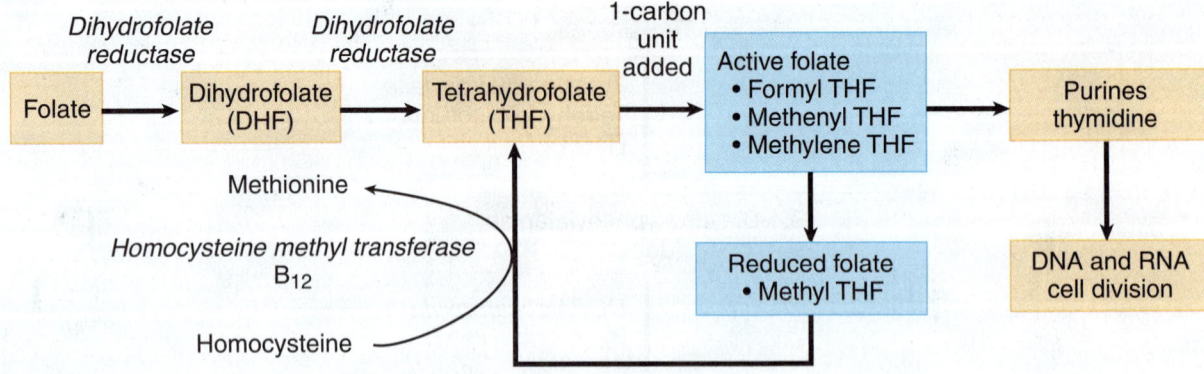

Figure 17-5. Folate Metabolism

Cobalamin

The vitamin cobalamin (vitamin B_{12}) is reduced and activated in the body to two forms, adenosylcobalamin, used by methylmalonyl-CoA mutase, and methylcobalamin, formed from N^5-methyl-THF in the N-methyl THF-homocysteine methyltransferase reaction. These are the only two enzymes that use vitamin B_{12} (other than the enzymes that reduce and add an adenosyl group to it).

Cobalamin deficiency can create a secondary deficiency of active THF by preventing its release from the storage pool through the N-methyl THF-homocysteine methyltransferase reaction, and thus also result in megaloblastic anemia. Progressive peripheral neuropathy also results from cobalamin deficiency. Treating a cobalamin deficiency with folate corrects the megaloblastic anemia but does not halt the neuropathy.

The most likely reason for cobalamin deficiency is pernicious anemia (failure to absorb vitamin B_{12} in the absence of intrinsic factor from parietal cells). Vitamin B_{12} absorption also decreases with aging and in individuals with chronic pancreatitis. Less common reasons for B_{12} deficiency include a long-term completely vegetarian diet (plants don't contain vitamin B_{12}) and infection with *Diphyllobothrium latum,* a parasite found in raw fish. Excess vitamin B_{12} is stored in the body, so deficiencies develop slowly.

Bridge to Pathology

Vitamin B_{12} deficiency causes demyelination of the posterior columns and lateral corticospinal tracts in the spinal cord.

Deficiencies of folate and cobalamin are compared in Table 17-1.

Table 17-1. Comparison of Folate and Vitamin B$_{12}$ Deficiencies

Folate Deficiency	Vitamin B$_{12}$ (Cobalamin) Deficiency
Megaloblastic anemia	Megaloblastic anemia
• Macrocytic	• Macrocytic
• MCV greater than 100 femtolitres (fL)	• MCV greater than 100 femtolitres (fL)
• PMN nucleus more than 5 lobes	• PMN nucleus more than 5 lobes
Homocysteinemia with risk for cardiovascular disease	Homocysteinemia with risk for cardiovascular disease
	Methylmalonic aciduria
	Progressive peripheral neuropathy
Deficiency develops in 3–4 months	Deficiency develops in years
Risk factors for deficiency:	Risk factors for deficiency:
• Pregnancy (neural tube defects in fetus may result)	• Perni cious anemia
• Alcoholism	• Gastric resection
• Severe malnutrition	• Chronic pancreatitis
• Gastric or terminal ileum resection	• Severe malnutrition
	• Vegan
	• Infection with *D. latum*
	• Ageing
	• Bacterial overgrowth of the terminal ileum
	• *H. pylori* infection

SPECIALIZED PRODUCTS DERIVED FROM AMINO ACIDS

The following table identifies some important products formed from amino acids.

Table 17-2. Products of Amino Acids

Amino Acid	Products
Tyrosine	Thyroid hormones T$_3$ and T$_4$
	Melanin
	Catecholamines
Tryptophan	Serotonin NAD, NADP
Arginine	Nitric oxide (NO)
Glutamate	γ-Aminobutyric acid (GABA)
Histidine	Histamine

HEME SYNTHESIS

Heme synthesis occurs in almost all tissues because heme proteins include not only hemoglobin and myoglobin but all the cytochromes (electron transport chain, cytochrome P-450, cytochrome b_5), as well as the enzymes catalase, peroxidase, and the soluble guanylate cyclase stimulated by nitric oxide. The pathway producing heme, shown in Figure 17-6, is controlled independently in different tissues. In liver, the rate-limiting enzyme δ-aminolevulinate synthase (ALA) is repressed by heme.

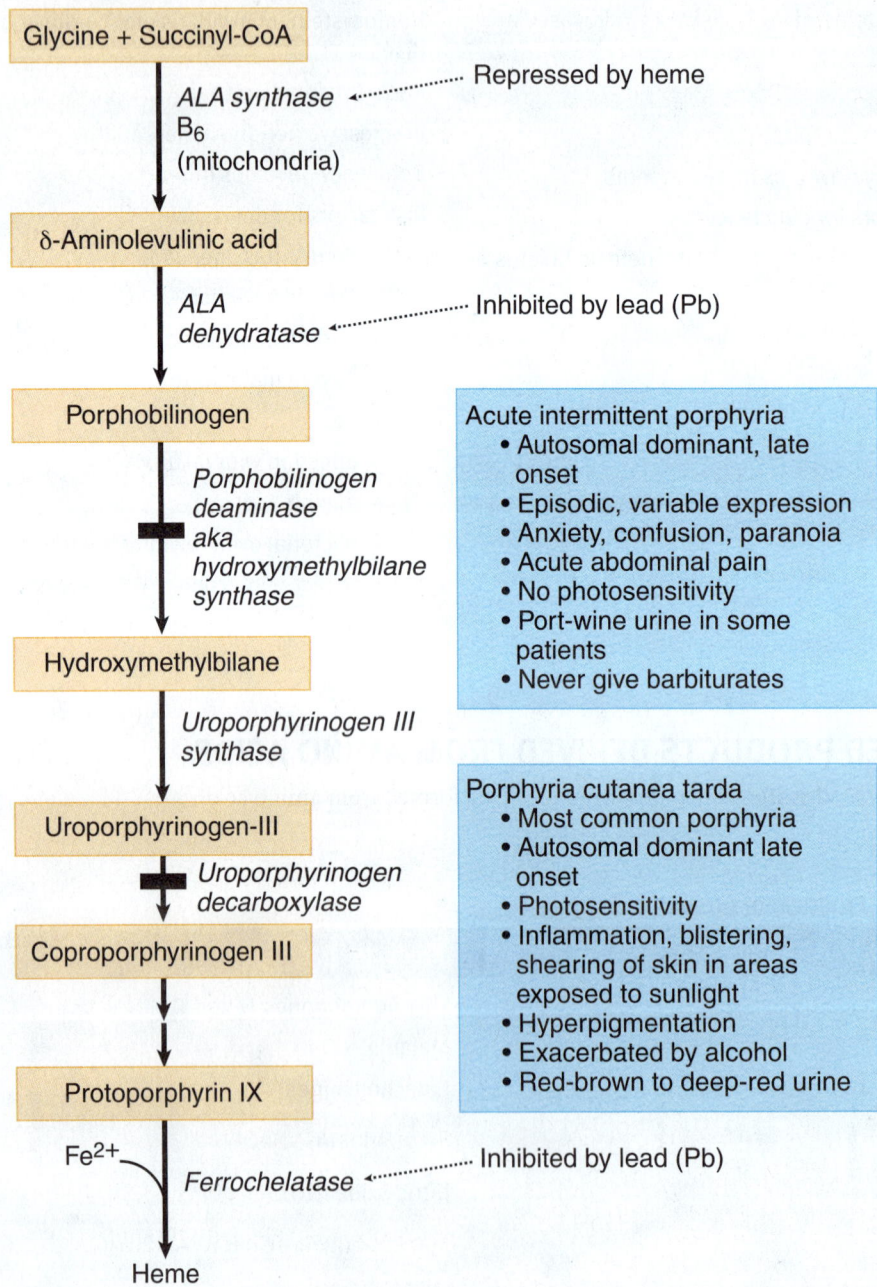

Figure 17-6. Heme Synthesis

Vitamin B$_6$ Deficiency

ALA synthase, the rate-limiting enzyme, requires pyridoxine (vitamin B$_6$). Deficiency of pyridoxine is associated with isoniazid therapy for tuberculosis and may cause sideroblastic anemia with ringed sideroblasts.

Iron Deficiency

The last enzyme in the pathway, heme synthase (ferrochelatase), introduces the Fe^{2+} into the heme ring. Deficiency of iron produces a microcytic hypochromic anemia.

Lead Poisoning

Lead inactivates many enzymes including ALA dehydrase and ferrochelatase (heme synthase), and can produce a microcytic sideroblastic anemia with ringed sideroblasts in the bone marrow. Other symptoms include:

- Coarse basophilic stippling of erythrocytes
- Headache, nausea, memory loss
- Abdominal pain, diarrhea (lead colic)
- Lead lines in gums
- Lead deposits in abdomen and epiphyses of bone seen on radiograph
- Neuropathy (claw hand, wrist-drop)
- Increased urinary ALA
- Increased free erythrocyte protoporphyrin

Vitamin B$_6$ deficiency, iron deficiency, and lead poisoning all can cause anemia. These three conditions are summarized and compared in the following table.

Table 17-3. Comparison of Vitamin B$_6$ Deficiency, Iron Deficiency, and Lead Poisoning

Vitamin B$_6$ (Pyridoxine) Deficiency	Iron Deficiency	Lead Poisoning
Microcytic	Microcytic	Microcytic Coarse basophilic stippling in erythrocyte
Ringed sideroblasts in bone marrow		Ringed sideroblasts in bone marrow
Protoporphyrin: ↓	Protoporphyrin: ↑	Protoporphyrin: ↑
δ-ALA: ↓	δ-ALA: Normal	δ-ALA: ↑
Ferritin: ↑	Ferritin: ↓	Ferritin: ↑
Serum iron: ↑	Serum iron: ↓	Serum iron: ↑
Isoniazid for tuberculosis	Dietary iron insufficient to compensate for normal loss	Lead paint Pottery glaze Batteries (Diagnose by measuring blood lead level)

IRON TRANSPORT AND STORAGE

Iron (Fe^{3+}) released from hemoglobin in the histiocytes is bound to ferritin and then transported in the blood by transferrin, which can deliver it to tissues for synthesis of heme. Important proteins in this context are:

- Ferroxidase (also known as ceruloplasmin, a Cu^{2+} protein) oxidizes Fe^{2+} to Fe^{3+} for transport and storage (Figure 17-7).

- Transferrin carries Fe^{3+} in blood.

- Ferritin itself oxidizes Fe^{2+} to Fe^{3+} for storage of normal amounts of Fe^{3+} in tissues. Loss of iron from the body is accomplished by bleeding and shedding epithelial cells of the mucosa and skin. The body has no mechanism for excreting iron, so controlling its absorption into the mucosal cells is crucial. No other nutrient is regulated in this manner.

- Hemosiderin binds excess Fe^{3+} to prevent escape of free Fe^{3+} into the blood, where it is toxic.

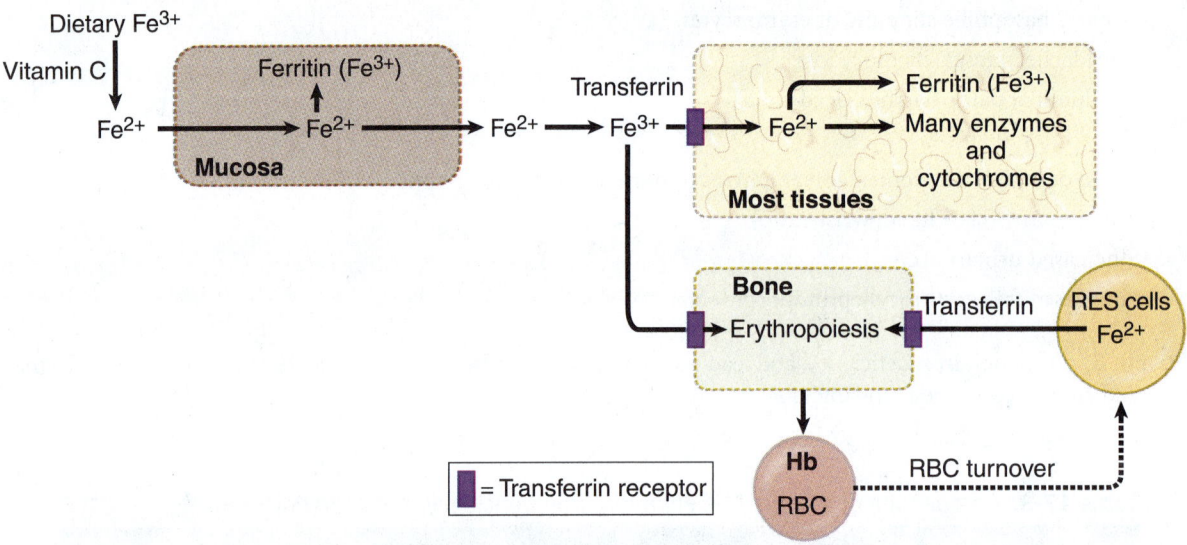

Figure 17-7. Iron Metabolism

BILIRUBIN METABOLISM

Subsequent to lysis of older erythrocytes in the spleen, heme released from hemoglobin is converted to bilirubin in the histiocytes. This sequence is shown in Figure 17-8.

- Bilirubin is not water soluble and is therefore transported in the blood attached to serum albumin.

- Hepatocytes conjugate bilirubin with glucuronic acid, increasing its water solubility.

- Conjugated bilirubin is secreted into the bile.

- Intestinal bacteria convert conjugated bilirubin into urobilinogen.

- A portion of the urobilinogen is further converted to bile pigments (stercobilin) and excreted in the feces, producing their characteristic red-brown color. Bile duct obstruction results in clay-colored stools.

- Some of the urobilinogen is converted to urobilin (yellow) and excreted in urine.

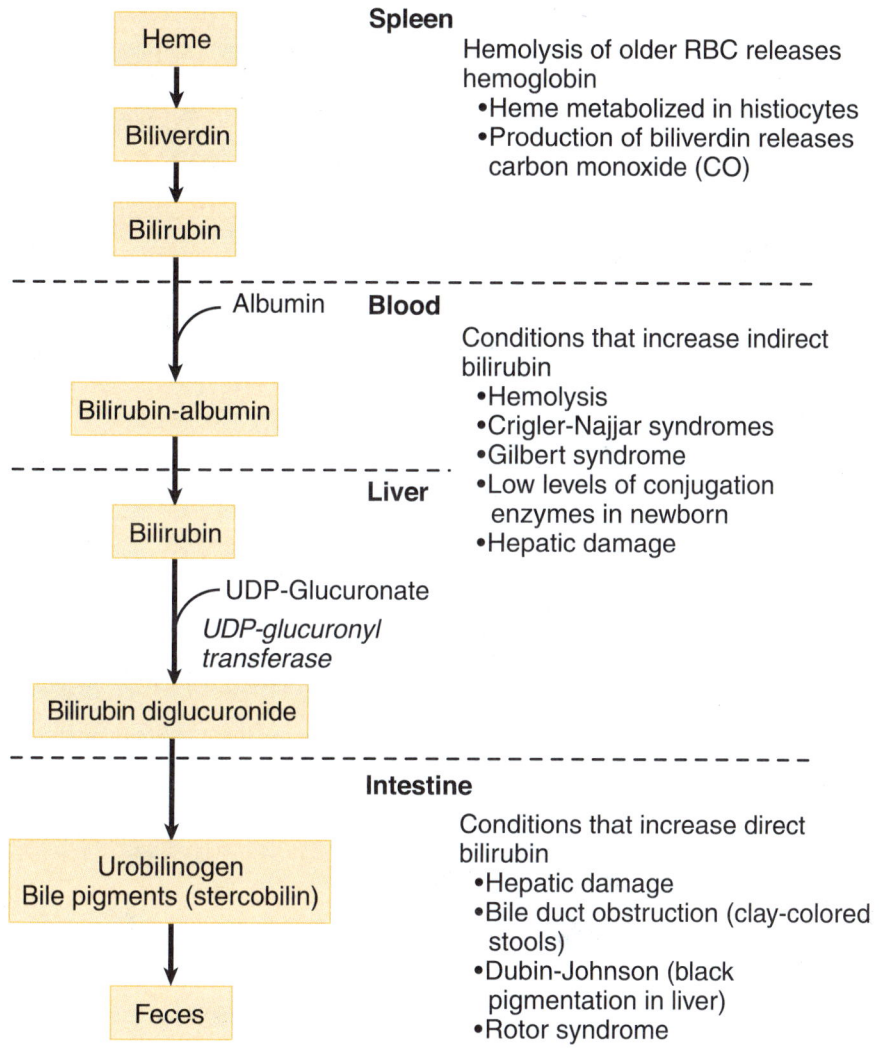

Figure 17-8. Heme Catabolism and Bilirubin

Spleen
Hemolysis of older RBC releases hemoglobin
- Heme metabolized in histiocytes
- Production of biliverdin releases carbon monoxide (CO)

Blood
Conditions that increase indirect bilirubin
- Hemolysis
- Crigler-Najjar syndromes
- Gilbert syndrome
- Low levels of conjugation enzymes in newborn
- Hepatic damage

Liver

Intestine
Conditions that increase direct bilirubin
- Hepatic damage
- Bile duct obstruction (clay-colored stools)
- Dubin-Johnson (black pigmentation in liver)
- Rotor syndrome

Clinical Correlates

Excessive RBC destruction in hemolytic anemia results in excessive conversion of bilirubin to urobilinogen in the intestine. Higher-than-normal absorption of the urobilinogen and its subsequent excretion in the urine results in a deeper-colored urine.

At very high levels, lipid-soluble bilirubin may cross the blood-brain barrier and precipitate in the basal ganglia, causing irreversible brain damage (kernicterus).

Bilirubin and Jaundice

Jaundice (yellow color of skin, whites of the eyes) may occur when blood levels of bilirubin exceed normal (icterus). Jaundice may be characterized by an increase in unconjugated (indirect) bilirubin, conjugated (direct) bilirubin, or both. Accumulation of bilirubin (usually unconjugated) in the brain (kernicterus) may result in death. When conjugated bilirubin increases, it may be excreted, giving a deep yellow-red color to the urine. Examples of conditions associated with increased bilirubin and jaundice include hemolytic crisis, UDP-glucuronyl transferase deficiency, hepatic damage, and bile duct occlusion.

Purine and Pyrimidine Metabolism 18

Learning Objectives

❏ Explain information related to pyrimidine synthesis

❏ Use knowledge of pyrimidine catabolism

❏ Explain information related to purine synthesis

❏ Demonstrate understanding of purine catabolism and the salvage enzyme HGPRT

OVERVIEW

Nucleotides are needed for DNA and RNA synthesis (DNA replication and transcription) and for energy transfer. Nucleoside triphosphates (ATP and GTP) provide energy for reactions that would otherwise be extremely unfavorable in the cell.

Ribose 5-phosphate for nucleotide synthesis is derived from the hexose monophosphate shunt and is activated by the addition of pyrophosphate from ATP, forming phosphoribosyl pyrophosphate (PRPP) using PRPP synthetase. Cells synthesize nucleotides in two ways, *de novo* synthesis and salvage pathways (Figure 18-1). In *de novo* synthesis, which occurs predominantly in the liver, purines and pyrimidines are synthesized from smaller precursors, and PRPP is added to the pathway at some point. In the salvage pathways, preformed purine and pyrimidine bases can be converted into nucleotides by salvage enzymes distinct from those of *de novo* synthesis. Purine and pyrimidine bases for salvage enzymes may arise from:

- Synthesis in the liver and transport to other tissues
- Digestion of endogenous nucleic acids (cell death, RNA turnover)

In many cells, the capacity for *de novo* synthesis to supply purines and pyrimidines is insufficient, and the salvage pathway is essential for adequate nucleotide synthesis. In patients with Lesch-Nyhan disease, an enzyme for purine salvage (hypoxanthine guanine phosphoribosyl pyrophosphate transferase, HPRT) is absent or deficient. People with this genetic deficiency have CNS deterioration, mental retardation, and spastic cerebral palsy associated with compulsive self-mutilation. Cells in the basal ganglia of the brain (fine motor control) normally have very high HPRT activity. These patients also all have hyperuricemia because purines cannot be salvaged, causing gout.

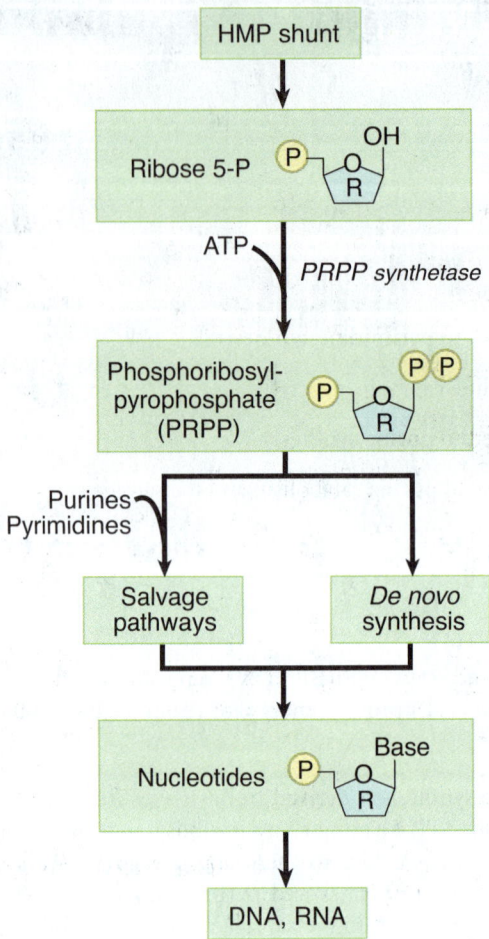

Figure 18-1. Nucleotide Synthesis by Salvage and De Novo Pathways

PYRIMIDINE SYNTHESIS

Pyrimidines are synthesized *de novo* in the cytoplasm from aspartate, CO_2, and glutamine, as shown in Figure 18-2. Synthesis involves a cytoplasmic carbamoyl phosphate synthetase that differs from the mitochondrial enzyme with the same name used in the urea cycle.

Orotic Aciduria

Several days after birth, an infant was observed to have severe anemia, which was found to be megaloblastic. There was no evidence of hepatomegaly or splenomegaly. The pediatrician started the newborn on a bottle-fed regimen containing folate, vitamin B_{12}, vitamin B_6, and iron. One week later, the infant's condition did not improve. The pediatrician noted that the infant's urine contained a crystalline residue, which was analyzed and determined to be orotic acid. Laboratory tests indicated no evidence of hyperammonemia. The infant was given a formula that contained uridine. Shortly thereafter, the infant's condition improved significantly.

Orotic aciduria is an autosomal recessive disorder caused by a defect in uridine monophosphate (UMP) synthase. This enzyme contains two activities, orotate phosphoribosyltransferase and orotidine decarboxylase. The lack of pyrimidines impairs nucleic acid synthesis needed for hematopoiesis, explaining the megaloblastic anemia in this infant. Orotic acid accumulates and spills into the urine, resulting in orotic acid crystals and orotic acid urinary obstruction. The presence of orotic acid in urine might suggest that the defect could be ornithine transcarbamylase (OTC) deficiency, but the lack of hyperammonemia rules out a defect in the urea cycle. Uridine administration relieves the symptoms by bypassing the defect in the pyrimidine pathway. Uridine is salvaged to UMP, which feedback-inhibits carbamoyl phosphate synthase-2, preventing orotic acid formation.

Note

Two Orotic Acidurias

1. Hyperammonemia

   No megaloblastic anemia
   - Pathway: Urea cycle
   - Enzyme deficient: OTC

2. Megaloblastic anemia

   No hyperammonemia
   - Pathway: Pyrimidine synthesis
   - Enzyme deficient: UMP synthase

Folate and vitamin B_{12} deficiency: megaloblastic anemia, but no orotic aciduria

---

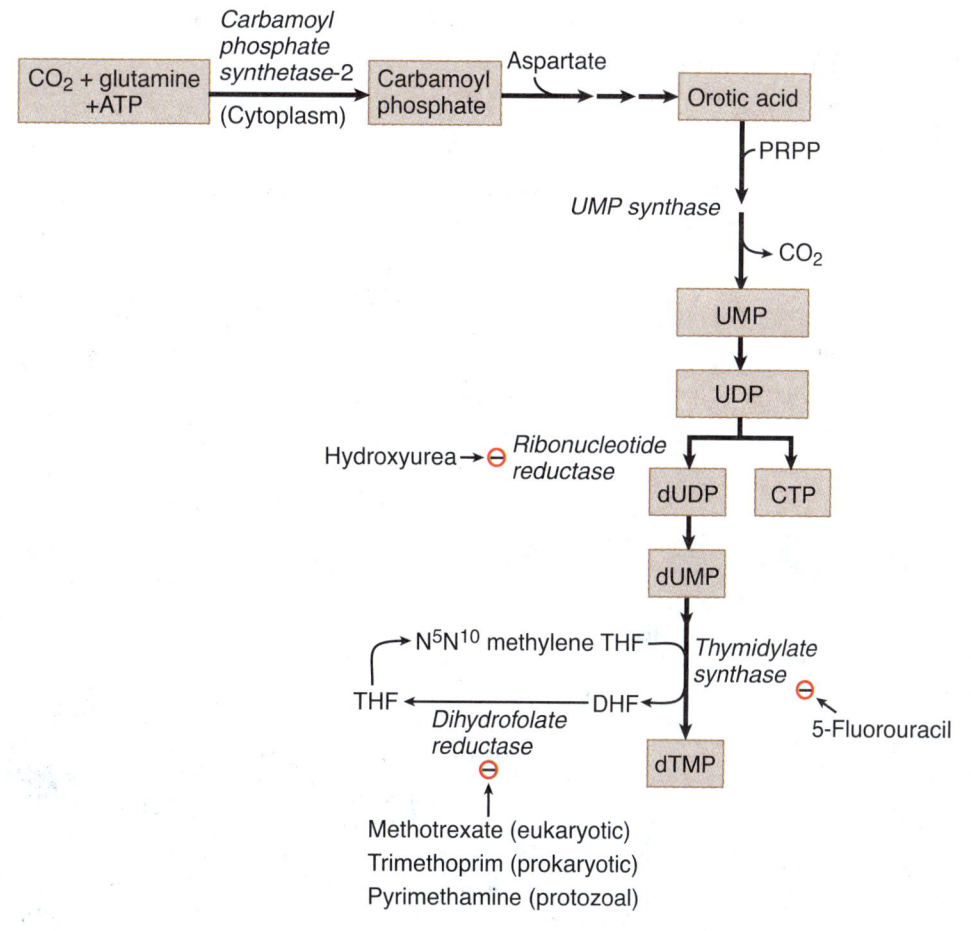

Figure 18-2. *De Novo* Pyrimidine Synthesis

The primary end product of pyrimidine synthesis is UMP. In the conversion of UMP to dTMP, three important enzymes are ribonucleotide reductase, thymidylate synthase, and dihydrofolate reductase. All three enzymes are targets of antineoplastic drugs and are summarized in the following table.

Table 18-1. Important Enzymes of Pyrimidine Synthesis

Enzyme	Function	Drug
Ribonucleotide reductase	Reduces all NDPs to dNDPs for DNA synthesis	Hydroxyurea (S phase)
Thymidylate synthase	Methylates dUMP to dTMP Requires THF	5-Fluorouracil (S phase)
Dihydrofolate reductase (DHFR)	Converts DHF to THF Without DHFR, thymidylate synthesis will eventually stop	Methotrexate (eukaryotic) (S phase) Trimethoprim (prokaryotic) Pyrimethamine (protozoal)

Ribonucleotide Reductase

Ribonucleotide reductase is required for the formation of the deoxyribonucleotides for DNA synthesis. Figure 18-2 shows its role in dTMP synthesis, and Figure 18-3 shows all four nucleotide substrates:

- All four nucleotide substrates must be diphosphates.
- dADP and dATP strongly inhibit ribonucleotide reductase.
- Hydroxyurea, an anticancer drug, blocks DNA synthesis indirectly by inhibiting ribonucleotide reductase.

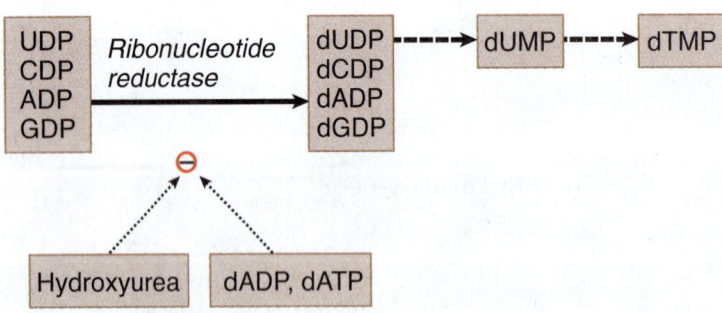

Figure 18-3. Ribonucleotide Reductase

PYRIMIDINE CATABOLISM

Pyrimidines may be completely catabolized (NH_4^+ is produced) or recycled by pyrimidine salvage enzymes.

PURINE SYNTHESIS

Purines are synthesized *de novo* beginning with PRPP as shown in 18-4. The most important enzyme is PRPP amidotransferase, which catalyzes the first and rate-limiting reaction of the pathway. It is inhibited by the three purine nucleotide end products AMP, GMP, and IMP.

The drugs allopurinol (used for gout) and 6-mercaptopurine (antineoplastic) also inhibit PRPP amidotransferase. These drugs are purine analogs that must be converted to their respective nucleotides by HGPRT within cells. Also note that:

- The amino acids glycine, aspartate, and glutamine are used in purine synthesis.
- Tetrahydrofolate is required for synthesis of all the purines.
- Inosine monophosphate (contains the purine base hypoxanthine) is the precursor for AMP and GMP.

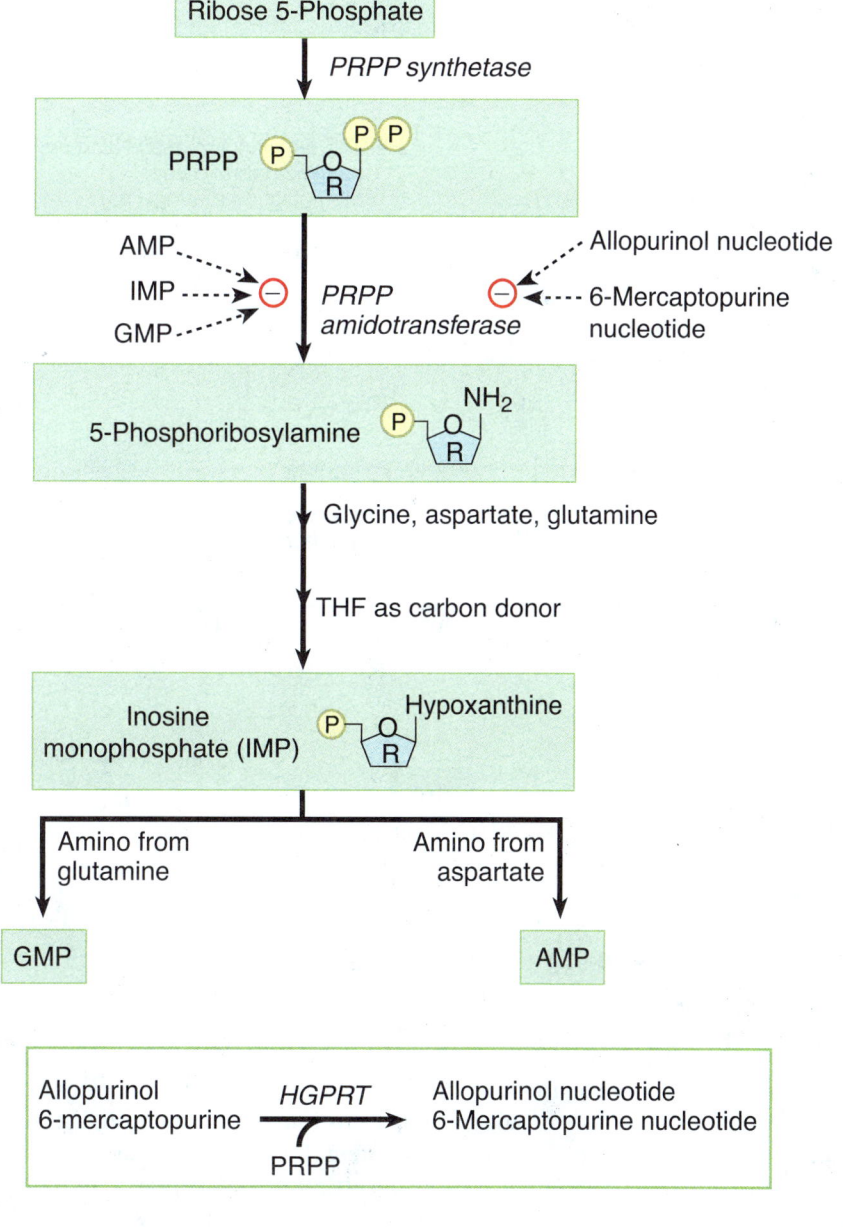

Figure 18-4. *De Novo* Purine Synthesis

PURINE CATABOLISM AND THE SALVAGE ENZYME HGPRT

Excess purine nucleotides or those released from DNA and RNA by nucleases are catabolized first to nucleosides (loss of P_i) and then to free purine bases (release of ribose or deoxyribose). Excess nucleoside monophosphates may accumulate when:

- RNA is normally digested by nucleases (mRNAs and other types of RNAs are continuously turned over in normal cells).
- Dying cells release DNA and RNA, which is digested by nucleases.
- The concentration of free P_i decreases as it may in galactosemia, hereditary fructose intolerance, and glucose-6-phosphatase deficiency.

Salvage enzymes recycle normally about 90% of these purines, and 10% are converted to uric acid and excreted in urine. When purine catabolism is increased significantly, a person is at risk for developing hyperuricemia and potentially gout.

Purine catabolism to uric acid and salvage of the purine bases hypoxanthine (derived from adenosine) and guanine are shown in the following figure.

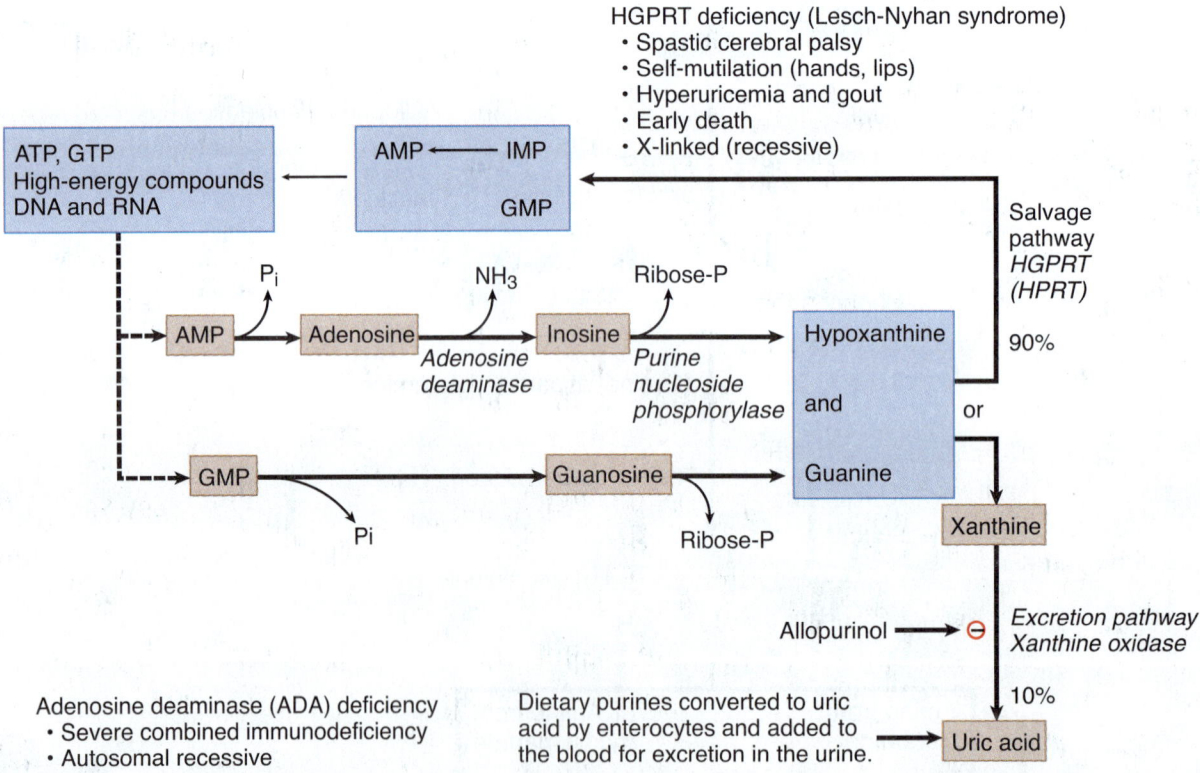

Figure 18-5. Purine Excretion and Salvage Pathways

Hyperuricemia and Gout

Hyperuricemia may be produced by overproduction of uric acid or underexcretion of uric acid by the kidneys. Hyperuricemia may progress to acute and chronic gouty arthritis if uric acid (monosodium urate) is deposited in joints and surrounding soft tissue, where it causes inflammation. Uric acid is produced from excess endogenous purines as shown in Figure 18-5, and is also produced from dietary purines (digestion of nucleic acid in the intestine) by intestinal epithelia. Both sources of uric acid are transported in the blood to the kidneys for excretion in urine.

Allopurinol inhibits xanthine oxidase and also can reduce purine synthesis by inhibiting PRPP amidotransferase, provided HGPRT is active (see Figure 18-4). Hyperuricemia and gout often accompany the following conditions:

- Lesch-Nyhan syndrome (no purine salvage)
- Partial deficiency of HGPRT
- Alcoholism (lactate and urate compete for same transport system in the kidney)
- Glucose 6-phosphatase deficiency
- Hereditary fructose intolerance (aldolase B deficiency)
- Galactose 1-phosphate uridyl transferase deficiency (galactosemia)
- Mutations in PRPP synthetase that lower K_m

In the last two diseases, phosphorylated sugars accumulate, decreasing the available Pi and increasing AMP (which cannot be phosphorylated to ADP and ATP). The excess AMP is converted to uric acid.

Clinical Correlate

Gout

Acute gouty arthritis, seen most commonly in males, results from precipitation of monosodium urate crystals in joints. The crystals, identified as negatively birefringent and needle-shaped, initiate neutrophil-mediated and acute inflammation, often first affecting the big toe. Chronic gout may manifest over time as tophi (deposits of monosodium urate) develop in soft tissue around joints, leading to chronic inflammation involving granulomas.

Single-Gene Disorders 19

Learning Objectives

❏ Interpret scenarios about basic definitions

❏ Use knowledge of major modes of inheritance

❏ Use knowledge of important principles that can characterize single-gene diseases

BASIC DEFINITIONS

Chromosomes

Humans are composed of two groups of cells:

- **Gametes.** Ova and sperm cells, which are haploid, have one copy of each type of chromosome (1–22, X or Y). This DNA is transmitted to offspring.
- **Somatic cells** (cells other than gametes). Nearly all somatic cells are diploid, having two copies of each type of autosome (1–22) and either XX or XY.

Diploid cells

- **Homologous chromosomes.** The two chromosomes in each diploid pair are said to be homologs, or homologous chromosomes. They contain the same genes, but because one is of paternal origin and one is of maternal origin, they may have different alleles at some loci.
- **X and Y chromosomes,** or the sex chromosomes, have some homologous regions but the majority of genes are different. The regions that are homologous are sometimes referred to as pseudoautosomal regions. During meiosis-1 of male spermatogenesis, the X and Y chromosomes pair in the pseudoautosomal regions, allowing the chromosomes to segregate into different cells.

Genes

- **Gene.** Physically a gene consists of a sequence of DNA that encodes a specific protein (or a nontranslated RNA; for example: tRNA, rRNA, or snRNA).
- **Locus.** The physical location of a gene on a chromosome is termed a locus.
- **Alleles.** Variation (mutation) in the DNA sequence of a gene produces a new allele at that locus. Many genes have multiple alleles. Although this term has been used most frequently with genes, noncoding DNA can also have alleles of specific sequences.
- **Polymorphism.** When a specific site on a chromosome has multiple alleles in the population, it is said to be polymorphic (many forms).

For example, the β-globin gene encodes a protein (β-globin). It has been mapped to chromosome 11p15.5 indicating its locus, a specific location on chromosome 11. Throughout human history there have been many mutations in the β-globin gene, and each mutation has created a new allele in the population. The β-globin locus is therefore polymorphic. Some alleles cause no clinical disease, but others, like the sickle cell allele, are associated with significant disease. Included among the disease-causing alleles are those associated with sickle cell anemia and several associated with β-thalassemia.

Genotype

The specific DNA sequence at a locus is termed a genotype. In diploid somatic cells a genotype may be:

- **Homozygous** if the individual has the same allele on both homologs (homologous chromosomes) at that locus.
- **Heterozygous** if the individual has different alleles on the two homologs (homologous chromosomes) at that locus.

Phenotype

The phenotype is generally understood as the expression of the genotype in terms of observable characteristics.

Mutations

A *mutation* is an alteration in DNA sequence (thus, mutations produce new alleles). When mutations occur in cells giving rise to gametes, the mutations can be transmitted to future generations. *Missense* mutations result in the substitution of a single amino acid in the polypeptide chain (e.g., sickle cell disease is caused by a missense mutation that produces a substitution of valine for glutamic acid in the β-globin polypeptide). *Nonsense* mutations produce a stop codon, resulting in premature termination of translation and a truncated protein. Nucleotide bases may be inserted or deleted. When the number of inserted or deleted bases is a multiple of three, the mutation is said to be *in-frame*. If not a multiple of three, the mutation is a *frameshift*, which alters all codons downstream of the mutation, typically producing a truncated or severely altered protein product. Mutations can occur in promoter and other regulatory regions or in genes for transcription factors that bind to these regions. This can decrease or increase the amount of gene product produced in the cell. (For a complete description of these and other mutations, see Section I, Chapter 4: Translation; Mutations.)

Mutations can also be classified according to their phenotypic effects. Mutations that cause a missing protein product or cause decreased activity of the protein are termed *loss-of-function*. Those that produce a protein product with a new function or increased activity are termed *gain-of-function*.

Recurrence risk

The *recurrence risk* is the probability that the offspring of a couple will express a genetic disease. For example, in the mating of a normal homozygote with a heterozygote who has a dominant disease-causing allele, the recurrence risk for each offspring is 1/2, or 50%. It is important to remember that each reproductive event is statistically independent of all previous events. Therefore, the recurrence risk remains the same regardless of the number of previously affected or unaffected offspring. Determining the mode of inheritance of a disease (e.g., autosomal dominant versus autosomal recessive) enables one to assign an appropriate recurrence risk for a family.

Pedigrees

A patient's family history is diagrammed in a pedigree (see symbols in the following figure). The first affected individual to be identified in the family is termed the **proband**.

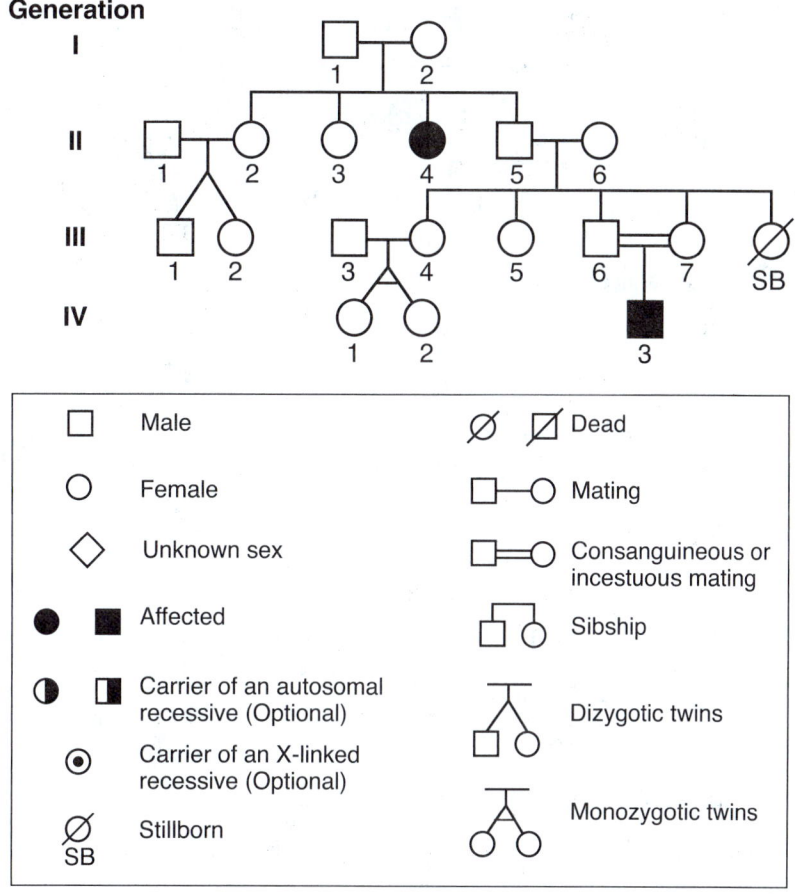

Figure 19-1. Pedigree Nomenclature

MAJOR MODES OF INHERITANCE

Autosomal Dominant Inheritance

A number of features in a pedigree help identify autosomal dominant inheritance:

- Because affected individuals must receive a disease-causing gene from an affected parent, the disease is typically observed in multiple generations of a pedigree (see Figure 19-2).

- Skipped generations are not typically seen because two unaffected parents cannot transmit a disease-causing allele to their offspring (an exception occurs when there is reduced penetrance, discussed below).

- Because these genes are located on autosomes, males and females are affected in roughly equal frequencies.

Autosomal dominant alleles are relatively rare in populations, so the typical mating pattern is a heterozygous affected individual (Aa genotype) mating with a homozygous normal individual (aa genotype), as shown in Figure 19-3. Note that, by convention, the dominant allele is shown in uppercase (A) and the recessive allele is shown in lowercase (a). The recurrence risk is thus 50%, and half the children, on average, will be affected with the disease. If both parents are heterozygous, the recurrence risk is 75%.

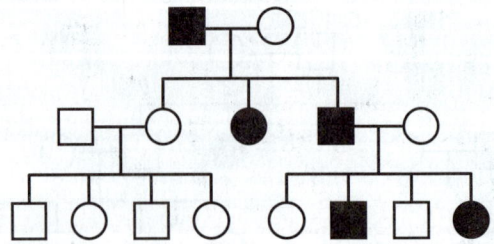

Figure 19-2. Autosomal Dominant Inheritance

	A	a
a	Aa	aa
a	Aa	aa

A Punnett square: Affected offspring (Aa) are shaded.

Figure 19-3. Recurrence Risk for the Mating of Affected Individual (Aa) with a Homozygous Unaffected Individual (aa) using a Punnett Square

Note

Autosomal Dominant Diseases

- Familial hypercholesterolemia (LDL receptor deficiency)
- Huntington disease
- Neurofibromatosis type 1
- Marfan syndrome
- Acute intermittent porphyria

Autosomal Recessive Inheritance

Important features that distinguish autosomal recessive inheritance:

- Because autosomal recessive alleles are clinically expressed only in the homozygous state, the offspring must inherit one copy of the disease-causing allele from each parent.
- In contrast to autosomal dominant diseases, autosomal recessive diseases are typically seen in only one generation of a pedigree (see Figure 19-4).
- Because these genes are located on autosomes, males and females are affected in roughly equal frequencies.

Most commonly, a homozygote is produced by the union of two heterozygous (*carrier*) parents. The recurrence risk for offspring of such matings is 25% (see Figure 19-5).

Consanguinity(the mating of related individuals) is sometimes seen in recessive pedigrees because individuals who share common ancestors are more likely to carry the same recessive disease-causing alleles.

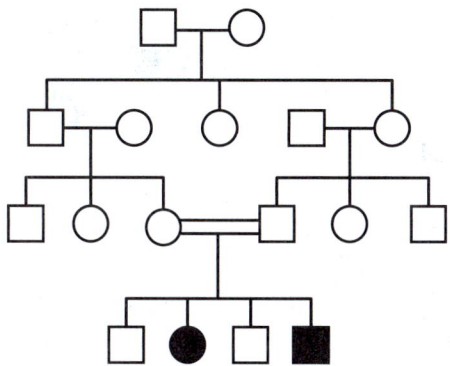

A consanguineous mating has produced two affected offspring.

Figure 19-4. Pedigree for an Autosomal Recessive Disease

	A	a
A	AA	Aa
a	Aa	aa

The affected genotype (aa) is shaded.

Figure 19-5. Recurrence Risk for the Mating of Two Heterozygous Carriers (Aa) of a Recessive Mutation

Determining the Recurrence Risk for an Individual Whose Phenotype Is Known. In Figure 19-4, Individual IV-1 may wish to know his risk of being a carrier. Because his phenotype is known, there are only three possible genotypes he can have, assuming complete penetrance of the disease-producing allele. He cannot be homozygous for the recessive allele (aa). Two of the remaining three possibilities are carriers (Aa and aA), and one is homozygous normal (AA). Thus, his risk of being a carrier is 2/3, or 0.67 (67%).

Note

Autosomal Recessive Diseases

Examples include:

- Sickle cell anemia
- Cystic fibrosis
- Phenylketonuria (PKU)
- Tay-Sachs disease (hexosaminidase A deficiency)

X-linked Recessive Inheritance

Properties of X-linked recessive inheritance

Because males have only one copy of the X chromosome, they are said to be **hemizygous** (*hemi* = "half") for the X chromosome. If a recessive disease-causing mutation occurs on the X chromosome, a male will be affected with the disease.

- Because males require only one copy of the mutation to express the disease and females require two copies, X-linked recessive diseases are seen much more commonly in males than in females (see Figure 19-6).

- Skipped generations are commonly seen because an affected male can transmit the disease-causing mutation to a heterozygous daughter, who is unaffected but who can transmit the disease-causing allele to her sons.

- Male-to-male transmission is not seen in X-linked inheritance; this helps distinguish it from autosomal inheritance.

Note

X-Linked Recessive Diseases

- Duchenne muscular dystrophy
- Lesch-Nyhan syndrome (hypoxanthine-guanine phosphoribosyltransferase [HGPRT] deficiency)
- Glucose-6-phosphate dehydrogenase deficiency
- Hemophilia A and B
- Red-green color blindness
- Menke's disease
- Ornithine transcarbamoylase (OTC) deficiency
- SCID (IL-receptor γ-chain deficiency)

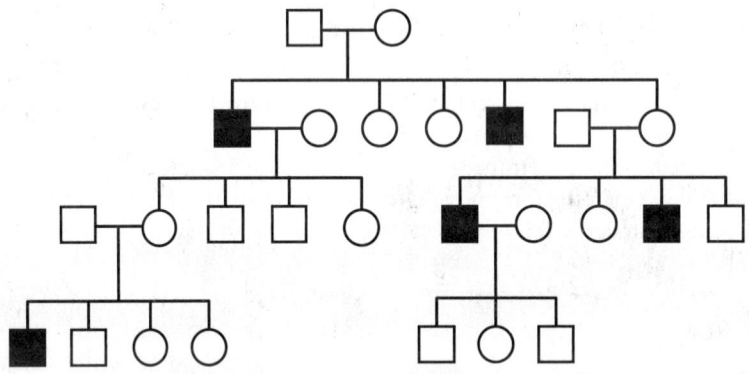

Figure 19-6. X-Linked Recessive Inheritance

Recurrence Risks. Figure 19-7 shows the recurrence risks for X-linked recessive diseases.

- Affected male–homozygous normal female: All of the daughters will be heterozygous carriers; all of the sons will be homozygous normal.

- Normal male–carrier female: On average, half of the sons will be affected and half of the daughters will be carriers. Note that in this case, the recurrence rate is different depending on the sex of the child. If the fetal sex is known, the recurrence rate for a daughter is 0, and that for a son is 50%. **If the sex of the fetus is not known, then the recurrence rate is multiplied by 1/2, the probability that the fetus is a male versus a female. Therefore if the sex is unknown, the recurrence risk is 25%.**

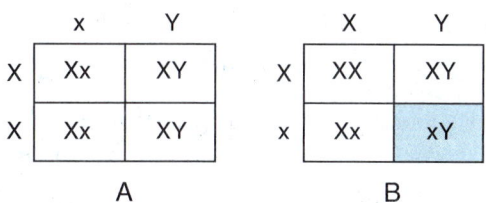

A. Affected male–homozygous normal female
   (X chromosome with mutation is in lower case)

B. Normal male–carrier female

Figure 19-7. Recurrence Risks for X-Linked Recessive Diseases

X inactivation

Normal males inherit an X chromosome from their mother and a Y chromosome from their father, whereas normal females inherit an X chromosome from each parent. Because the Y chromosome carries only about 50 protein-coding genes and the X chromosome carries hundreds of protein-coding genes, a mechanism must exist to equalize the amount of protein encoded by X chromosomes in males and females. This mechanism, termed X inactivation, occurs in the blastocyst (~100 cells) during the development of female embryos (Figure 19-8). When an X chromosome is inactivated, its DNA is not transcribed into mRNA, and the chromosome is visualized under the microscope as a highly condensed *Barr body* in the nuclei of interphase cells. X inactivation has several important characteristics:

- It is *random*—in some cells of the female embryo, the X chromosome inherited from the father is inactivated, and in others the X chromosome inherited from the mother is inactivated. Like coin tossing, this is a random process. As shown in Figure 19-6, most women have their paternal X chromosome active in approximately 50% of their cells and the maternal X chromosome active in approximately 50% of their cells. Thus, females are said to be *mosaics* with respect to the active X chromosome.

- It is *fixed*—once inactivation of an X chromosome occurs in a cell, the same X chromosome is inactivated in all descendants of the cell.

- It is *incomplete*—there are regions throughout the X chromosome, including the tips of both the long and short arms, that are not inactivated.

- X-chromosome inactivation is permanent in somatic cells and reversible in developing germ line cells. Both X chromosomes are active during oogenesis.

- All X chromosomes in a cell are inactivated except one. For example, females with three X chromosomes in each cell have two X chromosomes inactivated in each cell (thus, two Barr bodies can be visualized in an interphase cell).

Note

Genetic Mosaicism

Genetic mosaicism is the presence of 2 or more cell lines with different karyotypes in an individual. It arises from mitotic nondisjunction. The number of cell lines that develop and their relative proportions are influenced by the *timing* of nondisjunction during embryogenesis and the *viability* of the aneuploid cells produced.

Mechanisms Associated with X Inactivation

X-chromosome inactivation is thought to be mediated by more than one mechanism.

- A gene called *XIST* has been identified as the primary gene that causes X inactivation. *XIST* produces an RNA product that coats the chromosome, helping produce its inactivation.
- Condensation into heterochromatin
- Methylation of gene regions on the X chromosome

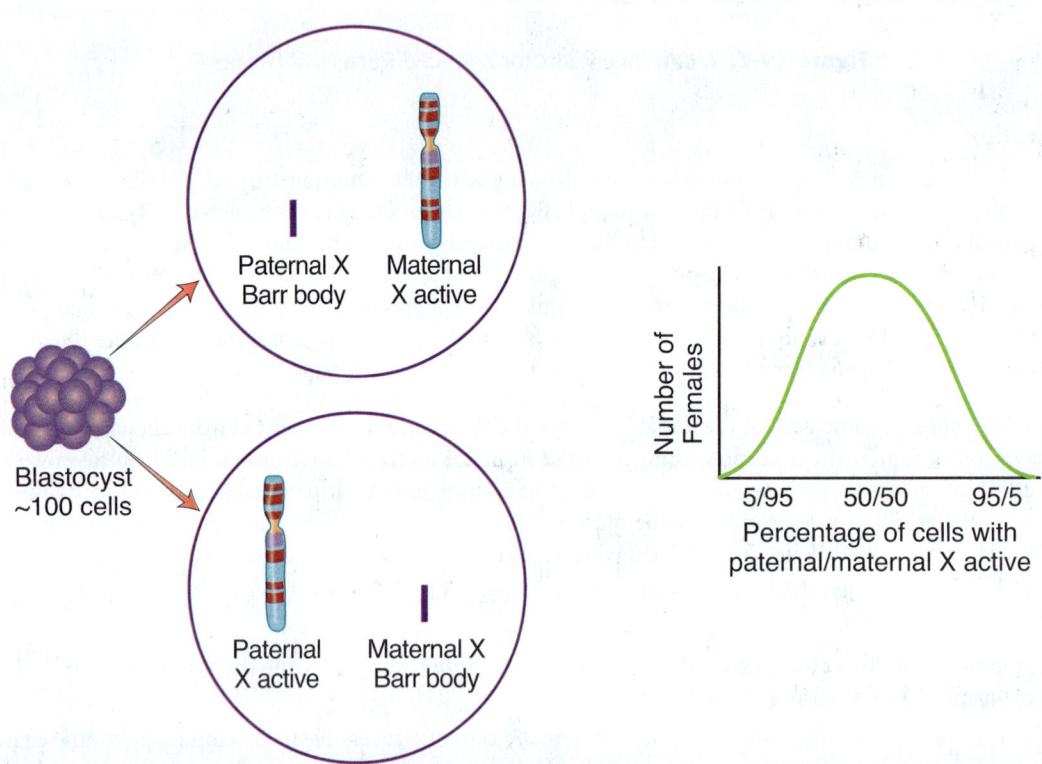

Figure 19-8. Inactivation of the X Chromosome during Embryogenesis Is a Random Process

Manifesting (female) heterozygotes

Normal females have two copies of the X chromosome, so they usually require two copies of the mutation to express the disease. However, because X inactivation is a random process, a heterozygous female will occasionally express an X-linked recessive mutation because, by random chance, most of the X chromosomes carrying the normal allele have been inactivated. Such females are termed *manifesting heterozygotes*. Because they usually have at least a small population of active X chromosomes carrying the normal allele, their disease expression is typically milder than that of hemizygous males.

Y Chromosome Highlights

- The *SRY* (sex determining region) gene is a transcription factor that initiates male development.
- The q arm of Y chromosomes contains a large block of heterochromatin.
- Microdeletions of Yq in males result in nonobstructive azoospermia.

X-Linked Dominant Inheritance

There are relatively few diseases whose inheritance is classified as X-linked dominant. Fragile X syndrome is an important example. In this condition, females are differently affected than males, and whereas penetrance in males is 100%, that in females is approximately 60%. The typical fragile X patient described is male.

Clinical Correlate

Fragile X Syndrome

Males: 100% penetrance

- Mental retardation
- Large ears
- Prominent jaw
- Macro-orchidism (usually postpubertal)

Females: 60% penetrance

- Mental retardation

As in X-linked recessive inheritance, male–male transmission of the disease-causing mutation is not seen (see Figure 19-9).

- Heterozygous females are affected. Because females have two X chromosomes (and thus two chances to inherit an X-linked disease-causing mutation) and males have only one, X-linked dominant diseases are seen about twice as often in females as in males.
- As in autosomal dominant inheritance, the disease phenotype is seen in multiple generations of a pedigree; skipped generations are relatively unusual.
- Examine the children of an affected male (II-1 in Figure 19-9). None of his sons will be affected, but all of his daughters have the disease (assuming complete penetrance).

Note

Penetrance in Genetic Diseases

The penetrance of a disease-causing mutation is the percentage of individuals who are known to have the disease-causing genotype who display the disease phenotype (develop symptoms).

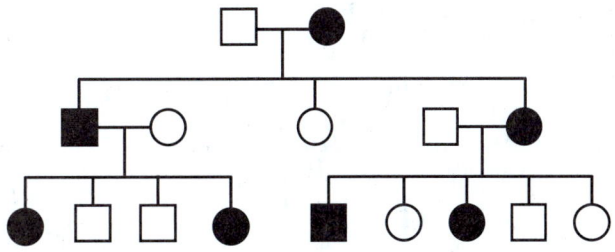

Figure 19-9. X-Linked Dominant Inheritance

Recurrence Risks

Figure 19-10 shows the recurrence risks for X-linked dominant inheritance.

- Affected male–homozygous normal female: None of the sons are affected; all of the daughters are affected. Note that in this case, the recurrence rate is different depending on the sex of the child. If the fetal sex is known, the recurrence rate for a daughter is 100%, and that for a son is 0%. **If the sex of the fetus is not known, then the recurrence rate is multiplied by 1/2, the probability that the fetus is a male versus a female. Therefore if the sex is unknown, the recurrence risk is 50%.**

- Normal male–heterozygous affected female: On average, 50% of sons are affected and 50% of daughters are affected.

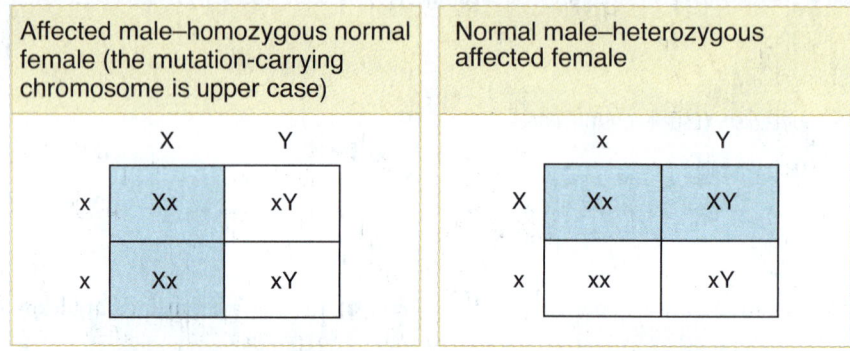

Figure 19-10. Recurrence Risks for X-Linked Dominant Inheritance

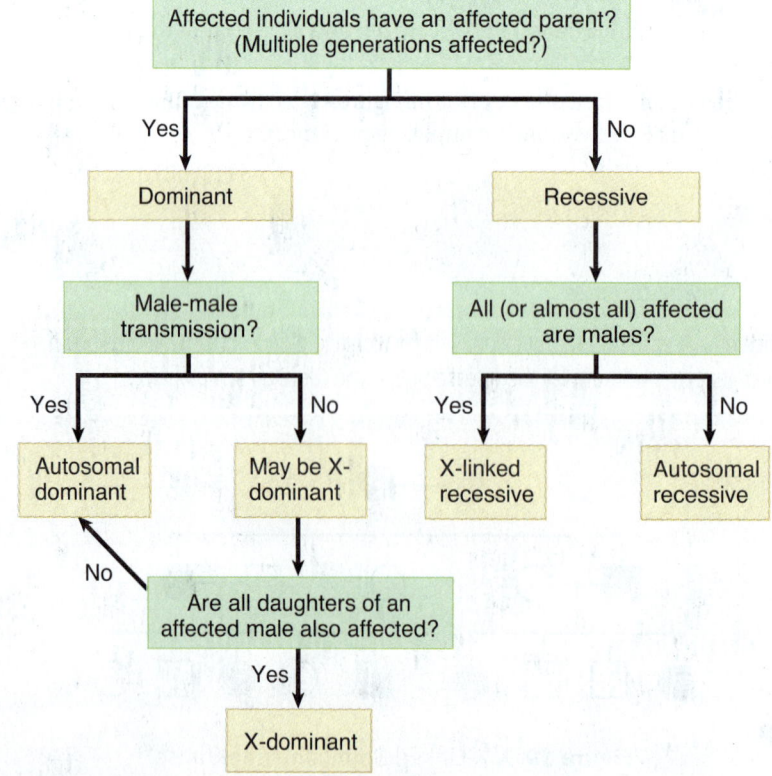

Note: If transmission occurs *only* through affected mothers and never through affected sons, the pedigree is likely to reflect mitochondrial inheritance.

Figure 19-11. A Basic Decision Tree for Determining the Mode of Inheritance in a Pedigree

Mitochondrial Inheritance

Mitochondria, which are cytoplasmic organelles involved in cellular respiration, have their own chromosomes, each of which contains 16,569 DNA base pairs (bp) arranged in a circular molecule. This DNA encodes 13 proteins that are subunits of complexes in the electron transport and oxidative phosphorylation processes (see Section I, chapter 13). In addition, mitochondrial DNA encodes 22 transfer RNAs and 2 ribosomal RNAs.

Because a sperm cell contributes no mitochondria to the egg cell during fertilization, mitochondrial DNA is inherited exclusively through females. Pedigrees for mitochondrial diseases thus display a distinct mode of inheritance: Diseases are transmitted only from affected females to their offspring (see Figure 19-12).

- Both males and females are affected.
- Transmission of the disease is only from a female.
- All offspring of an affected female are affected.
- None of the offspring of an affected male is affected.
- Diseases are typically neuropathies and/or myopathies (see margin note).

Heteroplasmy

A typical cell contains hundreds of mitochondria in its cytoplasm, and each mitochondrion has its own copy of the mitochondrial genome. When a specific mutation occurs in some of the mitochondria, this mutation can be unevenly distributed into daughter cells during cell division: Some cells may inherit more mitochondria in which the normal DNA sequence predominates, while others inherit mostly mitochondria with the mutated, disease-causing gene. This condition is known as *heteroplasmy*. Variations in heteroplasmy account for substantial variation in the severity of expression of mitochondrial diseases.

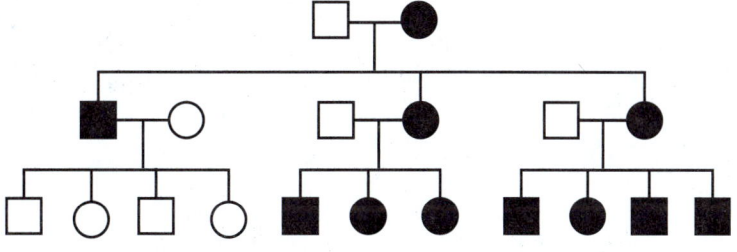

Figure 19-12. Pedigree for a Mitochondrial Disease

Population Genetics 20

Learning Objectives

❑ Solve problems concerning definition

❑ Solve problems concerning genotype and allele frequencies

❑ Explain information related to Hardy-Weinberg equilibrium

❑ Interpret scenarios about factors responsible for genetic variation in/among populations

DEFINITION

Population genetics is the study of genetic variation in populations. Basic concepts of population genetics allow us to understand how and why the prevalence of various genetic diseases differs among populations.

GENOTYPE AND ALLELE FREQUENCIES

An essential step in understanding genetic variation is to measure it in populations. This is done by estimating genotype and allele frequencies.

Genotype Frequencies

For a given locus, the genotype frequency measures the proportion of each genotype in a population. For example, suppose that a population of 100 individuals has been assayed for an autosomal restriction fragment length polymorphism (RFLP; see chapter 7 in Section I). If the RFLP has two possible alleles, labeled 1 and 2, there are three possible genotypes: 1-1, 1-2, and 2-2. Visualization of a Southern blot allows us to determine the genotype of each individual in our population, and we find that the genotypes are distributed as follows:

Table 20-1. Genotype Frequency

Genotype	Count	Genotype Frequency
1-1	49	0.49
1-2	42	0.42
2-2	9	0.09
Total	100	1.00

The genotype frequency is then obtained by dividing the count for each genotype by the total number of individuals. Thus, the frequency of genotype 1-1 is 49/100 = 0.49, and the frequencies of genotypes 1-2 and 2-2 are 0.42 and 0.09, respectively.

Allele Frequencies

The allele frequency measures the proportion of chromosomes that contain a specific allele. To continue the RFLP example given above, we wish to estimate the frequencies of alleles 1 and 2 in our population. Each individual with the 1-1 genotype has two copies of allele 1, and each heterozygote (1-2 genotype) has one copy of allele 1. Because each diploid somatic cell contains two copies of each autosome, our denominator is 200. Thus, the frequency of allele 1 in the population is:

$$\frac{(2 \times 49) + 42}{200} = 0.7$$

The same approach can be used to estimate the frequency of allele 2, which is 0.3. A convenient shortcut is to remember that the allele frequencies for all of the alleles of a given locus must add up to 1. Therefore, we can obtain the frequency of allele 2 simply by subtracting the frequency of allele 1 (0.7) from 1.

HARDY-WEINBERG EQUILIBRIUM

If a population is large and if individuals mate at random with respect to their genotypes at a locus, the population should be in Hardy-Weinberg equilibrium. This means that there is a constant and predictable relationship between genotype frequencies and allele frequencies. This relationship, expressed in the Hardy-Weinberg equation, allows one to estimate genotype frequencies if one knows allele frequencies, and vice versa.

The Hardy-Weinberg Equation

$$p^2 + 2pq + q^2 = 1$$

In this equation:

p = frequency of allele 1 (conventionally the most common, normal allele)

q = frequency of allele 2 (conventionally a minor, disease-producing allele)

p^2 = frequency of genotype 1-1 (conventionally homozygous normal)

$2pq$ = frequency of genotype 1-2 (conventionally heterozygous)

q^2 = frequency of genotype 2-2 (conventionally homozygous affected)

In most cases where this equation is used, a simplification is possible. Generally p, the normal allele frequency in the population, is very close to 1 (e.g., most of the alleles of this gene are normal). In this case, we may assume that $p \sim 1$, and the equation simplifies to:

$$1 + 2q + q^2 \sim 1$$

The frequency of the disease-producing allele, q, in question is a very small fraction. This simplification would not necessarily be used in actual medical genetics practice, but for answering test questions, it works quite well. However, if the disease prevalence is greater than 1/100, e.g., q is greater than 1/10, the complete Hardy-Weinberg equation should be used to obtain an accurate answer. In this case, $p = 1 - q$. Although the Hardy-Weinberg equation applies equally well to autosomal dominant and recessive alleles, genotypes, and diseases, the equation is most frequently used with autosomal recessive conditions. In these instances, a large percentage of the disease-producing allele is "hidden" in heterozygous carriers who cannot be distinguished phenotypically (clinically) from homozygous normal individuals.

A Practical Application of the Hardy-Weinberg Principle

A simple example is illustrated by the following case.

> A 20-year-old female college student is taking a course in human genetics. She is aware that she has an autosomal recessive genetic disease that has required her lifelong adherence to a diet low in natural protein with supplements of tyrosine and restricted amounts of phenylalanine. She also must avoid foods artificially sweetened with aspartame (Nutrasweet™). She asks her genetics professor about the chances that she would marry a man with the disease-producing allele.

The geneticist tells her that the known prevalence of PKU in the population is 1/10,000 live births, but the frequency of carriers is much higher, approximately 1/50. Her greatest risk comes from marrying a carrier for two reasons. First, the frequency of carriers for this condition is much higher than the frequency of affected homozygotes, and second, an affected person would be identifiable clinically. The geneticist used the Hardy-Weinberg equation to estimate the carrier frequency from the known prevalence of the disease in the following way:

Disease prevalence = q^2 = 1/10,000 live births

Carrier frequency = $2q$ (to be calculated)

q = square root of 1/10,000, which is 1/100

$2q$ = 2/100, or **1/50, the carrier frequency**

The woman now asks a second question: "Knowing that I have a 1/50 chance of marrying a carrier of this allele, what is the probability that I will have a child with PKU?"

The geneticist answers, "The chance of you having a child with PKU is 1/100." This answer is based on the joint occurrence of two nonindependent events:

- The probability that she will marry a heterozygous carrier (1/50), and
- If he is a carrier, the probability that he will pass his PKU allele versus the normal allele to the child (1/2).

These probabilities would be multiplied to give:

- 1/50 × 1/2 = **1/100, the probability that she will have a child with PKU** .

In summary, there are three major terms one usually works with in the Hardy-Weinberg equation applied to autosomal recessive conditions:

- q^2, the disease prevalence
- $2q$, the carrier frequency
- q, the frequency of the disease-causing allele

When answering questions involving Hardy-Weinberg calculations, it is important to identify which of these terms has been given in the stem of the question and which term you are asked to calculate.

This exercise demonstrates two important points:

- The Hardy-Weinberg principle can be applied to estimate the prevalence of heterozygous carriers in populations when we know only the prevalence of the recessive disease.
- For autosomal recessive diseases, such as PKU, the prevalence of heterozygous carriers is much higher than the prevalence of affected homozygotes. In effect, the vast majority of recessive genes are hidden in the heterozygotes.

FACTORS RESPONSIBLE FOR GENETIC VARIATION IN/AMONG POPULATIONS

Although human populations are typically in Hardy-Weinberg equilibrium for most loci, deviations from equilibrium can be produced by new mutations, the introduction of a new mutation into a population from outside (founder effect), nonrandom mating (for example, consanguinity), the action of natural selection, genetic drift, and gene flow. Although these factors are discussed independently, often more than one effect contributes to allele frequencies in a population.

Mutation

Mutation, discussed previously, is ultimately the source of all new genetic variation in populations. In general, mutation rates do not differ very much from population to population.

Founder Effect. In some cases, a new mutation can be introduced into a population when someone carrying the mutation is one of the early founders of the community. This is referred to as a founder effect. As the community rapidly expands through generations, the frequency of the mutation can be affected by natural selection, by genetic drift (*see* below), and by consanguinity.

Natural Selection

Natural selection acts upon genetic variation, increasing the frequencies of alleles that promote survival or fertility (referred to as fitness) and decreasing the frequencies of alleles that reduce fitness. The reduced fitness of most disease-producing alleles helps explain why most genetic diseases are relatively rare. Dominant diseases, in which the disease-causing allele is more readily exposed to the effects of natural selection, tend to have lower allele frequencies than do recessive diseases, where the allele is typically hidden in heterozygotes.

Sickle Cell Disease and Malaria

Sickle cell disease affects 1/600 African Americans and up to 1/50 individuals in some parts of Africa. How could this highly deleterious disease-causing mutation become so frequent, especially in Africa? The answer lies in the fact that the falciparum malaria parasite, which has been common in much of Africa, does not survive well in the erythrocytes of sickle cell heterozygotes. These individuals, who have no clinical signs of sickle cell disease, are thus protected against the lethal effects of malaria. Consequently, there is a heterozygote advantage for the sickle cell mutation, and it maintains a relatively high frequency in some African populations.

There is now evidence for heterozygote advantages for several other recessive diseases that are relatively common in some populations. Examples include:

- Cystic fibrosis (heterozygote resistance to typhoid fever)
- Hemochromatosis (heterozygote advantage in iron-poor environments)
- Glucose-6-phosphate dehydrogenase deficiency, hemolytic anemia (heterozygote resistance to malaria)

Genetic Drift

Mutation rates do not vary significantly from population to population, although they can result in significant differences in allele frequencies when they occur in small populations or are introduced by a founder effect. Mutation rates and founder effects act along with genetic drift to make certain genetic diseases more common (or rarer) in small, isolated populations than in the world at large. Consider the pedigrees (very small populations) shown in the following figure.

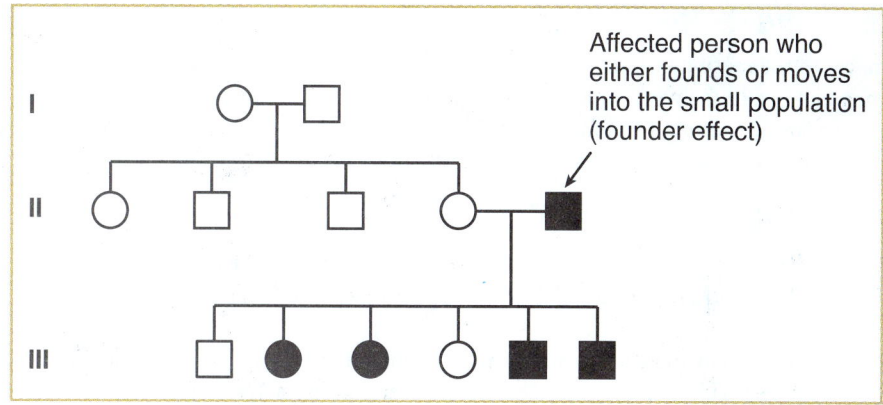

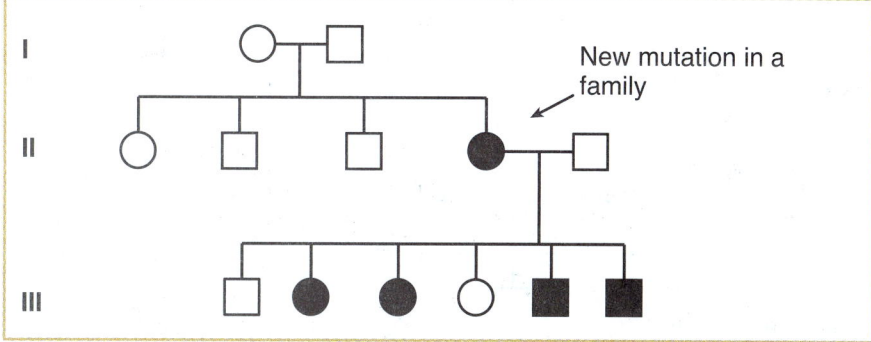

Genetic drift begins. In both examples the frequency of affected persons in generation III is 2/3, higher than the 1/2 predicted by statistics.

Figure 20-1. Genetic Drift in Two Small Populations (Illustrated with a Dominant Disease)

If the woman and the affected man (II-5) in Panel A had 1,000 children rather than 6, the prevalence of the disease in their offspring (Generation III) would be closer to 1/2, the statistical mean. Although genetic drift affects populations larger than a single family, this example illustrates two points:

- When a new mutation or a founder effect occurs in a small population, genetic drift can make the allele more or less prevalent than statistics alone would predict.

- A relatively large population in Hardy-Weinberg equilibrium for an allele or many alleles can be affected by population "bottlenecks" in which natural disaster or large-scale genocide dramatically reduces the size of the population. Genetic drift may then change allele frequencies and a new Hardy-Weinberg equilibrium is reached.

Gene Flow

Gene flow refers to the exchange of genes among populations. Because of gene flow, populations located close to one another often tend to have similar gene frequencies. Gene flow can also cause gene frequencies to change through time: The frequency of sickle cell disease is lower in African Americans in part because of gene flow from other sectors of the U.S. population that do not carry the disease-causing mutation; in addition, the heterozygote advantage for the sickle cell mutation (*see* text box) has disappeared because malaria has become rare in North America.

Consanguinity and Its Health Consequences

Consanguinity refers to the mating of individuals who are related to one another (typically, a union is considered to be consanguineous if it occurs between individuals related at the second-cousin level or closer). Figure 20-2 illustrates a pedigree for a consanguineous union. Because of their mutual descent from common ancestors, relatives are more likely to share the same disease-causing genes. Statistically,

- Siblings (II-2 and II-3 or II-4) share 1/2 of their genes.
- First cousins (III-3 and III-4) share 1/8 of their genes ($1/2 \times 1/2 \times 1/2$).
- Second cousins (IV-1 and IV-2) share 1/32 of their genes ($1/8 \times 1/2 \times 1/2$).

These numbers are referred to as the coefficients of relationship. Thus, if individual III-1 carries a disease-causing allele, there is a 1/2 chance that individual III-3 (his brother) has it and a 1/8 chance that individual III-4 (his first cousin) has it.

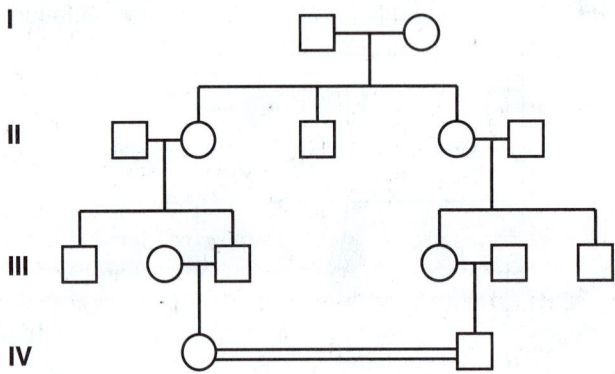

Figure 20-2. A Pedigree Illustrating Consanguinity

Consequently, there is an increased risk of genetic disease in the offspring of consanguineous matings. Dozens of empirical studies have examined the health consequences of consanguinity, particularly first-cousin matings. These studies show that the offspring of first-cousin matings are approximately twice as likely to present with a genetic disease as are the offspring of unrelated matings. The frequency of genetic disease increases further in the offspring of closer unions (e.g., uncle/niece or brother/sister matings).

Learning Objectives

❏ Interpret scenarios about basic definitions and terminology

❏ Solve problems concerning numerical chromosome abnormalities

❏ Demonstrate understanding of structural chromosome abnormalities

❏ Demonstrate understanding of other chromosome abnormalities

❏ Solve problems concerning advances in molecular cytogenetics

OVERVIEW

This chapter reviews diseases that are caused by microscopically observable alterations in chromosomes. These alterations may involve the presence of extra chromosomes or the loss of chromosomes. They may also consist of structural alterations of chromosomes. Chromosome abnormalities are seen in approximately 1 in 150 live births and are the leading known cause of mental retardation. The vast majority of fetuses with chromosome abnormalities are lost prenatally: Chromosome abnormalities are seen in 50% of spontaneous fetal losses during the first trimester of pregnancy, and they are seen in 20% of fetuses lost during the second trimester. Thus, chromosome abnormalities are the leading known cause of pregnancy loss.

Note
X chromosome contains ~1,200 genes
Y chromosome contains ~50 genes

BASIC DEFINITIONS AND TERMINOLOGY

Karyotype

Chromosomes are most easily visualized during the metaphase stage of mitosis, when they are maximally condensed. They are photographed under the microscope to create a karyotype, an ordered display of the 23 pairs of human chromosomes in a typical somatic cell. In Figure 21-1A, a karyogram represents a drawing of each type of chromosome; the presentation is haploid (only one copy of each chromosome is shown). Figure 21-1B is a karyotype of an individual male. It is diploid, showing both copies of each autosome, the X and the Y chromosome. Chromosomes are ordered according to size, with the sex chromosomes (X and Y) placed in the lower right portion of the karyotype.

Metaphase chromosomes can be grouped according to size and to the position of the centromere, but accurate identification requires staining with one of a variety of dyes to reveal characteristic banding patterns.

Chromosome banding

To visualize chromosomes in a karyotype unambiguously, various stains are applied so that banding is evident.

- **G-banding.** Mitotic chromosomes are partially digested with trypsin (to digest some associated protein) and then stained with Giemsa, a dye that binds DNA.

G-banding reveals a pattern of light and dark (G-bands) regions that allow chromosomes to be accurately identified in a karyotype. There are several other stains that can be used in a similar manner. The chromosomes depicted in the following figure have been stained with Giemsa.

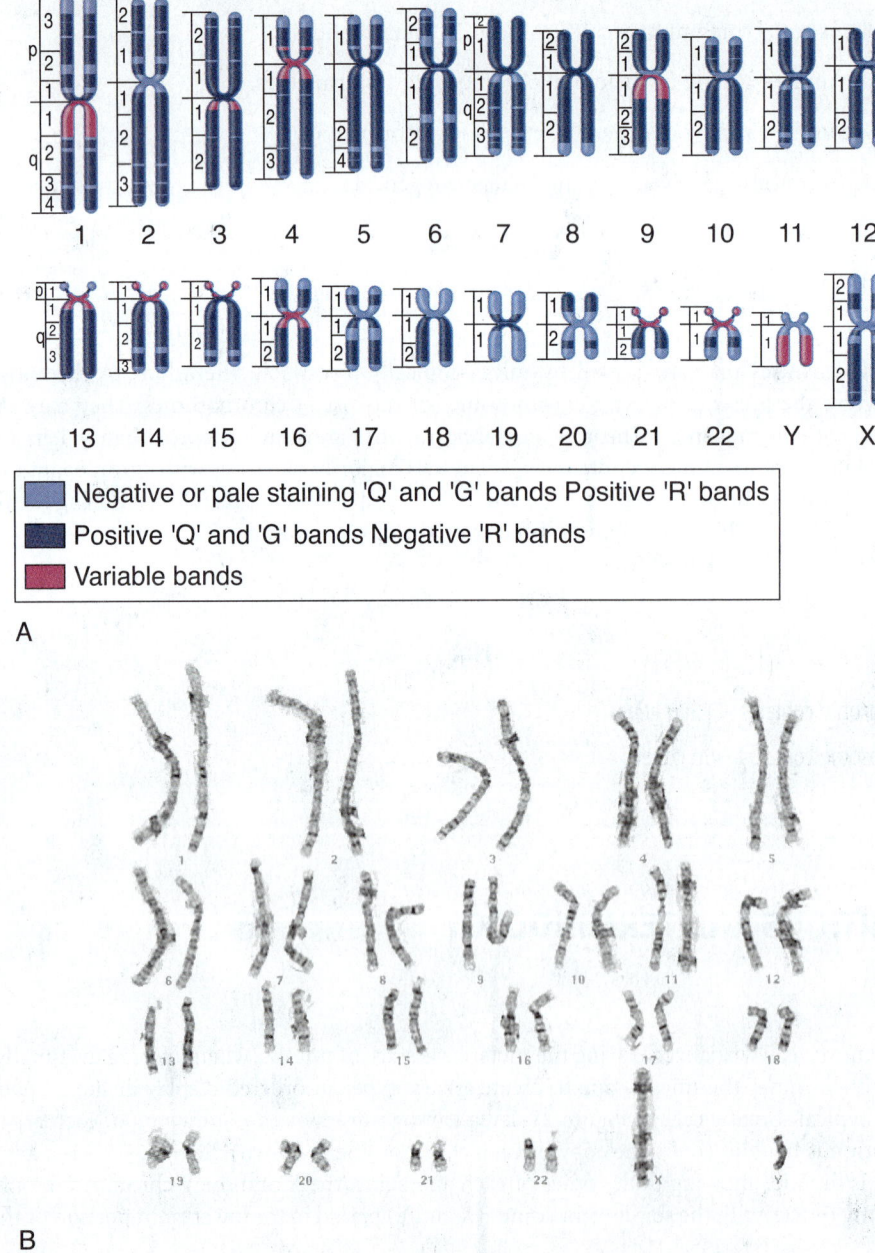

Figure 21-1. Human Metaphase Chromosomes. (*A*) Idealized Drawing (Karyogram) and (*B*) Photograph of Metaphase Chromosomes (Karyotype)

Chromosome abnormalities in some cases can be identified visually by looking at the banding pattern, but this technique reveals differences (for instance, larger deletions) only to a resolution of about 4 Mb. Smaller abnormalities (microdeletions) must be identified in other ways (FISH), discussed at the end of the chapter.

Chromosome nomenclature

Each mitotic chromosome contains a centromere and two sister chromatids because the cell has gone through interphase and has entered mitosis when the karyotype analysis is performed (metaphase). The long arm of the chromosome is labeled q, and the short arm is labeled p. One of the characteristics described is the relative position of the centromere.

- **Metacentric** chromosomes (for instance, chromosome 1) have the centromere near the middle. The p and q arms are of roughly equal length.

- **Submetacentric** chromosomes have the centromere displaced toward one end (for example, chromosome 4). The p and q arms are evident.

- **Acrocentric** chromosomes have the centromere far toward one end. In these chromosomes, the p arm contains little genetic information, most of it residing on the q arm. Chromosomes 13, 14, 15, 21, and 22 are the acrocentric chromosomes. Only the acrocentric chromosomes are involved in **Robertsonian translocations**, which will be discussed in this chapter.

The tips of the chromosomes are termed telemeres.

The following table contains some standard nomenclature applied to chromosomes.

Table 21-1. Common Symbols Used in Karyotype Nomenclature

1-22	Autosome number
X, Y	Sex chromosomes
(+) or (–)	When placed before an autosomal number, indicates that chromosome is extra or missing
p	Short arm of the chromosome
q	Long arm of the chromosome
t	Translocation
del	Deletion

NUMERICAL CHROMOSOME ABNORMALITIES

Euploidy

When a cell has a multiple of 23 chromosomes, it is said to be **euploid**. Gametes (sperm and egg cells) are euploid cells that have 23 chromosomes (one member of each pair); they are said to be **haploid**. Most somatic cells are **diploid**, containing both members of each pair, or 46 chromosomes. Two types of euploid cells with abnormal numbers of chromosomes are seen in humans: triploidy and tetraploidy.

Triploidy. Triploidy refers to cells that contain three copies of each chromosome (69 total). Triploidy, which usually occurs as a result of the fertilization of an ovum by two sperm cells, is common at conception, but the vast majority of these conceptions are lost prenatally. However, about 1 in 10,000 live births is a triploid. These babies have multiple defects of the heart and central nervous system, and they do not survive.

Tetraploidy. Tetraploidy refers to cells that contain four copies of each chromosome (92 total). This lethal condition is much rarer than triploidy among live births: Only a few cases have been described.

Aneuploidy

Aneuploidy, a deviation from the euploid number, represents the gain (+) or loss (−) of a specific chromosome. Two major forms of aneuploidy are observed:

- Monosomy (loss of a chromosome)
- Trisomy (gain of a chromosome)

Autosomal aneuploidy

Two generalizations are helpful:

- All autosomal monosomies are inconsistent with a live birth.
- Only three autosomal trisomies (trisomy 13, 18, and 21) are consistent with a live birth.

Trisomy 21 (47,XY,+21 or 47,XX,+21); Down Syndrome

- Most common autosomal trisomy
- Mental retardation
- Short stature
- Hypotonia
- Depressed nasal bridge, upslanting palpebral fissures, epicanthal fold
- Congenital heart defects in approximately 40% of cases
- Increased risk of acute lymphoblastic leukemia
- Alzheimer disease by fifth or sixth decade (*amyloid precursor protein, APP* gene on chromosome 21)
- Reduced fertility
- Risk increases with increased maternal age

Trisomy 18 (47,XY,+18 or 47,XX,+18); Edward Syndrome

- Clenched fist with overlapping fingers
- Inward turning, "rocker-bottom" feet
- Congenital heart defects
- Low-set ears, micrognathia (small lower jaw)
- Mental retardation
- Very poor prognosis

Trisomy 13 (47,XY,+13 or 47,XX,+13); Patau Syndrome

- Polydactyly (extra fingers and toes)
- Cleft lip, palate
- Microphthalmia (small eyes)
- Microcephaly, mental retardation
- Cardiac and renal defects
- Very poor prognosis

Sex chromosome aneuploidy

Aneuploidy involving the sex chromosomes is relatively common and tends to have less severe consequences than does autosomal aneuploidy. Some generalizations are helpful:

- At least one X chromosome is required for survival.
- If a Y chromosome is present, the phenotype is male (with minor exceptions).
- If more than one X chromosome is present, all but one will become a Barr body in each cell.

The two important sex chromosome aneuploidies are Turner syndrome and Klinefelter syndrome.

Klinefelter Syndrome (47,XXY)

- Testicular atrophy
- Infertility
- Gynecomastia
- Female distribution of hair
- Low testosterone
- Elevated FSH and LH
- High-pitched voice

Turner Syndrome (45,X or 45,XO)

- Only monosomy consistent with life
- 50% are 45,X
- Majority of others are mosaics for 45,X and one other cell lineage (46,XX, 47,XXX, 46,XY)
- Females with 45,X;46,XY are at increased risk for gonadal blastoma.
- Short stature
- Edema of wrists and ankles in newborn
- Cystic hygroma *in utero* resulting in excess nuchal skin and "webbed" neck
- Primary amenorrhea
- Coarctation of the aorta or other congenital heart defect in some cases
- Infertility
- Gonadal dysgenesis

Note

Genetic Mosaicism in Turner Syndrome

Genetic mosaicism is defined as a condition in which there are cells of different genotypes or chromosome constitutions within a single individual. Some women with Turner syndrome have somatic cells that are 45,X and others that are 46,XX or 47,XXX. Mosaicism in Turner syndrome is thought to arise in early embryogenesis by mechanisms that are not completely understood.

Nondisjunction is the usual cause of aneuploidies

Germ cells undergo meiosis to produce the haploid egg or sperm. The original cell is diploid for all chromosomes, although only one homologous pair is shown in the figure for simplicity. The same events would occur for each pair of homologs within the cell.

Nondisjunction of one homologous pair (for example, chromosome 21) during meiosis 1. All other homologs segregate (disjoin) normally in the cell. Two of the gametes are diploid for chromosome 21. When fertilization occurs, the conception will be a trisomy 21 with Down syndrome. The other gametes with no copy of chromosome 21 will result in conceptions that are monosomy 21, a condition incompatible with a live birth.

When nondisjunction during meiosis 2 occurs, the sister chromatids of a chromosome (for example, chromosome 21) fail to segregate (disjoin). The sister chromatids of all other chromosomes segregate normally. One of the gametes is diploid for chromosome 21. When fertilization occurs, the conception will be a trisomy 21 with Down syndrome. One gamete has no copy of chromosome 21 and will result in a conception that is a monosomy 21. The remaining two gametes are normal haploid ones.

Some important points to remember:

- Nondisjunction is the usual cause of aneuploidies including Down, Edward, and Patau syndromes, as well as Turner and Klinefelter syndromes.
- Nondisjunction is more likely to occur during oogenesis than during spermatogenesis.
- Nondisjunction is more likely with increasing maternal age. No environmental agents (e.g., radiation, alcohol) have been shown to have measurable influence.
- Nondisjunction is more likely in meiosis I than meiosis II.

Clinical Correlate

Maternal Age, Risk of Down Syndrome, and Prenatal Diagnosis

Surveys of babies with trisomy 21 show that approximately 90–95% of the time, the extra copy of the chromosome is contributed by the mother (similar figures are obtained for trisomies of the 18th and 13th chromosomes). The increased risk of Down syndrome with maternal age is well documented. The risk of bearing a child with Down is less than 1/1,000 for women age <30. The risk increases to about 1/400 at age 35, 1/100 at age 40, and 3–4% or age >45. This increase reflects an elevated rate of nondisjunction in older ova (recall that all of a woman's egg cells are formed during her fetal development, and they remain suspended in prophase I until ovulation). There is no corresponding increase in risk with advanced paternal age; sperm cells are generated continuously throughout the life of the male.

The increased risk of trisomy with advanced maternal age motivates more than half of pregnant women in North America to undergo prenatal diagnosis (most commonly, amniocentesis or chorionic villus sampling, discussed in Chapter 6). Down syndrome can also be screened by assaying maternal serum levels of α-fetoprotein, chorionic gonadotropin, and unconjugated estriol. This so-called *triple screen* can detect approximately 70% of fetuses with Down.

STRUCTURAL CHROMOSOME ABNORMALITIES

Structural alterations of chromosomes occur when chromosomes are broken by agents termed **clastogens** (e.g., radiation, some viruses, and some chemicals). Some alterations may result in a loss or gain of genetic material and are called **unbalanced** alterations; **balanced** alterations do not result in a gain or loss of genetic material and usually have fewer clinical consequences. As with other types of mutations, structural alterations can occur either in the germ line or in somatic cells. The former can be transmitted to offspring. The latter, although not transmitted to offspring, can alter genetic material such that the cell can give rise to cancer.

Translocations

Translocations occur when chromosomes are broken and the broken elements reattach to other chromosomes. Translocations can be classified into two major types: reciprocal and Robertsonian.

Reciprocal translocation

Reciprocal translocations occur when genetic material is exchanged between nonhomologous chromosomes; for example, chromosomes 2 and 8. If this happens during gametogenesis, the offspring will carry the reciprocal translocation in all his or her cells and will be called a **translocation carrier**. The karyotype would be 46,XY,t(2p;8p) or 46,XX,t(2p;8p). Because this individual has all of the genetic material (balanced, albeit some of it misplaced because of the translocation), there are often no clinical consequences other than during reproduction.

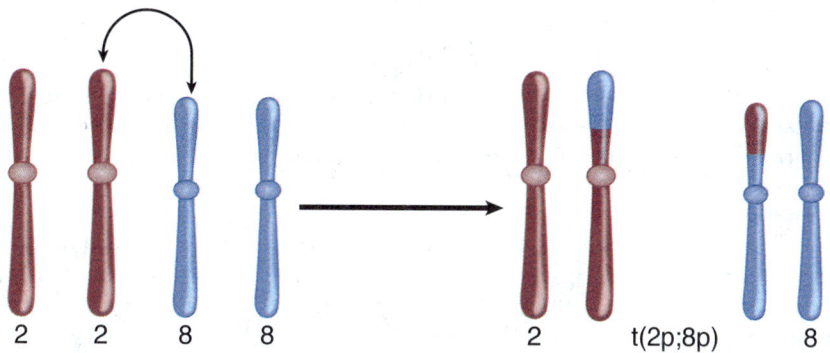

Figure 21-2. A Reciprocal Translocation

In a translocation carrier, during gametogenesis and meiosis, unbalanced genetic material can be transmitted to the offspring, causing partial trisomies and partial monosomies typically resulting in pregnancy loss. During meiosis 1, the translocated chromosomes may segregate as chromosome 8 or as chromosome 2, producing a variety of possible gametes with respect to these chromosomes.

Sperm that contain balanced chromosomal material (labeled alternate segregation in the diagram) produce either a normal diploid conception or another translocation carrier. Both are likely to be live births.

Sperm that contain unbalanced chromosomal material (labeled adjacent segregation in the diagram) produce conceptions that have partial monosomies and partial trisomies. These conceptions are likely to result in pregnancy loss.

Robertsonian translocations

These translocations are much more common than reciprocal translocations and are estimated to occur in approximately 1 in 1,000 live births. They occur only in the acrocentric chromosomes (13, 14, 15, 21, and 22) and involve the loss of the short arms of two of the chromosomes and subsequent fusion of the long arms. An example of a Robertsonian translocation involving chromosomes 14 and 21 is shown in Figure 21-3. The karyotype of this (male) translocation carrier is designated 45,XY,−14,−21,+t(14q;21q). Because the short arms of the acrocentric chromosomes contain no essential genetic material, their loss produces no clinical consequences, and the translocation carrier is not clinically affected.

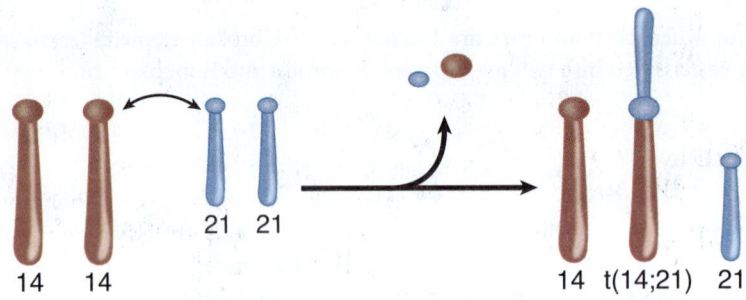

Figure 21-3. A Robertsonian Translocation

When the carrier's germ cells are formed through meiosis, the translocated chromosome must pair with its homologs. If **alternate segregation** occurs, the offspring will inherit either a normal chromosome complement or will be a normal carrier like the parent. If **adjacent segregation** occurs, the offspring will have an unbalanced chromosome complement (an extra or missing copy of the long arm of chromosome 21 or 14). Because only the long arms of these chromosomes contain genetically important material, the effect is equivalent to a trisomy or monosomy.

Robertsonian Translocation and Down Syndrome. Approximately 5% of Down syndrome cases are the result of a Robertsonian translocation affecting chromosome 14 and chromosome 21. When a translocation carrier produces gametes, the translocation chromosome can segregate with the normal 14 or with the normal 21. A diagram can be drawn to represent the six possible gametes that could be produced. Shows the diagram, the six sperm (in this example, the translocation carrier is a male), and the outcome of conception with a genetically normal woman.

Although adjacent segregation usually results in pregnancy loss, one important exception is that which produces trisomy 21. This may be a live birth, resulting in an infant with Down syndrome.

One can determine the mechanism leading to Down syndrome by examining the karyotype. Trisomy 21 due to nondisjunction during meiosis (95% of Down syndrome cases) has the karyotype 47,XX,+21 or 47,XY,+21. In the 5% of cases where Down syndrome is due to a Robertsonian translocation in a parent, the karyotype will be 46,XX,−14,+t(14q;21q) or 46,XY,−14,+t(14q;21q). The key difference is 47 versus 46 chromosomes in the individual with Down syndrome.

Although the recurrence risk for trisomy 21 due to nondisjunction during meiosis is very low, the recurrence risk for offspring of the Robertsonian translocation carrier parent is significantly higher. The recurrence risk (determined empirically) for female translocation carriers is 10–15%, and that for male translocation carriers is 1–2%. The reason for the difference between males and females is not well understood. The elevated recurrence risk for translocation carriers versus noncarriers underscores the importance of ordering a chromosome study when Down syndrome is suspected in a newborn.

Down syndrome (nondisjunction during meiosis)	Down syndrome (parent carries a Robertsonian translocation)
• 47,XX,+21 or 47,XY.+21 • No association with prior • pregnancy loss • Older mother • Very low recurrence rate	• 46,XX,−14,+t(14;21), or • 46,XY,−14,+t(14;21) • *May* be associated with prior pregancy loss • *May* be a younger mother • Recurrence rate 10–15% if mom is translocation carrier; 1–2% if dad is translocation carrier

Deletions

A deletion occurs when a chromosome loses some of its genetic information. Terminal deletions (the end of the chromosome is lost) and interstitial deletions (material within the chromosome is lost) may be caused by agents that cause chromosome breaks and by unequal crossover during meiosis.

Deletions can be large and microscopically visible in a stained preparation. The following figure shows both an interstitial deletion and a terminal deletion of 5p. Both result in Cri-du-chat syndrome.

- 46,XX or 46,XY, del(5p)
- High-pitched, cat-like cry
- Mental retardation, microcephaly
- Congenital heart disease

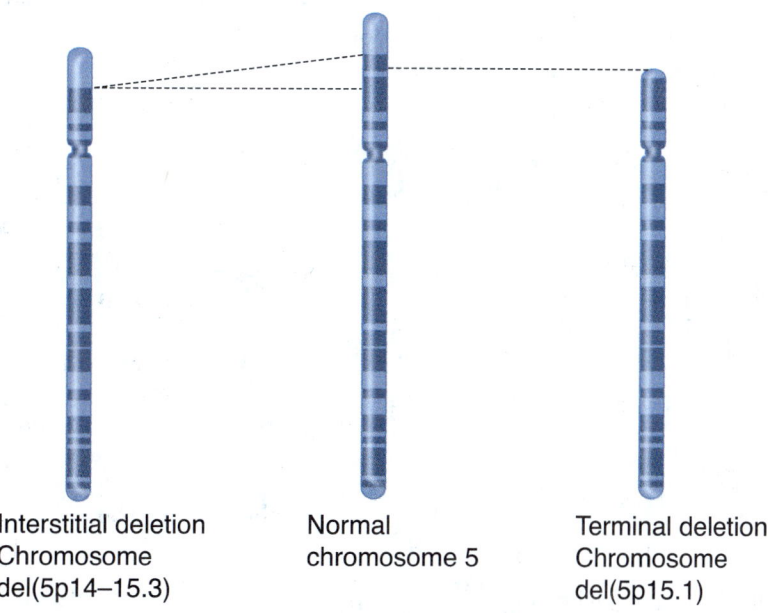

Interstitial deletion
Chromosome
del(5p14–15.3)

Normal
chromosome 5

Terminal deletion
Chromosome
del(5p15.1)

Figure 21-4. Terminal and Interstitial Deletions of Chromosome 5p

Microdeletions

Some deletions may be so small that they are not readily apparent microscopically without special fluorescent probes (FISH). Examples include:

- Prader-Willi syndrome
- Angelman syndrome

If a microdeletion includes several contiguous genes, a variety of phenotypic outcomes may be part of the genetic syndrome. Examples are

- DiGeorge syndrome: congenital absence of the thymus and parathyroids, hypocalcemic tetany, T-cell immunodeficiency, characteristic facies with cleft palate, heart defects
- Wilms tumor: aniridia, genital abnormalities, mental retardation (WAGR)
- Williams syndrome: hypercalcemia, supravalvular aortic stenosis, mental retardation, characteristic facies

OTHER CHROMOSOME ABNORMALITIES

Several other types of structural abnormalities are seen in human karyotypes. In general, their frequency and clinical consequences tend to be less severe than those of translocations and deletions.

Inversions

Inversions occur when the chromosome segment between two breaks is reinserted in the same location but in reverse order. Inversions that include the centromere are termed **pericentric**, whereas those that do not include the centromere are termed **paracentric**. The karyotype of the inversion shown in Figure 21-5, extending from 3p21 to 3q13 is 46,XY,inv(3)(p21;q13). Inversion carriers still retain all of their genetic material, so they are usually unaffected (although an inversion may interrupt or otherwise affect a specific gene and thus cause disease). Because homologous chromosomes must line up during meiosis, inverted chromosomes will form loops that, through recombination, may result in a gamete that contains a deletion or a duplication, which may then be transmitted to the offspring.

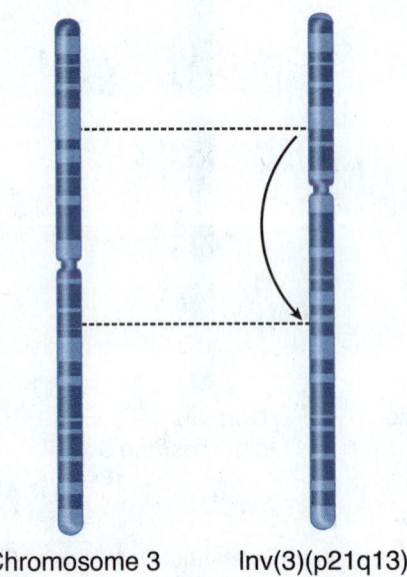

Chromosome 3   Inv(3)(p21q13)

Figure 21-5. A Pericentric Inversion of Chromosome 3

Ring Chromosome

A ring chromosome can form when a deletion occurs on both tips of a chromosome and the remaining chromosome ends fuse together. The karyotype for a female with a ring chromosome X would be 46,X,r(X). An example of this chromosome is shown in Figure 21-6. Ring chromosomes are often lost, resulting in a monosomy (e.g., loss of a ring X chromosome would produce Turner syndrome). These chromosomes have been observed at least once for each human chromosome.

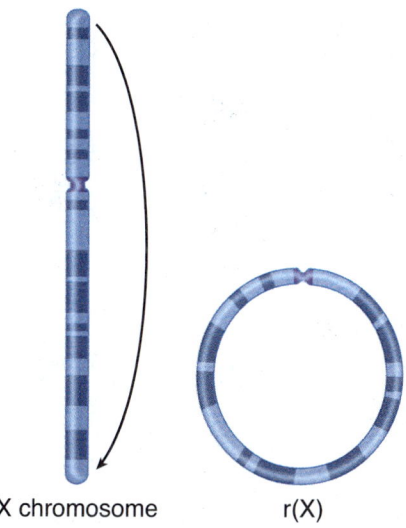

X chromosome   r(X)

Figure 21-6. Ring X-Chromosome

Isochromosome

When a chromosome divides along the axis perpendicular to its normal axis of division, an **isochromosome** is created (i.e., two copies of one arm but no copy of the other). Because of the lethality of autosomal isochromosomes, most isochromosomes that have been observed in live births involve the X chromosome, as shown in Figure 21-7. The karyotype of an isochromosome for the long arm of the X chromosome would be 46,X,i(Xq); this karyotype results in an individual with Turner syndrome, indicating that most of the critical genes responsible for the Turner phenotype are on Xp.

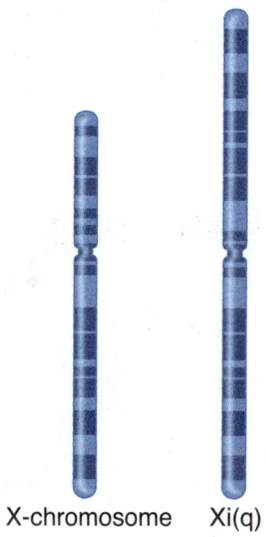

X-chromosome   Xi(q)

Figure 21-7. Isochromosome Xq

Physiology

Fluid Distribution and Edema 1

Learning Objectives

❏ Interpret scenarios on distribution of fluids within the body

❏ Answer questions about review and integration

❏ Use knowledge of microcirculation

❏ Interpret scenarios on edema (pathology integration)

❏ Interpret scenarios on volume measurement of compartments

DISTRIBUTION OF FLUIDS WITHIN THE BODY

Total Body Water

- Intracellular fluid (ICF):approximately 2/3 of total of body water
- Extracellular fluid (ECF):approximately 1/3 of total body water
- Interstitial fluid (ISF): approximately 3/4 of the extracellular fluid
- Plasma volume (PV):approximately 1/4 of the extracellular fluid
- Vascular compartment:contains the blood volume which is plasma and the cellular elements of blood, primarily red blood cells

It is important to remember that membranes can serve as barriers. The two important membranes are illustrated in the following figure. The **cell membrane** is a relative barrier for Na$^+$, while the **capillary membrane** is a barrier for plasma proteins.

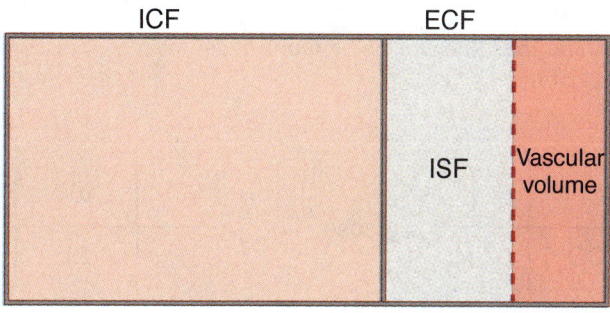

Figure 1-1. Solid-line division represents cell membrane. Dashed line division represents capillary membranes.

Osmosis

The distribution of fluid is determined by the osmotic movement of water. Osmosis is the diffusion of water across a semipermeable or selectively permeable membrane. Water diffuses from a region of higher water concentration to a region of lower water concentration. The concentration of water in a solution is determined by the concentration of solute. The greater the solute concentration is, the lower the water concentration will be.

The osmotic properties are defined by:

- **Osmolarity:**

  mOsm (milliosmoles)/L = concentration of particles per liter of solution

- **Osmolality:**

  mOsm/kg = concentration of particles per kg of solvent (water being the germane one for physiology/ medicine)

It is the **number of particles** that is crucial. The basic principles are demonstrated in the following figure.

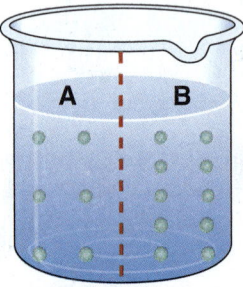

Figure 1-2.

This figure shows two compartments separated by a membrane that is permeable to water but not to solute. Side B has the greater concentration of solute (circles) and thus a lower water concentration than side A. As a result, water diffuses from A to B, and the height of column B rises, and that of A falls.

Effective osmole: If a solute doesn't easily cross a membrane, then it is an "effective" osmole for that compartment. In other words, it creates an osmotic force for water. For example, plasma proteins do not easily cross the capillary membrane and thus serve as effective osmoles for the vascular compartment. Sodium does not easily penetrate the cell membrane, but it does cross the capillary membrane, thus it is an effective osmole for the extracellular compartment.

Extracellular Solutes

The figure below represents a basic metabolic profile/panel (BMP). These are the common labs provided from a basic blood draw. The same figure to the right represents the normal values corresponding to the solutes. Standardized exams provide normal values and thus knowing these numbers is not required. However, knowing them can be useful with respect to efficiency of time.

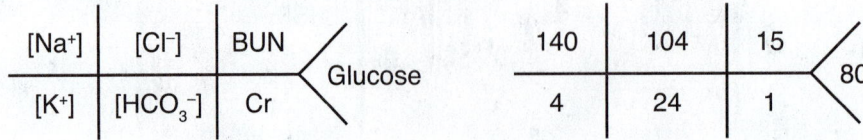

Figure 1-3.

Osmolar Gap

The osmolar gap is defined as the difference between the **measured** osmolality and the **estimated** osmolality using the equation below. Using the data from the BMP, we can estimate the extracellular osmolality using the following formula:

$$\textbf{ECF Effective osmolality} = 2\left(\textbf{Na}^{+}\right)\textbf{mEq}/\textbf{L} + \frac{\textbf{glucose mg \%}}{\textbf{18}} + \frac{\textbf{urea mg \%}}{\textbf{2.8}}$$

The basis of this calculation is:

- Na^+ is the most abundant osmole of the extracellular space.
- Na^+ is doubled because it is a positive charge and thus for every positive charge there is a negative charge, chloride being the most abundant, but not the only one.
- The 18 and 2.8 are converting glucose and BUN into their respective osmolarities (note: their units of measurement are mg/dL).
- Determining the osmolar gap (normal ≤15) aids in narrowing the differential diagnosis. While many things can elevate the osmolar gap, some of the more common are:ethanol, methanol, ethylene glycol, acetone, and mannitol. Thus, an inebriated patient has an elevated osmolar gap.

Graphical Representation of Body Compartments

It is important to understand how body osmolality and the intracellular and extracellular volumes change in clinically relevant situations. Figure 1-4 is one way to present this information. The y axis is solute concentration or osmolality. The x axis is the volume of intracellular (2/3) and extracellular (1/3) fluid.

If the solid line represents the control state, the dashed lines show a decrease in osmolality and extracellular volume but an increase in intracellular volume.

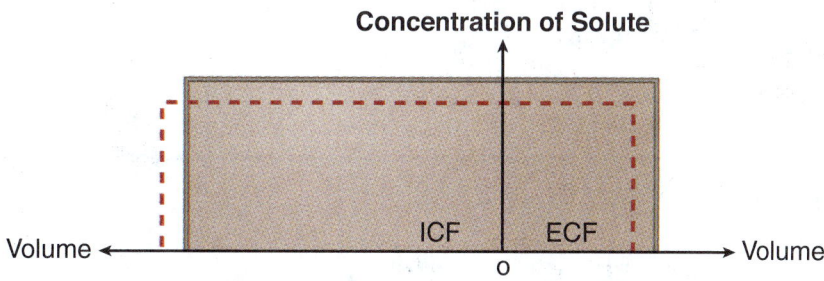

Figure 1-4. Darrow-Yannet Diagram

- **Extracellular volume**

  When there is a net gain of fluid by the body, this compartment always enlarges. A net loss of body fluid decreases extracellular volume.

- **Concentration of solutes**

  This is equivalent to body osmolality. At steady-state, the intracellular concentration of water equals the extracellular concentration of water (cell membrane is not a barrier for water). Thus, the intracellular and extracellular osmolalities are the same.

- **Intracellular volume**

    This varies with the effective osmolality of the extracellular compartment. Solutes and fluids enter and leave the extracellular compartment first (sweating, diarrhea, fluid resuscitation, etc.). Intracellular volume is only altered if extracellular osmolality changes.

- If ECF osmolality increases, cells lose water and shrink. If ECF osmolality decreases, cells gain water and swell.

Below are 6 Darrow-Yannet diagrams illustrating changes in volume and/or osmolality. You are encouraged to examine the alterations and try to determine what occurred and how it could have occurred. Use the following to approach these alterations (answers provided on subsequent pages):

Does the change represent net water and/or solute gain or loss?

Indicate various ways in which this is likely to occur from a clinical perspective, i.e., the patient is hemorrhaging, drinking water, consuming excess salt, etc.

Changes in volume and concentration (dashed lines)

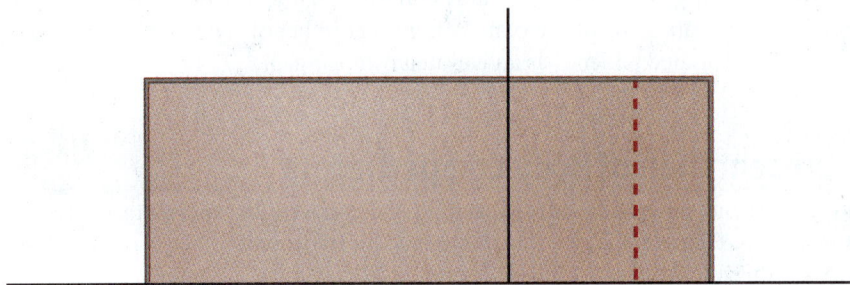

Figure 1-5. Patient shows isotonic fluid loss of extracellular volume with no change in osmolality. Since extracellular osmolality is the same, then intracellular volume is unchanged. This represents an isotonic fluid loss (equal loss of fluid and osmoles). Possible causes are hemorrhage, isotonic urine, or the immediate consequences of diarrhea or vomiting.

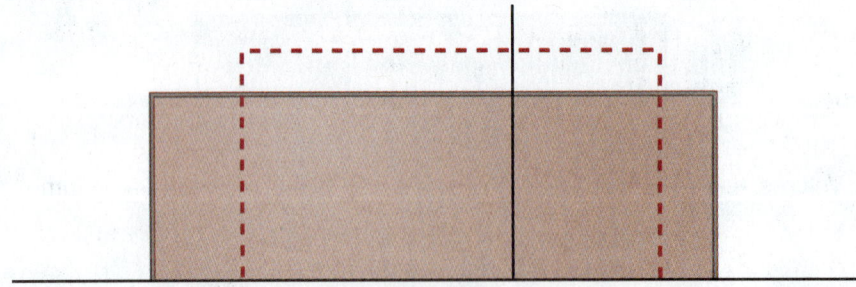

Figure 1-6. Patient shows loss of extracellular and intracellular volume with rise in osmolality. This represents a net loss of water (greater loss of water than osmoles). Possible causes are inadequate water intake or sweating. Pathologically, this could be hypotonic water loss from the urine resulting from diabetes insipidus.

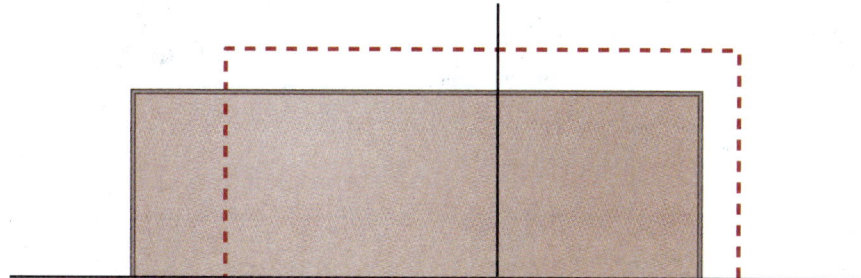

Figure 1-7. Patient shows gain of extracellular volume, increase in osmolality, and a decrease in intracellular volume. The rise in osmolality shifted water out of the cell. This represents a net gain of solute (increase in osmoles greater than increase in water). Possible causes are ingestion of salt, hypertonic infusion of solutes that distribute extracellularly (saline, mannitol), or hypertonic infusion of colloids. Colloids, e.g., dextran, don't readily cross the capillary membrane and thus expand the vascular compartment only (vascular is part of extracellular compartment).

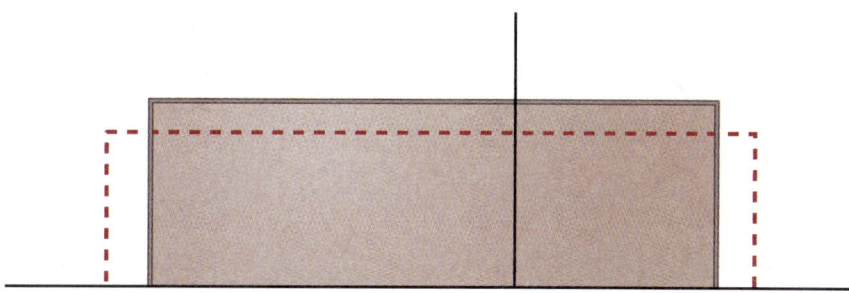

Figure 1-8. Patient shows increase in extracellular and intracellular volumes with a decrease in osmolality. The fall in osmolality shifted water into the cell. Thus, this represents net gain of water (more water than osmoles). Possible causes are drinking significant quantities of water (could be pathologic primary polydipsia), drinking significant quantities of a hypotonic fluid, losshypotonic fluid, or a hypotonic fluid infusion (saline, dextrose in water). Pathologically this could be abnormal water retention such as that which occurs with syndrome of inappropriate ADH.

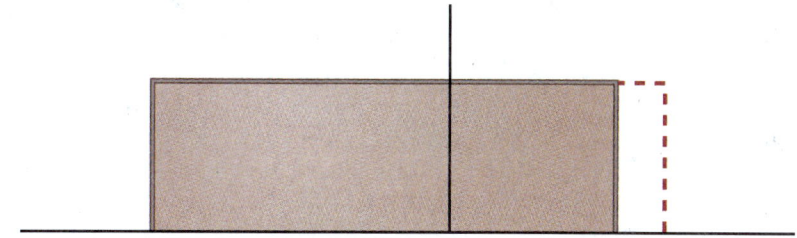

Figure 1-9. Patient shows increase in extracellular volume with no change in osmolality or intracellular volume. Since extracellular osmolality didn't change, then intracellular volume is unaffected. This represents a net gain of isotonic fluid (equal increase fluid and osmoles). Possible causes are isotonic fluid infusion (saline), drinking significant quantities of an isotonic fluid, or infusion of an isotonic colloid. Pathologically this could be the result of excess aldosterone. Aldosterone is a steroid hormone that causes Na^+ retention by the kidney. At first glance one would predict excess Na^+ retention by aldosterone would increase the concentration of Na^+ in the extracellular compartment. However, this is rarely the case because water follows Na^+, and even though the total body mass of Na^+ increases, its concentration doesn't.

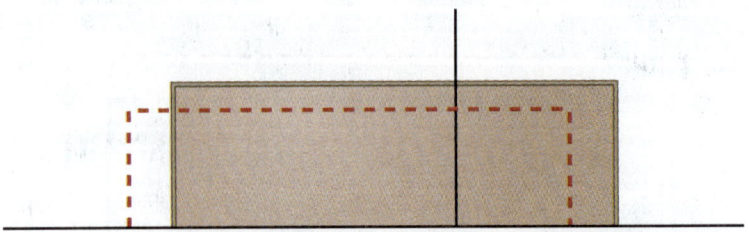

Figure 1-10. Patient shows decrease in extracellular volume and osmolality with an increase in intracellular volume. The rise in intracellular volume is the result of the decreased osmolality. This represents a net loss of hypertonic fluid loss (more osmoles lost than fluid). The only cause to consider is the pathologic state of adrenal insufficiency. Lack of mineralcorticoids, e.g., aldosterone, causes excess Na^+ loss.

Table 1-1. Summary of Volume Changes and Body Osmolarity Following Changes in Body Hydration

	ECF Volume	Body Osmolarity	ICF Volume	D-Y Diagram
Loss of isotonic fluid Hemorrhage Diarrhea Vomiting	↓	no change	no change	
Loss of hypotonic fluid Dehydration Diabetes insipidus Alcoholism	↓	↑	↓	
Gain of isotonic fluid Isotonic saline	↑	no change	no change	
Gain of hypotonic fluid Hypotonic saline Water intoxication	↑	↓	↑	
Gain of hypertonic fluid Hypertonic saline Hypertonic mannitol	↑	↑	↓	

ECF = extracellular fluid; ICF = intracellular fluid; D-Y = Darrow-Yannet

MICROCIRCULATION

Filtration and Absorption

Fluid flux across the capillary is governed by the two fundamental forces that cause water flow:

- Hydrostatic, which is simply the pressure of the fluid
- Osmotic (oncotic) forces, which represents the osmotic force created by solutes that don't cross the membrane (discussed earlier in this section)

Each of these forces exists on both sides of the membrane. Filtration is defined as the movement of fluid from the plasma into the interstitium, while absorption is movement of fluid from the interstitium into the plasma. The interplay between these forces is illustrated here

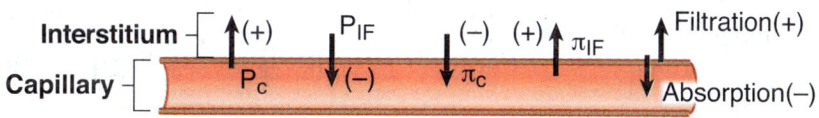

Figure 1-11. Starling Forces
P = Hydrostatic pressure; π = Osmotic (oncotic) pressure (mainly proteins)

Forces for filtration

P_C = hydrostatic pressure (blood pressure) in the capillary

This is directly related to:

- Blood flow (regulated at the arteriole)
- Venous pressure
- Blood volume

π_{IF} = oncotic (osmotic) force in the interstitium

- This is determined by the concentration of protein in the interstitial fluid.
- Normally the small amount of protein that leaks to the interstitium is minor and is removed by the lymphatics.
- Thus, under most conditions this is not an important factor influencing the exchange of fluid.

Forces for absorption

π_C = oncotic (osmotic) pressure of plasma

- This is the oncotic pressure of plasma solutes that cannot diffuse across the capillary membrane, i.e., the plasma proteins.
- Albumin, synthesized in the liver, is the most abundant plasma protein and thus the biggest contributor to this force.

P_{IF} = hydrostatic pressure in the interstitium

- This pressure is difficult to determine.
- In most cases it is close to zero or negative (subatmospheric) and is not a significant factor affecting filtration versus reabsorption.
- However, it can become significant if edema is present or it can affect glomerular filtration in the kidney (pressure in Bowman's space is analogous to interstitial pressure).

Starling Equation

These four forces are often referred to as Starling forces. Grouping the forces into those that favor filtration and those that oppose it, and taking into account the properties of the barrier to filtration, the formula for fluid exchange is the following:

$$Qf = k \left[(P_c + \pi_{IF}) - (P_{IF} + \pi_C) \right]$$

Qf = fluid movement
k = filtration coefficient

The filtration coefficient depends upon a number of factors but for our purposes permeability is most important. As indicated below, a variety of factors can increase permeability of the capillary resulting in a large flux of fluid from the capillary into the interstitial space.

A positive value of Qf indicates net filtration; a negative value indicates net absorption. In some tissues (e.g., renal glomerulus), filtration occurs along the entire length of the capillary; in others (intestinal mucosa), absorption normally occurs along the whole length. In other tissues, filtration may occur at the proximal end until the forces equilibrate.

Lymphatics

The lymphatics play a pivotal role in maintaining a low interstitial fluid volume and protein content. Lymphatic flow is directly proportional to interstitial fluid pressure, thus a rise in this pressure promotes fluid movement out of the interstitium via the lymphatics.

The lymphatics also remove proteins from the interstitium. Recall that the lymphatics return their fluid and protein content to the general circulation by coalescing into the lymphatic ducts, which in turn empty into to the subclavian veins.

EDEMA (PATHOLOGY INTEGRATION)

Edema is the accumulation of fluid in the interstitial space. It expresses itself in peripheral tissues in two different forms:

- **Pitting edema**: In this type of edema, pressing the affected area with a finger or thumb results in a visual indentation of the skin that persists for some time after the digit is removed. This is the "classic," most common type observed clinically. It generally responds well to diuretic therapy.
- **Non-pitting edema**: As the name implies, a persistent visual indentation is absent when pressing the affected area. This occurs when interstitial oncotic forces are elevated (proteins for example). This type of edema does not respond well to diuretic therapy.

Primary Causes of Peripheral Edema

Significant alterations in the Starling forces which then tip the balance toward filtration, increase capillary permeability (k), and/or interrupted lymphatic function can result in edema. Thus:

- **Increased capillary hydrostatic pressure (P_C)**: causes can include the following:
  - Marked increase in blood flow, e.g., vasodilation in a given vascular bed
  - Increasing venous pressure, e.g., venous obstruction or heart failure
  - Elevated blood volume (typically the result of Na^+ retention), e.g., heart failure

- **Increased interstitial oncotic pressure (π_{IF})**: primary cause is thyroid dysfunction (elevated mucopolysaccharides in the interstitium)
  - These act as osmotic agents resulting in fluid accumulation and a non-pitting edema. Lymphedema (see below) can also increase π_{IF}.

- **Decreased vascular oncotic pressure (π_C):** causes can include the following:
  - Liver failure
  - Nephrotic syndrome

- **Increased capillary permeability (k):** Circulating agents, e.g., tumor necrosis factor alpha (TNF-alpha), bradykinin, histamine, cytokines related to burn trauma, etc., increase fluid (and possibly protein) filtration resulting in edema.

- **Lymphatic obstruction/removal (lymphedema):** causes can include the following:
  - Filarial (*W. bancrofti*—elephantitis)
  - Bacterial lymphangitis (streptococci)
  - Trauma
  - Surgery
  - Tumor

  Given that one function of the lymphatics is to clear interstitial proteins, lymphedema can produce a non-pitting edema because of the rise in π_{IF}.

Pulmonary Edema

Edema in the interstitium of the lung can result in grave consequences. It can interfere with gas exchange, thus causing hypoxemia and hypercapnia (see Respiration section). A low hydrostatic pressure in pulmonary capillaries and lymphatic drainage helps "protect" the lungs against edema. However, similar to peripheral edema, alterations in Starling forces, capillary permeability, and/or lymphatic blockage can result in pulmonary edema. The most common causes relate to elevated capillary hydrostatic pressure and increased capillary permeability.

- **Cardiogenic (elevated P_C)**
  - Most common form of pulmonary edema
  - Increased left atrial pressure, increases venous pressure, which in turn increases capillary pressure
  - Initially increased lymph flow reduces interstitial proteins and is protective
  - First patient sign is often orthopnea (dyspnea when supine), which can be relieved when sitting upright
  - Elevated pulmonary wedge pressure provides confirmation
  - Treatment: reduce left atrial pressure, e.g., diuretic therapy

- **Non-cardiogenic (increased permeability): adult respiratory distress syndrome (ARDS)**
  - Due to direct injury of the alveolar epithelium or after a primary injury to the capillary endothelium
  - Clinical signs are severe dyspnea of rapid onset, hypoxemia, and diffuse pulmonary infiltrates leading to respiratory failure
  - Most common causes are sepsis, bacterial pneumonia, trauma, and gastric aspirations
  - Fluid accumulation as a result of the loss of epithelial integrity
  - Presence of protein-containing fluid in the alveoli inactivates surfactant causing reduced lung compliance
  - Pulmonary wedge pressure is normal or low

VOLUME MEASUREMENT OF COMPARTMENTS

To measure the volume of a body compartment, a tracer substance must be easily measured, well distributed within that compartment, and not rapidly metabolized or removed from that compartment. In this situation, the volume of the compartment can be calculated by using the following relationship:

$$V = \frac{A}{C}$$

V = volume of the compartment to be measured
C = concentration of tracer in the compartment to be measured
A = amount of tracer

For example, 300 mg of a dye is injected intravenously; at equilibrium, the concentration in the blood is 0.05 mg/mL. The volume of the compartment that contained the dye is $\text{volume} = \dfrac{300 \text{ mg}}{0.05 \text{ mg}/\text{mL}} = 6,000 \text{ mL}$.

This is called the volume of distribution (VOD).

Properties of the tracer and compartment measured

Tracers are generally introduced into the vascular compartment, and they distribute throughout body water until they reach a barrier they cannot penetrate. The two major barriers encountered are **capillary membranes** and **cell membranes**. Thus, tracer characteristics for the measurement of the various compartments are as follows:

- Plasma: tracer not permeable to capillary membranes, e.g., albumin
- ECF: tracer permeable to capillary membranes but not cell membranes, e.g., inulin, mannitol, sodium, sucrose
- Total body water: tracer permeable to capillary and cell membranes, e.g., tritiated water, urea

Blood Volume versus Plasma Volume

Blood volume represents the plasma volume plus the volume of RBCs, which is usually expressed as hematocrit (fractional concentration of RBCs).

The following formula can be utilized to convert plasma volume to blood volume:

$$\textbf{Blood volume} = \frac{\textbf{plasma volume}}{\textbf{1 - hematocrit}}$$

For example, if the hematocrit is 50% (0.50) and plasma volume = 3 L, then:

$$\text{Blood volume} = \frac{3\text{L}}{1 - 0.5} = 6 \text{ L}$$

If the hematocrit is 0.5 (or 50%), the blood is half RBCs and half plasma. Therefore, blood volume is double the plasma volume.

Blood volume can be estimated by taking 7% of the body weight in kgs. For example, a 70 kg individual has an approximate blood volume of 5.0 L.

The distribution of intravenously administered fluids is as follows:

- Vascular compartment: whole blood, plasma, dextran in saline
- ECF: saline, mannitol
- Total body water: D5W–5% dextrose in water
  - Once the glucose is metabolized, the water distributes 2/3 ICF, 1/3 ECF

Ionic Equilibrium and Resting Membrane Potential 2

Learning Objectives

❏ Explain information related to overview of excitable tissue

❏ Interpret scenarios on ion channels

❏ Explain information related to equilibrium potential

OVERVIEW OF EXCITABLE TISSUE

Figure 2-1 provides a basic picture of excitable cells and the relative concentration of key electrolytes inside versus outside the cell. The intracellular proteins have a negative charge.

In order to understand and apply what governs the conductance of ions as it relates to the function of excitable tissue (nerves and muscle), it is important to remember this relative difference in concentrations for these ions. In addition, it is imperative to understand the following five key principles.

1. **Membrane potential (E_m)**
   - There is a separation of charge across the membrane of excitability tissue at rest. This separation of charge means there is the potential to do work and is measured in volts. Thus, E_m represents the measured value.

2. **Electrochemical gradient**
   - Ions diffuse based upon chemical (concentration) gradients (high to low) and electrical gradients (like charges repel, opposites attract). Electrochemical gradient indicates the combination of these two forces.

3. **Equilibrium potential**
   - This is the membrane potential that puts an ion in electrochemical equilibrium, i.e., the membrane potential that results in no NET diffusion of an ion. If reached, the tendency for an ion to diffuse in one direction based upon the chemical gradient is countered by the electrical force in the opposite direction. The equilibrium potential for any ion can be calculated by the Nernst equation (see below).

4. **Conductance (g)**
   - Conductance refers to the flow of an ion across the cell membrane. Ions move across the membrane via channels (see below). Open/closed states of channels determine the relative permeability of the membrane to a given ion and thus the conductance. Open states create high permeability and conductance, while closed states result in low permeability and conductance.

5. **Net force (driving force)**
   - This indicates the relative "force" driving the diffusion of an ion. It is estimated by subtracting the ions equilibrium potential from the cell's membrane potential. In short, it quantitates how far a given ion is from equilibrium at any membrane potential.

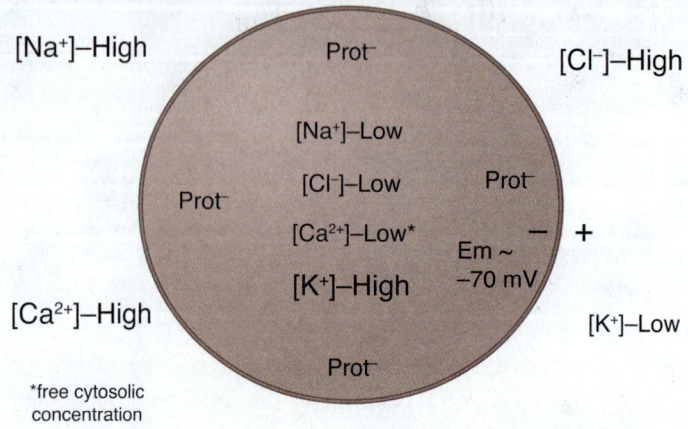

Figure 2-1. Basic Schematic of an Excitable Cell

ION CHANNELS

Ions diffuse across the membrane via ion channels. There are three basic types of ion channels.

Ungated (leak)

- Always open
- Direction the ion moves depends upon electrochemical forces
- Important for determining resting membrane potential of a cell

Voltage-gated

- Open/closed state is determined primarily by membrane potential (voltage)
- Change in membrane potential may open or close the channel

Ligand-gated

- Channel contains a receptor
- State of the channel (open or closed) is influenced by the binding of a ligand to the receptor
- Under most circumstances, the binding of the ligand opens the channel

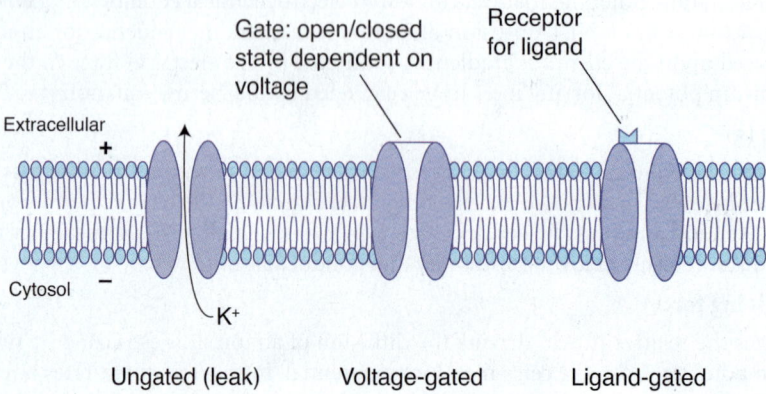

Figure 2-2. Classes of Ion Channels

NMDA Receptor (Exception to the Rule)

Above, we defined the three basic classes into which ion channels fall. The NMDA (N-methyl-D-aspartic acid) is an exception because it is both voltage- and ligand-gated.

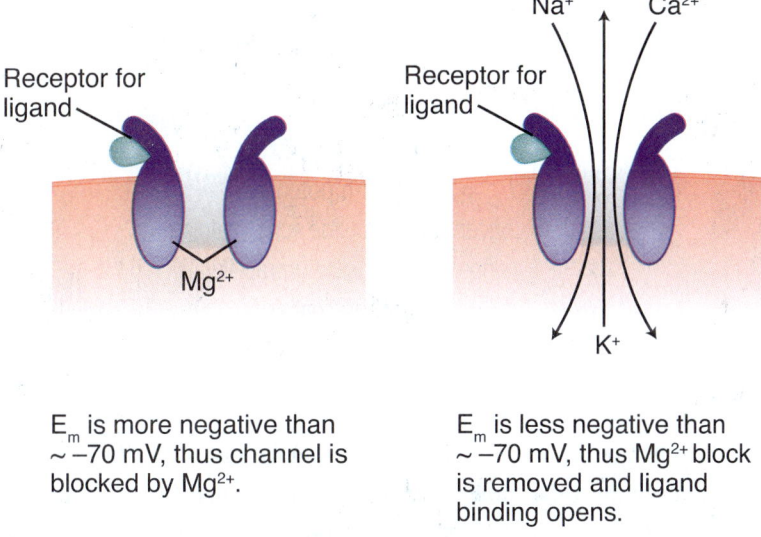

E_m is more negative than ~ −70 mV, thus channel is blocked by Mg^{2+}.

E_m is less negative than ~ −70 mV, thus Mg^{2+} block is removed and ligand binding opens.

Figure 2-3. NMDA Receptor

Voltage-gated

- The pore of the NMDA receptor is blocked by Mg^{2+} if E_m is more negative than ~ −70 mV.
- This Mg^{2+} block is removed if E_m becomes less negative than ~ −70 mV.
- Thus, the NMDA receptor exhibits characteristics of a voltage-gated channel.

Ligand-gated

Glutamate and aspartate are the endogenous ligands for this receptor. Binding of one of the ligands is **required** to open the channel, thus it exhibits characteristics of a ligand-gated channel.

- If E_m is more negative than ~ −70 mV, binding of the ligand does **not** open the channel (Mg^{2+} block related to voltage prevents).
- If E_m is less negative than ~ −70 mV, binding of the ligand opens the channel (even though no Mg^{2+} block at this E_m, channel will not open without ligand binding).

The NMDA receptor is a non-selective cation channel (Na^+, K^+, and Ca^{2+} flux through it). Thus, opening of this channel results in depolarization. Although the NMDA receptor is likely involved in a variety of functions, the two most important are (1) memory and (2) pain transmission. With respect to memory, NMDA has been shown to be involved in long-term potentiation of cells, thought to be an important component of memory formation. With respect to pain transmission, NMDA is expressed throughout the CNS and has been proven in numerous studies to play a pivotal role in the transmission and ultimate perception of pain.

EQUILIBRIUM POTENTIAL

Equilibrium potential is the membrane potential that puts an ion in electrochemical equilibrium, and it can be calculated using the **Nernst equation**. This equation computes the equilibrium potential for any ion based upon the concentration gradient.

$$E_{x^+} = \frac{60}{Z} \log_{10} \frac{[X^+]_o}{[X^+]_i}$$

> $E_X{}^+$ = equilibrium potential
> $[X^+]_o$ = concentration outside (extracellular)
> $[X^+]_i$ = concentration inside (intracellular)
> Z = value of the charge

Key points regarding the Nernst equation:

- The ion always diffuses in a direction that brings the E_m toward its equilibrium.
- The overall conductance of the ion is directly proportional to the net force and the permeability (determined by ion channel state) of the membrane for the ion.
- The E_m moves toward the E_X of the most permeable ion.
- The number of ions that actually move across the membrane is negligible. Thus, opening of ion channels does not alter intracellular or extracellular concentrations of ions under normal circumstances.

Approximate Equilibrium Potentials for the Important Ions

It is difficult to measure the intracellular concentration of the important electrolytes, thus equilibrium potentials for these ions will vary some across the various references. The following represent reasonable equilibrium potentials for the key electrolytes:

$E_{K+} \sim -95\ mV$ $E_{Na+} \sim +70\ mV$

$E_{Cl-} \sim -76\ mV$ $E_{Ca2}{}^+ \sim +125\ mV$

Definitions

In **depolarization**, E_m becomes less negative (moves toward zero). In **hyperpolarization**, E_m becomes more negative (further from zero).

Resting Membrane Potential

Potassium (K$^+$)

There is marked variability in the resting membrane potential (rE$_m$) for excitable tissues, but the following generalizations are applicable.

- rE$_m$ for nerves is ~ -70 mV while rE$_m$ for striated muscle is ~ -90 mV.
- Excitable tissue has a considerable number of leak channels for K$^+$, but not for Cl$^-$, Na$^+$, or Ca^{2+}. Thus, K$^+$ conductance (g) is high in resting cells.
- Because of this high conductance, rE$_m$ is altered in the following ways by changes in the extracellular concentration of K$^+$:
  - **Hyperkalemia depolarizes the cell.** If acute, excitability of nerves is increased (nerve is closer to threshold for an action potential) and heart arrhythmias may occur.
  - **Hypokalemia hyperpolarizes the cell.** This decreases the excitability of nerves (further from threshold) and heart arrhythmias may occur.

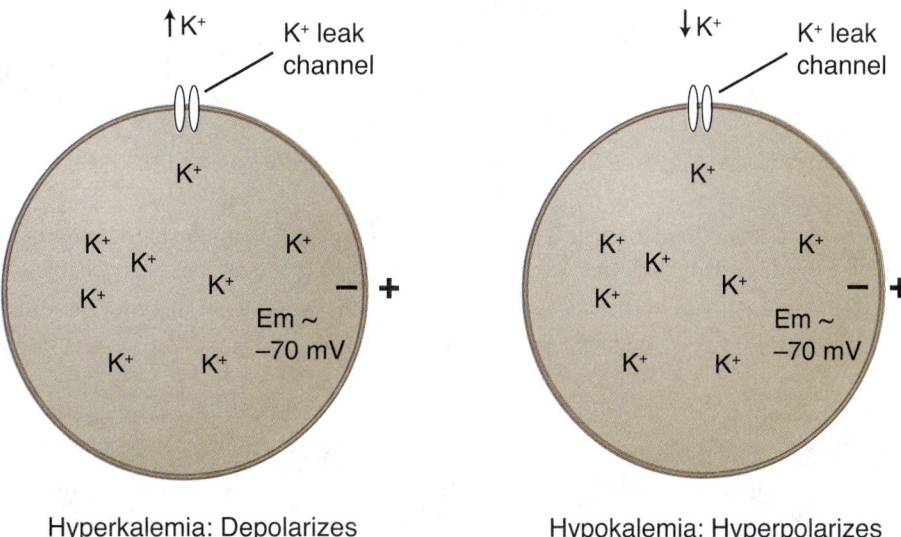

Figure 2-4. Effect of Changes in Extracellular K$^+$ on Resting Membrane Potential

Altering the g for K$^+$ has the following effects:

- Increasing g causes K$^+$ to leave the cell, resulting in hyperpolarization of the cell. Recall that increasing g for an ion causes the E$_m$ to move toward the equilibrium potential for that ion. Thus, the cell will move from -70 mV toward -95 mV.
- Decreasing g depolarizes the cell (cell moves away from K$^+$ equilibrium). This applies to K$^+$ because of its high resting g.

The Na$^+$/K$^+$ ATPase

Although the cell membrane is relatively impermeable to Na$^+$, it is not completely impervious to it. Thus, some Na$^+$ does leak into excitable cells. This Na$^+$ leak into the cells is counterbalanced by pumping it back out via the Na$^+$/K$^+$ ATPase. Important attributes of this pump are:

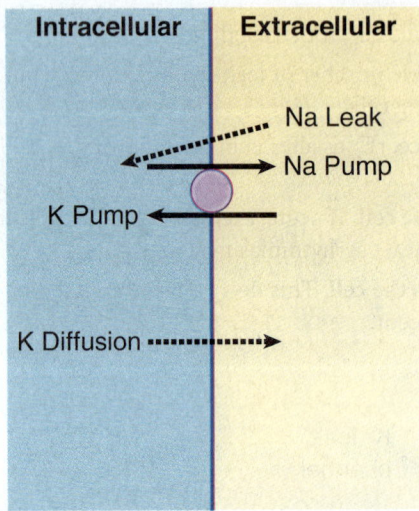

Figure 2-5. Steady-State Resting Relationship between Ion Diffusion and Na/K-ATPase Pump

- The stoichiometry is 3 Na$^+$ out, 2 K$^+$ in. This means the pump is electrogenic because more positive charges are removed from inside the cell than are replaced. This helps maintain a negative charge inside the cell.

- Three solutes are pumped out in exchange for two solutes. This causes a net flux of water out of the cell. This pump is important for volume regulation of excitable tissue.

Chloride (Cl$^-$)

- Cl$^-$ g is low at rest. Thus, decreasing g or changing the extracellular concentration has minimal effect on rE_m.
- Assuming rE_m is −70 mV, increasing Cl$^-$ g hyperpolarizes the cell (E_m moves toward equilibrium for Cl$^-$, which is −76 mV, see also Figure 2-6).
- If rE_m is −80 mV or more negative, increasing Cl$^-$ g depolarizes the cell.

Sodium (Na$^+$)

- Na$^+$ g is very low at rest. Thus decreasing g or changing the extracellular concentration has no effect on rE$_m$.
- Increasing Na$^+$ g depolarizes the cell (E$_m$ moves to equilibrium for Na$^+$, which is +70 mV, see also Figure 2-6).

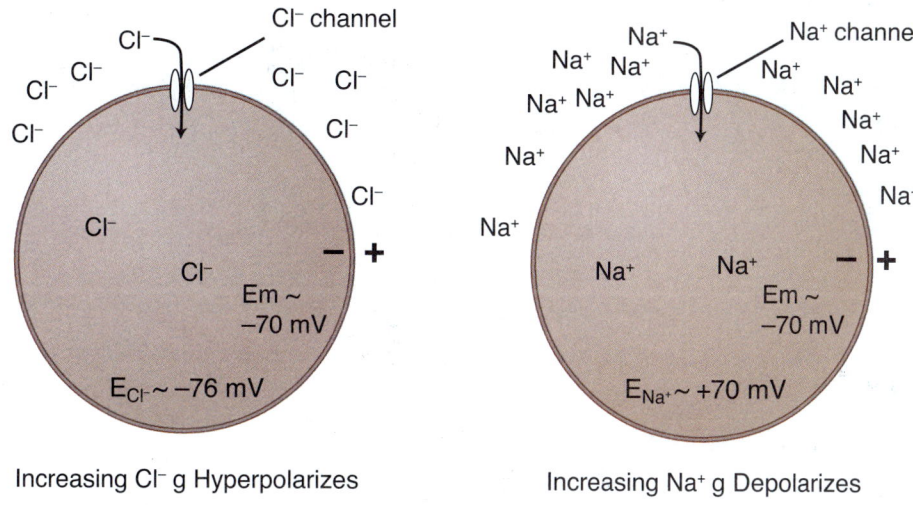

Figure 2-6. Effect of Increase Cl$^-$ g (left) or Na$^+$ g (right)

Calcium (Ca^{2+})

- Similar to Na$^+$, Ca^{2+} g is very low at rest. Thus decreasing g or changing the extracellular concentration has no effect on rE$_m$.
- Increasing Ca^{2+} g depolarizes the cell (E$_m$ moves toward equilibrium for Ca^{2+}, which is +125 mV).

The Neuron Action Potential and Synaptic Transmission

Learning Objectives

❏ Explain information related to overview of the action potential

❏ Solve problems concerning voltage-gated ion channels

❏ Demonstrate understanding of the action potential

❏ Answer questions about synaptic transmission

❏ Interpret scenarios on review and integration

OVERVIEW OF THE ACTION POTENTIAL

The action potential is a rapid depolarization followed by a repolarization (return of membrane potential to rest). The function is:

- **Nerves**: conduct neuronal signals
- **Muscle**: initiate a contraction

Figure 3-1 shows the action potential from three types of excitable cells. Even though there are many similarities, there are differences between these cell types, most notably the duration of the action potential. In this chapter, we discuss the specific events pertaining to the nerve action potential, but the action potential in skeletal muscle is virtually the same. Thus, what is stated here can be directly applied to skeletal muscle. Because the cardiac action potential has several differences, it will be discussed in the subsequent chapter.

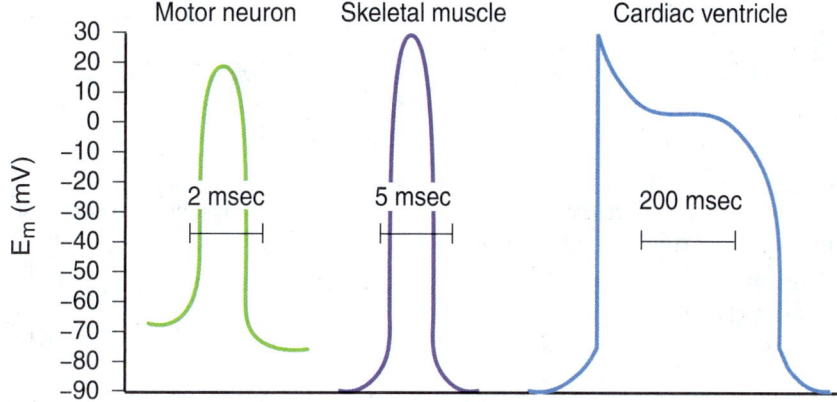

Figure 3-1. Action Potentials from 3 Vertebrate Cell Types. Note the different time scales.
(Redrawn from Flickinger, C.J., et al.: Medical Cell Biology, Philadelphia, 1979, W.B. Saunders Co.)

VOLTAGE-GATED ION CHANNELS

In order to understand how the action potential is generated, we must first discuss the ion channels involved.

Voltage-gated (fast) Na$^+$ Channels

The opening of these channels is responsible for the rapid depolarization phase (upstroke) of the action potential. Figure 3-2 shows the details of the fast Na$^+$ channel. It has two gates and three conformational states:

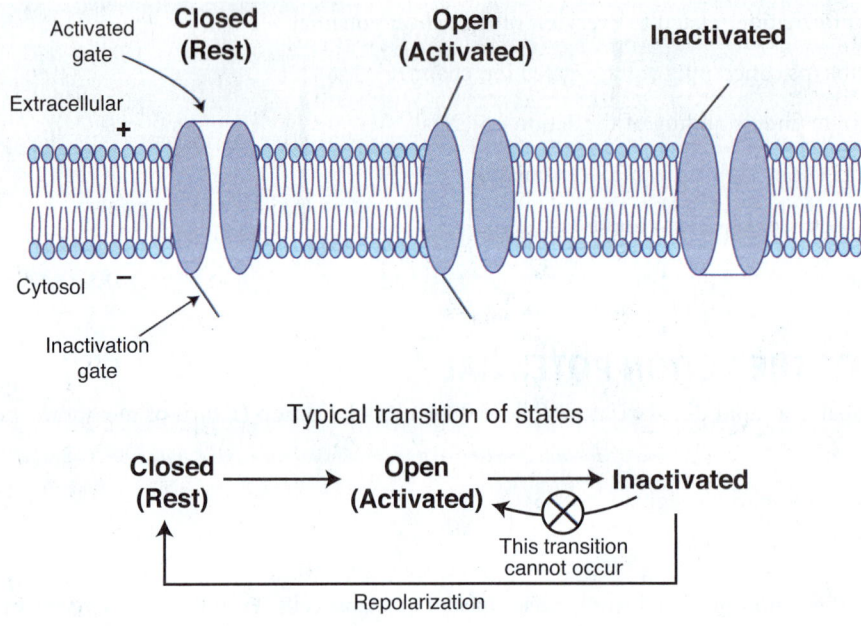

Figure 3-2. Voltage-gated (fast) Na$^+$ Channel

- **Closed:** In the closed state, the activation gate (m-gate) is closed and the inactivation gate (h-gate) is open. Because the activation gate is closed, Na$^+$ conductance (g) is low.

- **Open:** Depolarization causes the channel to transition to the open state, in which both gates are open and thus Na$^+$ g increases. The elevated Na$^+$ g causes further depolarization, which in turn opens more Na$^+$ channels, causing further depolarization. In short, a positive-feedback cycle can be initiated if enough Na$^+$ channels open at or near the same time. Bear in mind, there are numerous fast Na$^+$ channels in every cell, and each one has its own threshold voltage for opening.

- **Inactivated:** After opening, the fast Na$^+$ channel typically transitions to the inactivated state. In this state, the activation gate is open and inactivation gate (h-gate) is closed. Under normal circumstances, this occurs when membrane potential becomes positive as a result of the action potential.

- Once the cell repolarizes, the fast Na$^+$ channel transitions back to the closed state, and is thus ready to reopen to cause another action potential.

Key point: Once a Na$^+$ channel inactivates, it cannot go back to the open state until it transitions to the closed state (see Figure 3-2). The transition to the closed state typically occurs when the cell repolarizes. However, there are conditions in which this transition to the closed state doesn't occur.

Important fact: Extracellular Ca^{2+} blocks fast Na$^+$ channels.

Voltage-gated K+ Channels

- Closed at resting membrane potential
- Depolarization opens, but kinetics are much slower than fast Na+ channels
- Primary mechanism for repolarization

THE ACTION POTENTIAL

Subthreshold Stimulus

The blue and purple lines in Figure 3-3 show changes in membrane potential (E_m) to increasing levels of stimuli, but neither result in an action potential. Thus, these are subthreshold stimuli. Important points regarding these stimuli are:

- The degree of depolarization is related to the magnitude of the stimulus.
- The membrane repolarizes (returns to rest).
- It can summate, which means if another stimulus is applied before repolarization is complete, the depolarization of the second stimulus adds onto the depolarization of the first (the two depolarizations sum together).

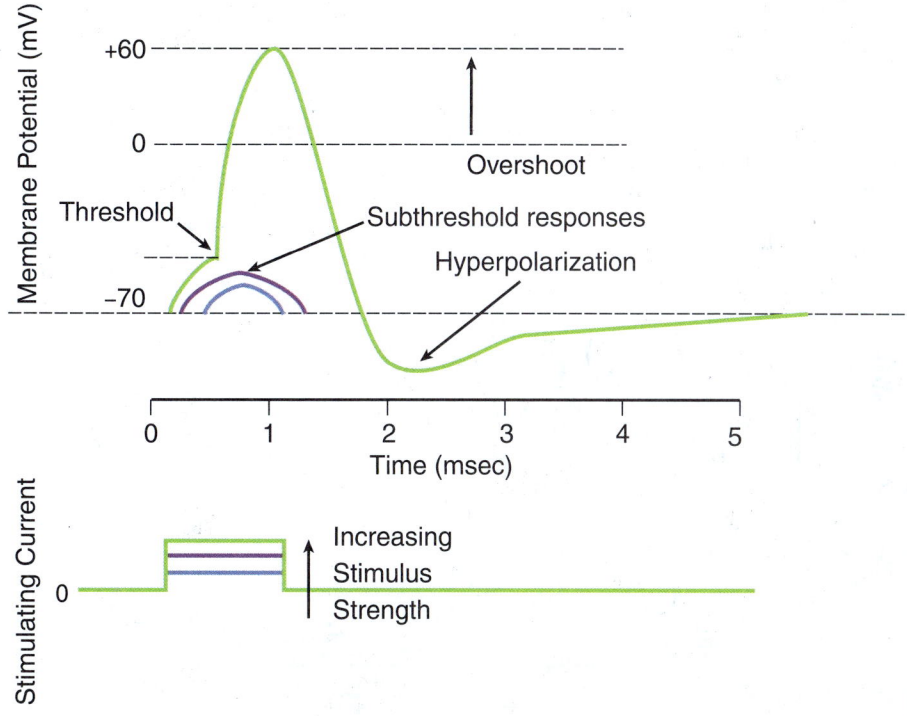

Figure 3-3. The Neuron Action Potential

Threshold Stimulus

The green line in Figure 3-3 depicts the action potential. Provided the initial stimulus is great enough to depolarize the neuron to threshold, then an action potential results. The following represents the events that occur during an action potential, which is an application of the aforementioned discussion on ion channels.

- At threshold, a critical mass of fast Na+ channels open, resulting in further depolarization and the opening of more fast Na+ channels.

- Because Na$^+$ g is high (see also Figure 3-4), the E$_m$ potential rapidly approaches the equilibrium potential for Na$^+$ ($\sim$ +70 mV)
- As membrane potential becomes positive, fast Na$^+$ channels begin to inactivate (see above), resulting in a rapid reduction in Na$^+$ conductance (see also Figure 3-4).
- Voltage-gated K$^+$ channels open in response to the depolarization, but since their kinetics are much slower, the inward Na$^+$ current (upstroke of the action potential) dominates initially.
- K$^+$ g begins to rise as more channels open. As the rise in E$_m$ approaches its peak, fast Na$^+$ channels are inactivating, and now the neuron has a high K$^+$ g and a low Na$^+$ g (see also Figure 3-4).
- The high K$^+$ g drives E$_m$ toward K$^+$ equilibrium ($\sim$ −95 mV) resulting in a rapid repolarization.
- As E$_m$ becomes negative, K$^+$ channels begin to close, and K$^+$ g slowly returns to its original level. However, because of the slow kinetics, a period of hyperpolarization occurs.

Key Points

- The upstroke of the action potential is mediated by a Na$^+$ current (fast Na$^+$ channels).
- Although the inactivation of fast Na$^+$ channels participates in repolarization, the dominant factor is the high K$^+$ g due to the opening of voltage-gated K$^+$ channels.
- The action potential is all or none: Occurs if threshold is reached, doesn't occur if threshold is not reached.
- The action potential cannot summate.
- Under normal conditions, the action potential regenerates itself as it moves down the axon, thus it is propagated (magnitude is unchanged).

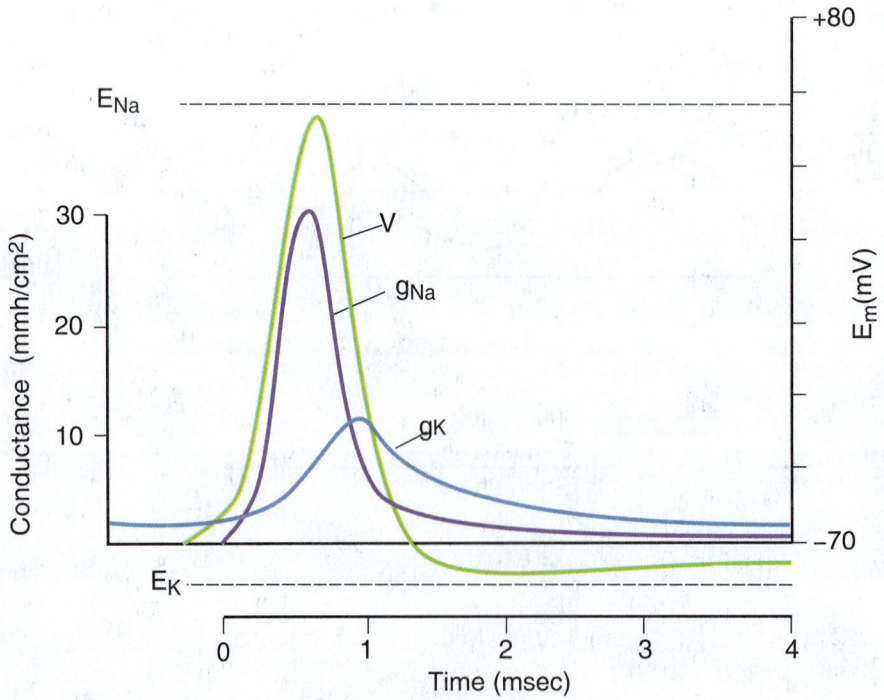

Figure 3-4. Axon Action Potential and Changes in Conductance. V = Membrane potential (action potential); gNa = Sodium ion conductance; gK = Potassium conductance.

PROPERTIES OF ACTION POTENTIALS

Refractory Periods

Absolute refractory period

The absolute refractory period is the period during which no matter how strong the stimulus, it cannot induce a second action potential. The mechanism underlying this is the fact that during this time, most fast Na^+ channels are either open or in the inactivated state. The approximate duration of the absolute refractory period is illustrated in Figure 3-5. The length of this period determines the maximum frequency of action potentials.

Relative refractory period

The relative refractory period is that period during which a greater than threshold stimulus is required to induce a second action potential (see approximate length in Figure 3-5). The mechanism for this is the elevated K^+ g.

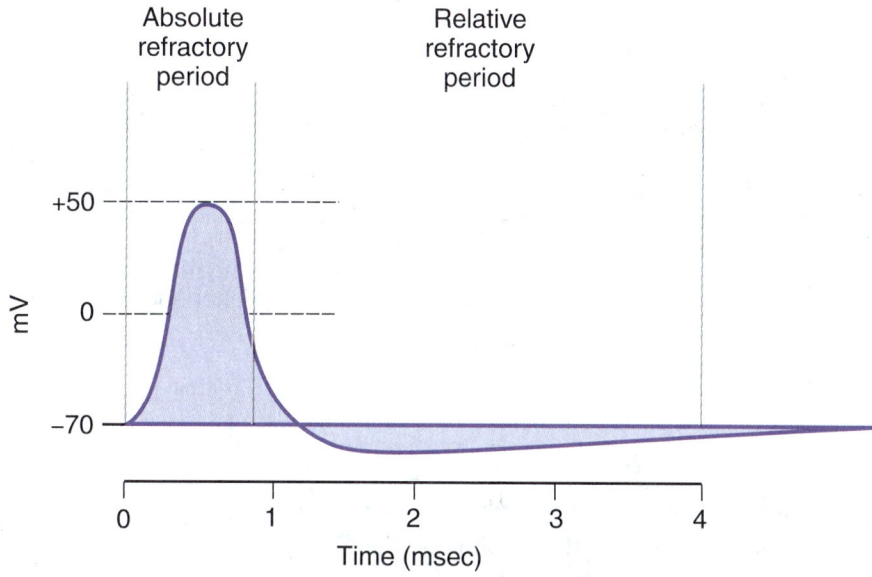

Figure 3-5. Refractory Periods

Conduction Velocity of the Action Potential

The two primary factors influencing conduction velocity in nerves are:

- **Cell diameter**: The greater the cell diameter, the greater the conduction velocity. A greater cross-sectional surface area reduces the internal electrical resistance.

- **Myelination**: Myelin provides a greater electrical resistance across the cell membrane, thereby reducing current "leak" through the membrane. The myelination is interrupted at the nodes of Ranvier where fast Na^+ channels cluster. Thus, the action potential appears to "bounce" from node to node with minimal decrement and greater speed (saltatory conduction).

SYNAPTIC TRANSMISSION

Neuromuscular Junction (NMJ)

The synapse between the axons of an alpha-motor neuron and a skeletal muscle fiber is called the neuromuscular junction (NMJ). The terminals of alpha-motor neurons contain acetylcholine (Ach), thus the synaptic transmission at the neuromuscular junction is one example of cholinergic transmission. The basics of neurotransmitter release described in this section are applicable to synaptic transmission for all synapses.

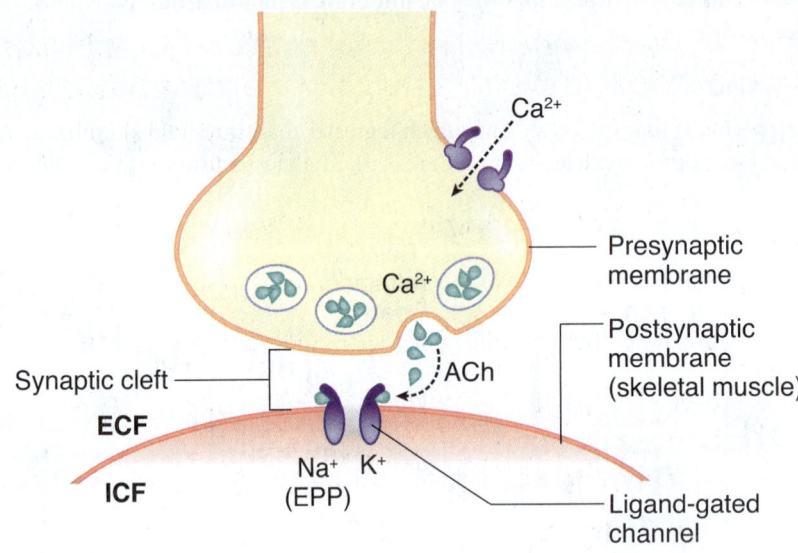

Figure 3-6. Neuromuscular Transmission and Nicotinic Synapses

Sequence of events

1. The action potential travelling down the motor neuron depolarizes the presynaptic membrane.

2. This depolarization opens voltage-gated Ca^{2+} channels in the presynaptic membrane, resulting in Ca^{2+} influx into the presynaptic terminal.

3. The rise in Ca^{2+} causes synaptic vesicles to release their contents, in this case, Ach. The amount of neurotransmitter release is **directly related** to the rise in cytosolic Ca^{2+}, i.e., the more Ca^{2+} that enters, the more neurotransmitter released.

4. Ach binds to a nicotinic receptor located on the muscle membrane (N_M receptor). The N_M receptor is a non-selective monovalent cation channel (both Na^+ and K^+ can traverse). Given that Na^+ has a much greater net force (see Chapter 1 of this section), depolarization occurs. This depolarization is called an end-plate potential (EPP). The magnitude of the EPP is directly related to the amount of Ach released.

5. The resulting depolarization opens fast Na^+ channels on the muscle membrane (sarcolemma) causing an action potential in the sarcolemma. Under normal circumstances, an action potential in the motor neuron releases enough Ach to cause an EPP that is at least threshold for the action potential in the skeletal muscle cell. In other words, there is a one-to-one relationship between an action potential in the motor neuron and an action potential in the skeletal muscle cell.

6. The actions of Ach are terminated by acetylcholinesterase (AchE), an enzyme located on the postsynaptic membrane that breaks down Ach into choline and acetate. Choline is taken back into the presynaptic terminal (reuptake), hence providing substrate for re-synthesis of Ach.

Bridge to Pathology

Two important pathologies related to neuromuscular junctions are **myasthenia gravis** and **Lambert-Eaton** syndrome. The most common form of myasthenia gravis is an autoimmune condition in which antibodies are created that block the N_M receptor. Lambert-Easton is also an autoimmune condition, but the antibodies block the presynaptic voltage-gated Ca^{2+} channels.

Other cholinergic synapses

Neuronal nicotinic (N_N) receptors

Outside of the CNS, these primarily reside in autonomic ganglia. Recall that preganglionic neurons are cholinergic and these fibers synapse on nicotinic receptors in the ganglia.

Muscarinic receptors

Muscarinic receptors are G-protein coupled receptors. These reside in target tissues innervated by parasympathetic postganglionic neurons.

Synapses Between Neurons

Figure 3-7 illustrates synaptic junctions between neurons. In general, the synaptic potentials produced are either excitatory or inhibitory (see below) and are produced by **ligand-gated ion channels.** Some other important aspects associated with these synapses are:

- Synapses are located on the cell body and dendrites.
- The currents produced at these synapses travel along the dendritic and cell body membranes.
- The axon hillock–initial segment region has a high density of fast Na^+ channels and is the origin for the action potential of the axon.
- The closer the synapse is to this region, the greater its influence in determining whether an action potential is generated.
- If the sum of all the inputs reaches threshold, an action potential is generated and conducted along the axon to the nerve terminals.

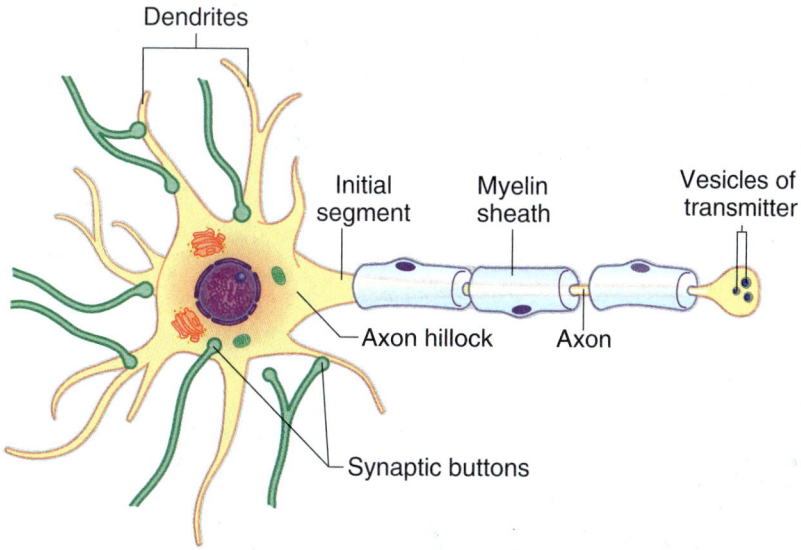

Figure 3-7. Synapse Transmission between Neurons

Excitatory postsynaptic potential (EPSP)

EPSP is excitatory if it increases the excitability of the postsynaptic neuron, i.e., it is more likely to fire an action potential.

- It is primarily the result of increased Na^+ g.
- It is similar to the EPP found at the neuromuscular junction.
- Important receptors that produce:
  - Nicotinic: Endogenous ligand is Ach and include N_M and N_N.
  - Non-NMDA (N-methyl-D-aspartic acid): Endogenous ligands are glutamate and aspartate (excitatory amino acid transmitters), and Na^+ g is increased when they bind.
  - NMDA: Endogenous ligands are the excitatory amino acids and it is a non-selective cation channel (discussed in the preceding chapter).

Inhibitory postsynaptic potential (IPSP)

IPSP is inhibitory if it decreases the excitability of the postsynaptic neuron, i.e., it is less likely to fire an action potential.

- It is primarily the result of increased Cl^- g.
- Important receptors that produce:
  - $GABA_{A\&C}$: Endogenous ligand is GABA (gamma-aminobutryic acid).
  - Glycine: Endogenous ligand is glycine.

Electrical Synapses

- In contrast to chemical synaptic transmission, there is a direct flow of current from cell to cell.
- This cell-to-cell communication occurs via gap junctions; because the cells are electrically coupled, there is no synaptic delay.
- Cardiac and single-unit smooth muscle cells have these electrical synapses.

Electrical Activity of the Heart 4

Learning Objectives

❏ Use knowledge of properties of cardiac tissue

❏ Answer questions about cardiac action potentials

❏ Use knowledge of control of nodal excitability

❏ Answer questions about electrocardiology

❏ Explain information related to arrhythmias/ECG alterations

PROPERTIES OF CARDIAC TISSUE

Different cells within the heart are specialized for different functional roles. In general, these specializations are for automaticity, conduction, and/or contraction.

Automaticity

Cardiac cells initiate action potentials spontaneously. Further, the cells are electrically coupled via gap junctions. Thus, when a cell fires an action potential, it typically sweeps throughout the heart. Although all cardiac tissue shows spontaneous depolarization, only the following three are germane.

- **Sinoatrial (SA) node cells** are specialized for automaticity. They spontaneously depolarize to threshold and have the highest intrinsic rhythm (rate), making them the pacemaker in the normal heart. Their intrinsic rate is ~ 100/min.

- **Atrioventricular (AV) node cells** have the second highest intrinsic rhythm (40-60/min). Often, these cells become the pacemaker if SA node cells are damaged.

- Although not "specialized" for automaticity per se, **Purkinje cells** do exhibit spontaneous depolarizations with a rate of ~ 35/min.

Conduction

All cardiac tissue conducts electrical impulses, but the following are particularly specialized for this function.

- AV node: These cells are specialized for slow conduction. They have small diameter fibers, a low density of gap junctions, and the rate of depolarization (phase 0, see below) is slow in comparison to tissue that conducts fast.

- Purkinje cells: These cells are specialized for rapid conduction. Their diameter is large, they express many gap junctions, and the rate of depolarization (phase 0, see below) is rapid. These cells constitute the HIS-Purkinje system of the ventricles.

Contraction

Although myocytes have a spontaneous depolarization and they conduct electrical impulses, they contain the protein machinery to contract.

Conduction Pathway

Because cells are electrically coupled via gap junctions, excitation to threshold of one cell typically results in the spread of this action potential throughout the heart. In the normal heart, the SA node is the pacemaker because it has the highest intrinsic rhythm. Below is the normal conduction pathway for the heart.

atrial muscle

SA node ⟶ internodal fibers ⟶ AV node (delay) ⟶ Purkinje fibers ⟶ ventricular muscle

CARDIAC ACTION POTENTIALS

Resting Membrane Potential (Non-Nodal Cells)

Potassium conductance is high in resting ventricular or atrial myocytes. This is also true for Purkinje cells. Because of this, resting membrane potential is close to K$^+$ equilibrium potential. This high-resting K$^+$ conductance is the result to two major types of channels.

Ungated potassium channels

Always open and unless the membrane potential reaches the potassium equilibrium potential ($\sim$ –95 mV), a potassium flux (efflux) is maintained through these channels.

Inward K$^+$ rectifying channels (IK$_1$)

- Voltage-gated channels that are open at rest.
- Depolarization closes.
- They open again as the membrane begins to repolarize.

Action Potential (Non-Nodal Cells)

Understanding the ionic basis of cardiac action potentials is important for understanding both cardiac physiology and the electrocardiogram (ECG), which is a recording of the currents produced by these ionic changes. In addition, antiarrhythmic drugs exert their effects by binding to the channels that produce these ionic currents.

In this section, we go through the various phases of the action potentials that occur in myocytes and Purkinje cells. Action potentials generated by nodal cells (SA and AV) are discussed later. Although there are slight differences in the action potentials generated by atrial and ventricular myocytes, as well as Purkinje cells, these differences are not included here. Furthermore, it is important to remember that cardiac cells are electrically coupled by gap junctions. Thus, when a cell fires an action potential, it spreads and is conducted by neighboring cells.

The following figure shows the labeled phases of the action potential from a ventricular myocyte and the predominant ionic currents related to the various phases.

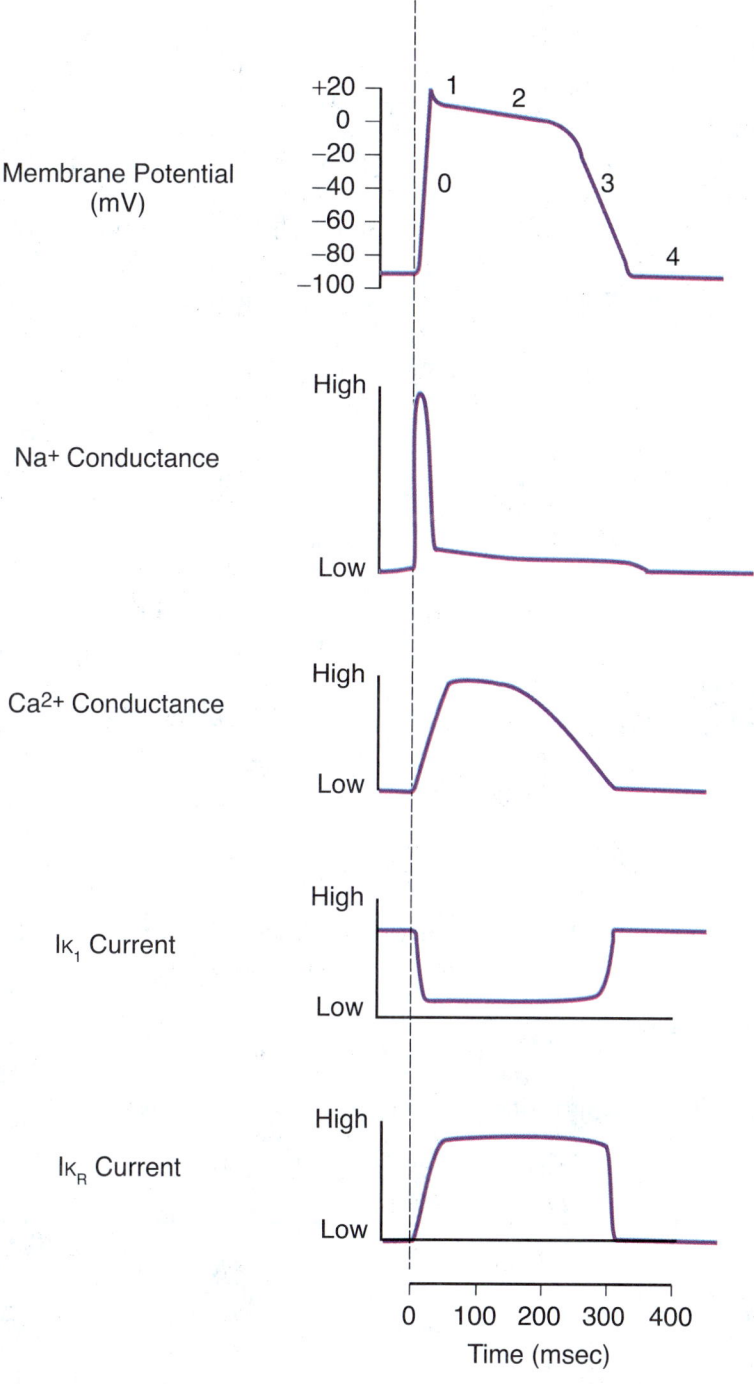

Figure 4-1. Action Potential in a Ventricular Myocyte

Phase 0

- Upstroke of the action potential
- Similar to nerve and skeletal muscle, mediated by the opening of voltage-gated, fast Na$^+$ channels (note high Na$^+$ conductance)
- Conduction velocity is directly related to rate of change in potential (slope). Stimulation of β-1 receptors, e.g., epinephrine and norepinephrine, increases the slope and thus increases conduction velocity.
- Creates the QRS complex of the ECG

Phase 1

- Slight repolarization mediated by a transient potassium current
- Sodium channels transition to the inactivated state (note reduction in Na^+ conductance).

Phase 2 (plateau)

- Depolarization opens voltage-gated Ca^{2+} channels (primarily L-type) and voltage-gated K^+ channels (IK_R current being one example).
- The inward Ca^{2+} current offset by the outward K^+ current results in little change in membrane potential (plateau).
- The influx of Ca^{2+} triggers the release of Ca^{2+} from the SR (Ca^{2+} induced Ca^{2+} release), resulting in cross-bridge cycling and muscle contraction (see next chapter).
- Creates the ST segment of the ECG
- The long duration of the action potential prevents tetany in cardiac muscle (see next chapter).

Phase 3

- Repolarization phase
- L-type channels begin closing, but rectifying K^+ currents (IK_R current being one example) still exist resulting in repolarization.
- IK_1 channels reopen and aid in repolarization.
- Creates the T wave of the EKG

Phase 4

- Resting membrane potential
- Fast Na^+, L-type Ca^{2+}, and rectifying K^+ channels (IK_R) close, but IK_1 channels remain open.

Action Potential (Nodal Cells)

Nodal tissue (SA and AV) lacks fast Na^+ channels. Thus, the upstroke of the action potential is mediated by a Ca^{2+} current rather than an Na^+ current. In addition, note that phases 1 and 2 are absent.

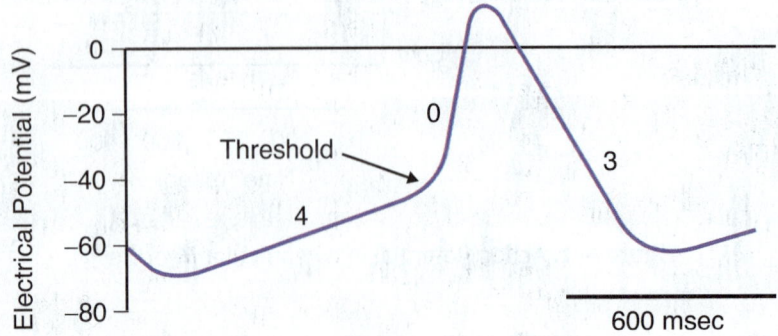

Figure 4-2. SA Nodal (Pacemaker) Action Potential

Phase 4

- Resting membrane potential
- Given this tissue is specialized for automaticity (see above), these cells show a spontaneous depolarization at rest. This spontaneous depolarization is referred to as the "pacemaker" potential and results from:

— **Inward Ca^{2+} current:** Primarily related to T-type Ca^{2+} channels. These differ from the L-type in that they open at a more negative membrane potential ($\sim$ −70 mV).

— **Inward Na$^+$ current:** This inward Na$^+$ current is referred to as the "funny" current (I_f) and the channel involved is a hyperpolarization-activated cyclic nucleotide-gated (HCN) channel. HCN are non-selective monovalent cation channels and thus conduct both Na$^+$ and K$^+$. However, opening of these channels evokes a sodium-mediated depolarization (similar to nicotinic receptors, see previous chapter). These channels open when the membrane repolarizes (negative membrane potential), and they close in response to the depolarization of the action potential.

— **Outward K$^+$ current:** There is a reduced outward K$^+$ current as the cell repolarizes after the action potential. Reducing this current helps to produce the pacemaker potential.

Phase 0

- Upstroke of the action potential
- Mediated by opening of L-type (primarily) Ca^{2+} channels
- Note the time scale: the slope of phase 0 is not steep in nodal tissue like it is in ventricular myocytes or the upstroke of the action potential in nerves. This is part of the reason conduction velocity is slow in the AV node.

Phase 3

- Repolarization phase
- Mediated by voltage-gated K$^+$ channels

CONTROL OF NODAL EXCITABILITY

Catecholamines

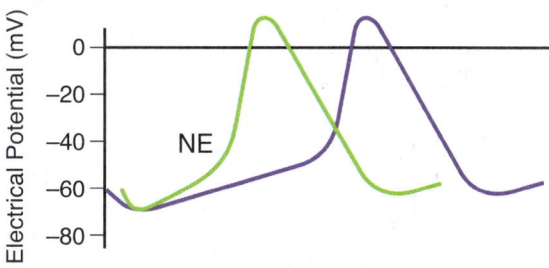

Figure 4-3. Sympathetic Effects on SA Nodal Cells

- Norepinephrine (NE) from postganglionic sympathetic nerve terminals and circulating epinephrine (Epi)
- β-1 receptors; Gs—cAMP; stimulates opening of HCN and Ca^{2+} channels
- Increased slope of pacemaker potential (gets to threshold sooner)
- Functional effect
  - Positive chronotropy (SA node): increased HR
  - Positive dromotropy (AV node): increased conduction velocity through the AV node

Parasympathetic

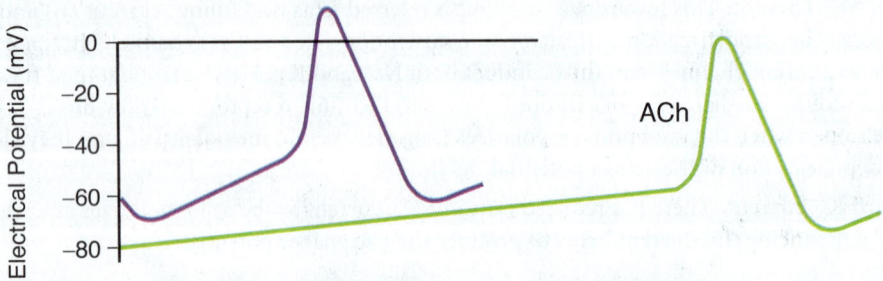

Figure 4-4. Parasympathetic Effects on SA Nodal Cells

- Ach released from post-ganglionic fibers.
- M_2 receptor; Gi-Go; Opens K^+ channels and inhibits cAMP
- Hyperpolarizes; reduced slope of pacemaker potential
- Functional effect
  - Negative chronotropy (SA node): Decreased HR
  - Negative dromotropy (AV node): Decreased conduction velocity through the AV node

ELECTROCARDIOLOGY

The Electrocardiogram (EKG or ECG)

The normal pattern is demonstrated here.

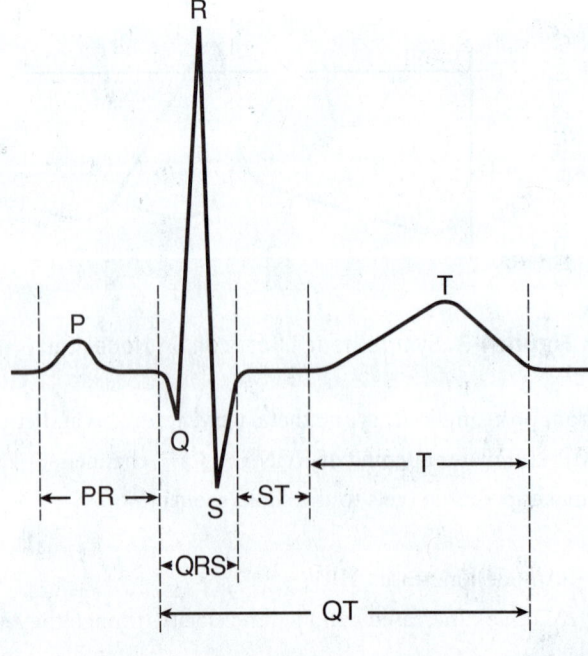

Figure 4-5. Normal Pattern of an ECG

P wave: atrial depolarization

QRS complex: ventricular depolarization (40–100 msec)

R wave: first upward deflection after the P wave

S wave: first downward deflection after an R wave

T wave: ventricular repolarization

PR interval: start of the P wave to start of the QRS complex (120–200 msec); mostly due to conduction delay in the AV node

QT interval: start of the QRS complex to the end of the T wave; represents duration of the action potential (see Figure 4-6)

ST segment: ventricles are depolarized during this segment; roughly corresponds to the plateau phase of the action potential

J point: end of the S wave; represents isoelectric point

Note: Height of waves is directly related to (a) mass of tissue, (b) rate of change in potential, and (c) orientation of the lead to the direction of current flow.

Figure 4-6 further illustrates the alignment of the cardiac action potential and the ECG recording. To recap:

- Phase 0 produces the QRS complex.
- Phase 3 produces the T wave.
- The ST segment occurs during phase 2.
- The QT interval represents the duration of the action potential and this interval is inversely related to heart rate. For example, stimulation of sympathetics to the heart increases heart rate and reduces the duration of the action potential, thus decreasing the QT interval.

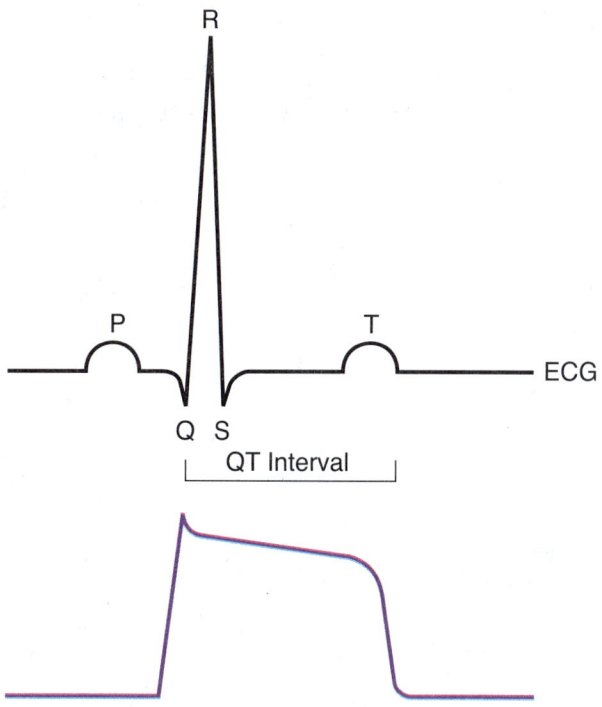

Figure 4-6. Ventricular Action Potential Versus ECG

Excitation-Contraction Coupling 5

Learning Objectives

❏ Interpret scenarios on skeletal muscle structure-function relationships

❏ Interpret scenarios on regulation of cytosolic calcium

❏ Interpret scenarios on altering force in skeletal muscle

❏ Interpret scenarios on comparison of striated muscles (skeletal vs. cardiac)

SKELETAL MUSCLE STRUCTURE–FUNCTION RELATIONSHIPS

Ultrastructure of a Myofibril

- A muscle is made up of individual cells called muscle fibers.
- Longitudinally within the muscle fibers, there are bundles of myofibrils. A magnified portion is shown in the figure below.
- A myofibril can be subdivided into individual sarcomeres. A sarcomere is demarked by a Z lines.
- Sarcomeres are composed of filaments creating bands as illustrated below.
- Contraction causes no change in the length of the A band, a shortening of the I band, and a shortening in the H zone (band).
- Titin anchors myosin and is an important component of striated muscle's elasticity.

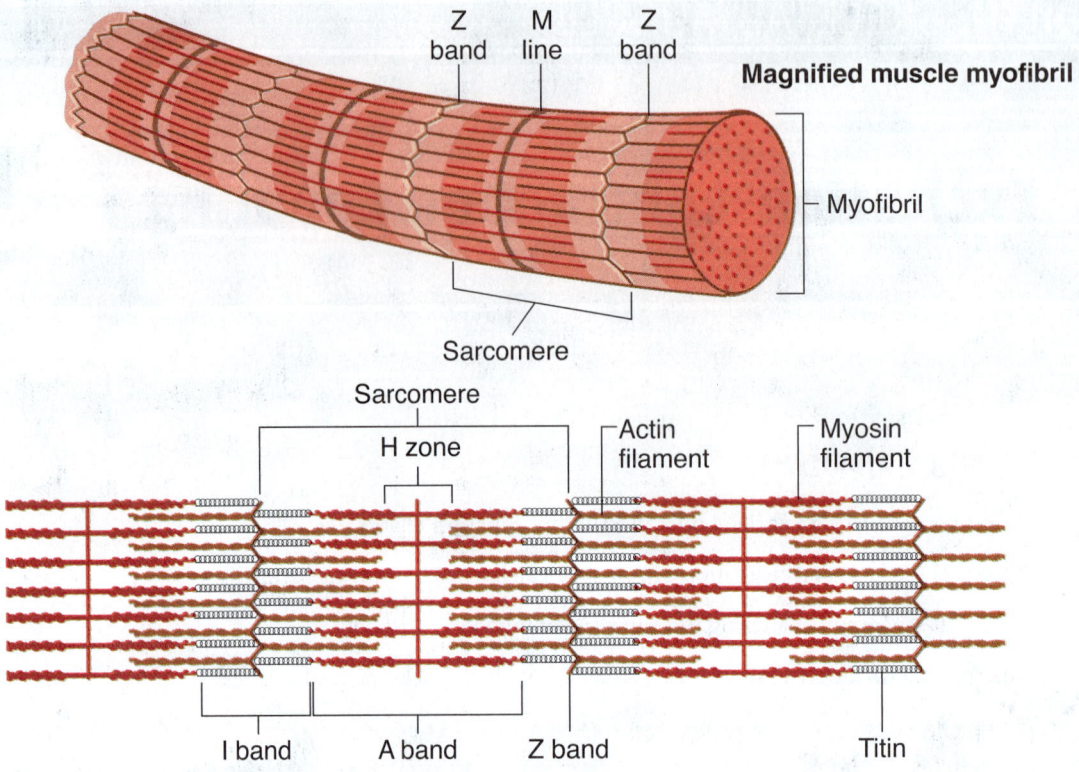

Figure 5-1. Organization of Sarcomeres

Ultrastructure of the Sarcoplasmic Reticulum

The external and internal membrane system of a skeletal muscle cell is displayed below.

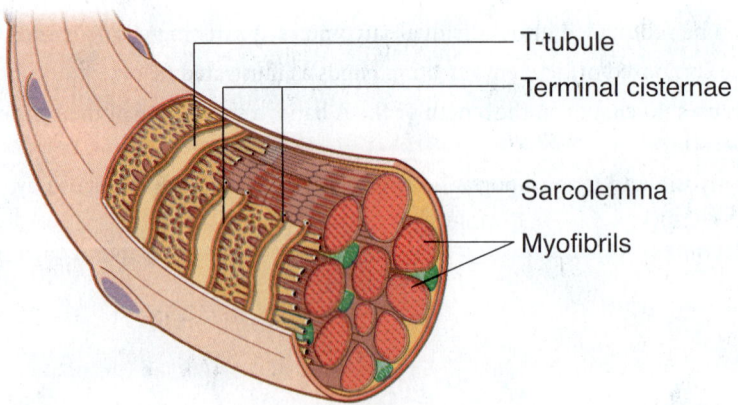

Figure 5-2. Skeletal Muscle Cell Membranes

T-tubule membranes are extensions of the surface membrane; therefore, the interiors of the T tubules are part of the extracellular compartment.

Terminal cisternae: The sarcoplasmic reticulum is part of the internal membrane system, one function of which is to store calcium. In skeletal muscle, most of the calcium is stored in the terminal cisternae close to the T-tubule system.

Functional Proteins of the Sarcomere

The following figure shows the relationships among the various proteins that make up the thin and thick filaments in striated muscle (skeletal and cardiac) and the changes that occur with contraction.

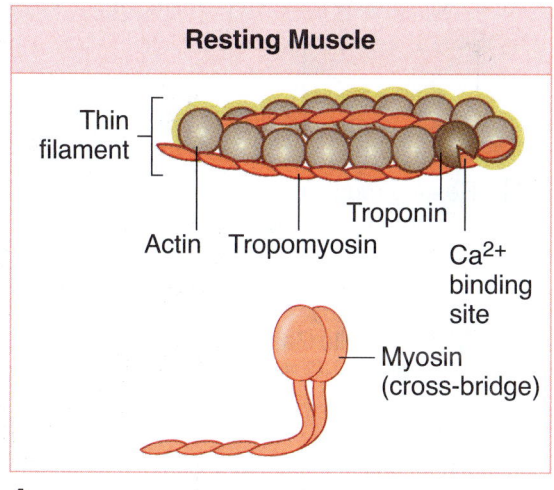

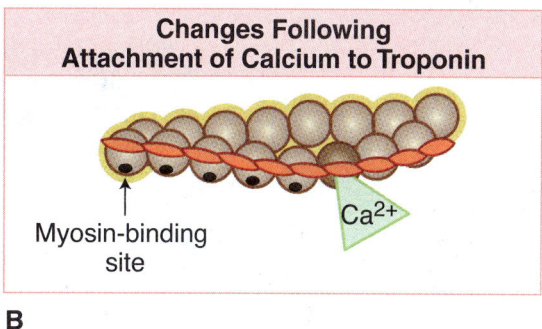

Figure 5-3. Regulation of Actin by Troponin

Proteins of the thin filaments

- **Actin** is the structural protein of the thin filament. It possesses attachment sites for myosin.
- **Tropomyosin** blocks myosin binding sites on actin.
- **Troponin** is composed of three subunits: **troponin-T** (binds to tropomyosin), **troponin-I** (binds to actin and inhibits contraction), and **troponin-C** (binds to calcium).
  - Under resting conditions, no calcium is bound to the troponin, preventing actin and myosin from interacting.
  - When calcium binds to troponin-C, the troponin-tropomyosin complex moves, exposing actin's binding site for myosin. (Figure 5-3B)

Proteins of the thick filaments

Myosin has ATPase activity. The splitting of ATP puts myosin in a "high energy" state; it also increases myosin's affinity for actin.

- Once myosin binds to actin, the chemical energy is transferred to mechanical energy, causing myosin to pull the actin filament. This generates active tension in the muscle and is commonly referred to as "the power stroke."
- If the force generated by the power stroke is sufficient to move the load (see next chapter), then the muscle shortens (isotonic contraction).
- If the force generated is not sufficient to move the load (see next chapter), then the muscle doesn't shorten (isometric contraction).

Cross-Bridge Interactions (Chemical-Mechanical Transduction)

The following figure illustrates the major steps involved in cross-bridge cycling in a contracting muscle.

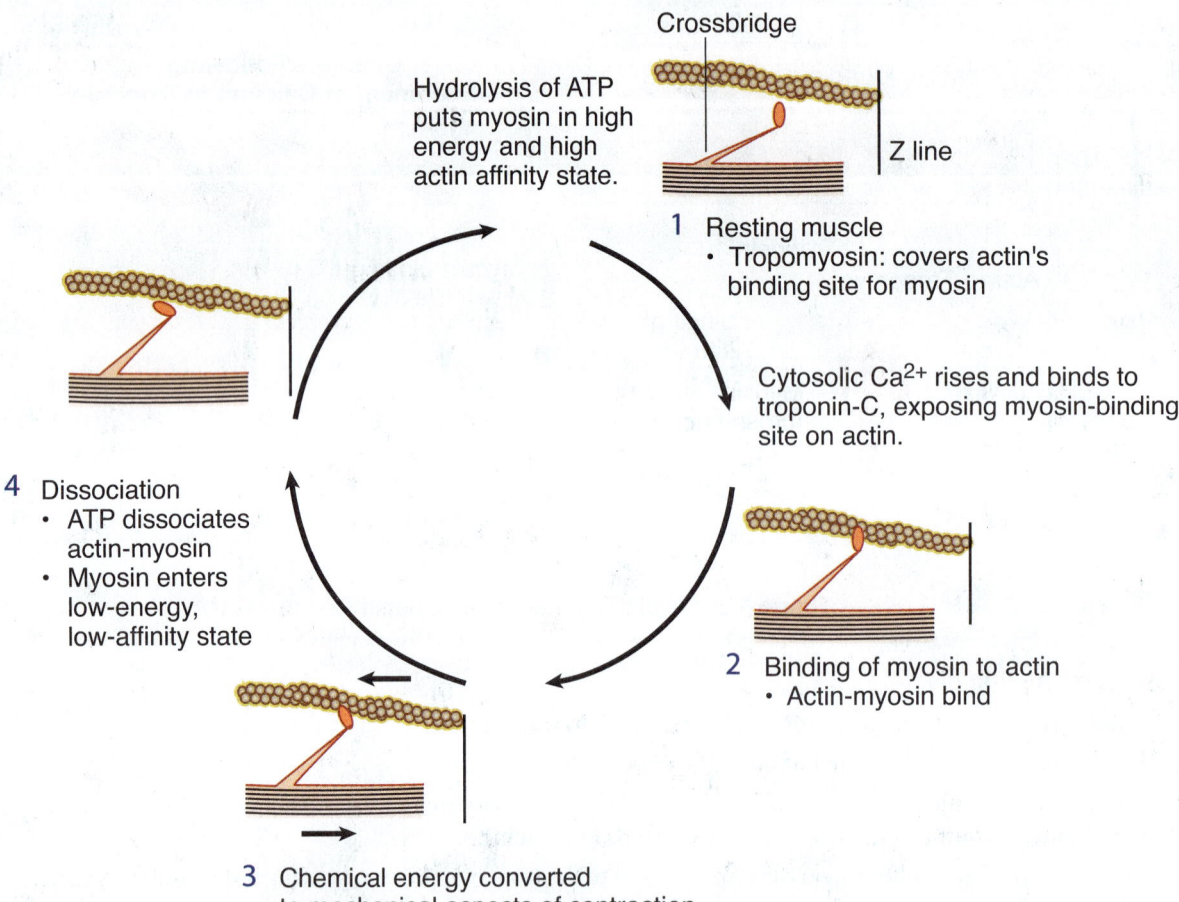

Figure 5-4. Crossbridge Cycling During Contraction

- Cross-bridge cycling starts when free calcium is available and attaches to troponin, which in turn moves tropomyosin so that myosin binds to actin.
- Contraction is the continuous cycling of cross-bridges.
- ATP is not required to form the cross-bridge linking to actin but is required to break the link with actin.
- Cross-bridge cycling (contraction) continues until either of the following occurs:
  - Withdrawal of Ca^{2+}: cycling stops at position 1 (normal resting muscle)
  - ATP is depleted: cycling stops at position 3 (rigor mortis; this would not occur under physiologic conditions)

REGULATION OF CYTOSOLIC CALCIUM

The sarcoplasmic reticulum (SR) has a high concentration of Ca^{2+}. Thus, there is a strong electrochemical gradient for Ca^{2+} to diffuse from the SR into the cytosol. There are two key receptors involved in the flux of Ca^{2+} from the SR into the cytosol: dihydropyridine (DHP) and ryanodine (RyR).

Dihydropyridine (DHP)

- DHP is a voltage-gated Ca^{2+} channel located in the sarcolemmal membrane
- Although it is a voltage-gated Ca^{2+} channel, Ca^{2+} **does not** flux through this receptor in skeletal muscle. Rather, DHP functions as a voltage-sensor.
- When skeletal muscle is at rest, DHP blocks RyR.

Ryanodine Receptor (RyR)

- RyR is a calcium channel on the SR membrane.
- When the muscle is in the resting state, RyR is blocked by DHP. Thus, Ca^{2+} is prevented from diffusing into the cytosol.

Sequence

1. Skeletal muscle action potential is initiated at the neuromuscular junction.
2. The action potential travels down the T-tubule.
3. The voltage change causes a conformation shift in DHP (voltage sensor), removing its block of RyR (Figure 5-5B).
4. Removal of the DHP block allows Ca^{2+} to diffuse into the cytosol (follows its concentration gradient).
5. The rise in cytosolic Ca^{2+} opens more RyR channels (calcium-induced calcium release).
6. Ca^{2+} binds to troponin-C, which in turn initiates cross-bridge cycle, creating active tension.
7. Ca^{2+} is pumped back into the SR by a calcium ATPase on the SR membrane called sarcoplasmic endoplasmic reticulum calcium ATPase (SERCA).
8. The fall in cytosolic Ca^{2+} causes tropomyosin to once again cover actin's binding site for myosin and the muscle relaxes, provided of course ATP is available to dissociate actin and myosin.

Key Points

- Contraction-relaxation states are determined by cytosolic levels of Ca^{2+}.
- The source of the calcium that binds to the troponin-C in skeletal muscle is solely from the cell's sarcoplasmic reticulum. Thus, no extracellular Ca^{2+} is involved.
- Two ATPases are involved in contraction:
  - **Myosin ATPase** supplies the energy for the mechanical aspects of contraction by putting myosin in a high energy and affinity state.
  - **SERCA** pumps Ca^{2+} back into the SR to terminate the contraction, i.e., causes relaxation.

ALTERING FORCE IN SKELETAL MUSCLE

Mechanical Response to a Single Action Potential

The following figure illustrates the mechanical contraction of skeletal muscle and the action potential on the same time scale.

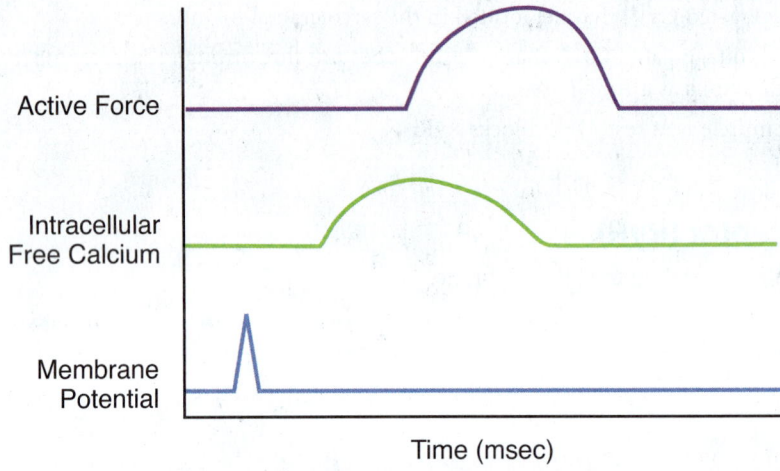

Figure 5-5. The Time Course of Events During Contraction

- Note the sequence of events: action potential causes Ca^{2+} release.
- Release of Ca^{2+} evokes muscle contraction (twitch).
- Note that the muscle membrane has completely repolarized well before the start of force development.

Summation and Recruitment

Under normal circumstances, enough Ca^{2+} is released by a single muscle action potential to completely saturate all the troponin-C binding sites. This means all available cross-bridges are activated and thus force cannot be enhanced by increasing cytosolic Ca^{2+}. Instead, peak force in skeletal muscle is increased in two ways: summation and recruitment.

Summation

- Because the membrane has repolarized well before force development, multiple action potentials can be generated prior to force development.
- Each action potential causes a pulse of Ca^{2+} release.
- Each pulse of Ca^{2+} initiates cross-bridge cycling and because the muscle has not relaxed, the mechanical force adds onto (summates) the force from the previous action potential (Figure 5-7).
- This summation can continue until the muscle tetanizes in which case there is sufficient free Ca^{2+} so that cross-bridge cycling is continuous.

Recruitment

- A single alpha motor neuron innervates multiple muscle fibers. The alpha motor neuron and all the fibers it innervates is called a motor-unit.

- Recruitment means activating more motor units, which in turn engage more muscle fibers, causing greater force production.

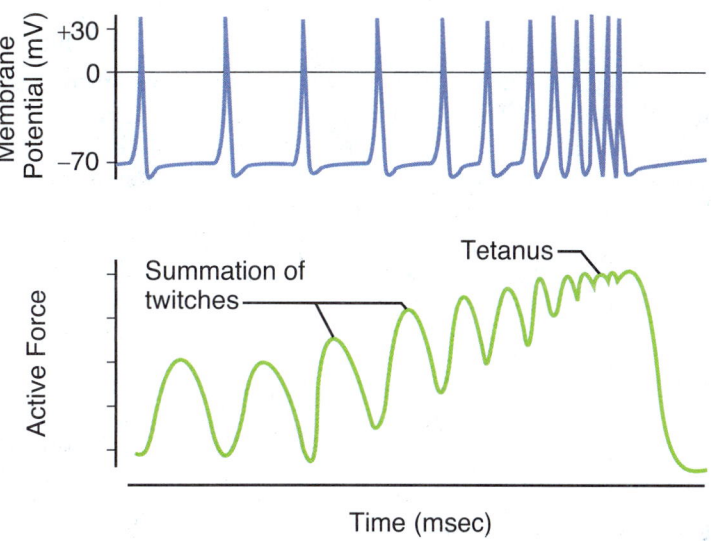

Figure 5-6. Summation of Individual Twitches and Fusion into Tetanus

COMPARISON OF STRIATED MUSCLES (SKELETAL VS. CARDIAC)

Skeletal and cardiac muscle are both striated muscle and share many similarities. Nevertheless, there are important differences.

Similarities

- Both have the same functional proteins, i.e., actin, tropomyosin, troponin, myosin, and titin.
- A rise in cytosolic Ca^{2+} initiates cross-bridge cycling thereby producing active tension.
- ATP plays the same role.
- Both have SERCA.
- Both have RyR receptors on the SR and thus show calcium-induced calcium release.

Differences

- Extracellular Ca^{2+} is involved in cardiac contractions, but not skeletal muscle. This extracellular Ca^{2+} causes calcium-induced calcium release in cardiac cells.

- Magnitude of SR Ca^{2+} release can be altered in cardiac (see section on cardiac mechanics), but not skeletal muscle.

- Cardiac cells are electrically coupled by gap junctions, which do not exist in skeletal muscle.

- Cardiac myocytes remove cytosolic Ca^{2+} by two mechanisms: SERCA and a Na^+—Ca^{2+} exchanger (3 Na^+ in, 1 Ca^{2+} out) on the sarcolemmal membrane. Skeletal muscle only utilizes SERCA.

- Cardiac cells have a prolonged action potential (Figure 5-7). This figure illustrates that the twitch tension is already falling (muscle starting to relax) while the action potential is still in the absolute refractory period. Thus, a second action potential cannot be evoked before the mechanical event is almost completed. This approximately equal mechanical and electrical event prevents summation of the force and if the muscle can't summate, it can't tetanize.

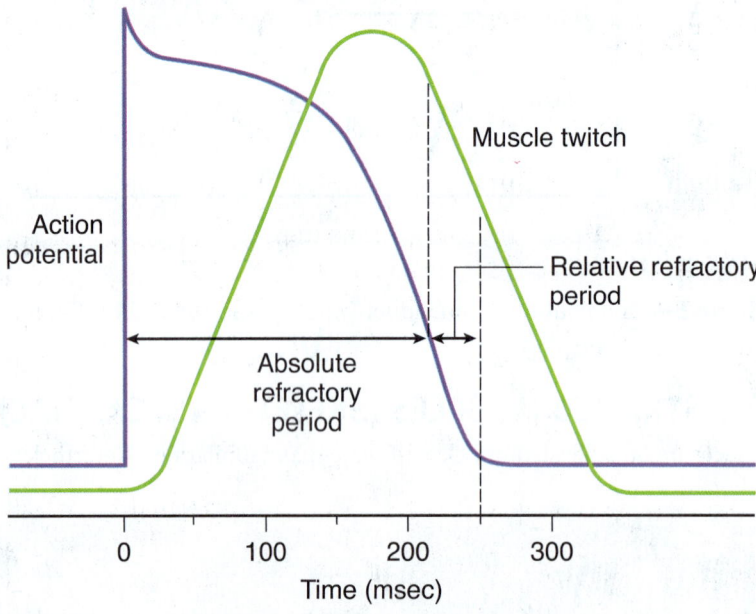

Figure 5-7. Force and Refractory Periods

Skeletal Muscle Mechanics

6

Learning Objectives

❏ Use knowledge of overview of muscle mechanics

❏ Interpret scenarios on length-tension curves

❏ Use knowledge of relationship between velocity and load

❏ Demonstrate understanding of properties of white vs. red muscle

❏ Solve problems concerning comparison of muscle types

OVERVIEW OF MUSCLE MECHANICS

Preload

Preload is the load on a muscle in a relaxed state, i.e., before it contracts. Applying preload to muscle does two things:

- Stretches the muscle: This in turn, stretches the sarcomere. **The greater the preload, the greater the stretch of the sarcomere.**

- Generates passive tension in the muscle: Muscle is elastic (see titin, previous chapter) and thus "resists" the stretch applied to it. Think of the "snap-back" that occurs when one stretches a rubber band. The force of this resistance is measured as passive tension. **The greater the preload, the greater the passive tension in the muscle.**

Afterload

Afterload is the load the muscle works against. If one wants to lift a 10 Kg weight, then this weight represents the afterload. Using the 10 kg weight example, two possibilities exist:

- If the muscle generates more than 10 kg of force, then the weight moves as the muscle shortens. This is an **isotonic contraction**.

- If the muscle is unable to generate more than 10 kg of force, then the muscle won't shorten. This is an **isometric contraction**.

- Types of tension
  - Passive: Produced by the preload
  - Active: Produced by cross-bridge cycling (described in previous chapter)
  - Total: The sum of active and passive tension

LENGTH–TENSION CURVES

Length–tension curves are important for understanding both skeletal and cardiac muscle function. The graphs that follow are all generated from skeletal muscle in vitro, but the information can be applied to both skeletal muscle and heart muscle in vivo.

Passive Tension Curve

The green line in Figure 6-1 shows that muscle behaves like a rubber band. The elastic properties of the muscle resist this stretch and the resulting tension is recorded. There is a direct (non-linear) relationship between the degree of stretch and the passive tension created that resists this stretch.

Point A: No preload, thus no stretch and no passive tension

Point B: Preload of 1 g stretches muscle, thus increasing its resting length, resulting in ~1 g of passive tension

Point C: Preload of 5 g increases muscle stretch, producing a greater resting length and thus a greater passive tension

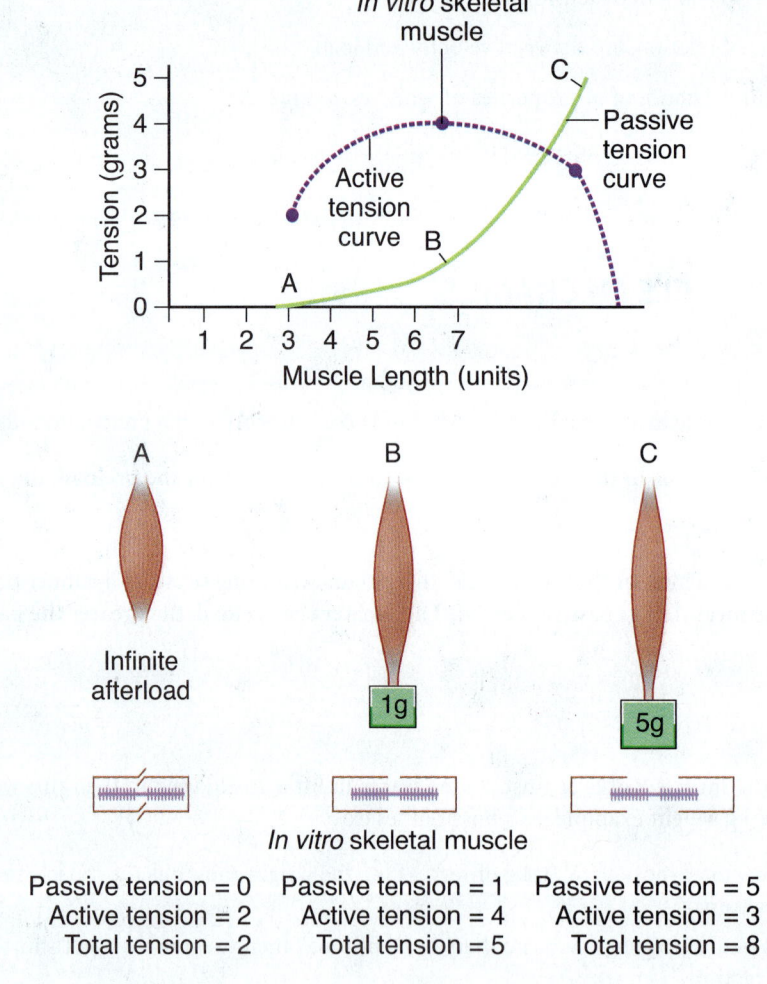

Figure 6-1. Preload, Active and Passive Tension: The Length–Tension Relationship

Active Tension

The purple line in Figure 6-1 shows the tension developed by stimulating the muscle to contract at the different preloads. In this example, the contraction is a **maximal isometric contraction**, i.e., the contraction produces tension, but the afterload is much greater than the tension the muscle develops and thus the muscle doesn't shorten. Recall that active tension represents the force generated by cross-bridge cycling. It is important to note the shape (bell-shaped) of the active tension curve.

- Preload of A: When there is no preload, the evoked muscle contraction develops ~2 g of active tension.

- Preload of B: At this preload, the active tension produced by stimulation of the muscle is greater, ~4 g.

- Preload of C: This preload results in less active tension than the previous preload. Thus, active tension increases as the muscle is stretched, up to a point. If stretched beyond this point, then active tension begins to fall.

- Optimal length (L_o): L_o represents the muscle length (preload) that produces the greatest active tension. In Figure 6-1, this occurs at the preload designated by B.

Explanation of Bell-shaped Active Tension Curve

Figure 6-1 shows a simplified picture of a sarcomere. Actin is the thin brown line, while myosin is depicted in purple. The magnitude of active tension depends on the number of actin-myosin cross-bridges that can form (directly related).

- Preload A: actin filaments overlap
  - Thus, the force that can be exerted by myosin tugging the actin is compromised and the active tension is less.
- Preload B (L_o): all myosin heads can bind to actin, and there is separation of actin filaments
  - Thus, active tension generated is greatest here because there is optimal overlap of actin and myosin.
- Preload C: the stretch is so great that actin has been pulled away from some of the myosin filament, and thus fewer actin-myosin interactions are available, resulting in diminished active tension.
  - If taken to the extreme, greater stretch could pull actin such that no actin-myosin interactions can occur, and thus no active tension results (active tension curve intersects the X-axis). This is an experimental, rather than physiologic phenomenon.
- Total tension: sum of passive and active tension (bottom of Figure 6-1)

RELATIONSHIP BETWEEN VELOCITY AND LOAD

The following graph shows that the maximum velocity of shortening (Vmax) occurs when there is no afterload on the muscle. Increasing afterload decreases velocity, and when afterload exceeds the maximum force generated by the muscle, shortening does not occur (isometric contraction).

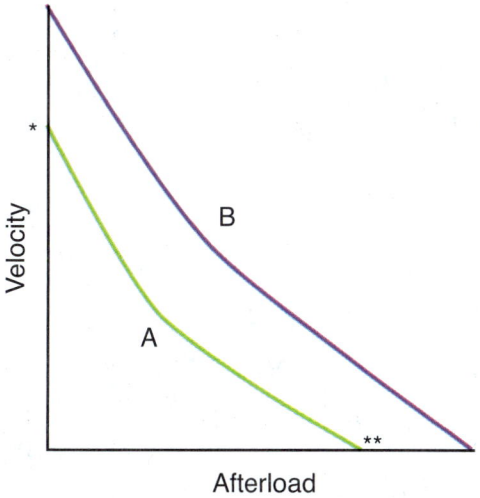

Figure 6-2. Force–Velocity Curve

In Figure 6-2:

*Maximum velocity (Vmax) is determined by the muscle's ATPase activity. It is the ATPase activity that determines a fast versus a slow muscle.

**Maximum force generated by a muscle. This occurs when summation is maximal (complete summation) and all motor units for the given muscle are fully recruited. The absolute amount of force is directly related to muscle mass and preload, with the greatest force occurring when the preload is at L_o.

Muscle A: a smaller, slower muscle (red muscle)

Muscle B: a larger, faster muscle (white muscle)

As load increases, the distance shortened during a single contraction decreases. So, with increased afterload, both the velocity of contraction and the distance decrease.

PROPERTIES OF WHITE VS. RED MUSCLE

White Muscle

Generally, this is the large (powerful) muscle that is utilized short-term, e.g., ocular muscles, leg muscles of a sprinter. Major characteristics are as follows:

- Large mass per motor unit
- High ATPase activity (fast muscle)
- High capacity for anaerobic glycolysis
- Low myoglobin

Red Muscle

Generally, this is the smaller (less powerful) muscle utilized long-term (endurance muscle), e.g., postural muscle. Major characteristics are as follows:

- Small mass per motor unit
- Lower ATPase activity (slower muscle)
- High capacity for aerobic metabolism (mitochondria)
- High myoglobin (imparts red color)

COMPARISON OF MUSCLE TYPES

Table 6-1. Histologic Features of Skeletal, Cardiac, and Smooth Muscle

Skeletal	Cardiac	Smooth
Striated	Striated	Nonstriated
Actin and myosin form sarcomeres	Actin and myosin form sarcomeres	Actin and myosin not organized into sarcomeres
Sarcolemma lacks junctional complexes between fibers	Junctional complexes between fibers including gap junctions	Gap junctions
Each fiber innervated	Electrical syncytium	Electrical syncytium
Troponin to bind calcium	Troponin to bind calcium	Calmodulin to bind calcium
High ATPase activity (fast muscle)	Intermediate ATPase activity	Low ATPase activity (slow muscle)
Extensive sarcoplasmic reticulum	Intermediate sarcoplasmic reticulum	Limited sarcoplasmic reticulum
T tubules form triadic contacts with reticulum at A-I junctions	T tubules form dyadic contact with reticulum near Z lines	Lack T tubules, SR controlled by second messengers
Surface membrane lacks calcium channels	Voltage-gated calcium channels	Voltage-gated calcium channels

Cardiac Muscle Mechanics **7**

Learning Objectives

❏ Answer questions about systolic performance of the ventricle

❏ Explain information related to ventricular function curves

❏ Solve problems concerning chronic changes: systolic and diastolic dysfunction

SYSTOLIC PERFORMANCE OF THE VENTRICLE

Systolic performance actually means the overall force generated by the ventricular muscle during systole. The heart does two things in systole: pressurizes and ejects blood. An important factor influencing this systolic performance is the number of cross-bridges cycling during contraction.

The greater the number of cross-bridges cycling, the greater the force of contraction.

Systolic performance is determined by three independent variables:

- Preload
- Contractility
- Afterload

These three factors are summed together to determine the overall systolic performance of the ventricle. Recent work has demonstrated that they are not completely independent, but the generalizations made here will apply to the physiologic and clinical setting.

Preload

As in skeletal muscle, preload is the load on the muscle in the relaxed state.

More specifically, it is the load or prestretch on ventricular muscle at the end of diastole.

Preload on ventricular muscle is not measured directly; rather, indices are utilized.

The best indices of preload on ventricular muscle are those measured directly in the ventricles. Indices of left ventricular preload:

- Left ventricular end-diastolic volume (LVEDV)
- Left ventricular end-diastolic pressure (LVEDP)

Possibly somewhat less reliable indices of left ventricular preload are those measured in the venous system.

- Central venous pressure (CVP)
- Pulmonary capillary wedge pressure (PCWP)
- Right atrial pressure (RAP)

Pulmonary wedge pressure, sometimes called pulmonary capillary wedge pressure, is measured from the tip of a Swan-Ganz catheter, which, after passing through the right heart, has been wedged in a small pulmonary artery. The tip is pointing downstream toward the pulmonary capillaries, and the pressure measured at the tip is probably very close to pulmonary capillary pressure. Since the vessel is occluded and assuming minimal flow, the pressure is probably also very close to left atrial pressure as well. A rise in pulmonary capillary wedge pressure is evidence of an increase in preload on the left ventricle. In some cases, such as in mitral stenosis, it is not a good index of left ventricular preload.

Along similar lines, measurement of systemic central venous pressure is used as an index of preload.

Preload factor in systolic performance (Frank-Starling mechanism)

The preload effect can be explained on the basis of a change in sarcomere length. This is illustrated in the following graphs.

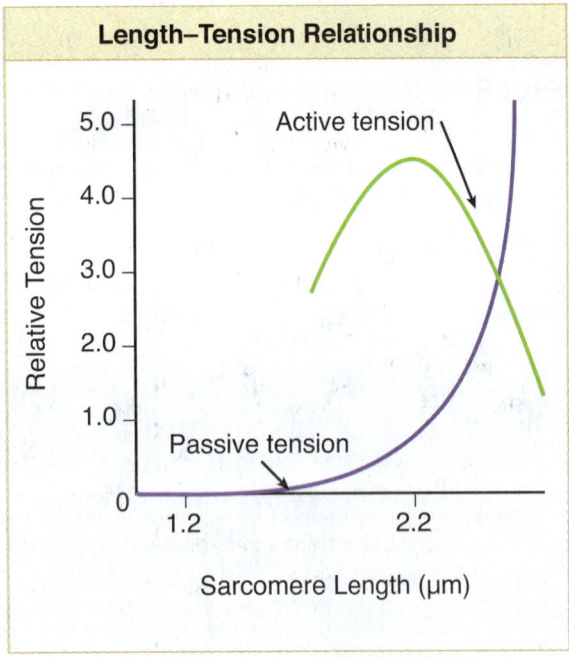
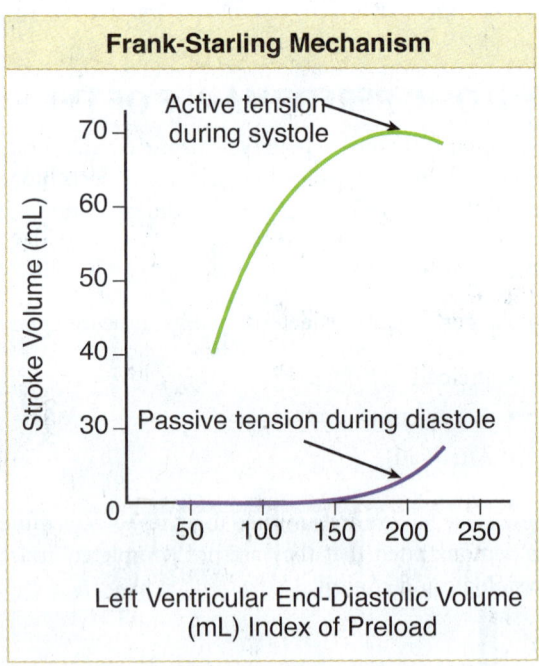

Figure 7-1. Length–Tension Relationships in Skeletal and Cardiac Muscle

The resting length of skeletal muscle *in vivo* is at a sarcomere length close to the optimum for maximal cross-bridge linking between actin and myosin during contraction (L_o).

Heart muscle at the end of diastole is below this point. Thus, in a normal heart, increased preload increases sarcomere length toward the optimum actin-myosin overlap. This results in more cross-linking and a more forceful contraction during systole.

Contractility (Inotropic State)

An acceptable definition of *contractility* would be a change in performance at a given preload and afterload. Thus, contractility is a change in the force of contraction at any given sarcomere length.

- Acute changes in contractility are due to changes in the intracellular dynamics of calcium.
- Drugs that increase contractility usually provide more calcium and at a faster rate to the contractile machinery.
- More calcium increases the availability of cross-link sites on the actin, increasing cross-linking and the force of contraction during systole.
- Calcium dynamics do not explain chronic losses in contractility, which in most cases are due to overall myocyte dysfunction.

Afterload

Afterload is defined as the "load" that the heart must eject blood against. Exactly what constitutes afterload to the heart is the subject of much debate. Probably, the best "marker" of afterload is systemic vascular resistance (SVR), also called total peripheral resistance (TPR). However, TPR is not routinely calculated clinically and thus arterial pressure (diastolic, mean, or systolic) is often used as the index of afterload.

Afterload is increased in three main situations:

1. When aortic pressure is increased (elevated mean arterial pressure); for example, when hypertension increases the afterload, the left ventricle has to work harder to overcome the elevated arterial pressures.
2. When systemic vascular resistance is increased, resulting in increased resistance and decreased compliance
3. In aortic stenosis, resulting in pressure overload of the left ventricle

In general, when afterload increases, there is an initial fall in stroke volume.

VENTRICULAR FUNCTION CURVES

Ventricular function curves are an excellent graphical depiction of the effects of preload versus contractility and afterload.

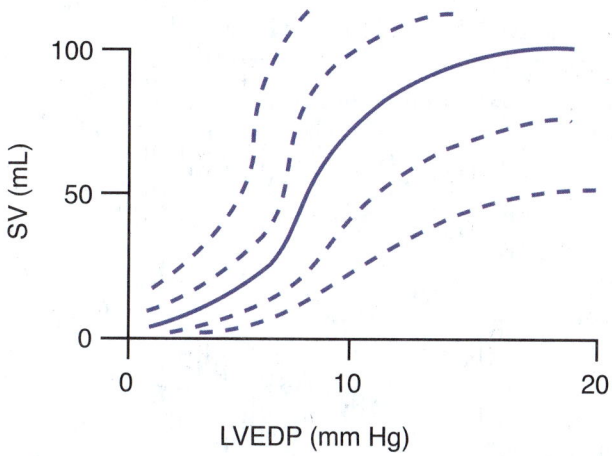

Figure 7-2. Family of Frank-Starling Curves

Changes in afterload and contractility shift the curve up or down, left or right.

There is no single Frank-Starling curve on which the ventricle operates. There is actually a family of curves, each of which is defined by the afterload and the inotropic state of the heart:

- Increasing afterload and decreasing contractility shift the curve down and to the right.
- Decreasing afterload and increasing contractility shift the curve up and to the left.

Ventricular Volumes

End-diastolic volume (EDV): volume of blood in the ventricle at the end of diastole

End-systolic volume (ESV): volume of blood in the ventricle at the end of systole

Stroke volume (SV): volume of blood ejected by the ventricle per beat

$$SV = EDV - ESV$$

Ejection Fraction (EF): EF = SV/EDV

(should be greater than 55% in a normal heart)

CHRONIC CHANGES: SYSTOLIC AND DIASTOLIC DYSFUNCTION

Systolic dysfunction can be defined as an abnormal reduction in ventricular emptying due to impaired contractility or excessive afterload.

Diastolic dysfunction is a decrease in ventricular compliance during the filling phase of the cardiac cycle due to either changes in tissue stiffness or impaired ventricular relaxation. The consequence is a diminished Frank-Starling mechanism.

Pressure Overload

- Examples of a pressure overload on the left ventricle include hypertension and aortic stenosis.
- Initially, there is no decrease in cardiac output or an increase in preload since the cardiac function curve shifts to the left (increased performance due to increased contractility).
- Chronically, in an attempt to normalize wall tension (actually internal wall stress), the ventricle develops a concentric hypertrophy. There is a dramatic increase in wall thickness and a decrease in chamber diameter.
- The consequence of concentric hypertrophy (new sarcomes laid down in parallel, i.e., the myofibril thickens) is a decrease in ventricular compliance and diastolic dysfunction, followed eventually by a systolic dysfunction and ventricular failure.

Volume Overload

- Examples of a volume overload on the left ventricle include mitral and aortic insufficiency and patent ductus arteriosus.
- Fairly well tolerated if developed slowly. A large acute volume overload less well tolerated and can precipitate heart failure.
- Due to the LaPlace relationship, a dilated left ventricle must develop a greater wall tension to produce the same ventricular pressures.

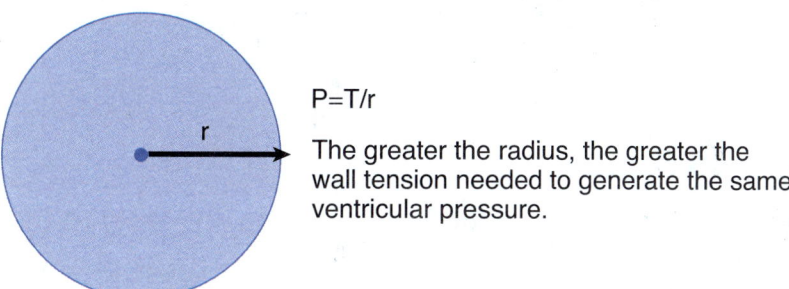

$P=T/r$

The greater the radius, the greater the wall tension needed to generate the same ventricular pressure.

Figure 7-3.

- Chronically, in an attempt to normalize wall tension (actually external wall stress), the ventricle develops an eccentric hypertrophy (new sarcomeres laid down end-to-end, i.e., the myofibril lengthens). As cardiac volumes increase, there is a modest increase in wall thickness that does not reduce chamber size.

- Compliance of the ventricle is not compromised and diastolic function is maintained.

- Eventual failure is usually a consequence of systolic dysfunction.

General Aspects of the Cardiovascular System

8

Learning Objectives

❑ Demonstrate understanding of overview of the cardiovascular system

❑ Demonstrate understanding of hemodynamics and wall tension

❑ Use knowledge of vessel compliance

❑ Answer questions about characteristics of systemic arteries

❑ Answer questions about baroreceptor reflex and the control of blood pressure

OVERVIEW OF THE CARDIOVASCULAR SYSTEM

The following figure illustrates the general organization of the cardiovascular system.

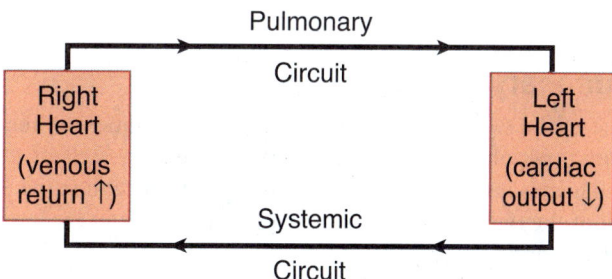

Figure 8-1. Overview of Circulatory System

In a Nutshell

The function of the heart is to transport blood and deliver oxygen in order to maintain adequate tissue perfusion. It also removes waste products, e.g., CO_2 created by tissue metabolism.

Because the heart is a "demand pump" that pumps out whatever blood comes back into it from the venous system, it is effectively the amount of blood returning to the heart that determines how much blood the heart pumps out.

The cardiovascular system consists of two pumps (left and right ventricles) and two circuits (pulmonary and systemic) connected in series.

- When circuits are connected in series, flow must be equal in the two circuits.
- Cardiac output is the output of either the left or right ventricle, and because of the series system, they are equal.
- The chemical composition of pulmonary venous blood is very close to the chemical composition of systemic arterial blood.
- Systemic mixed venous blood entering the right atrium has the same composition as pulmonary arterial blood.

Table 8-1. Pressure Differential

Pressures in the Pulmonary Circulation		Pressures in the Systemic Circulation	
Right ventricle	25/0 mm Hg	Left ventricle	120/0 mm Hg
Pulmonary artery	25/8 mm Hg	Aorta	120/80 mm Hg
Mean pulm. art.	15 mm Hg	Mean art. blood p	93 mm Hg
Capillary	7–9 mm Hg	Capillary: skeletal renal glomerular	30 mm Hg 45–50 mm Hg
Pulmonary venous	5 mm Hg	Peripheral veins	15 mm Hg
Left atrium	5–10 mm Hg	Right atrium (central venous)	0 mm Hg
Pressure gradient	15–5 = 10 mm Hg	Pressure gradient	93–0 = 93 mm Hg

Systemic versus Pulmonary Circuit

Cardiac output and heart rate of the two circuits are equal, so stroke volumes are the same. Despite this, all pressures are higher in the systemic (peripheral) circuit. This shows that the vessels of the circuits are very different. The systemic circuit has much higher resistance and much lower compliance than the pulmonary circuit. The lower pressures mean that the work of the right ventricle is much lower. In addition, the lower capillary pressure protects against the development of pulmonary edema.

Structure–Function Relationships of the Systemic Circuit

The following figure shows that the systemic circuit is a branching circuit. It begins as a large single vessel, the aorta, and branches extensively into progressively smaller vessels until the capillaries are reached. The reverse then takes place in the venous circuit.

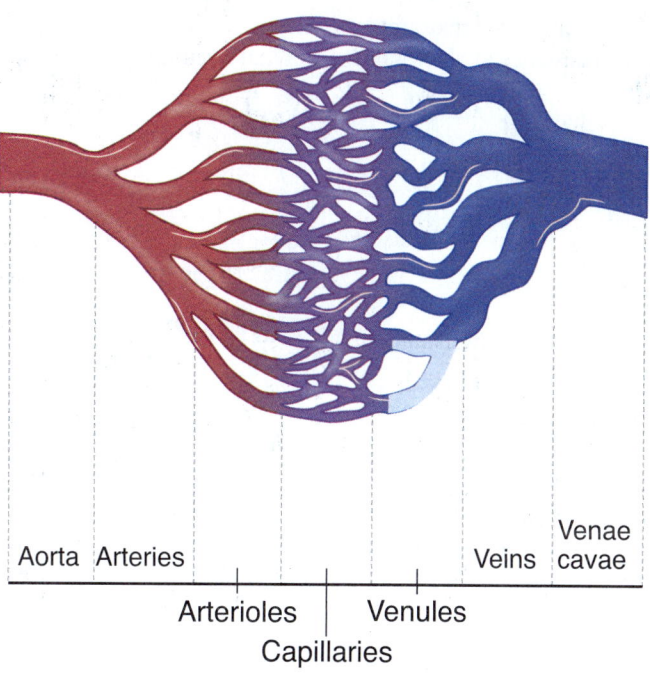

Figure 8-2. Organization of the Systemic Vessels

HEMODYNAMICS

Pressure, Flow, Resistance

The Poiseuille equation represents the relationship of flow, pressure, and resistance.

$$Q = \frac{P_1 - P_2}{R}$$

Q: flow (mL/min)
P_1: upstream pressure (pressure head) for segment or circuit (mm Hg)
P_2: pressure at the end of the segment or circuit (mm Hg)
R: resistance of vessels between P_1 and P_2 (mm Hg/mL/min)

It can be applied to a single vessel (Figure 8-3), an organ, or an entire circuit.

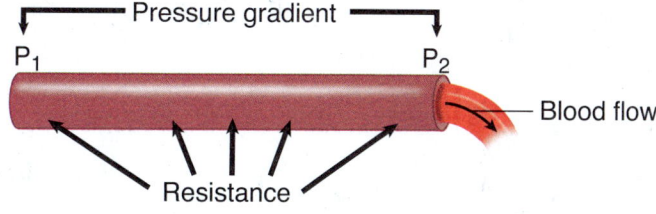

Figure 8-3. Poiseuille Equation Applied to Single Vessel

The flow to an organ such as the kidney, for example, could be calculated as mean arterial pressure minus renal venous pressure divided by the resistance of all vessels in the renal circuit.

Determinants of Resistance

$$\text{Resistance} = \frac{P_1 - P_2}{Q}$$

$$\text{Units of Resistance} = \frac{\text{mm Hg}}{\text{mL} / \text{min}} = \frac{\text{pressure}}{\text{volume} / \text{time}}$$

The resistance of a vessel is determined by 3 major variables: $R \propto \dfrac{\upsilon L}{r^4}$

Vessel Radius (r)

The most important factor determining resistance is the radius of the vessel. If resistance changes, then the following occurs:

- Increased resistance decreases blood flow, increases upstream pressure, and decreases downstream pressure.
- Decreased resistance increases blood flow, decreases upstream pressure and increases downstream pressure.
- The pressure "drop" (difference between upstream and downstream) is directly related to the resistance. There is a big pressure drop when resistance is a high and minimal pressure drop when resistance is a low.

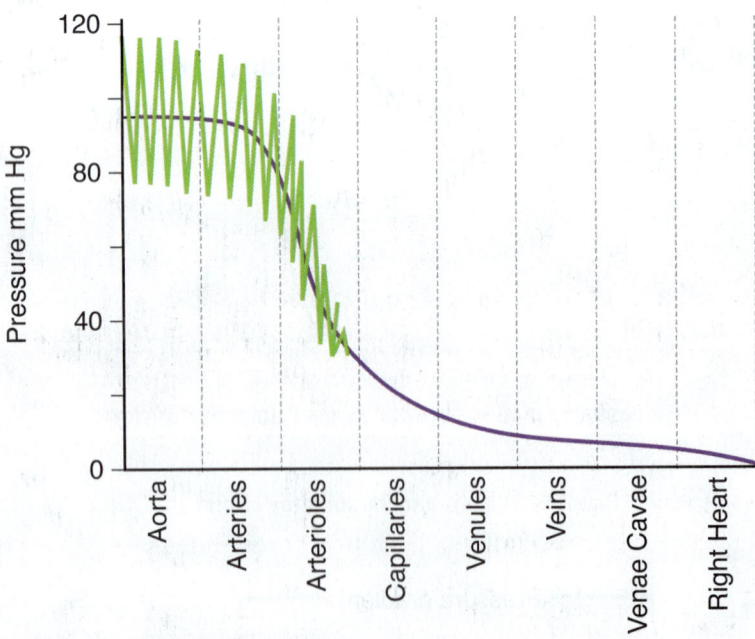

Figure 8-4. Systemic System Pressures

Whole body application of resistance

- Figure 8-4 shows, in a horizontal subject, the phasic and mean pressures from the aorta to the vena cava.
- Mean arterial pressure (MAP) is measured in the aorta and is about 93 mm Hg (time weighted average because more time is spent in diastole). This represents the pressure head (upstream pressure) for the systemic circulation.

- The pressure dissipates as the blood flows down the circulatory tree because of resistance. The amount of pressure lost in a particular segment is proportional to the resistance of that segment.

- There is a small pressure drop in the major arteries (low-resistance segment); the largest drop is across the arterioles (highest resistance segment), and another small pressure drop occurs in the major veins (low-resistance segment).

- Dilation of arterioles decreases arteriolar resistance, which increases flow, decreases upstream pressure (MAP), and increases downstream pressure (capillary pressure).

- Likewise, constriction of arterioles increases arteriolar resistance, which in turn decreases flow, increases upstream pressure (MAP), and decreases downstream pressure (capillary pressure).

- Since blood flows from high pressure to low pressure, the sequence of the vessels in any system or part of a system will also be the sequence of pressures, from highest to lowest.

Blood Viscosity (v)

Viscosity is a property of a fluid that is a measure of the fluid's internal resistance to flow:

- The greater the viscosity, the greater the resistance.
- The prime determinant of blood viscosity is the hematocrit.

    Figure 8-5 shows how viscosity varies with hematocrit.

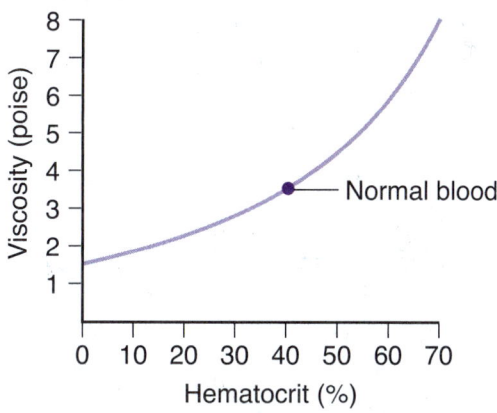

Figure 8-5. Effect of Hematocrit on Blood Viscosity

Anemia decreases viscosity. Polycythemia increases viscosity.

Note

What is the Hematocrit?

If a blood sample from an adult is centrifuged in a graduated test tube, the relative volume of packed red cells is termed the *hematocrit*. For a normal adult this volume is about 40–45% of the total, meaning the red cells occupy about 40–45% of the blood in the body. The white blood cells are less dense than the red blood cells and form a thin layer (the so-called buffy coat). This is why the hematocrit is a major determinant of blood viscosity.

Vessel Length (L)

The greater the length, the greater the resistance.

- If the length doubles, the resistance doubles.
- If the length decreases by half, the resistance decreases by half.
- Vessel length is constant; therefore, changes in length are not a physiologic factor in regulation of resistance, pressure, or flow.

Velocity

Velocity refers to the rate at which blood travels through a blood vessel. Although velocity is directly related to blood flow, it is different in that it refers to a rate, e.g., cm/sec. Mean linear velocity is equal to flow divided by the cross-sectional area (CSA). Thus, velocity is directly related to flow, but if CSA changes, then velocity is affected. The important functional applications of this are:

- CSA is high in capillaries, but low in the aorta.
- Velocity is therefore high in the aorta and low in the capillaries.
- The functional consequence of this is that low velocity in the capillaries optimizes exchange.
- The potential pathology of this is that because the aorta has high velocity and a large diameter, turbulent blood flow can occur here (see below).

Laminar versus Turbulent Flow

There can be two types of flow in a system: laminar and turbulent.

Characteristics of laminar flow:

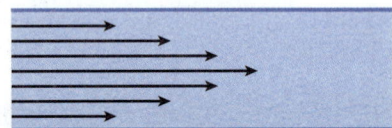

Figure 8-6. Laminar Flow

- As shown in Figure 8-6, laminar flow is flow in layers.
- Laminar flow occurs throughout the normal cardiovascular system, excluding flow in the heart.
- The layer with the highest velocity is in the center of the tube.

Characteristics of turbulent flow:

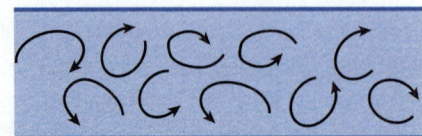

Figure 8-7. Turbulent Flow
>2,000 = turbent flow; <2,000 = laminar flow

As shown in Figure 8-7, turbulent flow is nonlayered flow.

- It creates murmurs. These are heard as bruits in vessels with severe stenosis.
- It produces more resistance than laminar flow.

Bridge to Pathology

Sepsis, anaphylaxis, and neurogenic shock are examples of uncontrolled vasodilation in the periphery, leading to diminished MAP.

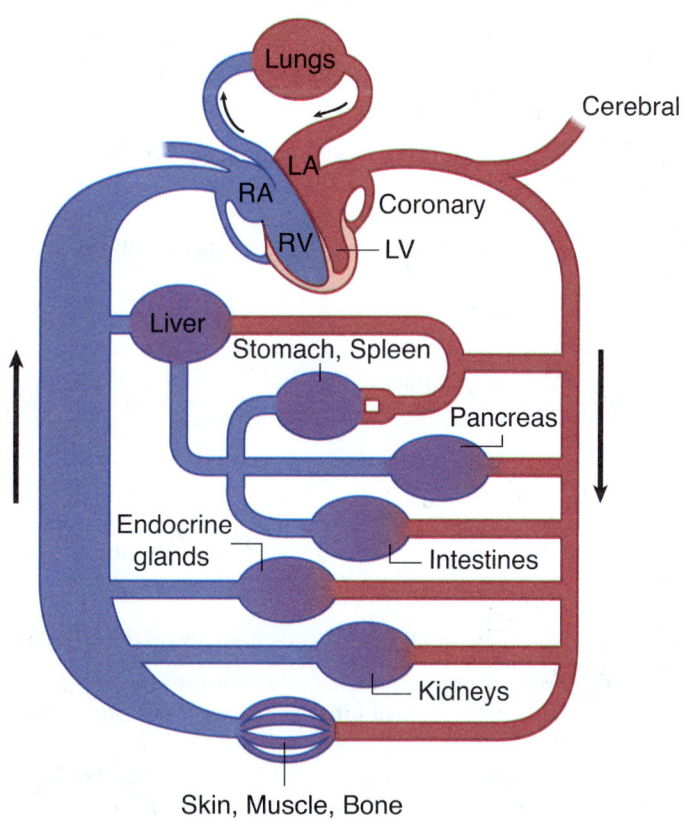

Figure 8-8. Systemic Circuit

WALL TENSION

LaPlace relationship:

$$\mathbf{T} \propto \mathbf{Pr}$$

T = wall tension
P = pressure
r = radius

The aorta is the artery with the greatest wall tension (greatest pressure and radius).

VESSEL COMPLIANCE

$$C = \frac{V}{P}$$

Compliance of a vessel can be calculated, but the resulting number is, for all practical purposes, meaningless. It is much more important to simply have a good concept of compliance and understand the differences in compliance among the vessels that make up the cardiovascular system.

- Compliance is essentially how easily a vessel is stretched. If a vessel is easily stretched, it is considered very compliant. The opposite is noncompliant or stiff.
- Elasticity is the inverse of compliance. A vessel that has high elasticity (a large tendency to rebound from a stretch) has low compliance.

Systemic Veins

Systemic veins are about 20 times more compliant than systemic arteries.

- Veins also contain about 70% of the systemic blood volume and thus represent the major blood reservoir.
- If blood is in the veins, then it is not available for the heart to pump and is thus not contributing to the circulating blood volume.

In short: When considering whole-body hemodynamics, compliance resides in the venous system. One must not forget the functional implications of arterial compliance, particularly with respect to arterial pressures (see below), but for the circulation as a whole, compliance is in the venous system.

Venous Return

To understand vascular function and thus ultimately the regulation of cardiac output, one can "split" the circulation into two components (Figure 8-9):

- Cardiac output (CO): flow of blood exiting the heart (down arrow on the arterial side).
- Venous return (VR): flow of blood returning to the heart (up arrow on the venous side). Because this is the flow of blood to the heart, it determines preload for the ventricles (assuming normal ventricular function).

Because the circulation is a closed system, these flows are intertwined and must be the same when one examines it "over time" or at steady-state. In addition, each flow is "dependent" on the other. For example:

- If CO fell to zero, then ultimately VR would become zero.
- If one were to stop VR, there would ultimately be no CO.

These are extreme examples to illustrate the point that altering one ultimately alters the other and a variety of factors can transiently or permanently alter each of the variables, resulting in the other variable being impacted to the same degree. In Section IV, chapter 1, we discussed ventricular function, which plays a pivotal role in CO. In this section, we discuss the regulation of VR. **VR represents vascular function** and thus understanding its regulation sets the stage for understanding CO regulation.

VR is the flow of blood back to the heart and it determines preload. Since it is a flow, it must follow the hemodynamic principles described above, i.e., it is directly proportional to the pressure gradient and inversely related to the resistance.

- **Right atrial pressure (RAP):** blood is flowing to the right atrium, thus RAP is the downstream pressure.
- **Mean systemic filling pressure (Psf):** represents the upstream pressure (pressure head) for VR.

Mean systemic filling pressure (Psf): Although not a "theoretical" pressure (as per numerous experiments, Psf is typically ~7 mm Hg prior to endogenous compensations), this is not a pressure that can be conveniently measured, particularly in a patient. However, because it is the pressure when no flow exists, it is primarily determined by volume and compliance (see Vessel Compliance above):

- Blood volume: There is a direct relation between blood volume and Psf. The greater the blood volume, the higher the Psf and vice versa.
- Venous compliance: There is an inverse relation between venous compliance and Psf. The more compliant the veins, the lower the Psf and vice versa.

Note
Engaging the muscle pump also increases Psf.

Because Psf is the pressure head (upstream pressure) driving VR, then VR is directly related to Psf. If all other factors are unchanged, it follows that:

- An increase in blood volume increases VR.
- A decrease in blood volume decreases VR.
- A decrease in venous compliance (sympathetic stimulation; muscle pump) increases VR.
- An increase in venous compliance (sympathetic inhibition; venodilators; alpha block) decreases VR.

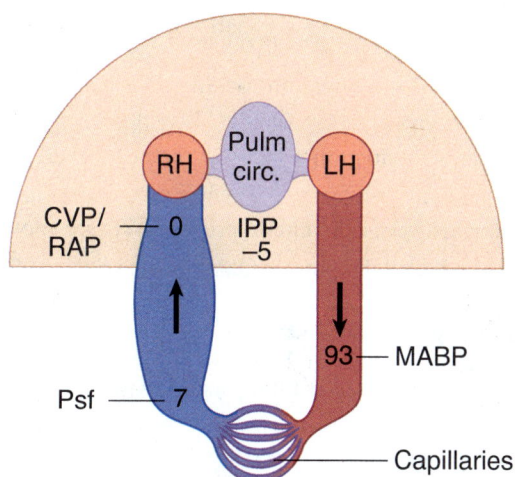

Figure 8-9. Pressure Gradients in the Circulatory System

CVP: central venous pressure
IPP: intrapleural pressure
LH: left heart
MABP: mean arterial blood pressure
Psf: mean systemic filling pressure
RH: right heart
RAP: right atrial pressure

DETERMINANTS OF CARDIAC OUTPUT

Because VR plays an important role in determining CO, we can now discuss the regulation of CO. The key point to remember is that **steady-state CO** is the interplay between **ventricular function** (see ventricular function curves in the previous chapter) and **vascular function**, which is defined by VR curves. The four determinants are:

- Heart rate
- Contractility
- Afterload
- Preload (determined by VR)

The latter three factors can be combined on CO/VR curves, which are illustrated and discussed later. Let's first start with heart rate.

Heart Rate (HR)

$$CO = HR \times SV \text{ (stroke volume)}$$

Although HR and CO are directly related, the effect of changes in HR on CO is complicated because the other variable, SV must be considered (Figure 8-10). High heart rates decrease filling time for the ventricles, and thus can decrease SV. In short, the effect of HR on CO depends upon the cause of the rise in HR.

Endogenously mediated tachycardia, e.g., exercise

In exercise, the rise in HR increases CO. Although filling time is reduced, a variety of changes occur that prevent SV from falling. These are:

- Sympathetic stimulation to the heart increases contractility. This helps maintain stroke volume. In addition, this decreases the systolic interval (see previous chapter) thus preserving some of the diastolic filling time.
- Sympathetic stimulation increases conduction velocity in the heart, thereby increasing the rate of transmission of the electrical impulse.
- Sympathetic stimulation venoconstricts, which helps preserve VR (see above) and ventricular filling.
- The skeletal muscle pump increases VR, helping to maintain ventricular filling.

Pathologically mediated tachycardia, e.g., tachyarrhythmias

- The sudden increase in HR curtails ventricular filling resulting in a fall in CO (Figure 8-10).
- Although the fall in CO decreases MAP and activates the sympathetic nervous system, this occurs "after the fact" and is thus unable to compensate.
- There is no muscle pump to increase VR.

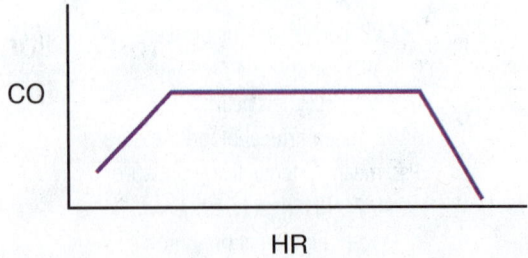

Figure 8-10.

Contractility

Contractility was discussed in depth in chapter 7 of Section IV. There is a direct relation between contractility and ventricular output, thus there is typically a direct relation between contractility and CO.

Afterload

Afterload is the load the heart works against and the best marker of afterload is TPR. This was also discussed in chapter 7. There is an inverse relation between afterload and ventricular output, thus there is generally an inverse relation between afterload and CO.

Preload

As discussed in chapter 7, there is a direct relation between preload and ventricular output (Frank-Starling). Presuming there is no change in contractility or afterload, increasing preload increases CO and vice versa.

Cardiac Output (CO)/Venous Return (VR) Curves

CO/VR curves (Figure 8-11) depict the interplay between ventricular and vascular function indicated in the venous return section above. Steady-state CO is determined by this interplay.

Ventricular function (solid line of Figure 8-11)

- X-axis is RAP, a marker of preload.
- Y-axis is CO.
- This curve shows that RAP has a positive impact on CO (Frank-Starling mechanism)

Vascular function (dashed line of Figure 8-11)

- X-axis is RAP, the downstream pressure for VR.
- Y-axis is VR.
- The curve shows that as RAP increases, VR decreases. This is because RAP is the downstream pressure for VR. As RAP increases, the pressure gradient for VR falls, which in turn decreases VR. Thus, RAP has a negative impact on VR.
- X-intercept for the VR curve is Psf (point B on the graph). This is the pressure in the circulation when there is no flow (see section on venous return). Psf is the pressure head (upstream pressure) for VR. Thus, when RAP = Psf, flow (VR) is zero.

Steady-state CO

- The intersection of the ventricular and vascular function curves determines steady-state CO (point A in Figure 8-11). In other words, point A represents the interplay between ventricular and vascular function.
- Discounting HR, the only way steady-state CO can change is if ventricular function, or vascular function, or both change.

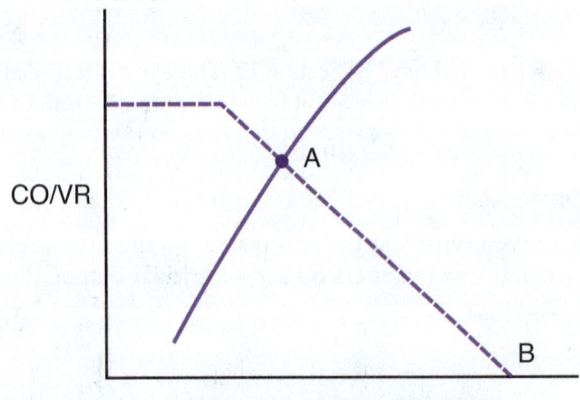

Figure 8-11.
A = steady-state cardiac output. All individuals operate at the intersection of the ventricular function and venous return curves. **B = mean systemic filling pressure (Psf).** This is directly related to vascular volume and inversely related to venous compliance.

Resistance

- The primary site of resistance for the circulation is the arterioles.
- If arterioles vasodilate (decreased resistance), VR increases (line A of Figure 8-12). Recall that VR is a flow, and thus decreasing resistance increases flow. Note that this vasodilation provides more VR (move up the Frank-Starling curve).

  Although not depicted in the graph, vasodilation decreases afterload and thus shifts the ventricular function curve up and to the left. In short, arteriolar vasodilation enhances both ventricular and vascular function.

- If arterioles vasoconstrict (increased resistance), VR falls (line B of Figure 8-12). Note that this vasoconstriction reduces VR, and steady-state CO falls as one moves down the Frank-Starling curve.

  Although not depicted in the graph, vasoconstriction increases afterload, shifting the ventricular function curve down and to the right. Thus, arteriolar vasoconstriction reduces both ventricular and vascular function.

Psf

- As indicated above (venous return section), Psf is directly related to blood volume and inversely related to venous compliance.
- Increasing vascular volume (infusion; activation of RAAS) or decreasing venous compliance (sympathetic stimulation; muscle pump; exercise; lying down) increases Psf, causing a right shift in the VR curve (line C of Figure 8-12). Thus, either of these changes enhances filling of the ventricles (move up the Frank-Starling curve) and CO.
- Decreasing vascular volume (hemorrhage; burn trauma; vomiting; diarrhea) or increasing venous compliance (inhibit sympathetics; alpha block; venodilators; standing upright) decreases Psf, causing a left shift in the VR curve (line D of Figure 8-12). Thus, either of these changes reduces filling of the ventricles (move down the Frank-Starling curve) and CO.

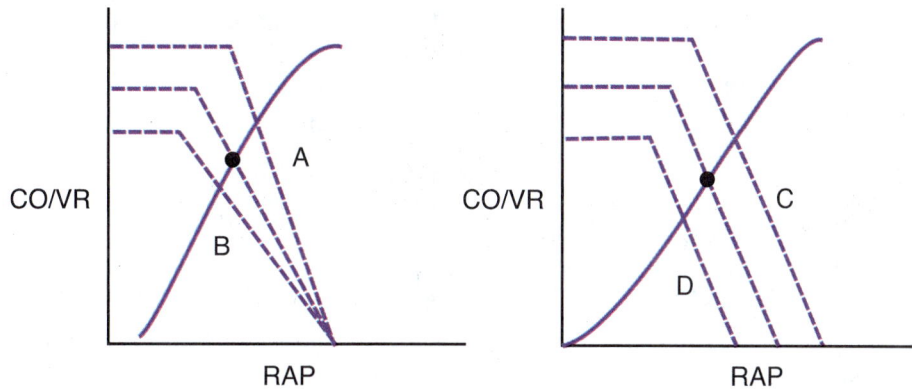

Figure 8-12. Solid circles represent starting CO.

A = arteriolar dilation
B = arteriolar constriction
C = increased vascular volume; decreased venous compliance
D = decreased vascular volume; increased venous compliance

THE EFFECT OF GRAVITY

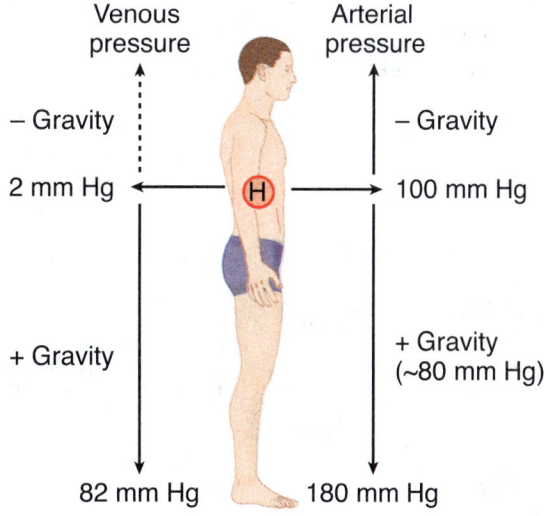

Figure 8-13. Effect of Gravity

Below heart level, there are equal increases in systemic arterial and venous pressures (assuming no muscular action). Thus, the pressure difference between arteries and veins does not change.

Because veins are very compliant vessels, the higher pressures in the dependent veins mean a significant pooling of blood, a volume that is not contributing to cardiac output. Although venous compliance doesn't "technically" increase, gravity's impact is functionally the same as an increase in venous compliance.

When a person goes from supine to an upright posture, the following important changes take place:

- Pressure in the dependent veins increases.
- Blood volume in the dependent veins increases.
- VR decreases.
- If no compensations occurred, then MAP would fall because of the diminished SV.

The initial compensation arises from stretch receptors in the heart, great veins, and pulmonary artery. Collectively, these receptors are called **cardiopulmonary mechanoreceptors** (cardiopulmonary baroreceptors).

- Afferent activity from these receptors is directly related to the volume of blood in the heart. In other words, they respond to changes in preload.
- If preload increases, then the resultant activation of these receptors stimulates parasympathetics and inhibits sympathetic. Activation of these receptors also inhibits the release of antidiuretic hormone (see chapter 22).
- Conversely, if preload falls, then reduced activity of these receptors inhibits parasympathetics and stimulates sympathetics.

The reflex activation of the sympathetic nervous system causes:

- Arteriolar vasoconstriction (TPR increases)
- Increase in HR
- Venoconstriction

If MAP falls, then the arterial baroreceptors also participate in the reflex changes.

Above heart level, systemic arterial pressure progressively decreases. Because venous pressure at heart level is close to zero, venous pressure quickly becomes subatmospheric (negative).

Surface veins above the heart cannot maintain a significant pressure below atmospheric and will collapse; however, deep veins and those inside the cranium supported by the tissue can maintain a pressure that is significantly below atmospheric. A consequence of the preceding is that a severed or punctured vein above heart level has the potential for introducing air into the system.

Bridge to Pathology and Pharmacology

The inability to maintain MAP when standing upright is called orthostatic intolerance. In this condition, the fall in MAP reduces cerebral blood flow, causing the patient to feel dizzy or light-headed. This can lead to a syncope event. One of the more common causes for this is reduced vascular volume. The low volume reduces VR and the added fall in VR (due to venous pooling) overwhelms the compensatory mechanisms. Other factors that can lead to orthostatic intolerance are venodilators, poor ventricular function such as heart failure or cardiac transplant, and dysautonomias.

CHARACTERISTICS OF SYSTEMIC ARTERIES

The following figure shows a pressure pulse for a major systemic artery.

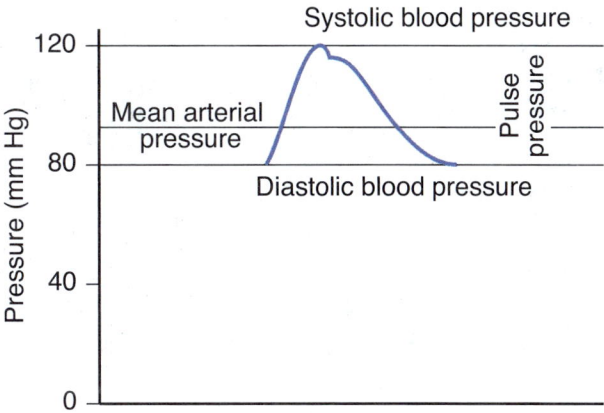

Figure 8-14. Pulse Pressure and Mean Pressure

Pulse pressure equals systolic – diastolic, so here, pulse pressure is 120 – 80 = 40 mm Hg.

Factors Affecting Systolic Pressure

- Systolic blood pressure is the highest pressure in the systemic arteries during the cardiac cycle.
- The main factor determining systolic blood pressure on a beat-to-beat basis is stroke volume.
- An increase in stroke volume increases systolic blood pressure and a decrease in stroke volume decreases systolic blood pressure.
- Systolic blood pressure is also directly related to ventricular contractility. In addition, the rate of pressure change in the aorta is directly related to contractility. Thus, if contractility increases, then the rate of pressure and the absolute level of aortic pressure increases, and vice-versa.
- In chronic conditions, a decrease in the compliance of the systemic arteries (age-related arteriosclerosis) also increases systolic blood pressure.

Factors Affecting Diastolic Pressure

- Diastolic blood pressure (DBP) is directly related to the volume of blood left in the aorta at the end of diastole.
- One important factor determining DBP is total peripheral resistance (TPR).
- Dilation of the arterioles decreases DBP and constriction of the arterioles increases DBP.
- HR is the second key factor influencing diastolic pressure and they are directly related: increased HR increases DBP, while decreased HR decreases DBP.
- DBP is also directly related to SV, but this is typically not a major factor.

Factors Affecting Pulse Pressure

The following increase (widen) pulse pressure:

- An increase in stroke volume (systolic increases more than diastolic)
- A decrease in vessel compliance (systolic increases and diastolic decreases)

The aorta is the most compliant artery in the arterial system. Peripheral arteries are more muscular and less compliant. Based on the preceding information, in Figure 8-15 the pressure record on the left best represents the aorta, whereas the one on the right best represents the femoral artery.

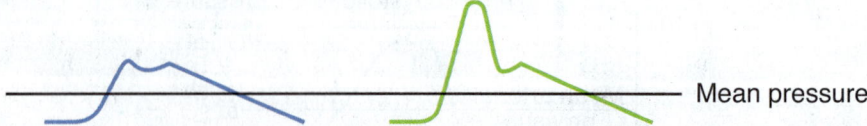

Figure 8-15. Compliance and Pulse Pressure

The figure demonstrates that a compliant artery has a small pulse pressure and that a stiff artery has a large pulse pressure. Also, pulse pressure increases with age because compliance is decreasing. This can produce isolated systolic hypertension, in which mean pressure is normal because the elevated systolic pressure is associated with a reduced diastolic pressure.

Note

Theoretically, the **systemic pulse pressure** can be conceptualized as being proportional to stroke volume, or the amount of blood ejected from the left ventricle during systole, and inversely proportional to the compliance of the aorta.

Factors Affecting Mean Pressure

Mean pressure is pressure averaged over time. It is not the arithmetic mean and is closer to diastolic pressure than to systolic pressure.

Mean pressure can be approximated by the following formulas:

For a blood pressure of 120/80 mm Hg:

$$\text{Mean pressure} = \text{diastolic} + \tfrac{1}{3} \text{ pulse pressure}$$

$$80 + \tfrac{1}{3}(40) = 93 \text{ mm Hg}$$

$$= \tfrac{2}{3} \text{ diastolic pressure} + \tfrac{1}{3} \text{ systolic pressure}$$

$$\tfrac{2}{3}(80) + \tfrac{1}{3}(120) = 93 \text{ mm Hg}$$

Any formula that calculates mean pressure must give a value between systolic and diastolic but closer to diastolic than systolic.

Factors that affect mean pressure (application of hemodynamics discussed above):

Q = cardiac output

P_1 = aortic pressure (mean arterial pressure)

P_2 = pressure at the entrance of the right atrium

R = resistance of all vessels in the systemic circuit. This is referred to as total peripheral resistance (TPR).

Because the major component of TPR is the arterioles, TPR can be considered an index of arteriolar resistance.

Because P_1 is a very large number (93 mm Hg) and P_2 is a very small one (~0 mm Hg), that doesn't change dramatically in most situations, we can simplify the equation if we approximate P_2 as zero. Then:

$$CO = \frac{MAP}{TPR} \text{ or } MAP = CO \times TPR$$

MAP = mean arterial pressure
CO = cardiac output
TPR = total peripheral resistance

This equation simply states that:

- Mean arterial pressure (MAP) is determined by only t variables: cardiac output and TPR.
- CO is the circulating volume. The blood stored in the systemic veins and the pulmonary circuit would not be included in this volume.
- TPR is the resistance of all vessels in the systemic circuit. By far the largest component is the resistance in the arterioles.
- However, if venous or right atrial pressure (RAP) is severely increased, it must be taken into account when estimating TPR. In this case, the formula is:

$$\left(MAP - RAP\right) = CO \times TPR$$

or rearranged to solve for resistance: $TPR = \dfrac{\left(MAP - RAP\right)}{CO}$

BARORECEPTOR REFLEX AND THE CONTROL OF BLOOD PRESSURE

The baroreceptor reflex is the short-term regulation of blood pressure. The renin-angiotensin-aldosterone system is the long-term regulation of blood pressure. The following figure illustrates the main features of the baroreceptor reflex.

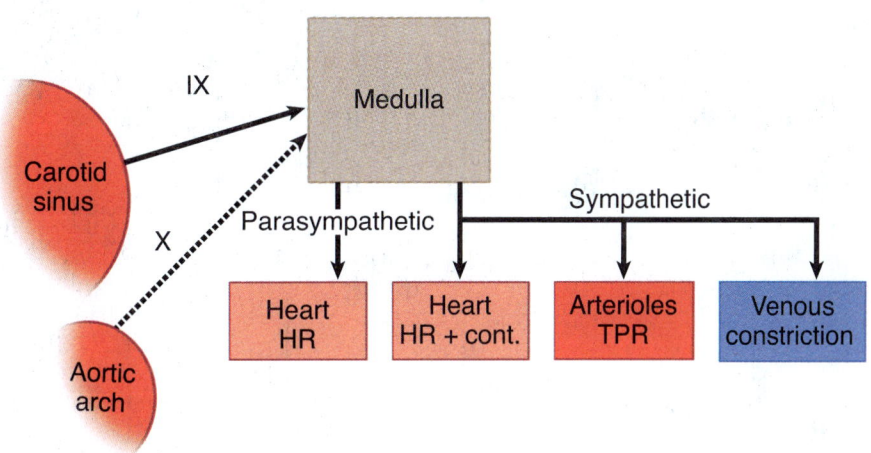

Figure 8-16. Baroreflexes

$$MAP = CO \times TPR$$

Key points regarding arterial baroreceptors:

- Mechanoreceptors imbedded in the walls of the aortic arch and carotid sinus that are stimulated by a rise in intravascular pressure.
- Afferent activity is relayed to the medulla via cranial nerves IX (carotid sinus) and X (aortic arch).
- Baroreceptor activity exists at the person's resting arterial blood pressure.
- Afferent activity stimulates the parasympathetic nervous system and inhibits the sympathetic nervous system.
- A fall in arterial blood pressure evokes a reflex decrease in parasympathetic activity and increase in sympathetic activity. This is a negative feedback system to bring blood pressure back to its original level.
- A rise in arterial blood pressure evokes a reflex increase in parasympathetic activity and fall in sympathetic activity. This is a negative feedback system to bring blood pressure back to its original level.
- Activation of arterial baroreceptors inhibits the secretion of ADH.

Clinical Correlate

Increasing vagal outflow to the heart can be beneficial for patients with supraventricular tachycardia. Because it increases baroreceptor afferent activity, carotid massage is one maneuver that increases vagal outflow to the heart.

Table 8-2. Reflex Changes for Specific Maneuvers

Condition	Afferent Activity	Parasympathetic Activity	Sympathetic Activity		
BP increase	↑	↑	↓		
BP decrease	↓	↓	↑	**BP**	**HR**
Carotid occlusion	↓	↓	↑	↑	↑
Carotid massage	↑	↑	↓	↓	↓
Cut afferents	↓	↓	↑	↑	↑
• Lying to stand • Orthostatic hypotension • Fluid loss	↓	↓	↑	↑ toward normal	↑
• Volume load • Weightlessness	↑	↑	↓	↓ toward normal	↓

Learning Objectives

❏ Demonstrate understanding of Fick principle of blood flow

❏ Interpret scenarios on blood flow regulation

❏ Explain information related to blood flow to the various organs

❏ Demonstrate understanding of fetal circulation

❏ Explain information related to cardiovascular stress: exercise

FICK PRINCIPLE OF BLOOD FLOW

The Fick principle can be utilized to calculate the blood flow through an organ.

Calculation of flow through the pulmonary circuit provides a measure of the CO.

$$\text{Flow} = \frac{\text{uptake}}{\text{A} - \text{V}}$$

Required data are: oxygen consumption of the organ

A – V oxygen content (concentration) difference across the organ (not PO_2)

Pulmonary venous (systemic arterial)

oxygen content
= 20 vol%
= 20 volumes O_2 per 100 volumes blood
= 20 mL O_2 per 100 mL blood
= 0.2 mL O_2 per mL blood

If pulmonary vessel data are not available, you may substitute arterial oxygen content for pulmonary venous blood and use venous oxygen content in place of pulmonary artery values.

The following figure illustrates the situation in a normal resting individual.

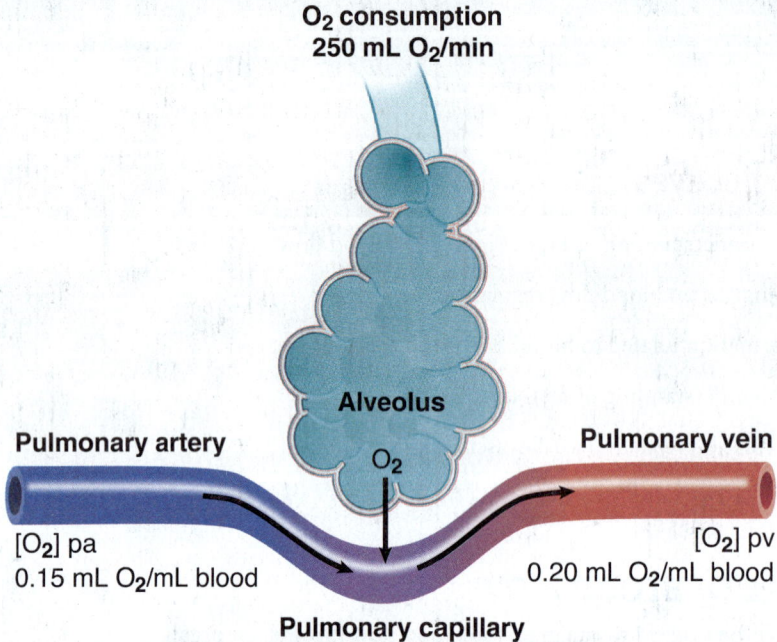

Figure 9-1. Alveolar Oxygen Uptake

$$Q(\text{flow}) = \frac{\text{oxygen consumption}}{[O_2]\text{pv} - [O_2]\text{pa}}$$

$$= \frac{250 \text{ mL} / \text{min}}{0.20 \text{ mL} / \text{mL} - 0.15 \text{ mL} / \text{mL}} = 5{,}000 \text{ mL} / \text{min}$$

$$\text{Cardiac index} = \frac{\text{cardiac output}}{\text{body surface area}}$$

This would normalize the value for body size.

Application of the Fick Principle

Rearranging the Fick Principle to O_2 consumption $= Q \times (CaO_2 - CvO_2)$ can be applied to important concepts regarding homeostatic mechanisms and pathologic alterations (Figure 9-2). $CaO_2 - CvO_2$ represents the extraction of O_2 by the tissue.

O_2 consumption

- O_2 consumption is dependent upon flow and the extraction of O_2.
- If tissue O_2 consumption increases, then flow or extraction or both must increase.
- The rise in flow in response to a rise in tissue O_2 consumption is the result of increased production of vasodilator metabolites (see metabolic mechanism below).
- In short, this change in flow and extraction represents homeostatic mechanisms designed to ensure adequate O_2 availability and thus sufficient ATP production.

O₂ delivery

- O_2 delivery $= Q \times CaO_2$
  - The "first part" of the Fick Principle indicates that delivery of O_2 to the tissue is dependent upon Q and the total amount of O_2 in the blood (CaO_2).
- For any given tissue O_2 consumption, reduced delivery of O_2 results in increased lactic acid production and possible hypoxic/ischemic damage to tissues.
- For any given tissue O_2 consumption, if O_2 delivery decreases, then PvO_2 and SvO_2% fall.
- Clinical application
  - A fall in PvO_2 or SvO_2% indicates the patient's O_2 consumption increased and/or there was a fall in Q or CaO_2 or both.

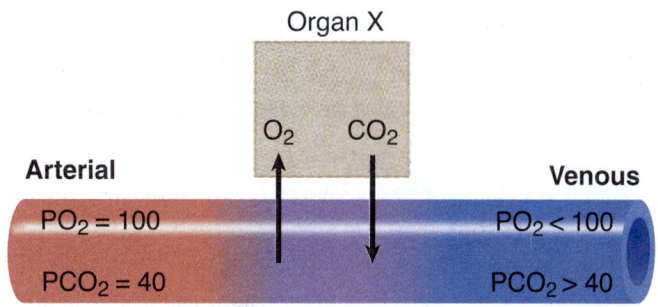

Figure 9-2. Application of the Fick Principle

BLOOD FLOW REGULATION

Flow is regulated by constricting and dilating the smooth muscle surrounding the arterioles.

Intrinsic Regulation (Autoregulation)

The control mechanisms regulating the arteriolar smooth muscle are entirely within the organ itself.

- What is regulated is blood flow, not resistance. It is more correct to say that resistance is changed in order to regulate flow.
- No nerves or circulating substances are involved in autoregulation. Thus, the autonomic nervous system and circulating epinephrine have nothing to do with autoregulation.

There are two main mechanisms to explain autoregulation.

Metabolic mechanism

- Tissue produces a vasodilatory metabolite that regulates flow, e.g., adenosine, CO_2, H^+, and K^+.
- A dilation of the arterioles is produced when the concentration of these metabolites increases in the tissue. The arterioles constrict if the tissue concentration decreases.

Myogenic mechanism

- Increased perfusing pressure causes stretch of the arteriolar wall and the surrounding smooth muscle.
- Because an inherent property of the smooth muscle is to contract when stretched, the arteriole radius decreases, and flow does not increase significantly.

Major Characteristics of an Autoregulating Tissue

Blood flow should be independent of blood pressure.

This phenomenon is demonstrated for a theoretically perfect autoregulating tissue in Figure 9-3. The range of pressure over which flow remains nearly constant is the **autoregulatory range**.

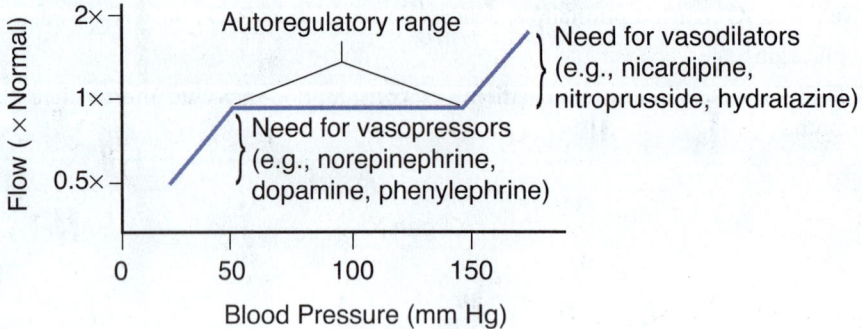

Figure 9-3. Autoregulation

Blood flow in most cases is proportional to tissue metabolism.

Blood flow is independent of nervous reflexes (e.g., carotid sinus) or circulating humoral factors.

Autoregulating tissues include (tissues least affected by nervous reflexes):

- Cerebral circulation
- Coronary circulation
- Skeletal muscle vasculature during exercise

Extrinsic Regulation

These tissues are controlled by nervous and humoral factors originating outside the organ, e.g., resting skeletal muscle. Extrinsic mechanisms were covered in the previous chapter and thus will only be briefly reviewed here.

The following figure illustrates an arteriole in skeletal muscle and the factors regulating flow under resting conditions.

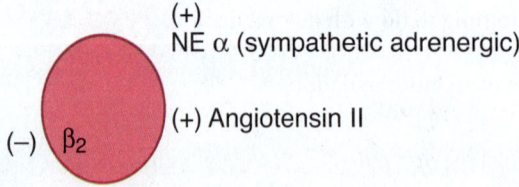

Figure 9-4. Resting Skeletal Muscle Blood Flow

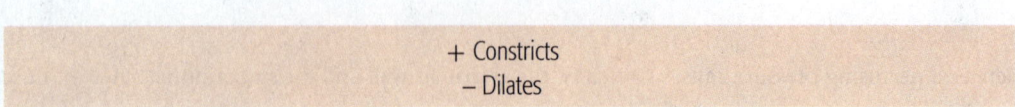

+ Constricts
− Dilates

The key points for extrinsic regulation are:

- Norepinephrine (NE) released from sympathetic nerves has a tonic influence on arteriolar tone (α receptors) in resting skeletal muscle and skin vasculature in a thermo-neutral environment.
- In times of stress, sympathetic activation can evoke substantial vasoconstriction in the aforementioned tissues, but can also greatly affect renal and splanchnic circulations.
- Epinephrine can evoke vasodilation by binding to vascular $\beta2$ receptors.
- With the exception of the penis, the parasympathetic nervous system does not affect arteriolar tone.

Control of Resting versus Exercising Muscle

Resting muscle

Flow is controlled mainly by increasing or decreasing sympathetic-adrenergic activity.

Exercising muscle

The elevated metabolism in exercising skeletal muscle demands an increase in blood flow (see application of the Fick principle). In addition, the increased tissue O_2 consumption results in a fall the PvO_2 of blood leaving the working muscle. The primary mechanisms for increasing flow are:

- Production of vasodilator metabolites, e.g., adenosine, CO_2, H^+, and K^+ causes marked vasodilation. In addition, these metabolites diminish NE's ability to vasoconstrict the arterioles. Further, the increased endothelial shear-stress of the high flow liberates NO.
- Muscle pump

BLOOD FLOW TO THE VARIOUS ORGANS

Coronary Circulation

Coronary flow patterns

Characteristics of left coronary flow (flow to the left ventricular myocardium):

Left ventricular contraction causes severe mechanical compression of subendocardial vessels. Therefore:

- Very little if any blood flow occurs during systole.
- Most of the blood flow is during diastole.
- Some subepicardial flow occurs during systole.

Characteristics of right coronary blood flow (flow to the right ventricular myocardium):

Right ventricular contraction causes modest mechanical compression of intramyocardial vessels. Therefore:

- Significant flow can occur during systole.
- The greatest flow under normal conditions is still during diastole.

Oxygenation

In the coronary circulation, the tissues extract almost all the oxygen they can from the blood, even under "basal" conditions. Therefore:

- The venous PO_2 is extremely low. It is the lowest venous PO_2 in a resting individual.
- Because the extraction of oxygen is almost maximal under resting conditions, increased oxygen delivery to the tissue can be accomplished only by increasing blood flow (Fick principle).
- In the coronary circulation, flow must match metabolism.
- Coronary blood flow is most closely related to cardiac tissue oxygen consumption and demand.

Pumping action

Coronary blood flow (mL/min) is determined by the pumping action, or **stroke work** times heart rate, of the heart.

Increased pumping action means increased metabolism, which increases the production of vasodilatory metabolites. In turn, coronary flow increases.

Increased pump function occurs with:

- An increase in any of the parameters that determine CO:
  - HR
  - Contractility
  - Afterload
  - Preload
- HR, contractility, and afterload (often called pressure work) are more metabolically costly than the work associated with preload (volume work).
- Thus, conditions in which HR, contractility, and/or afterload increase, e.g., hypertension, aortic stenosis, and exercise require a greater increase in flow compared to conditions that only increase volume work (supine, aortic regurgitation, volume loading).

Cerebral Circulation

Flow is proportional to arterial PCO_2. Under normal conditions, arterial PCO_2 is an important factor regulating cerebral blood flow.

- Hypoventilation increases arterial PCO_2, thus it increases cerebral blood flow.
- Hyperventilation decreases arterial PCO_2, thus it decreases cerebral blood flow.

As long as arterial PO_2 is normal or above normal, cerebral blood flow is regulated via arterial PCO_2. Therefore:

- If a normal person switches from breathing room air to 100% oxygen, there is no significant change in cerebral blood flow.
- However, a (large) decrease in arterial PO_2 increases cerebral blood flow; an example is high-altitude pulmonary edema (HAPE). Under these conditions, it is the low arterial PO_2 that is determining flow.
- Baroreceptor reflexes do not affect flow.

Intracranial pressure is an important pathophysiologic factor that can affect cerebral blood flow.

Cutaneous Circulation

- Almost entirely controlled via sympathetic adrenergic nerves
- Large venous plexus innervated by sympathetics
- A-V shunts innervated by sympathetics
- Sympathetic stimulation to the skin causes:
  - Constriction of arterioles and a decrease in blood flow, which is one reason why physicians use a central line to administer vasopressors to prevent distal necrosis
  - Constriction of the venous plexus and a decrease in blood volume in the skin
- Sympathetic activity to the skin varies mainly with the body's need for heat exchange with the environment.

Increased skin temperature directly causes vasodilation, which increases heat loss.

Temperature regulation

There are temperature-sensitive neurons in the anterior hypothalamus, whose firing rate reflects the temperature of the regional blood supply.

- Normal set point: oral 37°C (rectal + 0.5°C)
- Circadian rhythm: low point, morning; high point, evening

As illustrated in the following figure, the body does not lose the ability to regulate body temperature during a fever. It simply regulates body temperature at a higher set point.

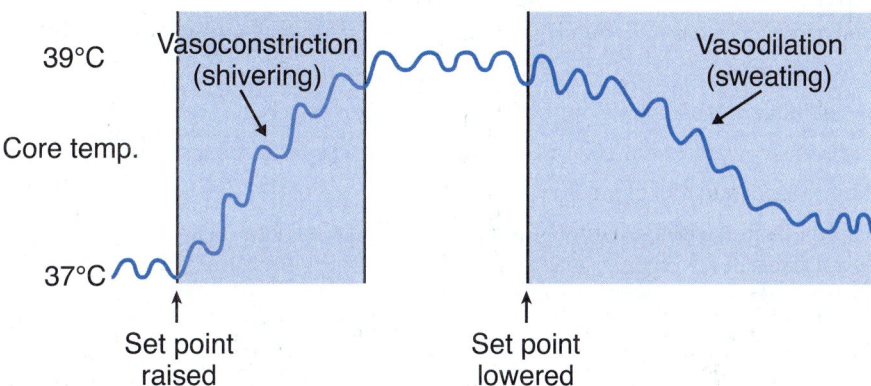

Figure 9-5. Temperature Regulation

When a fever develops, body temperature rises toward the new higher set point. Under these conditions, heat-conserving and heat-generating mechanisms include:

- Shivering
- Cutaneous vasoconstriction

After a fever "breaks," the set point has returned to normal, and body temperature is decreasing. Heat-dissipating mechanisms include:

- Sweating (sympathetic cholinergics)
- Cutaneous vasodilation

Renal and Splanchnic Circulation

- A small change in blood pressure invokes an autoregulatory response to maintain renal and splanchnic blood flows.
- Thus, under normal conditions, the renal and splanchnic circulations demonstrate autoregulation.
- Situations in which there is a large increase in sympathetic activity (e.g., hypotension) usually cause vasoconstriction and a decrease in blood flow.
- Renal circulation is greatly overperfused in terms of nutrient requirements, thus the venous PO_2 is high.
- About 25% of the CO goes to the splanchnic circulation, thus it represents an important reservoir of blood in times of stress.
- Splanchnic blood flow increases dramatically when digesting a meal.

Bridge to Anatomy

The **splanchnic circulation** is composed of the gastric small intestinal, colonic, pancreatic, hepatic, and splenic circulations, arranged in parallel with one another. The three major arteries that supply the splanchnic organs are the celiac, superior, and inferior mesenteric arteries.

Pulmonary Circuit

Characteristics

- Low-pressure circuit, arterial = 15 mm Hg, venous = 5 mm Hg; small pressure drop indicates a low resistance.
- High flow, receives entire CO
- Very compliant circuit; both arteries and veins are compliant vessels
- Hypoxic vasoconstriction (low alveolar PO_2 causes local arteriolar vasoconstriction)
- Blood volume proportional to blood flow
  - Because of the very compliant nature of the pulmonary circuit, large changes in the output of the right ventricle are associated with only small changes in pulmonary pressures.

Pulmonary response to exercise

- A large increase in cardiac output means increased volume pumped into the circuit. This increases pulmonary intravascular pressures.
- Because of the compliant nature of the circuit, the pulmonary arterial system distends.
- In addition, there is recruitment of previously unperfused capillaries. Because of this recruitment and distension, the overall response is a large decrease in pulmonary vascular resistance (PVR).
- Consequently, when CO is high, e.g., during exercise, there is only a slight increase in pulmonary pressures.
  - Without this recruitment and distension, increasing CO would result in a very high pulmonary artery pressure.

Pulmonary response to hemorrhage

- A large decrease in CO reduces intravascular pulmonary pressures.
- Because these vessels have some elasticity, pulmonary vessels recoil. In addition, there is derecruitment of pulmonary capillaries, both of which contribute to a rise in PVR.
- Consequently, during hemorrhage, there is often only a slight decrease in pulmonary artery pressure.
- Vessel recoil also means less blood is stored in this circuit.

CARDIOVASCULAR STRESS: EXERCISE

The following assumes the person is in a steady state, performing moderate exercise at sea level.

Pulmonary Circuit

- Blood flow (CO): large increase
- Pulmonary arterial pressure: slight increase
- Pulmonary vascular resistance: large decrease
- Pulmonary blood volume: increase
- Number of perfused capillaries: increase
- Capillary surface area: increase, i.e., increased rate of gas exchange

Systemic Circuit

Arterial system

- PO_2: no significant change, hemoglobin still fully saturated
- PCO_2: no significant change, increase in ventilation proportional to increase in metabolism
- pH: no change or a decrease due mainly to the production of lactic acid
- Mean arterial pressure: slight increase
- Body temperature: slight increase
- Vascular resistance (TPR): large decrease, dilation of skeletal muscle beds

Venous system

- PO_2: decrease
- PCO_2: increase

Regional Circulations

Exercising skeletal muscle

- Vascular resistance decreases.
- Blood flow increases.
- Capillary pressure increases.
- Capillary filtration increases.
- Lymph flow increases.
- As predicted by the Fick principle, oxygen extraction increases and venous PO_2 falls.

Cutaneous blood flow

Initial decrease, then an increase to dissipate heat

Coronary blood flow

Increase due to increased work of the heart

Cerebral blood flow

No significant change (arterial CO_2 remains unchanged)

Renal and GI blood flow

Both decrease

Physical conditioning

- Regular exercise increases maximal oxygen consumption ($\dot{V}O_2$ max) by:
    - Increasing the ability to deliver oxygen to the active muscles. It does this by increasing the CO.
    - The resting conditioned heart has a lower heart rate but greater stroke volume (SV) than does the resting unconditioned heart.
    - At any level of exercise, stroke volume is elevated.
    - However, the maximal heart rate remains similar to that of untrained individuals.
- Regular exercise also increases the ability of muscles to utilize oxygen. There are:
    - An increased number of arterioles, which decreases resistance during exercise.
    - An increased capillary density, which increases the surface area and decreases diffusion distance.
    - An increased number of oxidative enzymes in the mitochondria.

Cardiac Cycle 10

Learning Objectives

❏ Interpret scenarios on normal cardiac cycle

❏ Interpret scenarios on pressure-volume loops

NORMAL CARDIAC CYCLE

Figure 10-1 illustrates the most important features of the cardiac cycle.

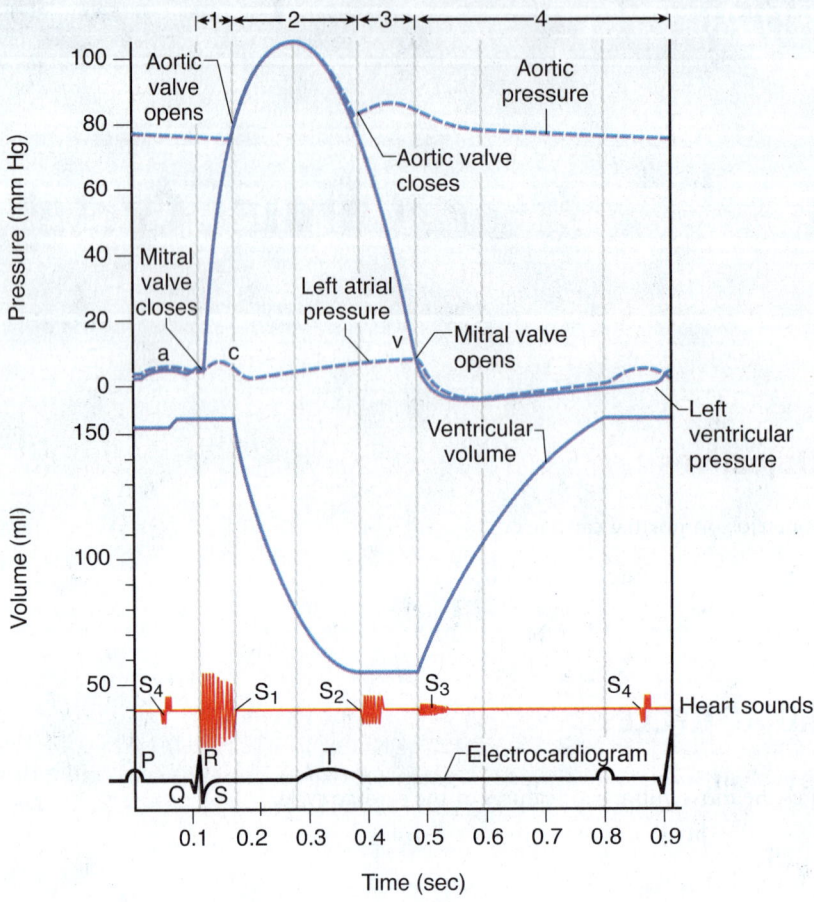

Figure 10-1. Cardiac Cycle

The most important aspects of Figure 10-1 are the following:

- → QRS → contraction of ventricle → rise in ventricular pressure above atrial pressure → closure of mitral valve
- It is always a pressure difference that causes the valves to open or close.
- Closure of the mitral valve terminates the ventricular filling phase and begins iso-volumetric contraction.
- Isovolumetric contraction—no change in ventricular volume, and both valves (mitral, aortic) closed. Ventricular pressure increases, and volume is equivalent to end-diastolic volume.
- Opening of the aortic valve terminates isovolumetric contraction and begins the ejection phase. The aortic valve opens because pressure in the ventricle slightly exceeds aortic pressure.
- Ejection Phase—ventricular volume decreases, but most rapidly in early stages. Ventricular and aortic pressures increase initially but decrease later in phase.
- Closure of the aortic valve terminates the ejection phase and begins isovolumetric relaxation. The aortic valve closes because pressure in the ventricle goes below aortic pressure. Closure of the aortic valve creates the dicrotic notch.
- Isovolumetric relaxation—no change in ventricular volume, and both valves (mitral, aortic) closed. Ventricular pressure decreases, and volume is equivalent to end-systolic volume.
- Opening of the mitral valve terminates isovolumetric relaxation and begins the filling phase. The mitral valve opens because pressure in the ventricle goes below atrial pressure.
- Filling Phase—the final relaxation of the ventricle occurs after the mitral valve opens and produces a rapid early filling of the ventricle. This rapid inflow will in some cases induce the third heart sound. The final increase in ventricular volume is due to atrial contraction, which is responsible for the fourth heart sound.

- In a young, healthy individual, atrial contraction doesn't provide significant filling of the ventricle. However, the contribution of atrial contraction becomes more important when ventricular compliance is reduced.

Heart Sounds

The systolic sounds are due to the sudden closure of the heart valves. Normally the valves on the left side of the heart close first. Valves on the right side open first.

Systolic sounds

S1: Produced by the closure of the mitral and tricuspid valves. The valves close with only a separation of about 0.01 seconds which the human ear can appreciate only as a single sound.

S2: Produced by the closure of the aortic (A2 component) and pulmonic valves (P2 component). They are heard as a single sound during expiration but during inspiration the increased output of the right heart causes a physiological splitting. The following figure illustrates several situations where splitting of the second heart sound may become audible.

Venous Pulse

The following figure provides an example of a normal jugular venous pulse tracing. The jugular pulse is generated by changes on the right side of the heart. The pressures will generally vary with the respiratory cycle and are generally read at the end of expiration when intrapleural pressure is at its closest point to zero.

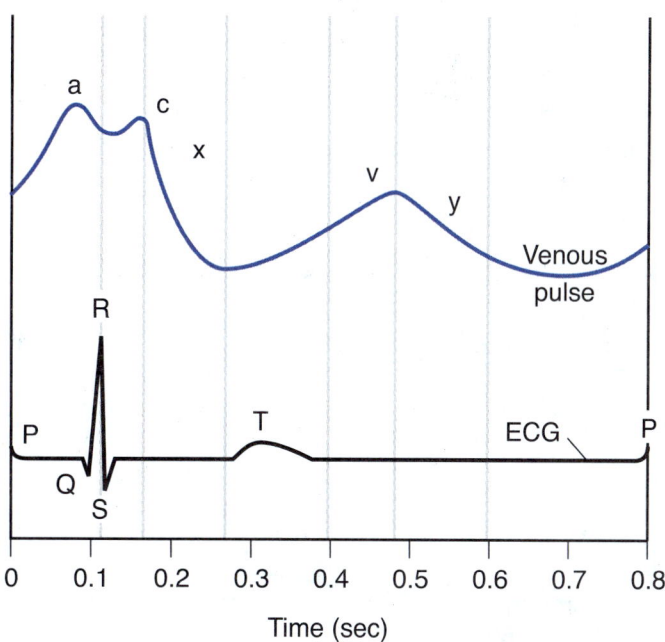

Figure 10-2. Venous Pulse and the ECG

a wave

- Highest deflection of the venous pulse and produced by the contraction of the right atrium
- Correlates with the PR interval (see figure)
- Is prominent in a stiff ventricle, pulmonic stenosis, and insufficiency
- Is absent in atrial fibrillation

c wave

- Mainly due to the bulging of the tricuspid valve into the atrium (rise in right atrial pressure)
- Occurs near the beginning of ventricular contraction (is coincident with right ventricular isovolumic contraction)
- Is often not seen during the recording of the venous pulse

x descent

- Produced by a decreasing atrial pressure during atrial relaxation
- Separated into two segments when the c wave is recorded
- Alterations occur with atrial fibrillation and tricuspid insufficiency

v wave

- Produced by the filling of the atrium during ventricular systole when the tricuspid valve is closed
- Corresponds to T wave of the EKG
- A prominent v wave would occur in tricuspid insufficiency and right heart failure

y descent

- Produced by the rapid emptying of the right atrium immediately after the opening of the tricuspid valve
- A more prominent wave in tricuspid insufficiency and a blunted wave in tricuspid stenosis.

PRESSURE-VOLUME LOOPS

The following figure shows the major features of a left ventricular pressure–volume loop.

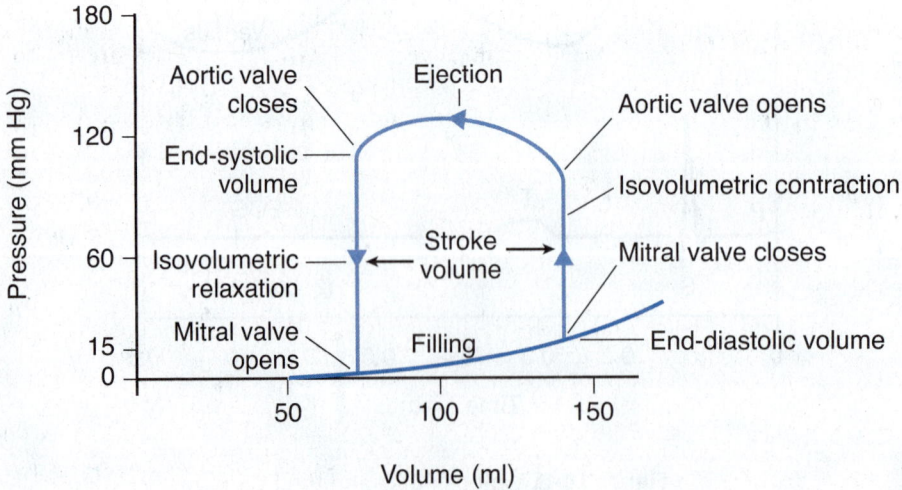

Figure 10-3. Left Ventricular Pressure–Volume Loop

- Most of the energy consumption occurs during isovolumetric contraction.
- Most of the work is performed during the ejection phase.

Lung Mechanics 11

Learning Objectives

❑ Interpret scenarios on lung volumes and capacities

❑ Use knowledge of lung mechanics

❑ Solve problems concerning positive-pressure ventilation

❑ Use knowledge of lung compliance

❑ Interpret scenarios on airway resistance

Tidal volume (Vt): amount of air that enters or leaves the lung in a single respiratory cycle (500 mL)

Functional residual capacity (FRC): amount of gas in the lungs at the end of a passive expiration; the neutral or equilibrium point for the respiratory system (2,700 mL) ; it is a marker for lung compliance

Inspiratory capacity (IC): maximal volume of gas that can be inspired from FRC (4,000 mL)

Inspiratory reserve volume (IRV): additional amount of air that can be inhaled after a normal inspiration (3,500 mL)

Expiratory reserve volume (ERV): additional volume that can be expired after a passive expiration (1,500 mL)

Residual volume (RV): amount of air in the lung after a maximal expiration (1,200 mL)

Vital capacity (VC): maximal volume that can be expired after a maximal inspiration (5,500 mL)

Total lung capacity (TLC): amount of air in the lung after a maximal inspiration (6,700 mL)

OVERVIEW OF THE RESPIRATORY SYSTEM

The purpose of understanding lung mechanics is to view them in the big clinical picture of pulmonary function test (PFT) interpretation. The PFT is the key diagnostic test for the pulmonologist, just as the EKG is to the cardiologist. PFTs consist of three individual tests (covered in greater detail in the *Respiratory* section):

1. Measurements of static lung compartments (meaning lung volumes)
2. Airflow used to evaluate dynamic compliance using a spirometer
3. Alveolar membrane permeability using carbon monoxide as a marker of diffusion

LUNG VOLUMES AND CAPACITIES

Figure 11-1 shows the relationships among the various lung volumes and capacities. Clinical measurements of specific volumes and capacities provide insights into lung function and the origin of disease processes. Those that provide the greatest information display a *.

The values for the volumes and capacities given below are typical for a 70 kg male.

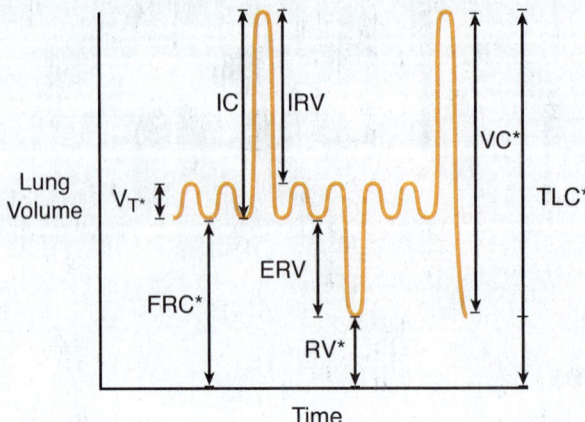

Figure 11-1. Lung Volumes and Capacities

A spirometer can measure only changes in lung volume. As such, it cannot measure the residual volume (RV) or any capacity containing RV. Thus, TLC and FRC cannot be measured using simple spirometry; an indirect method must be used. Three common indirect methods are helium dilution, nitrogen washout, and plethysmography.

VENTILATION

Total Ventilation

Total ventilation is also referred to as minute volume or minute ventilation. It is the total volume of air moved in or out (usually the volume expired) of the lungs per minute.

$$\dot{V}_E = V_T \times f$$

$\dot{V}_E$ = total ventilation

V_T = tidal volume

f = respiratory rate

Normal resting values would be:

V_T = 500 mL

f = 15

500 mL × 15/min = 7,500 mL/min

Dead Space

Regions of the respiratory system that contain air but are not exchanging O_2 and CO_2 with blood are considered dead space.

Anatomic dead space

Airway regions that, because of inherent structure, are not capable of O_2 and CO_2 exchange with the blood. Anatomic dead space ($anatV_D$) includes the conducting zone, which ends at the level of the terminal bronchioles. Significant gas exchange (O_2 uptake and CO_2 removal) with the blood occurs only in the alveoli.

The size of the $anatV_D$ in mL is approximately equal to a person's weight in pounds. Thus a 150-lb individual has an anatomic dead space of 150 mL.

Composition of the anatomic dead space and the respiratory zone

The respiratory zone is a very constant environment. Under resting conditions, rhythmic ventilation introduces a small volume into a much larger respiratory zone. Thus, the partial pressure of gases in the alveolar compartment changes very little during normal rhythmic ventilation.

Composition at the End of Expiration (Before Inspiration)

- At the end of an expiration, the $anatV_D$ is filled with air that originated in the alveoli or respiratory zone.
- Thus, the composition of the air in the entire respiratory system is the same at this static point in the respiratory cycle.
- This also means that a sample of expired gas taken near the end of expiration (end tidal air) is representative of the respiratory zone.
- This situation is illustrated in the following figure.

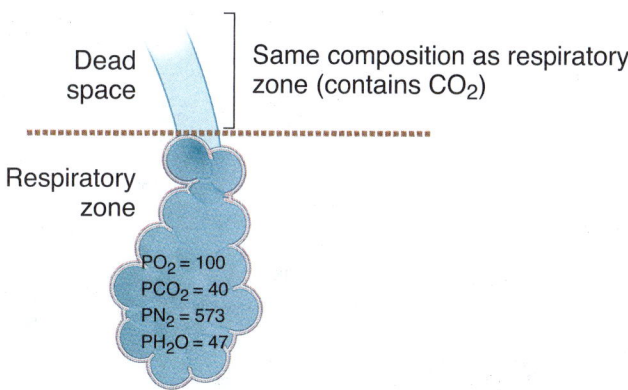

Figure 11-2. End of Expiration

Composition at the End of Inspiration (Before Expiration)

- The first 150 mL of air to reach the alveoli comes from the $anatV_D$.
- It is air that remained in the dead space at the end of the previous expiration and has the same composition as alveolar gas.
- After the first 150 mL enters the alveoli, room air is added to the respiratory zone.
- At the end of inspiration the $anatV_D$ is filled with room air.
- The presence of the $anatV_D$ implies the following: in order to get fresh air into the alveoli, one must always take a tidal volume larger than the volume of the $anatV_D$. This is illustrated in the Figure 11-3.

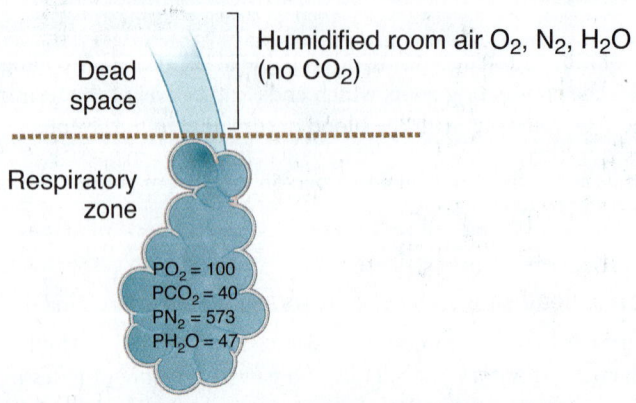

Figure 11-3. End of Inspiration

Alveolar dead space

Alveolar dead space (alvV_D) refers to alveoli containing air but without blood flow in the surrounding capillaries. An example is a pulmonary embolus.

Physiologic dead space

Physiologic dead space (physioIV_D) refers to the total dead space in the lung system (anatV_D + alvV_D). When the physiol V_D is greater than the anatV_D, it implies the presence of alvV_D, i.e., somewhere in the lung, alveoli are being ventilated but not perfused.

Total Ventilation

$V = VT \, (f)$

$= 500 \, (15)$

$= 7,500 \text{ mL/min}$

Minute ventilation ($\dot{V}$) is the total volume of air entering the lungs per minute.

Alveolar Ventilation

Alveolar ventilation $\dot{V}A$ represents the room air delivered to the respiratory zone per breath.

- The first 150 mL of each inspiration comes from the anatomic dead space and does not contribute to alveolar ventilation.
- However, every additional mL beyond 150 does contribute to alveolar ventilation.

$$\dot{V}A = (V_T - V_D) \, f$$

$$= (500 \text{ mL} - 150 \text{ mL}) \, 15 = 5250 \text{ mL/min}$$

$\dot{V}E$ = alveolar ventilation
V_T = tidal volume
V_D = dead space
f = respiratory rate

The alveolar ventilation per inspiration is 350 mL. This equation implies that the volume of fresh air that enters the respiratory zone per minute depends on the pattern of breathing (how large a V_T and the rate of breathing).

Increases in the Depth of Breathing

There are equal increases in total and alveolar ventilation per breath, since dead space volume is constant.

If the depth of breathing increases from a depth of 500 mL to a depth of 700 mL, the increase in total and alveolar ventilation is 200 mL per breath.

Increases in the Rate of Breathing

There is a greater increase in total ventilation per minute than in alveolar ventilation per minute, because the increased rate causes increased ventilation of dead space and alveoli.

For every additional inspiration with a tidal volume of 500 mL, total ventilation increases 500 mL, but alveolar ventilation only increases by 350 mL (assuming dead space is 150 mL).

For example, given the following, which person has the greater alveolar ventilation?

	Tidal Volume	**Rate**	**Total Ventilation**
Person A	600 mL	10/min	6,000 mL/min
Person B	300 mL	20/min	6,000 mL/min

Answer: Person A. Person B has rapid, shallow breathing. This person has a large component of dead-space ventilation (first 150 mL of each inspiration). Even though total ventilation may be normal, alveolar ventilation is decreased. Therefore, the individual is hypoventilating.

In rapid, shallow breathing, total ventilation may be above normal, but alveolar ventilation may be below normal.

LUNG MECHANICS

Muscles of Respiration

Inspiration

The major muscle of inspiration is the diaphragm. Contraction of the diaphragm enlarges the vertical dimensions of the chest. Also utilized are the external intercostal muscles of the chest wall. Contraction of these muscles causes the ribs to rise and thus increases the anterior-posterior dimensions of the chest.

Expiration

Under resting conditions, expiration is normally a passive process, i.e., it is due to the relaxation of the muscles of inspiration and the elastic recoil of the lungs. For a forced expiration, the muscles of the abdominal wall and the internal intercostals contract. This compresses the chest wall down and forces the diaphragm up into the chest.

Included would be external oblique, rectus abdominal, internal oblique, and transverse abdominal muscles.

Forces Acting on the Lung System

Units of pressure

In respiratory physiology, they are usually given as cm H_2O.

$$1 \text{ cm } H_2O = 0.74 \text{ mm Hg } (1 \text{ mm Hg} = 1.36 \text{ cm } H_2O)$$

Lung recoil and intrapleural pressure

Understanding lung mechanics mainly involves understanding the main forces acting on the respiratory system.

Lung Recoil

- Represents the inward force created by the elastic recoil properties of alveoli.
- As the lung expands, recoil increases; as the lung gets smaller, recoil decreases.
- Recoil, as a force, always acts to collapse the lung.

Chest Wall Recoil

- Outward force of the chest wall
- FRC represents the point where this outward recoil of the chest wall is counterbalanced by the inward recoil of the lung.

Intrapleural Pressure (IPP)

- Represents the pressure inside the thin film of fluid between the visceral pleura, which is attached to the lung, and the parietal pleura, which is attached to the chest wall.
- The outward recoil of the chest and inward recoil of the lung create a negative (subatmospheric) IPP.
- IPP is the outside pressure for all structures inside the chest wall.

Transmural Pressure Gradient (P_{TM})

- Represents the pressure gradient across any tube or sphere
- Calculated as inside pressure minus outside pressure
- If positive (inside greater than outside), it is a net force pushing out against the walls of the structure
- If negative (outside greater than inside), it is a net force pushing in against the walls of the structure; depending upon the structural components, the tube/sphere can collapse if P_{TM} is negative or zero
- At FRC, IPP is negative, and thus P_{TM} is positive. This positive outward force prevents alveolar collapse (atelectasis).
- For the entire lung, P_{TM} is called the transpulmonary pressure (TPP) .

Before Inspiration

The glottis is open, and all respiratory muscles are relaxed (FRC). This is the neutral or equilibrium point of the respiratory system (Figure 11-4). Intrapleural pressure is negative at FRC because the inward elastic recoil of the lungs is opposed by the outward-directed recoil of the chest wall. Because no air is flowing through the open glottis, alveolar pressure must be zero. By convention, the atmospheric pressure is set to equal zero.

Intrapleural pressure = −5 cm H$_2$O
PTM = 5
Alveolar pressure = O

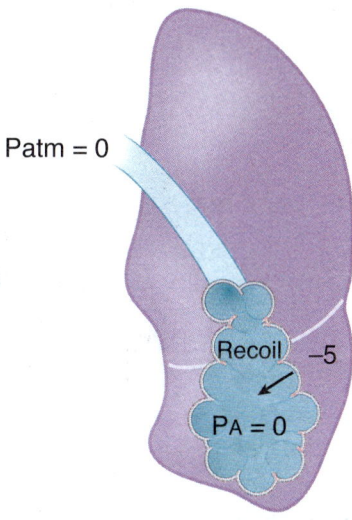

Patm = 0

Recoil −5

P$_A$ = 0

Figure 11-4. Lung Force Relationships at FRC

During Inspiration

1. Inspiration is induced by the contraction of the diaphragm and external intercostal muscles that expand the chest wall. The net result is to make intrapleural pressure more negative.

2. The more negative IPP causes P$_{TM}$ (TPP) to increase, which in turn causes expansion of the lungs. The greater the contraction, the greater the change in intrapleural pressure and the larger the P$_{TM}$ (TPP) expanding the lung.

3. The expansion of the lung increases alveolar volume. Based upon Boyle's law, the rise in volume causes pressure to decrease, resulting in a negative (subatmospheric) alveolar pressure.

4. Because alveolar pressure is now less than atmospheric, air rushes into the lungs.

Figure 11-5 illustrates the situation at some point during inspiration.

End of Inspiration

1. The lung expands until alveolar pressure equilibrates with atmospheric pressure. The lungs are at their new, larger volume.

2. Under resting conditions, about 500 mL of air flows into the lung system in order to return alveolar pressure back to zero.

Figure 11-6 illustrates the situation at the end of a normal inspiration.

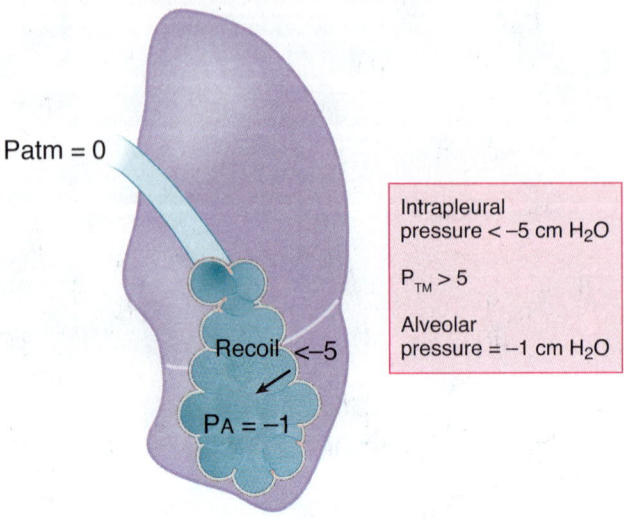

Figure 11-5. Lung Forces during Inspiration

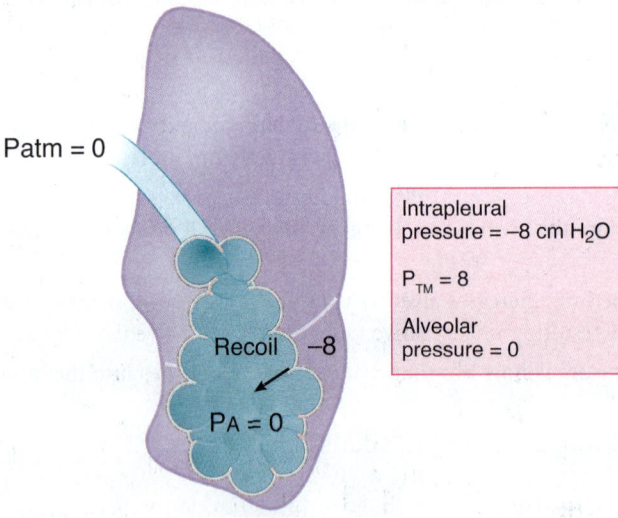

Figure 11-6. Lung Forces at End of Inspiration

Expiration

1. Expiration under resting conditions is produced simply by the relaxation of the muscles of inspiration.

2. Relaxation of the muscles of inspiration causes intrapleural pressure to return to −5 cm H_2O.

3. This decreases IPP back to its original level of −5 cm H_2O, resulting in a decreased P_{TM}.

4. The drop in P_{TM} reduces alveolar volume, which increases alveolar pressure (Boyle's law). The elevated alveolar pressure causes air to flow out of the lungs.

5. The outflowing air returns alveolar pressure toward zero, and when it reaches zero, airflow stops. The lung system returns to FRC.

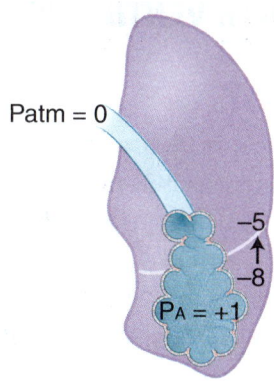

Figure 11-7. Lung Forces During Expiration

Intrapleural pressure during a normal respiratory cycle

The intrapleural pressure during a normal respiratory cycle is illustrated in Figure 11-8. Under resting conditions, it is always a subatmosphere pressure.

Intraalveolar pressure during a normal respiratory cycle

The intraalveolar pressure during a normal respiratory cycle is illustrated below.

- Intraalveolar pressure is slightly negative during inspiration and slightly positive during expiration.
- No matter how large a breath is taken, intraalveolar pressure always returns to 0 at the end of inspiration and expiration. By convention, total atmospheric pressure = 0.

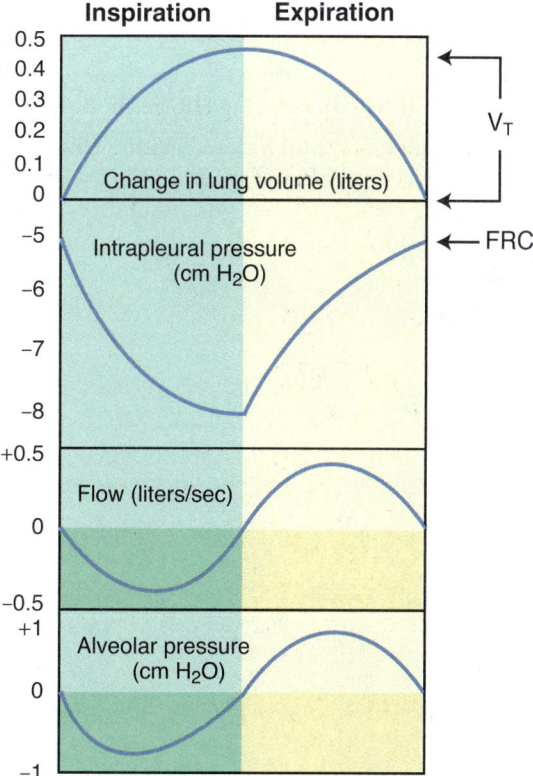

Figure 11-8. Essentials of Pulmonary Events during a Breath

CARDIOVASCULAR CHANGES WITH VENTILATION

Inspiration

- **Intrapleural pressure becomes more negative (decreases).**
- This increases the P_{TM} across the vasculature, causing the great veins and right atrium to expand.
- This expansion decreases intravascular pressure, thereby increasing the pressure gradient driving VR to the right heart.
- Systemic venous return and right ventricular output are increased.
- An increase in the output of the right ventricle delays closing of the pulmonic valves and typically results in a splitting of the second heart sound.
- Pulmonary vessels expand, and the volume of blood in the pulmonary circuit increases. In addition, because pulmonary vascular resistance (PVR) is lowest at FRC, it increases.
- In turn, venous return to the left heart, and the output of the left ventricle is decreased, causing decreased systemic arterial pressure (drop in systolic most prominent).
- This inspiration reduces vagal outflow to the heart (mechanism debatable) resulting in a slight rise in heart rate (respiratory sinus arrhythmia). This is why patients are asked to hold their breath, if clinically possible, when an EKG is taken.

Expiration

- In short, reverse the above processes.
- **Intrapleural pressure becomes more positive (increases)**, i.e., returns to original negative value.
- P_{TM} returns to its original level, thereby decreasing the pressure gradient for VR.
- Systemic venous return and output of the right ventricle are decreased.
- Pulmonary vessels are compressed, and the volume of blood in the pulmonary circuit decreases.
- The return of blood and output of the left ventricle increases, causing systemic arterial pressure to rise (primarily systolic).
- Vagal outflow increases (mechanism debated), reducing HR (respiratory sinus arrhythmia).
- A Valsalva maneuver is a forced expiration against a closed glottis. This forced expiration creates a positive IPP (see later in this chapter), which compresses the great veins in the chest. This in turn reduces VR.

LUNG COMPLIANCE

The following graph represents a static isolated lung inflation curve.

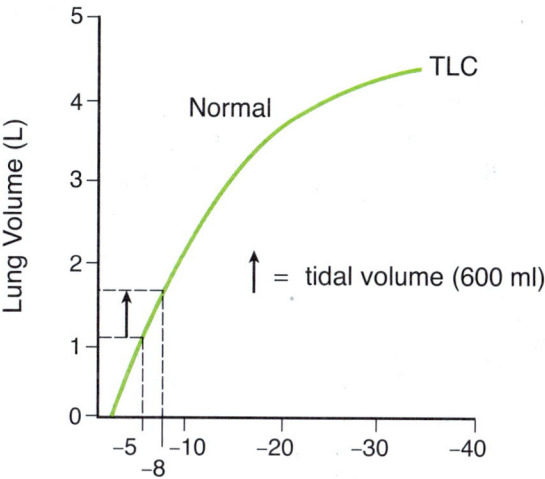

Figure 11-9. Lung Inflation Curve

Lung compliance is the change in lung volume (tidal volume) divided by the change in surrounding pressure. This is stated in the following formula:

$$\text{Compliance} = \frac{\Delta V}{\Delta P}$$

The following graph shows pathologic states in which lung compliance changes.

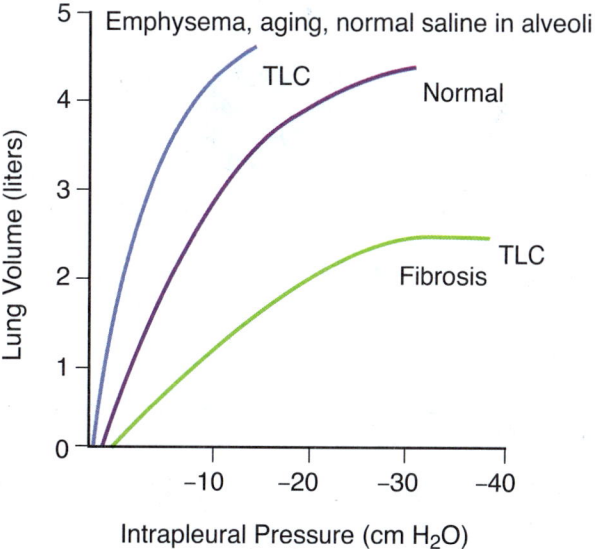

Figure 11-10. Lung Compliance

Increased lung compliance also occurs with aging and with a saline-filled lung.

In summary:

- Compliance is an index of the effort required to expand the lungs (to overcome recoil). It does not relate to airway resistance.
- Compliance decreases as the lungs are inflated because the curve is not a straight line.
- For any given fall in intrapleural pressure, large alveoli expand less than small alveoli.
- Very compliant lungs (easy to inflate) have low recoil. Stiff lungs (difficult to inflate) have a large recoil force.

Components of Lung Recoil

Lung recoil has the following components:

- **The tissue itself;** more specifically, the collagen and elastin fibers of the lung.

  The larger the lung, the greater the stretch of the tissue and the greater the recoil force.
- **The surface tension forces in the fluid lining the alveoli.** Surface tension forces are created whenever there is a liquid–air interface (Figure 11-11).

  Surface tension forces tend to reduce the area of the surface and generate a pressure. In the alveoli, they act to collapse the alveoli; therefore, these forces contribute to lung recoil.
- **Surface tension forces are the greatest component of lung recoil.**

  The relationship between the surface tension and the pressure inside a bubble is given by the law of LaPlace.

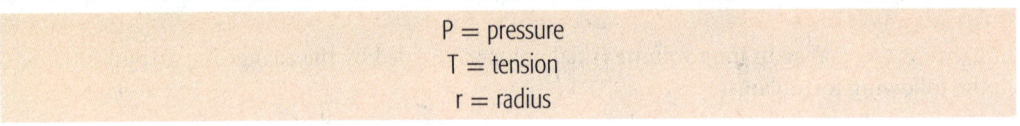

P = pressure
T = tension
r = radius

$$P \propto \frac{T}{r}$$

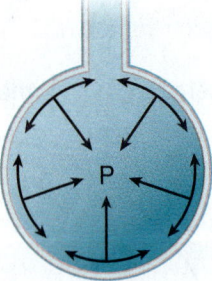

Figure 11-11. Surface Tension

If wall tension is the same in two bubbles, the smaller bubble will have the greater pressure.

Although the situation is more complex in the lung, it follows that small alveoli tend to be unstable. They have a great tendency to empty into larger alveoli and collapse (creating regions of atelectasis). This is illustrated in the following figure. Collapsed alveoli are difficult to reinflate.

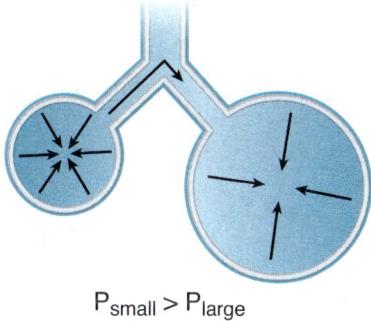

$$P_{small} > P_{large}$$

Figure 11-12. Atelectasis

If the alveoli were lined with a simple electrolyte solution, lung recoil would be so great that lungs theoretically should not be able to inflate. This is prevented by a chemical (produced by alveolar type II cells), surfactant, in the fluid lining a normal lung.

Surfactant has two main functions:

- It lowers surface tension forces in the alveoli. In other words, surfactant lowers lung recoil and increases compliance.
- It lowers surface tension forces more in small alveoli than in large alveoli. This promotes stability among alveoli of different sizes by decreasing the tendency of small alveoli to collapse (decreases the tendency to develop atelectasis).

AIRWAY RESISTANCE

Radius of an Airway

$$\text{Resistance} = \frac{1}{\text{radius}^4}$$

In the branching airway system of the lungs, it is the first and second bronchi that represent most of the airway resistance.

- Parasympathetic nerve stimulation produces bronchoconstriction. This is mediated by M3 receptors. In addition, M3 activation increases airway secretions.
- Circulating catecholamines produce bronchodilation. Epinephrine is the endogenous agent and it bronchodilates via b2 receptors.

Mechanical Effect of Lung Volume

The following graph demonstrates the mechanical effect of lung volume.

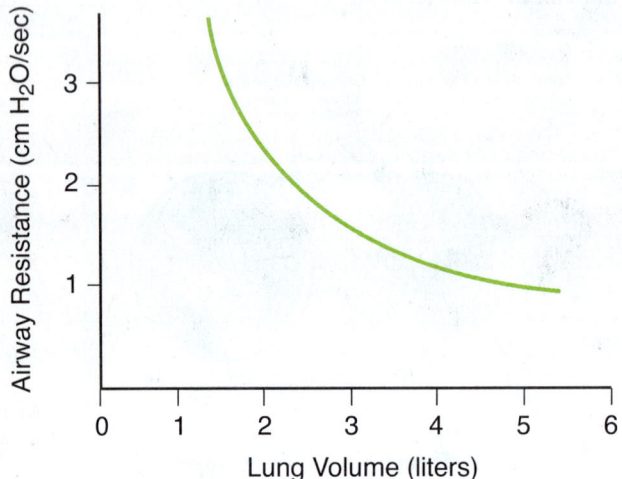

Figure 11-13. Airway Resistance

As lung volume increases, airway resistance decreases. The mechanisms for this are:

- P_{TM}: To get to high lung volumes, IPP becomes more and more negative. This increases the P_{TM} across small airways, causing them to expand. The result is decreased resistance.

- **Radial traction:** The walls of alveoli are physically connected to small airways. Thus, as alveoli expand, they pull open small airways. The result is decreased resistance.

Alveolar–Blood Gas Exchange 12

Learning Objectives

❏ Answer questions about the normal lung

❏ Solve problems concerning factors affecting alveolar PCO_2

❏ Use knowledge of factors affecting alveolar PO_2

❏ Interpret scenarios on alveolar-blood gas transfer: Fick law of diffusion

❏ Use knowledge of diffusing capacity of the lung

THE NORMAL LUNG

Partial Pressure of a Gas in Ambient Air

$$Pgas = Fgas \times Patm$$

Patm = atmospheric pressure
Pgas = partial pressure of a gas
Fgas = concentration of a gas

By convention, the partial pressure of the gas is expressed in terms of its dry gas concentration. For example, the PO_2 in ambient air is:

$$PO_2 = 0.21 \times 760 = 160 \text{ mm Hg}$$

Partial Pressure of a Gas in Inspired Air

Inspired air is defined as air that has been inhaled, warmed to 37°C, and completely humidified, but has not yet engaged in gas exchange. It is the fresh air in the anatV_D that is about to enter the respiratory zone.

The partial pressure of H_2O is dependent only on temperature and at 37°C is 47 mm Hg. Humidifying the air reduces the partial pressure of the other gases present.

$$PIgas = Fgas(Patm - PH_2O)$$

PIgas = partial pressure of inspired gas
PH_2O = partial pressure of H_2O vapor

For example, the PO_2 of inspired air is:

$$PIO_2 = 0.21(760 - 47) = 150 \text{ mm Hg}$$

Figure 12-1 shows the pressures of oxygen and carbon dioxide in the alveolar, pulmonary end capillary, and systemic arterial blood.

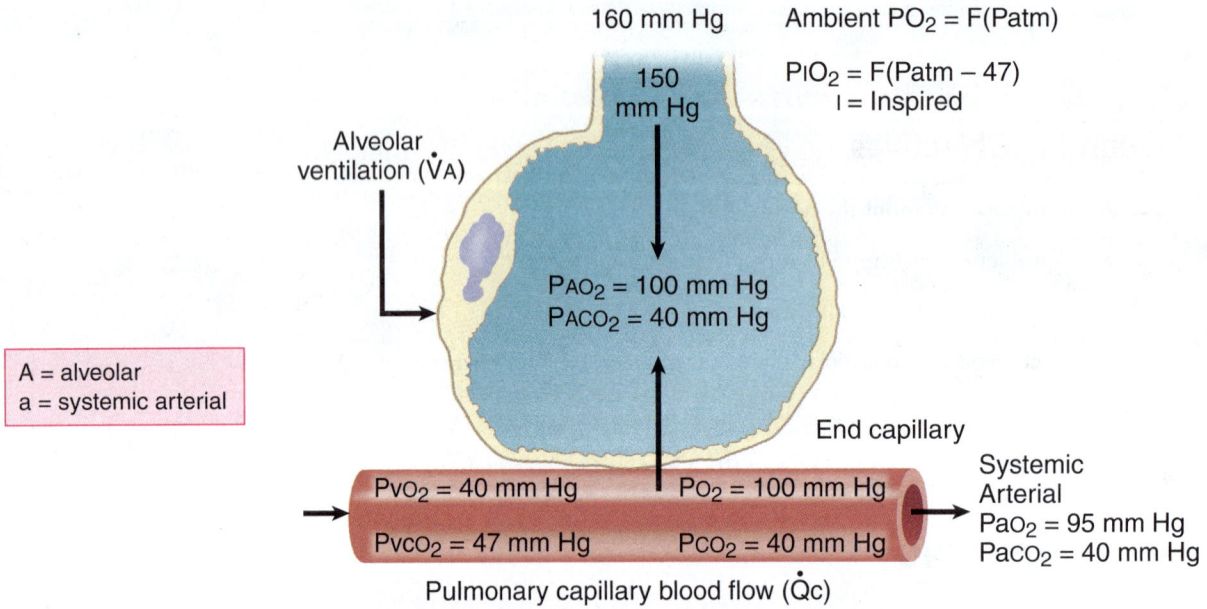

Figure 12-1. Pulmonary Capillary Gases

- Under normal conditions, the PO_2 and PCO_2 in the alveolar compartment and pulmonary end capillary blood are the same (perfusion-limited).
- There is a slight change ($PO_2\downarrow$) between the end capillary compartment and systemic arterial blood because of a small but normal shunt through the lungs.
- Alveolar–systemic arterial PO_2 differences = A – a-gradient.
- This difference (5–10 mm Hg) often provides information about the cause of a hypoxemia.

In a Nutshell

Dalton's law of partial pressures states that the total pressure exerted by a mixture of gases is the sum of the pressures exerted independently by each gas in the mixture. Also, the pressure exerted by each gas (its partial pressure) is directly proportional to its percentage in the total gas mixture.

FACTORS AFFECTING ALVEOLAR PCO$_2$

Only two factors affect alveolar PCO_2: metabolic rate and alveolar ventilation.

$$PACO_2 \propto = \frac{\text{metabolic } CO_2 \text{ production}}{\text{alveolar ventilation}}$$

At rest, unless there is fever or hypothermia, CO_2 production is relatively constant; so you can use changes of $PACO_2$ to evaluate alveolar ventilation.

Alveolar Ventilation

There is an inverse relationship between $PACO_2$ and alveolar ventilation. This is the main factor affecting alveolar PCO_2. Therefore, if ventilation increases, $PACO_2$ decreases; if ventilation decreases, $PACO_2$ increases.

Hyperventilation

During hyperventilation, there is an inappropriately elevated level of alveolar ventilation, and $PACO_2$ is depressed.

If $\dot{V}A$ is doubled, then $PACO_2$ is decreased by half.

e.g., $PACO_2 = 40$ mm Hg

$2 \times \dot{V}A$; $PACO_2 = 20$ mm Hg

Hypoventilation

During hypoventilation, there is an inappropriately depressed level of alveolar ventilation, and $PACO_2$ is elevated.

If $\dot{V}A$ is halved, then $PACO_2$ is doubled.

e.g., $PACO_2 = 40$ mm Hg

$1/2\ \dot{V}A$; $PACO_2 = 80$ mm Hg

Metabolic Rate

There is a direct relationship between alveolar PCO_2 and body metabolism. For $PaCO_2$ to remain constant, changes in body metabolism must be matched with equivalent changes in alveolar ventilation.

- If $\dot{V}A$ matches metabolism, then $PACO_2$ remains constant.
- For example, during exercise, if body metabolism doubles, then $\dot{V}A$ must double if $PaCO_2$ is to remain constant.
- If body temperature decreases and there is no change in ventilation, $PaCO_2$ decreases, and the individual can be considered to be hyperventilating.

FACTORS AFFECTING ALVEOLAR PO_2

Alveolar Air Equation

The alveolar air equation includes all the factors that can affect alveolar PO_2.

$$PAO_2 = (Patm - 47)FiO_2 - \frac{PACO_2}{RQ}$$

Practical application of the equation includes differential diagnosis of hypoxemia by evaluating the alveolar arterial (A–a) gradient of oxygen.

Three important factors can affect PAO_2:

Patm = atmospheric pressure, at sea level 760 mm Hg

An increase in atmospheric pressure (hyperbaric chamber) increases alveolar PO_2, and a decrease (high altitude) decreases alveolar PO_2.

FiO_2 = fractional concentration of oxygen, room air 0.21

An increase in inspired oxygen concentration increases alveolar PO_2.

$PaCO_2$ = alveolar pressure of carbon dioxide, normally 40 mm Hg

An increase in alveolar PCO_2 decreases alveolar PO_2, and a decrease in alveolar PCO_2 increases alveolar PO_2. For most purposes, you can use arterial carbon dioxide $(PaCO_2)$ in the calculation.

The fourth variable is RQ.

$$RQ = \text{respiratory exchange ratio} = \frac{CO_2 \text{ produced mL / min}}{O_2 \text{ consumed mL / min}} ; \text{normally } 0.8$$

For example, a person breathing room air at sea level would have:

$$PAO_2 = (760 - 47)\, 0.21 - 40/0.8 = 100 \text{ mm Hg}$$

Effect of $PACO_2$ on PAO_2

PIO_2 = P inspired O_2, i.e., the PO_2 in the conducting airways during inspiration

Because $PaCO_2$ affects alveolar PO_2, hyperventilation and hypoventilation also affect PaO_2.

Hyperventilation (e.g., $PaCO_2$ = 20 mm Hg)

$PaO_2 = PiO_2 - PaCO_2$ (assume R = 1)
normal = 150 − 40 = 110 mm Hg
hyperventilation = 150 − 20 = 130 mm Hg

Hypoventilation (e.g., $PaCO_2$ = 80 mm Hg)

normal = 150 − 40 = 110 mm Hg
hypoventilation = 150 − 80 = 70 mm Hg

ALVEOLAR–BLOOD GAS TRANSFER: FICK LAW OF DIFFUSION

Simple diffusion is the process of gas exchange between the alveolar compartment and pulmonary capillary blood. Thus, those factors that affect the rate of diffusion also affect the rate of exchange of O_2 and CO_2 across alveolar membranes. (An additional point to remember is that each gas diffuses independently.)

$$\dot{V}\,\text{gas} = \frac{A}{T} \times D \times (P_1 - P_2)$$

$\dot{V}\,\text{gas} = $ rate of gas diffusion

Two structural factors and two gas factors affect the rate of diffusion.

Structural Features That Affect the Rate of Diffusion

A = surface area for exchange, ↓ in emphysema, ↑ in exercise

T = thickness of the membranes between alveolar gas and capillary blood, ↑ in fibrosis and many other restrictive diseases

A structural problem in the lungs is any situation in which there is a loss of surface area and/or an increase in the thickness of the membrane system between the alveolar air and the pulmonary capillary blood. In all cases, the rate of oxygen and carbon dioxide diffusion decreases. The greater the structural problem, the greater the effect on diffusion rate.

Factors Specific to Each Gas Present

D (diffusion constant) = main factor is solubility

The only clinically significant feature of D is solubility. The more soluble the gas, the faster it diffuses across the membranes. CO_2 is the most soluble gas with which we will be dealing. The great solubility of CO_2 is the main reason why it diffuses faster across the alveolar membranes than O_2.

Gradient across the membrane

$(P_1 - P_2)$: This is the gas partial pressure difference across the alveolar membrane. The greater the partial pressure difference, the greater the rate of diffusion.

Under resting conditions, when blood first enters the pulmonary capillary, the gradient for O_2 is:

$$100 - 40 = 60 \text{ mm Hg}$$

An increase in the PO_2 gradient across the lung membranes helps compensate for a structural problem. If supplemental O_2 is administered, alveolar PO_2 increases, because of the elevated gradient. However, supplemental O_2 does not improve the ability of the lungs to remove CO_2 from blood. This increased gradient helps return the rate of O_2 diffusion toward normal. The greater the structural problem, the greater the gradient necessary for a normal rate of O_2 diffusion.

The gradient for CO_2 is $47 - 40 = 7$ mm Hg.

Even though the gradient for CO_2 is less than for O_2, CO_2 still diffuses faster because of its greater solubility.

DIFFUSING CAPACITY OF THE LUNG (DLCO)

There are two terms that describe the dynamics of the transfer of individual substances between the interstitium and the capillary:

- If the substance equilibrates between the capillary and interstitium, it is said to be in a **perfusion-limited situation**.
- If the substance does not equilibrate between the capillary and interstitium, it is said to be in a **diffusion-limited situation**.

Carbon monoxide is a unique gas in that it typically doesn't equilibrate between the alveolar air and the capillary blood. Thus, it is a diffusion-limited gas. This is taken advantage of clinically, and the measurement of the uptake of CO in mL/min/mm Hg is referred to as the diffusing capacity of the lung. It is an index of the lung's structural features.

Transport of O₂ and CO₂ and the Regulation of Ventilation

Learning Objectives

❏ Interpret scenarios on transport of oxygen

❏ Answer questions about transport of carbon dioxide

❏ Interpret scenarios on neural regulation of alveolar ventilation

❏ Answer questions about respiratory stress: unusual environments

TRANSPORT OF OXYGEN

Units of Oxygen Content

Oxygen content   = concentration of oxygen in the blood, e.g., arterial blood

= 20 volumes %

= 20 volumes of oxygen per 100 volumes of blood

= 20 mL of oxygen per 100 mL of blood

= 0.2 mL of oxygen per mL of blood

Dissolved Oxygen

Oxygen dissolves in blood and this dissolved oxygen exerts a pressure. Thus, PO_2 of the blood represents the pressure exerted by the dissolved gas, and this PO_2 is directly related to the amount dissolved.

The amount dissolved (PO_2) is the primary determinant for the amount of oxygen bound to hemoglobin (Hb).

There is a direct linear relationship between PO_2 and dissolved oxygen. When PO_2 is 100 mm Hg, 0.3 mL O_2 is dissolved in each 100 mL of blood (0.3 vol%). Maximal hyperventilation can increase the PO_2 in blood to 130 mm Hg (0.4 vol%).

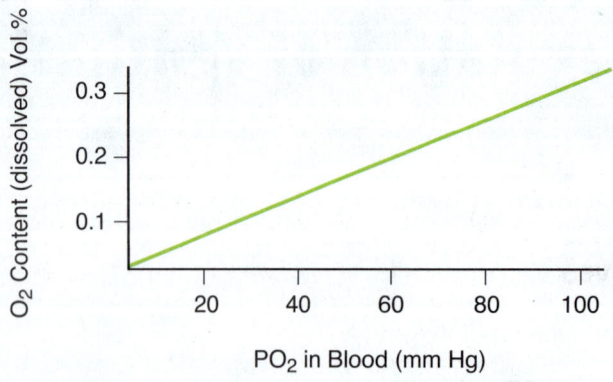

Figure 13-1. Dissolved Oxygen in Plasma

Oxyhemoglobin

Each Hb molecule can attach and carry up to four oxygen molecules. Binding sites on Hb have different affinities for oxygen. Also, the affinity of a site can and does change as oxygen is loaded or unloaded from the Hb molecule and as the chemical composition of the plasma changes.

Site 4 – O_2 attached when the minimal $PO_2 \cong 100$ mm Hg

systemic arterial blood = 97% saturated

Site 3 – O_2 attached when the minimal $PO_2 \cong 40$ mm Hg

systemic venous blood = 75% saturated (resting state)

Site 2 – O_2 attached when the minimal $PO_2 \cong 26$ mm Hg

P50 for arterial blood. P_{50} is the PO_2 required for 50% saturation

Site 1 – O_2 usually remains attached under physiologic conditions. Under physiologic conditions, only sites 2, 3, and 4 need to be considered.

Most of the oxygen in systemic arterial blood is oxygen attached to Hb. The only significant form in which oxygen is delivered to systemic capillaries is oxygen bound to Hb.

Hemoglobin O$_2$ Content

The number of mL of oxygen carried in each 100 mL of blood in combination with Hb depends on the Hb concentration [Hb]. Each gram of Hb can combine with 1.34 mL of O_2.

If the [Hb] is 15 g/100 mL (15 g%), then the maximal amount of O_2 per 100 mL (100% saturation) in combination with Hb is:

$1.34([Hb]) = 1.34(15) = 20$ mL O_2/100 mL blood = 20 vol%

This volume represents the "carrying capacity" of the blood.

The Hb in systemic arterial blood is about 97% saturated with oxygen, which means slightly less than 20 vol% is carried by Hb.

When blood passes through a systemic capillary, it is the dissolved oxygen that diffuses to the tissues. However, if dissolved oxygen decreases, PO_2 also decreases, and there is less force to keep oxygen attached to Hb. Oxygen comes off Hb and dissolves in the plasma to maintain the flow of oxygen to the tissues.

Hyperventilation or supplementing the inspired air with additional oxygen in a normal individual can significantly increase the PaO_2 but has effect on total oxygen content. For example:

	Dissolved O₂	HbO₂	Total O₂ Content
If PaO₂ = 100 mm Hg	0.3	≅ 19.4	≅ 19.7 vol%
If PaO₂ = 130 mm Hg (hyperventilation)	0.4	≅ 19.4	≅ 19.8 vol%

Oxygen–Hb Dissociation Curves

The following figure represents three major points on the oxygen–hemoglobin dissociation curve. The numbered sites refer to the hemoglobin site numbers discussed just previously.

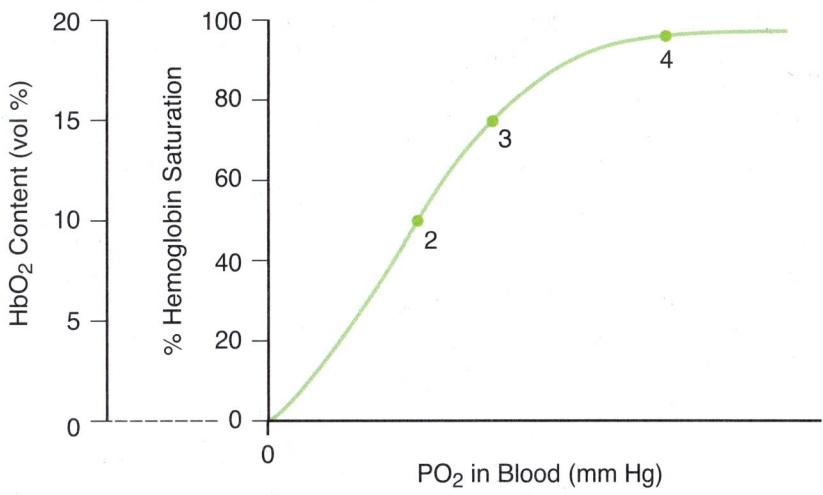

Figure 13-2. Oxygen–Hb Dissociation Curves

Shifting the curve

The following factors shift the curve to the right: increased CO_2 (Bohr effect), increased hydrogen ion (decrease pH), increased temperature, increased 2,3-bisphosphoglycerate (2,3-BPG).

In each case, the result can be explained as a reduced affinity of the Hb molecule for oxygen. However, carrying capacity is not changed, and systemic arterial blood at a PO_2 of 100 mm Hg is still close to 100% saturation.

The opposite chemical changes shift the curve to the left.

The following figure shows the result of a shift in the O_2–Hb dissociation curve. Note that only points on the steep part of the curve are affected.

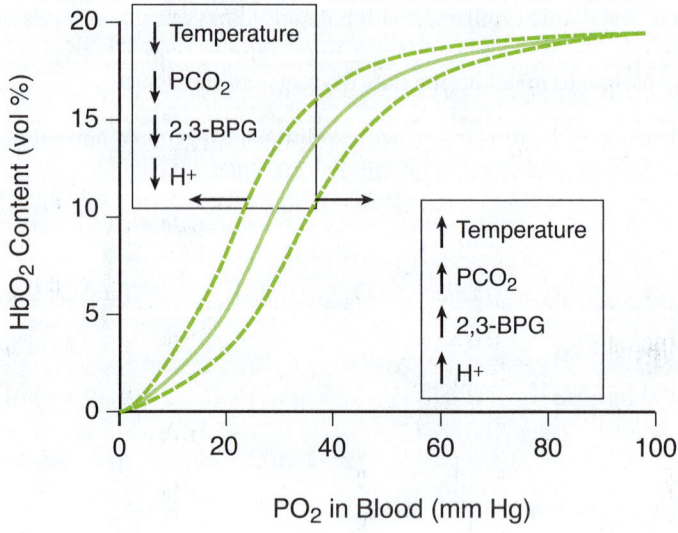

Figure 13-3. Shifts in Hb-O$_2$ Dissociation Curve

Shift to the Right	Shift to the Left
Easier for tissues to extract oxygen	More difficult for tissues to extract oxygen
Steep part of curve, O$_2$ content decreased	Steep part of curve, O$_2$ content increased
P$_{50}$ increased	P$_{50}$ decreased

Stored outdated blood loses 2,3-bisphosphoglycerate, causing a shift to the left. Fetal hemoglobin is also shifted to the left.

Hb Concentration Effects

Anemia

Characterized by a reduced concentration of Hb in the blood.

Polycythemia

Characterized by a higher than normal concentration of Hb in the blood.

P$_{50}$

In simple anemia and polycythemia, the P$_{50}$ does not change without tissue hypoxia; e.g., a PO$_2$ of 26 mm Hg produces 50% saturation of arterial hemoglobin.

The following figure illustrates the effects of an increase and a decrease in hemoglobin concentration. The main change is the plateau or carrying capacity of the blood. Note that the point halfway up each curve, the P$_{50}$, is still close to 26 mm Hg.

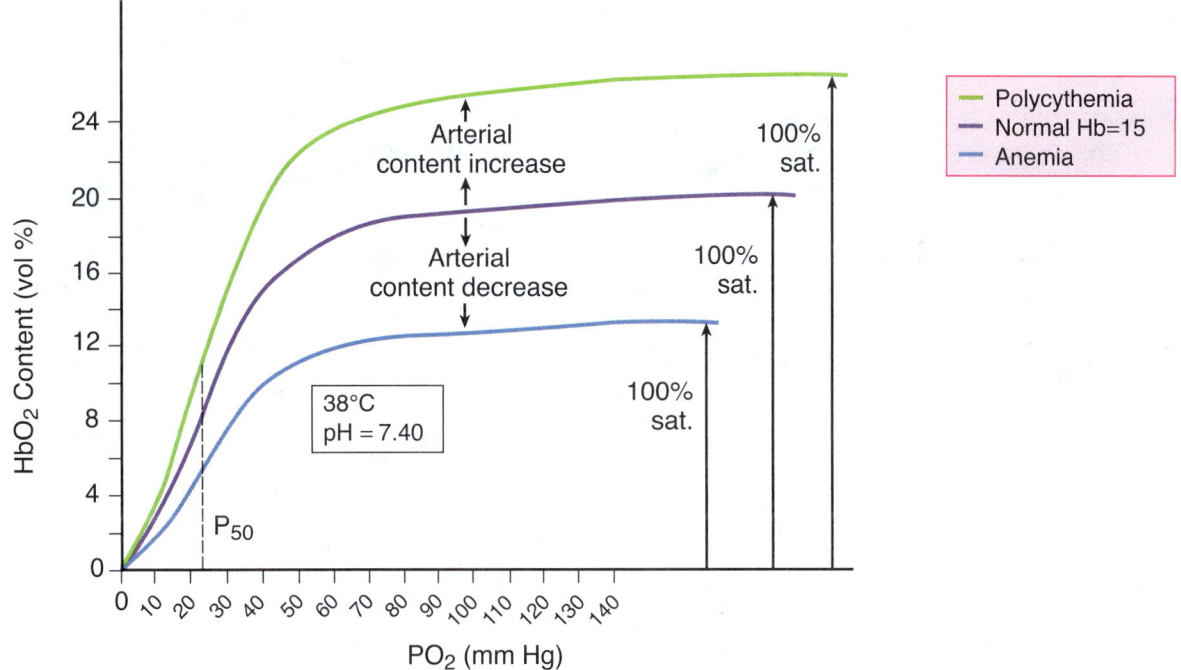

Figure 13-4. Effect of Hemoglobin Content on O$_2$ Content

Effects of Carbon Monoxide

Carbon monoxide (CO) has a greater affinity for Hb than does oxygen (240 times greater). The following figure shows that with CO the O$_2$–Hb dissociation curve is shifted to the left (CO increases the affinity of Hb for O$_2$) and HbO$_2$ content is reduced.

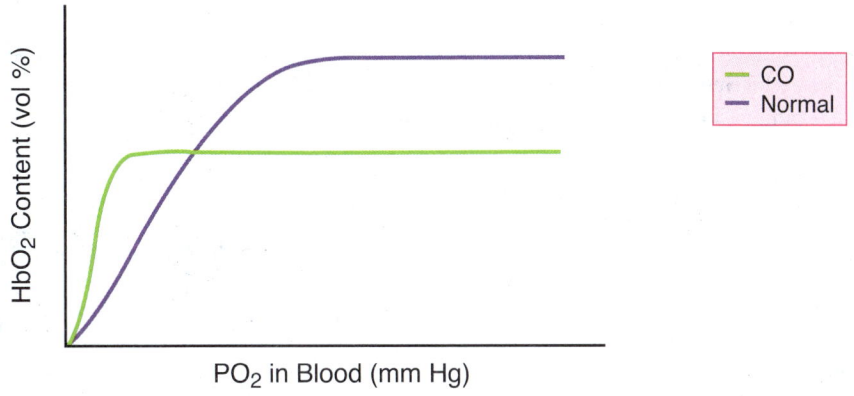

Figure 13-5. Carbon Monoxide Poisoning

The following table is a summary of the effects of anemia, polycythemia, and carbon monoxide poisoning.

Table 13-1. Systemic Arterial Blood

	PO₂	Hb Concentration	O₂ per g Hb	O₂ Content
Anemia	N	↓	N	↓
Polycythemia	N	↑	N	↑
CO poisoning (acute)	N	N	↓	↓

N = normal; O_2 per g Hb = % saturation.

In **anemia**, hemoglobin is saturated but arterial oxygen content is depressed because of the reduced concentration of hemoglobin.

In **polycythemia**, arterial oxygen content is above normal because of an increased hemoglobin concentration.

In **CO poisoning**, arterial PO₂ is normal, but oxygen saturation of hemoglobin is depressed.

TRANSPORT OF CARBON DIOXIDE

Dissolved Carbon Dioxide

Carbon dioxide is 24 times more soluble in blood than oxygen is. Even though the blood has a PCO_2 of only between 40 and 47 mm Hg, about 5% of the total CO_2 is carried in the dissolved form.

Carbamino Compounds

Carbon dioxide reacts with terminal amine groups of proteins to form carbamino compounds. The protein involved appears to be almost exclusively hemoglobin. About 5% of the total CO_2 is carried as carbamino compounds. The attachment sites that bind CO_2 are different from the sites that bind O_2.

Bicarbonate

About 90% of the CO_2 is carried as plasma bicarbonate. In order to convert CO_2 into bicarbonate or the reverse, carbonic anhydrase (CA) must be present.

$$CO_2 + H_2O \overset{CA}{\leftrightarrow} H_2CO_3 \leftrightarrow H^+ + HCO_3^-$$

The following people illustrates the steps in the conversion of CO_2 into bicarbonate in a systemic capillary.

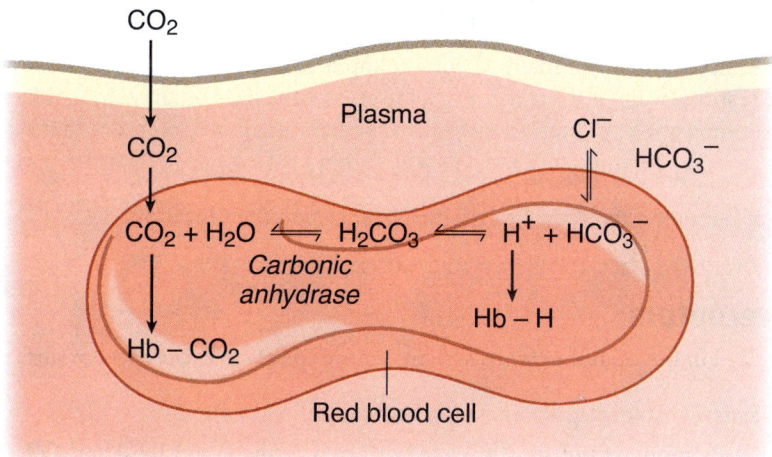

Figure 13-6. Formation of Bicarbonate Ion

Plasma contains no carbonic anhydrase; therefore, there can be no significant conversion of CO$_2$ to HCO$_3^-$ in this compartment.

Because deoxygenated Hb is a better buffer, removing oxygen from hemoglobin shifts the reaction to the right and thus facilitates the formation of bicarbonate in the red blood cells (Haldane effect).

To maintain electrical neutrality as HCO$_3^-$ moves into the plasma, Cl$^-$ moves into the red blood cell (chloride shift).

In summary:

- Bicarbonate is formed in the red blood cell but it is carried in the plasma compartment.
- The PCO$_2$ determines the volume of CO$_2$ carried in each of the forms listed above. The relationship between the PCO$_2$ and the total CO$_2$ content is direct and nearly linear, as shown in Figure 13-7.
- Thus, hyperventilation not only lowers the PCO$_2$ (mm Hg), it also lowers the CO$_2$ content (vol%).

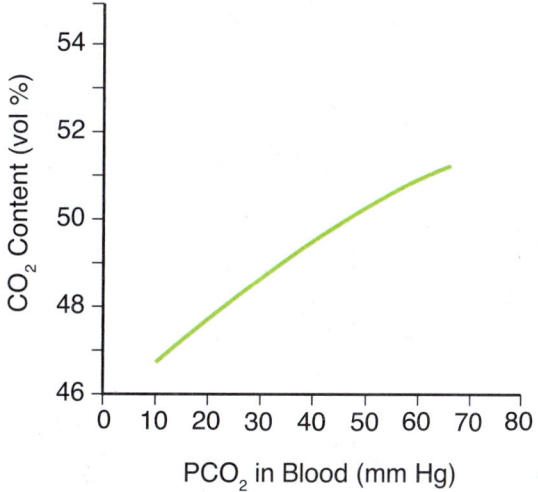

Figure 13-7. CO$_2$ Content in Blood

NEURAL REGULATION OF ALVEOLAR VENTILATION

The level of alveolar ventilation is driven mainly from the input of specific chemoreceptors to the central nervous system. The stronger the stimulation of these receptors, the greater the level of alveolar ventilation. Chemoreceptors monitor the chemical composition of body fluids. In this system, there are receptors that respond to pH, PCO_2, and PO_2.

There are two groups of receptors, and they are classified based upon their location.

Central Chemoreceptors

These receptors are located in the central nervous system—more specifically, close to the surface of the medulla.

- Stimulation of central chemoreceptors increases ventilation.
- The receptors directly monitor and are stimulated by cerebrospinal fluid $[H^+]$ and CO_2. The stimulatory effect of increased CO_2 may be due to the local production of H^+ from CO_2.
- Because the blood–brain barrier is freely permeable to CO_2, the activity of these receptors changes with increased or decreased systemic arterial PCO_2.
- H^+ does not easily penetrate the blood-brain barrier. Thus, an acute rise in arterial H^+, not of CO_2 origin, does not stimulate central chemoreceptors.
- These receptors are very sensitive and represent the main drive for ventilation under normal resting conditions at sea level.
- Therefore, the main drive for ventilation is CO_2 (H^+) on the central chemoreceptors.

This figure illustrates the relationship between the central chemoreceptors and the systemic arterial blood.

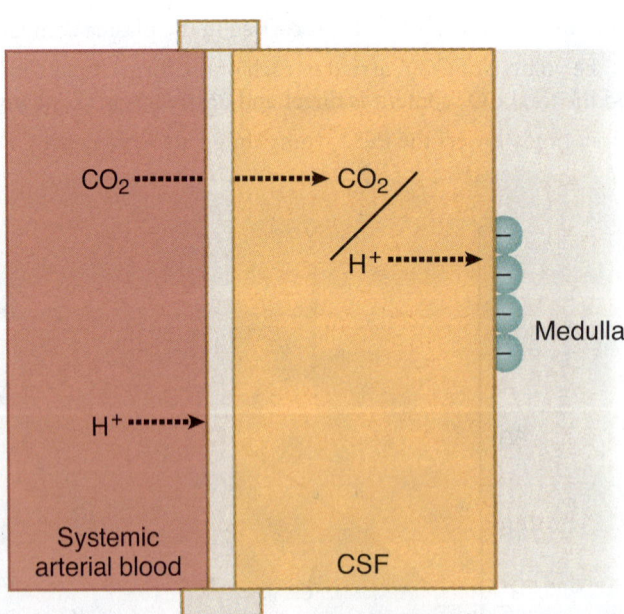

Figure 13-8. Central Chemoreceptors

The system does adapt, usually within 12 to 24 hours. The mechanism of adaptation may be the normalization of CSF H^+ by the pumping of HCO_3^- into or out of the CSF. There are no central PO_2 receptors.

Peripheral Chemoreceptors

These receptors are found within small bodies at two locations:

> **Carotid bodies:** near carotid sinus, afferents to CNS in glossopharyngeal nerve IX
> **Aortic bodies:** near aortic arch, afferents to CNS in vagus nerve X

The peripheral chemoreceptors are bathed in arterial blood, which they monitor directly. These bodies have two different receptors:

- **H$^+$/CO$_2$ receptors**
  - These receptors are less sensitive than the central chemoreceptors, but they still contribute to the normal drive for ventilation.
  - Therefore, under normal resting conditions at sea level, for all practical purposes, the total drive for ventilation is CO$_2$, mainly via the central chemoreceptors but with a small contribution via the peripheral chemoreceptors.
- **PO$_2$ receptors**
  - The factor monitored by these receptors is PO$_2$, not oxygen content.
  - Because they respond to PO$_2$, they are actually monitoring dissolved oxygen and not oxygen on Hb.
  - When systemic arterial PO$_2$ is close to normal ($\cong$100 mm Hg) or above normal, there is little if any stimulation of these receptors.
- They are strongly stimulated only by a dramatic decrease in systemic arterial PO$_2$.
- Sensitivity to hypoxia increases with CO$_2$ retention.

These receptors do not adapt.

Clinical Correlate

Although oxygen content is reduced in anemia, the PaO$_2$ is normal; thus, anemia does not directly stimulate ventilation. However, the reduced oxygen delivery can cause excess lactic acid production, which would in turn stimulate peripheral chemoreceptors.

Central Respiratory Centers

Medullary centers

Site of the inherent rhythm for respiration.

- Inspiratory center
- Expiratory center

For spontaneous breathing, an intact medulla must be connected to the diaphragm (via the phrenic nerve). Thus a complete C1 or C2 lesion will prevent diaphragmatic breathing but not a complete C6 or lower lesion.

The following figure illustrates the main features involved in the central control of ventilation.

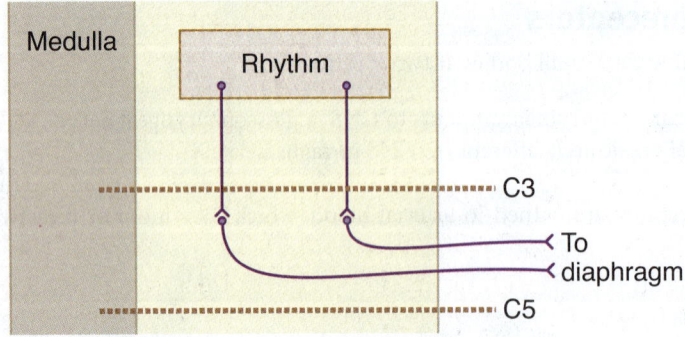

Figure 13-9. CNS Respiratory Centers

RESPIRATORY STRESS: UNUSUAL ENVIRONMENTS

High Altitude

At high altitude, atmospheric pressure is reduced from 760 mm Hg of sea level. Because atmospheric pressure is a factor that determines room air and alveolar PO_2, these two values are also reduced. These two values are permanently depressed unless enriched oxygen is inspired.

Therefore, PAO_2 <100 mm Hg, PaO_2 <100 mm Hg, and the low arterial PO_2 stimulates the peripheral chemoreceptors and increases alveolar ventilation. At high altitude, then, the main drive for ventilation changes from CO_2 on the central chemoreceptors at sea level to a low PO_2 drive of the peripheral chemoreceptors, and hyperventilation ensues.

Table 13-2. Acute Changes and Long-Term Adaptations (Acclimatization)

	Acute Changes	Acclimatization
PAO_2 and PaO_2	decreased	remains decreased
$PACO_2$ and $PaCO_2$	decreased	remains decreased
Systemic arterial pH	increased	decreases to normal via renal compensation
Hb concentration	no change	increases (polycythemia)
Hb % sat	decreased	remains decreased
Systemic arterial O_2 content	decreased	increases to normal

At high altitude, hypoxia can develop, resulting in increased circulating levels of erythropoietin. Erythropoietin increases red blood cell production and eventually causes an adaptive polycythemia.

Transport of O_2 and CO_2 and the Regulation of VentilationChapter 13 ● Transport of O_2 and CO_2 and the Regulation of Ventilation

Causes and Evaluation of Hypoxemia

14

Learning Objectives

❏ Demonstrate understanding of ventilation-perfusion differences in the lung

❏ Demonstrate understanding of review of the normal lung

❏ Answer questions about causes of hypoxemia

❏ Use knowledge of left-to-right shunts

VENTILATION–PERFUSION DIFFERENCES IN THE LUNG

Regional Differences in Intrapleural Pressure (IPP)

At FRC, the mean value for intrapleural pressure is –5 cm H_2O. However, there are regional differences, and the reason for these differences is gravity.

- Recall that the pleura is a fluid-filled space.
- Similar to the cardiovascular system, it is subject to gravitational influences
  - (P = height × gravity × density)
- Thus, IPP is higher (less negative) at the base (bottom) of the lung compared to the apex (top).

Regional Difference in Ventilation

- Because IPP is higher (less negative) at the base, the P_{TM} is less, resulting in less distension of alveoli, i.e., there is less volume.
- In contrast, IPP is more negative at the apex, thus the P_{TM} is higher, resulting in a greater volume in alveoli near the apex.
- As described in chapter 11, alveolar compliance decreases as lung volume increases. Thus, alveoli near the base are more compliant than alveoli near the apex. Stated another way, alveoli near the base are on a much steeper portion of the pressure-volume curve than alveoli near the apex.
- Because alveoli near the base are more compliant, there is more ventilation in this region compared to the apex.

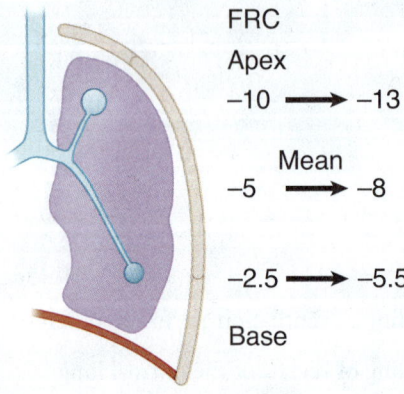

Figure 14-1. Upright Posture

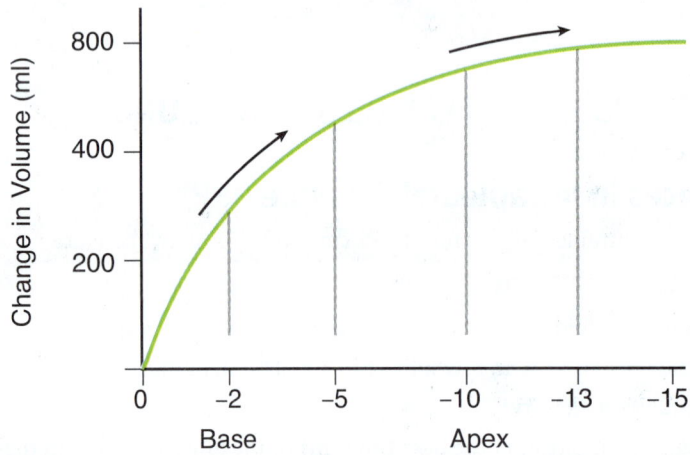

Figure 14-2. Regional Ventilation

Regional Differences in Blood Flow

Even in a normal individual, there are regional differences in blood flow through the pulmonary circuit. These differences, for the most part, can be attributed to the effect of gravity.

- Moving toward the base (with gravity), pressure in the pulmonary arteries is higher compared to pressure in the pulmonary arteries of the apex (against gravity).

- Since the intravascular pressure in arteries is higher, there is more blood flow to the base of the lung compared to the apex.

Ventilation–Perfusion Relationships

The partial pressures of O_2 and CO_2 in alveoli are determined by the combination of ventilation (adding O_2, removing CO_2) and perfusion (removing O_2 and adding CO_2). However, it is not the absolute amount of either that determines the composition of alveolar gases. Instead, it is the relative relationship between ventilation and perfusion that ultimately determines the alveolar gases. This is **ventilation-perfusion matching.**

In the normal situation, it would be "ideal" if ventilation and perfusion (blood flow) matched, i.e., the ventilation-perfusion ratio is one (Figure 14-3). If this were the case, then:

- $P_AO_2 = 100$ mm Hg
- $P_ACO_2 = 40$ mm Hg
- The blood draining the alveolus would have a pH = 7.40 (normal blood pH)

Although the above is "ideal," it is not often encountered. Figure 14-3 illustrates ventilation, blood flow (Q) or perfusion, and the relative ventilation-perfusion relationship for an **upright individual**. Toward the base of the lung:

- Alveolar ventilation is high relative to the apex (described above).
- Q is high relative to the apex (described above).
- However, relative to one another, Q is higher than alveolar ventilation, thus the ventilation-perfusion relationship is less than 1.0.
- In short, the alveoli are under-ventilated relative to the perfusion. If alveolar ventilation is inadequate, then it follows that PO_2 falls, PCO_2 rises, and blood pH falls (remember that CO_2 generates H^+).
- Thus, the PaO_2 at the base is <100 mm Hg and the $PaCO_2$ is >40 mm Hg.

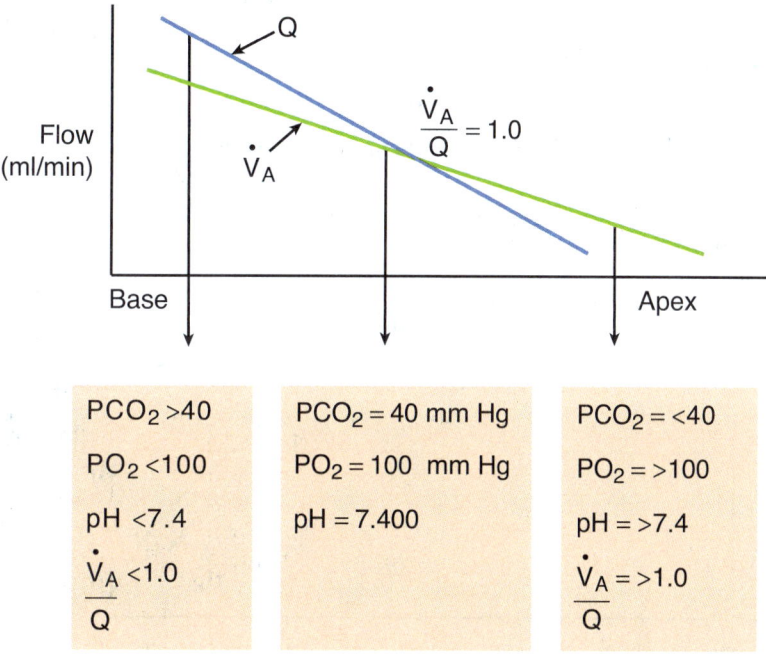

Figure 14-3. Ventilation–Perfusion Relationships

Moving toward the apex, the situation reverses:

- Alveolar ventilation is less relative to the base (described above).
- Q is less relative to the base (described above).
- However, relative to one another, Q is less than alveolar ventilation, thus the ventilation-perfusion relationship is greater than 1.0.
- In short, the alveoli are over-ventilated relative to the perfusion. If alveolar ventilation is excessive, then it follows that PO_2 rises, PCO_2 falls, and blood pH increases (remember that CO_2 generates H^+).
- Thus, the PaO_2 at the apex is >100 mm Hg and $PaCO_2$ is <40 mm Hg.

The effect of the ventilation-perfusion relationship is a continuum, which is illustrated in Figure 14-4.

- As $\dot{V}A/Q$ **falls**, PO_2 falls and PCO_2 rises.
- As $\dot{V}A/Q$ **rises**, PO_2 rises and PCO_2 falls.

Extremes of $\dot{V}A/Q$ Mismatch

- **Shunt:** If ventilation is zero but there is blood flow, then $\dot{V}A/Q = 0$.
  - This is a right-to-left shunt, and the blood gases leaving the alveoli are the same as venous blood (low PO_2, and high PCO_2; Y-axis intercept in Figure 14-4). This causes arterial hypoxemia, which is discussed later in this chapter.
- **Alveolar dead space:** If blood flow is zero but there is ventilation, then $\dot{V}A/Q = \infty$.
  - This is alveolar dead space, and alveolar gases become the same as inspired (high PAO_2 and $PACO_2 = 0$; X-axis intercept in Figure 14-4).

To summarize:

- As $\dot{V}A/Q$ falls, PO_2 falls and PCO_2 rises. The extreme is a shunt.
  - Remember, however, that the lower the $\dot{V}A/Q$, the more it "behaves" as a shunt, i.e., the alveolar and blood gases get closer and closer to venous gases. Similar to a shunt, this can lead to arterial hypoxemia, both of which are discussed later in this chapter.
- As $\dot{V}A/Q$ rises, PO_2 rises and PCO_2 falls. The extreme is alveolar dead space.
  - Similar to above, the higher the $\dot{V}A/Q$, the more the situation looks like alveolar dead space.

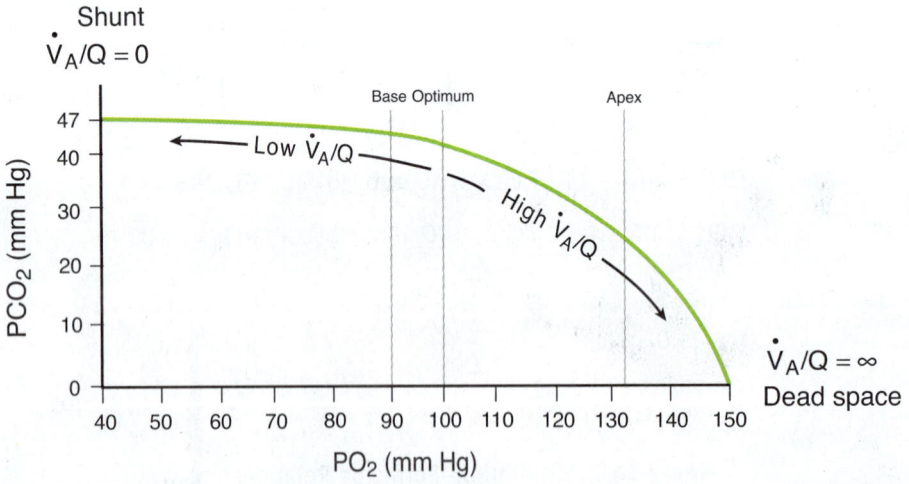

Figure 14-4. Shunt and Dead Space

Hypoxic Vasoconstriction

This is a clinically important phenomenon that is unique to the pulmonary circulation. Whenever there is a decrease in alveolar PO_2, a local vasoconstriction of pulmonary blood vessels is produced. The result is a lowering of blood flow through that lung unit and a redistribution of blood to better-ventilated units.

Exercise

In exercise, there is increased ventilation and pulmonary blood flow. However, during exercise, ventilation increases more than cardiac output and $\dot{V}_A/Q$ goes well above 1.0 as one approaches maximal oxygen consumption. Also, the base–apex flows are more uniform.

REVIEW OF THE NORMAL LUNG

Before discussing the causes of hypoxemia let's review the normal state using standard values:

- The blood entering the alveolar-capillary unit is mixed venous blood.
    - $PO_2 = 40$ and $PCO_2 = 45$ mm Hg
- $PaO_2 = 100$ mm Hg and $PaCO_2 = 40$ mm Hg
- Both gases are perfusion-limited and thus their partial pressures at the end of the capillary are the same as alveolar.
- Arterial blood gas (ABG) sample shows $PaO_2 = 95$ mm Hg, and $PaCO_2 = 40$ mm Hg.
    - The A–a gradient is 5 mm Hg (ranges 5-10 mm Hg but is influenced by age; see Clinical Correlate) and is primarily the result of anatomic shunts.

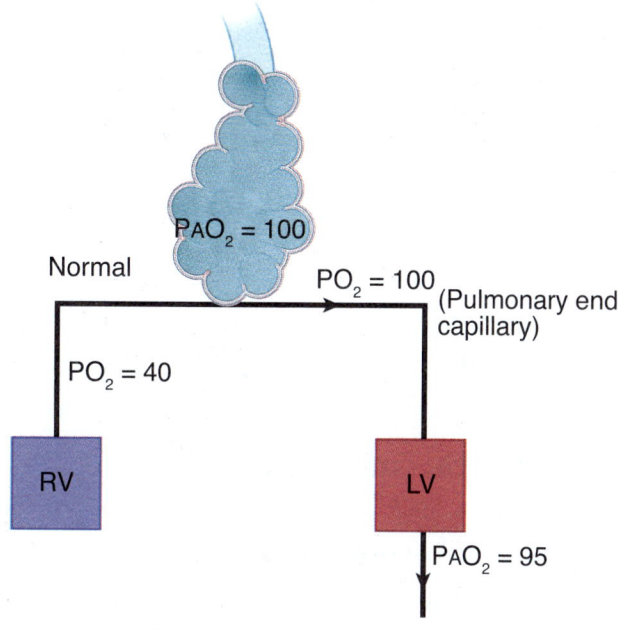

Figure 14-5. Normal State

CAUSES OF HYPOXEMIA

Hypoventilation

Hypoventilation of the entire lung elevates alveolar PCO_2, and the increase in PCO_2 decreases PO_2. For example, if alveolar ventilation decreases by 50%, alveolar PCO_2 becomes 80 mm Hg (an increase of 40 mm Hg). Assuming a respiratory ratio close to 1.0, alveolar PO_2 decreases by about 40 mm Hg to 60 mm Hg. If no other problem exists, pulmonary end capillary and systemic arterial PO_2 also decreases by 40 mm Hg.

Hypoventilation is characterized as an equal decrease in PO_2 in all three compartments. **As a result, A–a is normal and end-tidal PO_2 is still be a good index of systemic arterial PO_2** (provided A–a gradient is taken into consideration).

The hypoxemia can be relieved by increasing the inspired oxygen, however CO_2 remains elevated because ventilation is unchanged.

In summary

- There is no increase in the A–a oxygen gradient.
- Supplemental oxygen can relieve the hypoxemia.
- End-tidal air still reflects the systemic arterial compartment.
- The problem is not within the lung itself.

Diffusion Impairment

Diffusion impairment means a structural problem in the lung. As described in chapter 12, this can be produced by a decreased surface area and/or increased thickness of lung membranes. The consequences of diffusion impairment are illustrated and summarized in the following figure.

In marked diffusion impairment, pulmonary end capillary PO_2 is less than alveolar PO_2. End-tidal PO_2 is not a good index of systemic arterial PO_2.

In diffusion impairment, supplemental oxygen corrects the hypoxemia. Note that although the arterial PO_2 may be restored to normal, or even be above normal by supplemental oxygen, there is still an abnormally large A–a gradient.

In summary

- There is an increase in A–a oxygen gradient.
- Supplemental oxygen can relieve the hypoxemia.
- End-tidal air does not reflect the arterial values.
- It is characterized by a decrease in DLCO.

Ventilation-Perfusion Mismatch: Low $\dot{V}_A/Q$ Units

If ventilation to a significant portion of the lungs is markedly compromised, then $\dot{V}_A/Q$ is $<< 1.0$. As described earlier, low $\dot{V}_A/Q$ creates alveolar and end-pulmonary capillary blood gases that are approaching venous gases (low PO_2, and high CO2). The blood from these low $\dot{V}_A/Q$ units mixes in with blood draining normal alveolar-capillary units, resulting in systemic hypoxemia.

Because PaO_2 is normal in areas that don't have low $\dot{V}_A/Q$, the A–a gradient is elevated. Supplemental oxygen corrects the hypoxemia because the problem regions still have some ventilation—it is just much lower than normal. Similar to diffusion impairment described above, the increased A–a gradient means end-tidal PO_2 is not reflective of PaO_2.

In summary

- There is an increased A–a oxygen gradient.
- Supplemental oxygen corrects the hypoxemia.
- End-tidal air does not reflect the arterial values.

Renal Structure and Glomerular Filtration

15

Learning Objectives

❏ Use knowledge of overview of the renal system

❏ Demonstrate understanding of nephron hemodynamics

❏ Demonstrate understanding of glomerular filtration

OVERVIEW OF THE RENAL SYSTEM

Functions of the Kidney

- Excretes waste products: urea, uric acid, creatinine
- Water and electrolyte balance
- Acid/base balance
- Secretes the hormone erythropoietin and the enzyme, renin into the circulation
- Hydroxylates 25-hydroxy-Vit D to form the active form of Vitamin D (1,25 dihydroxy-Vit D)

Functional Organization of the Kidney

Figure 15-1 illustrates the cortical versus the medullary organization of the kidney. Nephrons (the funcionting unit of the kidney) with glomeruli in the outer cortex have short loops of Henle (cortical nephrons). Those with glomeruli in the inner cortex have long loops of Henle that penetrate the medullary region (juxtamedullary nephrons).

- 7/8 of all nephrons are cortical nephrons
- 1/8 of all nephrons are juxtamedullary nephrons

Nephron structures in the medulla consist of the long loops of Henle and the terminal regions of the collecting ducts. All other structures, including the first section of the collecting ducts, are in the cortex.

- In the cortex, the proximal and distal tubules, as well as the initial segment of the collecting duct, are surrounded by a capillary network, and the interstitium is close to an isotonic environment (300 mOsm/kg).
- The medullary region has capillary loops organized similar to the loops of Henle, known as the vasa recta.
- The slow flow through these capillary loops preserves the osmolar gradient of the interstitium.
- However, this slow flow also keeps the PO_2 of the medulla lower than that in the cortex and even though the metabolic rate of the medulla is lower than in the cortex, it is more susceptible to ischemic damage.

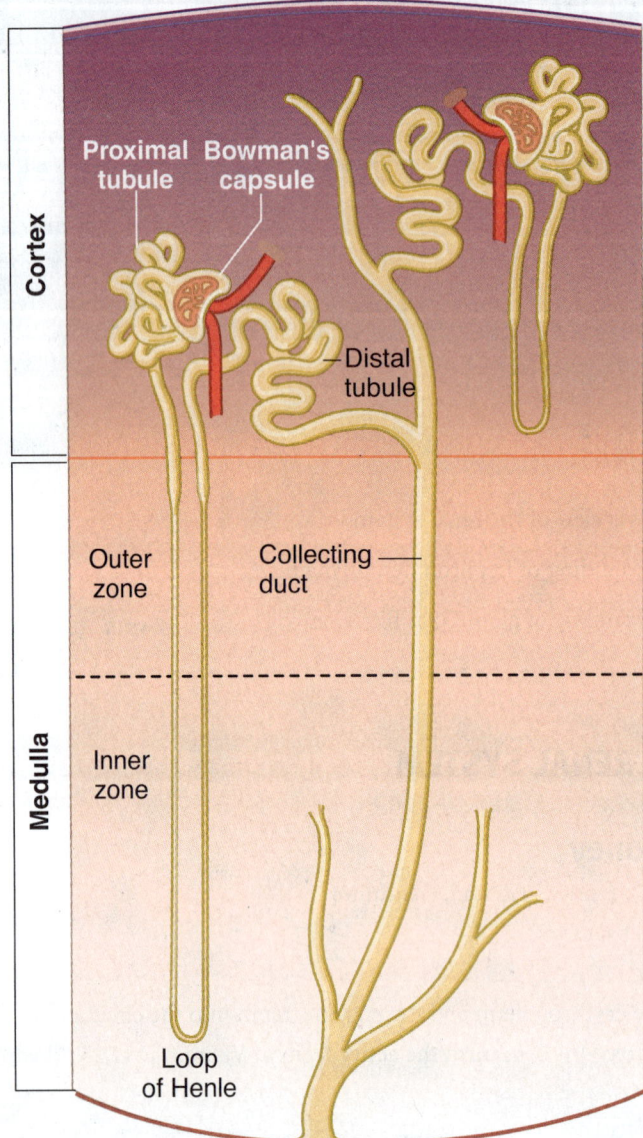

Figure 15-1. Nephron Structures

Function of the Nephron

There are four basic renal processes (Figure 15-2): filtration, reabsorption, secretion, and excretion.

Filtration

- Blood is filtered by nephrons, the functional units of the kidney.
- Each nephron begins in a renal corpuscle (site of filtration), which is composed of a glomerulus enclosed in a Bowman's capsule.
- An ultrafiltrate resembling plasma enters Bowman's space.
- Filtration is driven by Starling forces.
- The ultrafiltrate is passed through, in turn, the proximal convoluted tubule, the loop of Henle, the distal convoluted tubule, and a series of collecting ducts to form urine.
- Filtration rate or filtered load is the amount of a substance (in mg) that is filtered at the glomeruli in a min (mg/min; see chapter 16 for more details).

Reabsorption

- Tubular reabsorption is the process by which solutes and water are removed from the tubular fluid that was formed in Bowman's space and transported into the blood.
- Reabsorption rate is the amount (in mg) that is reabsorbed from the ultrafiltrate in a min (mg/min; see chapter 16 for more details).

Secretion

- Tubular secretion is the transfer of materials from peritubular capillaries to the renal tubular lumen.
- Tubular secretion is primarily the result of active transport.
- Usually only a few substances are secreted.
- Many drugs are eliminated by tubular secretion.
- Secretion rate is the amount (in mg) that is secreted into the ultrafiltrate in a min (mg/min; see chapter 16 for more details).

Excretion

- Substances that are in the urine are excreted.
- A substance that is filtered and not completely reabsorbed is excreted in the urine.
- A substance that is filtered and then secreted is excreted in large amounts in the urine because it comes from two places in the nephron.
- Excretion rate is the amount (in mg) that is excreted in the urine in a min (mg/min; see chapter 16 for more details).

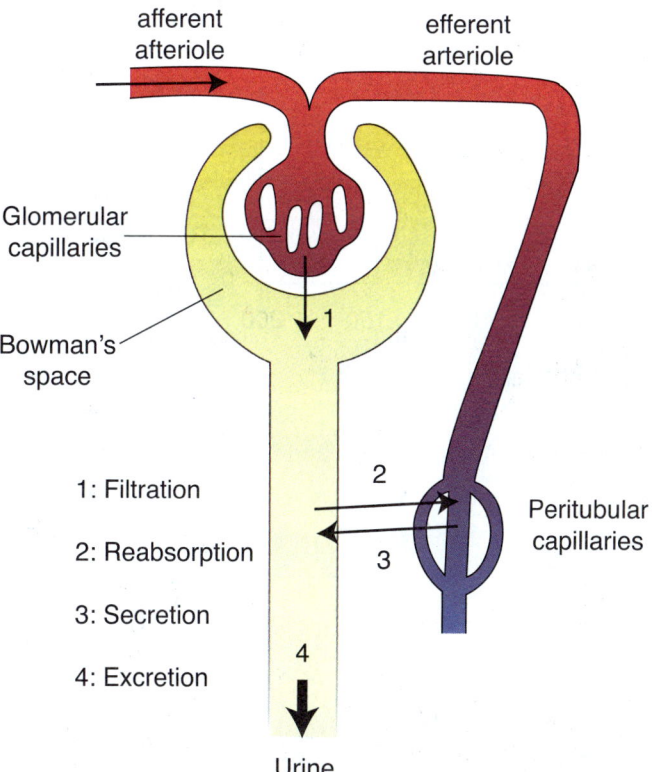

Excretion = (filtration − reabsorption) + secretion

Figure 15-2. Renal Processes

The following equation is central to understanding renal physiology and will be addressed in detail in a later chapter.

$$\text{Excretion rate (ER)} = (\text{filtration rate} - \text{reabsorption rate}) + \text{secretion rate}$$

Blood flow throughout the kidney: renal artery → arcuate artery → afferent arteriole → glomerular capillaries → efferent arterioles → peritubular capillaries → vasa recta → arcuate vein → renal vein

The kidneys are very effective in autoregulating blood flow (Figure 15-3). This is primarily due to changes in the resistance of the afferent arterioles, for which two mechanisms are involved:

- **Myogenic responses**

    - The intrinsic property of smooth muscle is to contract when stretched (see also CV chapter)

- **Tubuloglomerular feedback (TGF)**

    - Increased MAP leads to an increase in RBF and GFR

    - High delivery of sodium ions to the macula densa (the part of the nephron where the thick ascending loop of Henle connects with the beginning of the distal tubule) → adenosine and ATP secretion → vasoconstriction of the afferent arteriole → decreases renal blood flow and GFR.

    - Decreased delivery of sodium to the macula densa dilates the arteriole and leads to an increase in renal blood flow and GFR.

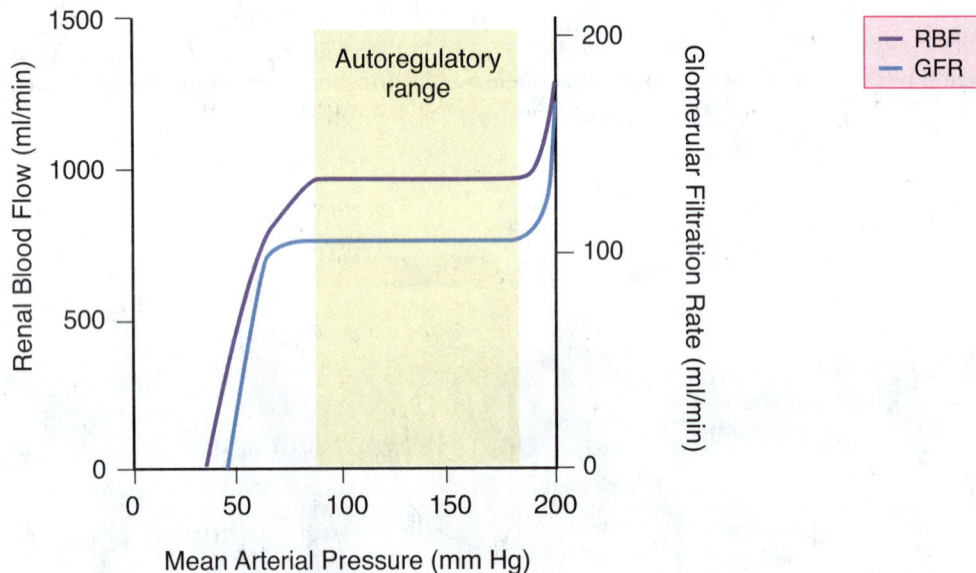

Figure 15-3. Autoregulation and the Renal Function Curve

NEPHRON HEMODYNAMICS

Series Hemodynamics

The individual nephrons that make up both kidneys are connected in parallel. However, the flow through a single nephron represents two arterioles and two capillary beds connected in series.

Flow must be equal at all points in any series system. If flow changes, it changes equally at all points in the system.

For a brief review of CV hemodynamics, refer back to section V, chapter 8.

Flow (Q) = pressure gradient / resistance (R) = (upstream pressure-downstream pressure)

Blood flows from high pressure to low pressure. Two factors decrease flow:

- Decreasing the pressure gradient (decreasing the upstream pressure or increasing the downstream pressure)
- Increasing resistance at any point throughout the circuit

Therefore, when considering blood flow through the nephron as a series circuit, if resistance increases (vasoconstriction) at the afferent arteriole or efferent arteriole, renal plasma flow decreases.

When an arteriole vasoconstricts, this increases the resistance at that arteriole and there are two changes to consider:

- Flow across the entire circuit **decreases**
- Pressure builds up or **increases** before (upstream) the point of resistance **and** pressure **decreases** after (downstream) the point of resistance

When an arteriole vasodilates, this decreases the resistance at that arteriole, and there are two changes to consider:

- Flow across the entire circuit **increases**
- Pressure **decreases** before (upstream) the point of resistance **and** pressure **rises** after (downstream) the point of resistance

---

Clinical Correlate

A patient with essential hypertension has increased renal artery pressure leading to vasoconstriction of the afferent arterioles and vasodilation of the efferent arterioles.

- High pressure of the juxtaglomerular apparatus leads to decreased renin secretion → low angiotensin II → vasodilation of the efferent arterioles.

A patient with renal artery stenosis has low renal artery pressures, leading to low pressures at the afferent arterioles.

- Vasodilation of the afferent arterioles and vasoconstriction of the efferent arterioles (increased renin secretion leads to increased angiotensin II).

Hemodynamics of a single nephron

Figure 15-4 represents the hemodynamics of a single nephron. Connected in series are the high-pressure filtering capillaries of the glomerulus and the low-pressure reabsorbing peritubular capillaries.

The glomerular capillaries have a very high hydrostatic pressure because the efferent arterioles are very narrow and thus have a very high resistance. Likewise, there is a large pressure drop as blood flows past this high resistant arteriole and the peritubular capillaries have very low hydrostatic pressure.

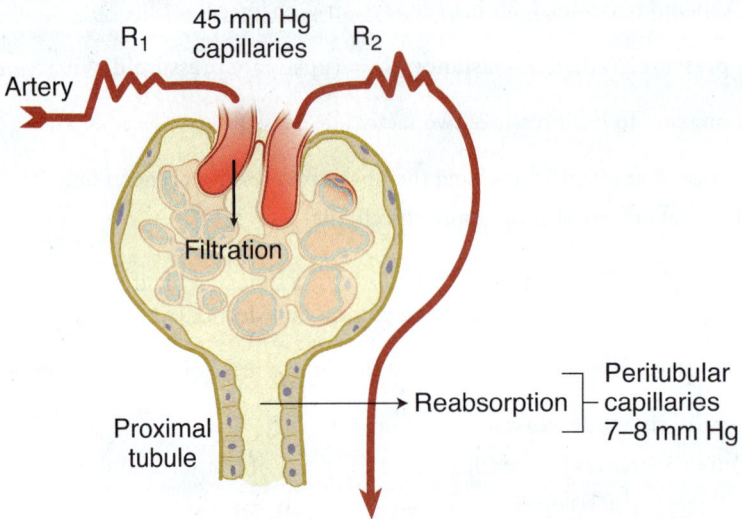

Figure 15-4. Glomerular Hemodynamics
R_1 = Afferent arteriole; R_2 = Efferent arteriole.

Independent response of the afferent and efferent arterioles

The following table illustrates the expected consequences of independent isolated constrictions or dilations of the afferent and efferent arterioles.

Table 15-1. Consequences of Independent Isolated Constrictions or Dilations of the Afferent and Efferent Arterioles

	Glomerular Cap Pressure	Peritubular Cap Pressure	Nephron Plasma Flow
Constrict efferent	↑	↓	↓
Dilate efferent	↓	↑	↑
Constrict afferent	↓	↓	↓
Dilate afferent	↑	↑	↑

GLOMERULAR FILTRATION

Glomerular filtration rate (GFR) is the rate at which fluid is filtered into Bowman's capsule. The units of filtration are volume filtered per unit time, e.g., mL/min or liters/day; in a young healthy adult it is about 120 mL/min or 180 L/day.

If one kidney is removed (half of the functioning nephrons lost), GFR decreases only about 25% because the other nephrons compensate.

The Four Factors Determining Net Filtration Pressure

The following figure illustrates the role of the four factors that determine net filtration pressure.

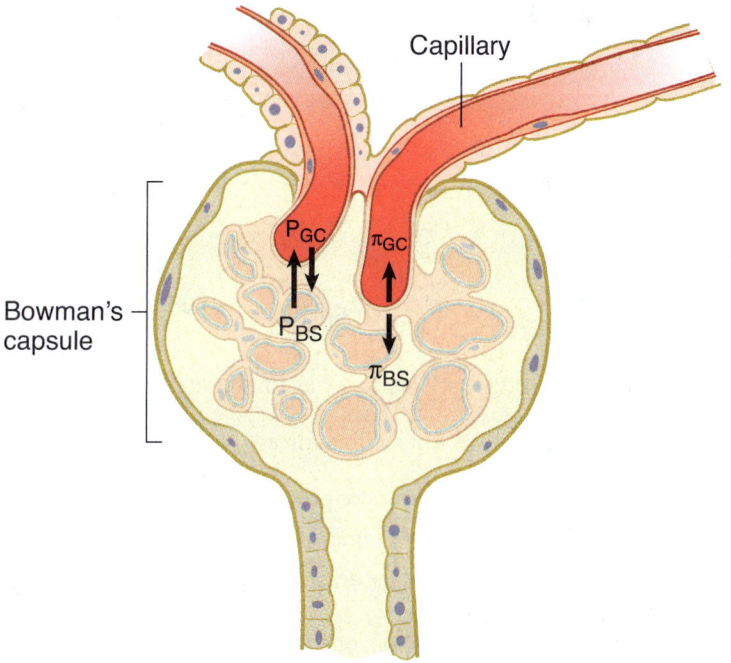

Figure 15-5. Determinants of Filtration

$$P_{GC} = \text{Hydrostatic pressure of glomerular capillary}$$
$$\pi_{GC} = \text{Oncotic pressure of glomerular capillary}$$
$$P_{BS} = \text{Hydrostatic pressure of Bowman's space}$$
$$\pi_{BS} = \text{Oncotic pressure of Bowman's space}$$

Hydrostatic pressure of the glomerular capillaries

PGC: The hydrostatic pressure of the glomerular capillaries is the only force that promotes filtration. Under normal conditions, this is the main factor that determines GFR.

Oncotic pressure of the plasma

πGC: The oncotic pressure of the plasma varies with the concentration of plasma proteins. Because fluid is filtered but not protein, oncotic pressure, which opposes filtration, increases from the beginning to the end of the glomerular capillaries.

Hydrostatic pressure in Bowman's space

PBS: The hydrostatic pressure in Bowman's capsule opposes filtration. Normally, it is low and fairly constant and does not affect the rate of filtration. However, it increases and reduces filtration whenever there is an obstruction downstream, such as a blocked ureter or urethra (postrenal failure).

Protein or oncotic pressure in Bowman's space

πBS: This represents the protein or oncotic pressure in Bowman's space. Very little if any protein is present, and for all practical purposes this factor can be considered zero.

> **Normal Values**
>
> PBS = 8 mm Hg
>
> PGC = 45 mm Hg
>
> πBS = 0 mm Hg
>
> πGC = 24 mm Hg

Net filtration pressure = PGC − πGC − PBS = 45 − 24 − 8 = 13 mm Hg

To summarize, filtration at the glomeruli depends on starling forces:

- The glomerular capillaries have very high hydrostatic pressures → this is why filtration occurs here
- Increasing the glomerular hydrostatic pressure → increases GFR
- Decreasing the glomerular hydrostatic pressure → decreases GFR

Oncotic pressure opposes GFR →↑ plasma protein →↑ oncotic pressure →↓ GFR (no effect on RPF) ↓ plasma protein →↓ oncotic pressure →↑ GFR (no effect on RPF)

The increased concentration of protein (increase oncotic pressure) is carried into the peritubular capillaries and promotes a greater net force of reabsorption.

Important: If the main driving force for GFR is the hydrostatic pressure, what is the main driving force the reabsorption at the proximal tubule? The force that is driving reabsorption at the proximal tubule is the oncotic pressure in the peritubular capillaries.

Filtering Membrane

The membrane of the glomerulus consists of three main structures:

- Capillary endothelial wall with fenestrations that have a magnitude greater than proteins; in addition, the wall is covered with negatively charged compounds
- Glomerular basement membrane made up of a matrix of extracellular negatively charged proteins and other compounds
- Epithelial cell layer of podocytes next to Bowman's space; the podocytes have foot processes bridged by filtration slit diaphragms

Around the capillaries is the mesangium, containing mesangial cells similar to monocytes.

The capillary wall with its fenestrated endothelium, the basement membrane with hydrated spaces, and the interdigitating foot processes of the podocytes combined with an overall large surface area, create a high hydraulic conductivity (permeable to water and dissolved solutes). Passage of large proteins is restricted because of negative charge of the membrane system.

In addition to the net hydraulic force, GFR depends on both the permeability and the surface area of the filtering membrane. The decrease in GFR in most diseased states is due to a reduction in the membrane surface area. This also includes a decrease in the number of functioning nephrons.

Bridge to Pathology

In nephrotic syndrome, there is marked disruption of the filtering membrane. As a result, plasma proteins now pass through the membrane and are eliminated in the urine. This is typically associated with a non-inflammatory injury to the glomerular membrane system. The most common clinical signs are:

- Marked proteinuria >3.5 gm/day (because of disrupted glomerular membrane system)
- Edema (loss of plasma oncotic pressure)
- Hypoalbuminemia (albumin lost in urine)
- Lipiduria (disrupted membrane system and proteins in urine)
- Hyperlipidemia (increased lipid synthesis in liver)

In nephritic syndrome, there is an inflammatory disruption of the glomerular membrane system. This disruption allows proteins and cells to cross the filtering membrane. The most common clinical signs are:

- Proteinuria <3.5 gm/day (evidence of disrupted membrane)
- Hematuria (disrupted membrane)
- Oliguria (inflammatory infiltrates reduce fluid movement across the membrane)
- Hypertension (inability of kidney to regulate the extracellular volume)
- Azotemia (inability to filter and excrete urea)

Materials Filtered

The following are easily or freely filtered:

- Major electrolytes: sodium, chloride, potassium, bicarbonate
- Metabolic waste products: urea, creatinine
- Metabolites: glucose, amino acids, organic acids (ketone bodies)
- Nonnatural substances: inulin, PAH (p-aminohippuric acid)
- Lower-weight proteins and peptides: insulin, myoglobin

The following are not freely filtered:

- Albumin and other plasma proteins
- Lipid-soluble substances transported in the plasma attached to proteins, such aslipid-soluble bilirubin, T4 (thyroxine), other lipid-soluble hormones; unbound lipid-soluble substances such as free-cortisol are filtered and can appear in the urine

As blood flows though the glomerular capillary, plasma is filtered, but albumin is not, so the plasma albumin concentration and oncotic pressure increase.

Fluid Entering Bowman's Capsule

The fluid entering Bowman's space is an ultrafiltrate of plasma; that is, the filtrate has the same concentration of dissolved substances as plasma, except proteins. The osmolality of the filtrate is 300 mOsm/Kg. The criteria for effective osmolality are the same as those previously stated for extracellular fluid (section I).

If a substance is freely filtered by the kidney, the ratio of the filtrate concentration to plasma concentration TF/P = 1.0. This means the concentrations in Bowman's space and the plasma is the same.

Filtration Fraction

The following formula for filtration fraction (FF) and the normal values given should be memorized.

$$FF = \text{fraction of the material entering the kidney that is filtered normally 0.20 or 20\% for a freely filtered substance}$$

$$FF = \frac{GFR}{RPF} \qquad \begin{array}{l} GFR = 120 \text{ mL/min} \\ RPF \text{ (renal plasma flow)} = 600 \text{ mL/min} \end{array}$$

$$= \frac{120 \text{ mL/min}}{600 \text{ mL/min}} = 0.20 \text{ or } 20\%$$

- FF affects oncotic pressure in the peritubular capillary (πPC). The greater the FF, the higher the oncotic pressure in the peritubular capillaries; that is because FF represents loss of protein-free fluid into Bowman's space, thereby increasing the concentration of protein in the plasma.
- If FF decreases, then πPC decreases
- Only 20% of the renal plasma flow is filtered. Every minute 600 ml of plasma enters the kidneys. That is the renal plasma flow.
- 20% or 120 mL of plasma is filtered hence a GFR of 120 mL.

Factors Affecting FF

Based on the preceding discussion, the following should be expected for afferent versus efferent constriction:

	Afferent Constriction	Efferent Constriction
Glomerular filtration pressure	↓	↑
GFR	↓	↑
RPF	↓	↓
FF	↔	↑

Effects of Sympathetic Nervous System

Stimulation of the sympathetic neurons to the kidney causes vasoconstriction of the arterioles, but has a greater effect on the afferent arteriole. As a consequence:

- RPF decreases
- PGC decreases
- GFR decreases
- FF increases
- PPC decreases
- πPC increases
- ↑ forces promoting reabsorption in the peritubular capillaries because of a lower peritubular capillary hydrostatic pressure and an increase in plasma oncotic pressure (FF increases)

Effects of Angiotensin II

Angiotensin II (Ang II) is a vasoconstrictor. It constricts both the afferent and efferent arterioles, but is has a bigger effect on the efferent arteriole. As a consequence:

- RPF decreases
- PGC increases
- GFR increases
- FF increases
- PPC decreases
- πPC increases
- ↑ forces promoting reabsorption in the peritubular capillaries because of a lower peritubular capillary hydrostatic pressure and an increase in plasma oncotic pressure (FF increases)

During a stress response, there is an increase in both sympathetic input and very high levels of circulating angiotensin II. As a consequence:

- Increased sympathetic tone to the kidneys and very high levels of angiotensin II vasoconstrict both the afferent and the efferent arterioles. Because both arterioles constrict, there is a large drop in the RPF and only a small drop in the GFR.
- The net effect is an increase in FF.
- The increase in FF → increase in oncotic pressure → increase in the reabsorption in proximal tubules
- Overall, less fluid is filtered and a greater percentage of that fluid is reabsorbed in the proximal tubule, leading to preservation of volume in a volume depleted state
- There is also an increase in ADH due to the low volume state
- Activation of the sympathetic nervous system also directly increases renin release

The net effect of angiotensin II is to preserve GFR in volume-depleted state. In a volume-depleted state, a decrease in GFR is beneficial because less fluid filtered results in less fluid excretion (however, a very large decrease in GFR prevents removal of waste products like creatinine and urea). Angiotensin II prevents a large decrease in GFR.

Solute Transport: Reabsorption and Secretion

Solute Transport: Reabsorption and Secretion

16

Learning Objectives

❏ Interpret scenarios on solute transport

❏ Interpret scenarios on quantifying renal processes (mass balance)

❏ Demonstrate understanding of clearance

❏ Answer questions about TM tubular reabsorption and TM tubular secretion

❏ Use knowledge of the renal handling of some important solutes

SOLUTE TRANSPORT

Transport proteins in the cell membranes of the nephron mediate the reabsorption and secretion of solutes and water transport in the kidneys. Acquired defects in transport proteins are the cause of many kidney diseases.

In addition the transport proteins are important drug targets.

Transport Mechanisms

Simple diffusion

- Net movement represents molecules or ions moving down their electrochemical gradient.
- This doesn't require energy.

Facilitated diffusion (facilitated transport)

- A molecule or ion moving across a membrane down its concentration gradient attached to a specific membrane-bound protein.
- This doesn't require energy.

Active transport

- A protein-mediated transport that uses ATP as a source of energy to move a molecule or ion against its electrochemical gradient.

Dynamics of Protein-Mediated Transport

Uniport

- Transporter moves a single molecule or ion as in the uptake of glucose into skeletal muscle or adipose tissue. This is an example of facilitated diffusion.

Symport (cotransport)

- A coupled protein transport of two or more solutes in the same direction as in Na-glucose, Na-amino acid transporters.

Antiport (countertransport)

- A coupled protein transport of two or more solutes in the opposite direction.

Generally, protein carriers transport substances that cannot readily diffuse across a membrane. There are no transporters for gases and most lipid-soluble substances because those substances readily move across membranes by simple diffusion.

Characteristics common to all protein-mediated transport

Rate of transport

A substance is transported more rapidly than it would be by diffusion, because the membrane is not usually permeable to any substance for which there is a transport protein.

Saturation kinetics

- As the concentration of the substance initially increases on one side of the membrane, the transport rate increases.
- Once the transporters become saturated, transport rate is maximal (TM = transport maximum). Rate of transport is dependent upon:
  - Concentration of solute
  - Number of functioning transporters; the only way to increase TM is to add more protein carriers to the membrane
- Once all the protein carriers are saturated, the solutes are transported across the membrane at a constant rate. This constant rate is TM.
- There is no TM is simple diffusion.

Chemical specificity

To be transported, the substance must have a certain chemical structure. Generally, only the natural isomer is transported (e.g., D-glucose but not L-glucose).

Competition for carrier

Substances of similar chemical structure may compete for the same transporter. For example, glucose and galactose generally compete for the same transport protein.

Primary and secondary transport

- In primary active transport, ATP is consumed directly by the transporting protein, (e.g., the Na/K-ATPase pump, or the calcium-dependent ATPase of the sarcoplasmic reticulum).
- Secondary active transportdepends indirectly on ATP as a source of energy, as in the cotransport of Na-glucose in the proximal tubule. This process depends on ATP utilized by the Na/K-ATPase pump.
- Glucose moves up a concentration gradient via secondary active transport.

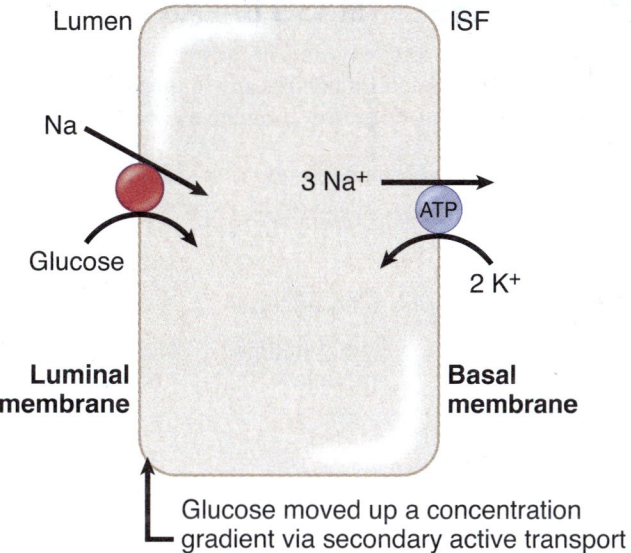

Figure 16-1. Renal Tubule or Small Intestine

This figure represents a renal proximal tubular cell. The Na/K-ATPase pump maintains a low intracellular sodium concentration, which creates a large gradient across the cell membrane. It is this sodium gradient across the luminal membrane that drives secondary active transport of glucose.

In summary, the secondary active transport of glucose:

- Depends upon luminal sodium
- Is stimulated by luminal sodium (via increased sodium gradient)
- Is linked to the uptake of sodium
- Depends upon rate of metabolic ATP production

Another example of secondary active transport is the counter transport of Na–H^+ also in the proximal tubule. This process depends on the Na/K-ATPase pump.

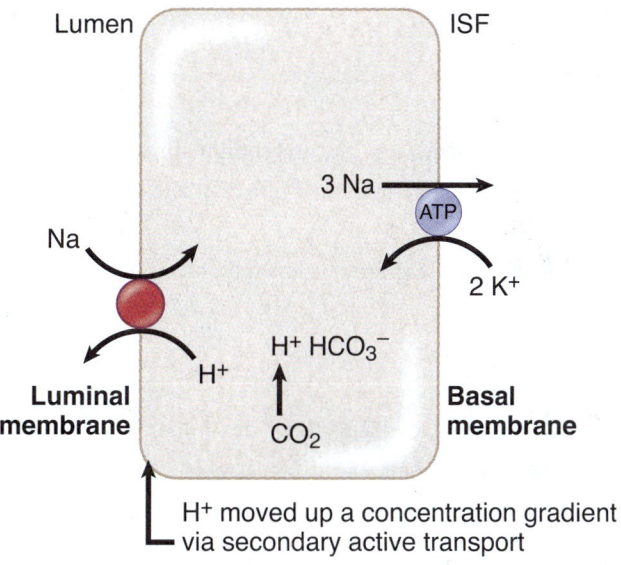

Figure 16-2. Proximal Tubule

QUANTIFYING RENAL PROCESSES (MASS BALANCE)

As indicated in the previous chapter, there are four processes in the nephron: filtration, reabsorption, secretion, and excretion. Figure 16-3 illustrates that how the nephron handles any solute, on a net basis, can be derived because the rate at which it enters (filtered load) and its rate of excretion can be measured.

Both variables are expressed as an amount of substance per unit time, and the units are the same, e.g., mg/min.

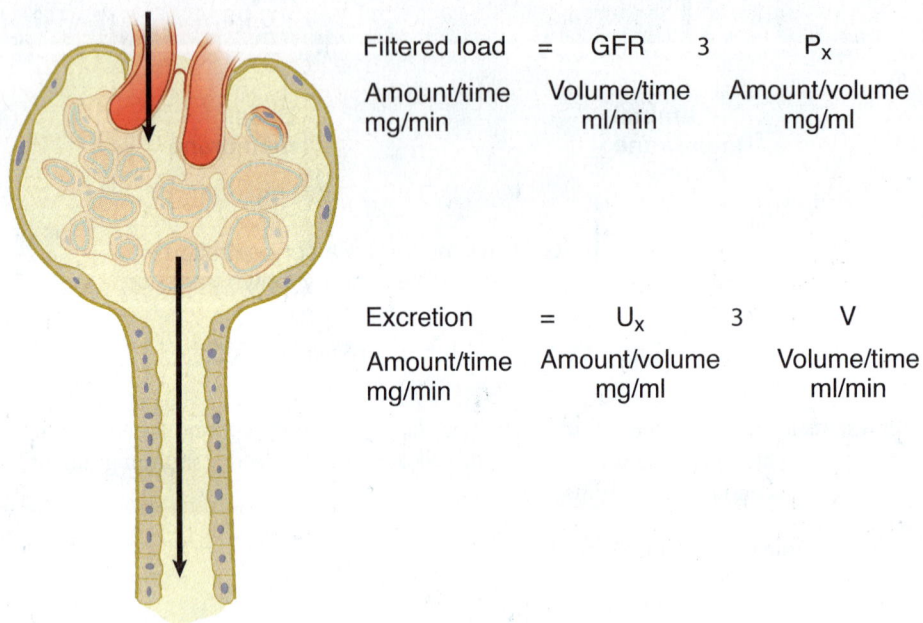

Filtered load $=$ GFR $\times$ P_x

| Amount/time | Volume/time | Amount/volume |
| mg/min | ml/min | mg/ml |

Excretion $=$ U_x $\times$ V

| Amount/time | Amount/volume | Volume/time |
| mg/min | mg/ml | ml/min |

Figure 16-3. Relationship of Filtered Load and Excretion
U_x = urine concentration of substance; V = urine flow rate

No Net Tubular Modification

- Filtered load = excretion rate
- The amount filtered and amount excreted per unit time are always the same, e.g., inulin, mannitol.

Net Reabsorption

- Filtered load > excretion
- Excretion is always less than filtered load, e.g., glucose, sodium, urea.
- If the substance is completely reabsorbed, the rate of filtration and the rate of reabsorption are equal.
- Excretion rate is 0.
- If the substance is partially reabsorbed, excretion is less than filtration.

Net Secretion

- Filtered load < excretion
- Excretion is always greater than filtered load, e.g., PAH, creatinine.
- Creatinine is freely filtered, and a very small amount is secreted.

CLEARANCE

Clearance refers to a theoretical volume of plasma from which a substance is removed over a period of time. Applying the principles of mass balance above, if a solute has an ER, then it is cleared by the kidney. In other words, if it is filtered and not fully reabsorbed or is secreted, then it appears in the urine and is thus cleared from the body.

If, on the other hand, it is filtered and then all is reabsorbed, the ER and clearance is zero, and it is not cleared by the kidney.

For example, if the concentration of substance x is 4 molecules per liter and the excretion of x is 4 molecules per minute, the volume of plasma cleared of x is 1 L per minute. If the excretion of x decreases to 2 molecules per minute, the volume cleared of x is only 0.5 L per minute. If the concentration of x decreases to 2 molecules per liter of plasma and excretion is maintained at 2 molecules per minute, the cleared volume is back to 1 L per minute. These numbers are summarized in the following table.

Table 16-1. Example Calculations of Clearance Values

Plasma Concentration (molecules/L)	Excretion Rate (molecules/minute)	Volume Cleared (L/minute)
4	4	1.0
4	2	0.5
2	2	1.0

TM TUBULAR REABSORPTION

Glucose

The following figure graphically represents the dynamics of glucose filtration, reabsorption, and excretion. It is the application of the principle of mass balance and clearance discussed above. Many substances are reabsorbed via a TM system, and glucose serves as our prototypical example.

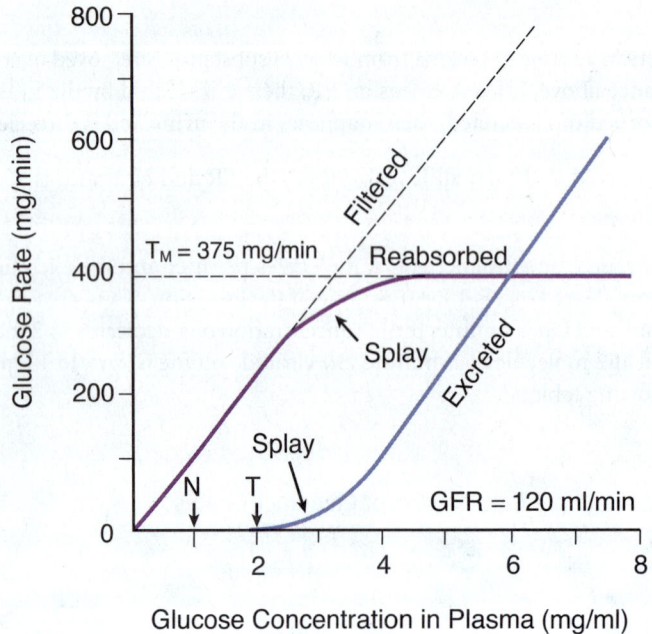

Figure 16-4. Transport Maximum Reabsorption of Glucose

N = normal plasma glucose concentration
T = plasma (renal) threshold

Note the X-axis is glucose rate (mg/min). As was just discussed, there are 3 rates: filtration (dashed line), excretion (blue line); and reabsorption (purple line), which is filtered load (filtration rate) – excretion rate (ER).

- At low plasma levels, the filtration and reabsorption rates of glucose are equal, thus glucose does not appear in the urine and the clearance is zero.

- TM is the maximal reabsorption rate of glucose, i.e., the rate when all the carriers (SGLT-2/1; see chapter 18) are saturated. TM can be used as an index of the number of functioning nephrons.

- The rounding of the reabsorption curve into the plateau is called **splay**. Splay occurs because some nephrons reach TM before others. Thus, TM for the entire kidney is not reached until after the region of splay.

- Plasma (or renal) threshold is the plasma glucose concentration at which glucose first appears in the urine. This occurs at the beginning of splay. Before splay, all of the glucose that is filtered is reabsorbed and the ER is 0.

TM TUBULAR SECRETION

p-aminohippuric acid (PAH) secretion

- PAH secretion from the peritubular capillaries into the proximal tubule is an example of a transport maximum system.

- As a TM system, it has the general characteristics discussed for the reabsorption of glucose except for the direction of transport.

Figure 16-5 illustrates the renal handling of PAH at low plasma concentrations.

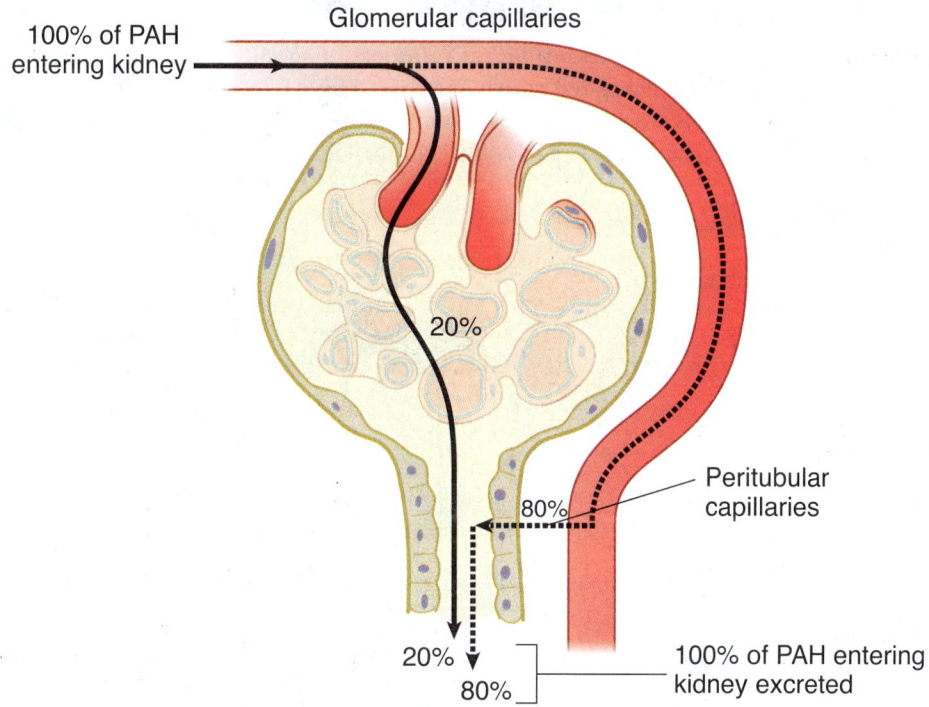

Figure 16-5. Secretion of PAH

Normal values:

Renal plasma flow = 600 mL/min

GFR = 120 mL/min

FF = .20

- The renal plasma flow (RPF) is the volume of plasma that enters the kidney in a minute (600 mL/min).
- The RPF contains the total concentration of PAH dissolved in plasma in mg/ml entering the PAH.
- Of the RPF, 20% (120 mL) is typically filtered, regardless of the total amount of PAH entering the kidney (in the RPF).
- Whatever is filtered is excreted, it is NOT reabsorbed; therefore, that 20% is **always** cleared (removed from the plasma) and excreted (placed in the urine)!!

What happens to the rest of the PAH (the 480 mL [80%] of plasma that was not filtered)? That depends on the concentration of PAH in the RPF:

- If the RPF has a low concentration of PAH, 20% of the PAH in the RPF is filtered and the rest of PAH (the remaining 80% of the RPF) is secreted; 100% of PAH in the RPF is excreted in the urine right arrow; therefore, 100% is cleared.
- **All** of the PAH that enters the kidney is removed and is excreted in the urine; it is all cleared from the plasma. If you looked at the renal vein, it would have no PAH.
- When the PAH concentration is below the transport maximum, we can use the clearance of PAH to calculate the estimated RPF.

Remember:

- If it is in the renal vein, it was not cleared.
- If it is in the urine, it was cleared.

THE RENAL HANDLING OF SOME IMPORTANT SOLUTES

The illustrations in the following figure represent the net transport of specific types of substances for a normal individual on a typical Western diet (contains red meat). The dashed lines represent the route followed by the particular substance. Quantitative aspects are not shown. For example, in B, 20% of the substance entering the kidney is filtered and excreted, and the remaining 80% passes through the kidneys and back into the general circulation without processing.

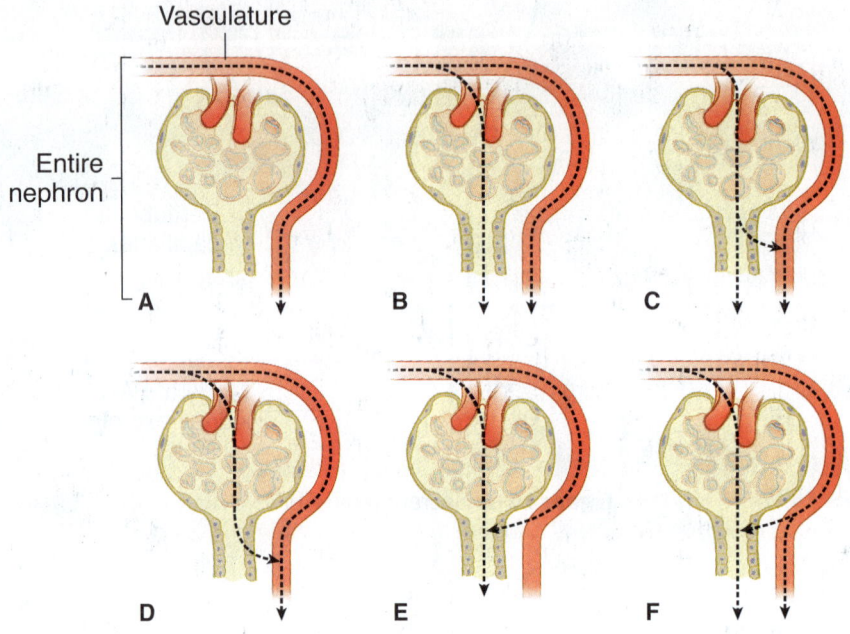

Figure 16-6. Graphical Representation of Transport
A = protein; **B** = inulin; **C** = potassium, sodium, urea; **D** = glucose, bicarbonate; **E** = PAH; **F** = creatinine

---

Note

These illustrations are meant to show overall net transport only.

Clinical Estimation of GFR and Patterns of Clearance

17

Learning Objectives

❏ Use knowledge of clearance as an estimator of GFR

❏ Demonstrate understanding of clearance curves for some characteristic substances

❏ Solve problems concerning free water clearance

❏ Use knowledge of sodium and urea clearance

CLEARANCE AS AN ESTIMATOR OF GFR

Estimates of GFR are used clinically as an index of renal function and to assess the severity and the course of renal disease. A fall in GFR means the disease is progressing, whereas an increase in GFR suggests a recovery. In many cases a fall in GFR may be the first and only clinical sign of renal dysfunction. Estimations of GFR rely on the concept of clearance.

Substances having the following characteristics can be used to estimate GFR.

- Stable plasma concentration that is easily measured
- Freely filtered into Bowman's space
- Not reabsorbed, secreted, synthesized, or metabolized by the kidney

Ideal substances include inulin, sucrose, and mannitol. Even though the clearance of inulin is considered the gold standard for the measurement of GFR, it is not used clinically. Instead clinical estimates of GFR rely on creatinine.

Creatinine is released from skeletal muscle at a constant rate proportional to muscle mass. Muscle mass decreases with age but GFR also normally decreases with age. Creatinine is freely filtered and not reabsorbed by the kidney, though a very small amount is secreted into the proximal tubule.

$$\text{Creatinine production} = \text{creatinine excretion} = \text{filtered load of creatinine} = P_{cr} \times GFR$$

Thus, if creatinine production remains constant, a decrease in GFR increases plasma creatinine concentration, while an increase in GFR decreases plasma creatinine concentration.

Plasma creatinine, however, is not a very sensitive measure of reduced GFR. It only reveals large changes in GFR. As shown in Figure 17-1, a significant reduction of GFR only produces a modest elevation of plasma or serum creatinine concentration.

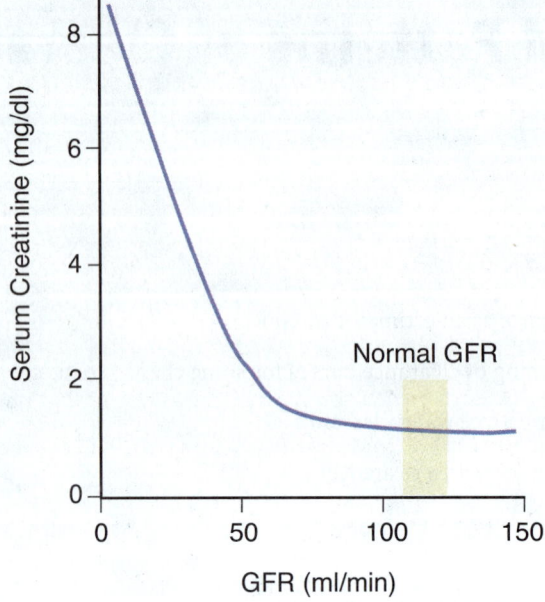

Figure 17-1. Serum Creatinine as Index of GFR

The only practical numerical estimate is the calculated clearance of creatinine. The following is all that is needed:

- Plasma creatinine concentration
- Timed collection of urine and the urine concentration of creatinine

CLEARANCE CURVES FOR SOME CHARACTERISTIC SUBSTANCES

The following graph plots clearance versus increasing plasma concentration for four substances. A description of each curve follows the figure.

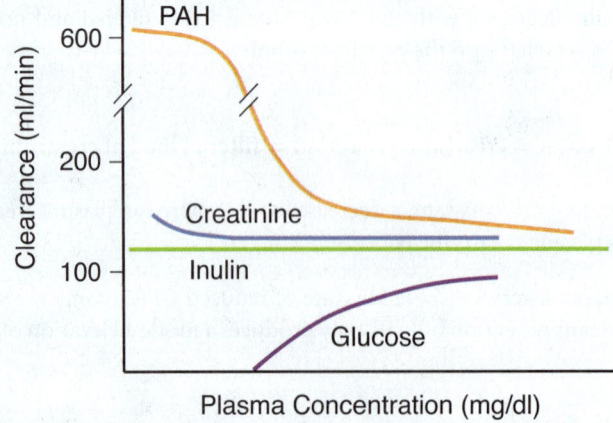

Figure 17-2. Clearance Curves

Inulin

- The clearance of inulin is independent of the plasma concentration, thus plotting it on the graph produces a line parallel to the X-axis. This is because a rise in the plasma concentration produces a corresponding rise in filtered load and thus a corresponding rise in ER (recall that inulin is neither secreted nor reabsorbed). In other words, the numerator and denominator of the clearance equation for inulin change in proportion, leaving the quotient (clearance) unchanged.

- It is always parallel to the X-axis, and the point of intersection with the y axis is always GFR.

- If GFR increases, the line shifts upward; likewise, if GFR decreases, the line shifts down.

Glucose

- At low plasma levels, the clearance of glucose is zero because all of the FL is reabsorbed.

- As the plasma levels rise, the FL exceeds the TM in some nephrons and as a result, glucose appears in the urine and thus has a clearance.

- The plasma level at which glucose first appears in the urine is called the plasma (or renal) threshold.

- As the plasma level rises further, the clearance increases and approaches that of inulin. The clearance never equals inulin because some glucose is always reabsorbed.

Creatinine

- Because there is some secretion of creatinine, the clearance is always greater than the clearance of inulin.

- However, because only a small amount is secreted, creatinine clearance parallels inulin clearance and is independent of production rate (excretion rises as plasma concentration increases).

- Because it is endogenously produced, it is not necessary to infuse it to get a clearance measurement, as has to be done to measure inulin clearance. Therefore, the clearance of creatinine is the preferred clinical method for determining GFR.

PAH

- At low plasma concentrations, the clearance equals renal plasma flow.

- As the plasma concentration rises, the carriers in some nephrons hit TM, resulting in some PAH appearing in the renal venous plasma.

- Plasma concentrations above TM reduce the clearance of PAH (described in chapter 16)

- As the plasma level rises further, the clearance approaches but never equals GFR because some PAH is always secreted.

Summary of the highest clearance to the lowest clearance:

$$PAH > creatinine > inulin > urea > sodium > glucose = albumin$$

Remember, if it is in the renal vein, it is not cleared. This could be because it was not filtered (like albumin) or it was filtered and all reabsorbed (like glucose).

FREE WATER CLEARANCE

Free water clearance is the best measure of the balance between solute and water excretion. Its use is to determine whether the kidneys are responding appropriately to maintain normal plasma osmolality. Free water clearance is how much solute-free water is being excreted; it is as if urine consisted of plasma (with solutes) plus or minus pure water.

- If urine osmolality is 300 mOsm/kg (isotonic urine), free water clearance is zero.
- If plasma osmolality is too low, urine osmolality should be lower still (positive free water clearance) in order to compensate.
- Positive-free water clearance tends to cause increased plasma osmolality; negative free water clearance causes reduced plasma osmolality.
- C_{H_2O} (+) = hypotonic urine is formed (osmolality <300 mOsm/kg)
- C_{H_2O} (−) = hypertonic urine is formed (osmolality >300 mOsm/kg)

$$C_{H_2O} = V - \frac{U_{osm}V}{P_{osm}}$$

$$V = C_{H_2O} + C_{osm}$$

V = urine flow rate
U_{osm} = urine osmolarity
P_{osm} = plasma osmolarity

SODIUM AND UREA CLEARANCE

Sodium

- Sodium always appears in the urine, thus sodium always has a positive clearance.
- The fractional excretion of Na^+ ($F_E Na^+$; equation not shown) indicates the fraction (percentage) of the filtered Na^+ that is excreted. It is very useful in differentiating prerenal from intrarenal acute renal failure (see next chapter).
- Since almost the entire filtered load of sodium is reabsorbed its clearance is just above zero. Aldosterone, by increasing the reabsorption of sodium, decreases the $FeNa^+$. Atrial natriuretic factor increases the $FeNa^+$ by causing a sodium diuresis.

Urea

- Urea is freely filtered but partially reabsorbed.
- Because some urea is always present in the urine, you always clear a portion of the 120 mL/min filtered into Bowman's space.
- Since urea tends to follow the water and excretion is flow dependent, a diuresis increases urea clearance and an antidiuresis decreases urea clearance.
- ADH increases reabsorption of urea in the medullary collecting duct → increase in BUN → decrease in clearance → if the plasma concentration is increasing in the renal venous plasma, less is cleared from the plasma
- With a small volume of concentrated urine, the concentration of urea is relatively high, but the excretion is less than in a diuresis that has a much lower concentration of urea. It is the large volume in the diuresis that increases the urea excretion and clearance.

Regional Transport 18

Learning Objectives

❏ Solve problems concerning the proximal tubule

❏ Explain information related to loop of Henle

❏ Use knowledge of distal tubule and collecting duct

❏ Use knowledge of collecting duct

❏ Answer questions about renal tubular acidosis and renal failure

❏ Explain information related to disorders of potassium homeostasis

THE PROXIMAL TUBULE

The fluid that enters the proximal tubule is an isotonic ultrafiltrate (300 mOsm/kg). The concentration of a freely filtered substance in this fluid equals its plasma concentration. Figure 18-1 illustrates the main cellular transport processes of the proximal tubular cells.

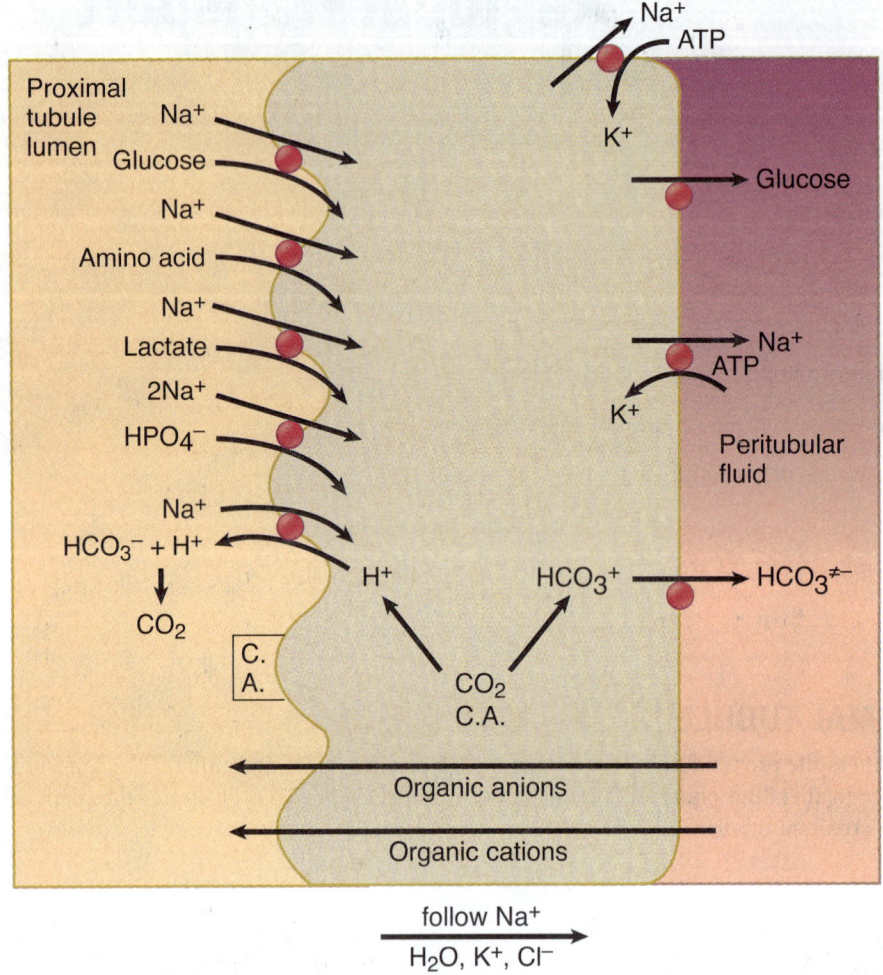

Figure 18-1. Transport in Proximal Tubule

Proximal Tubule (PT) Changes

Sodium

- Approximately two-thirds of the filtered sodium is reabsorbed in the proximal tubule (PT). The basolateral Na^+-K^+ ATPase creates the gradient for Na^+ entry into the cell and its removal from the cell back into the bloodstream.

- Although it can be modified some, the PT captures two-thirds of the filtered sodium (referred to as glomerulotubular balance). Recapturing two-thirds of the sodium helps protect extracellular volume despite any changes that may occur in GFR.

- Catecholamine and angiotensin II stimulate the basolateral ATPase and thus enhance the fraction of sodium reabsorbed in the proximal tubule.

Water and electrolytes

- About two-thirds of the filtered H_2O, K^+ and almost two-thirds of the filtered Cl^- follow the sodium (leaky system to these substances), and the osmolality at the end of the proximal tubule remains close to 300 mOsm/kg (isosmotic reabsorption). The chloride concentration rises slightly through the proximal tubule because of the large percentage of bicarbonate reabsorbed here.

- Therefore, at the end of the proximal tubule, osmolality and the concentrations of Na^+ and K^+ have not changed significantly from plasma, but only one-third of the amount originally filtered remains.

Metabolites

- Normally, all of the filtered glucose is reabsorbed in the PT via secondary active transport linked to sodium. This transporter is termed the sodium glucose-linked transporter (SGLT) and type 2 (SGLT-2) is the predominant form in the kidney.
- In addition, all proteins, peptides, amino acids, and ketone bodies are reabsorbed here via secondary active transport (requires luminal sodium, linked to sodium reabsorption).
- Therefore, the concentration of the above should be zero in the tubular fluid leaving the proximal tubule (clearance is zero).

Bicarbonate

About 80% of the filtered bicarbonate is reabsorbed here. The mechanism for this reabsorption is:

- Bicarbonate combines with free H^+ in lumen and is converted into CO_2 and H_2O, catalyzed by the luminal carbonic anhydrase enzyme (CA). H^+ is pumped into the lumen in exchange with sodium (antiporter). Although not pictured, there is a H^+--ATPase on the luminal membrane that contributes to pumping H^+ into the lumen.
- CO_2, being very soluble, crosses the luminal membrane where it combines with water to reform H^+ and bicarbonate (note CA in the cell). The H^+ is then pumped back into the lumen, while bicarbonate exits the baslolateral membrane to complete its reabsorption.
- Because of this mechanism, bicarbonate reabsorption is dependent upon H^+ secretion and the activity of CA.
- The most important factor for H^+ secretion is the concentration of H^+ in the cell. Thus, H^+ secretion and bicarbonate reabsorption are increased during an acidosis and they decrease with an alkalosis.
- Angiotensin II stimulates the Na^+--H^+ antiporter. Thus, in volume-depleted states, the amount of bicarbonate reabsorption in the PT increases. This is thought to be the mechanism preventing bicarbonate loss when a patient develops a contraction alkalosis.

The small amount of bicarbonate that leaves the proximal tubule is normally reabsorbed in subsequent segments.

Urate (uric acid)

The details of the renal handling of urate are too complex for the scope of this book. In short:

- Urate is formed by the breakdown of nucleotides
- Xanthine oxidase is the enzyme that catalyzes the final reaction to form urate.
- About 90% of the filtered urate is reabsorbed by the proximal tubule.
- If the FL of urate is high enough and the luminal pH is low, then more of the urate exists as uric acid, which can precipitate and form a kidney stone.
  - This is not the most common type of kidney stone, but it can occur in patients with gout.

Secretion

The proximal tubule is where many organic anions and cations are secreted and cleared from the circulation including PAH, penicillin, atropine, and morphine.

Energy requirements

Notice that all of the active processes illustrated in Figure 18-1 are powered by the Na/K-ATPase primary active pump. This pump is located in the proximal tubule basal and basolateral borders and is directly or indirectly responsible for most of the water and electrolyte reabsorption in the nephron. It thus represents the most energy-demanding process of the nephron.

The following figure depicts the ratio of the concentration of the substance in the proximal tubular fluid (TF) to the concentration in the plasma (P), beginning in Bowman's space through the end of the PT.

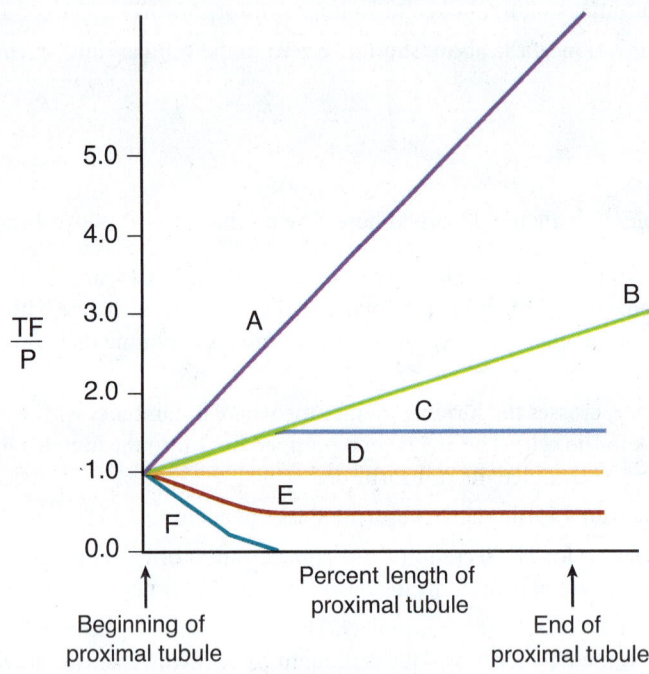

Figure 18-2.

Proximal Tubule Transport **A** = PAH; **B** = Inulin; **C** = Substance reabsorbed somewhat less rapidly than water, e.g., chloride; **D** = Major electrolytes such as sodium, potassium; **E** = Substance reabsorbed somewhat more rapidly than water; **F** = Substance completely reabsorbed in proximal tubule, e.g., glucose

Concentration of Inulin in the Nephron Tubule

- The concentration of inulin along the nephron tubule is an index of water reabsorption.
- Inulin is freely filtered; thus, its concentration in Bowman's space is the same as it is in the plasma. Because water is reabsorbed but inulin is not, the concentration of inulin increases throughout the nephron. The greater the water reabsorption, the greater the increase in inulin concentration.
- Since two-thirds of the water is reabsorbed in the proximal tubule, the inulin concentration should triple TF/P = 3.0. Its concentration should further increase in the descending limb of the loop of Henle, distal tubule, and the collecting duct (assuming ADH is present).
- The segment of the nephron with the highest concentration of inulin is the terminal collecting duct. The segment of the nephron with the lowest concentration of inulin is Bowman's space.

LOOP OF HENLE

- Fluid entering the loop of Henle is isotonic (300 mOsm/kg), but the volume is only one-third the volume originally filtered into Bowman's space.
- The loop of Henle has countercurrent flow and it acts as a countercurrent multiplier, the details of which are not imperative to learn. In short, the loop of Henle creates a concentrated medullary interstitium.
- The osmolality of the medulla can reach a maximum of about 1200 mOsm/kg, and the predominant osmoles are NaCl and urea.
- Juxtamedullary nephrons are responsible for this extremely high medullary osmolality. They are surrounded by vasa recta and slow flow in the vasa recta is crucial for maintaining the concentrated medullary interstitium.

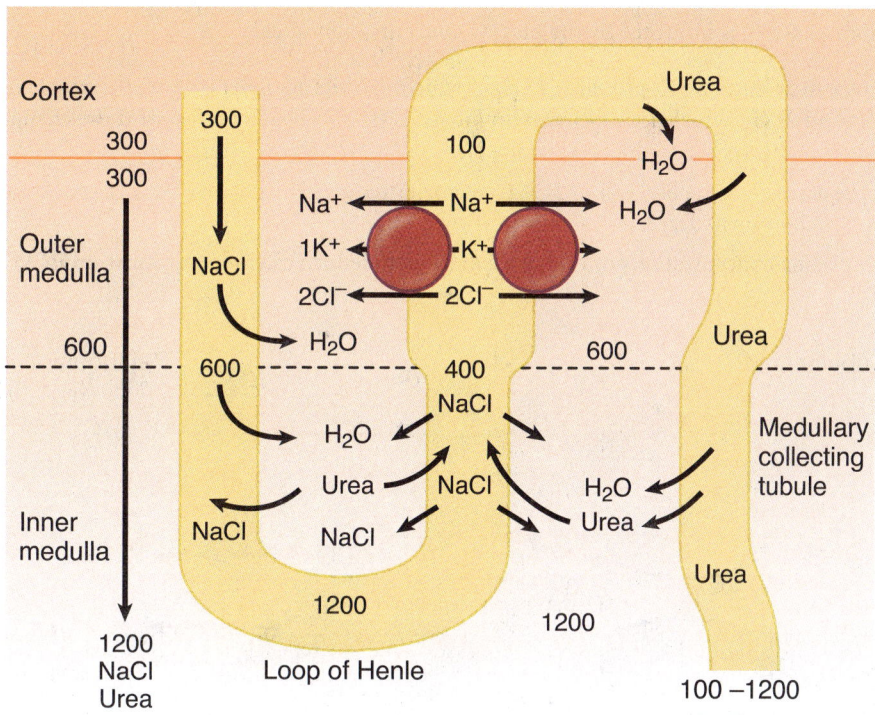

Figure 18-3. Countercurrent and the Loop of Henle

Descending Limb

- Permeable to water (about 15% of filtered is reabsorbed here)
- Relatively impermeable to solute

Ascending Limb

- Impermeable to water
- Solutes transported out

Figure 18-4 shows a typical cell in the ascending thick limb (ATL) of the loop of Henle. Similar to the PT, there is a luminal Na^+-H^+ antiporter and bicarbonate is reabsorbed here.

Na$^+$--K$^+$--2Cl$^-$ transporter

This is an electroneutral transport resulting in the reabsorption of about 25% of the filtered sodium, chloride, and potassium.

- The luminal membrane contains a K$^+$ channel (Figure 18-4), allowing diffusion of this ion back into lumen (recall that the concentration of K$^+$ inside cells is very high compared to the extracellular concentration).

- This back diffusion of K$^+$ into the lumen creates a positive luminal potential, which in turn, promotes calcium and magnesium reabsorption (about 25% of FL) via a paracellular pathway (primarily). This positive luminal potential also causes sodium reabsorption via a paracellular pathway.

Calcium-sensing receptor (CaSR)

The basolateral membrane of cells in ATL contain CaSR, which is a G-protein coupled receptor. Because it is on the basolateral membrane, CaSR is influence by the plasma concentration of calcium.

- CaSR couples to at least two G-proteins: 1) G$_{I/O}$, which inhibits adenylyl cyclase, thereby reducing intracellular cAMP, and 2) G$_q$, which activates protein kinase C (PKC). The net effect of these changes in intracellular signaling pathways is an inhibition of the Na$^+$--K$^+$--2Cl$^-$ transporter.

- Reducing the activity of the Na$^+$--K$^+$--2Cl$^-$ transporter reduces the positive luminal potential (less K$^+$ back diffusion), which in turn, decreases calcium reabsorption.

- Thus, high plasma concentrations of calcium can directly reduce calcium reabsorption in ATL.

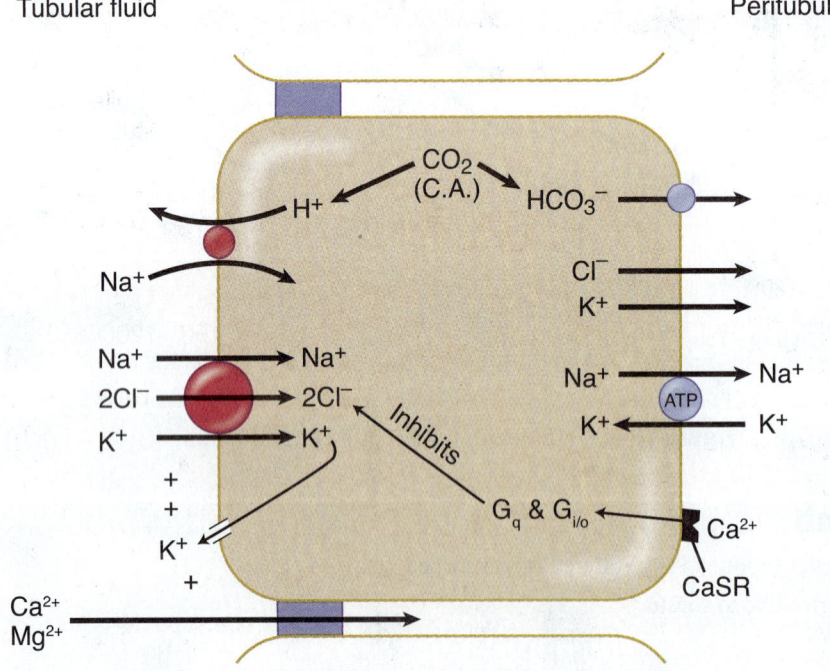

Figure 18-4. Loop of Henle

DISTAL TUBULE

The early distal tubule reabsorbs Na$^+$, Cl$^-$, and Ca^{2+}. Transporters in the distal tubule are summarized in Figure 18-5.

NaCl

- NaCl crosses the apical membrane via a Na^+-Cl^- symporter.
- The Na^+ is pumped across the basal membrane via the Na/K-ATPase proteins and Cl^- diffuses down its electrochemical gradient through channels.
- This section is impermeable to water. Thus, osmolality decreases further. In fact, the ultrafiltrate in the early distal tubule has the lowest osmolality of the entire nephron.

Calcium

- Calcium enters the cell from the luminal fluid passively through calcium channels.
- The opening of these channels is primarily regulated by parathyroid hormone (PTH).
- Calcium is actively extruded into the peritubular fluid via Ca^{2+}-ATPase or a $3Na^+$-Ca^{2+} antiporter.
- These cells also express the calcium binding protein, calbindin, which facilitates calcium reabsorption. Calbindin synthesis is increased by the active form of vitamin D, and thus vitamin D enhances PTH's action on the distal tubule.

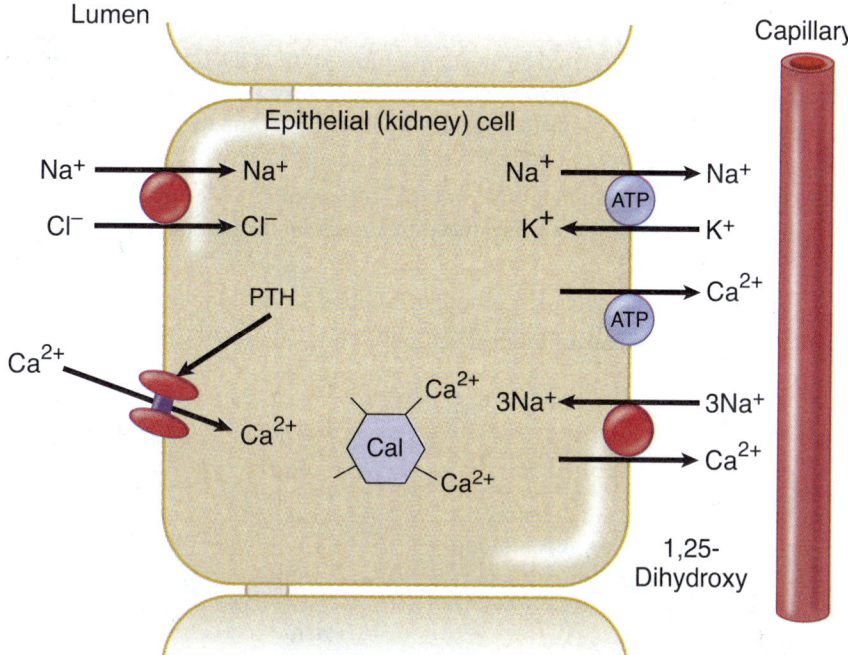

Figure 18-5. Transporters in Distal Tubule
Cal: calbindin

COLLECTING DUCT

The collecting duct (DC) is composed of principal cells and intercalated cells, both of which are illustrated in Figure 18-6.

Principal Cells

- The luminal membrane of principal cells contains sodium channels, commonly referred to as epithelial Na^+ channels (ENaC). Because of these channels, sodium follows its electrochemical gradient (created by the basolateral Na^+-K^+ ATPase) into the cell.

- Some chloride does not follow the sodium, thus the reabsorption of sodium produces a negative luminal potential. This negative luminal potential causes potassium secretion.

- Thus, the reabsorption of sodium and secretion of potassium are linked.

- Mineralcorticoids such as aldosterone exert an important effect on these cells. Activation of the mineralcorticoid receptor increases the number of luminal ENaC channels, increases their open time, and induces synthesis and trafficking of the basolateral Na^+--K^+ ATPase. The net effect is increased sodium reabsorption and potassium secretion.

- Although not illustrated on the slide, principal cells express aquaporins, which are regulated by anti-diuretic hormone (ADH), also known as arginine vasopressin (AVP). ADH acts on V2 (Gs—cAMP) receptors to cause insertion of aquaporins, which in turn, causes water (and urea) reabsorption.

Intercalated Cells

- Intercalated cells are intimately involved in acid-base regulation. The amount of fixed acid generated by an individual is mainly determined by diet. A high percentage of animal protein in the diet generates more fixed acid than a vegetarian-based diet.

- The luminal membrane contains a H^+--ATPase, which pumps H^+ into the lumen. Although free H^+ is pumped into the lumen, luminal pH can only go so low before it causes damage to cells, and thus most of the H^+ is eliminated from the body via buffers, phosphate and ammonia being the two most common.

- Monoprotonated phosphate is freely filtered at the glomerulus. About 80% is reabsorbed in the PT and another 10% is reabsorbed in the distal tubule. The remaining phosphate serves as a buffer for the secreted H^+. The H^+ pumped into the lumen binds to phosphate to form diprotonated phosphate, which is poorly reabsorbed, thus eliminating H^+ from the body. Phosphate is the primary titratable acid.

- In addition, the H^+ pumped into the lumen can combine with ammonia to form ammonium, which is not reabsorbed and is thus excreted. Ammonia is produced by the catabolism of glutamine and this occurs in cells of the PT.

- For every H^+ excreted by the above buffers, bicarbonate is added to the body (new bicarbonate).

- Aldosterone stimulates the H^+--ATPase of intercalated cells. Thus, excess aldosterone results in a metabolic alkalosis.

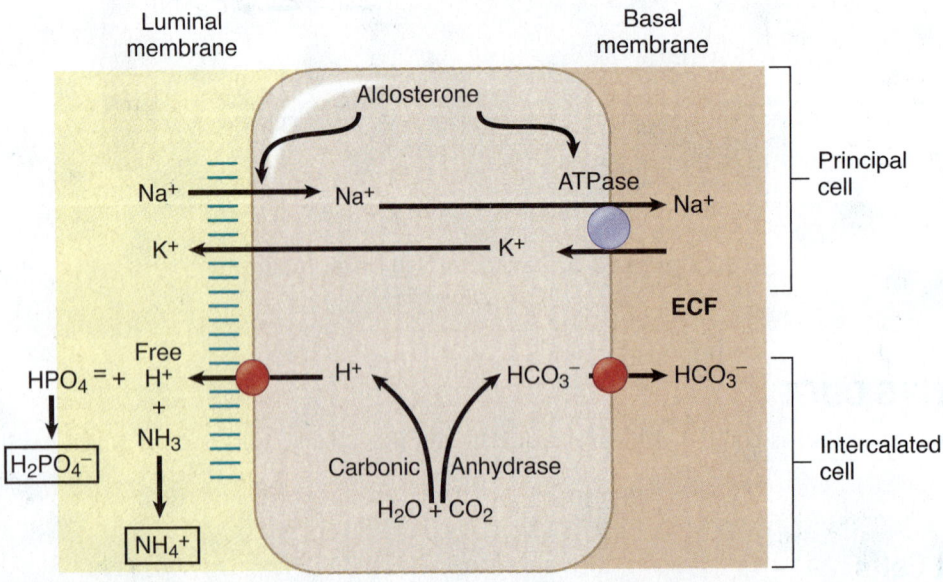

Figure 18-6. Late Distal Tubule and Collecting Duct

Acid–Base Disturbances **19**

Learning Objectives

❏ Interpret scenarios on buffering systems

❏ Explain information related to three-question method

❏ Solve problems concerning the four primary disturbances

❏ Solve problems concerning plasma anion gap diagnosis

❏ Solve problems concerning supplemental information

BUFFERING SYSTEMS

The following shows the CO_2-bicarbonate buffer system. This is one of the major buffers systems of the blood and the one we focus on in this chapter.

$$H_2O + CO_2 \underset{\longleftarrow}{\overset{CA}{\longrightarrow}} H_2CO_3 \rightleftharpoons H^+ + HCO_3^-$$

Figure 19-1. Production of Carbonic Acid

To demonstrate the changes in the major variables during acid–base disturbances, the scheme can be simplified to the following:

$$CO_2 \longleftrightarrow H^+ + HCO_3^-$$

Recall that the respiratory system plays the key role in regulating CO_2, while the kidneys serve as the long-term regulators of H^+ and HCO_3^-. Thus, these two organ systems are paramount in our discussion of acid-base regulation.

FORMULATING A DIAGNOSIS

Acid-base disturbances can be diagnosed from arterial blood gases (ABGs) using a three-step approach. Given that arterial blood is the source for the diagnostic data, one is actually determining an acidemia or alkalemia. However, an acidemia or alkalemia is typically indicative of an underlying acidosis or alkalosis, respectively.

An overview of this approach is provided here to lay the framework for remainder of the chapter.

THREE-QUESTION METHOD

Question 1: What is the osis?

- If pH <7.35, then acidosis
- If pH >7.45, then alkalosis

The normal value of pH is 7.4 (see below), with the normal range 7.35–7.45, thus the basis of the above numbers. However, one can in fact have an underlying acid-base disorder even though pH is in the normal range.

Question 2: What is the cause of the osis?

To answer this, one looks at bicarbonate next. In the section that follows, we will go into more detail.

Question 3: Was there compensation?

A calculation must be performed to answer this final question, and this will be covered in detail below. However, bear in mind the following:

- For respiratory disturbances, the kidneys alter total bicarbonate; whether or not compensation has occurred is based upon the patient's measured bicarbonate versus a calculated value of bicarbonate.
- The respiratory system responds quickly and it is important to determine if it has responded appropriately; respiratory compensation compares the patient's measured PCO_2 versus a calculated (predicted) value.

THE FOUR PRIMARY DISTURBANCES

There are four primary acid-base disturbances, each of which results in an altered concentration of H^+. The basic deviations from normal can be an acidosis (excess H^+) or an alkalosis (deficiency of H^+), either of which may be caused by a respiratory or metabolic problem.

- **Respiratory acidosis**: too much CO_2
- **Metabolic acidosis**: addition of H^+ (not of CO_2 origin) and/or loss of bicarbonate from the body
- **Respiratory alkalosis**: not enough CO_2
- **Metabolic alkalosis**: loss of H^+ (not of CO_2 origin) and/or addition of base to the body

Normal systemic arterial values are as follows:

$$pH = 7.4$$

$$HCO_3^- = 24 \text{ mEq/L}$$

$$PCO_2 = 40 \text{ mm Hg}$$

Follow the Bicarbonate Trail

Question 2 asks for the cause of the osis. To answer this, look at the bicarbonate concentration and remember the basic CO_2–bicarbonate reaction, applying mass action. The table below shows the 4 primary disturbances with the resultant bicarbonate changes.

$$CO_2 \leftrightarrow H^+ + HCO_3^-$$

Table 19-1. Summary of Acute Changes in pH/HCO_3^-

	pH	HCO_3^-
Respiratory acidosis	↓	↑
Metabolic acidosis	↓	↓↓
Respiratory alkalosis	↑	↓
Metabolic alkalosis	↑	↑↑

Respiratory acidosis is characterized by too much CO_2.

- Increasing CO_2 drives the reaction to the right, thereby increasing HCO_3^-.
  - For every 1 mm Hg rise in $PaCO_2$, there is a 0.1 mEq/L increase in HCO_3^-, as a result of the chemical reaction.
  - Thus, there is a **1: 0.1 ratio** of CO_2 increase to HCO3$^-$ increase for an **acute (uncompensated) respiratory acidosis.**

Metabolic acidosis causes a marked decrease in HCO_3^- because the addition of H^+ consumes bicarbonate (drives reaction to the left).

- Alternatively, the acidosis could be caused by loss of base (HCO_3^-).

Respiratory alkalosis is characterized by a reduced CO_2.

- Decreasing CO_2 drives the reaction to the left, thereby reducing HCO_3^-.
  - For every 1 mm Hg fall in $PaCO_2$, there is a 0.2 mEq/L decrease in HCO_3^- as a result of the chemical reaction.
  - Thus, there is a **1: 0.2 ratio** of CO_2 decrease to HCO_3^- decrease for an **acute (uncompensated) respiratory alkalosis.**

Metabolic alkalosis causes a rise in HCO_3^- because the loss of H^+ drives the reaction to the right.

- Alternatively, an alkalosis can be caused by addition of base (bicarbonate) to the body.

COMPENSATION

Respiratory Acidosis

The kidneys compensate by increasing HCO_3^- and eliminating H^+, but the kidneys take days to fully compensate.

- For every 1 mm Hg increase in $PaCO_2$, HCO_3^- increases 0.35 mEq/L as a result of kidney compensation. Thus, there is a **1:0.35 ratio of CO_2 increase to HCO_3^- increase in a chronic (compensated) respiratory acidosis.**

Metabolic Acidosis

Metabolic acidosis is characterized by low pH and HCO_3^-. The drop in pH stimulates ventilation via peripheral chemoreceptors, thus the respiratory system provides the first, rapid compensatory response.

- Winter's equation is used to determine if the respiratory response is adequate.

$$\text{Predicted } PaCO_2 = (1.5 \times HCO_3^-) + 8$$

- The patient's $PaCO_2$ should be within $2(\pm)$ of this predicted value, and if so, then respiratory compensation has occurred.

Respiratory Alkalosis

The kidneys compensate by eliminating HCO_3^- and conserving H^+, but the kidneys take days to fully compensate.

- For every 1 mm Hg drop in $PaCO_2$, HCO_3^- decreases 0.5 mEq/L as a result of kidney compensation. Thus, there is a **1:0.5 ratio** of CO_2 decrease to HCO_3^- decrease **in a chronic (compensated) respiratory alkalosis.**
- The maximum low for HCO_3^- is 15 mEq/L.

Metabolic Alkalosis

Similar to a metabolic acidosis, the respiratory system is the first-line compensatory mechanism. Ventilation decreases to retain CO_2.

- The following equation is used to determine if compensation occurred. It computes the $PaCO_2$, which denotes appropriate compensation.

$$\text{Expected } PaCO_2 = (0.7 \times \text{rise in } HCO_3^-) + 40$$

- The patient's $PaCO_2$ should be within $2(\pm)$ of the computed value, but should not exceed 55 mm Hg. The 40 represents the normal $PaCO_2$ (see above).

Additional Important Points

- The body never overcompensates.
  - If it appears that a patient "overcompensated" for a primary disorder, there is likely a second disorder.
- If CO_2 and HCO_3^- go in opposite directions, there is a combined disturbance—either a combined (mixed) respiratory and metabolic acidosis or a combined (mixed) respiratory and metabolic alkalosis.
- Although the opposite direction rule is true, do not presume that it is **required** for someone to have a combined disturbance, i.e., a combined disturbance can still exist even if CO_2 and HCO_3^- go in the same direction.
- Too much CO_2 is a respiratory acidosis.
- Too little CO_2 is a respiratory alkalosis.

General Aspects of the Endocrine System

20

Learning Objectives

❏ Demonstrate understanding of overview of hormones

❏ Answer questions about disorders of the endocrine system

OVERVIEW OF HORMONES

Lipid- Versus Water-Soluble Hormones

The following figure demonstrates several major differences between the lipid-soluble hormones and the water-soluble hormones.

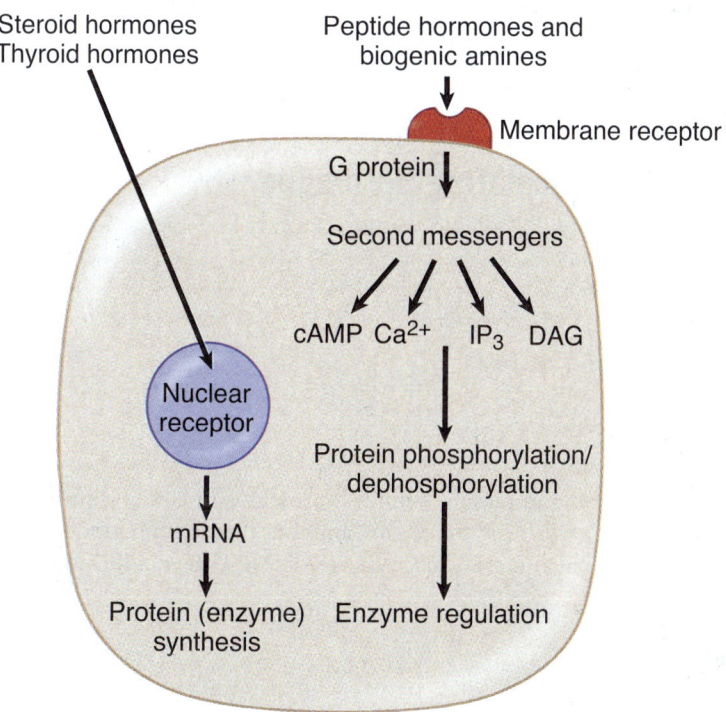

Figure 20-1. Signal Transduction Mechanisms
IP_3 = inositol triphosphate; DAG = diacylglycerol

Table 20-1. Differences Between the 2 Major Classes of Hormones

	Lipid-Soluble Hormones (steroids, thyroid hormones)	Water-Soluble Hormones (peptides, proteins)
Receptors	Inside the cell, usually in nucleus	Outer surface of the cell membrane
Intracellular action	Stimulates synthesis of specific new proteins	• Production of second messengers, e.g., cAMP • Insulin does not utilize cAMP, instead activates membrane-bound tyrosine kinase • Second messengers modify action of intracellular proteins (enzymes)
Storage	• Synthesized as needed • Exception: thyroid hormones	• Stored in vesicles • In some cases, prohormone stored in vesicle along with an enzyme that splits off the active hormone
Plasma transport	• Attached to proteins that serve as carriers • Exception: adrenal androgens	Dissolved in plasma (free, unbound)
Half-life	Long (hours, days) $\propto$ to affinity for protein carrier	Short (minutes) $\propto$ to molecular weight

Protein-Bound and Free Circulating Hormones

The liver produces proteins that bind lipid-soluble hormones, e.g.:

- cortisol-binding globulin
- thyroid-binding globulin
- sex hormone-binding globulin (SHBG)

Equilibrium

The lipid-soluble hormone circulating in plasma bound to protein is in equilibrium with a small amount of free hormone. It is the free form that is available to the tissues, and thus the free unbound form normally determines the plasma activity. It is the free form that also creates negative feedback. This equilibrium is shown here

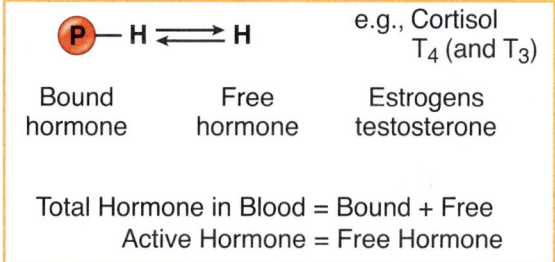

Figure 20-2. Transport of Lipid-Soluble Hormones

Role of the liver

If the liver changes its production and release of binding proteins, the circulating level of **bound hormone will change.** However, under most conditions the level of **free hormone will remain constant.**

Modulation

Liver dysfunction and androgens can decrease and estrogens can increase the circulating level of binding proteins. For example, a rise in circulating estrogen causes the release of more binding protein by the liver, which binds more free hormone. The transient decrease in free hormone reduces negative feedback to the hormone-secreting tissue. The increased secretion of free hormone quickly returns the plasma free hormone to normal.

This explains why during pregnancy and other states with a rise in estrogen levels:

- Total plasma lipid-soluble hormone increases.
- Free plasma hormone remains constant at a normal level; thus, the individual does not show signs of hyperfunction.

Hormone Receptors

Hormone specificity

A hormone affects only cells that possess receptors specific to that particular hormone.

For example, both adrenocorticotropic hormone (ACTH) and luteinizing hormone (LH) increase the secretion of steroid hormones. However, ACTH does so only in the adrenal cortex and LH only in gonadal tissue.

Hormone activity

Under normal conditions, receptors are not saturated; that is, extra receptors exist. Therefore:

- Normally, the number of hormone receptors is not rate-limiting for hormone action.
- The plasma concentration of free hormone is usually indicative of activity.

Resistance to hormone action

- Abnormalities in receptors or events distal to the ligand-receptor interaction, often due to chronic elevation of circulating hormone (e.g., type II diabetes) or drug therapy.
- Under these conditions receptors are often saturated.
- Reduction of hormone levels often produces some recovery in sensitivity.
- The clinical presentation is often one of normal or elevated hormone levels but with reduced or absent peripheral manifestations of the hormone and a failure of replacement therapy to correct the problem.

Permissive action

A phenomenon in which one type of hormone must be present before another hormone can act; for example, cortisol must be present for glucagon to carry out gluconeogenesis and prevent hypoglycemia.

Measurement of Hormone Levels

Plasma analysis

- Provides information at the time of sampling only and may not reflect the overall secretion rate
- When hormone secretion is episodic, single sampling may reflect peaks (erroneous hyperfunction) or nadirs (erroneous hypofunction). Pulsatile secretion, diurnal and cyclic variation, age, sleep entrainment, and hormone antagonism must all be considered in evaluating circulating levels.
  - Growth hormone is secreted in pulses and mainly at night. This is not reflected in a fasting morning sample. However, growth hormone stimulates the secretion of IGF-I which circulates attached to protein and has a long half-life (20 hours). Plasma IGF-I measured at any time during the day is usually a good index of overall growth hormone secretion.
  - Thyroid is a fairly constant system and T4 has a half-life of about 6–7 days. Thus, a random measurement of total T4 is usually a good estimate of daily plasma levels.

Urine analysis

- Restricted to the measurement ofcatecholamines, steroid hormones, and water-soluble hormones such as hCG and LH.
- A distinct advantage of urine analysis is that it provides an integrated sample.
  - A "24-hour urine free cortisol" is often necessary to pick up a low-level Cushing's syndrome and to eliminate the highs and lows of the normal circadian rhythm.

DISORDERS OF THE ENDOCRINE SYSTEM

Primary versus Secondary Disorders

- A primary disordermeans dysfunction originating in the endocrine gland itself, either hyper- or hypo-function. Examples of a primary disorder include:
  - excess cortisol from an adrenal adenoma (Conn's disease)
  - decreased thyroid secretion (Hashimoto's thyroiditis)
  - reduced ADH secretion (central diabetes insipidus)
- A secondary disorder indicates that a disturbance has occurred causing the gland secrete more or less of the hormone. Examples of a secondary disorder include:
  - Cushing disease (pituitary adenoma secreting ACTH) resulting in hypercortisolism
  - a dehydrated patient with elevated plasma osmolality causing high ADH levels

Hypofunction

- Can be caused by autoimmune disease (e.g., type I diabetes, hypothyroidism, primary adrenal insufficiency, gonadal failure), tumors, hemorrhage, infection, damage by neoplasms
- Evaluated by a stimulation test
  - Hypothalamic hormones test anterior pituitary reserve
  - Injection of the pituitary trophic hormone (e.g., ACTH) tests target gland reserve.
  - Failure of growth hormone release after arginine injection

Hyperfunction

- Caused by hormone-secreting tumors, hyperplasia, autoimmune stimulation, ectopically produced peptide hormones (e.g., ACTH, ADH)
- Evaluated by a suppression test
  - Failure of glucose to suppress growth hormone diagnostic for acromegaly
  - Failure of dexamethasone (low dose) to suppress cortisol diagnostic for hypercortisolism
  - Multiple endocrine neoplasia (MEN) represents a group of inheritable syndromes characterized by multiple benign or malignant tumors.
    - MEN 1: hyperparathyroidism, endocrine pancreas, and pituitary adenomas
    - MEN 2A: medullary carcinoma of the thyroid, pheochromocytoma, hyperparathyroidism
    - MEN 2B: medullary carcinoma of the thyroid, pheochromocytoma, hyperparathyroidism typically absent.

Gland Structure and Size

- When an endocrine gland does not receive its normal stimulus, it generally undergoes a reversible atrophy.
  - Long-term high doses of glucocorticoids suppress the ACTH-adrenal axis. Withdrawal of therapy can require up to a year for complete recovery.
- Overstimulation of endocrine tissue can cause cell proliferation or hypertrophy in addition to hormone overproduction.
  - In Graves' disease, overstimulation of the thyroid tissues causes cell proliferation and this polyclonal expansion creates a goiter in addition to hyperthyroidism.
- Tumors, which are generally monoclonal expansions, may also create a hyperfunction. Others produce little if any hormone but are still disease-producing because of the compressive (mass) effect of the additional tissue.

Hypothalamic–Anterior Pituitary System 21

Learning Objectives

❑ Solve problems concerning hypothalamic-anterior pituitary axis

❑ Solve problems concerning disorders of the hypothalamic-anterior pituitary axis

HYPOTHALAMIC–ANTERIOR PITUITARY AXIS

- The hormones in this system are all water-soluble.
- The hypothalamic hormones are synthesized in the neuron cell body, packaged in vesicles, and transported down the axon to be stored and released from the nerve terminals.
- Pituitary is located in the bony sella turcica at the base of the skull. It hangs from the hypothalamus by a stalk (the infundibulum) and is controlled by the hypothalamus. The dura membrane (diaphragm sellae) separates it from and prevents cerebrospinal fluid from entering the sella turcica.
- Optic chiasm is 5–10 mm above this diaphragm.
- In the hypothalamic–anterior pituitary system, hormonal release is mainly pulsatile. A possible exception is the thyroid system.
- The pulsatile release of GnRH prevents downregulation of its receptors on the gonadotrophs of the anterior pituitary. A constant infusion of GnRH will cause a decrease in the release of both LH and FSH.

The hypothalamic–anterior pituitary system is summarized in the following figure.

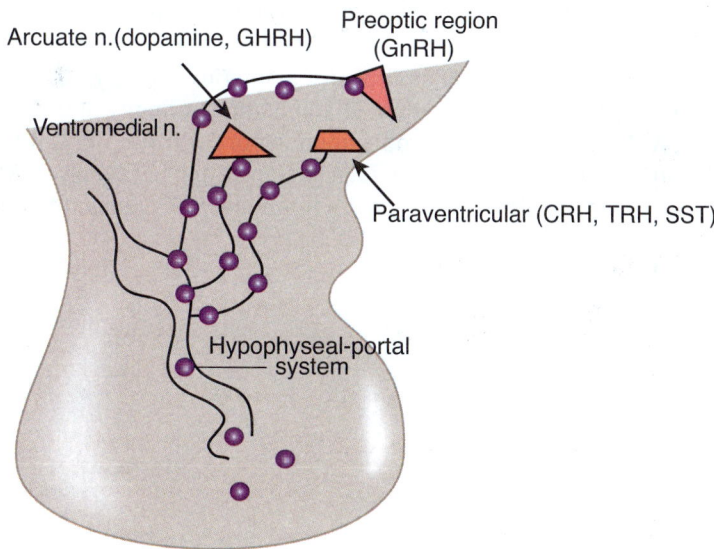

Figure 21-1. Hypothalamic–Anterior Pituitary Axis

- The hypothalamic hormones, thyrotropin-releasing hormone (TRH), corticotropin-releasing hormone (CRH), growth hormone–releasing hormone (GHRH), somatostatin (SST), and dopamine are synthesized in neuronal cell bodies in the arcuate and paraventricular nuclei; gonadotropin-releasing hormone (GnRH) is synthesized in the preoptic nucleus.

- The nerve endings all come together in the median eminence region of the hypothalamus. The hormones are then secreted into the hypophyseal-portal system and transported to the anterior pituitary.

- Hypothalamic hormones bind to receptors on cells of the anterior pituitary and modify the secretion of thyroid-stimulating hormone (TSH) (thyrotropin), corticotropin (ACTH), luteinizing hormone (LH), follicle-stimulating hormone (FSH), growth hormone (GH), and prolactin.

Effect of Each Hypothalamic Hormone on Anterior Pituitary

+ = releaser
− = inhibitor

Hypothalamus	Pituitary Target	Secretion
TRH ———+———→	Thyrotrophs (10%)	TSH
CRH ———+———→	Corticotrophs (10–25%)	ACTH
GnRH* ———+———→	Gonadotrophs (10–15%)	LH, FSH
GHRH** ———+———→ SST ———−———→	Somatotrophs (50%)	GH
Dopamine*** ———−———→ TRH (elevated) ———+———→	Lactotrophs (10–15%)	Prolactin

*High frequency pulses favor LH, low frequency pulses favor FSH

**The fact that eliminating hypothalamic input causes a decrease in growth hormone secretion indicates that GHRH is the main controlling factor.

***When the connection between the hypothalamus and the anterior pituitary is severed (e.g., there is damage to the pituitary stalk), secretion of all anterior pituitary hormones decreases, except prolactin, which increases. The secretion of prolactin increases because a chronic source of inhibition (dopamine) has been removed.

Figure 21-2. Control of the Anterior Pituitary

TRH = thyrotropin-releasing hormone; **TSH** = thyroid-stimulating hormone or thyrotropin; **CRH** = corticotropin-releasing hormone; **ACTH** = adrenocorticotropic hormone or corticotropin; **GnRH** = gonadotropin-releasing hormone; **LH** = luteinizing hormone; **FSH** = follicle-stimulating hormone; **GHRH** = growth hormone-releasing hormone; **GH** = growth hormone; **SST** = somatostatin

Learning Objectives

❏ Answer questions about hormones of the posterior pituitary

❏ Explain information related to regulation of ECF volume and osmolarity

❏ Answer questions about pathophysiologic changes in ADH secretion

HORMONES OF THE POSTERIOR PITUITARY

- Made up of distal neuron terminals
- Secreted hormones; arginine vasopressin (ADH), oxytocin — both are peptide hormones.
- Cell bodies located in the supraoptic nucleus and paraventricular nucleus of the hypothalamus.
- ADH is a major controller of water excretion and regulator of extracellular osmolarity.
- The osmoreceptor neurons in the hypothalamus are extremely sensitive and are able to maintain ECF osmolarity within a very narrow range.
- There is a downward shift in plasma osmolarity regulation in pregnancy, the menstrual cycle, and with volume depletion. In the latter case osmoregulation is secondary to volume regulation; a return of circulating volume occurs even though osmolarity decreases.
- Volume receptors are less sensitive than osmoreceptors and a change of 10–15% in volume is required to produce a measurable change in ADH.
- Angiotensin II and CRH can stimulate the release of ADH.

Figure 22-1 illustrates the neural control mechanisms that regulate secretion of ADH by the posterior pituitary. The principal inputs are inhibition by baroreceptor and cardiopulmonary mechanoreceptors (see Section V, Chapter 8) and stimulation by osmoreceptors.

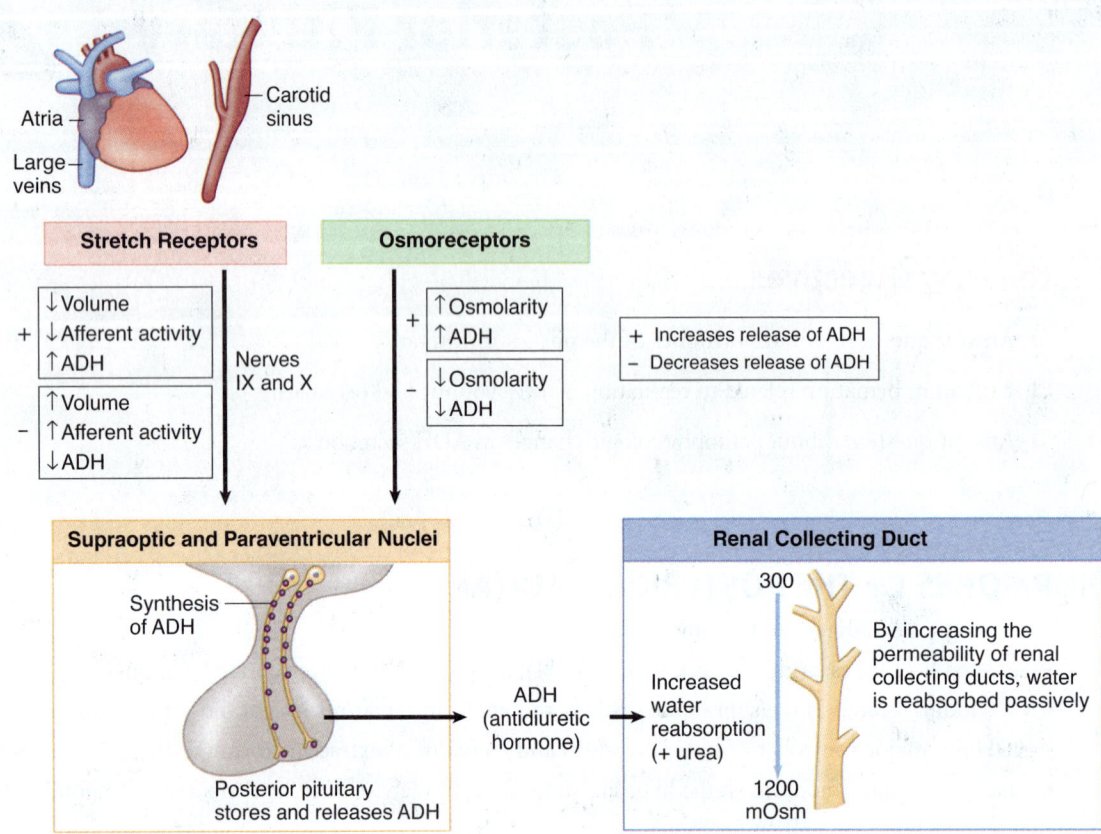

Figure 22-1. Neural Control Mechanism

Synthesis and Release of ADH

- ADH is synthesized in the supraoptic (SO) and paraventricular (PVN) nuclei of the hypothalamus; it is stored and released from the posterior pituitary.

- Osmoreceptorsare neurons that respond to increased plasma osmolarity, principally plasma sodium concentration. They synapse with neurons of the SO and PVN and stimulate them to secrete ADH from the posterior pituitary. They also stimulate consumption of water through hypothalamic centers that regulate thirst.

- The SO and PVN also receive input from cardiopulmonary mechanoreceptors, as well as arterial baroreceptors. High blood volume or blood pressure tends to inhibit secretion of ADH.

- Secretion of ADH is most sensitive to plasma osmolarity (1%); however, if blood volume decreases by 10% (such as hemorrhage) or cardiac output falls, high levels of ADH are secreted even if it causes abnormal plasma osmolarity.

Note
ADH is also stimulated by Ang II and CRH.

Action of ADH

- The main target tissue is the renal collecting duct (V2 receptors).
- ADH increases the permeability of the duct to water by placing water channels (aquaporins) in the luminal membrane.
- ADH, acting via the V1 receptor, contracts vascular smooth muscle.

REGULATION OF ECF VOLUME AND OSMOLARITY

Osmoregulation

- An increase of only 1% in the osmolality of the ECF bathing the hypothalamic osmoreceptors evokes an increased in ADH secretion.
- A similarly sized decrease in osmolality decreases ADH secretion.
- In this manner, ECF osmolality is kept very close to 285 mOsm/Kg.

Volume Regulation

- Stimuli arising from stretch receptors act to chronically inhibit ADH secretion.
- Decreases in blood volume cause venous and arterial stretch receptors to send fewer signals to the CNS, decreasing chronic inhibition of ADH secretion.
- This mechanism is especially important for restoring ECF volume following a hemorrhage.

Effect of Alcohol and Weightlessness on ADH Secretion

Ingesting ethyl alcohol or being in a weightless environment suppresses ADH secretion. In weightlessness, there is a net shift of blood from the limbs to the abdomen and chest. This results in greater stretch of the volume receptors in the large veins and atria, thus suppressing ADH secretion.

Atrial Natriuretic Peptide (ANP)

ANP is the hormone secreted by the heart. ANP is found throughout the heart but mainly in the right atrium. The stimuli that release ANP (two peptides are released) are:

- Stretch, an action independent of nervous involvement
- CHF and all fluid overload states

ANP increases sodium loss (natriuresis) and water loss by the kidney because of, in part, an increase in glomerular filtration rate due to:

- ANP-mediated dilation of the afferent arteriole
- ANP-mediated constriction of the efferent arteriole

ANP also increases sodium loss (natriuresis) and water loss (diuresis) by the kidney because it inhibits aldosterone release as well as the reabsorption of sodium and water in the collecting duct.

The physiologic importance of ANP is not known because it has not been possible to identify or produce a specific deficiency state in humans. However, ANP secretion increases in weightlessness (submersion to the neck in water), while renin, aldosterone, and ADH secretion decrease. It may play a role in normal regulation of the ECF osmolality and volume.

ANP tends to antagonize the effects of aldosterone and ADH.

A normal ANP level is used to exclude CHF as a cause of dyspnea.

PATHOPHYSIOLOGIC CHANGES IN ADH SECRETION

Diabetes Insipidus

The consequences can be explained on the basis of the lack of an effect of ADH on the renal collecting ducts.

Central diabetes insipidus (CDI)

- Sufficient ADH is not available to affect the renal collecting ducts.
- Causes include familial, tumors (craniopharyngioma), autoimmune, trauma
- Pituitary trauma – transient diabetes insipidus
- Sectioning of pituitary stalk – triphasic response: diabetes insipidus, followed by SIADH, followed by a return of diabetes insipidus
- Destruction of the hypothalamus from any cause can lead to diabetes insipidus. Forms of hypothalamic destruction are stroke, hypoxia, head trauma, infection, cancer or mass lesions.
- CDI = ADH deficiency. CDI is treated with replacing ADH as vasopressin or DDAVP (desmopressin).

Nephrogenic diabetes insipidus

- Due to inability of the kidneys to respond to ADH
- Causes include familial, acquired, drugs (lithium)
- Hypokalemia
- Hypercalcemia

Lithium, low potassium, and high calcium all diminish ADH's effectiveness on principal cells. The precise mechanism is still unclear, but it may involve disruption in the ability to traffic aquaporins to the luminal membrane of principal cells of the kidney.

Table 22-1. Differential Diagnosis Following Water Deprivation

	Plasma Osm	Urine Osm	Plasma ADH	Urine Osm Post Desmopressin
Normal	297	814	↑	815
Central DI*	342	102	↓	622
Nephrogenic	327	106	↑	118

*Patients with partial central DI will concentrate their urine somewhat but will achieve an additional boost following desmopressin.

Learning Objectives

- ❏ Demonstrate understanding of biosynthetic pathways of steroid hormone synthesis
- ❏ Interpret scenarios on physiologic actions of glucocorticoids
- ❏ Solve problems concerning control of adrenocorticotropin and cortisol secretion
- ❏ Explain information related to control of aldosterone secretion
- ❏ Explain information related to glucocorticoid disorders and mineralocorticoid disorders

FUNCTIONAL REGIONS OF THE ADRENAL GLAND

The following figure summarizes each adrenal region.

- ACTH controls the release of both cortisol and adrenal androgens.
- Aldosterone is stimulated by a rise in angiotensin II and/or K^+.

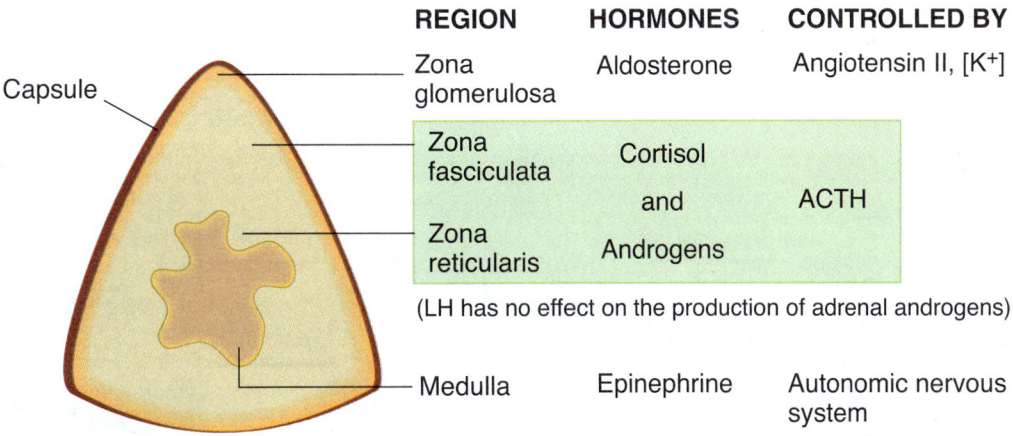

REGION	HORMONES	CONTROLLED BY
Zona glomerulosa	Aldosterone	Angiotensin II, [K^+]
Zona fasciculata	Cortisol and Androgens	ACTH
Zona reticularis		

(LH has no effect on the production of adrenal androgens)

| Medulla | Epinephrine | Autonomic nervous system |

Figure 23-1. Adrenal Cortex Regions

Consequences of the Loss of Regional Adrenal Function

Zona glomerulosa: The **absence of the mineralocorticoid, aldosterone**, results in:

- Loss of Na$^+$
- Decreased volume of the ECF
- Low blood pressure
- Circulatory shock
- Death

Zona fasciculata, zona reticularis: The **absence of the glucocorticoid, cortisol,** contributes to:

- Circulatory failure, because without cortisol, catecholamines do not exert their normal vasoconstrictive action.
- An inability to readily mobilize energy sources (glucose and free fatty acids) from glycogen or fat. Under normal living conditions, this is not life-threatening; however, under stressful situations, severe problems can arise. For example, fasting can result in fatal hypoglycemia.

If problems develop with anterior pituitary secretion, glucocorticoid secretion may be affected, but the mineralocorticoid system remains intact.

BIOSYNTHETIC PATHWAYS OF STEROID HORMONE SYNTHESIS

Synthetic Pathways

Figure 23-2 shows a composite of the synthetic pathways in all steroid hormone-producing tissues. A single tissue has only the pathways necessary to produce the hormones normally secreted by that particular tissue. For example, the zona glomerulosa has only the pathways of the first column because the main output of the zona glomerulosa is aldosterone. Cholesterol is pulled off circulating LDL or made de novo by acetate.

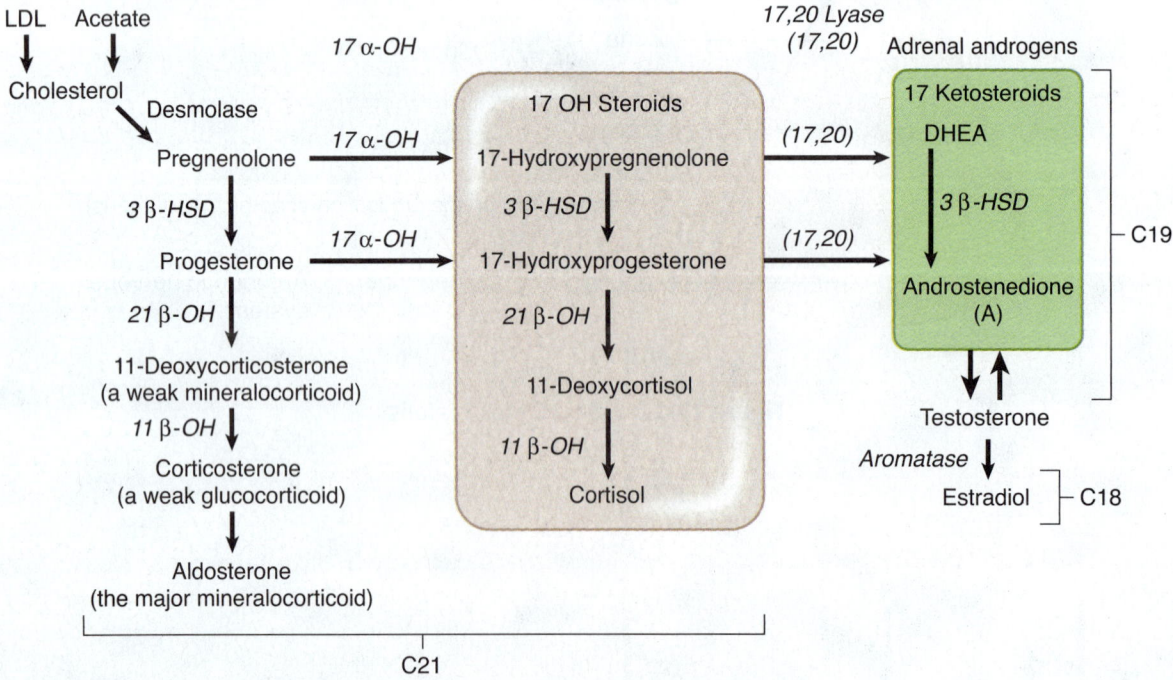

Figure 23-2. Pathways of Adrenal Steroid Synthesis
HSD = hydroxysteroid dehydrogenase; **OH** = hydroxylase

C21 steroids (21 carbon atoms)

C21 steroids with an OH at position 17 are called 17-hydroxysteroids. The only 17 OH steroid with hormonal activity is cortisol.

The lipid-soluble 17 OH steroids are metabolized to water-soluble compounds before they are filtered and excreted in the urine. The pathway for cortisol is shown here:

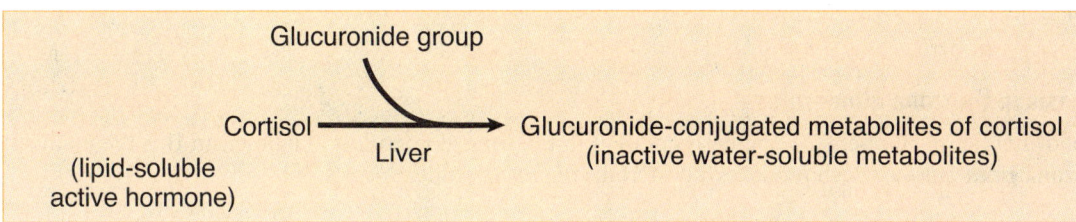

Figure 23-3. Metabolism of Cortisol

Urinary 17 OH steroids have in the past been measured as an index of cortisol secretion. This has been replaced by the measurement of the 24-hour urine-free cortisol.

C19 steroids (19 carbon atoms)

Adrenal Androgens

- Have a keto group at position 17 and are therefore called 17-ketosteroids.
- Are conjugated with sulfate in the adrenal cortex, making them water soluble. As water-soluble metabolites, they circulate in the bloodstream, are filtered by the kidney, and are excreted in the urine. The sulfated form is not produced in the gonads and is thus considered an index of androgen production by the adrenals.
- The major secreted form is dehydroepiandrosterone (DHEA).
- DHEA, DHEA sulfate, and androstenedione have very low androgenic activity. They function primarily as precursors for the peripheral conversion to the more potent testosterone and dihydrotestosterone (men and women).
- In adult males, excessive production of adrenal androgens has no clinical consequences. In prepubertal males it causes premature penile enlargement and early development of secondary sexual characteristics. In women excessive adrenal androgens cause hirsutism and virilization.

Testosterone

- Produced mainly by the Leydig cells of testes
- The active hormone is lipid-soluble and not a 17-ketosteroid.
- When metabolized, it is converted to a 17-ketosteroid and conjugated to become water soluble. In this form, it is filtered and excreted by the kidney.

Urinary Excretion

- Urinary 17-ketosteroids are an index of all androgens, adrenal and testicular.
- In females and prepubertal males, urinary 17-ketosteroids are an index of adrenal androgen secretion.
- In adult males (postpuberty), urinary 17-ketosteroids are 2/3 adrenal and 1/3 testicular, and thus mainly an index of adrenal secretion.

C18 steroids—estrogens (e.g., estradiol)

- Aromatase converts androgen into estrogen.

Regional Synthesis

Conversion of cholesterol to pregnenolone

The starting point in the synthesis of all steroid hormones is the transport of cholesterol into the mitochondria by steroidogenic acute regulatory protein (StAR). This is the rate-limiting step.

The enzyme catalyzing the conversion of cholesterol to pregnenolone is sidechain cleavage enzyme (SCC, also called desmolase.).

Synthesis in the zona glomerulosa

The following figure represents the pathways present in the zona glomerulosa. Angiotensin II is the main stimulus to the zona glomerulosa, which produces aldosterone, the major mineralocorticoid.

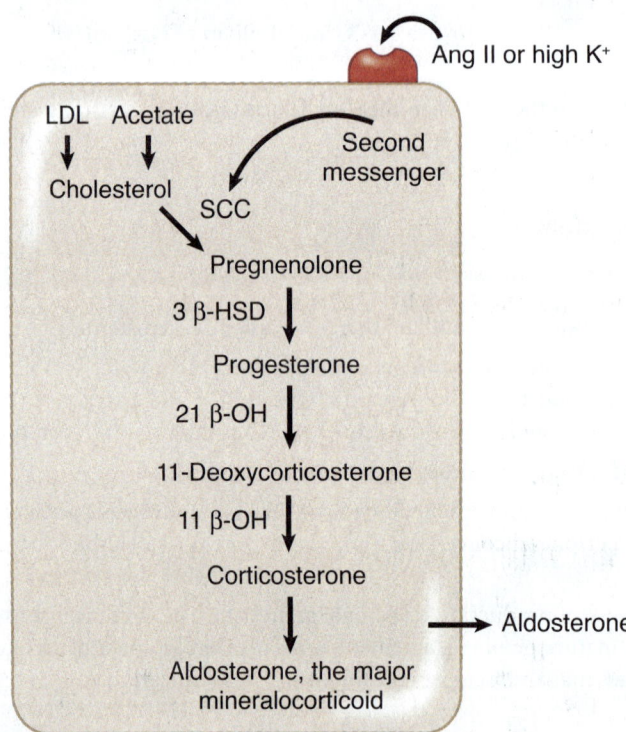

Figure 23-4. Pathway to Aldosterone Synthesis

Synthesis in the zona fasciculata and the zona reticularis

Normal hormonal output of the zona fasciculata and zona glomerulosa consists of the following:

- 11-Deoxycorticosterone: Under normal conditions, this weak mineralocorticoid is not important. Almost all mineralocorticoid activity is due to aldosterone.

- Corticosterone: Also not important under normal conditions. Almost all glucocorticoid activity is due to cortisol.

- Cortisol: Main glucocorticoid secreted by the adrenal cortex, responsible for most of the hypothalamic and anterior pituitary negative feedback control of ACTH secretion.

Normal hormonal output of the zona reticularis consists of the following

- Adrenal androgens: These weak water-soluble androgens represent a significant secretion; however, they produce masculinizing characteristics only in women and prepubertal males when secretion is excessive.

PHYSIOLOGIC ACTIONS OF GLUCOCORTICOIDS

Stress

Stress includes states such as trauma, exposure to cold, illness, starvation, and exercise. The capacity to withstand stress is dependent on adequate secretion of the glucocorticoids.

Stress hormones usually act to mobilize energy stores. The stress hormones are:

- **Growth hormone:** mobilizes fatty acids by increasing lipolysis in adipose tissue
- **Glucagon:** mobilizes glucose by increasing liver glycogenolysis
- **Cortisol:** mobilizes fat, protein, carbohydrate (see below)
- **Epinephrine**, in some forms of stress such as exercise: mobilizes glucose via glycogenolysis and fat via lipolysis

All stress hormones raise plasma glucose. Severe hypoglycemia is a crisis and causes a rapid increase in all stress hormones. By definition, because these hormones raise plasma glucose, they are referred to as counterregulatory hormones (opposite to insulin).

A deficiency in a stress hormone may cause hypoglycemia.

Metabolic Actions of Cortisol

Cortisol promotes the mobilization of energy stores, specifically:

- **Protein:** Cortisol promotes degradation and increased delivery of hepatic gluconeogenic precursors.
- **Lipids:** Cortisol promotes lipolysis and increased delivery of free fatty acids and glycerol.
- **Carbohydrate:** Cortisol raises blood glucose, making more glucose available for nervous tissue. Two mechanisms are involved:
  - Cortisol counteracts insulin's action in most tissues (muscle, lymphoid, and fat).
  - Cortisol increases hepatic output of glucose by regulating the enzymes involved in gluconeogenesis, particularly phosphoenolpyruvate carboxykinase (PEPCK) (not from liver glycogenolysis).

Permissive Actions of Cortisol

Cortisol enhances the capacity of glucagon and catecholamines, hence the adjective *permissive* aptly describes many of the actions of cortisol.

Glucagon

Promotes glycogenolysis in the liver (some lipolysis from adipocytes as well). Without cortisol, fasting hypoglycemia rapidly develops. Cortisol permits glucagon to raise blood glucose.

Catecholamines

Promotes both alpha and beta receptor expression. Beta receptor function involves glucose regulation, lipolysis (see next chapter), and bronchodilation. Alpha receptor function is pivotal for blood pressure regulation. Without cortisol, blood pressure decreases.

CONTROL OF ADRENOCORTICOTROPIN (ACTH) AND CORTISOL SECRETION

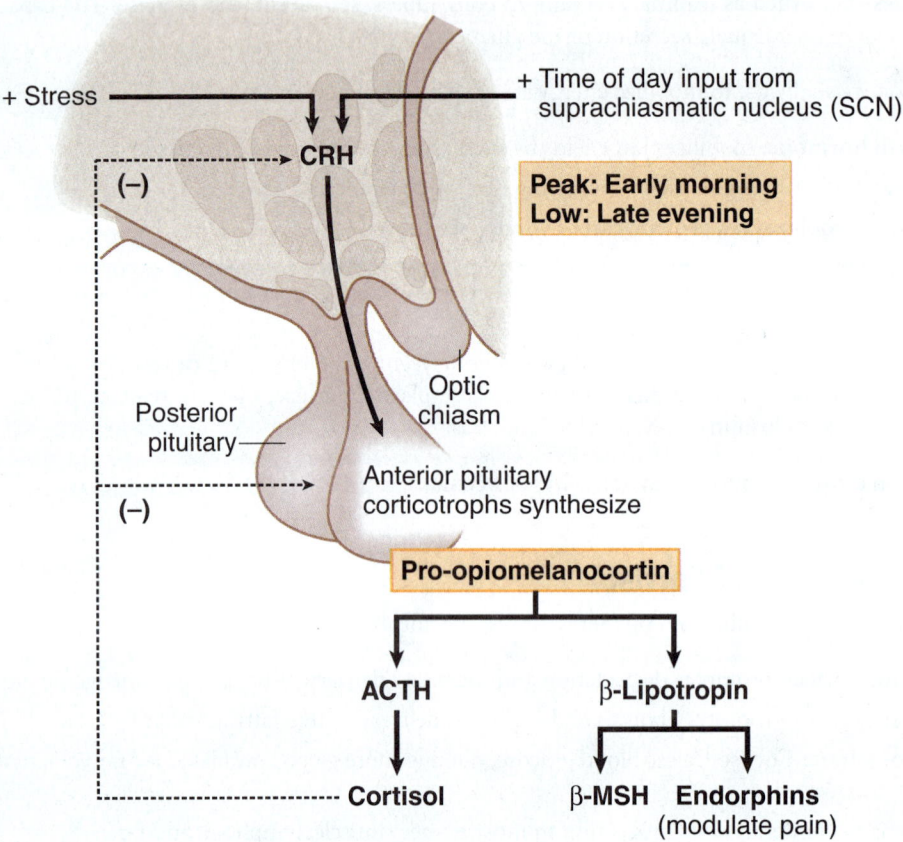

Figure 23-5. Control of ACTH and Cortisol
CRH = hypothalamic corticotropin-releasing hormone

Role of the Specific Modulators

Corticotropin-Releasing Hormone (CRH)

Secretion of CRH increases in response to stress and in the early morning:

- Peak cortisol secretion occurs early in the morning between the 6th and 8th hours of sleep. Secretion then declines slowly during the day and reaches a low point late in the evening.
- Increased AM CRH = increased AM cortisol
- Increased AM cortisol = increased AM blood sugar and lipid levels
- Increased AM sugar and lipid levels help get you out of bed

ACTH

Stimulates the secretion of cortisol (and adrenal androgens) of adrenal cortex. Cortisol suppresses the release of ACTH by acting on the hypothalamus and anterior pituitary.

Excessive secretion of ACTH (e.g., primary adrenal insufficiency) causes darkening of the skin. This is due to the melanocyte-stimulating hormone (α-MSH) sequence within the ACTH molecule, and the β-MSH activity of β-lipotropin.

β-Lipotropin

- Role not well understood
- Precursor to β-MSH and endorphins. Endorphins modulate the perception of pain.

PHYSIOLOGIC ACTIONS OF ALDOSTERONE

The primary target tissue for aldosterone is the kidney, where it increases Na^+ reabsorption by the principal cells of the kidney's collecting ducts. Because water is reabsorbed along with the Na^+, aldosterone can be considered to control the amount of Na^+ rather than the concentration of Na^+ in the ECF.

Aldosterone also promotes the secretion of H^+ by the intercalated cells of the collecting duct, and K^+ secretion by the principal cells. The Na^+-conserving action of aldosterone is also seen in salivary ducts, sweat glands, and the distal colon.

The following figure shows the overall effects of aldosterone. This is a generalized representation of the effect of aldosterone on the renal distal tubule/collecting duct region.

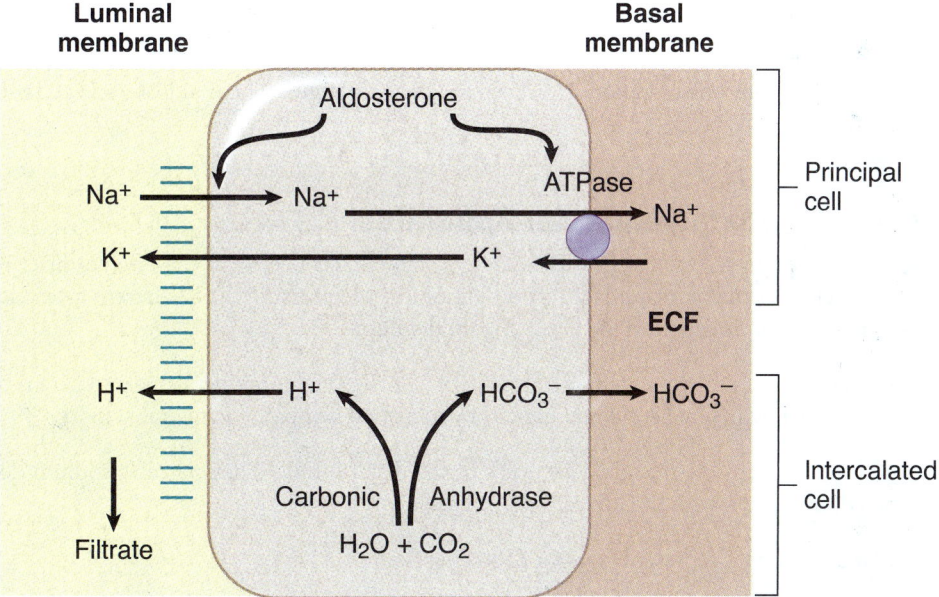

Figure 23-6. Late Distal Tubule and Collecting Duct

Specific Actions of Aldosterone

Aldosterone promotes the activity of Na/K-ATPase–dependent pump that moves Na^+ into the renal ECF in exchange for K^+. In addition, aldosterone enhances epithelial Na^+ channels (ENaC) in the luminal membrane of principal cells. The net effect is to increase Na^+ reabsorption, which in turn increases water reabsorption. Aldosterone regulates Na^+ to regulate extracellular volume.

The reabsorption of Na^+ creates a negative luminal potential promoting K^+ excretion.

Aldosterone stimulates H^+ secretion by intercalated cells. Thus, excess aldosterone causes alkalosis, while insufficient aldosterone causes acidosis (type IV RTA).

Table 23-1. Actions of Aldosterone

	Renal	
Na^+	reabsorption	↑ total body Na^+
K^+	secretion	↓plasma $[K^+]$
H^+	secretion	promotes metabolic alkalosis
HCO_3^-	production	promotes metabolic alkalosis
H_2O	reabsorption	volume expansion

CONTROL OF ALDOSTERONE SECRETION

Controlling Factors

Acutely, ACTH increases aldosterone secretion. However, the primary regulators of aldosterone secretion are circulating levels of Ang II and K^+.

Sensory Input—the Juxtaglomerular Apparatus

The main sensory cells are the granular cells (also called juxtamedullary cells) of the afferent arteriole. They are modified smooth-muscle cells that surround and directly monitor the pressure in the afferent arteriole. This signal in many cases is in response to a reduction in circulating fluid volume.

These cells are also innervated and stimulated by sympathetic neurons via norepinephrine and beta receptors. Thus the release of renin induced by hypovolemia is enhanced by increased sympathetic neural activity.

Additional sensory input is from the macula densa cells of the distal tubule. They perceive sodium delivery to the distal nephron and communicate with the juxtaglomerular cells.

The juxtaglomerular apparatus is represented in the following figure.

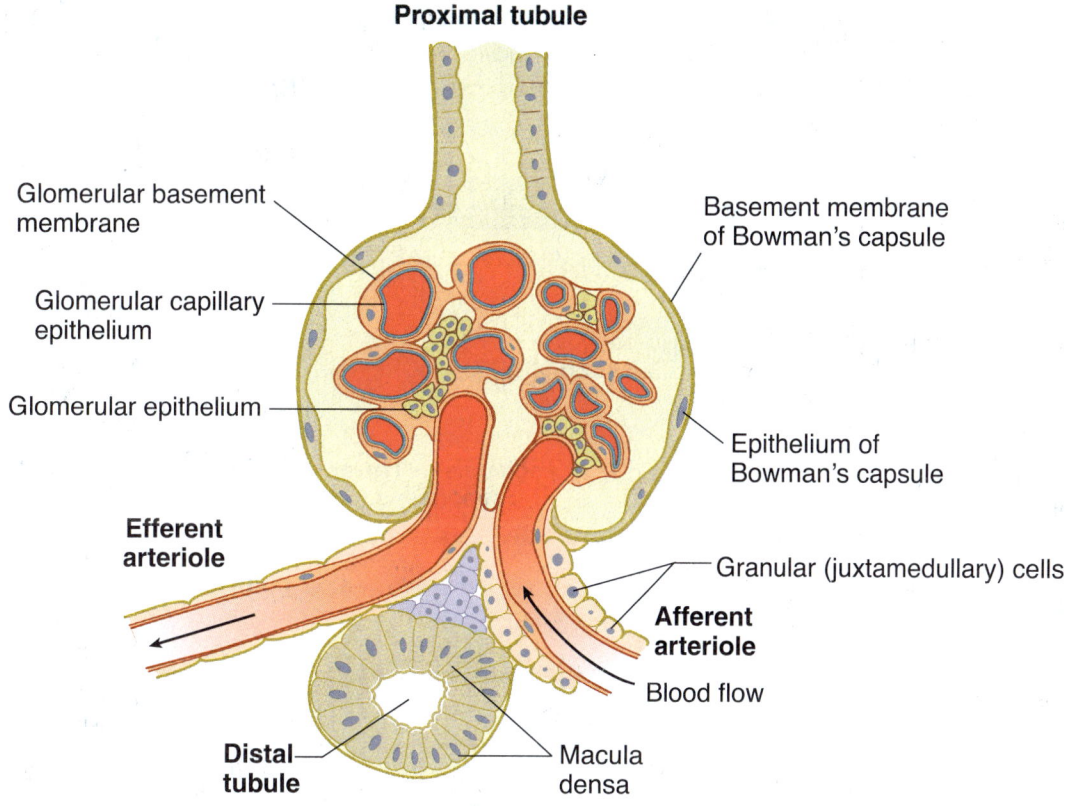

Figure 23-7. Renal Corpuscle and Juxtaglomerular Apparatus

Long-term Regulation of Blood Pressure and Cardiac Output by the Renin-Angiotensin-Aldosterone System

Long-term regulation of blood pressure and cardiac output is accomplished by the renin-angiotensin-aldosterone system.

Blood pressure is monitored by the juxtaglomerular apparatus. When renal perfusion pressure decreases, secretion of renin increases; conversely, when pressure increases, renin secretion is suppressed. Renin is an enzyme that converts a circulating protein produced in the liver, **angiotensinogen** into **angiotensin I**. Angiotensin converting enzyme (ACE), found mainly in endothelial cells of pulmonary vessels, converts angiotensin I into **angiotensin II**. Angiotensin II has potent effects to stimulate secretion of aldosterone and to cause arteriolar vasoconstriction. It also directly stimulates reabsorption of sodium in the proximal tubule.

$$MAP = CO \times TPR$$

This system regulates both resistance, via vasoconstriction, and cardiac output, via preload. Since aldosterone also causes increased renal excretion of potassium, it affects plasma potassium concentration. Plasma potassium strongly stimulates secretion of aldosterone, so this constitutes a negative-feedback control system for plasma potassium concentration.

Volume-depleted states tend to produce metabolic alkalosis, in part because aldosterone increases to compensate for the volume loss; the aldosterone increase stimulates excretion of acid and addition of bicarbonate to the plasma.

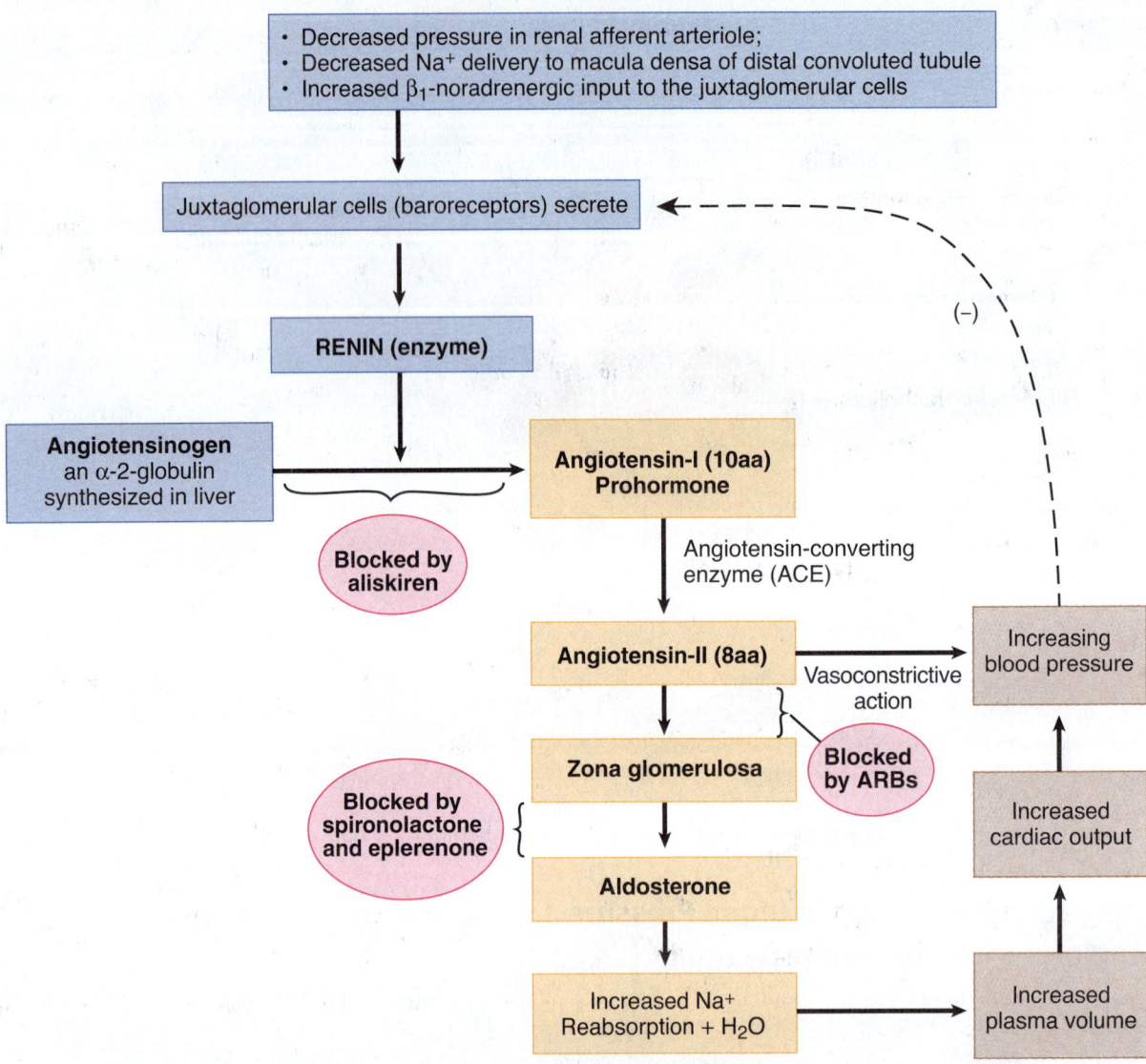

Figure 23-8. Feedback Control of Blood Pressure by Renin-Angiotensin-Aldosterone System

Any of the three stimuli listed at the top of the figure produces an increase in the secretion of renin and circulating angiotensin II. Angiotensin II raises blood pressure by two independent actions:

- The direct vasoconstrictive effects of angiotensin II increase total peripheral resistance.
- It stimulates the adrenal cortex to secrete aldosterone, resulting in increased reabsorption of Na^+.

As Na^+ reabsorption is increased, so is water. This increases the volume of the ECF, thus raising cardiac output and blood pressure.

An increase in blood pressure suppresses the renin-angiotensin-aldosterone system (RAAS). This decrease in angiotensin II reduces total peripheral resistance. Reduced activity of aldosterone causes a urinary loss of sodium and water, lowering cardiac output.

In addition to its effects to serve as a direct vasoconstrictor and increase aldosterone secretion, angiotensin II also:

- Increases ADH release from posterior pituitary
- Increases thirst
- Increases sodium reabsorption in proximal tubule

Potassium Effect

Any condition that decreases arterial blood pressure (e.g., hemorrhage, prolonged sweating) reduces perfusion pressure to the kidney and activates RAAS. In addition, it activates the sympathetic nervous system, which also stimulates RAAS. Sympathetic and RAAS activation work to restore arterial blood pressure.

Physiologic Changes in Aldosterone Secretion

Increased aldosterone secretion

Increased aldosterone secretion is any condition that decreases pressure in the renal artery (e.g., hemorrhage, prolonged sweating) activates the renin-angiotensin system, increases aldosterone secretion, and increases sympathetic stimulation to return blood pressure toward normal.

Decreased aldosterone secretion

Decreased aldosterone secretion is any condition that increases blood pressure in the renal artery. This includes weightlessness, because blood no longer pools in the extremities when the individual is standing or sitting. A large portion of the redistributed blood ends up in the atria and large veins of the chest and abdomen. The increased distention of these vessels stimulates baroreceptors located there. Signals from these baroreceptors reach the vasomotor center, where they inhibit sympathetic output, including sympathetic signals that normally promote renin secretion by the juxtaglomerular cells. As a result, less renin, angiotensin II, and aldosterone are secreted, causing individuals to lose Na^+ and ECF volume.

GLUCOCORTICOID DISORDERS

Definitions

Cushing syndrome: hypercortisolism regardless of origin, including chronic glucocorticoid therapy

Cushing disease: hypercortisolism due to an adenoma of the anterior pituitary (microadenoma)

Note

Hypercortisolism and an ACTH that is in the normal range or high is a secondary condition. Via negative feedback, a high cortisol should produce a low ACTH. If ACTH is in the "normal" range, then it is "inappropriately" normal (meaning it is too high) and is thus the cause of the hypercortisolism.

Hypercortisolism

Primary hypercortisolism (adrenal source)

- ACTH independent
- Cortisol elevated, ACTH depressed
- Most are benign adrenocorticol adenomas
- Adrenal adenoma usually unilateral and secretes only cortisol; decreased adrenal androgen and deoxycorticosterone (hirsutism absent)
- Presence of androgen or mineralocorticoid excess suggests a carcinoma.

Secondary hypercortisolism (pituitary vs. ectopic source)

- ACTH dependent
- Hypersecretion of ACTH results in bilateral hyperplasia of the adrenal zona fasciculata and reticularis
- Elevated ACTH, cortisol, adrenal androgen, deoxycorticosterone
- Two main subcategories:
  - **Pituitary adenoma,** usually a microadenoma (< 1 cm dia.)
    - This is Cushing disease
    - Increased ACTH not sufficient to cause hyperpigmentation
    - Dexamethasone suppressible
  - **Ectopic ACTH syndrome:**
    - Most frequently in patients with small cell carcinoma of the lung
    - Greater secretion of ACTH than in Cushing disease and hyperpigmentation often present
    - Ectopic site nonsupressible with dexamethasone

Differential diagnosis

- Hypercortisolism established by lack of cortisol suppression to 1 mg overnight dexamethasone and/or elevated 24-hour urine free cortisol
- Decreased plasma ACTH: Adrenal is source (primary hypercortisolism)
- High-dose dexamethasone
  - ACTH suppressed = Cushing disease (pituitary source)
  - ACTH not suppressed = ectopic ACTH syndrome

Characteristics of Cushing Syndrome

- Obesity because of hyperphagia, classically central affecting mainly the face, neck, trunk, and abdomen: "moon facies" and "buffalo hump"
- Protein depletion as a result of excessive protein catabolism
- Inhibition of inflammatory response and poor wound healing
- Hyperglycemia leads to hyperinsulinemia and insulin resistance.
- Hyperlipidemia
- Bone breakdown and osteoporosis
- Thinning of the skin with wide purple striae located around abdomen and hips
- Increased adrenal androgens, when present in women, can result in acne, mild hirsutism, and amenorrhea. In men, decreased libido and impotence
- Mineralocorticoid effects of the high level of glucocorticoid and deoxycorticosteroid lead to salt and water retention (hypertension), potassium depletion, and a hypokalemic alkalosis.
- Increased thirst and polyuria
- Anxiety, depression, and other emotional disorders may be present.

Hypocortisolism

Primary Hypocortisolism (in primary adrenal insufficiency, Addison's disease)

Cortisol deficiency leads to weakness, fatigue, anorexia, weight loss, hypotension, hyponatremia, hypoglycemia. Increases in ACTH result in hyperpigmentation of skin and mucous membranes.

Aldosterone deficiency leads to sodium wasting and hyponatremia, potassium retention and hyperkalemia, dehydration, hypotension, and acidosis

- Autoimmune origin with slow onset in about 80% of cases
- Loss of 90% of both adrenals required before obvious clinical manifestations
- With gradual adrenal destruction, basal secretion is normal but secretion does not respond to stress, which may initiate an adrenal crisis.
- Bilateral hemorrhage as the origin results in an adrenal crisis. Hyperpigmentation, hyponatremia, and hyperkalemia usually absent
- Orthostatic intolerance due to diminished alpha-receptor function and low blood volume.
- Abnormalities in GI function
- Loss of axillary and pubic hair in women due to loss of androgens, amenorrhea
- Insufficient glucocorticoids leads to hypoglycemia and an inability of the kidney to excrete a water load
- Severe hypoglycemia in children but rare in adults

Secondary hypocortisolism (secondary adrenal insufficiency)

- Most commonly due to sudden withdrawal of exogenous glucocorticoid therapy
- Trauma, infection, and infarction most common natural origin of ACTH deficiency
- In the early stages baseline hormone values are normal but ACTH reserve compromised and stress response subnormal (glucocorticoids administered presurgery)
- May be associated with the loss of other anterior pituitary hormones (panhypopituitarism) or adenomas secreting prolactin or growth hormone
- Atrophy of the zona fasciculata and zona reticularis
- Zona glomerulosa and aldosterone normal; no manifestations of mineralocorticoid deficiency
- Consequences as stated for cortisol deficiency
- Severe hypoglycemia and severe hypotension unusual (RAAS is still intact)
- Hyponatremia due to water retention

Summary

Table 23-2. Primary and Secondary Disorders of Cortisol Secretion

Disorder	Plasma Cortisol	Plasma ACTH	Hyperpigmentation
Primary hypercortisolism	↑	↓	no
Secondary hypercortisolism			
Cushing disease	↑	normal or ↑	no
Ectopic ACTH	↑	↑	yes (maybe)
Primary hypocortisolism	↓	↑	yes
Secondary hypocortisolism	↓	↓	no

MINERALOCORTICOID DISORDERS

Hyperaldosteronism with Hypertension

Primary hyperaldosteronism (Conn's syndrome)

- Most common cause is a small unilateral adenoma, on either side
- Remainder mostly bilateral adrenal hyperplasia (idiopathic hyperaldosteronism)
- Rarely due to adrenal carcinoma
- Increased whole body sodium, fluid, and circulating blood volume
- Hypernatremia is infrequent.
- Increased peripheral vasoconstriction and TPR
- Blood pressure from borderline to severe hypertension
- Edema rare (sodium escape*)
- Modest left ventricular hypertrophy
- Potassium depletion and hypokalemia create symptoms of weakness and fatigue.
- Detection of hypertension with hypokalemia is often the initial clue for Conn's syndrome
- Increased hydrogen ion excretion and new bicarbonate create metabolic alkalosis.
- A positive Chvostek or Trousseau's sign is suggestive of alkalosis leading to low calcium levels.
- Cortisol is normal.
- Suppression of renin a major feature

Secondary hyperaldosteronism refers to a state in which there is an appropriate increase in aldosterone in response to activation of the renin-angiotensin system.

Secondary hyperaldosteronism with hypertension

- In most cases a primary over-secretion of renin secondary to a decrease in renal blood flow and/or pressure
- Renal arterial stenosis, narrowing via atherosclerosis, fibromuscular hyperplasia.
- Renin-secreting tumor rare
- Modest to highly elevated renin
- Modest to highly elevated aldosterone
- Hypokalemia and metabolic alkalosis

Differential diagnosis

- Hypokalemia in a hypertensive patient not taking diuretics
- Hyposecretion of renin with elevated aldosterone that fails to respond to a volume contraction – Conn's syndrome
- Hypersecretion of renin with elevated aldosterone – renal vascular

---

*A major increase in sodium and water retention is prevented by "sodium escape" in primary hyperaldosteronism. The mechanism for this escape is still unclear.

Hyperaldosteronism with Hypotension

Secondary hyperaldosteronism with hypotension

Sequestration of blood on the venous side of the systemic circulation is a common cause of secondary hyperaldosteronism. This results in decreased cardiac output and thus decreased blood flow and pressure in the renal artery. The following conditions produce secondary hyperaldosteronism through this mechanism:

- Congestive heart failure
- Constriction of the vena cava
- Hepatic cirrhosis

Table 23-3. Summary of Secondary Hyperaldosteronism

The cause in all cases is a decrease in blood pressure.	
1. Plasma renin and angiotensin II activity: The increased angiotensin II activity will drive the secondary hyperaldosteronism.	↑
2. Total body sodium:	↑
3. ECF volume:	↑
4. Plasma volume:	↑
5. Edema*:	yes

*Na$^+$ escape prevents peripheral edema in primary but not secondary hyperaldosteronism. Also note that the increased ECF volume remains mainly on the venous side of the circulation, accentuating the venous congestion and preventing a return of circulating blood volume to normal.

Learning Objectives

❏ Answer questions about hormones of the adrenal medulla

❏ Demonstrate understanding of major metabolic actions of epinephrine

❏ Interpret scenarios on pheochromocytomas

HORMONES OF THE ADRENAL MEDULLA

- Secretion of the adrenal medulla is 20% norepinephrine and 80% epinephrine.
- Phenylethanolamine-N-methyltransferase (PMNT) converts norepinephrine into epinephrine.
- Half-life of the catecholamines is only about two minutes. Metabolic endproducts include metanephrines and vanillylmandelic acid (VMA) both of which can be measured in plasma and urine
- Removal of the adrenal medulla reduces plasma epinephrine to very low levels but does not alter plasma norepinephrine. Most circulating norepinephrine arises from postganglionic sympathetic neurons.
- Because many of the actions of epinephrine are also mediated by norepinephrine, the adrenal medulla is not essential for life.
- The vasoconstrictive action of norepinephrine is essential for the maintenance of normal blood pressure, especially when an individual is standing. Plasma norepinephrine levels double when one goes from a lying to a standing position. People with inadequate production of norepinephrine suffer from orthostatic hypotension.
- Epinephrine is a stress hormone and rapidly increases in response to exercise, exposure to cold, emergencies, and hypoglycemia.

MAJOR METABOLIC ACTIONS OF EPINEPHRINE

- Liver: Epinephrine increases the activity of liver and muscle phosphorylase, promoting glycogenolysis. This increases glucose output by the liver.
- Skeletal muscle: Epinephrine promotes glycogenolysis but because muscle lacks glucose-6-phosphatase, glucose cannot be released by skeletal muscle; instead, it must be metabolized at least to lactate before being released into the circulation.
- Adipose tissue: Epinephrine increases lipolysis in adipose tissue by increasing the activity of hormone-sensitive lipase. Glycerol from TG breakdown is a minor substrate for gluconeogenesis.
- Epinephrine increases the metabolic rate. This will not occur without thyroid hormones or the adrenal cortex.

Metabolic Actions of Epinephrine on CHO and Fat

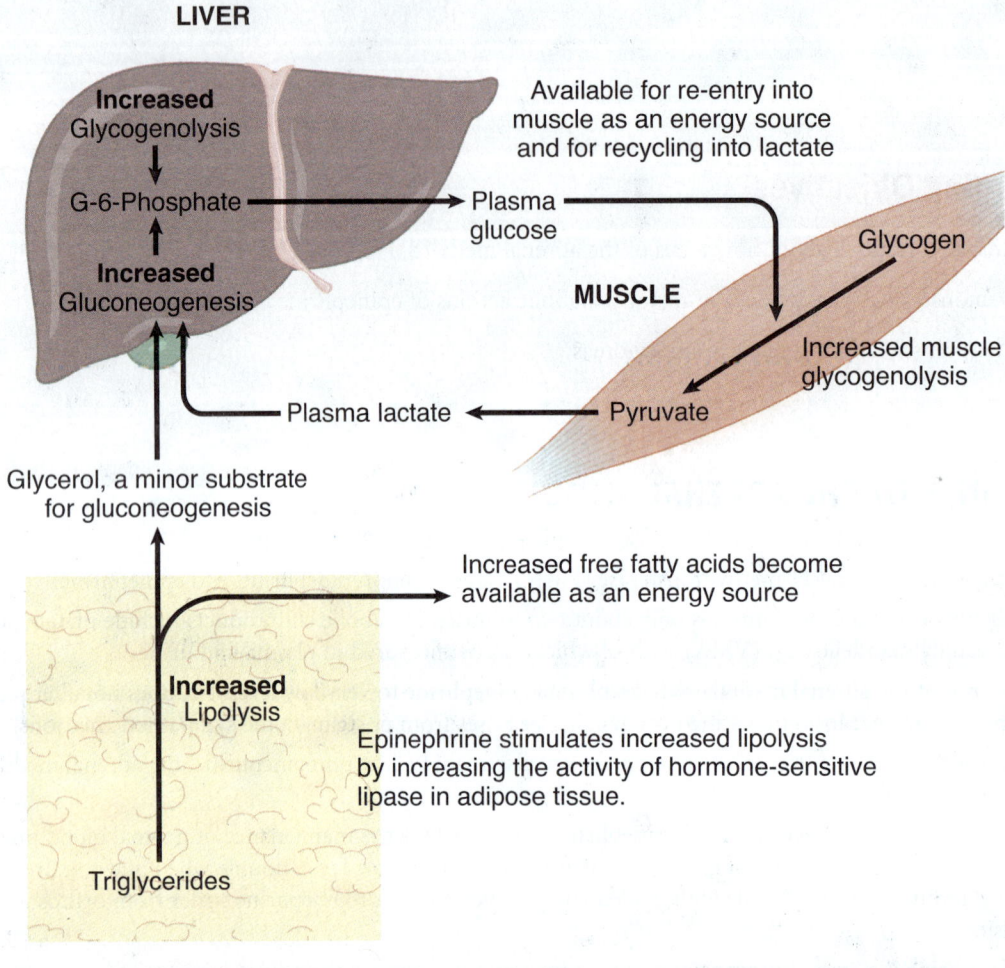

Figure 24-1. Actions of Catecholamines

PHEOCHROMOCYTOMAS

- Adrenal tumors that secrete epinephrine and norepinephrine in various ratios
- Usually unilateral benign tumors
- Characteristic of MEN 2A and MEN 2B
- Paragangliomas are extra-adrenal pheochromocytomas of sympathetic ganglia located primarily within the abdomen and that secrete norepinephrine.
- Most consistent feature is hypertension. Symptoms include headache, diaphoresis, palpitations, and anxiety. Increased metabolic rate and hyperglycemia also occur.
- Pheochromocytomas are highly vascular and encapsulated.
- Episodic release of hormone, particularly when it is mainly norepinephrine, can abruptly cause a hypertensive crisis. Can be induced by physical stimuli that displaces abdominal contents.
- Most reliable initial test is plasma metanephrines or 24-hour urine catecholamines or metanephines.
- Usually curable but can be fatal if undiagnosed
- Treat with alpha blocker followed by surgical removal.

Learning Objectives

❏ Use knowledge of hormones of the islets of Langerhans

❏ Use knowledge of control of insulin secretion

❏ Explain information related to actions of glucagon

❏ Answer questions about control of glucagon secretion

❏ Answer questions about pancreatic endocrine-secreting tumors

HORMONES OF THE ISLETS OF LANGERHANS

The location and proportion of each major hormone-secreting cell type of the islets of Langerhans are shown in Figure 25-1. The local inhibitory paracrine action of each islet hormone is shown by dashed arrows. The diameter of each circle approximately represents the proportion of that cell type present in the islets.

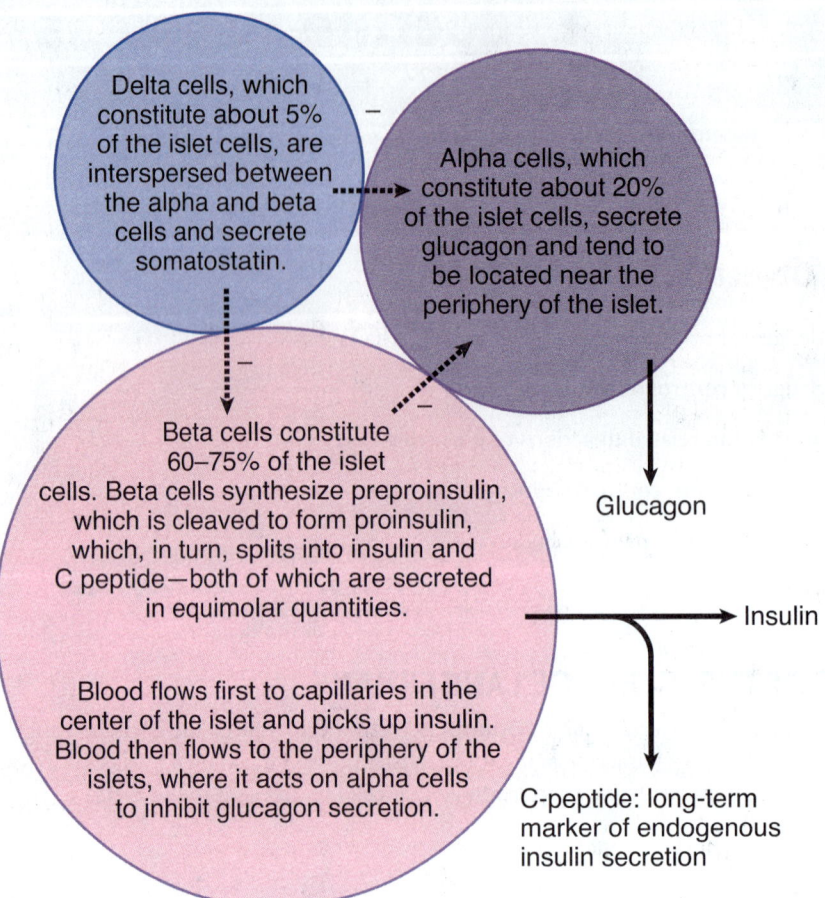

Figure 25-1. Hormones of the Pancreatic Islets

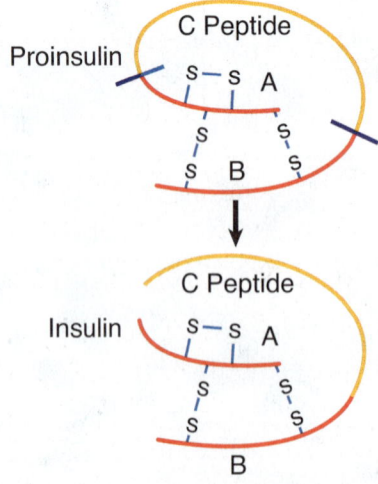

Figure 25-2. Insulin

ACTIONS OF INSULIN

Insulin Receptor

- The portion of the insulin receptor that faces externally has the hormone-binding domain.
- The portion of the insulin receptor that faces the cytosol has tyrosine kinase activity.
- When occupied by insulin, the receptor phosphorylates itself and other proteins.

Peripheral Uptake of Glucose

Glucose is taken up by peripheral tissues by facilitated diffusion. Insulin facilitates this uptake in some tissues. Typically the insulin receptor causes the insertion of glucose transporters in the membrane.

Tissues that require insulin for effective uptake of glucose are:

- Adipose tissue
- Resting skeletal muscle (although glucose can enter working muscle without the aid of insulin)
- Liver because of glucokinase stimulation

Tissues in which glucose uptake is not affected by insulin are:

- Nervous tissue
- Kidney tubules
- Intestinal mucosa
- Red blood cells
- β-cells of pancreas

Metabolic Actions of Insulin

Insulin is a major anabolic hormone, and it secreted in response to a carbohydrate- and/or protein-containing meal.

Anabolic hormones tend to promote protein synthesis (increase lean body mass). Other anabolic hormones include:

- Thyroid hormones
- Growth hormone/IGF I
- Sex steroids (androgens)

Effects of insulin on carbohydrate metabolism

Insulin increases the uptake of glucose and its metabolism in muscle and fat. By increasing glucose uptake in muscle, its metabolism increases, i.e., its conversion to carbon dioxide and water is increased.

Insulin increases glycogen synthesis in liver and muscle. The activity of enzymes that promote glycogen synthesis (glucokinase and glycogen synthetase) is increased. The activity of those enzymes that promote glycogen breakdown (phosphorylase and glucose-6-phosphatase) is decreased.

- Glucokinase and glucose-6-phosphatase are expressed by the liver but not by muscle.

Effects of insulin on protein metabolism

- Insulin increases amino acid uptake by muscle cells.
- Insulin increases protein synthesis.
- Insulin decreases protein breakdown (deficiency of insulin results in a breakdown of protein).

Effects of insulin on fat metabolism

Insulin increases:

- Glucose uptake by fat cells (increases membrane transporters). By increasing glucose uptake, insulin also makes triose phosphates available for triglyceride synthesis in adipose tissue.
- Triglyceride uptake by fat cells. It increases the activity of lipoprotein lipase. Lipoprotein lipase is located on the endothelium of capillaries, and it catalyzes the release of free fatty acids from triglycerides.
- Triglyceride synthesis (lipogenesis) in adipose tissue and liver by stimulating the rate-limiting step, namely the carboxylation of acetyl CoA to malonyl CoA. In other words, insulin stimulates the conversion of carbohydrate into fat.

Insulin decreases:

- Triglyceride breakdown (lipolysis) in adipose tissue by decreasing the activity of hormone-sensitive lipase. This enzyme is activated by stress hormones (i.e., cortisol, growth hormone, epinephrine [glucagon]).
- Formation of ketone bodies by the liver.

Insulin Effects on Potassium

Insulin promotes K^+ movement into cells. Although the overall process is not well understood, insulin increases the activity of Na/K-ATPase in most body tissues.

This K^+-lowering action of insulin is used to treat acute, life-threatening hyperkalemia. For example, sometimes the hyperkalemia of renal failure is successfully lowered by the simultaneous administration of insulin and glucose. (The glucose is given to prevent severe insulin-induced hypoglycemia from developing.)

It does not work as quickly as calcium chloride, which is instantaneous, in protecting the heart from arrhythmias. Insulin and glucose administration is faster than Na^+/K^+ cation exchange resins such as kayexalate. Kayexalate is taken into the GI tract orally but needs 6-12 hours to be effective in lowering potassium levels.

Summary

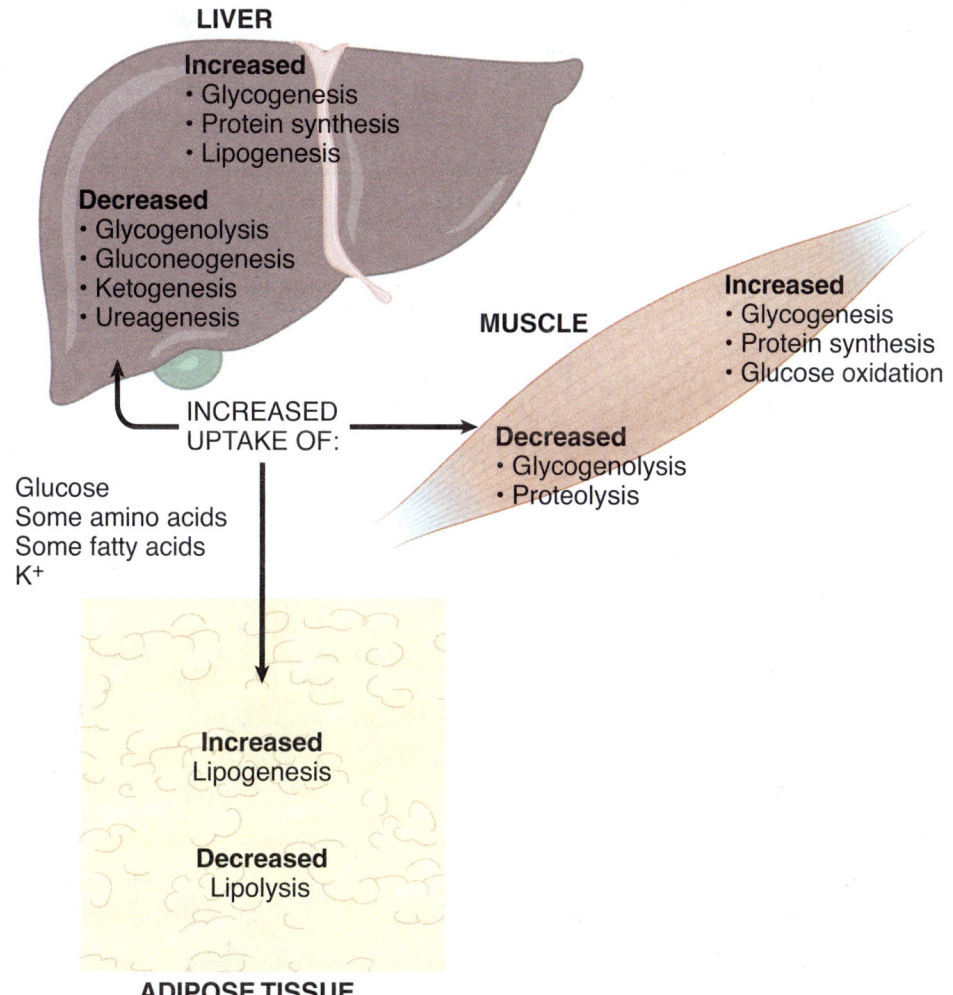

LIVER

Increased
• Glycogenesis
• Protein synthesis
• Lipogenesis

Decreased
• Glycogenolysis
• Gluconeogenesis
• Ketogenesis
• Ureagenesis

MUSCLE

Increased
• Glycogenesis
• Protein synthesis
• Glucose oxidation

Decreased
• Glycogenolysis
• Proteolysis

INCREASED
UPTAKE OF:

Glucose
Some amino acids
Some fatty acids
K+

Increased
Lipogenesis

Decreased
Lipolysis

ADIPOSE TISSUE

Figure 25-3. Major Actions of Insulin

CONTROL OF INSULIN SECRETION

The most important controller of insulin secretion is plasma glucose. Above a threshold of 100 mg%, insulin secretion is directly proportional to plasma glucose.

Glucose enters the cell, causing a rise in intracellular ATP that closes ATP-sensitive K^+ channels.

Closure of the ATP-sensitive K^+ channels results in depolarization, causing voltage-gated Ca^{2+} channels to open.

The rise in cytosolic Ca^{2+} causes exocytosis of the vesicles, which then secrete insulin and C-peptide into the blood.

All of the hormones or neurotransmitters named in Figure 25-5 attach to membrane receptors (R). In contrast, the metabolic substrates, glucose and amino acids, enter the β-cell.

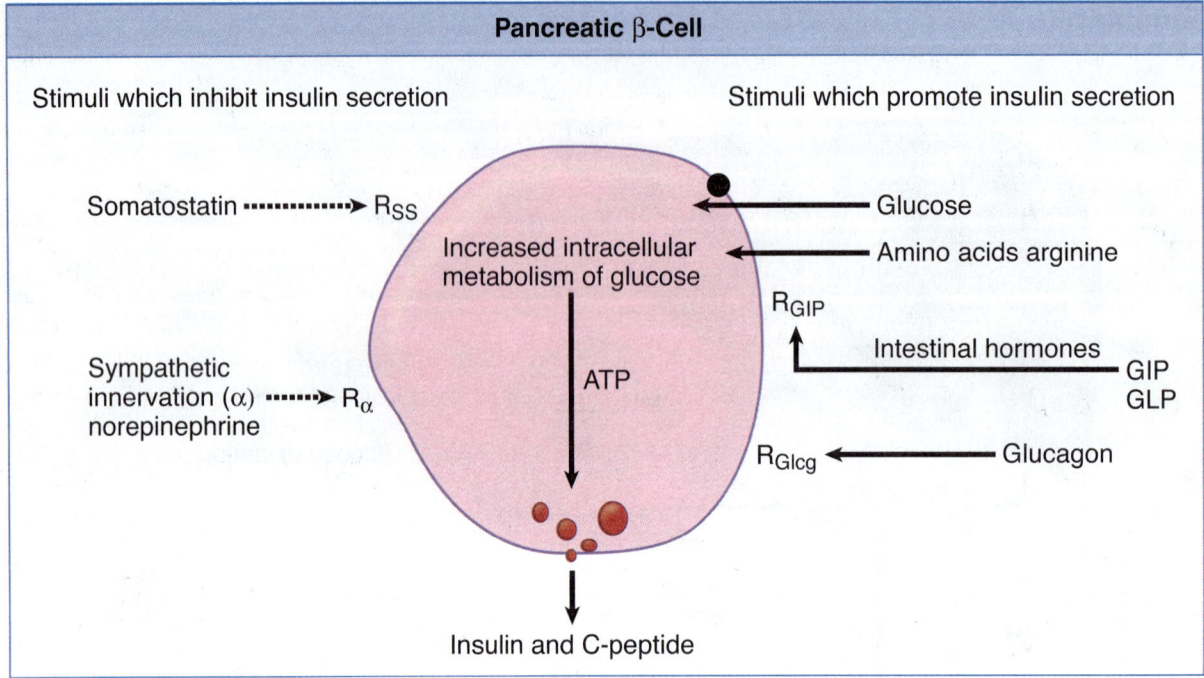

Figure 25-4. Control of Insulin Secretion

Incretin: GIP = gastric inhibitory peptide or glucose insulinotropic peptide; **GLP** = glucagon-like peptide

ACTIONS OF GLUCAGON

Glucagon is a peptide hormone. It is secreted by the α-cells of the pancreatic islets.

The primary target for glucagon action is the liver hepatocyte, where its action is mediated by an increase in the concentration of cAMP. The cAMP activates protein kinase A, which, by catalyzing phosphorylation, alters the activity of enzymes mediating the actions given below.

Note: Skeletal muscle is not a target tissue for glucagon.

Specific Actions of Glucagon on the Liver

1. Increases liver glycogenolysis.

   Glucagon activates glycogen phosphorylase, breaking down glycogen to glucose-1-phosphate. Glucagon inactivates glycogen synthetase, preventing the glucose-1-phosphate from being recycled back into glycogen.

2. Increases liver gluconeogenesis.

   Glucagon inhibits phosphofructokinase-2 (PFK-2), thereby reducing 2,6 bisphosphate, which in turn inhibits PFK-1 (an important enzyme driving glycolysis). Inhibition of PFK-1 aids gluconeogenesis. In addition, glucagon, along with cortisol, enhances phosphoenolpyruvate carboxykinase, a key enzyme in the gluconeogenic pathway. Finally, glucagon stimulates glucose-6-phosphatase, thereby releasing glucose into the blood (see Biochemistry notes).

3. Increases liver ketogenesis and decreases lipogenesis.

   Glucagon inhibits the activity of acetyl CoA carboxylase, decreasing the formation of malonyl CoA. When the concentration of malonyl CoA is low, ketogenesis is favored over lipogenesis.

4. Increases ureagenesis.

   It stimulates N-acetylglutamate synthesis, which stimulates the production of urea (see Biochemistry notes).

5. Increases insulin secretion.

   The amino acid sequence of glucagon is similar to that of the duodenal hormone, secretin. Like secretin (and most other gut hormones), glucagon stimulates insulin secretion.

6. Increases lipolysis in the liver.

   Glucagon activates hormone-sensitive lipase in the liver, but because the action is on the liver and not the adipocyte, glucagon is not considered a major fat-mobilizing hormone.

CONTROL OF GLUCAGON SECRETION

Major factors that control glucagon secretion are summarized in Figure 25-5. Stimuli that promote glucagon secretion are depicted on the right, and those that inhibit on the left. R designates a surface receptor for the particular hormone or neurotransmitter.

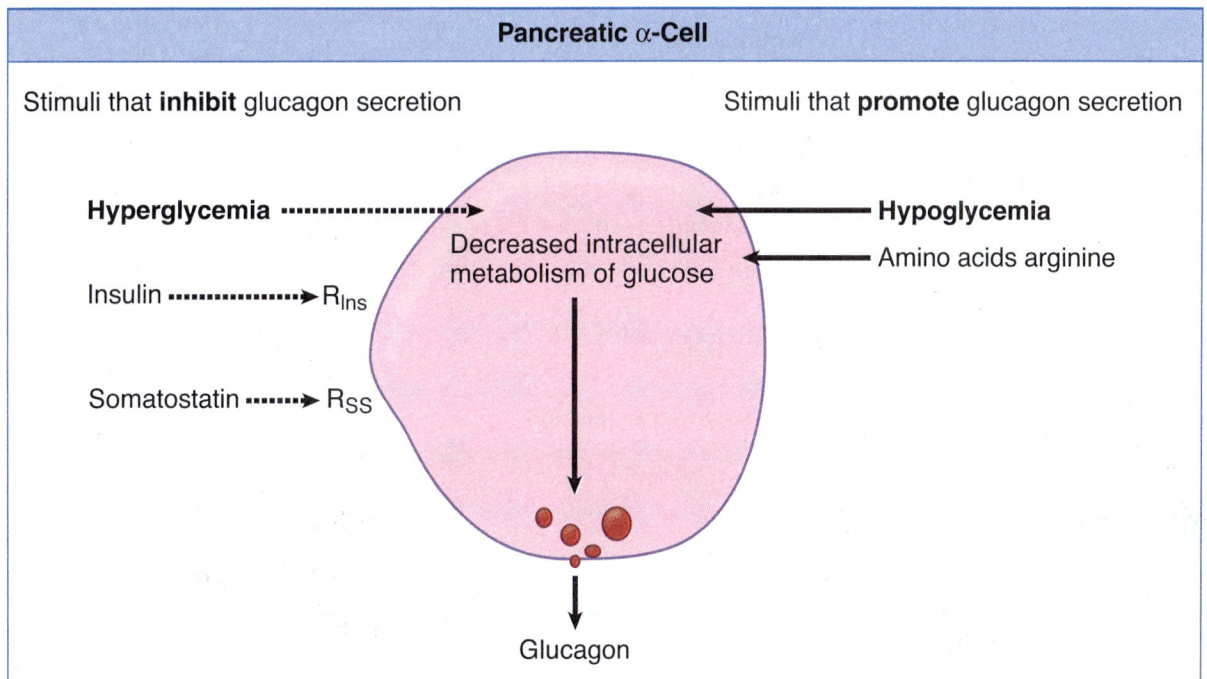

Figure 25-5. Control of Glucagon Secretion

Low plasma glucose (hypoglycemia) is the most important physiologic promoter for glucagon secretion, and elevated plasma glucose (hyperglycemia) the most important inhibitor.

Amino acids, especially dibasic amino acids (arginine, lysine), also promote the secretion of glucagon. Thus, glucagon is secreted in response to the ingestion of a meal rich in proteins.

Overall View of Glucose Counterregulation

Glucose counterregulation is the concept that plasma glucose concentration is regulated by insulin and by hormones that oppose, or counter, its actions. The following diagram shows glucose regulation in the postprandial and post-absorptive states.

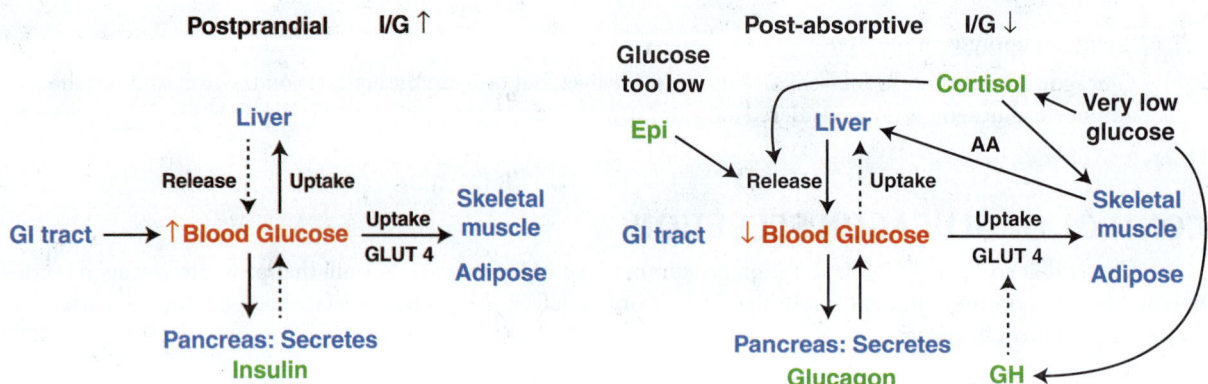

Figure 25-6. Insulin Actions in Liver
Stimulate/Increase ⟶
Inhibit/decrease ⇢

Insulin: Glucagon Ratio

- Insulin and glucagon: move substrates in opposite directions. The direction of substrate fluxes is very sensitive to this ratio.
- Normal postabsorptive ratio: 2.0
- States requiring mobilization of substrates ratio: 0.5 or less
- Carbohydrate meal, ratio 10 or more
- Protein meal or fat meal produces little change in the ratio.

DIABETES MELLITUS

In both types of diabetes mellitus, there is hyperglycemia, polyuria, increased thirst and fluid intake, hyperosmolar state, recurrent blurred vision, mental confusion, lethargy, weakness, and abnormal peripheral sensation. Coma, if it does occur, is due to the hyperosmotic environment, not the acidosis.

Type 2

- Accounts for about 90% of all the cases of diabetes
- Strong genetic component
- Body build is usually obese (particularly central or visceral).
- Usually, but not always, middle-aged or older
- The number of younger individuals in this category is increasing.
- Characterized by variable degrees of insulin resistance, impaired insulin secretion, and increased hepatic output of glucose. Insulin resistance precedes secretory defects and in the early stages hyperinsulinemia is able to overcome tissue resistance. Ultimately beta cell failure can occur.
- Insulin levels may be high, normal, or low.
- Resistance to insulin is not well understood. It is thought to be due to postreceptor defects in signaling, which ultimately lead to a decrease in the number of glucose transporters. Reducing plasma glucose and thus plasma insulin can increase receptor sensitivity toward normal.

- Plasma glucose good screening for type 2. Elevated glucose due to elevated hepatic output.
- With a controlled diet and exercise, the symptoms of type 2 diabetes often disappear without the necessity for pharmacologic therapy.
- Individuals tend to be ketosis resistant. The presence of some endogenous insulin secretion appears to protect from development of a ketoacidosis. If it does develop, it is usually the result of severe stress or infection (increased counterregulatory homones, suppressed insulin).
- In nonobese patients, a deficient insulin release by the pancreas is often the problem, but varying degrees of insulin resistance can also occur.

Metabolic Syndrome (Syndrome X)

A group of metabolic derangements that includes atherogenic dyslipidemia (low HDL) and high triglycerides, elevated blood glucose, hypertension, central obesity, prothrombotic state, and a proinflammatory state. The clustering of these risk factors increases the probability of developing cardiovascular disease and type 2 diabetes.

Type 1

- Genetic association less marked than in type 2
- Genetically predisposed individuals whose immune system destroys pancreatic beta cells
- Symptoms do not become evident until 80% of the beta cells are destroyed.
- Body build usually lean
- Usually, but not always, early age of onset
- Due to an absence of insulin production
- Increased glucagon secretion also generally occurs
- Three target tissues for insulin—liver, skeletal muscle, and adipose tissue—fail to take up absorbed nutrients (glucose, amino acids, and fatty acids), thus increasing their levels in the blood.

Metabolic effects in insulin-deficient individuals

CHO

- Increased blood glucose concentration
- Increased glycogen breakdown
- Decreased peripheral glucose use

Protein

- Increased protein breakdown
- Increased catabolism of amino acids
- Increased gluconeogenesis
- Increased ureagenesis
- Decreased protein synthesis

Fat

- Increased triglyceride breakdown
- Increased level of circulating free fatty acids
- Increased ketosis, resulting in ketoacidosis (metabolic acidosis)
- Decreased fatty acid synthesis
- Decreased triglyceride synthesis

Renal System

The failure to reabsorb all the filtered glucose in the proximal tube also prevents normal water and electrolyte reabsorption in this segment, resulting in an osmotic diuresis (polyuria). This causes loss of glucose, water, and electrolytes from the body. Thus, even though the electrolyte concentration of the urine is low, body stores of electrolytes, particularly Na^+ and K^+, are lost.

Potassium Ion

- Hydrogen ions move intracellularly to be buffered, and potassium ions leave the cell, reducing the intracellular concentration.
- There is a lack of the normal insulin effect of pumping potassium ion into cells.
- Consequently, hyperkalemia is typical, but plasma K^+ may be normal or low because of renal loss. Regardless, the body stores of K^+ are reduced because of the renal loss.
- Insulin replacement can produce severe hypokalemia, and potassium replacement is a normal part of therapy.

Sodium Ion

- Polyuria decreases total body sodium but dehydration may keep sodium within or close to the normal range.
- Hyperosmolar state due to the hyperglycemia. Thus, 2 times the sodium concentration is not a good index of osmolarity.

$$\text{Effective osmolarity} = 2(Na)\ mEq/L + \frac{glucose\ mg/dL}{18}$$

Hyperosmolar Coma

- Severe hyperglycemia shifts fluid from the intracellular to the extracellular space.
- Polyuria decreases volume of the extracellular space and leads to a decreased renal plasma flow and a reduced glucose excretion. Combined with the rise in counterregulatory hormones, the plasma glucose rises further.
- The severe loss of intracellular fluid from the brain causes the coma.
- Type 2 diabetics often present with the highest plasma glucose and greater states of dehydration. Thus these patients have a higher incidence of coma.

Diabetic Ketoacidosis (DKA)

- Without any insulin, excessive lipolysis provides fatty acids to the liver, where they preferentially converted to ketone bodies because of the unopposed action of glucagon.
- Blood pH and bicarbonate decrease due to the metabolic acidosis.
- Increased alveolar ventilation is the respiratory compensation for the metabolic acidosis. When the arterial pH decreases to about 7.20, ventilation becomes deep and rapid (Kussmaul breathing).
- An acidic urine results as the kidneys attempt to compensate for the acidosis.
- The severe acidosis is in addition to the dehydration and net decrease in total body sodium and potassium.
- Treatment is replacement of fluid and electrolytes and administration of insulin
- DKA treatment is first 2-3 liters of normal saline and IV insulin. Subcutaneous insulin may not be fully absorbed because of decreased skin perfusion. Hyponatremia is common because of hyperglycemia. For each 100 point increase in glucose above normal, there is a 1.6 decrease in sodium.

100 mg ELEVATION glucose = 1.6 meq DECREASE sodium

When hyponatremia is present with hyperglycemia, management is correction of the elevated glucose level. When glucose comes to normal, the sodium corrects.

Hypoglycemia

- In the diabetic, overdosing with insulin causes hypoglycemia.
- Type 1 diabetics are particularly prone to hypoglycemia. In these individuals the glucagon response to hypoglycemia is absent.
- Initial symptoms due to catecholamine release followed by the direct effects of hypoglycemia include slowed mental processes and confusion.

Summary

Table 25-1. Summary of Insulin-Related Pathophysiologic States

	Glucose	Insulin	C-peptide	Ketoacidosis
Type 2 diabetes	↑	↑, ↔	↑, ↔	−
Type 1 diabetes	↑	↓	↓	+
Insulinoma	↓	↑	↑	−
Factitious hypoglycemia (self-injection of insulin)	↓	↑	↓	−

Hormonal Control of Calcium and Phosphate

26

Learning Objectives

❏ Solve problems concerning overview of calcium and phosphate

❏ Solve problems concerning parathyroid hormone

❏ Demonstrate understanding of role of Vitamin D (Calcitriol) in calcium homeostasis

❏ Solve problems concerning disorders in calcium and phosphate

❏ Answer questions about metabolic bone disorders

OVERVIEW OF CALCIUM AND PHOSPHATE

- The percentage of dietary calcium absorbed from the gut is inversely related to intake.
- The dietary intake of and the percentage of calcium absorbed is diminished in the elderly.
- Ingested phosphate is also absorbed by the gut.
- Both calcium and phosphate absorption in the GI tract are stimulated by the active form of vitamin D (calcitriol).

The approximate percentage of the body's total calcium is given for each of the compartments in Figure 26-1. In addition, the fraction of calcium is indicated. The calcium concentration in the interstitial fluid is 103 to 104 times higher than the intracellular calcium concentration. The initiation of many cellular processes (secretion, movement of intracellular organelles, cell division) is linked to a sudden brief increase in intracellular (cytosolic) calcium.

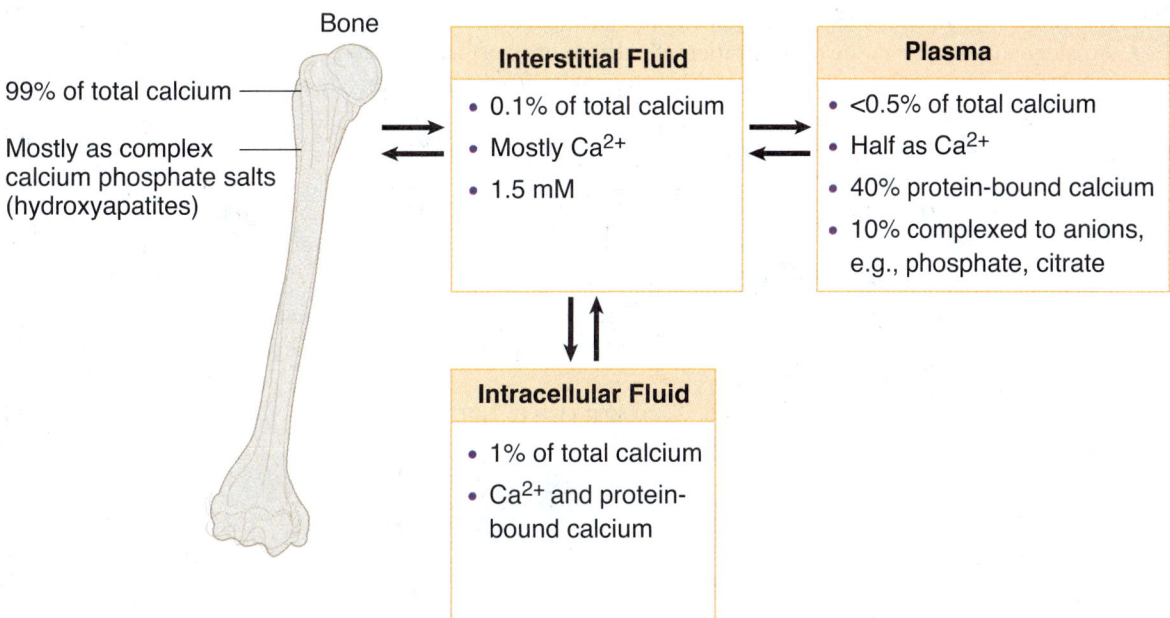

Figure 26-1. Calcium Distribution in the Body

Plasma Calcium

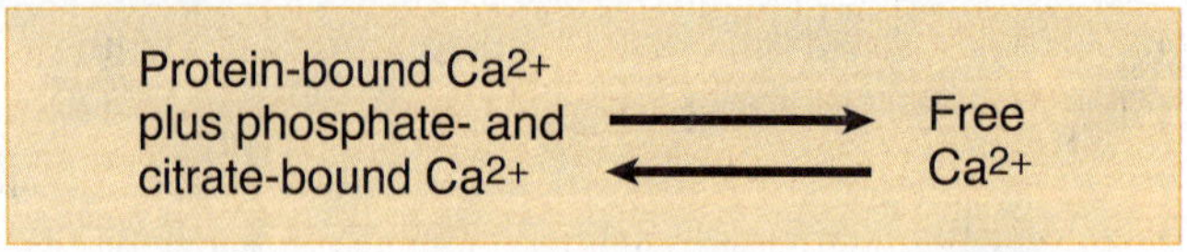

Protein-bound Ca^{2+} plus phosphate- and citrate-bound Ca^{2+} $\longrightarrow$ $\longleftarrow$ Free Ca^{2+}

Figure 26-2. Relationship of Bound and Free Calcium

- Plasma calcium represents 50% ionized free, 40% attached to protein, 10% associated with anions such as phosphate and citrate.
- The free calcium is the physiologically active and precisely regulated form.
- Alkalosis (hyperventilation) decreases and acidosis increases free plasma calcium by varying the amount bound to protein.
- Alkalosis lowers free calcium by increasing protein-binding, while acidosis raises free calcium by decreasing protein-binding.

Relationship Between Calcium and Phosphate

Bone is a complex precipitate of calcium and phosphate to which hydroxide and bicarbonate ions are added to make up the mature hydroxyapatite crystals, which are laid down in a protein (osteoid) matrix. Whether calcium and phosphate are laid down in bone (precipitate from solution) or are resorbed from bone (go into solution) depends on the product of their concentrations rather than on their individual concentrations.

When the product exceeds a certain number (solubility product or ion product), bone is laid down:

$$[Ca^{2+}] \times [PO_4^-] > \text{solubility product} = \text{bone deposition}$$

- Under normal conditions the ECF product of calcium times phosphate is close to the solubility product.
- Thus, an increase in the interstitial fluid concentration of either Ca^{2+} or phosphate increases bone mineralization.
- For example, an increase in plasma phosphate would increase the product of their concentrations, promote precipitation, and lower free calcium in the interstitial fluid.
- A malignant increase in the concentration of calcium or phosphate due to chronic renal disease or rhabdomyolysis can cause the precipitation of calcium phosphate within tissues.

When the product is below the solubility product, bone is resorbed:

$$[Ca^{2+}] \times [PO_4^-] < \text{solubility product} = \text{bone resorption}$$

- Thus, a decrease in the interstitial concentration of either Ca^{2+} or phosphate promotes the resorption of these salts from bone (demineralization).
- For example, a decrease in plasma phosphate alone would promote bone demineralization. Increasing renal excretion of phosphate would promote bone demineralization and a rise in interstitial free calcium.

It is the free Ca^{2+}, not the phosphate, that is regulated so precisely. Hormonal control of free Ca^{2+} levels is via a dual hormonal system; parathyroid hormone and vitamin D.

BONE REMODELING

- Bone is undergoing continual remodeling throughout life, although the turnover is faster in younger individuals. As many as 300,000 bone-remodeling sites are active in a normal person.

- Bone remodeling involves the interplay between bone-building cells (osteoblasts) and cells that break down bone (osteoclasts), as illustrated in Figure 26-3.

- Osteoblasts cause bone deposition and they secrete two proteins:

  - RANK-L (Receptor Activator of Nuclear KappaB Ligand): This protein binds to the RANK receptor, which is expressed on precursor cells resulting in their differentiation into active osteoclasts. Active osteoclasts also express the RANK receptor, which, when stimulated, activates osteoclastic activity.

  - OPG (osteoprotegerin): This protein binds RANK-L, thereby preventing it from binding onto precursor or osteoclast cells. This reduces differentiation and overall osteoclastic activity. Thus, OPG acts as a "decoy" for RANK-L.

- Bone remodeling is influenced by parathyroid hormone (PTH), and the active form of vitamin D, both of which are covered below. Estrogen is well known for conserving bone integrity and it does so by at least two mechanisms. First, it induces the synthesis of OPG. Second, it reduces the secretion of cytokines by T-Lymphocytes. These cytokines stimulate differentiation of precursor cells into active osteoclasts and they stimulate activity of mature osteocytes. By inhibiting these cytokines and increasing OPG, estrogen reduces the activity of osteoclasts.

- Glucocorticoids increase bone breakdown by inducing the synthesis and release of RANK-L and by inhibiting the synthesis of OPG.

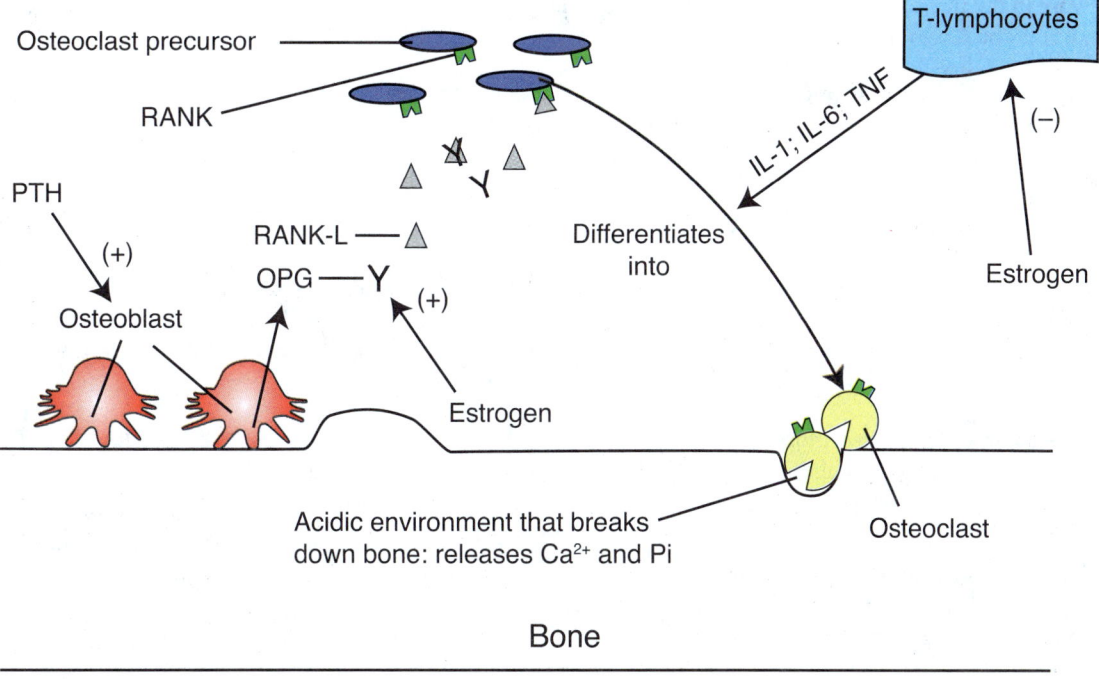

RANK = receptor activator of nuclear factor kappaB

RANK-L = receptor activator of nuclear factor kappaB ligand

OPG = osteoprotegerin (endogenous blocker of RANK-L)

Pi = phosphate

Figure 26-3. Relationship between Osteoblasts and Osteoclasts

Weight-Bearing Stress

Weight-bearing mechanical stress increases the mineralization of bone.

The absence of weight-bearing stress (being sedentary, bedridden, or weightless) promotes the demineralization of bone. Under these conditions, the following occurs:

- Plasma Ca^{2+} tends to be in the upper region of normal.
- Plasma PTH decreases.
- Urinary calcium increases.

Indices

Indices can be utilized to detect excess bone demineralization and remodeling:

- Increased serum osteocalcin and alkaline phosphatase are associated with osteoblastic activity.
- Increased urinary excretion of hydroxyproline is a breakdown product of collagen

PARATHYROID HORMONE (PTH)

Actions of PTH

A decrease in the free calcium is the signal to increase PTH secretion and the function of PTH is to raise free calcium, which it does by several mechanisms.

- Increases Ca^{2+} reabsorption in distal tubule of the kidney (section VIII, chapter 18)
- Inhibits phosphate (Pi) reabsorption in proximal tubule of the kidney.
- Stimulates the 1-alpha-hydroxylase enzyme in kidney, converting inactive vitamin D to its active form.
- Causes bone resorption, releasing Ca^{2+} and Pi into the blood.

Bone resorption

The mechanisms of PTH-induced bone resorption are complex and not fully understood. However, the following generalizations do apply.

- Osteoblasts express receptors for PTH. Binding of PTH stimulates the osteoblast to release RANK-L. This in turn, increases osteoclastic activity resulting in bone resorption and the release of calcium and phosphate into the blood, as shown in Figure 26-3.
- Although counterintuitive, intermittent spikes in PTH, e.g., intravenous or subcutaneous injection, stimulates osteoblastic activity resulting in bone deposition. Thus, PTH can be useful in treating osteoporosis in the clinical setting.

Parathyroid Hormone-Related Peptide

- PTHrP is a paracrine factor secreted by many tissues; e.g., lung, mammary tissue, placenta.
- It may have a role in fetal development. In postnatal life, its role is unclear.
- The majority of humoral hypercalcemias of malignancy are due to overexpression of PTHrP.
- PTHrP has a strong structural homology to PTH and binds with equal affinity to the PTH receptor.

Regulation of PTH Secretion

- PTH is a peptide hormone released from the parathyroid glands in response to lowered plasma free Ca^{2+} (Figure 26-4).

- Free Ca^{2+} in the plasma is the primary regulator of PTH.

- The negative feedback relationship between plasma calcium and PTH secretion is highly sigmoidal, with the steep portion of the curve representing the normal range of plasma free calcium.

- To sense the free calcium, the parathyroid cell depends upon high levels of expression of the calcium-sensing receptor (CaSR).

- In most cells, exocytosis depends on a rise in intracellular free calcium. In the parathyroid gland, a fall in intracellular free calcium causes release.

- Depletion of magnesium stores can create a reversible hypoparathyroidism.

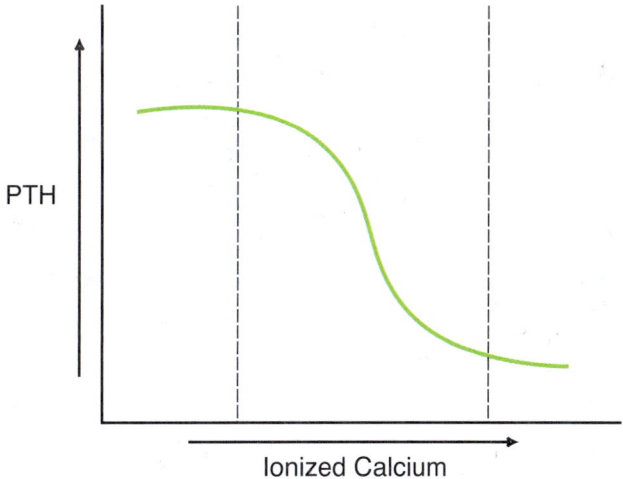

Figure 26-4. Relationship between Plasma Calcium and PTH
Normal range = region between dashed lines.

CALCITONIN

- Calcitonin (CT) is a peptide hormone secreted by the parafollicular cells (C cells) of the thyroid gland. It is released in response to elevated free calcium.

- Calcitonin lowers plasma calcium by decreasing the activity of osteoclasts, thus decreasing bone resorption. Calcitonin is useful in the treatment of Paget's disease, severe hypercalcemia, and osteoporosis.

- Calcitonin is not a major controller of Ca^{2+} in humans. Removing the thyroid (with the C cells) or excess of calcitonin via a C cell tumor (medullary carcinoma of the thyroid) has little impact on plasma calcium.

- No deficiency or excess disease has been described.

ROLE OF VITAMIN D (CALCITRIOL) IN CALCIUM HOMEOSTASIS

Sources and Synthesis

Vitamin D_2 (ergocalciferol) is a vitamin but can functionally be considered a prohormone. It is a normal dietary component. A slightly different form, vitamin D_3 (cholecalciferol), is synthesized in the skin. Its active form (1,25 di-OH D_3) is a hormone secreted by cells of the kidney's proximal tubule. The synthesis of 1,25 di-OH vitamin D (calcitriol) is outlined here:

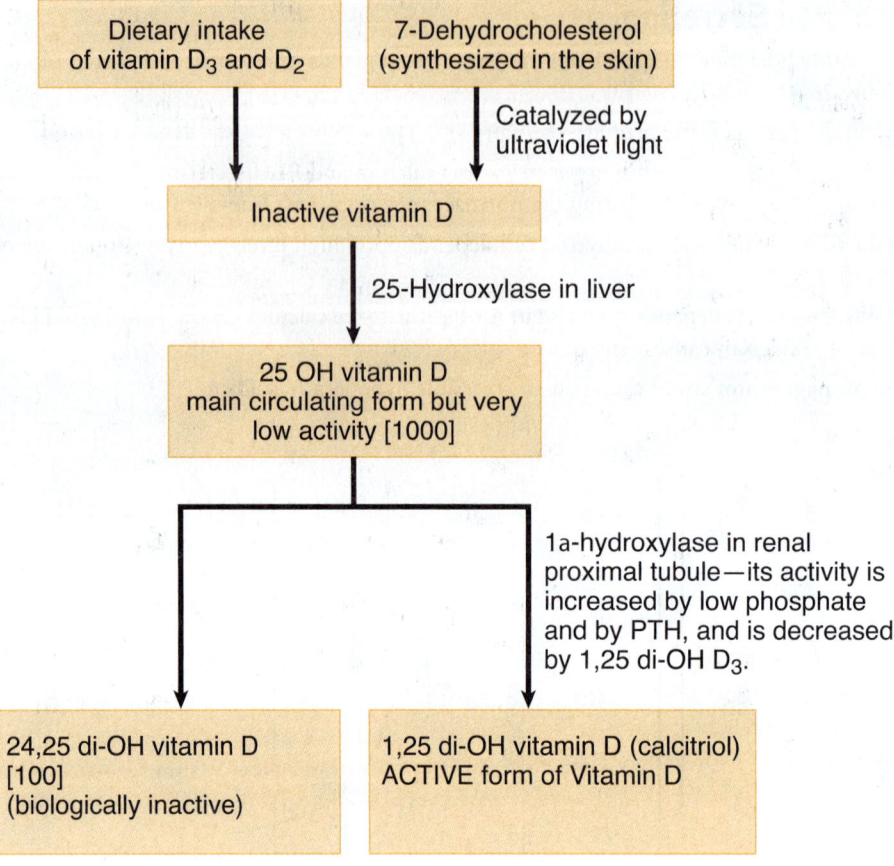

Figure 26-5. Vitamin D Metabolism

The synthesis of calcitriol occurs sequentially in the skin → liver → kidney. The relative numbers of molecules of each of the hydroxylated forms of D present in the blood of a normal person are given in brackets. After its conversion to the 25 OH form in the liver, it can be stored in fat tissue. The serum levels of 25 OH vitamin D represent the best measure of the body stores of vitamin D when a deficiency is suspected. Most of the 25 OH form, which is the immediate precursor of 1,25 di-OH D, is converted to the inactive metabolite, 24,25 di-OH D. Ultraviolet (UV) light also evokes skin tanning, decreasing the penetration of UV light, and thus decreases the subsequent formation of D_3. This mechanism may prevent overproduction of D_3 in individuals exposed to large amounts of sunlight.

Actions of Calcitriol

Under normal conditions, vitamin D acts to raise plasma Ca^{2+} and phosphate. Thus, vitamin D promotes bone deposition. This is accomplished by:

- Calcitriol increases the absorption of Ca^{2+} and phosphate by the intestinal mucosa by increasing the production of the Ca^{2+}-binding protein calbindin. The details of this process are poorly understood.
- The resulting high concentrations of Ca^{2+} and phosphate in the extracellular fluid exceed the solubility product, and precipitation of bone salts into bone matrix occurs.
- Calcitriol enhances PTH's action at the renal distal tubule.

At abnormally high activity levels calcitriol increases bone resorption and release . Receptors for calcitriol are on the nuclear membranes of osteoblasts. Through communication from osteoblasts, activated osteoclasts carry out the bone resorption. Calcitriol requires the concurrent presence of PTH for its bone-resorbing action.

The following figure provides an overview of regulation of calcium and phosphate by parathyroid hormone and vitamin D.

Summary

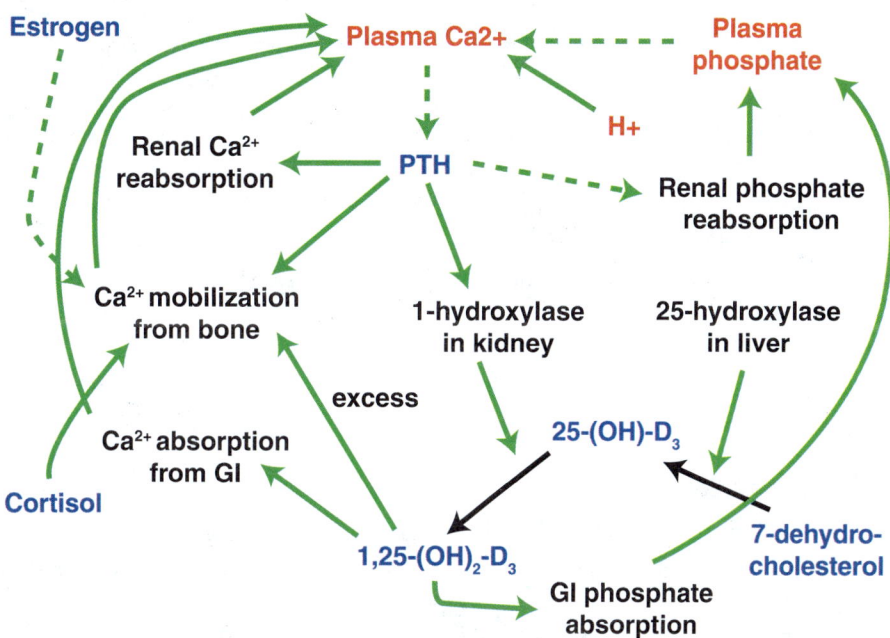

Figure 26-6. Regulation of Calcium and Phosphate
Stimulates ⟶
Inhibits ⇢

DISORDERS IN CALCIUM AND PHOSPHATE

Hypercalcemia

Hypercalcemia of primary hyperparathyroidism

- Initiating factor is primary hypersecretion of PTH
- Consequences include increased plasma calcium, decreased plasma phosphate, polyuria, hypercalciuria, and decreased bone mass
- 80% due to a single parathyroid adenoma
- High calcium can lead to nephrogenic diabetes insipidus. This is why there is massive volume deficit in hypercalcemia.
- High calcium makes it harder to depolarize neural tissue. This is why hypercalcemia causes lethargy, confusion, and constipation.
- 15% due to primary hyperplasia as in MEN 1 or MEN 2A
- Parathyroid carcinoma rare
- Ectopic hormonal hypercalcemia usually PTHrP.
- Most patients asymptomatic
- Symptoms include lethargy, fatigue, depression, neuromuscular weakness, and difficulty in concentrating

- Increased plasma alkaline phosphatase, osteocalcin and increased excretion of cAMP (second messenger for PTH in the kidney), and hydroxyproline
- Severe dehydration
- Bone manifestation is osteitis fibrosa cystica in which there are increased osteoclasts in scalloped areas of the surface bone and replacement of marrow elements with fibrous tissue. Increased alkaline phosphatase is due to high bone turnover.
- Hypercalcemia decreases QT interval and in some cases causes cardiac arrhythmias.

Related causes of hypercalcemia

- Lithium shifts the sigmoid Ca/PTH curve to the right. Higher calcium levels are thus needed to suppress PTH. Similarly, the CaSR is mutated in patients with familial hypocalciuric hypercalcemia (FHH; see Renal Physiology section, chapter 18), resulting in less PTH for any given calcium concentration in the plasma.
- Sarcoidosis and other granulomatous disorders (10%) due to increased activity of 1-alpha hydroxylase activity in granulomas.
- Thyrotoxicosis, milk-alkali syndrome
- Thiazide diuretics increase renal calcium absorption.

Differential diagnosis and treatment

- Elevated plasma calcium and PTH normal or elevated; conclusion is primary hyperparathyroidism
- Elevated plasma calcium and decreased PTH; conclusion is something other than primary hyperparathyroidism
- Treatment is usually surgery; i.e., removing the adenoma or with hyperplasia removing most of the parathyroid tissue
- Treat with high volume fluid replacement
- Bisphosphonates need 2-3 days to be fully effective
- Calcitonin rapidly inhibits osteoclastic activity

Hypocalcemia

Hypocalcemia of primary hypoparathyroidism

- Can be hereditary or autoimmune
- Caused by thyroid surgery or surgery to correct hyperparathyroidism
- The initiating factor is inadequate secretion of PTH by the parathyroid glands.
- The decrease in plasma calcium is accompanied by an increased plasma phosphate. Even though less phosphate is resorbed from bone, plasma phosphate increases because the normal action of PTH is to inhibit phosphate reabsorption and increase excretion by the kidney. Therefore, without PTH, more of the filtered load is reabsorbed.
- Symptoms focus on the hypocalcemic induced increased excitability of motor neurons creating muscular spasms and tetany
- Chvostek's sign is induced by tapping the facial nerve just anterior to the ear lobe.
- Trousseau's sign is elicited by inflating a pressure cuff on the upper arm. A positive response is carpal spasm.
- Hypomagnesemia prevents PTH secretion and induces hypocalcemia. This condition responds immediately to an infusion of magnesium.

Pseudohypoparathyroidism

- This is a rare familial disorder characterized by target tissue resistance to parathyroid hormone.
- Exhibits same signs and symptoms as primary hypoparathyroidism except PTH elevated
- It is usually accompanied by developmental defects: mental retardation, short and stocky stature, one or more metacarpal or metatarsal bones missing (short 4th or 5th finger).

Additional causes of hypocalcemia

- Acute hypocalcemia can occur even with intact homeostatic mechanisms. Included would be alkalosis via hyperventilation, transfusions of citrated blood, rhabdomyolysis or tumor lysis, and the subsequent hyperphosphatemia
- Hyperphosphatemia of chronic renal failure
- Failures with vitamin D system
- Congenital absence of parathyroids rare (DiGeorge's syndrome)
- Damaged muscle binds calcium. Rhabdomyolysis binds free calcium.

Predictive indices for a primary disorder

When plasma calcium and phosphate levels are changing in opposite directions, the cause is usually a primary disorder. An exception may be chronic renal failure. This state is not a primary disorder but is usually associated with hypocalcemia and hyperphosphatemia (hypocalcemic-induced secondary hyperparathyroidism).

Renal Failure and Secondary Hyperparathyroidism

- Most common cause of secondary hyperparathyroidism
- Loss of nephrons prevents kidneys from excreting phosphate (Pi)
- Elevated Pi lowers free Ca^{2+}, which in turn increases PTH

Vitamin D Deficiency and Secondary Hyperparathyroidism

- Causes include a diet deficient in vitamin D, inadequate sunlight exposure, malabsorption of vitamin D, enzyme deficiencies in the pathway to activation of vitamin D
- In all cases there is a decrease in plasma calcium, which elicits an increase in PTH secretion and a secondary hyperparathyroidism.
- A similar consequence is the increased demand for calcium as in pregnancy.
- Characterized by increased PTH, decreased plasma calcium, and decreased plasma phosphate. Even though the elevated PTH increases phosphate resorption from bone, PTH also inhibits phosphate reabsorption by the kidney, thereby promoting phosphate excretion and a drop in plasma phosphate.
- Bone mass is lost to maintain plasma calcium.
- Diagnostic test is a low plasma 25(OH) vitamin D.

Excess Vitamin D and Secondary Hypoparathyroidism

- An excessive intake of vitamin D raises plasma calcium, which elicits a decrease in PTH
- Characterized by decreased PTH, increased plasma calcium, and increased plasma phosphate but normal or decreased phosphate excretion. Because PTH increases the excretion of phosphate by inhibiting reabsorption in the proximal tubule, decreased PTH causes increased reabsorption of phosphate and elevated plasma levels.
- Excessive vitamin D promotes bone resorption and bone mass decreases.

Predictive indices for a secondary disorder

When the plasma calcium and phosphate are changing in the same direction, the origin is usually a secondary disorder.

- Secondary hyperparathyroidism: both decrease
- Secondary hypoparathyroidism: both increase

Note also that in either a deficiency or an excess of vitamin D, there is a decrease in bone mass but mechanism differs (high PTH in deficiency; direct effect of vitamin D with excess).

Thyroid Hormones 27

Learning Objectives

- ❏ Solve problems concerning overview of the thyroid gland
- ❏ Use knowledge of biosynthesis and transport of thyroid hormones
- ❏ Interpret scenarios on physiologic actions of thyroid hormones
- ❏ Answer questions about control of thyroid hormone secretion
- ❏ Answer questions about pathologic changes in thyroid hormone secretion

OVERVIEW OF THE THYROID GLAND

In mammals, thyroid hormones are essential for normal growth and maturation. Therefore, thyroid hormones are major anabolic hormones.

Dietary intake of about 500 µg per day is typical, mainly in the form of iodide (I^-) or iodine (I). To maintain normal thyroid hormone secretion, 150 µg is the minimal intake necessary. I^- is the form absorbed from the small intestine.

- The functional unit of the thyroid gland is the follicle.
- The lumen is filled with thyroglobulin, which contain large numbers of thyroid hormone molecules.
- Surrounding the lumen are the follicle cells, which function to both synthesize and release thyroid hormones.
- These relationships are schematically represented in the following figure.

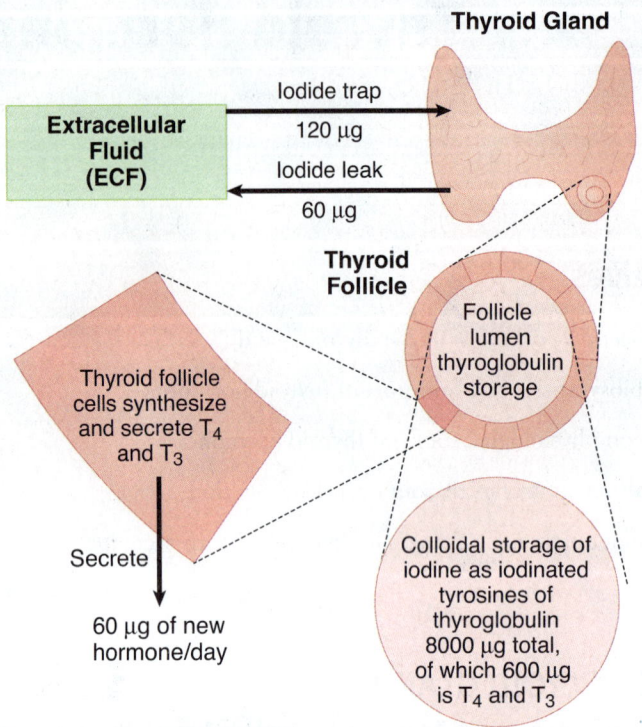

Figure 27-1. The Thyroid Follicle

BIOSYNTHESIS AND TRANSPORT OF THYROID HORMONE

Synthesis of Thyroid Hormones

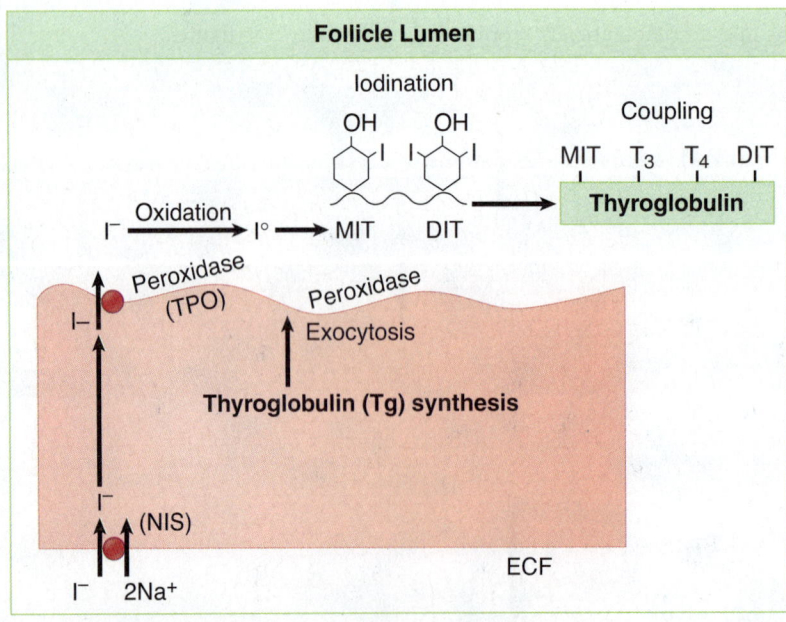

Figure 27-2. Steps in Thyroid Synthesis

Iodide transport

Iodine uptake is via a sodium/potassium pump powered sodium/iodide symporter on the basal membrane (NIS). This pump can raise the concentration of I⁻ within the cell to as much as 250 times that of plasma. The pump can be blocked by anions like perchlorate and thiocyanate, which compete with I.

Along the apical membrane, the I⁻ is transported into the lumen by an anion exchanger called pendrin.

The 24-hour iodine uptake by the thyroid is directly proportional to thyroid function.

Thyroglobulin synthesis

A high molecular weight protein (>300,000 daltons) is synthesized in ribosomes, glycosylated in the endoplasmic reticulum, and packaged into vesicles in the Golgi apparatus. The thyroglobin then enters the lumen via exocytosis.

Oxidation of I⁻ to I⁰

The enzyme thyroperoxidase (TPO), which is located at the apical border of the follicle cell, catalyzes oxidation. Peroxidase also catalyzes iodination and coupling.

Iodination

As thyroglobulin is extruded into the follicular lumen, a portion (<20%) of its tyrosine residues are iodinated. The catalyst for this reaction is peroxidase. The initial products of iodination are mono- and diiodotyrosine (MIT and DIT), respectively, with the latter form predominating, except when iodine is scarce.

Coupling

Peroxidase also promotes the coupling of iodinated tyrosine in the thyroglobulin molecule. When two DITs couple, tetraiodothyronine (T_4) is formed. When one DIT and one MIT combine, triiodothyronine (T_3) is formed. When iodine is abundant, mainly T_4 is formed. But when iodine becomes scarce, the production of T_3 increases.

Storage of thyroid hormones

Enough hormone is stored as iodinated thyroglobulin in the follicular colloid to last the body for 2-3 months.

Structure of Thyroid Hormones

The chemical structures of T_4, T_3, and reverse T_3 (rT_3) are shown in the following figure. Do not memorize structure; note the number and location of iodines, instead, attached to the tyrosine residues.

HO—[ring 3', 5']—O—[ring 3, 5]—CH_2—CH—$COOH$
|
NH_2
Thyroxine (T_4) 3,5,3',5',-tetra-iodothyronine

HO—[ring]—O—[ring]—CH_2—CH—$COOH$
|
NH_2
3,5,3'-tri-iodothyronine (T_3)
• More active form of hormone
• No 5' I

HO—[ring]—O—[ring]—CH_2—CH—$COOH$
|
NH_2
3,3',5'-tri-iodothyronine (reverse T_3)
• No activity
• No 5 I

Figure 27-3. Active and Inactive Forms of Thyroid Hormones

Secretion of Thyroid Hormone

The following figure illustrates the main steps in thyroglobulin degradation and the release of thyroid hormones.

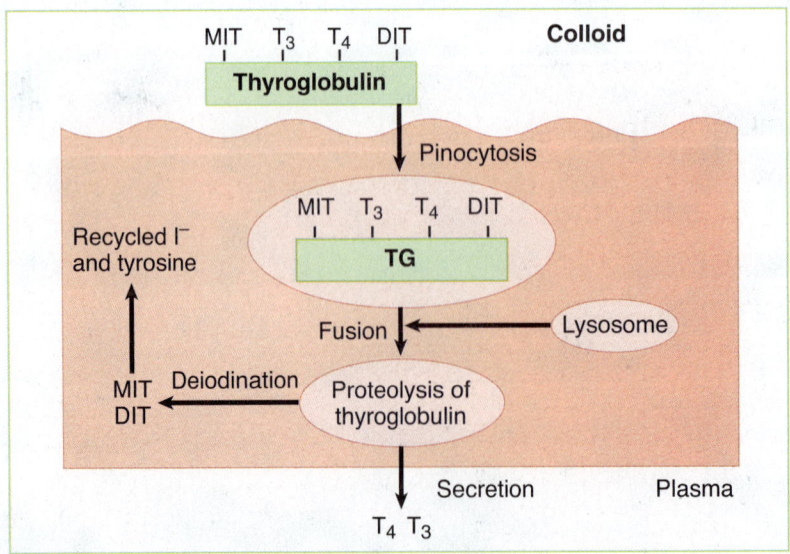

Figure 27-4. Secretion of Thyroid Hormone

Pinocytosis: Pieces of the follicular colloid are taken back into the follicle by endocytosis.

Fusion: The endocytosed material fuses with lysosomes, which transport it toward the basal surface of the cell.

Proteolysis of thyroglobulin: Within the lysosomes, the thyroglobulin is broken into free amino acids, some of which are T4, T3, DIT, and MIT.

Secretion: T4 and T3 are secreted into the blood, with the T4:T3 ratio being as high as 20:1. The thyroid has the same 5'-mono-deiodinase found in many peripheral tissues and in an iodine-deficient state more of the hormone can be released as T3.

Along with thyroid hormones a small amount of thyroglobulin is also released into the circulation. Its release is increased in a number of states including thyroiditis, nodular goiter, and by cancerous thyroid tissue. After the surgical removal of cancerous thyroid tissue, any residual thyroglobulin in the circulation indicates cancerous cells are still present.

Deiodination: A microsomal deiodinase removes the iodine from iodinated tyrosines (DIT and MIT) but not from the iodinated thyronines (T3 and T4). The iodine is then available for resynthesis of hormone. (Individuals with a deficiency of this enzyme are more likely to develop symptoms of iodine deficiency.)

Transport of Thyroid Hormones in Blood

There is an equilibrium between bound and free circulating thyroid hormone in the bloodstream. The following figure illustrates this equilibrium.

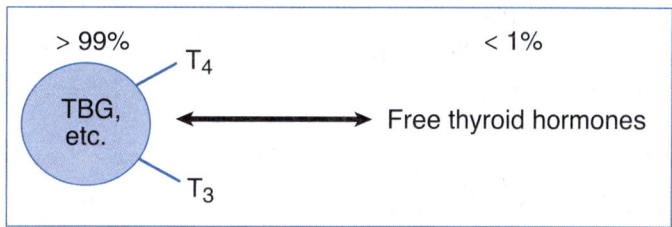

Figure 27-5. Plasma Transport of Thyroid Hormone
TBG = thyroid-binding globulin

About 70% of the circulating thyroid is bound to thyroid-binding globulin (TBG). The remainder of the bound protein is attached to thyroxine-binding prealbumin (transthyretin) and albumin. Large variations in TBG do not normally affect the free form. A rare congenital deficiency or excess of TBG drastically alters the bound fraction but because the free fraction is normal, the individuals are all euthyroid.

Also, T4 has the higher affinity for binding proteins; therefore, it binds more tightly to protein than does T3, and consequently has a greater half-life than T3. Most circulating thyroid hormone is T4. Normally, there is 50 times more T4 than T3.

- T4 half-life = 6 days
- T3 half-life = 1 day

The amount of circulating thyroid hormone is about 3 times the amount normally secreted by the thyroid gland each day. Thus, circulating protein-bound thyroid hormones act as a significant reserve.

Activation and Degradation of Thyroid Hormones

- T_3 and T_4 bind to the same nuclear receptor but T_3 binds with 10 times more affinity than T4.
- Thus, because it has greater affinity for the receptor, T_3 is the more active form of thyroid hormone.
- Many target tissues can regulate the conversion of T_4 to either T_3 or rT3, thereby locally controlling hormone activity.
- Most of the circulating T_3 is derived from the peripheral conversion of T_4 into T_3 and its release again into the circulation (e.g., liver, kidney, and skeletal muscle).
- This peripheral conversion of thyroid hormone is represented in the following chart.

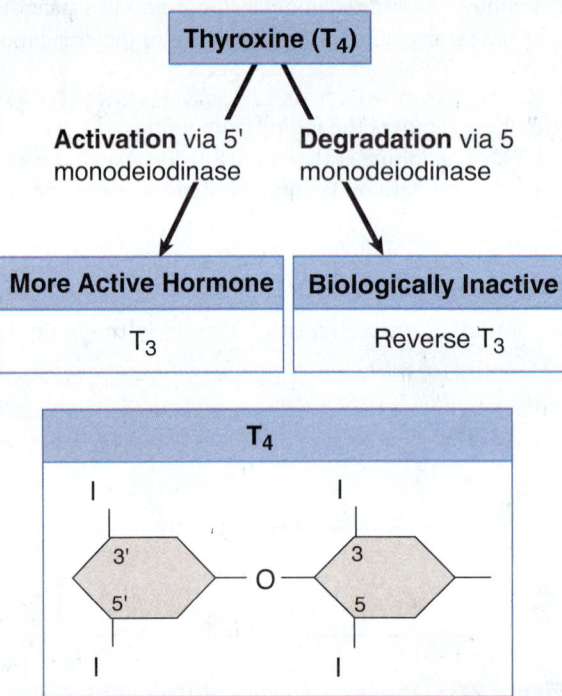

Figure 27-6. Peripheral Conversion of Thyroid Hormone

Certain clinical states are associated with a reduction in the conversion of T_4 into T_3, often with an enhanced conversion of T_4 into rT3 (low T_3 syndrome). Such states would include fasting, medical and surgical stresses, catabolic diseases, and even excess secretion of cortisol could be included here. The result is a reduction in metabolic rate and a conservation of energy resources. In the early stages, the circulating T_4 is normal but in many cases as the metabolic problem or stress becomes more severe, T_4 can fall as well.

PHYSIOLOGIC ACTIONS OF THYROID HORMONES

In many tissues, thyroid hormones are not the prime indicators or the major inhibitors of specific cellular processes. Rather, a multitude of processes function properly only when optimal amounts of thyroid hormones are present. This underscores the permissive nature of thyroid hormones.

Metabolic Rate

- Thyroid hormones increase metabolic rate, as evidenced by increased O_2 consumption and heat production.
- Thyroid hormones increase the activity of the membrane-bound Na/K⁻ATPase in many tissues, and it can be argued that it is the increased pumping of Na^+ that accounts for most of the increase in metabolic rate.
- The increase in metabolic rate produced by a single dose of T_4 occurs only after a latency of several hours but may last 6 days or more.
- Thyroid hormones are absolutely necessary for normal brain maturation and essential for normal menstrual cycles. Hypothyroidism leads to menstrual irregularities (menorrhagia) and infertility (anovulatory cycles).

Growth and Maturation (T4 and T3 Anabolic Hormones)

Fetal growth rates appear normal in the absence of thyroid hormone production (i.e., if the fetus is hypothyroid). However, without adequate thyroid hormones during the perinatal period, abnormalities rapidly develop in nervous system maturation.

- Synapses develop abnormally and there is decreased dendritic branching and myelination. These abnormalities lead to mental retardation.
- These neural changes are irreversible and lead to cretinism unless replacement therapy is started soon after birth.

Lipid Metabolism

- Thyroid hormone accelerates cholesterol clearance from the plasma.
- Thyroid hormones are required for conversion of carotene to vitamin A, and, as a consequence, hypothyroid individuals can suffer from night blindness and yellowing of the skin.

CHO Metabolism

- Thyroid hormone increases the rate of glucose absorption from the small intestine.

Cardiovascular Effects

- Thyroid hormones have positive inotropic and chronotropic effects on the heart.
- The increased contractility is partly direct and partly indirect: they increase the number and affinity of β-adrenergic receptors in the heart, thereby increasing the sensitivity to catecholamines.
- Acting on the SA node, they directly increase heart rate.
- Cardiac output is increased, and both heart rate and stroke volume are elevated.
- Systolic pressure increases are due to increased stroke volume, and diastolic pressure decreases are due to decreased peripheral resistance.
- Thyroid hormones in the normal range are required for optimum cardiac performance.

Additional Effects

- Thyroid hormones maintain the ventilatory response to hypoxia, increase erythropoietin, and increase gut motility and bone turnover.
- Hypothyroidism is associated with an increased prolactin. TRH in excess amounts will stimulate prolactin.

CONTROL OF THYROID HORMONE SECRETION

Feedback Relationships

The following figure shows the overall control of thyroid function.

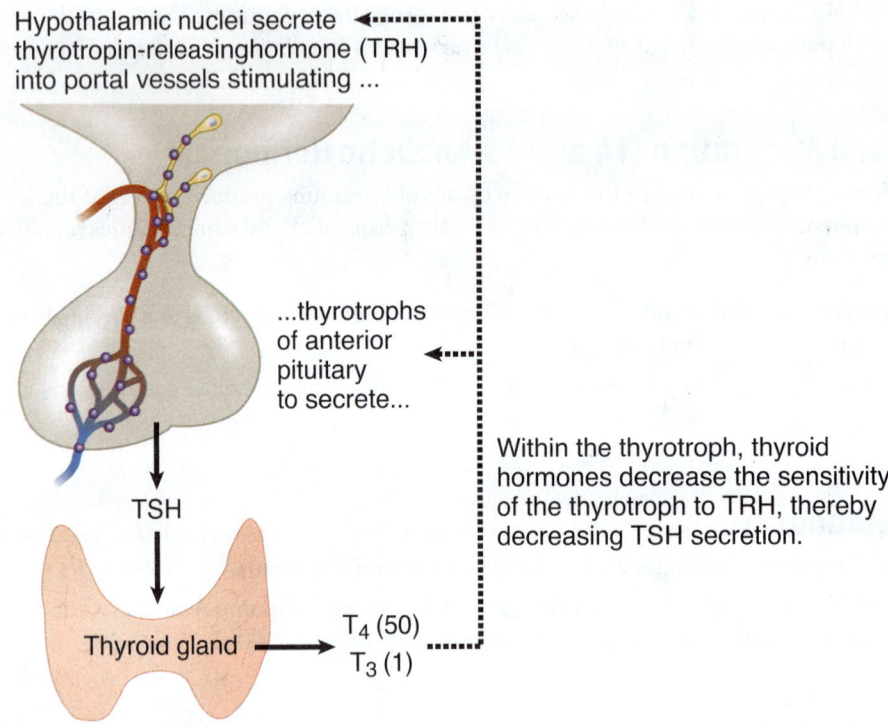

Hypothalamic nuclei secrete thyrotropin-releasinghormone (TRH) into portal vessels stimulating ...

...thyrotrophs of anterior pituitary to secrete...

TSH

Thyroid gland

T_4 (50)
T_3 (1)

Within the thyrotroph, thyroid hormones decrease the sensitivity of the thyrotroph to TRH, thereby decreasing TSH secretion.

Figure 27-7. Hypothalamic–Pituitary Control of Thyroid-Hormone Secretion

- TRH provides a constant and necessary stimulus for TSH secretion. In the absence of TRH, the secretion of TSH (and T_4) decreases to very low levels. The target tissue for TSH is the thyroid, where it increases the secretion mainly of T_4.

- Negative feedback of thyroid hormones is exerted mainly at the level of the anterior pituitary gland.

- Because the main circulating form is T_4, it is T_4 that is responsible for most of the negative feedback.

- However, within the thyrotrophs the T_4 is converted to T_3 before it acts to reduce the sensitivity of the thyrotroph to TRH.

- As long as circulating free T_4 remains normal, changes in circulating T_3 have minimal effects on TSH secretion. However, TSH secretion increases if there is a significant drop in circulating free T_4, even in the presence of an increase in circulating T_3.

Overall Effects of Thyrotropin (TSH) on the Thyroid

Rapidly induced TSH effects

TSH tends to rapidly increase (within minutes or an hour) all steps in the synthesis and degradation of thyroid hormones, including:

- Iodide trapping
- Thyroglobulin synthesis and exocytosis into the follicular lumen
- Pinocytotic reuptake of iodinated thyroglobulin back into the thyroid follicular cell
- Secretion of T4 into the blood

Slowly induced TSH effects

Changes that occur more slowly (hours or days) in response to TSH include:

- Increased blood flow to the thyroid gland
- Increased hypertrophy or hyperplasia of the thyroid cells, which initially leads to increased size of the gland or goiter

PATHOLOGIC CHANGES IN THYROID HORMONE SECRETION

Table 27-1. Changes in Feedback Relationships in Several Disorders

	T_4	TSH	TRH
Primary hypothyroidism	↓	↑	↑
Pituitary hypothyroidism (secondary)	↓	↓	↑
Pituitary hyperthyroidism (secondary)	↑	↑	↓
Graves' disease (autoimmune)	↑	↓	↓

A goiter can develop in all of the disorders shown in the preceding table except secondary and tertiary hypothyroidism.

Thyroidal Response to Low Intake of Iodine

In most cases, if iodine is deficient in the diet but not absent, the individual will remain euthyroid but will develop a goiter. The changes are shown in Figure 27-8. The adaptive sequence occurs when dietary intake of iodine is deficient. The sequence of events begins with 1 (decreased secretion of T_4) and proceeds through 4, the development of a goiter.

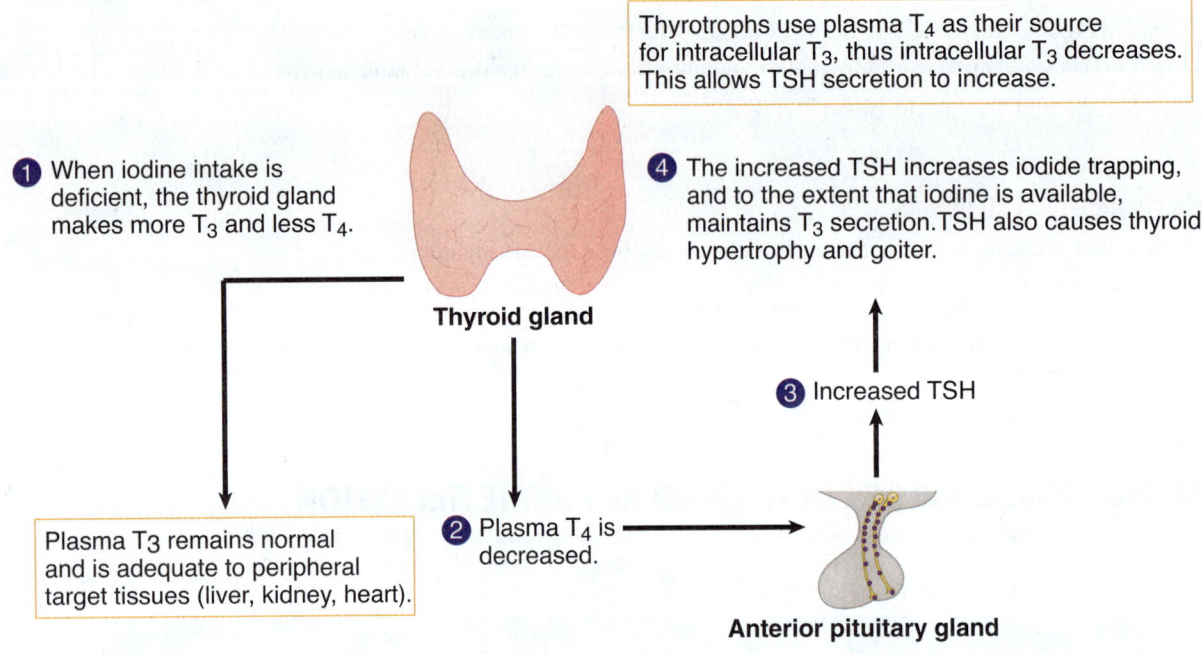

Thyrotrophs use plasma T_4 as their source for intracellular T_3, thus intracellular T_3 decreases. This allows TSH secretion to increase.

1. When iodine intake is deficient, the thyroid gland makes more T_3 and less T_4.

4. The increased TSH increases iodide trapping, and to the extent that iodine is available, maintains T_3 secretion. TSH also causes thyroid hypertrophy and goiter.

Thyroid gland

Plasma T_3 remains normal and is adequate to peripheral target tissues (liver, kidney, heart).

2. Plasma T_4 is decreased.

3. Increased TSH

Anterior pituitary gland

Figure 27-8. Iodine Deficiency

Primary Hypothyroidism

Primary changes and clinical presentation

- Most common cause is Hashimoto's thyroiditis, an autoimmune destruction of the thyroid with lymphocytic infiltration; ↑ TPO antibodies; early stages have a diffusely enlarged thyroid progressing in the later stages to a smaller atrophic and fibrotic gland.
- ↑ TSH, ↓ FT_4; in subclinical hypothyroidism the TSH is on the high side of normal and the FT_4 is on the low side of normal.
- Decreased basal metabolic rate and oxygen consumption
- Plasma cholesterol and other blood lipids tend to be elevated.
- Increased TRH drives a hyperprolactinemia. In women it may result in amenorrhea with galactorrhea; more often anovulatory cycles with menorrhagia. In men infertility and gynecomastia.
- Decreased GFR and an inability to excrete a water load, which may lead to hyponatremia.
- Inability to convert carotene to vitamin A may cause yellowing of the skin and night blindness.
- Slow thinking and lethargy; some patients have severe mental symptoms, dementia, or psychosis ("myxedema madness")
- Decreased food intake but individuals tend to be overweight
- Deep tendon reflexes with slow relaxation phase
- In the early stages, a decreased cardiac performance due to decreased loading conditions. In the later stages, cardiac features suggestive of cardiomyopathy

- Anemia, constipation, hoarseness in speech, and the skin is dry and cool
- A decreased ventilatory drive to hypercapnia and hypoxia
- Accumulation of subcutaneous mucopolysaccharides that give rise to a nonpitting edema (myxedema)
- Myxedema coma is the end stage of untreated hypothyroidism. The major features are hypoventilation, fluid and electrolyte imbalances, and hypothermia and ultimately shock and death.

Cretinism

- Untreated postnatal hypothyroidism results in cretinism, a form of dwarfism with mental retardation.
- Individuals often appear normal following delivery but may display some respiratory difficulty, jaundice, feeding problems, and hypotonia.
- Abnormalities rapidly develop in nervous system maturation, which are irreversible and result in mental retardation.
- Prepubertal growth, including bone ossification, is retarded in the absence of thyroid hormones. A stippled epiphysis is a sign of hypothyroidism in children.
- There is no evidence that thyroid hormones act directly on growth or bone formation. Rather, thyroid hormone appears to be permissive or act synergistically with growth hormone or growth factors acting directly on bone. Thyroid hormone is required for normal synthesis and secretion of growth hormone.
- Acquired hypothyroidism during childhood results in dwarfism but there is no mental retardation.
- At puberty, increased androgen secretion drives an increased growth hormone secretion. This will not occur with depressed levels of thyroid hormones.

Additional causes of hypothyroidism

- Secondary generally associated with panhypopituitarism
- Secondary or tertiary characterized by ↓ FT_4 and inappropriately normal TSH.
- Severe iodine deficiency (not in the United States)
- Drug induced, e.g. lithium
- Failure to escape from the Wolff-Chaikoff effect following excessive iodine intake
- Rarely there can be resistance to thyroid hormone

Primary Hyperthyroidism (Graves' Disease)

- Thyrotoxicosis by definition is the clinical syndrome whereby tissues are exposed to high levels of thyroid hormone (= hyperthyroidism)
- The most common cause of thyrotoxicosis is Graves' disease, a primary hyperthyroidism.
- Graves' disease is an autoimmune problem in which one antibody is directed against the thyroid receptor. It is referred to as the thyroid stimulating antibody (TSI or TSH-R).
- In addition TPO antibodies and those against thyroglobulin are also found in Graves' disease.
- ↑ FT4, ↓ TSH; it is the TSI stimulating the TSH receptor on the thyroid that is driving the hyperthyroidism.
- In Graves' disease the thyroid is symmetrically enlarged.
- Increased radioiodine uptake by the thyroid and decreased serum cholesterol.
- Only Graves' disease has thyroid-stimulating antibodies. The only types of hyperthyroidism with increased radioactive iodine uptake are Graves' disease and toxic nodular goiter.
  - Subacute thyroiditis and "silent" or "painless" thyroiditis do not have increased radioactive iodine uptake; they are "leaking" of thyroid hormone out of a gland damaged by antibodies.
- Increased metabolic rate and heat production. Individuals tend to seek a cool environment.

- Cardiac output, contractility, and heart rate are increased with possibly palpitations and arrhythmias (increased β-adrenergic stimulation)
- Many symptoms suggest a state of excess catecholamines but circulating catecholamines are usually normal.
- Weight loss with increased food intake, protein wasting, and muscle weakness.
- Tremor, nervousness, and excessive sweating.
- The wide-eyed stare (exophthalmos) in patients with Graves' is caused by an infiltration of orbital soft tissues and extraocular muscles and the resulting edema, and this process is caused by the antibodies.
- Untreated hyperthyroidism may decompensate into a condition called "thyroid storm."
- The end-stage of Graves' disease is often a hypothyroidism.

Additional origins of hyperthyroidism (thyrotoxicosis)

- Autonomously functioning thyroid adenoma
- Toxic multinodular goiter
- Subacute and silent thyroiditis
- TSH-secreting pituitary adenoma (secondary hyperthyroidism) (very rare)

Goiter

- A goiter is simply an enlarged thyroid and does not designate functional status. A goiter can be present in hypo-, hyper-, and euthyroid states. There is no correlation between thyroid size and function.
- A generalized enlargement of the thyroid is considered a "diffuse goiter."
- Diffuse enlargement often results from prolonged stimulation by TSH or TSH-like factor; e.g., Hashimoto's thyroiditis, Graves' disease, diet deficient in iodine
- An irregular or lumpy enlargement of the thyroid is considered a "nodular goiter."
- With time, excessive stimulation by TSH can result in a multinodular goiter e.g. iodine deficiency initially produces a diffuse nontoxic goiter. Long term however, focal hyperplasia with necrosis and hemorrhage results in the formation of nodules. Nodules vary from "hot nodules" that can trap iodine to "cold nodules" that cannot trap iodine.

Growth, Growth Hormone, and Puberty

28

Learning Objectives

❏ Explain information related to in-utero and prepubertal growth

❏ Explain information related to physiologic actions of growth hormone

❏ Use knowledge of control of growth hormone secretion

❏ Answer questions about puberty

❏ Use knowledge of acromegaly

IN-UTERO AND PREPUBERTAL GROWTH

Intrauterine Growth

- Important roles for growth hormone, IGF-II (early in gestation), IGF-I (later in gestation) and insulin
- Infants of diabetic mothers have increased insulin levels and are large.
- Smoking decreases vascularity of the placenta and decreases birth weight.
- Poor maternal nutrition leading cause of low birth weight worldwide.

Postnatal Growth

- Although fetal hypothyroidism does not decrease birth weight, hypothyroidism following delivery causes irreversible abnormalities in nervous system maturation, which in turn lead to mental retardation (cretinism).
- Growth hormone, insulin, and thyroid hormone play major roles. Acquired hypothyroidism later in childhood will slow growth and reduce bone advancement more than growth hormone deficiency, but will not cause mental retardation.
- Replacement of hormone deficiencies creates a period of catch-up growth, but it is soon replaced with a normal growth rate.
- There is no major role for gonadal sex steroids on prepubertal growth or for glucocorticoids but glucocorticoid excess will slow growth.
- Hypersecretion of growth hormone pre-puberty (pituitary adenoma) results in giantism. It also delays pubertal changes, and the subsequent hypogonadism contributes to the giantism.

Prepubertal Growth Hormone Deficiency

- Deficiencies can be congenital (decreased birth length), idiopathic (low GHRH), or acquired (hypothalamic-pituitary tumor).
- A deficiency causes dwarfism, which is characterized by: short stature, chubby, immature facial appearance, delayed skeletal maturation, and tendency to episodes of hypoglycemia.

- Tissue resistance to growth hormone (↑ growth hormone, ↓ IGF-I) results in Laron syndrome (Laron dwarfism).
- Stimulation test is with an arginine infusion.
- Growth hormone deficiency following puberty decreases lean body mass, and replacement therapy is now considered an acceptable treatment.
- Treatment of GH deficiency is simple replacement of GH.
- Treatment of Laron dwarfism (lack of GH receptor) is synthetic IGF. Mecasermin is the name of recombinant IGF.

PHYSIOLOGIC ACTIONS OF GROWTH HORMONE

Growth hormone is a major anabolic growth-promoting hormone and a stress hormone. All anabolic hormones (i.e., growth hormone, insulin, thyroid hormones, and androgens) are required for normal growth. The major stress and anabolic actions of growth hormone are shown in Figure 28-1. This figure shows that most of the direct actions of growth hormone are consistent with its actions as a stress hormone. A direct anabolic action is the promotion of amino acid entry into cells, thus making them more available for protein synthesis. However, most of the anabolic actions of growth hormone are indirect via the production of growth factors.

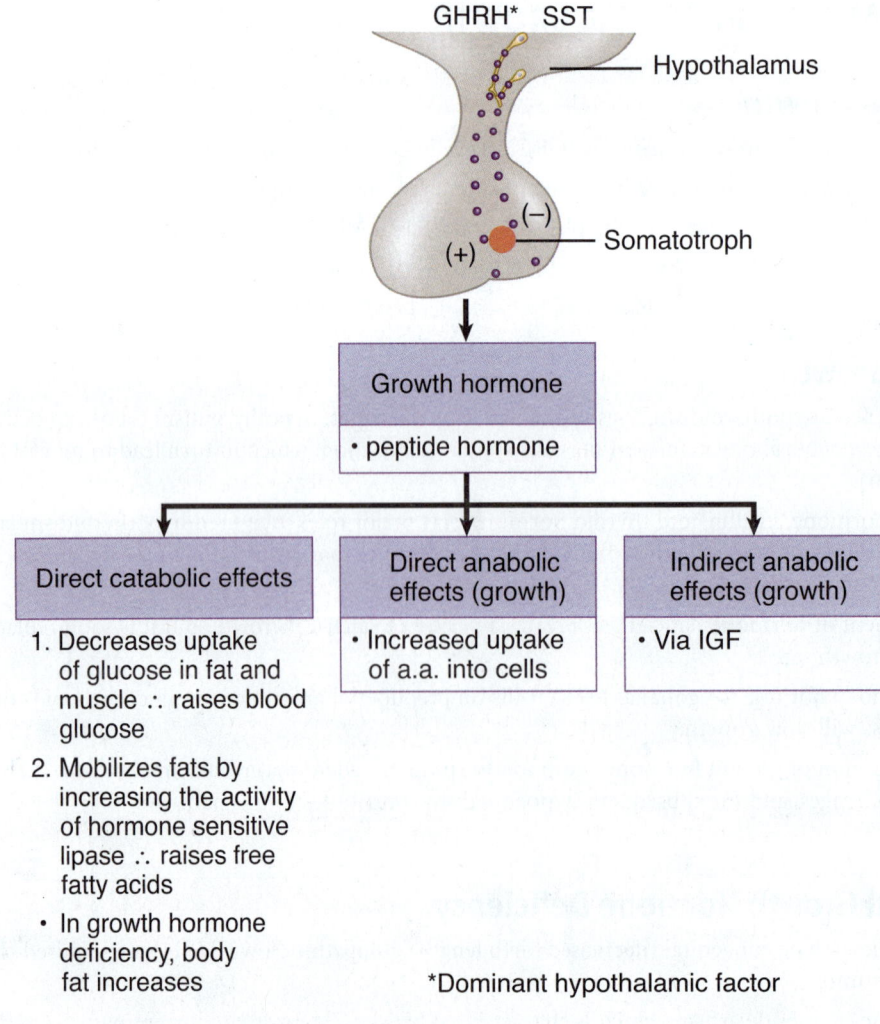

Figure 28-1. Overview of Growth Hormone
GHRH = growth hormone-releasing hormone; **SST** = somatostatin

Indirect Anabolic Actions of Growth Hormone

Most of the anabolic actions of growth hormone are an indirect result of increased production of insulin-like growth factors (IGFs). A major growth factor is IGF-I.

The steps in the production and release of IGF-I are shown here:

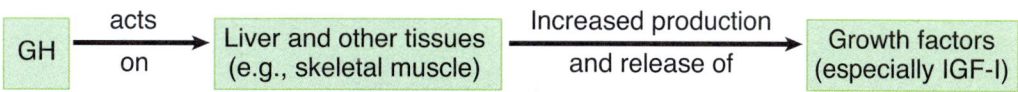

Figure 28-2. IGF-Mediated Effects of Growth Hormone

Specific Properties of the IGFs

IGF-I is a major anabolic growth factor. It has the following characteristics:

- Circulates peptide growth factor similar in structure to proinsulin and has some insulin-like activity
- Circulates in the blood tightly bound to a large protein, whose production is also dependent on growth hormone. Protein binding increases the half-life and thus serves as a better 24-hour marker of GH (half-life 15–20 minutes).
- The major known anabolic effect of IGF-I is that it increases the synthesis of cartilage (chondrogenesis) in the epiphyseal plates of long bones, thereby increasing bone length.
- It is also hypothesized that circulating IGFs increase lean body mass. The decreased lean body mass of aging may, in part, be due to the concomitant decrease in IGFs. IGFs also decrease in catabolic states, especially protein-calorie malnutrition.
- IGF-II is another growth factor, the importance of which is not well understood but may have a role in fetal development.

CONTROL OF GROWTH HORMONE (GH) SECRETION

- GH secretion is pulsatile. The secretory pulses are much more likely to occur during the night in stages III and IV (non-REM) of sleep than during the day.
- Secretion of GH requires the presence of normal plasma levels of thyroid hormones. GH secretion is markedly reduced in hypothyroid individuals.
- During the sixth decade of life and later, GH secretion diminishes considerably in both men and women. What initiates this decrease is unknown.

Each of the promoters could act by increasing GHRH secretion, decreasing SST secretion, or both.

Notice that most of the factors that regulate GH secretion are identical to those that regulate glucagon (except for those boxed). These factors are consistent with their shared role as stress hormones.

The inhibitory effect of IGF-I represents a negative feedback loop to the hypothalamus.

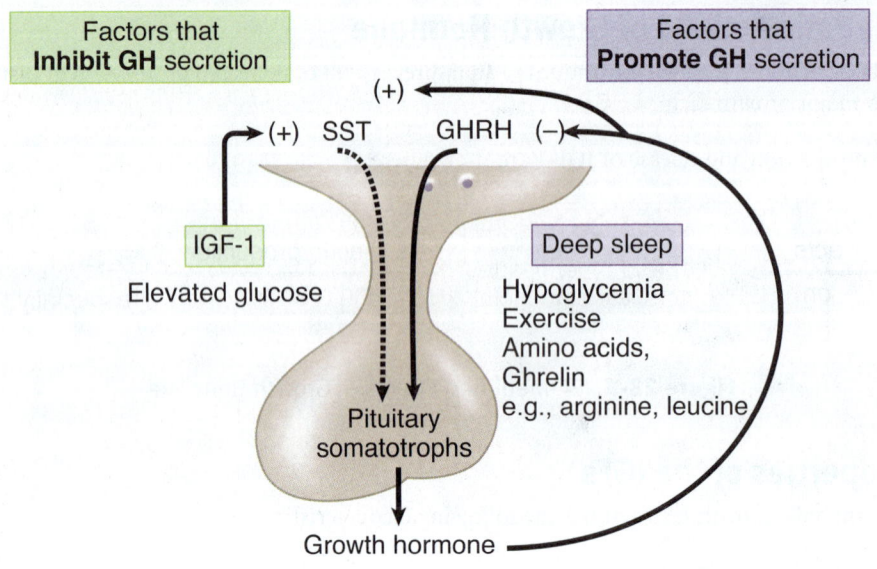

Figure 28-3. Control of Growth Hormone Secretion
SST = somatostatin

PUBERTY

Reproductive Changes

- Hypothalamic pulse generator increases activity just before physical changes at puberty.
- First noted sign in a female is breast development; first by estrogen (promotes duct growth) then progesterone (promotes development of milk-producing alveolar cells). First noted sign in a male is enlargement of the testes (mainly FSH stimulating seminiferous tubules).
- Pubic hair development in males and females is dependent on androgen.

Growth Changes

- During puberty, androgens promote the secretion in the following anabolic sequence:

At puberty, if T4 is normal, ↑ androgens drive ↑ growth hormone, which drives ↑ IGF-I.

- IGF-I is the major stimulus for cell division of the cartilage-synthesizing cells located in the epiphyseal plates of long bones.
- In males, the increased androgen arises from the testes (testosterone); in females, from the adrenals (adrenarche).
- Near the end of puberty, androgens promote the mineralization (fusion or closure) of the epiphyseal plates of long bones. Estrogen can also cause plate closure, even in men.
- In females, the growth spurt begins early in puberty and is near completion by menarche. In males, the growth spurt develops near the end of puberty.

ACROMEGALY

- It is caused by a post pubertal excessive secretion of growth hormone.
- It is almost always due to macroadenoma (> 1 cm dia) of the anterior pituitary and second in frequency to prolactinomas.
- There is a slow onset of symptoms, and the disease is usually present for 5 to 10 years before diagnosis.
- Ectopic GHRH secretion has been documented but is rare.
- Some tumors contain lactotrophs, and elevated prolactin can cause hypogonadism and galactorrhea.
- Increased IGF-I causes most of the deleterious effects of acromegaly but growth hormone excess directly causes the hyperglycemia and insulin resistance.
- There is characteristic proliferation of cartilage, bone and soft tissue, visceral, and cardiomegaly.
- Observable changes include enlargement of the hands and feet (acral parts) and coarsening of the facial features, including downward and forward growth of the mandible. Also, increased hat size.
- Measurement of IGF-I is a useful screening measure and confirms diagnosis with the lack of growth hormone suppression by oral glucose.
- Diagnosis: Treatment should only be done when 3 steps are completed:
  - Elevated IGF level
  - Failure of suppression of GH/IGF after giving glucose
  - MRI shows lesion in brain in pituitary

  Never start with a scan in endocrinology. Benign pituitary "incidentaloma" is common in 2–10% of the population. Always confirm the presence of an overproduction of a hormone before doing a scan. This is true for adrenal lesions as well.
- Treatment:
  - Surgical removal by trans-sphenoidal approach is first. Removal of an over-producing adenoma is the first treatment in most of endocrinology with the exception of prolactinoma.
  - If surgical removal fails, use the growth hormone receptor antagonist, pegvisomant, or octreotide. Octreotide is synthetic somatostatin. Cabergoline is a dopamine agonist used when other medications have failed.
  - Radiation is used last, only after surgery, pegvisomant, octreotide and cabergoline have failed.

Learning Objectives

❏ Solve problems concerning hypothalamic-pituitary-gonadal axis in males

❏ Solve problems concerning age-related hormonal changes in males

❏ Demonstrate understanding of erection, emission, and ejaculation

❏ Use knowledge of gonadal dysfunction in the male

HYPOTHALAMIC-PITUITARY-GONADAL (HPG) AXIS IN MALES

The factors involved in the overall control of adult male hormone secretion are summarized in the following figure.

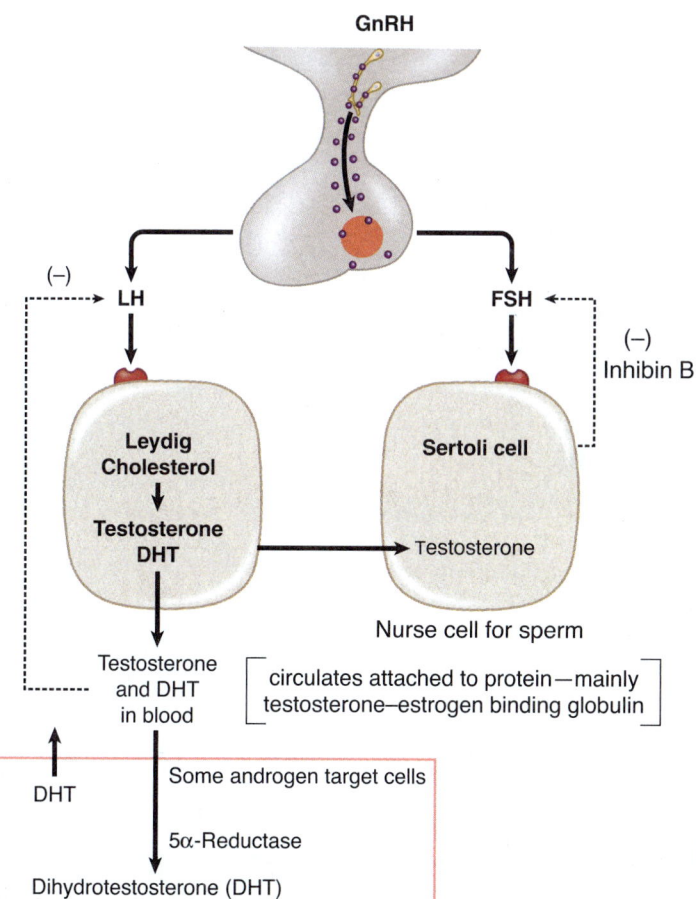

GnRH—synthesized in preoptic region of hypothalamus and secreted in pulses into hypophyseal portal vessels
- produces pulsatile release of LH and FSH
- pulsatile release of GnRH prevents downregulation of its receptors in anterior pituitary

LH and **FSH**—produced and secreted by gonadotrophs of anterior pituitary
- LH stimulates Leydig cells to produce testosterone.
- FSH stimulates Sertoli cells (see below).

Leydig cell testosterone—some diffuses directly to Sertoli cells, where it is required for Sertoli cell function.
- produces negative feedback for LH

Sertoli cell inhibin B—produces negative feedback for FSH

Figure 29-1. Control of Testes

LH/Leydig Cells

- Leydig cells express receptors for LH
- LH is a peptide hormone that activates Gs--cAMP, which in turn initiates testosterone production by activating steroidogenic acute regulatory protein (StAR).
- Testosterone diffuses into Sertoli cells (high concentration) and into the blood.
- Circulating testosterone provides negative feedback to regulate LH secretion at the level of the hypothalamus and anterior pituitary.

5α-reductase

Some target tissue express this enzyme, which converts testosterone into the more potent dihydrotestosterone. Some important physiologic effects primarily mediated by dihydrotestosterone are as follows:

- Sexual differentiation: differentiation to form male external genitalia
- Growth of the prostate
- Male-pattern baldness
- Increased activity of sebaceous glands
- Synthesis of NO synthase in penile tissue

FSH/Sertoli Cells

- FSH binds to Sertoli cells and activates a Gs--cAMP pathway.
- Sertoli cells release inhibin B, which has negative feedback on FSH secretion.

Hormonal Control of Testicular Function

Figure 29-2 illustrates the source and nature of the hormones controlling testicular function.

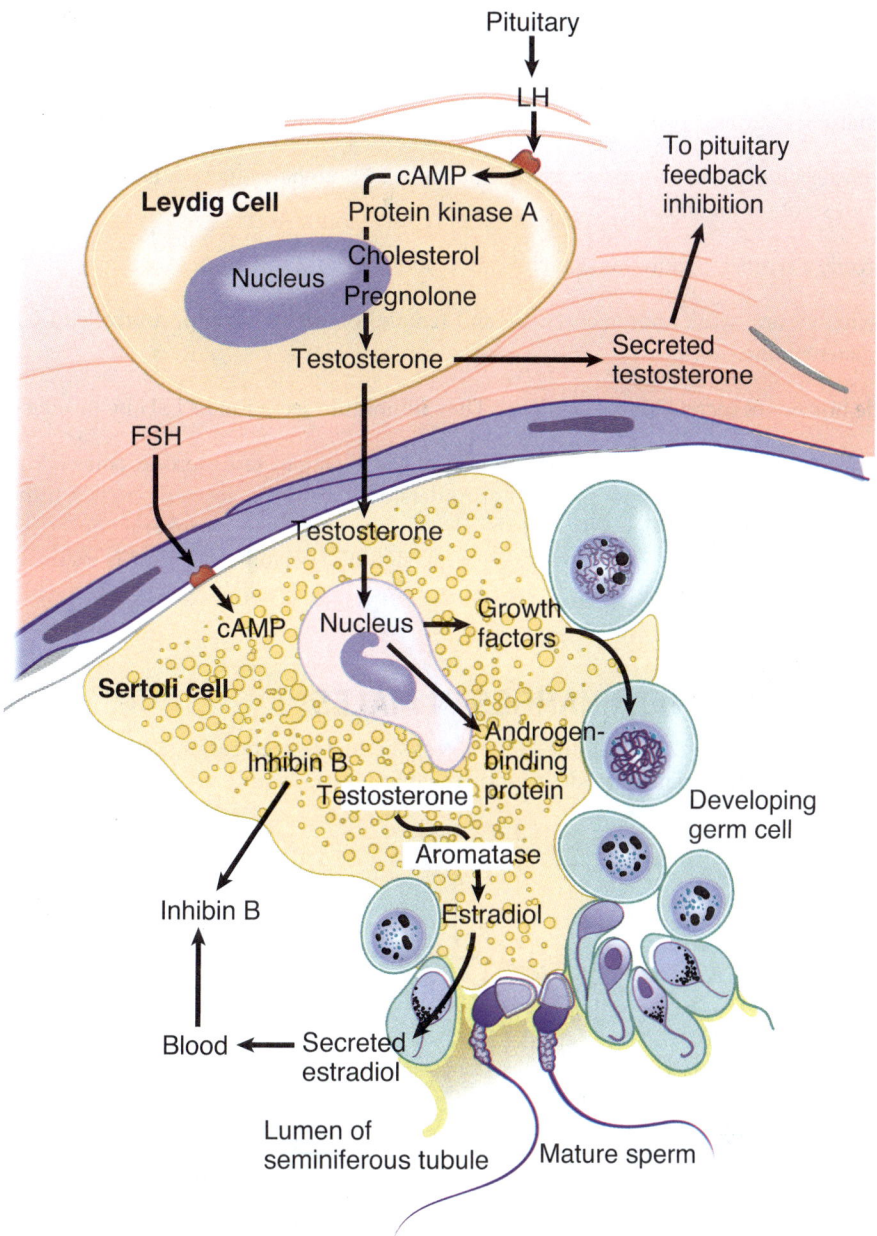

Figure 29-2. Endocrine Function of Testes

Note

Sertoli cells provide the nourishment that is required for normal spermatogenesis.

- FSH, along with a very high level of testosterone from the neighboring Leydig cells, produces growth factors necessary for growth and maturation of the sperm.

- FSH and testosterone induce the synthesis of androgen binding protein, which helps maintain high local levels of testosterone.

- FSH stimulates aromatase, which aromatizes testosterone into estradiol, an important hormone for growth and maturation of the sperm.

- Sertoli cells secrete inhibin B, which produces feedback regulation on FSH.

Definitions

Androgen: any steroid that controls the development and maintenance of masculine characteristics

Testosterone: a natural male androgen of testicular origin, controlled by the luteinizing hormone (LH)

Dihydrotestosterone: a more active form of testosterone made by 5-alpha-reductase. Dihydrotestosterone makes the penis, prostate, and scrotum on an embryo.

Methyl testosterone: a synthetic androgen, which is an anabolic steroid sometimes used by athletes

Adrenal androgens: natural weak androgens (male and female) of adrenal origin, controlled by ACTH. These are DHEA and androstenedione.

Inhibins: peptide hormones secreted into the blood. They inhibit the secretion of FSH by pituitary gonadotrophs.

Aromatase: an enzyme that stimulates the aromatization of the A-ring of testosterone, converting it into estradiol. The physiologic importance of this conversion is not understood; however, approximately a third of the estradiol in the blood of men arises from Sertoli cells, and the remainder arises from peripheral conversion of testosterone to estradiol by an aromatase present in adipose tissue. One sign of a Sertoli cell tumor is excessive estradiol in the blood of the affected man.

AGE-RELATED HORMONAL CHANGES IN MALES

The following figure depicts the relative plasma LH and testosterone concentrations throughout the life of the normal human male. The numbers refer to the descriptions that follow the figure.

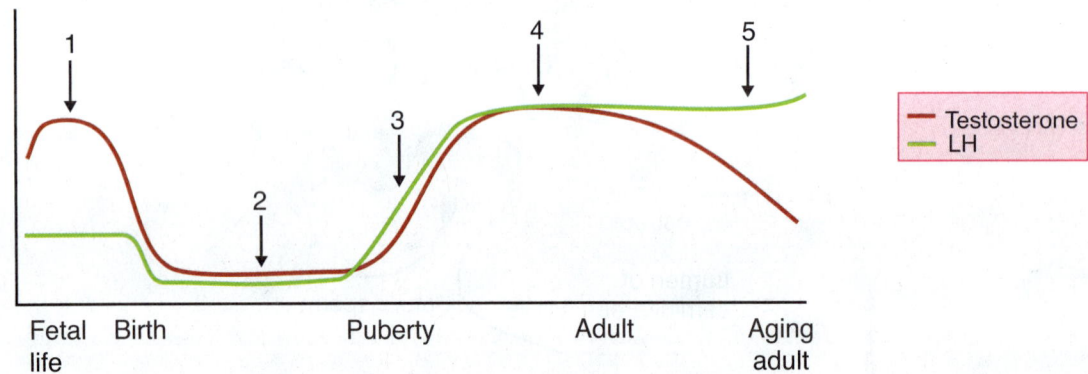

Figure 29-3. Development and Aging in Male Reproduction

1. Fetal life

The development of male and female internal and external structures depends on the fetal hormonal environment. The Wolffian and Müllerian ducts are initially present in both male and female fetuses. If there is no hormonal input (the situation in the normal female fetus), female internal and female external structures develop (Müllerian ducts develop, Wolffian ducts regress).

Normal male development requires the presence of three hormones: testosterone, dihydrotestosterone, and the Müllerian inhibiting factor (MIF).

1. (hCG) + LH → Leydig cells → testosterone → Wolffian ducts 5-α reductase

2. testosterone → dihydrotestosterone → urogenital sinus & genital organs

3. Sertoli cells → MIF → absence of female internal structures

MIF prevents the development of the Müllerian ducts, which would otherwise differentiate into female internal structures. In the absence of MIF, the Müllerian ducts develop. Thus, in addition to normal male structures, a uterus will be present.

- Wolffian ducts differentiate into the majority of male internal structures; namely, epididymis, vas deferens, and seminal vesicles.

  – In the absence of testosterone, the Wolffian ducts regress.

- Dihydrotestosterone induces the urogenital sinus and genital tubercle to differentiate into the external scrotum, penis, and prostate gland.

  – In the absence of dihydrotestosterone, female external structures develop.

2. Childhood

Within a few months after birth, LH and testosterone drop to low levels and remain low until puberty. The cause of this prolonged quiescence of reproductive hormone secretion during childhood is not known. Interestingly, LH secretion remains low in spite of low testosterone.

3. Puberty

Near the onset of puberty, the amplitude of the LH pulses becomes greater, driving the mean level of LH higher. Early in puberty, this potentiation of the LH pulses is especially pronounced during sleep. This increased LH stimulates the Leydig cells to again secrete testosterone.

4. Adult

During adulthood, LH secretion drives testosterone secretion. Thus, it is not surprising that the relative levels of the two hormones parallel one another.

5. Aging adult

Testosterone and inhibin secretions decrease with age. Men in their seventies generally secrete only 60–70% as much testosterone as do men in their twenties. Nevertheless, there is no abrupt decrease in testosterone secretion in men that parallels the relatively abrupt decrease in estrogen secretion that women experience at menopause. The loss of feedback will cause an increase in LH and FSH secretion.

Effect on Muscle Mass

The capacity of androgens to stimulate protein synthesis and decrease protein breakdown, especially in muscle, is responsible for the larger muscle mass in men as compared with women. Exogenous androgens (anabolic steroids) are sometimes taken by men and women in an attempt to increase muscle mass.

Spermatogenesis is Temperature Dependent

Effect on fertility

For unknown reasons, spermatogenesis ceases at temperatures typical of the abdominal cavity. Thus, when the testes fail to descend before or shortly after birth, and the condition (cryptorchidism) is not surgically corrected, infertility results.

Cooling mechanisms

Normally, the scrotum provides an environment that is 4°C cooler than the abdominal cavity. The cooling is accomplished by a countercurrent heat exchanger located in the spermatic cord. Also, the temperature of the scrotum and the testes is regulated by relative degree of contraction or relaxation of the cremasteric muscles and scrotal skin rugae that surround and suspend the testes.

Effect on FSH and LH

Sertoli cells, and therefore germ cell maturation, are adversely affected by the elevated temperatures of cryptorchid testes. In adults with bilaterally undescended testes, FSH secretion is elevated, probably as a result of decreased Sertoli cell production of inhibins. Testosterone secretion by the Leydig cells of cryptorchid testes also tends to be low, and as a result, LH secretion of adults with bilateral cryptorchidism is elevated.

Female Reproductive System 30

Learning Objectives

❏ Interpret scenarios on menstrual cycle

❏ Explain information related to female sex steroid metabolism and excretion

❏ Explain information related to pregnancy

❏ Solve problems concerning lactation

MENSTRUAL CYCLE

The Phases

The menstrual cycle (approximately 28 days) can be divided into the following phases or events. By convention, the first day of bleeding (menses) is called day 1 of the menstrual cycle.

- Follicular phase (first 2 weeks) is also called the proliferative or preovulatory phase. This phase is dominated by the peripheral effects of estrogen, which include the replacement of the endometrial cells lost during menses.

- Ovulation (approximately day 14) is preceded by the LH surge, which induces ovulation.

- Luteal phase (approximately 2 weeks) is dominated by the elevated plasma levels of progesterone, and along with lower levels of secreted estrogen, creates a secretory quiescent endometrium that prepares the uterus for implantation.

- Menses. Withdrawal of the hormonal support of the endometrium at this time causes necrosis and menstruation.

Follicular phase (approximately days 1 to 14)

- By convention, the first day of bleeding (menses) is called day 1 of the menstrual cycle.

- During the follicular phase, FSH secretion is slightly elevated, causing proliferation of granulosa cells and increased estrogen secretion within a cohort of follicles.

- One follicle has greater cellular growth and secretes more estradiol (dominant follicle). Estradiol promotes growth and increased sensitivity to FSH; thus the follicle continues to develop. The remaining follicles, lacking sufficient FSH, synthesize only androgen and become atretic (die).

Figures 30-1 through 30-4 illustrate the hormonal regulation of the menstrual cycle. The graphs represent the plasma hormonal levels throughout the cycle. The length of the menstrual cycle varies, but an average length is 28 days. Each of the plasma hormone concentrations is plotted relative to the day on which its concentration is lowest, i.e., just prior to menses (day 28). The accompanying diagram illustrates specific aspects of the phase under consideration.

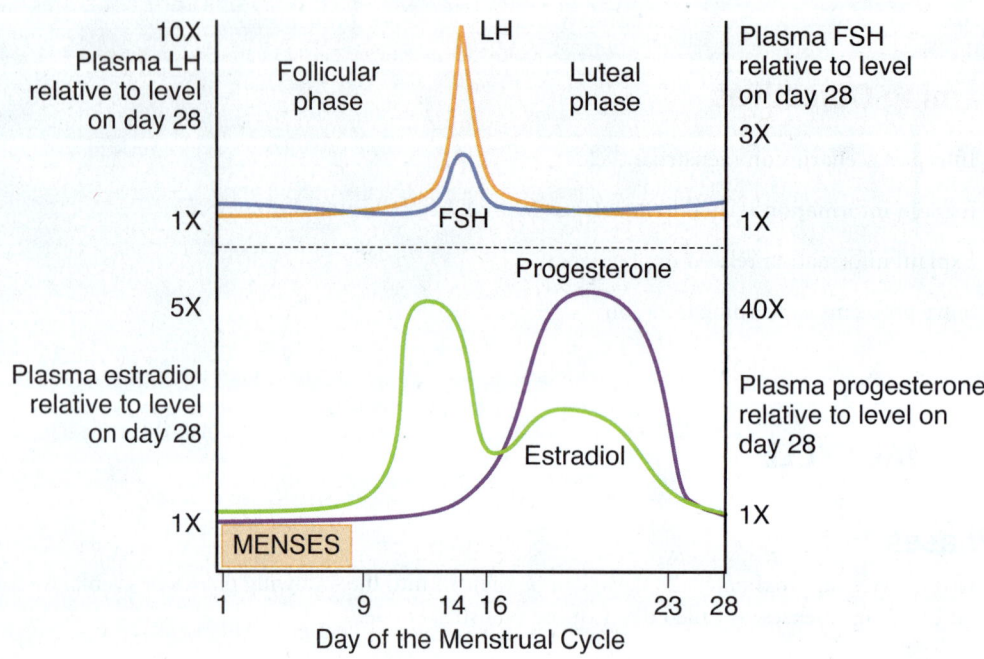

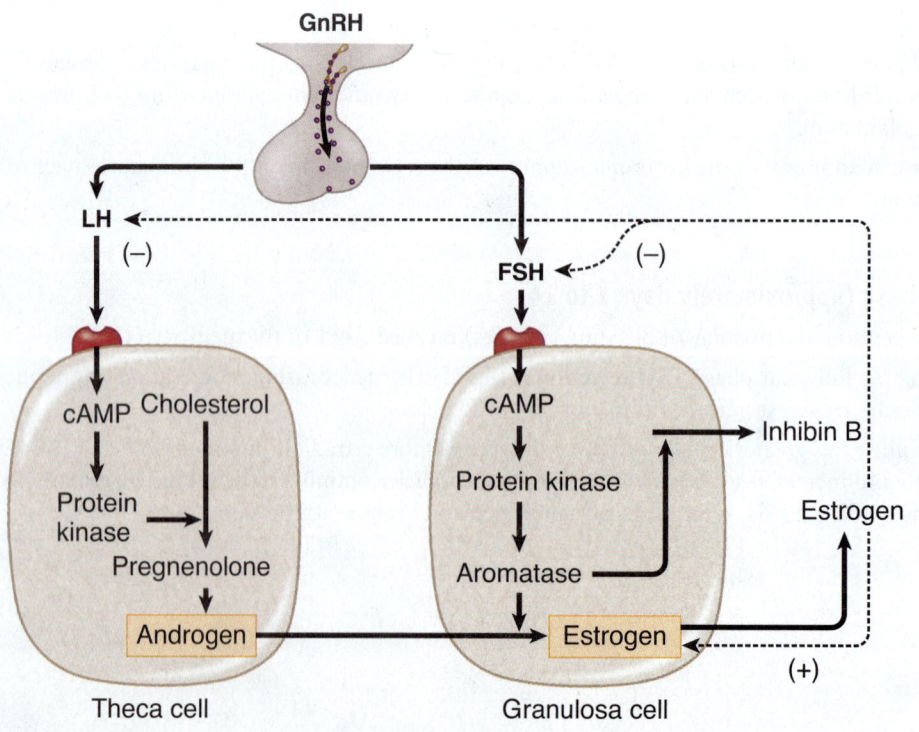

Figure 30-1. Follicular Phase Relationships Approximately Days 1 to 14

Theca Cells: Under LH stimulation, which acts intracellularly via cAMP, cholesterol is transported into the mitochondria (StAR is activated). The pathway continues through intermediates to androgens. Little androgen is secreted into the blood; most of the androgen enters the adjacent granulosa cells.

Granulosa Cells: Possess the follicle's only FSH receptors. When coupled to FSH, these act via cAMP to increase the activity of aromatase; aromatase converts the androgens to estrogens (mainly estradiol).

Estrogen: Some of the estrogen produced by the granulosa cells is released into the blood and inhibits the release of LH and FSH from the anterior pituitary. However, another fraction of the estrogen acts locally on granulosa cells, increasing their proliferation and sensitivity to FSH.

- This local positive effect of estrogens causes a rising level of circulating estrogens during the follicular phase, but at the same time FSH is decreasing because of the inhibitory effect of estrogen on FSH release.
- Granulosa cells also release inhibin B.
- Inhibin B inhibits the secretion of FSH by the pituitary but their role in the menstral cycle is poorly understood.

Peripheral effects of estrogen produced by the granulosa cells during the follicular phase include:

- Circulating estrogens stimulate the female sex accessory organs and secondary sex characteristics.
- Rising levels of estrogens cause the endometrial cells of the uterine mucosal layers to increase their rate of mitotic division (proliferate).
- Circulating estrogens cause the cervical mucus to be thin and watery, making the cervix easy for sperm to traverse.

Ovulation

Ovulation takes place approximately on day 14. This is an approximation. Since ovulation is always 14 days before the end of the cycle, you can subtract 14 from the cycle length to find the day of ovulation.

$$\text{Cycle length} - 14 = \text{ovulation day}$$

Estrogen Levels

As shown in Figure 30-2, near the end of the follicular phase, there is a dramatic rise in circulating estrogen. When estrogens rise above a certain level, they no longer inhibit the release of LH and FSH. Instead, they stimulate the release of LH and FSH (negative feedback loop to positive feedback loop).

This causes a surge in the release of LH and FSH. Only the LH surge is essential for the induction of ovulation and formation of the corpus luteum. Notice from the figure that the LH surge and ovulation occur after estrogen peaks. Therefore, if estrogens are still rising, ovulation has not occurred.

Follicular rupture occurs 24–36 hours after the onset of the LH surge. During this time interval, LH removes the restraint upon meiosis, which has been arrested in prophase for years. The first meiotic division is completed, and the first polar body is extruded.

Positive feedback loops are rare in the body. Only ovulation with estrogen and parturition with oxytocin represent positive feedback loops.

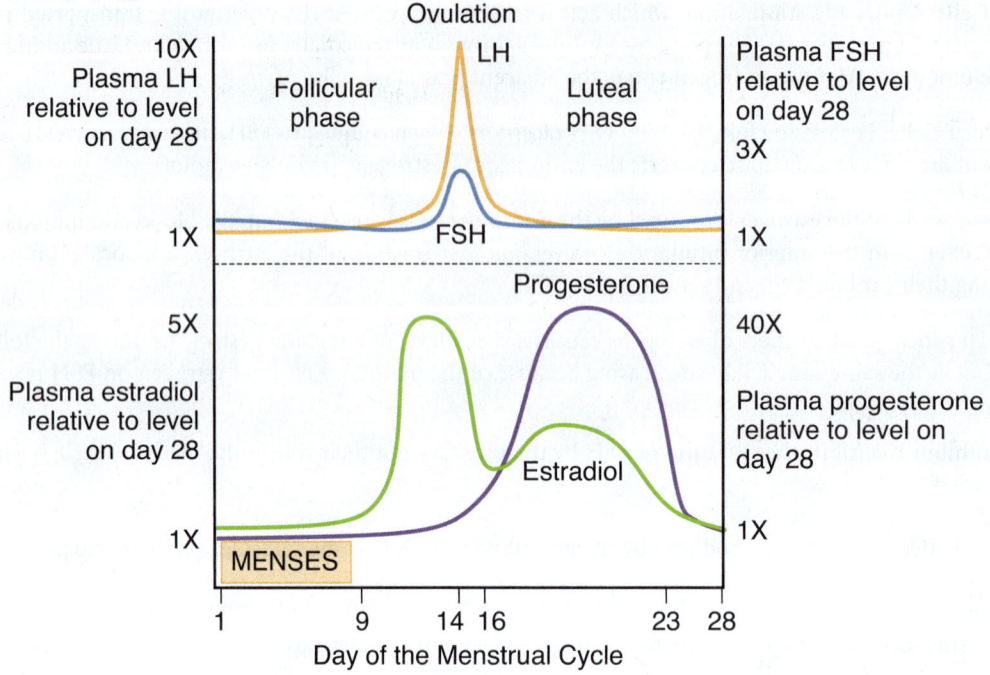

Ovulation occurs approximately day 14

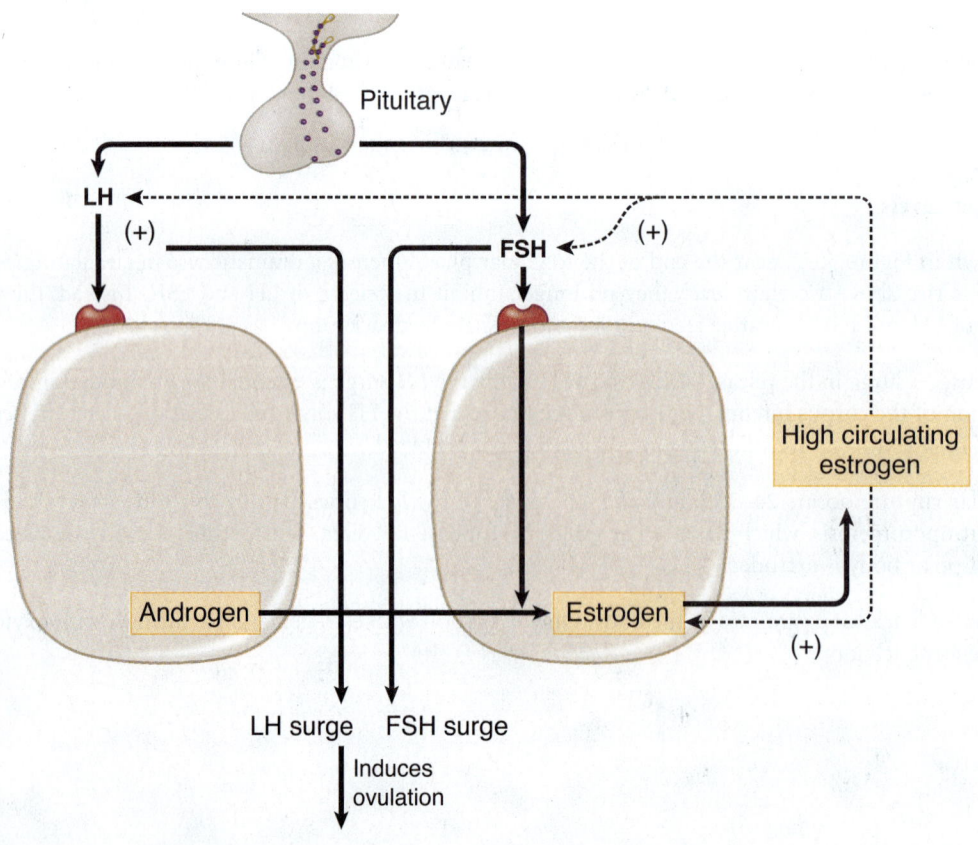

Figure 30-2. Pituitary-Ovarian Relationships at Ovulation

Luteal phase (approximately days 14 to 28)

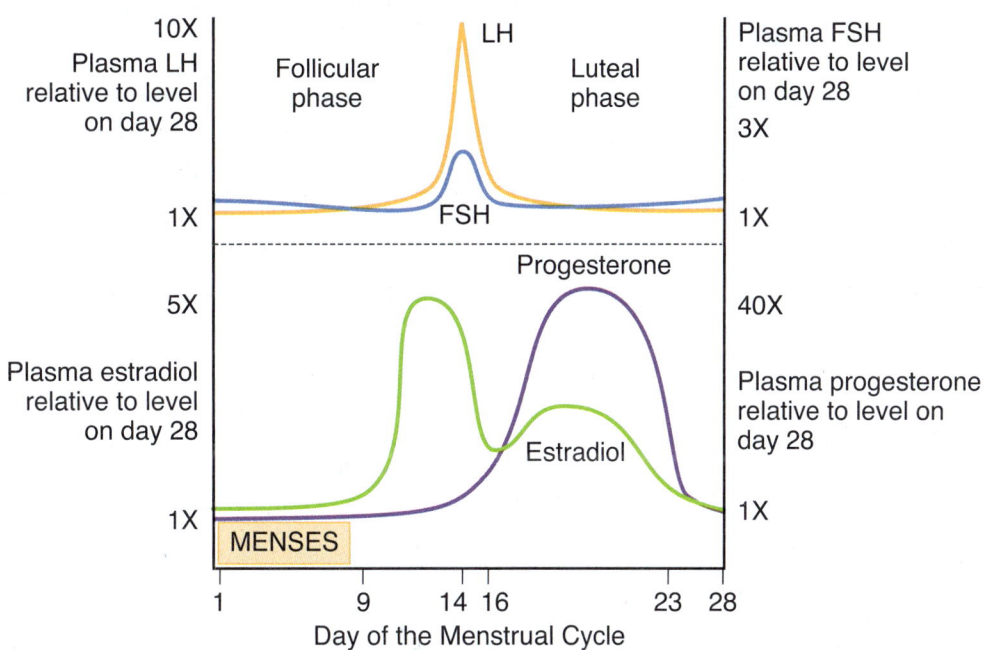

Luteinization of the preovulatory follicle

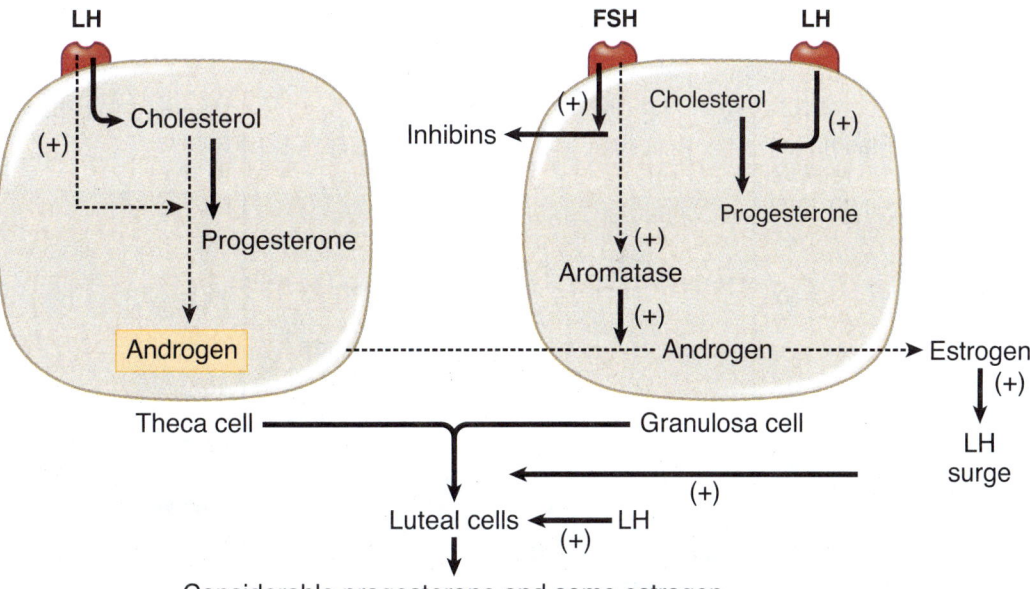

Figure 30-3. The Luteal Phase Reactions

Preovulatory Follicle

In the latter stages of the follicular phase, intracellular changes within the granulosa and theca cells occur in preparation for their conversion into luteal cells.

- Estradiol, in conjunction with FSH, causes the granulosa cells to produce LH receptors.
- The metabolic pathways are then altered to favor the production of progesterone.
- This would include a decrease in the activity of aromatase and a drop in estrogen production.

LH Surge

Induced by the elevated estrogens, it causes the granulosa cells and theca cells to be transformed into luteal cells and increases the secretion of progesterone.

Corpus Luteum

The process of luteinization occurs following the exit of the oocyte from the follicle. The corpus luteum is made up of the remaining granulosa cells, thecal cells, and supportive tissue. Once formed, the luteal cells are stimulated by LH to secrete considerable progesterone and some estrogen. Progesterone inhibits LH secretion (negative feedback). The corpus luteum secretes inhibin A, which has negative feedback on FSH.

The increased plasma level of progesterone has several actions:

- It causes the uterine endometrium to become secretory, providing a source of nutrients for the blastocyst.
- It causes the cervical mucus to become thick, sealing off the uterus from further entry of sperm or bacteria.
- It has thermogenic properties, causing the basal body temperature to increase by 0.5–1.0° F.

Menses

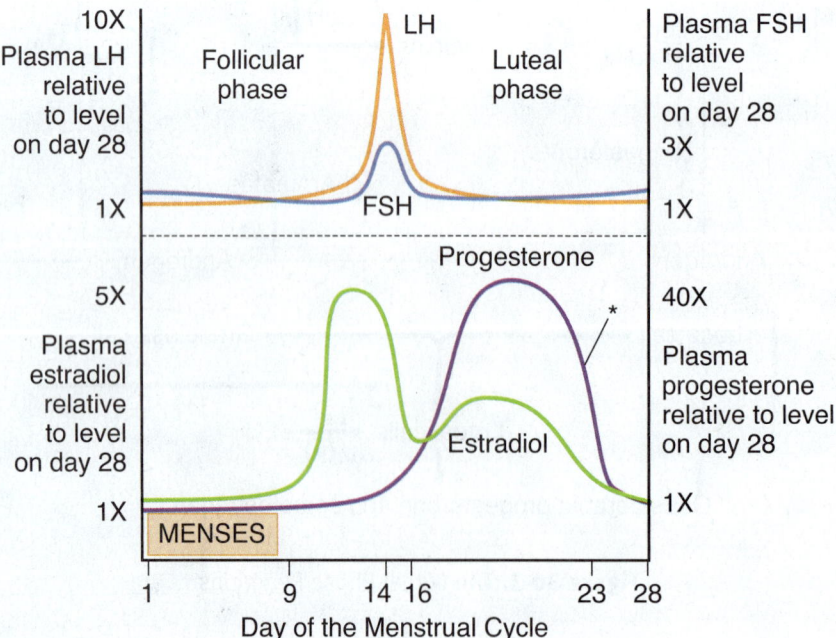

*The fall in sex steroids causes menses.

Figure 30-4. Onset of Menses

- The life of the corpus luteum is finite, hence the luteal phase is only 14 days.

- Initially, the corpus luteum is very responsive to LH. Over time however, as the corpus luteum becomes less functional, it becomes less responsive to LH.

- Progesterone exerts negative feedback on LH, which contributes to the demise of the corpus luteum.

- With the demise of the corpus luteum, progesterone and estradiol fall to levels that are unable to support the endometrial changes, and menses begins.

Menstruation is due to a lack of gonadal sex steroids.

FEMALE SEX STEROID METABOLISM AND EXCRETION

Solubilization and Excretion

The female sex steroids undergo oxidation or reduction in the liver (and other target tissues), and a glucuronide or sulfate group is attached to the steroidal metabolite. This "conjugation" increases the solubility of the steroids in water, and they thus become excretable in urine.

Estradiol can be excreted as a conjugate of estradiol, but most is first converted to estrone or estriol.

Progesterone is converted in the liver to pregnanediol and is excreted as pregnanediol glucuronide.

Monitoring the Menstrual Cycle

The amount of sex steroids excreted in the urine can be used to monitor the menstrual cycle. For example:

- Low progesterone metabolites and low but slowly rising estrogen metabolites characterize the early follicular phase.

- Low progesterone metabolites and rapidly rising estrogen metabolites characterize the latter part of the follicular phase just before ovulation.

- Elevated levels of progesterone metabolites characterize the luteal phase and pregnancy. In the early luteal phase progesterone is rising, in the latter half it is falling.

Estrogens and Androgen Formation

- Estrogen: Generic term for any estrus-producing hormone, natural or synthetic

- 17 β-Estradiol: Major hormone secreted by the ovarian follicle

- Estrone: Some is secreted from the ovary but much is formed in peripheral tissues such as adipose tissue from androgens. These androgens originate from both the ovary and the adrenal glands. This is the main circulating estrogen following menopause. Fat cells have aromatase. Adipose tissue creates modest levels of estrogen.

- Estriol: Major estrogen synthesized from circulating androgens by the placenta

- Potency: Estradiol > estrone > estriol

- Androgens: The follicles also secrete androgen; DHEA, androstenedione, and testosterone. Additional testosterone production is from the peripheral conversion of adrenal and ovarian androgen. Some testosterone is also converted via 5 α-reductase to dihydrotestosterone in the skin.

New Cycle

During the three days prior to and during menses, plasma levels of progesterone and estradiol are at their low point; negative feedback restraint for gonadotropin secretion is removed. FSH secretion rises slightly and initiates the next cycle of follicular growth.

The length of the follicular phase of the menstrual cycle is more variable than the length of the luteal phase. Long cycles are usually due to a prolonged follicular phase and short cycles to a short follicular phase. Once ovulation has occurred, menses generally follows in about 14 days. The length of the menstrual cycle in days minus 14 gives the most likely day of ovulation.

PREGNANCY

Ovum Pickup and Fertilization

In women, the ovum is released from the rupturing follicle into the abdominal cavity, where it is "picked up" by the fimbria of the oviduct. Failure of ovum pickup may result in ectopic pregnancy, i.e., the implantation of the blastocyst at any site other than the interior of the uterus.

Fertilization occurs in the upper end of the oviduct within 8–25 hours after ovulation. After this, the ovum loses its ability to be fertilized. Sperm retain their capacity to fertilize an ovum for as long as 72 hours after ejaculation. For about 48 hours around the time of ovulation the cervical mucus is copious and slightly alkaline. This environment represent a good conduit for the sperm.

Weeks of gestation (gestational age) to estimate the delivery date are commonly taken from the first day of the last menstrual period.

Sperm are transported from the vagina to the upper ends of the oviduct by contraction of the female reproductive tract. The swimming motions of the sperm are important for penetration of the granulosa cell layer (cumulus oophorus) and membranes surrounding the ovum.

Low sperm counts (<20 million/mL of ejaculate) are associated with reduced fertility because sperm from ejaculates with low counts often contain many sperm with poor motility and an abnormal morphology. The first step in infertility evaluation is semen analysis.

Implantation

At the time of implantation, which occurs about 5-7 days after fertilization, the development is at the blastocyst stage. The trophoblastic cells of the fetus now begin to secrete a peptide hormone, human chorionic gonadotropin (hCG). HCG starts 10 days after fertilization.

Fetal hCG possesses a β subunit similar to that of LH, and therefore it has considerable LH activity.

The presence of the beta subunit of hCG in the urine can be detected by a variety of test kits for the detection of pregnancy.

Hormonal Maintenance of the Uterine Endometrium

The following figure illustrates the production of estrogen and progesterone during pregnancy. The figure is divided into three phases:

- Part of the luteal phase before implantation
- Early pregnancy
- Late pregnancy

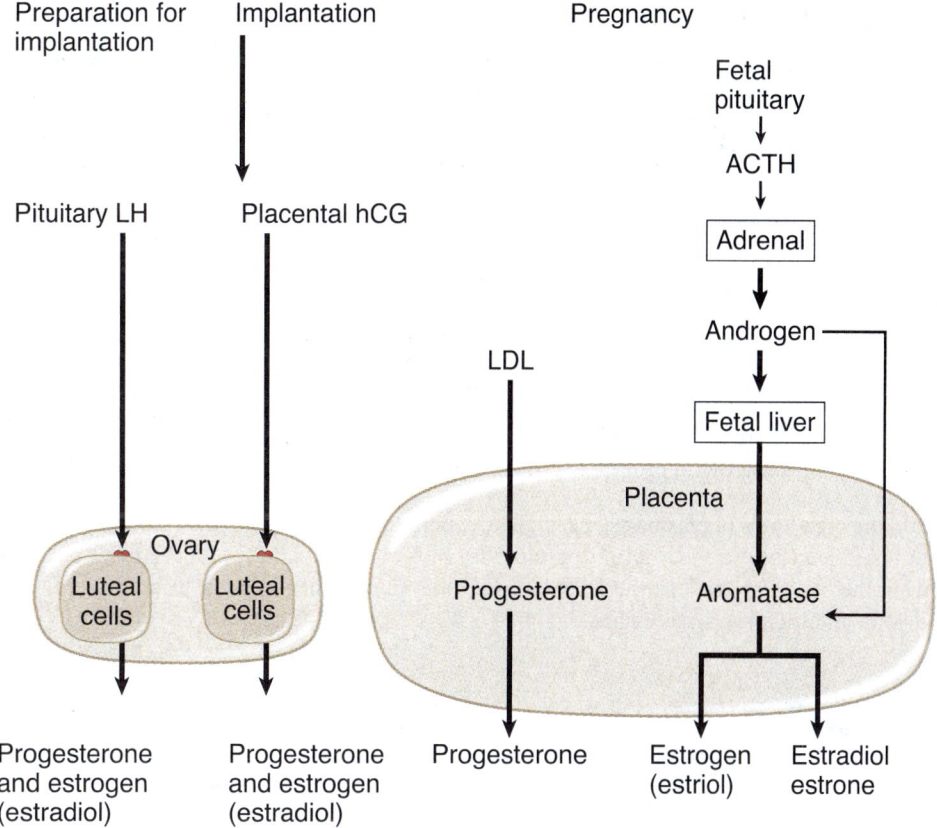

Figure 30-5. Steroids During Pregnancy

Preparation for implantation (luteal phase)

Pituitary LH stimulates luteal cells to secrete progesterone and some estrogen. Because the ovaries are the source of the estrogen, it is mainly estradiol.

Implantation to second month

- Within a week or two of fertilization, trophoblastic cells of the placenta begin secreting hCG. In short, hCG prevents regression of the corpus luteum, thus allowing it to continue producing estrogens and progesterone.
- hCG doubles in the early weeks of pregnancy. Because it maintains secretion of progesterone from the corpus luteum, progesterone is a sensitive marker of early fetal well-being.
- Loss of the corpus luteum during this period terminates the pregnancy. However, in lieu of the corpus luteum, exogenous progesterone would be a functional substitute.

Third month to term

- Placenta secretes enough progesterone and estrogen to maintain the uterus. This is not controlled by hCG. At this time, the ovaries (corpus luteum) can be removed and pregnancy continues.
- Progesterone secretion of the placenta is limited only by the amount of precursor (cholesterol) delivered by low-density lipoproteins (LDL) to the placenta. Progesterone maintains uterine quiescence during pregnancy.
- The secretion of estrogen involve both the fetus and the placenta.
- The fetal adrenal gland secretes dehydroepiandrosterone (DHEA). The fetal liver then converts DHEA to androstenodione (A) and testosterone.
- The placenta expresses aromatase. This enzyme converts the A and testosterone from the fetus into estrogens, estriol being the primary one. Thus, estriol becomes a good marker for fetal well-being.

Peripheral Effects of Hormonal Changes

The large amount of estrogen and progesterone secreted by the placenta during pregnancy stimulates the following important changes within the mother:

- Massive growth of the uterus, especially the myometrium
- Increased growth of all components (glands, stroma, and fat) of the breasts

LACTATION

Mammary Gland Growth and Secretion

Growth of mammary tissue is stimulated by the female sex steroids estrogen and progesterone. However, for these steroids to stimulate maximum growth, prolactin, growth hormone, and cortisol also must be present.

During pregnancy, the high levels of plasma estrogen greatly increase prolactin secretion, but milk synthesis does not occur because the high level of estrogen (and progesterone) blocks milk synthesis. At parturition, plasma estrogen drops, withdrawing the block on milk synthesis. As a result, the number of prolactin receptors in mammary tissue increases several-fold, and milk synthesis begins.

Maintaining Lactation

Suckling is required to maintain lactation.

The suckling of the baby at the mother's breast stimulates receptors in the mother's nipples. Signals from these receptors are transmitted to the hypothalamus and have the following effects:

- Oxytocin synthesis and secretion are increased. Oxytocin causes the myoepithelial basket cells that surround the alveoli to contract. Preformed milk is ejected into the ducts and out the openings of the nipple; that is, milk ejection is initiated.
- The release of dopamine by the hypothalamus into the hypophyseal portal vessels is inhibited. This removes a chronic restraint on prolactin secretion. Prolactin secretion increases, and milk secretion is stimulated each time the baby suckles.
- The secretion of GnRH into the hypophyseal portal vessels is inhibited; secretion of FSH and LH decreases. Thus, follicular growth, estrogen secretion, ovulation, and menses cease. High prolactin levels also contribute to the amenorrhea.

For the suckling stimulus to inhibit GnRH secretion completely, the stimulus must be prolonged and frequent. Supplementation of the mother's milk with other fluids or sources of energy reduces the baby's suckling and allows gonadotropin secretion, follicular growth, and ovulation to occur.

Women who do not wish to breastfeed their children are sometimes administered large doses of estrogen. The estrogen inhibits lactation (by its inhibitory action of milk synthesis), even though estrogen promotes increased prolactin secretion.

Breastfeeding is a form of contraceptive because it should stop ovulation.

Gastrointestinal Physiology 31

Learning Objectives

❏ Answer questions about overview of the gastrointestinal tract

❏ Explain information related to motility

❏ Demonstrate understanding of secretions

❏ Demonstrate understanding of digestion

❏ Demonstrate understanding of absorption

OVERVIEW OF THE GASTROINTESTINAL TRACT

Structure

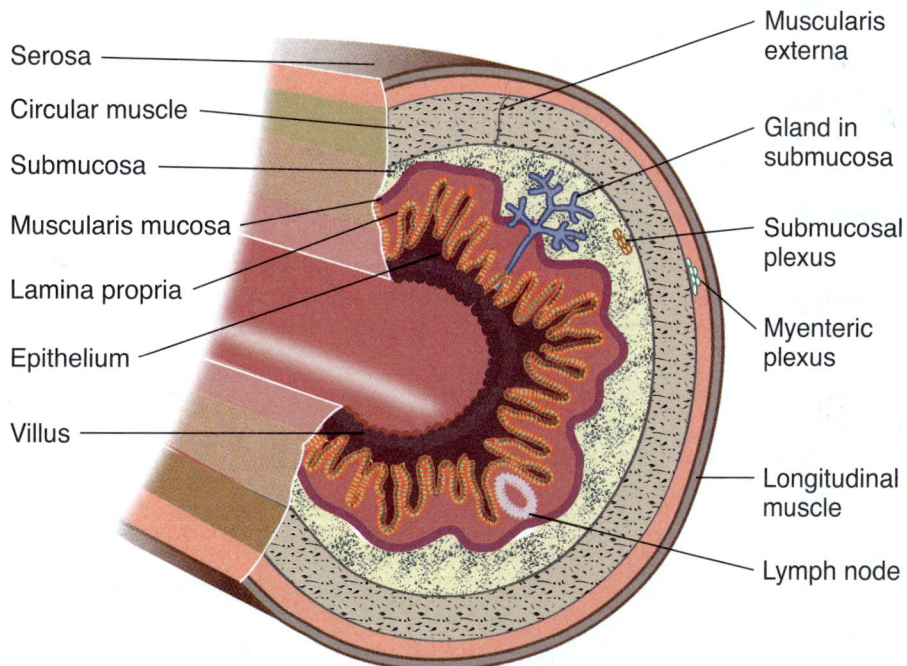

Figure 31-1. Gastrointestinal Tract

Mucosa

- Epithelium: consists of a single layer of specialized cells; some are involved in secretions and some release hormones
- Lamina propria: layer of connective tissue which contains glands, hormone-containing cells, lymph nodes, and capillaries
- Muscularis mucosa: a thin layer of muscle, the contraction of which causes folding and ridges in the mucosal layers

Submucosa

- A layer of connective tissue that contains glands, large blood vessels, and lymphatics.
- Outermost region has a nerve net called the submucosal (Meissner's) plexus.
- Meissner's plexus is part of the enteric nervous system and is involved in secretory activity.

Muscularis externa

- Inner layer of circular muscle
- Outer layer of longitudinal muscle
- Myenteric nerve plexus involved in motor activity is between the muscle layers.

Serosa

- Outermost layer of the GI tract
- Consists of connective tissue and a layer of epithelial cells
- Within this layer autonomic nerve fibers run and eventually synapse on target cells and the enteric nerve plexes

---

Note

Sympathetic regulation of the splanchnic circulation does not involve the enteric nervous system.

Nervous Control

Residing in the GI tract is a vast neural network called the enteric nervous system (Meissner's and myenteric plexi). Normal GI function is dependent on this neural network. The enteric nervous system is innervated by the autonomic nervous systems and serves as the final mediator for virtually all neurally mediated changes.

Sympathetic

The diagram below illustrates how the synaptic junction at the end of a nerve fiber secretes norepinephrine (NE), which then induces responses in the gastrointestinal (GI) system.

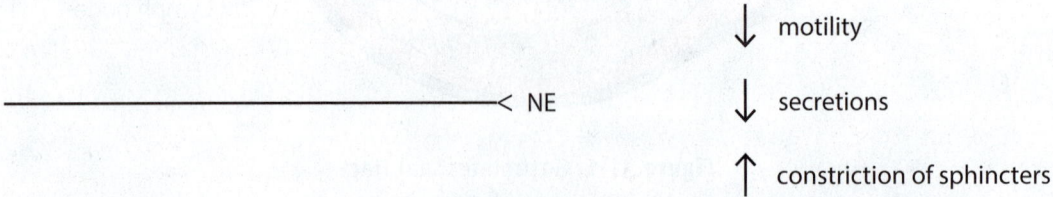

An increase in sympathetic activity slows processes.

Parasympathetic

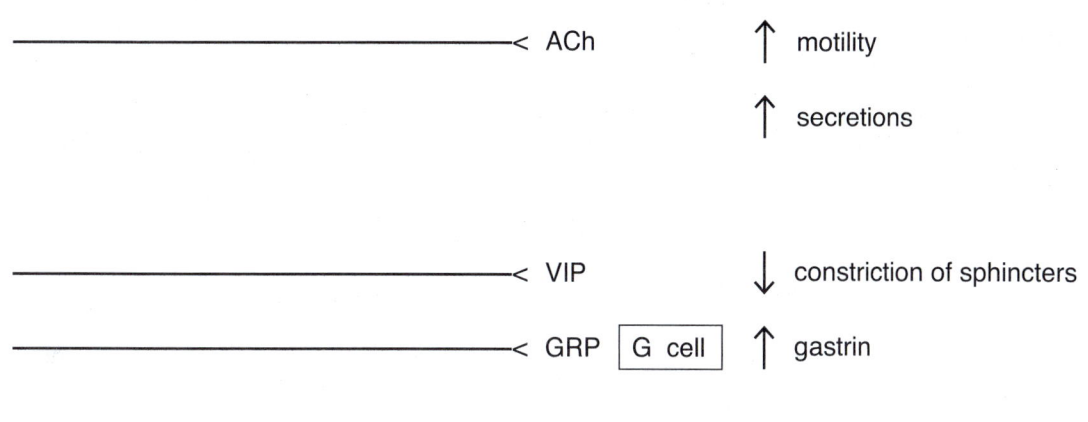

VIP = vasoactive intestinal peptide, an inhibitory parasympathetic transmitter
GRP = gastrin-releasing peptide; stimulates the release of gastrin from G cells

An increase in parasympathetic activity promotes digestive and absorptive processes.

Endocrine Control

Table 31-1. The Endocrine Control of the GI System

Hormone**	Source	Stimulus	Stomach Motility and Secretion	Pancreas	Gallbladder
Secretin	S cells lining duodenum	Acid entering duodenum	Inhibits	Stimulates fluid secretion (HCO_3^-)	
CCK	Cells lining duodenum	Fat and amino acids entering duodenum	Inhibits emptying	Stimulates enzyme secretion	1. Contraction 2. Relaxation sphincter (Oddi)
Gastrin	G cells of stomach	Stomach distension	Stimulates		
	Antrum	Parasym (GRP) Peptides			
	Duodenum	Stomach acid inhibits*			
GIP GLP	Duodenum	Fat, CHO, amino acids	Inhibits		Increases insulin Decreases glucagon

CCK = cholecystokinin; GIP = gastric inhibitory peptide (glucose insulinotropic peptide), GLP = glucagon-like peptide

*Note: In a non-acid-producing stomach (e.g., chronic gastritis), the reduced negative feedback increases circulating gastrin.

**All four hormones stimulate insulin release.

MOTILITY

Characteristics of Smooth Muscle

Electrical activity

- Resting membrane potential −40 to −65 mV. Close to depolarization.
- Oscillation of membrane potential is generated by interstitial cells (interstitial cells of Cajal) that act as pacemakers. This is referred to as slow waves or basic electrical rhythm, and if threshold is reached it generates action potentials.
- Action potentials are generated by the opening of slow channels that allow the entry of both sodium and calcium.
- The duodenum contracts the most often.

Note

Anticholinergic medications such as atropine or tricyclic antidepressants slow GI motility.

Motor activity

- Stretch produces a contractile response.
- Gap junctions create an electrical syncytium within the smooth muscle.
- Slow waves create low level contractions, and action potentials strengthen the contractions.
- Pacemaker activity from the interstitial cells creates the intrinsic motor activity.
- Tonic contraction at sphincters act as valves.

Note

Nerve gas increases GI and bronchial secretions.

Swallowing

Swallowing is a reflex controlled from the brain stem.

Efferent input is via the vagus nerve for all events:

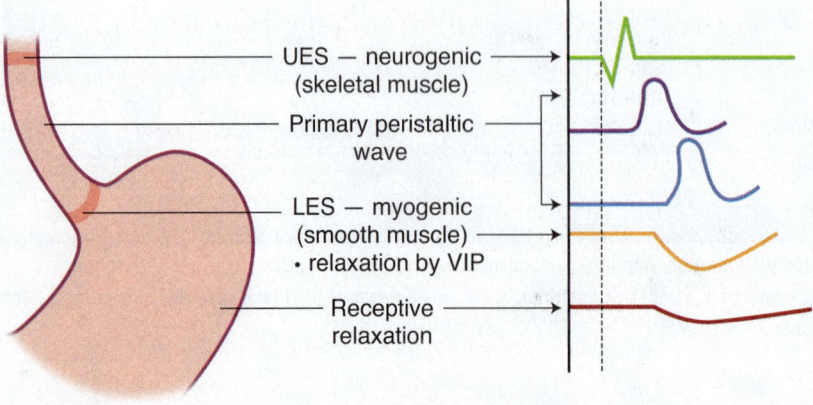

Figure 31-2. Swallowing, the Peristaltic Wave

An increase in sympathetic activity slows processes.

Events during swallowing:

- Relaxation of upper esophageal skeletal muscle sphincter (UES)
- Primary peristaltic wave
- Relaxation of lower esophageal smooth muscle sphincter (LES) via VIP acting as an inhibitory transmitter
- Relaxation of proximal stomach (receptive relaxation)

Bridge to Pathology

Barrett esophagus is the term used to describe alterations in the esophageal epithelium that accompany GERD.

If the primary peristaltic wave is not successful, a secondary peristaltic wave is initiated by local distension of the esophagus. The secondary wave is not "conscious."

Disorders of the Esophagus

Achalasia

- Failure of the LES to relax, resulting in swallowed food being retained in the esophagus
- Caused by abnormalities in the enteric nerves
- Peristaltic waves are weak

Gastroesophageal reflux disease (GERD)

- LES doesn't maintain tone
- Acid reflux damages esophageal epithelium

Diffuse esophageal spasm

- Spasms of esophageal muscle
- Presents with characteristics of a heart attack (e.g., chest pain)
- Barium swallow shows repeated, spontaneous waves of contraction

---

Note

Dysphagia refers to difficulty in swallowing.

Gastric Motility

The primary factors and additional aspects are illustrated in the following figure.

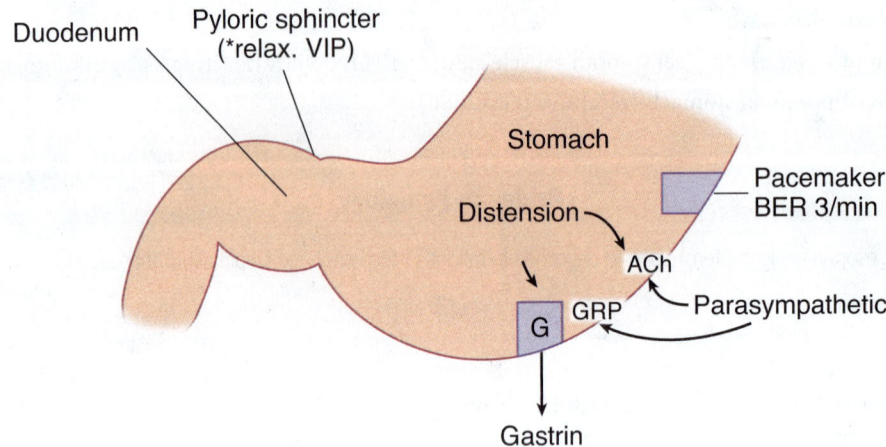

Figure 31-3. Endocrine and Neural Control of the Stomach

ACh = Acetylcholine; **BER** = Basic electrical rhythm; **GRP** = Gastrin-releasing peptide; **VIP** = Vasoactive intestinal polypeptide

Stimulation

- Acetylcholine released in response to activation of parasympathetics
- Local distension

Inhibition

- Low pH of stomach contents inhibits the release of gastrin
- Feedback from duodenal release of hormones (CCK, secretin, and GIP)

Stomach Emptying

- Liquids > CHO > protein > fat (> = faster than)
- The pyloris of the stomach acts as a sphincter to control the rate of stomach emptying. A wave of contraction closes the sphincter so that only a small volume is moved forward into the duodenum. CCK, GIP, and secretin increase the degree of pyloric constriction and slow stomach emptying.

Small Intestinal Motility

- Rhythmic contractions in adjacent sections create segmentation contractions, which are mixing movements.
- Waves of contractions preceded by a relaxation of the muscle (peristaltic movements) are propulsive.
- The ileocecal sphincter, or valve between the small and large intestine, is normally closed.
- Distension of the ileum creates a muscular wave that relaxes the sphincter.
- Distension of the colon creates a nervous reflex to constrict the sphincter.

Colon Motility

- Segmentation contractions create bulges (haustrations) along the colon.
- Mass movements, which are propulsive, are more prolonged than the peristaltic movements of the small intestine.

Migrating Motor Complex (MMC)

- A propulsive movement initiated during fasting that begins in the stomach and moves undigested material from the stomach and small intestine into the colon.
- Repeats every 90–120 minutes during fasting.
- When one movement reaches the distal ileum, a new one starts in the stomach.
- Correlated with high circulating levels of motilin, a hormone of the small intestine
- This movement prevents the backflow of bacteria from the colon into the ileum and its subsequent overgrowth in the distal ileum.

Defecation

- Defecation is a reflex involving the central nervous system.
- A mass movement in the terminal colon fills the rectum and causes a reflex relaxation of the internal anal sphincter and a reflex contraction of the external anal sphincter.
- Voluntary relaxation of the external sphincter accompanied with propulsive contraction of the distal colon complete defecation.
- Lack of a functional innervation of the external sphincter causes involuntary defecation when the rectum fills.

SECRETIONS

Salivary Secretions

- Parotid gland secretions are entirely serous (lack mucin).
- Submandibular and sublingual gland secretions are mixed mucus and serous.
- They are almost entirely under the control of the parasympathetic system, which promotes secretion.
- The initial fluid formation in the acinus is via an indirect chloride pump (secondary active transport powered by the Na/K ATPase pump), and the electrolyte composition is isotonic and similar to interstitial fluid.
- Note that structural details of salivary glands are described in the Dental Anatomy section.

Duct cells modify the initial acinar secretion.

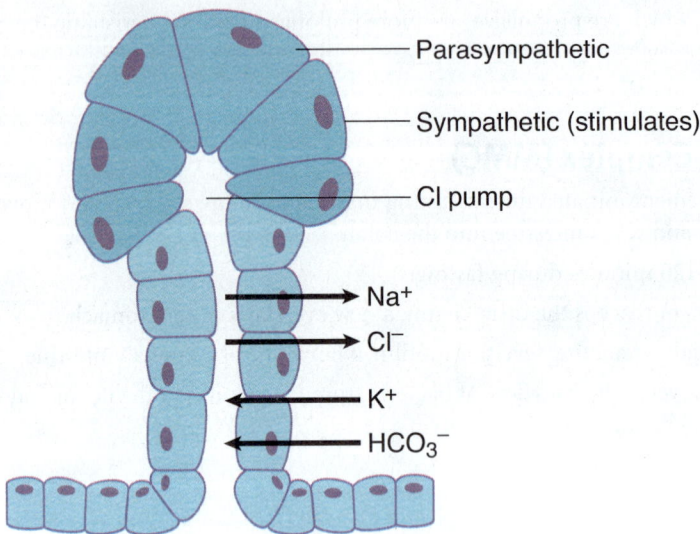

Figure 31-4. Salivary Secretion

Composition of salivary secretions

- Low in Na$^+$, Cl$^-$ because of reabsorption
- High in K$^+$, HCO$_3$ because of secretion (pH = 8)
- Low tonicity: Salivary fluid is hypotonic because of reabsorption of NaCl and impermeability of ducts to water.
- α-Amylase (ptyalin): secreted in the active form and begins the digestion of carbohydrates
- Mucus, glycoprotein
- Immunoglobulins and lysozymes

Gastric Secretions

- The epithelial cells that cover the gastric mucosa secrete a highly viscous alkaline fluid (mucin plus bicarbonate) that protects the stomach lining from the caustic action of HCl.
- Fluid needs both mucin and bicarbonate to be protective.
- Nonsteroidal anti-inflammatory drugs such as aspirin decrease the secretion of the mucin and bicarbonate.
- Surface of the mucosa studded with the openings of the gastric glands
- Except for the upper cardiac region and lower pyloric region whose glands secrete mainly a mucoid fluid, gastric glands secrete a fluid whose pH can be initially as low as 1.0.

Secretions of the main cells composing the oxyntic gastric glands

Parietal cells

- HCl
- Intrinsic factor combines with vitamin B$_{12}$ and is reabsorbed in the distal ileum. This is the only substance secreted by the stomach that is required for survival. It is released by the same stimuli that release HCl.

Chief Cells

Pepsinogen is converted to pepsin by H^+, as illustrated in the diagram below.

$$\text{Pepsinogen} \xrightarrow{\quad H^+ \quad} \text{pepsin (proteins to peptides)}$$

- Pepsinogen is initially converted to active pepsin by acid.
- Active pepsin continues the process.
- Pepsin is active only in the acid pH medium of the stomach.
- Pepsin begins the digestion of protein but is not essential for life.

Mucous Neck Cells

- Secrete the protective mucus, HCO_3 combination

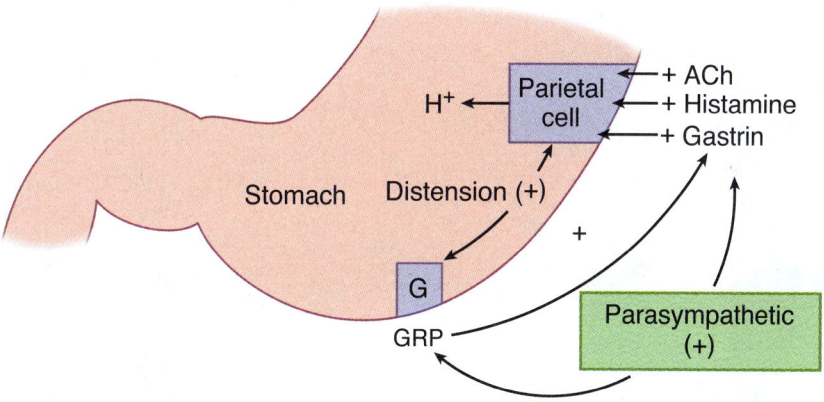

Figure 31-5. Control of Gastric Acid Secretion
+ Stimulates secretion
− Inhibits secretion

Control of acid secretion

There are three natural substances that stimulate parietal cells:

- Acetylcholine (ACh), acting as a transmitter; release is stimulated by sight/smell of food and reflexly in response to stomach distension (vagovagal reflex).
- Locally released histamine; stimulated by Ach and gastrin
- The hormone gastrin; stimulated by release of GRP

As stomach pH falls, somatostatin (SST) is released, which inhibits gastrin and reduces acid secretion (feedback regulation of acid secretion).

Cellular mechanisms of acid secretion

- Within the cell, carbonic anhydrase facilitates the conversion of CO_2 into H^+ and HCO_3^-.
- The demand for CO_2 can be so great following a meal that the parietal cells extract CO_2 from the arterial blood. This makes gastric venous blood the most basic in the body.

- Hydrogen ions are secreted by a H/K-ATPase pump similar to that in the distal nephron.
- The pumping of H^+ raises intracellular HCO_3^- and its gradient across the basal membrane and provides the net force for pumping Cl^- into the cell.
- The chloride diffuses through channels across the apical membrane, creating a negative potential in the stomach lumen.
- Because of the extraction of CO_2 and secretion of HCO_3^-, the venous blood leaving the stomach following a meal is alkaline.
- Compared with extracellular fluid, gastric secretions are high in H^+, K^+, Cl^-, but low in Na^+.
- The greater the secretion rate, the higher the H^+ and the lower the Na^+.
- Vomiting stomach contents produces a metabolic alkalosis and a loss of body potassium (hypokalemia mainly due to the alkalosis effect on the kidney).

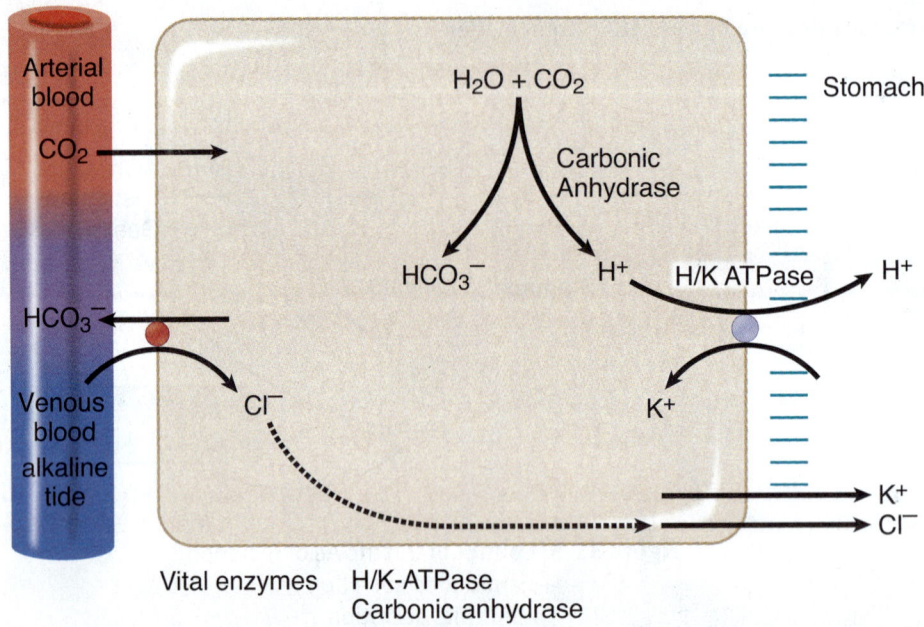

Figure 31-6. Regulation of Parietal Cell Secretion

Pancreatic Secretions

- Exocrine tissue is organized into acini and ducts very similar to that of the salivary glands.
- Cholinergic nerves to the pancreas stimulate the secretion of both the enzyme and aqueous component.
- Food in the stomach stimulates stretch receptors and, via vagovagal reflexes, stimulates a small secretory volume.
- Sympathetics inhibit secretion but are a minor influence.
- **Most of the control is via secretin and CCK.**

Enzymatic components

- Trypsin inhibitor, a protein present in pancreatic secretions, prevents activation of the proteases within the pancreas.

- In addition to the following groups of enzymes, pancreatic fluid contains ribonucleases and deoxyribonucleases.
- A diet high in one type of food (protein, CHO, fat) results in the preferential production of enzymes for that particular food.

Pancreatic amylases are secreted as active enzymes:

- Hydrolyze α-1,4-glucoside linkage of complex carbohydrates, forming three smaller compounds:
  - α-Limit dextrins: still a branched polysaccharide
  - Maltotriose, a trisaccharide
  - Maltose, a disaccharide
- Cannot hydrolyze β linkages of cellulose

Pancreatic lipases are mainly secreted as active enzymes. Glycerol ester lipase (pancreatic lipase) needs colipase to be effective. Colipase displaces bile salt from the surface of micelles. This allows pancreatic lipase to attach to the droplet and digest it, leading to formation of two free fatty acids and one monoglyceride (a 2-monoglyceride, i.e., an ester on carbon 2).

Cholesterol esterase (sterol lipase) hydrolyzes cholesterol esters to yield cholesterol and fatty acids. **Pancreatic proteases** are secreted as inactive zymogens. They include trypsinogen, chymotrypsinogen, and procarboxypeptidase.

Activation Sequence. The activation sequences are summarized below.

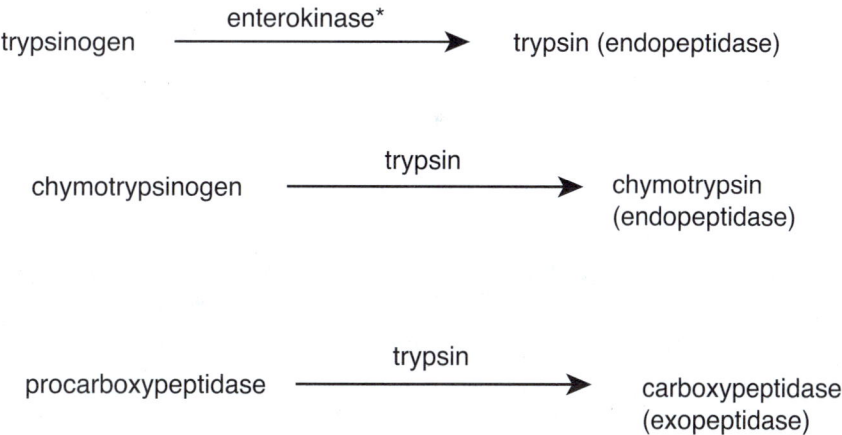

*Enterokinase (also known as enteropeptidase) is an enzyme secreted by the lining of the small intestine. It is not a brush border enzyme. It functions to activate some trypsinogen, and the active trypsin generated activates the remaining proteases.

Fluid and electrolyte components

- Aqueous component is secreted by epithelial cells which line the ducts.
- Fluid is isotonic due to the high permeability of the ducts to water and the concentrations of Na and K are the same as plasma.
- Duct cells secrete chloride into the lumen via the cystic fibrosis transmembrane conductance regulator (CFTR). This chloride is then removed from the lumen in exchange for bicarbonate. Thus, bicarbonate secretion is dependent upon chloride secretion.

- CFTR is activated by cAMP (see below).
- In cystic fibrosis there is a mutation in the gene that encodes this CFTR channel, resulting in less chloride and a reduced fluid component of pancreatic secretions. The smaller volume of highly viscous fluid may also contain few enzymes.

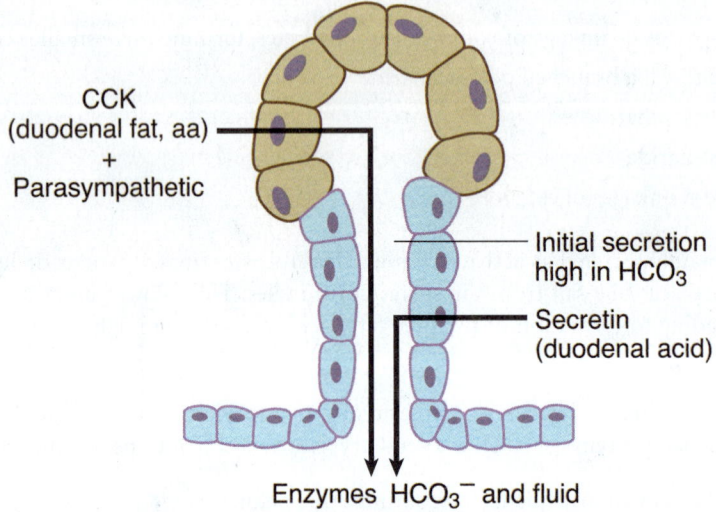

CCK
(duodenal fat, aa)
+
Parasympathetic

Initial secretion
high in HCO_3

Secretin
(duodenal acid)

Enzymes HCO_3^- and fluid

Figure 31-7. Control of the Exocrine Pancreas

Control of pancreatic secretions

Most of the regulation is via two hormones: secretin and cholecystokinin

Secretin

- Released from the duodenum in response to acid entering from the stomach.
- Action on the pancreas is the release of fluid high in HCO_3-. Secretin is a peptide hormone that stimulates chloride entry into the lumen from duct cells. Secretin activates Gs—cAMP, which in turn activates CFTR.
- This released HCO_3^--rich fluid is the main mechanism that neutralizes stomach acid entering the duodenum.

Cholecystokinin (CCK)

- Released from the duodenum in response to partially digested materials (e.g., fat, peptide, and amino acids)
- Action on the pancreas is the release of enzymes (amylases, lipases, proteases).

Composition and Formation of Bile

The following figure summarizes the major components of bile.

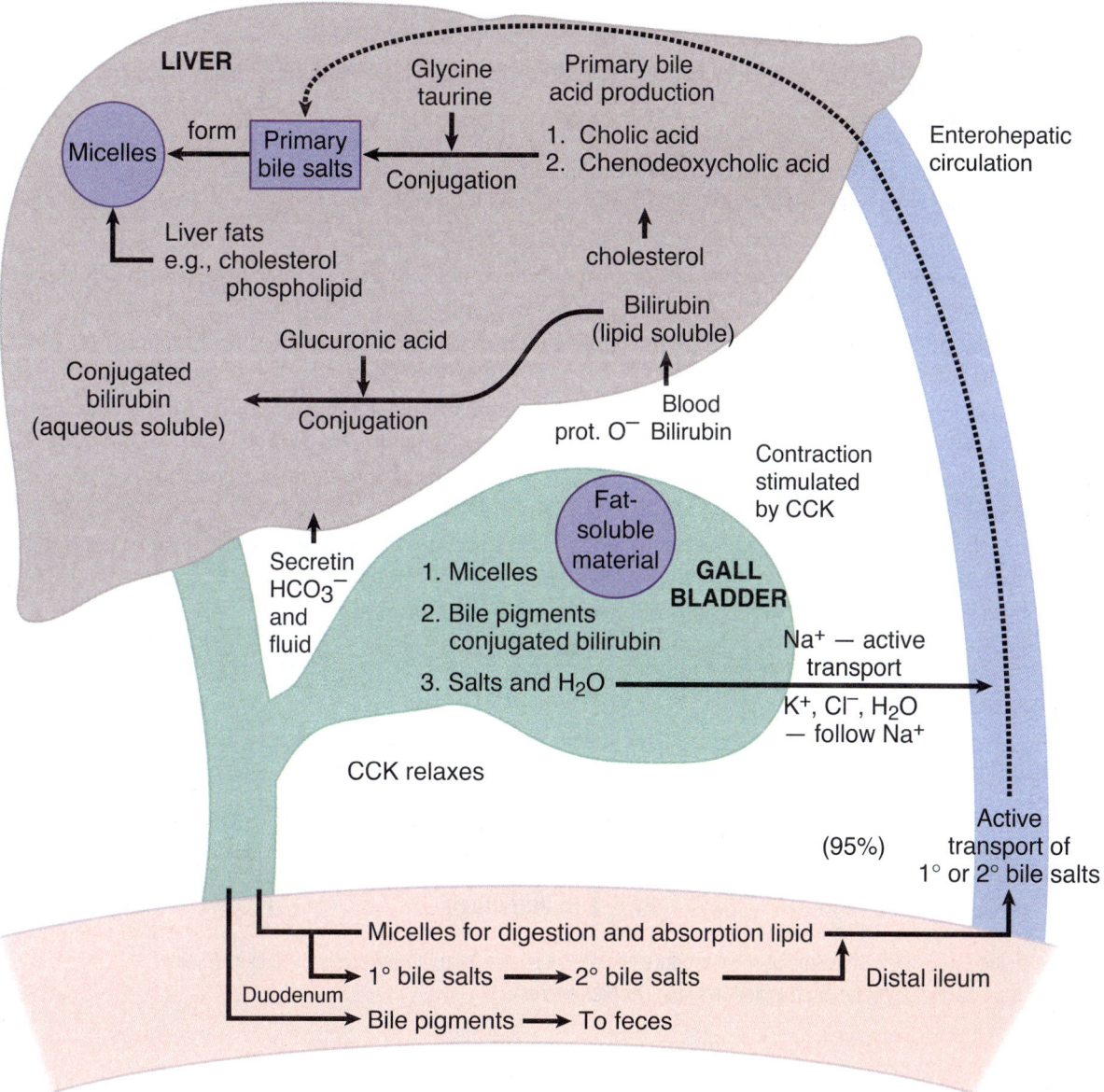

Figure 31-8. Production and Metabolism of Bile

Bile salts and micelles

- Primary bile acids known as cholic acid and chenodeoxycholic acid are synthesized by the liver from cholesterol.
- The lipid-soluble bile acids are then conjugated primarily with glycine.
- The conjugated forms are water-soluble but contain a lipid-soluble segment.
- Because they are ionized at neutral pH, conjugated bile acids exist as salts of cations (Na^+) and are, therefore, called bile salts.
- Bile salts are actively secreted by the liver.
- Secondary bile acids are formed by deconjugation and dehydroxylation of the primary bile salts by intestinal bacteria, forming deoxycholic acid (from cholic acid) and lithocholic acid (from chenodeoxycholic acid).
- Lithocholic acid has hepatotoxic activity and is excreted.
- When bile salts become concentrated, they form micelles. These are water-soluble spheres with a lipid-soluble interior.
- As such, they provide a vehicle to transport lipid-soluble materials in the aqueous medium of the bile fluid and the small intestine.
- Micelles are vital in the digestion, transport, and absorption of lipid-soluble substances from the duodenum to the distal ileum.
- In the distal ileum, and only in the distal ileum, can the bile salts be actively reabsorbed and recycled (enterohepatic circulation).
- Lack of active reabsorbing mechanisms (or a distal ileal resection) causes loss in the stool and a general deficiency in bile salts, as the liver has a limited capacity to manufacture them.
- This deficiency can lead to fat malabsorption and cholesterol gallstones.

Bile pigments

A major bile pigment, **bilirubin** is a lipid-soluble metabolite of hemoglobin. Transported to the liver attached to protein, it is then conjugated and excreted as water-soluble glucuronides. These give a golden yellow color to bile.

Stercobilin is produced from metabolism of bilirubin by intestinal bacteria. It gives a brown color to the stool.

Bridge to Pathology

Increased levels of plasma bilirubin produce jaundice. If severe, bilirubin can accumulate in the brain, producing profound neurological disturbances (kernicterus).

Salts and water

The HCO_3^- component is increased by the action of secretin on the liver.

The active pumping of sodium in the gallbladder causes electrolyte and water reabsorption, which concentrates the bile.

Bile pigments and bile salts are not reabsorbed from the gallbladder.

Phospholipids (mainly lecithin)

Insoluble in water but are solubilized by bile salt micelles

Cholesterol

Present in small amounts. It is insoluble in water and must be solubilized by bile salt micelles before it can be secreted in the bile.

Control of bile secretion and gallbladder contraction

- Secretin causes secretion of HCO_3^- and fluid into bile canalicular ducts.
- Secretion of bile salts by hepatocytes is directly proportional to hepatic portal vein concentration of bile salts.
- CCK causes gallbladder contraction and sphincter of Oddi relaxation.

Small Intestinal Secretions

- Most prominent feature of the small intestine is the villi.
- Surface epithelial cells display microvilli.
- Water and electrolyte reabsorption greatest at the villus tip.
- Water and electrolyte secretion greatest at the bottom in the crypts of Lieberkuhn.

Crypt secretion

- A Na^+-K^+-$2Cl^-$ transporter in the basolateral membrane facilitates the ion uptake by secondary active transport.
- Na^+ entry drives the entry of K^+ and Cl^- into the cell.
- The elevated intracellular Cl and negative intracellular potential drives the diffusion of chloride through channels on the apical membrane.
- Luminal Cl then pulls water, Na, and other ions into the lumen, creating the isotonic secretion. This is the general scheme of the chloride pump.
- Neurotransmitter secretagogues include VIP and ACh.
- The Cl^- channels are opened by increases in cytosolic Ca^{2+} and/or cAMP. The cAMP-dependent Ca^{2+} channels are CFTR channels.

DIGESTION

The following figure summarizes the regional entry of the major digestive enzymes proceeding from the mouth, stomach, and through the small intestine.

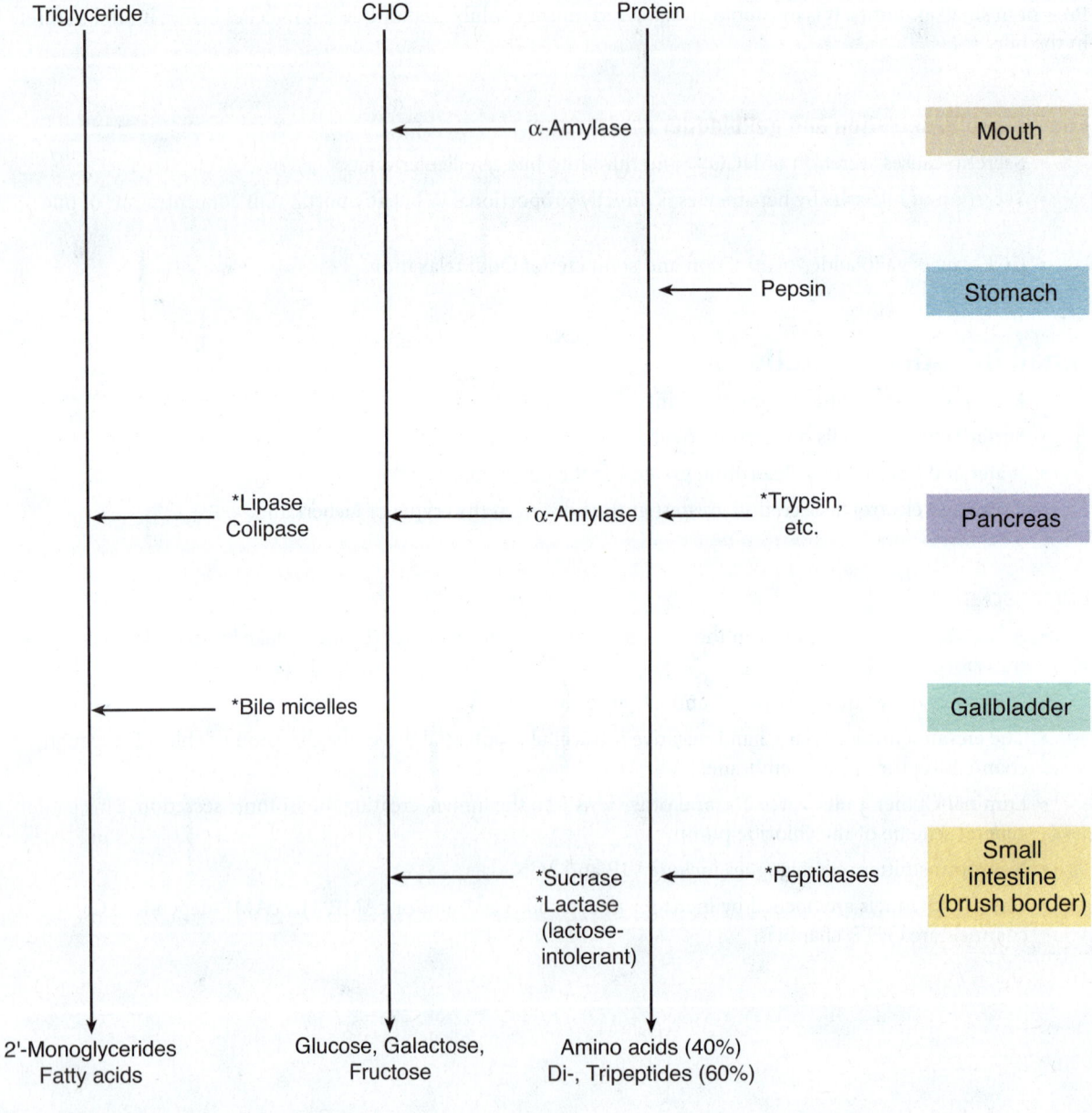

*Required for digestion

Figure 31-9. Summary of Digestive Processes

Digestive Enzymes and End Products

Triglycerides

Stomach: Fatty materials are pulverized to decrease particle size and increase surface area.

Small intestine: Bile micelles emulsify the fat, and pancreatic lipases digest it. Micelles and pancreatic lipase are required for triglyceride digestion. The major end products are 2-monoglycerides and fatty acids.

Carbohydrates

Mouth: Salivary α-amylase begins the digestion, and its activity continues in the stomach until acid penetrates the bolus; however, it is not a required enzyme.

Small intestine: Pancreatic α-amylase, a required enzyme for CHO digestion, continues the process. Hydrolysis of starch by α-amylase goes on in solution in the lumen of the small intestine, mostly in the duodenum. Further processing or splitting of these trisaccharides, disaccharides, and oligosaccharides is necessary but does not take place in solution; rather, it occurs on the brush border. The enzymes—α-dextrinase (or α-glucoamylase), isomaltase, and maltase—are all bound to the brush border (apical membrane of enterocytes). Brush border enzymes have their highest activity in the jejunum (upper). These brush border enzymes are required for digestion mainly because disaccharides—e.g., sucrose, lactose—are not absorbed from the gut.

- The α-dextrinase cleaves terminal α-1,4 bonds, producing free glucose.
- Lactase hydrolyzes lactose into glucose and galactose. Lactase deficiency (lactose intolerance) leads to osmotic diarrhea.
- Sucrase splits sucrose into glucose and fructose.
- Maltase (also a brush border enzyme) breaks down the maltose and maltotriose to form 2 and 3 glucose units, respectively.
- The monosaccharide end products—glucose, galactose, and fructose—are readily absorbed from the small intestine, also mainly in the jejunum.

Proteins

Stomach: Pepsin begins the digestion of protein in the acid medium of the stomach; however, it is not an essential enzyme.

Small intestine: Digestion continues with the pancreatic proteases (trypsin, chymotrypsin, elastase, and carboxypeptidases A and B), which are essential enzymes.

Protein digestion is completed by the small intestinal brush border enzymes, dipeptidases, and an aminopeptidase. The main end products are amino acids (40%) and dipeptides and tripeptides (60%).

Pancreatic enzymes are required for triglyceride, CHO, and protein digestion. Circulating CCK is almost totally responsible for their secretion following a meal.

ABSORPTION

Carbohydrate and Protein

The following figure illustrates the major transport processes carrying sugars and amino acids across the luminal and basal membranes of cells lining the small intestine.

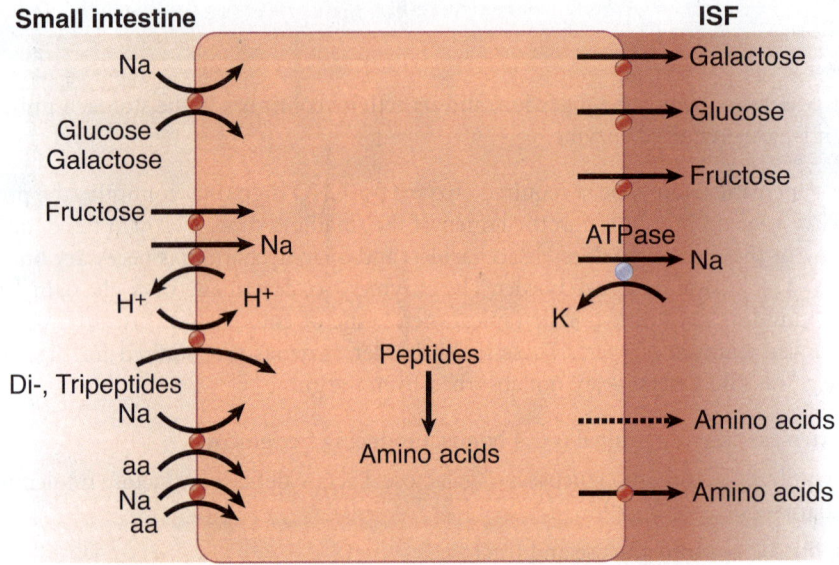

Figure 31-10. Absorption of Carbohydrates and Proteins

Bridge to Pathology

Celiac disease is an immune reaction to gluten (protein found in wheat) that damages intestinal cells; the end result is diminished absorptive capacity of the small intestine.

Carbohydrate

- **Luminal membrane:** Glucose and galactose are actively absorbed (secondary active transport linked to sodium) via the sodium-glucose linked transporter 1 (SGLT-1). Fructose is absorbed independently by facilitated diffusion.
- **Basal membrane:** The monosaccharides are absorbed passively mainly via facilitated diffusion.

Protein

- **Luminal membrane:** amino acids are transported by secondary active transport linked to sodium. Small peptides uptake powered by a Na-H antiporter.
- **Basal membrane:** simple diffusion of amino acids, although it is now known some protein-mediated transport also occurs.

Lipids

The end products of triglyceride digestion, 2-monoglycerides and fatty acids, remain as lipid-soluble substances that are then taken up by the micelles.

Digestive products of fats found in the micelles and absorbed from the intestinal lumen may include:

- Fatty acids (long chain)
- 2-Monoglyceride
- Cholesterol
- Lysolecithin
- Vitamins A, D, E, K
- Bile salts, which stabilize the micelles

Micelles diffuse to the brush border of the intestine. The diffusion through the unstirred layer is the rate-limiting step of fat absorption.

The digested lipids then diffuse across the brush border in the lipid matrix. In the mucosal cell, triglyceride is resynthesized and forms lipid droplets (chylomicrons). These leave the intestine via the lymphatic circulation (lacteals). They then enter the bloodstream via the thoracic duct. The more water-soluble short-chain fatty acids can be absorbed by simple diffusion directly into the bloodstream. The bile salts are actively reabsorbed in the distal ileum.

Electrolytes

The net transport of electrolytes along the length of the small and large intestine is summarized below.

Duodenum

- Hypertonic fluid enters this region, and following the movement of some water into the lumen, the fluid becomes and remains isotonic (see crypt secretion above).
- The absorption of most divalent ions and water-soluble vitamins begins here and continues through the small intestine.
- Injested iron and calcium tend to form insoluble salts. The acid environment of the stomach redissolves these salts, which facilitates their absorption in the small intestine. Iron and calcium absorption is diminished in individuals with a deficient stomach acid secretion.
- Calcium absorption is enhanced by the presence of calbindin in intestinal cells, and calcitriol (active vitamin D) induces the synthesis of this protein.
- Intestinal cells express the protein ferritin, which facilitates iron absorption.

Jejunum

- Overall, there is a net reabsorption of water and electrolytes.
- The cellular processes involved are almost identical to those described in the renal physiology section for the cells lining the nephron proximal tubule.

Ileum

- Net reabsorption of water, sodium, chloride, and potassium continues, but there begins a net secretion of bicarbonate.

- It is in the distal ileum, and only in the distal ileum, where the reabsorption of bile salts and intrinsic factor with vitamin B_{12} takes place.

Colon

- The colon does not have digestive enzymes or the protein transporters to absorb the products of carbohydrate and protein digestion.

- Also, because bile salts are reabsorbed in the distal ileum, very few lipid-soluble substances are absorbed in the colon.

- There is a net reabsorption of water and sodium chloride, but there are limitations.

- Most of the water and electrolytes must be reabsorbed in the small intestine, or the colon becomes overwhelmed.

- Most of the water and electrolytes are absorbed in the ascending and transverse colon; thereafter, the colon has mainly a storage function.

- The colon is a target for aldosterone, where it increases sodium and water reabsorption and potassium secretion.

- Because there is a net secretion of bicarbonate and potassium, diarrhea usually produces a metabolic acidosis and hypokalemia. It commonly presents as hyperchloremic, nonanion gap metabolic acidosis, as described in the acid-base section.

Diarrhea

Except for the infant where it can be hypotonic, diarrhea is a loss of isotonic fluid that is high in bicarbonate and potassium.

Anatomy

Gonad Development

1

Learning Objectives

- ❏ Explain information related to indifferent gonad
- ❏ Interpret scenarios on testis and ovary
- ❏ Answer questions about meiosis
- ❏ Interpret scenarios on spermatogenesis
- ❏ Solve problems concerning oogenesis

INDIFFERENT GONAD

Although sex is determined at fertilization, the gonads initially go through an **indifferent stage** between weeks 4 and 7 when there are no specific ovarian or testicular characteristics.

The indifferent gonads develop in a longitudinal elevation or ridge of **intermediate mesoderm** called the **urogenital ridge**.

Primordial Germ Cells

Primordial germ cells arise from the lining cells in the **wall of the yolk sac**.

At week 4, primordial germ cells migrate into the indifferent gonad.

Components of the Indifferent Gonad

- **Primordial germ cells** migrate into the gonad from the yolk sac and provide a critical inductive influence on gonad development.
- **Primary sex cords** are fingerlike extensions of the surface epithelium that grow into the gonad that are populated by the migrating primordial germ cells.
- **Mesonephric (Wolffian)** and the **paramesonephric (Mullerian)** ducts of the indifferent gonad contribute to the male and female genital tracts, respectively.

TESTIS AND OVARY

The indifferent gonad will develop into either the testis or ovary.

Testis

Development of the testis and male reproductive system is directed by:

- The **Sry gene** on the short arm of the **Y chromosome**, which encodes for **testis-determining factor** (TDF)
- **Testosterone,** which is secreted by the **Leydig cells**
- **Müllerian-inhibiting factor (MIF)**, which is secreted by the **Sertoli cells**
- **Dihydrotestosterone (DHT):** external genitalia

Ovary

Development of the female reproductive system requires estrogen.

MEIOSIS

Meiosis occurs within the testis and ovary. This is a specialized process of cell division that produces the male gamete (**spermatogenesis**) and female gamete (**oogenesis**). There are notable differences between spermatogenesis and oogenesis, discussed below.

Meiosis consists of two cell divisions, meiosis I and meiosis II.

Meiosis I

In meiosis I, the following events occur:

- **Synapsis**—the pairing of 46 homologous chromosomes
- **Crossing over**—the exchange of segments of DNA
- **Disjunction**—the separation of 46 homologous chromosome pairs (no centromere-splitting) into 2 daughter cells, each containing 23 chromosome pairs

Meiosis II

In meiosis II:

- Synapsis does not occur.
- Crossing over does not occur.
- Disjunction occurs **with** centromere-splitting.

SPERMATOGENESIS

- Primordial germ cells arrive in the indifferent gonad at week 4 and remain **dormant until puberty**.
- When a boy reaches puberty, primordial germ cells differentiate into **type A spermatogonia,** which serve as stem cells throughout adult life.
- Some type A spermatogonia differentiate into **type B spermatogonia.**
- Type B spermatogonia enter meiosis I to form **primary spermatocytes.**
- Primary spermatocytes form 2 **secondary spermatocytes.**
- Secondary spermatocytes enter meiosis II to form 2 **spermatids.**
- Spermatids undergo **spermiogenesis**, which is a series of morphological changes resulting in the mature **spermatozoa.**

OOGENESIS

- Primordial germ cells arrive in the indifferent gonad at week 4 and differentiate into oogonia.
- Oogonia enter meiosis I to form **primary oocytes**. All primary oocytes are formed by **month 5 of fetal life** and are **arrested the first time in prophase (diplotene) of meiosis I** and remain arrested until puberty.
- Primary oocyte arrested in meiosis I are present at birth.
- When a girl reaches puberty, during each monthly cycle a primary oocyte becomes unarrested and completes meiosis I to form a secondary oocyte and polar body.
- The secondary oocyte becomes **arrested the second time in metaphase of meiosis II** and is ovulated.
- At fertilization within the uterine tube, the secondary oocyte completes meiosis II to form a **mature oocyte** and **polar body.**

Learning Objectives

❏ Solve problems concerning beginning of development

BEGINNING OF DEVELOPMENT

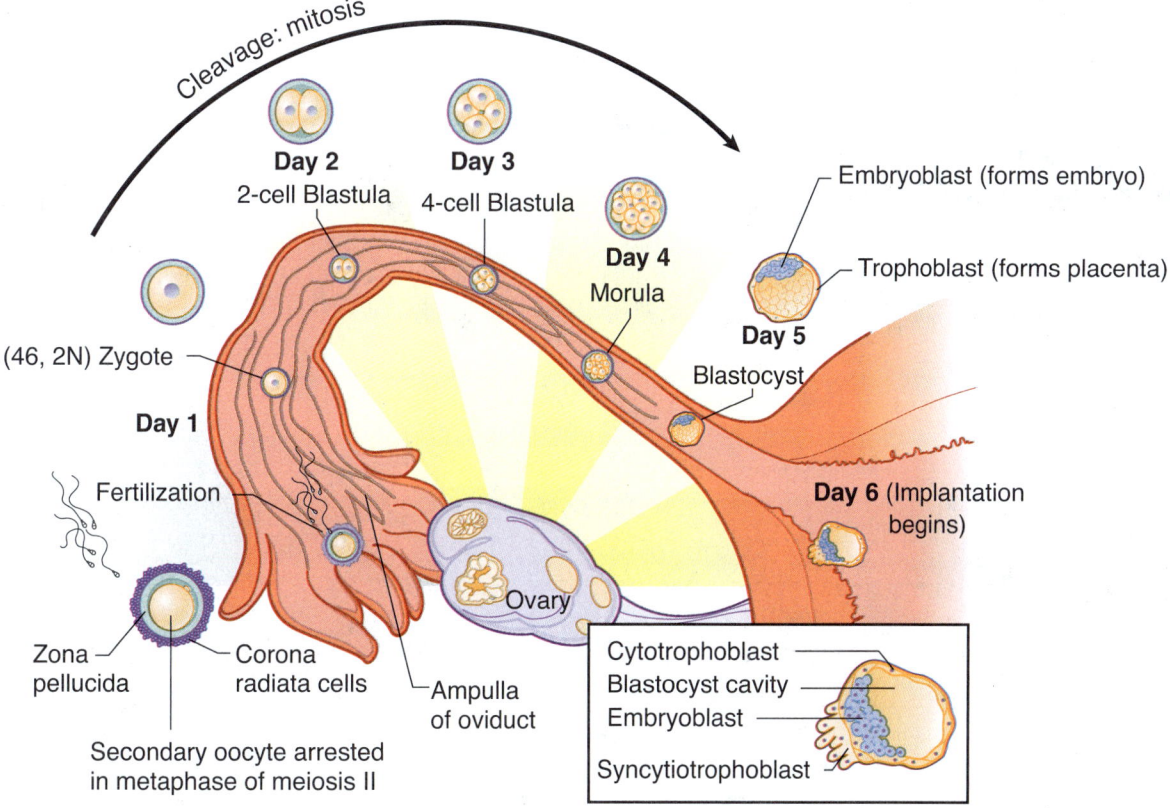

Figure 2-1. Week 1

Fertilization occurs in the **ampulla of the uterine tube** when the male and female pronuclei fuse to form a **zygote**. At fertilization, the secondary oocyte rapidly completes meiosis II.

Prior to fertilization, spermatozoa undergo changes in the female genital tract:

1. **Capacitation**: Occurs over about 7 hours in the female reproductive tract and consists of the removal of several proteins from the plasma membrane of the acrosome of the spermatozoa.
2. **Acrosome Reaction**: Release of hydrolytic enzymes from the acrosome used by the sperm to penetrate the zona pellucida. This results in a **cortical reaction** that prevents other spermatozoa penetrating the zona pellucida thus preventing polyspermy.

During the first 4 to 5 days of the first week, the zygote undergoes rapid mitotic division (**cleavage**) in the oviduct to form a **blastula**, consisting of increasingly smaller **blastomeres**. This becomes the **morula** (32-cell stage).

A **blastocyst** forms as fluid develops in the morula. The blastocyst consists of an inner cell mass known as the **embryoblast**, and the outer cell mass known as the **trophoblast**, which becomes the placenta.

At the end of the first week, the trophoblast differentiates into the **cytotrophoblast** and **syncytiotrophoblast** and then implantation begins (see below).

Implantation

The **zona pellucida** must degenerate for implantation to occur.

The blastocyst usually implants within the **posterior wall of the uterus.** The embryonic pole of the blastocyst implants first. The blastocyst implants within the **functional layer** of the endometrium during the **progestational phase** of the menstrual cycle.

Week 2: Formation of the Bilaminar Embryo

3

Learning Objectives

❏ Demonstrate understanding of the formation of the bilaminar embryo

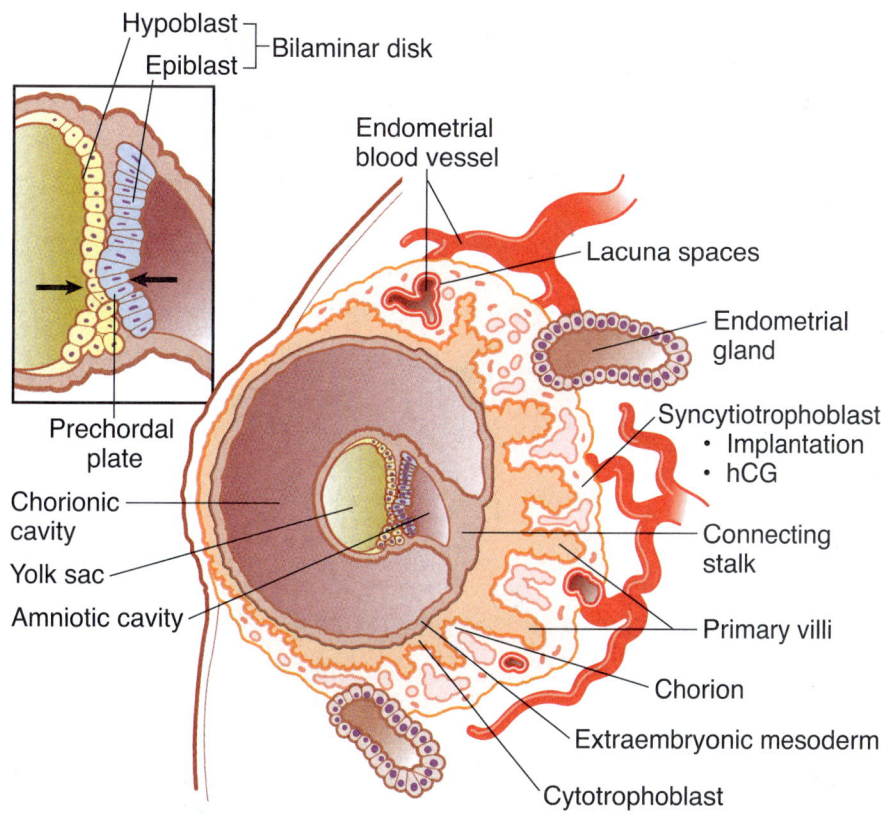

Figure 3-1. Week 2

- The embryoblast differentiates into the **epiblast** and **hypoblast**, forming a **bilaminar embryonic disk**.
- The epiblast forms the **amniotic cavity** and hypoblast cells migrate to form the **primary yolk sac**.
- The **prechordal plate**, formed from fusion of epiblast and hypoblast cells, is the site of the future **mouth**.

Extraembryonic mesoderm is derived from the epiblast. **Extraembryonic somatic mesoderm** lines the cytotrophoblast, forms the connecting stalk, and covers the amnion. **Extraembryonic visceral mesoderm** covers the yolk sac.

The connecting stalk suspends the conceptus within the chorionic cavity. The wall of the chorionic cavity is called the **chorion**, consisting of extraembryonic somatic mesoderm, the cytotrophoblast, and the syncytiotrophoblast.

The **syncytiotrophoblast** continues its growth into the endometrium to make contact with endometrial blood vessels and glands. **No mitosis occurs in the syncytiotrophoblast.** The cytotrophoblast is mitotically active.

Hematopoiesis occurs initially in the mesoderm surrounding the yolk sac (up to 6 weeks) and later in the fetal liver, spleen, thymus (6 weeks to third trimester), and bone marrow.

Learning Objectives

❑ Solve problems concerning embryonic period

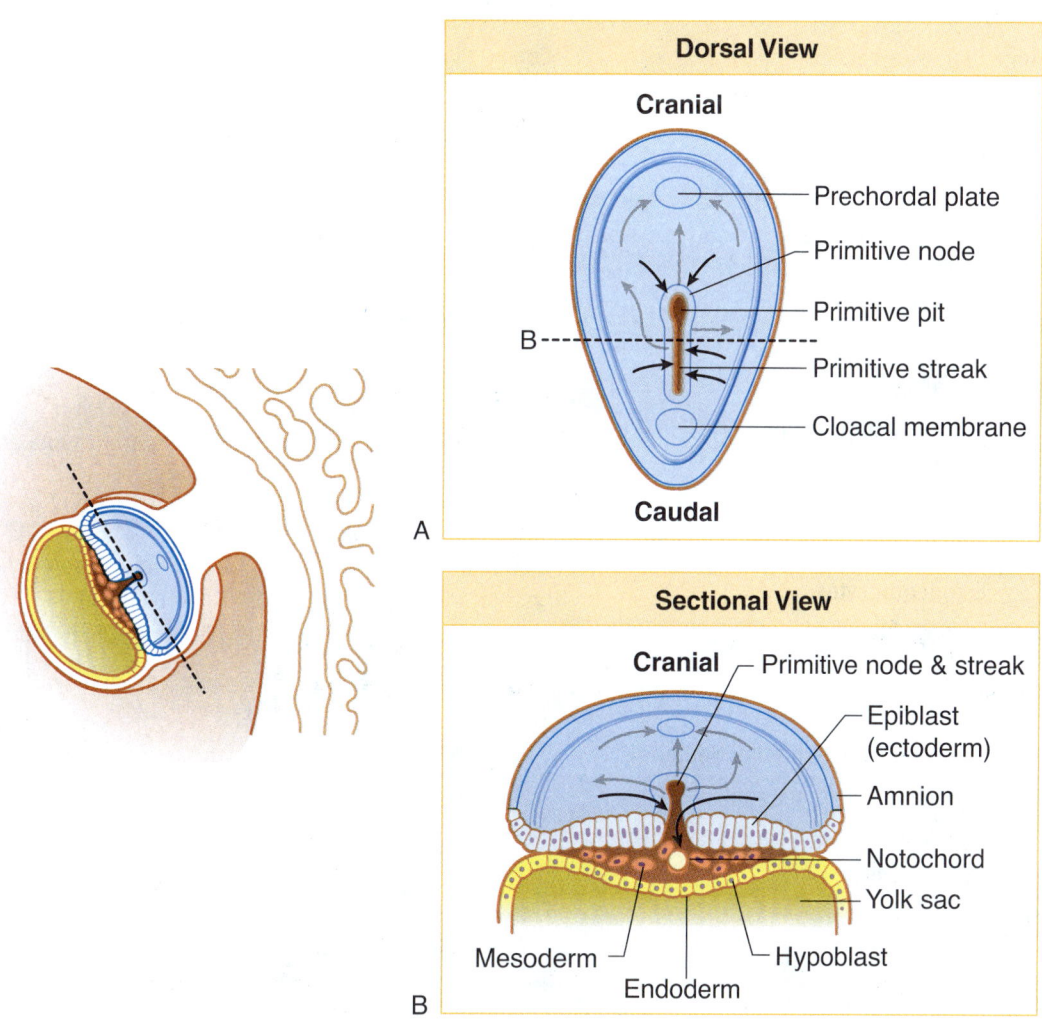

Figure 4-1. Week 3

- **Gastrulation**—process that produces the three primary germ layers: **ectoderm, mesoderm,** and **endoderm;** begins with the formation of the **primitive streak** within the epiblast
- Ectoderm forms **neuroectoderm** and **neural crest cells.**
- Mesoderm forms **paraxial mesoderm** (35 pairs of somites), **intermediate mesoderm,** and **lateral mesoderm.**

- All major organ systems begin to develop during the **embryonic period (weeks 3–8)**. By the end of this period, the embryo begins to look human.
- **Third week:** Gastrulation and early development of nervous and cardiovascular systems; corresponds to first missed period.

Table 4-1. Germ Layer Derivatives

Ectoderm	Mesoderm	Endoderm
Surface ectoderm	**Muscle**	**Forms epithelial lining of:**
Epidermis	Smooth	GI track: foregut, midgut, and hindgut
Hair	Cardiac	Lower respiratory system: larynx, trachea, bronchi, and lung
Nails	Skeletal	
Inner ear, external ear	Connective tissue	Genitourinary system: urinary bladder, urethra, and lower vagina
Enamel of teeth	All serous membranes	
Lens of eye	Bone and cartilage	Pharyngeal pouches:
Anterior pituitary (Rathke's pouch)	Blood, lymph, cardiovascular organs	• Auditory tube and middle ear
Parotid gland	Adrenal cortex	• Palatine tonsils
Anal canal below pectinate line	Gonads and internal reproductive organs	• Parathyroid glands
Neuroectoderm	Spleen	• Thymus
Neural tube	Kidney and ureter	**Forms parenchyma of:**
Central nervous system	Dura mater	• Liver
Retina and optic nerve	**Notochord**	• Pancreas
Pineal gland	Nucleus pulposus	• Submandibular and sublingual glands
Neurohypophysis		• Follicles of thyroid gland
Astrocytes		
Oligodendrocytes		
Neural crest ectoderm		
Adrenal medulla		
Ganglia		
Sensory—Pseudounipolar Neurons		
Autonomic—Postganglionic Neurons		
Pigment cells		
Schwann cells		
Meninges		
Pia and arachnoid mater		
Pharyngeal arch cartilage		
Odontoblasts		
Parafollicular (C) cells		
Aorticopulmonary septum		
Endocardial cushions		

Yolk sac derivatives:

  Primordial germ cells
  Early blood cells and blood vessels

Histology: Epithelia 5

Learning Objectives

❏ Demonstrate understanding of epithelial cells

❏ Use knowledge of epithelium

❏ Interpret scenarios on cytoskeletal elements

❏ Explain information related to cell adhesion molecules

❏ Answer questions about cell surface specializations

Histology is the study of normal tissues. Groups of cells make up tissues, tissues form organs, organs form organ systems, and systems make up the organism. Each organ consists of four different types of tissue: epithelial, connective, nervous, and muscular. Only certain aspects of epithelia will be reviewed in this section; other aspects of cell biology and histology are reviewed elsewhere.

EPITHELIAL CELLS

Epithelial cells are often polarized: the structure, composition, and function of the apical surface membrane differ from those of the basolateral surfaces. The polarity is established by the presence of tight junctions that separate these two regions. Internal organelles are situated symmetrically in the cell. Membrane polarity and tight junctions are essential for the transport functions of epithelia. Many simple epithelia transport substances from one side to the other (kidney epithelia transport salts and sugars; intestinal epithelia transport nutrients, antibodies, etc.). There are two basic mechanisms used for these transports:

1. A transcellular pathway through which larger molecules and a combination of diffusion and pumping in the case of ions that pass through the cell, and

2. A paracellular pathway that permits movement between cells.

Tight junctions regulate the paracellular pathway, because they prevent backflow of transported material and keep basolateral and apical membrane components separate.

Epithelial polarity is essential to the proper functioning of epithelial cells; and when polarity is disrupted, disease can develop. For example, epithelia lining the trachea, bronchi, intestine, and pancreatic ducts transport chloride from basolateral surface to lumen via pumps in the basolateral surface and channels in the apical surface. The transport provides a driving force for Na by producing electrical polarization of the epithelium. Thus NaCl moves across, and water follows. In cystic fibrosis the apical Cl channels do not open. Failure of water transport results in thickening of the mucus layer covering the epithelia.

Transformed cells may lose their polarized organization, and this change can be easily detected by using antibodies against proteins specific for either the apical or basolateral surfaces. Loss of polarity in the distribution of membrane proteins may eventually become useful as an early index of neoplasticity.

Epithelia are always lined on the basal side by connective tissue containing blood vessels. Since epithelia are avascular, interstitial tissue fluids provide epithelia with oxygen and nutrients.

Epithelia modify the two compartments that they separate by either secreting into or absorbing from them and by selective transport of solutes from one side of the barrier to the other.

Epithelia renew themselves continuously, some very rapidly (skin and intestinal linings), some at a slower rate. This means that the tissue contains stem cells that continuously proliferate. The daughter cells resulting from each cell division either remain in the pool of dividing cells or differentiate.

Epithelial Subtypes

- Simple cuboidal epithelium (e.g., renal tubules, salivary gland acini)
- Simple columnar epithelium (e.g., small intestine)
- Simple squamous epithelium (e.g., endothelium, mesothelium, epithelium lining the inside of the renal glomerular capsule)
- Stratified squamous epithelium
  – Nonkeratinized (e.g., esophagus)
  – Keratinizing (e.g., skin)
- Pseudostratified columnar epithelium (e.g., trachea, epididymis)
- Transitional epithelium (urothelium) (e.g., ureter and bladder)
- Stratified cuboidal epithelium (e.g., salivary gland ducts)

EPITHELIUM

Hematoxylin-and-Eosin Staining

The most common way to stain tissues for viewing in the light microscope is to utilize hematoxylin-and-eosin (H&E) staining.

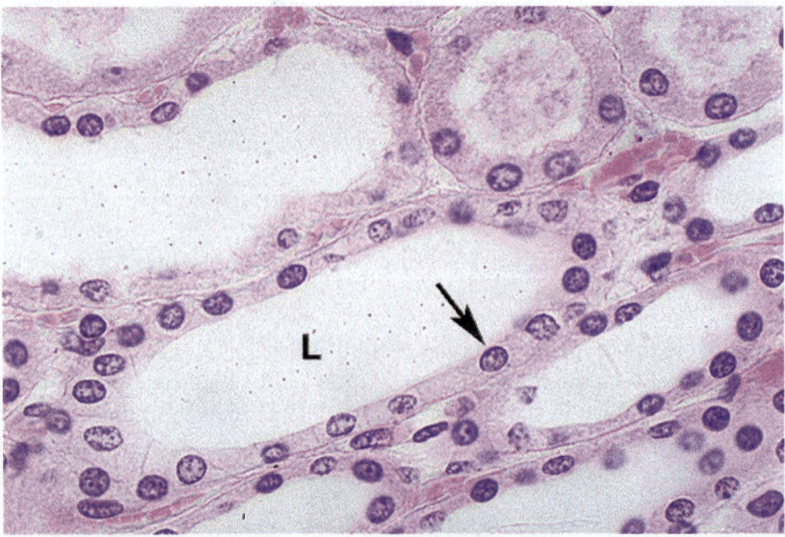

Copyright McGraw-Hill Companies. Used with permission.

Figure 5-1. Kidney tubule simple cuboidal epithelium (arrow) stained with H&E, L-lumen

Hematoxylin is a blue dye which stains basophilic substrates that are the acidic cellular components such as DNA and RNA. Hematoxylin stains nuclei blue, and may tint the cytoplasm of cells with extensive mRNA in their cytoplasm.

Eosin is a pink-to-orange dye which stains acidophilic substrates such as basic components of most proteins. Eosin stains the cytoplasm of most cells and many extracellular proteins, such as collagen, pink.

Epithelial Types

Simple columnar epithelium is found in the small and large intestine.

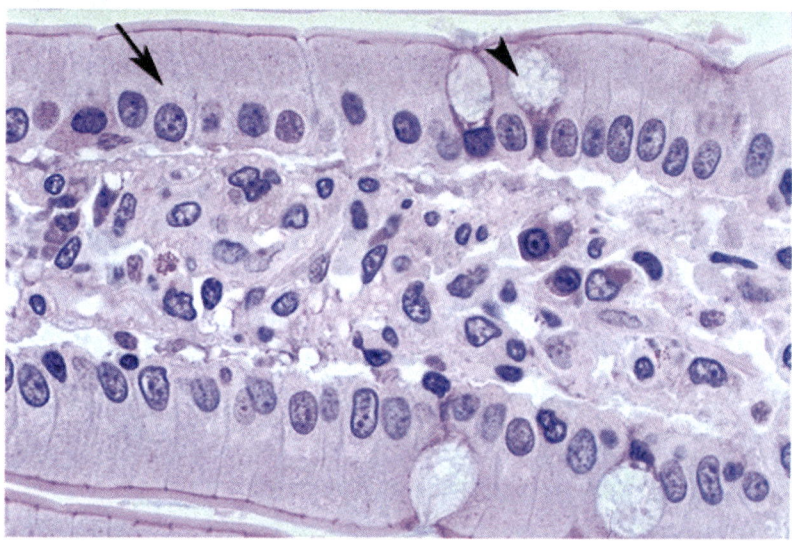

Copyright McGraw-Hill Companies. Used with permission.

Figure 5-2. Small Intestine Simple Columnar Epithelium
Enterocytes (arrow), Goblet cells (arrowhead)

Simple squamous epithelium forms an endothelium that lines blood vessels, a mesothelium that forms part of a serous membrane or forms the epithelium lining of the inside of the renal glomerular capsule.

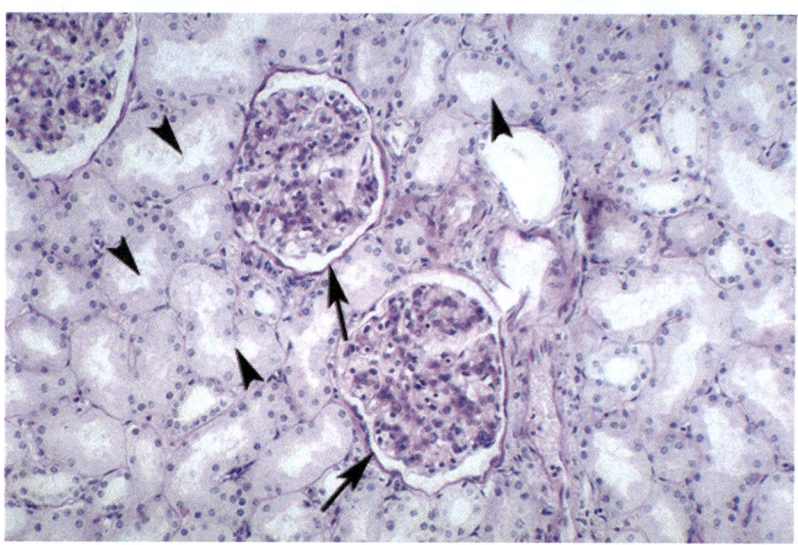

Copyright McGraw-Hill Companies. Used with permission.

Figure 5-3. Kidney simple squamous epithelium (arrows), simple cuboidal epithelium (arrowheads)

Pseudostratified columnar epithelium is found in the nasal cavity, trachea, bronchi, and epididymis.

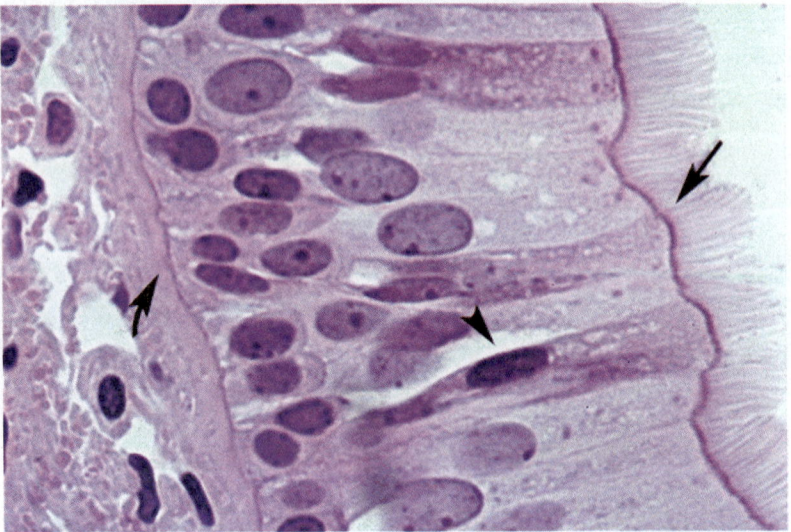

Figure 5-4. Trachea pseudostratified columnar epithelium with true cilia (arrow) and goblet cells (arrowhead), basement membrane (curved arrow)

Transitional epithelium is found in the ureter and bladder.

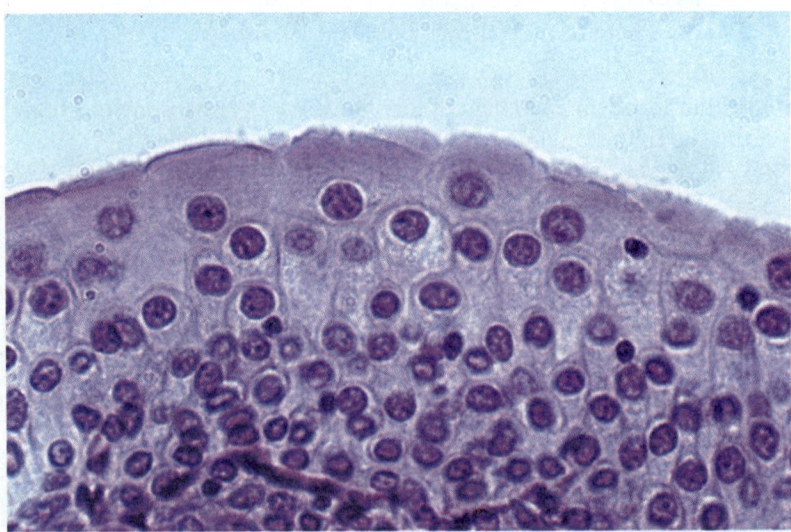

Figure 5-5. Bladder Transitional Epithelium

Stratified squamous epithelium is found in the oral cavity, pharynx, and esophagus (non-keratinized) and in the skin (keratinizing).

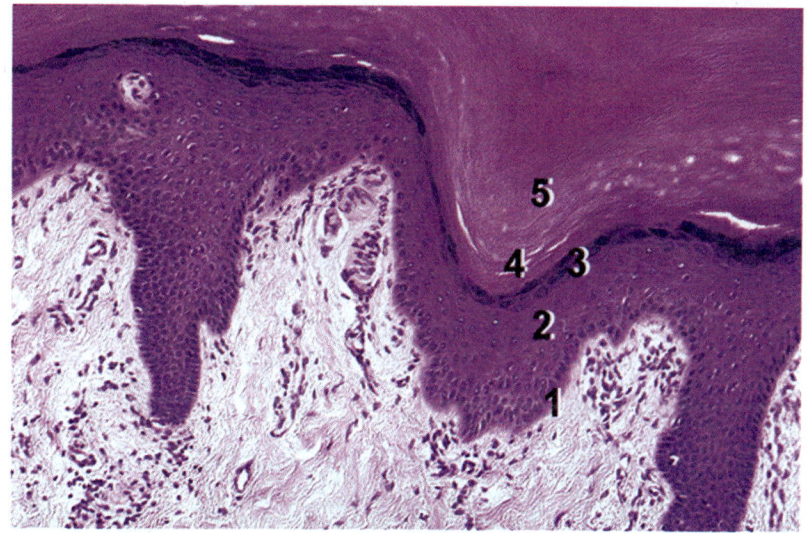

Figure 5-6. Stratified Squamous Epithelium (Thick Skin)
(1) stratum basale (2) stratum spinosum (3) stratum granulosum (4) stratum lucidum (5) stratum corneum

Simple cuboidal epithelium is the epithelium of the renal tubules and the secretory cells of salivary gland acini.

Stratified cuboidal epithelium is found in the ducts of salivary glands.

Note that more specific information on the salivary glands can be found in the Dental Anatomy section.

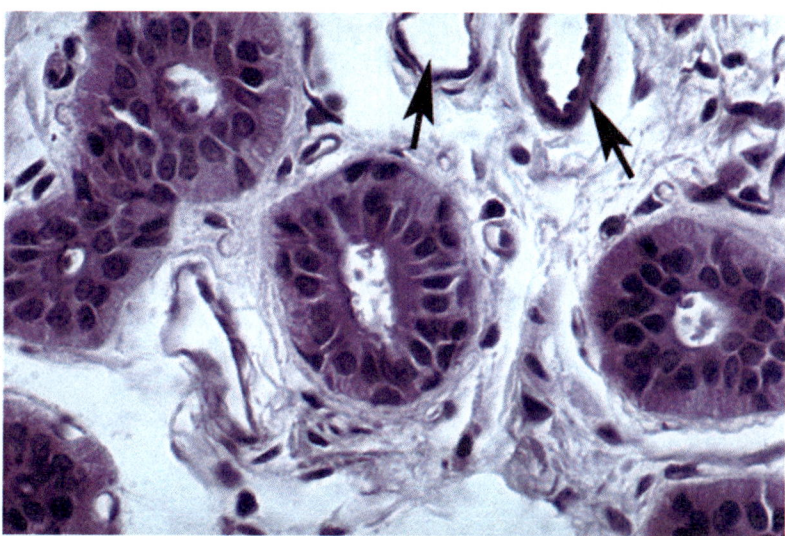

Figure 5-7. Ducts of salivary gland with stratified cuboidal epithelium small blood vessels with endothelium and smooth muscle (arrows)

Glands

- **Unicellular glands** are goblet cells found in the respiratory and GI epithelium.
- **Multicellular glands** may be exocrine (such as a salivary gland) or endocrine (as in the thyroid gland). All multicellular glands have tubules or acini formed mainly by a simple cuboidal epithelium. Only exocrine glands have ducts, which serve as conduits for glandular secretions to a body surface or to a lumen.

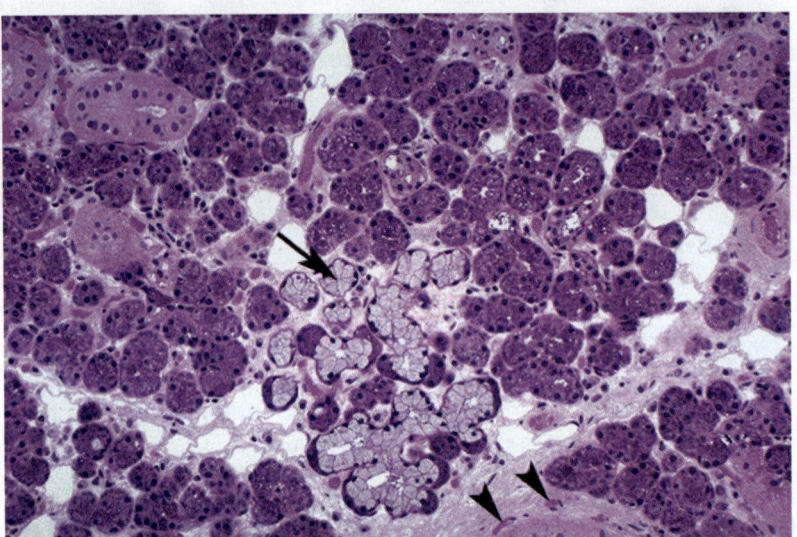

Copyright McGraw-Hill Companies. Used with permission.

Figure 5-8. Submandibular gland This gland is a mixed salivary gland with mucus acini (arrow) and darker staining serous acini; small blood vessels (arrowheads)

CYTOSKELETAL ELEMENTS

Microfilaments

Microfilaments are actin proteins. They are composed of globular monomers of G-actin that polymerize to form helical filaments of F-actin. Actin polymerization is ATP dependent. The F-actin filaments are 7-nm-diameter filaments that are constantly ongoing assembly and disassembly. F-actin has a distinct polarity. The barbed end (the plus end) is the site of polymerization and the pointed end is the site of depolymerization. Tread milling is the balance in the activity at the two ends.

In conjunction with myosin, actin microfilaments provide contractile and motile forces of cells including the formation of a contractile ring that provides a basis for cytokinesis during mitosis and meiosis. Actin filaments are linked to cell membranes at tight junctions and at the zonula adherens, and form the core of microvilli.

Intermediate Filaments

Intermediate filaments are 10-nm-diameter filaments that are usually stable once formed. These filaments provide structural stability to cells. There are four groups of intermediate filaments:

- **Type I** is keratins. Keratins are found in all epithelial cells.
- **Type II** is intermediate filaments comprising a diverse group.
  - Desmin is found in skeletal, cardiac, and gastrointestinal (GI) tract smooth muscle cells.
  - Vimentin is found in most fibroblasts, fibrocytes, endothelial cells, and vascular smooth muscle.
  - Glial fibrillary acidic protein is found in astrocytes and some Schwann cells.
  - Peripherin is found in peripheral nerve axons.
- **Type III** is intermediate filaments forming neurofilaments in neurons.
- **Type IV** is three types of lamins which form a meshwork rather than individual filaments inside the nuclear envelope of all cells.

Microtubules

Microtubules consist of 25-nm-diameter hollow tubes. Like actin, microtubules are undergoing continuous assembly and disassembly. They provide "tracks" for intracellular transport of vesicles and molecules. Such transport exists in all cells but is particularly important in axons. Transport requires specific ATPase motor molecules; **dynein** drives retrograde transport and **kinesin** drives anterograde transport. Microtubules are found in **true cilia and flagella**, and utilize dynein to convey motility to these structures. Microtubules form the mitotic spindle during mitosis and meiosis.

CELL ADHESION MOLECULES

Cell adhesion molecules are surface molecules that allow cells to adhere to one another or to components of the extracellular matrix. The expression of adhesion molecules on the surface of a given cell may change with time, altering its interaction with adjacent cells or the extracellular matrix.

Cadherin and selectin are adhesion molecules that are **calcium ion-dependent**. The extracellular portion binds to a cadherin dimer on another cell (trans binding). The cytoplasmic portions of cadherins are linked to cytoplasmic actin filaments by the catenin complex of proteins.

Integrins are adhesion molecules that are **calcium-independent**. They are transmembrane surface molecules with extracellular domains which bind to fibronectin and laminin, that are components of extracellular basement membrane. The cytoplasmic portions of integrins bind to actin filaments. Integrins form a portion of hemidesmosomes but are also important in interactions between leukocytes and endothelial cells.

CELL SURFACE SPECIALIZATIONS

Cell Adhesion

A cell must physically interact via cell surface molecules with its external environment, whether it be the extracellular matrix or **basement membrane**. The basement membrane is a sheet-like structure underlying virtually all epithelia, which consists of **basal lamina** (made of type IV collagen, glycoproteins [e.g., laminin], and proteoglycans [e.g., heparin sulfate]), and **reticular lamina** (composed of reticular fibers). Cell junctions anchor cells to each other, seal boundaries between cells, and form channels for direct transport and communication between cells. The three types of junctional complexes include **anchoring, tight,** and **gap junctions**.

Cell Junctions

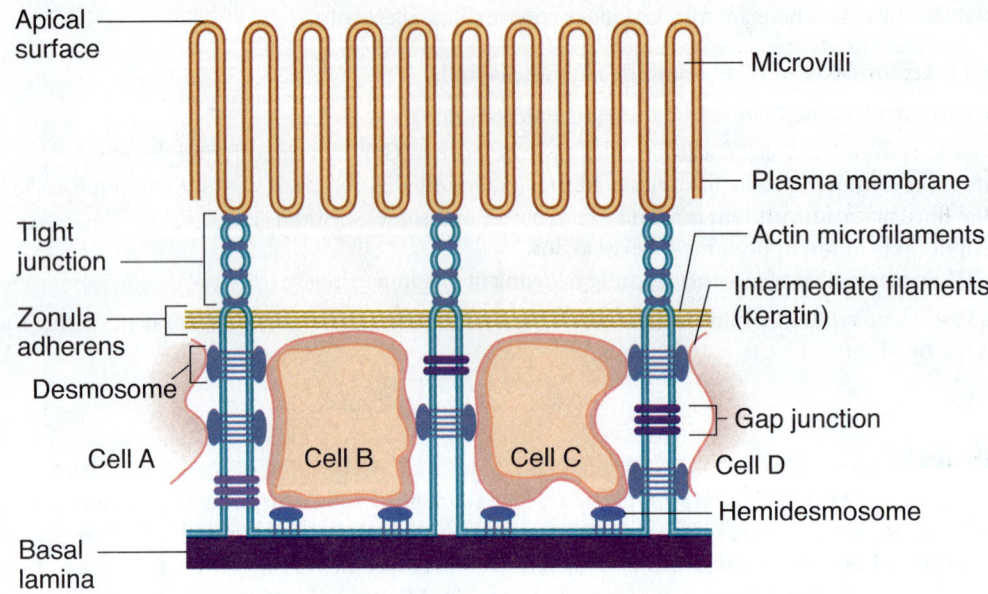

Figure 5-9. Junctions

Tight junctions (zonula occludens) function as barriers to diffusion and determine cell polarity. They form a series of punctate contacts of adjacent epithelial cells near the apical end or luminal surface of epithelial cells. The major components of tight junctions are occludins (ZO-1,2,3) and claudin proteins. These proteins span between the adjacent cell membranes and their cytoplasmic parts bind to actin microfilaments.

Zonula adherens forms a belt around the entire apicolateral circumference of the cell, immediately below the tight junction of epithelium. Cadherins span between the cell membranes. Like the tight junctions immediately above them, the cytoplasmic parts of cadherins are associated with actin filaments.

Desmosomes (macula adherens) function as anchoring junctions. Desmosomes provide a structural and mechanical link between cells. Cadherins span between the cell membranes of desmosomes and internally desmosomes are anchored to intermediate filaments in large bundles called tonofilaments.

Hemidesmosomes adhere epithelial cells to the basement membrane. The basement membrane is a structure that consists of the basal membrane of a cell and two underlying extracellular components, the basal lamina and the reticular lamina. The basal lamina is a thin felt-like extracellular layer composed of predominantly of type IV collagen associated with laminin, proteoglycans, and fibronectin that are secreted by epithelial cells. Fibronectin binds to integrins on the cell membrane, and fibronectin and laminin in turn bind to collagen in the basal lamina. Internally, like a desmosome, the hemidesmosomes are linked to intermediate filaments. Below the basal lamina is the reticular lamina, composed of reticular fibers.

Through the binding of extracellular components of hemidesmosomes to integrins, and thus to fibronectin and laminin, the cell is attached to the basement membrane and therefore to the extracellular matrix components outside the basement membrane. These interactions between the cell cytoplasm and the extracellular matrix have implications for permeability, cell motility during embryogenesis, and cell invasion by malignant neoplasms.

Clinical Correlate

Pemphigus Vulgaris (autoantibodies against desmosomal proteins in skin cells)

- Painful flaccid bullae (blisters) in oropharynx and skin that rupture easily
- Postinflammatory hyperpigmentation
- Treatment: corticosteroids

Bullous Pemphigoid (autoantibodies against basement-membrane hemidesmosomal proteins)

- Widespread blistering with pruritus
- Less severe than pemphigus vulgaris
- Rarely affects oral mucosa
- Can be drug-induced (e.g., middle-aged or elderly patient on multiple medications)
- Treatment: corticosteroids

Gap junctions (**communicating junctions**) function in cell-to-cell communication between the cytoplasm of adjacent cells by providing a passageway for ions such as calcium and small molecules such as cyclic adenosine monophosphate (cAMP). The transcellular channels that make up a gap junction consist of connexons, which are hollow channels spanning the plasma membrane. Each connexon consists of 6 connexin molecules. Unlike other intercellular junctions, gap junctions are not associated with any cytoskeletal filament.

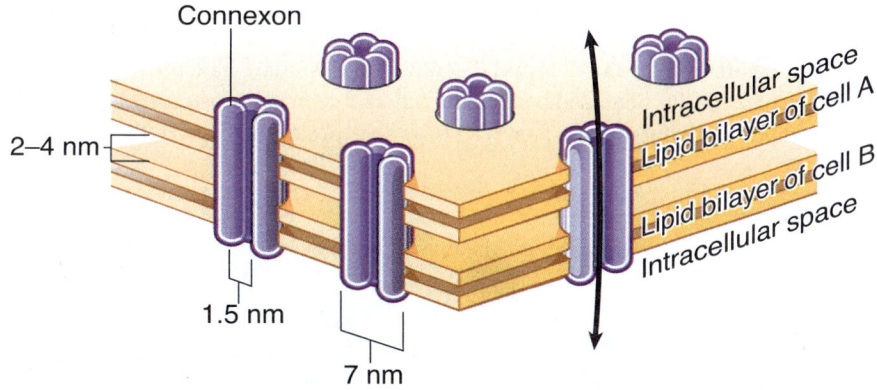

Figure 5-10. Gap junction

Gap junctions—direct passage for small particles and ions between cells via **connexon** channel proteins

Microvilli

Microvilli contain a core of actin microfilaments and function to increase the absorptive surface area of an epithelial cell. They are found in columnar epithelial cells of the small and large intestine, cells of the proximal tubule of the kidney and on columnar epithelial respiratory cells.

Stereocilia are long, branched microvilli that are found in the male reproductive tract (e.g., epididymis). Short stereocilia cap all sensory cells in the inner ear.

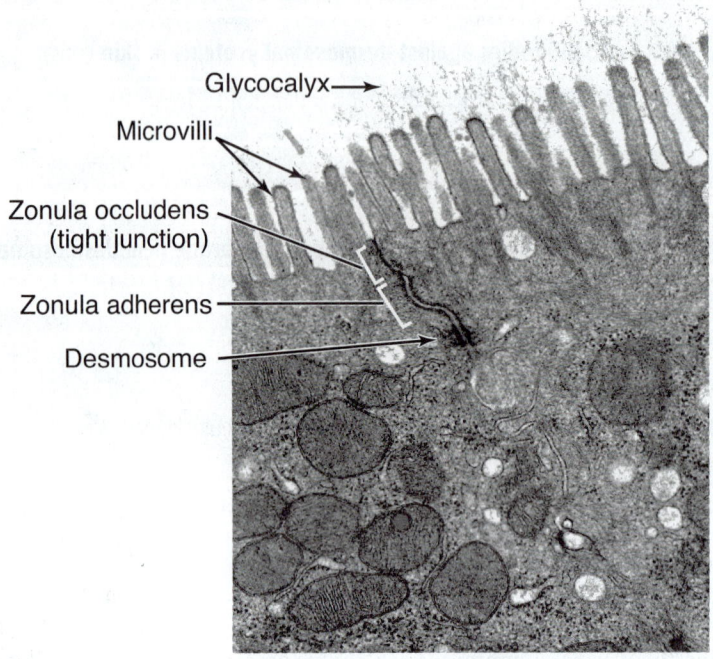

Figure 5-11. Apical cell surface/cell junctions

Cilia

Cilia contain 9 peripheral pairs of microtubules and 2 central microtubules. The microtubules convey motility to cilia through the ATPase dynein. Cilia bend and beat on the cell surface of pseudostratified ciliated columnar respiratory epithelial cells to propel overlying mucus. They also form the core of the flagella, the motile tail of sperm cells.

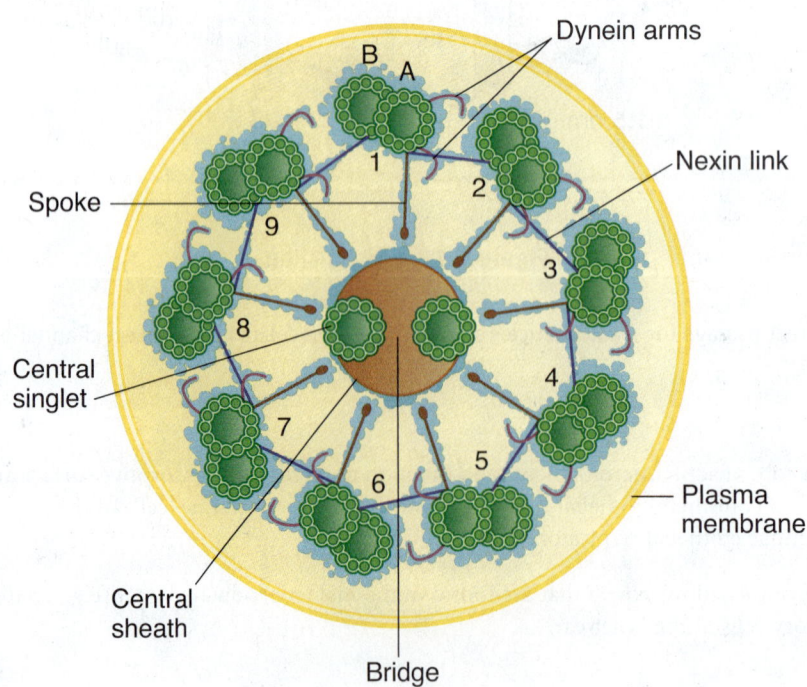

Figure 5-12. Structure of the axoneme of a cilium

Back and Autonomic Nervous System

6

Learning Objectives

❏ Solve problems concerning vertebral column

❏ Demonstrate understanding of spinal meninges

❏ Use knowledge of spinal nerves

❏ Use knowledge of autonomic nervous system

VERTEBRAL COLUMN

Embryology

During week 4, **sclerotome** cells of the somites (mesoderm) migrate medially to surround the spinal cord and notochord. After proliferation of the caudal portion of the sclerotomes, the vertebrae are formed, each consisting of the caudal part of one sclerotome and the cephalic part of the next.

Vertebrae

The vertebral column is the central component of the axial skeleton which functions in muscle attachments, movements, and articulations of the head and trunk.

- The vertebrae provide a flexible support system that transfers the weight of the body to the lower limbs and also provides protection for the spinal cord.
- The vertebral column is composed of 32–33 vertebrae (7 cervical, 12 thoracic, 5 lumbar, and the fused 5 sacral, and 3–4 coccygeal), intervertebral disks, synovial articulations (zygapophyseal joints) and ligaments.

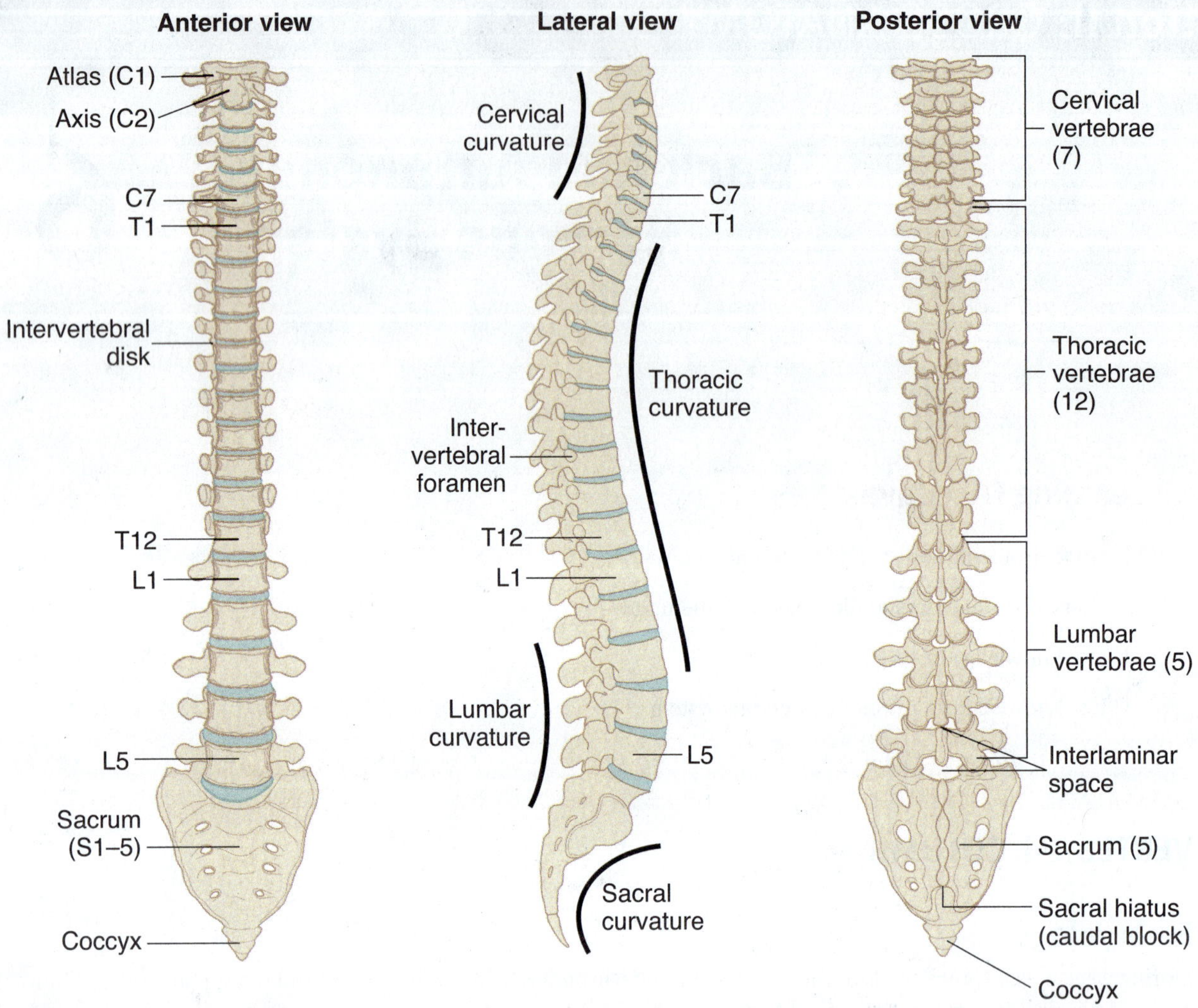

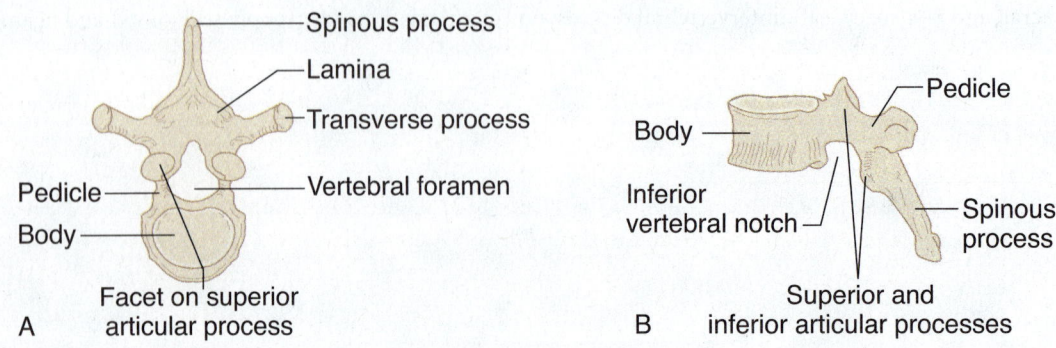

Anterior view

Atlas (C1)
Axis (C2)
C7
T1
Intervertebral disk
T12
L1
L5
Sacrum (S1–5)
Coccyx

Lateral view

Cervical curvature
C7
T1
Thoracic curvature
Inter-vertebral foramen
T12
L1
Lumbar curvature
L5
Sacral curvature

Posterior view

Cervical vertebrae (7)
Thoracic vertebrae (12)
Lumbar vertebrae (5)
Interlaminar space
Sacrum (5)
Sacral hiatus (caudal block)
Coccyx

Figure 6-1. Vertebral Column

~33 vertebrae
31 spinal nerves

A **typical vertebra** consists of an anterior **body** and a posterior **vertebral arch** consisting of 2 **pedicles** and 2 **laminae**. The vertebral arch encloses the **vertebral (foramen) canal** that houses the spinal cord. **Vertebral notches** of adjacent pedicles form **intervertebral foramina** that provide for the exit of the spinal nerves. The dorsal projecting **spines** and the lateral projecting **transverse processes** provide attachment sites for muscles and ligaments.

Spinous process
Lamina
Transverse process
Pedicle
Vertebral foramen
Body
Facet on superior articular process

A

Pedicle
Body
Inferior vertebral notch
Superior and inferior articular processes
Spinous process

B

Figure 6-2. Typical Vertebra

Intervertebral Disks

The **intervertebral disks** contribute to about 25% of the length of the vertebral column. They form the cartilaginous joints between the vertebral bodies and provide limited movements between the individual vertebrae.

- Each intervertebral disk is numbered by the vertebral body **above** the disk.
- Each intervertebral disk is composed of the following:
  - **Anulus fibrosus** consists of the outer concentric rings of fibrocartilage and fibrous connective tissue. The anuli connect the adjacent bodies and provide limited movement between the individual vertebrae.
  - **Nucleus pulposus** is an inner soft, elastic, compressible material that functions as a shock absorber for external forces placed on the vertebral column. The nucleus pulposus is the postnatal remnant of the **notochord.**

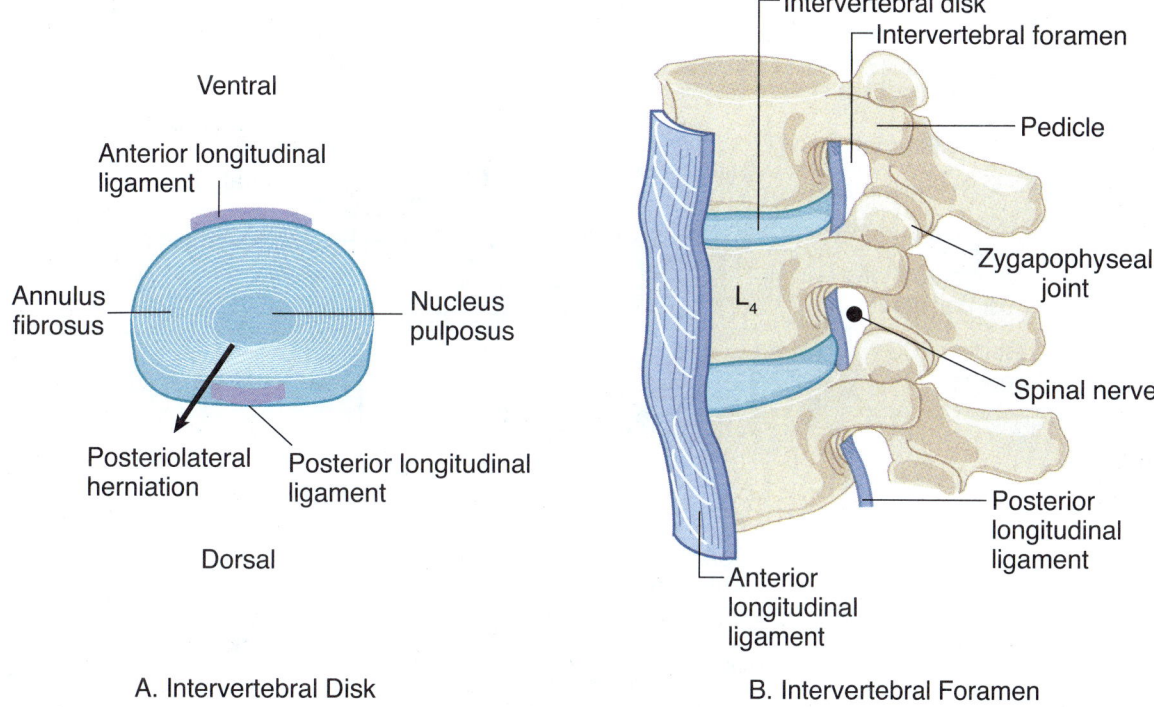

Figure 6-3. Intervertebral Disks

Ligaments of the Vertebral Column

The vertebral bodies are strongly supported by two longitudinal ligaments (Figure 6-3). Both ligaments are firmly attached to the intervertebral disks and to the bodies of the vertebrae.

- **Anterior longitudinal ligament**: The anterior ligament forms a broad band of fibers that connects the anterior surfaces of the bodies of the vertebrae between the cervical and sacral regions. It prevents **hyperextension** of the vertebrae and is often involved in "whiplash" accidents.
- **Posterior longitudinal ligament**: The posterior ligament connects the posterior surfaces of the vertebral bodies and is located in the vertebral canal. The posterior ligament limits **flexion** of the vertebral column. This ligament causes the herniation of a disk to be positioned **posterolaterally.**

Intervertebral Foramen

The intervertebral foramina (Figure 6-3B) are formed by successive intervertebral notches and provide for the passage of the **spinal nerve**. The boundaries of the foramina are:

- **Anterior: Bodies** of the vertebrae and **intervertebral disks**
- **Posterior:** Zygapophyseal joint and **articular processes**
- **Superior and inferior: Pedicles** of the vertebrae

SPINAL MENINGES

The spinal cord is protected and covered by three connective tissue layers within the vertebral canal: the pia mater, dura mater, and arachnoid.

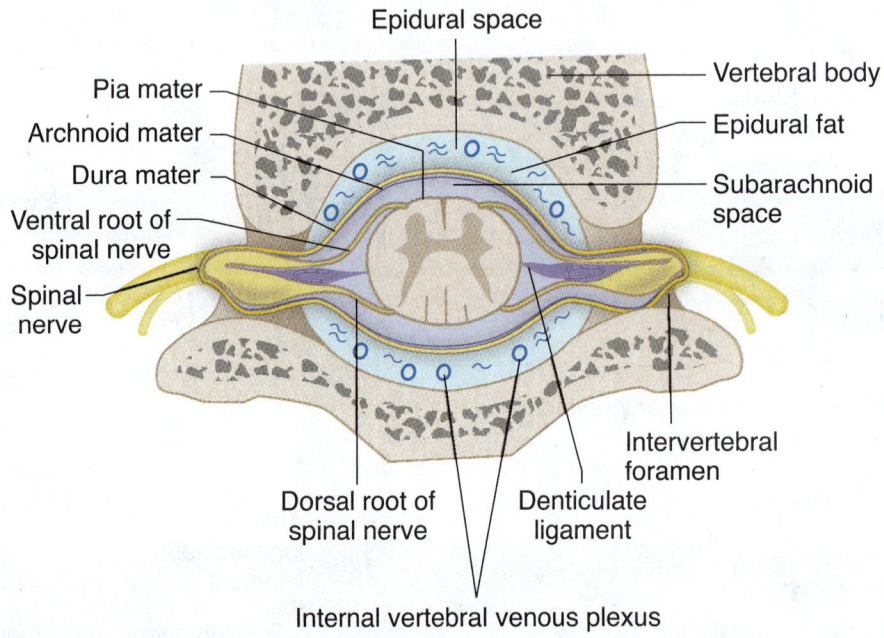

Figure 6-4. Cross-Section of Vertebral Canal

Pia Mater

The **pia mater** is tightly attached to the surface of the spinal cord and provides a delicate covering of the cord.

- The spinal cord, with its covering of pia mater, terminates at the **L1 or L2 vertebral levels** in the adult.
- There are two specializations of the pia mater that are attached to the spinal cord:
  - The **denticulate ligaments** are bilateral thickenings of pia mater that run continuously on the lateral sides of the midpoint of the cord. They separate the ventral and dorsal roots of the spinal nerves and anchor to the dura mater.
  - The **filum terminale** is a continuation of the pia mater distal to the lower end of the spinal cord. The filum terminale is part of the **cauda equina** which is composed of ventral and dorsal roots of lumbar and sacral nerves that extend below the inferior limit of the spinal cord.

Dura Mater

The **dura mater** is a tough, cylindrical covering of connective tissue forming a **dural sac** which envelops the entire spinal cord and cauda equina.

- The dura mater and dural sac terminate inferiorly at the **second sacral vertebra level**.
- Superiorly, the dura mater continues through the foramen magnum and is continuous with the meningeal layer of the cranial dura.

Arachnoid

The **arachnoid** is a delicate membrane which completely lines the inner surface of the dura mater and dural sac. It continues inferiorly and terminates at the **second sacral vertebra**.

Two Spaces Related to the Meninges

The **epidural space** is located between the inner walls of the vertebral canal and the dura mater. It contains fat and the **internal vertebral venous plexus.** The venous plexus runs the entire length of the epidural space and continues superiorly through the foramen magnum to connect with dural venous sinuses in the cranial cavity.

The **subarachnoid space** is a pressurized space located between the arachnoid and pia mater layers. It contains **cerebrospinal fluid (CSF)**, which bathes the spinal cord and spinal nerve roots within the dural sac, and terminates at the **second sacral vertebral level**.

Two Important Vertebral Levels

L1 or **L2** vertebrae: inferior limit of the **spinal cord** in adult (**conus medullaris**)

S2 vertebra: inferior limit of the **dural sac** and the **subarachnoid** space (cerebrospinal fluid)

SPINAL NERVES

There are 31 pairs of **spinal nerves** attached to each of the segments of the spinal cord: 8 cervical, 12 thoracic, 5 lumbar, 5 sacral, and 1 coccygeal. The spinal nerves with the cranial nerves form part of the **peripheral nervous system**.

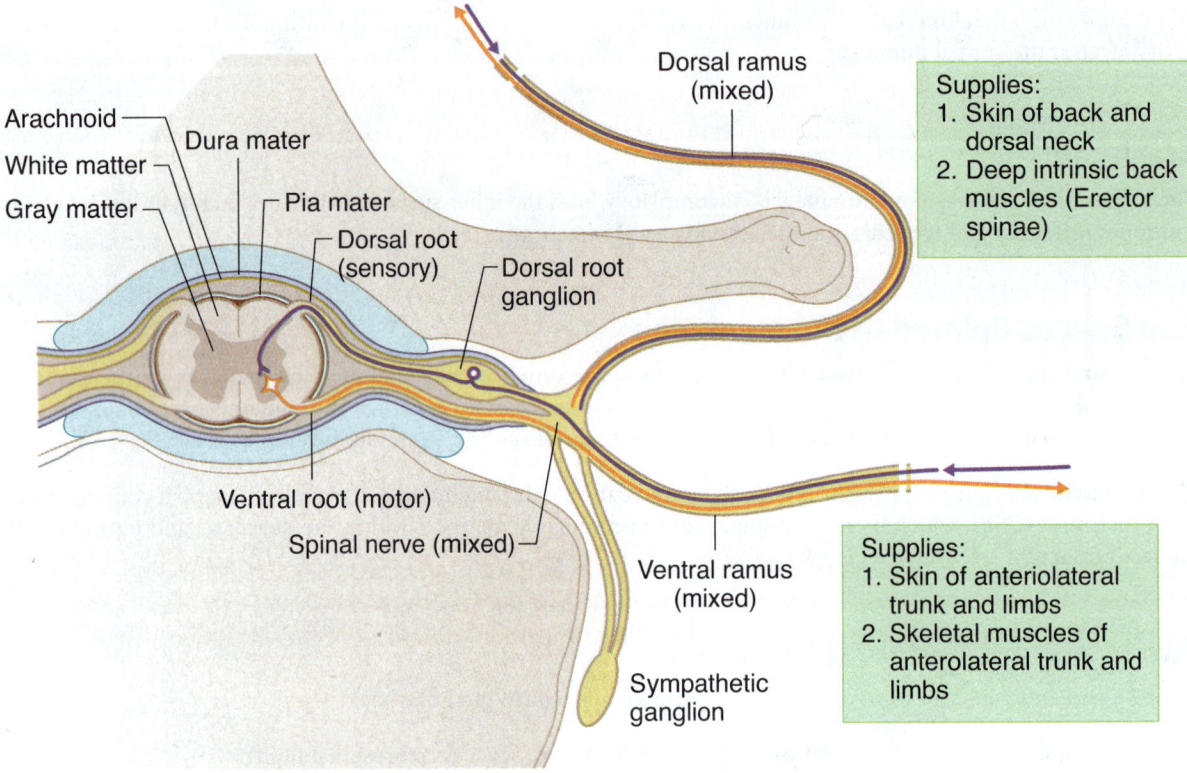

Figure 6-5. Cross Section of Spinal Cord and Parts of Spinal Nerve

Each spinal nerve is formed by the following components:

- **Dorsal root**: The dorsal root carries **sensory** fibers from the periphery into the dorsal aspect of the spinal cord. On each dorsal root there is a **dorsal root ganglion** (sensory) which contains the pseudounipolar cell bodies of the nerve fibers that are found in the dorsal root.

- **Ventral root**: The ventral root arises from the ventral aspect of the spinal cord and carries axons of **motor** neurons from the spinal cord to the periphery. The cell bodies of the axons in the ventral root are located in the ventral or lateral horns of the spinal- cord gray matter.

- **Spinal nerve**: The spinal nerve is formed by the union of the ventral and dorsal roots. The spinal nerve exits the vertebral column by passing through the intervertebral foramen.

- **Dorsal rami**: The dorsal rami innervate the skin of the dorsal surface of the back, neck, zygapophyseal joints, and intrinsic skeletal muscles of the deep back.

- **Ventral rami**: The ventral rami innervate the skin of the anterolateral trunk and limbs, and the skeletal muscles of the anterolateral trunk and limbs (ventral rami form the brachial and lumbosacral plexuses).

Relationship of Exit of Spinal Nerves and Vertebral Levels

The spinal nerves exit the vertebral column by a specific relationship to the vertebrae as described.

1. The cervical nerves C1–C7 exit the intervertebral foramina **superior** to the pedicles of the same-numbered vertebrae.

2. The C8 nerve exits the intervertebral foramen **inferior** to the C7 pedicle. This is the transition point.

3. All nerves beginning with T1 and below will exit the intervertebral foramina **inferior** to the pedicle of the same-numbered vertebrae.

AUTONOMIC NERVOUS SYSTEM

The autonomic nervous system (ANS) is concerned with the motor innervation of smooth muscle, cardiac muscle, and glands of the body.

Anatomically and functionally, the ANS is composed of two motor divisions: (1) **sympathetic** and (2) **parasympathetic** (Figure 6-6). In both divisions, two neurons form an autonomic pathway.

- **Preganglionic neurons** have their neuronal cell bodies in the **CNS** (formed by neuroectoderm); their axons exit in cranial and spinal nerves.
- **Postganglionic neurons** have cell bodies in **autonomic ganglia** in the **peripheral nervous system** (PNS) (formed by neural crest cells)

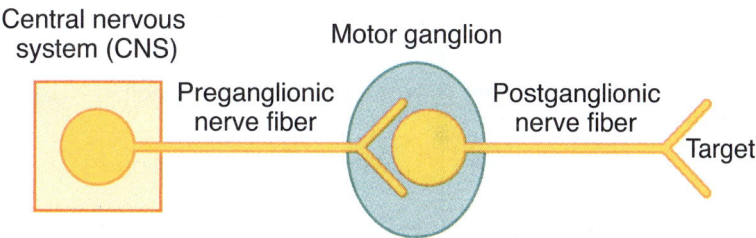

Figure 6-6. Autonomic Nervous System

Sympathetic Nervous System

The **preganglionic cell bodies** of the sympathetic nervous system are found in the **lateral horn** gray matter of spinal cord segments **T1–L2** (14 segments).

The **postganglionic cell bodies** of the sympathetic system are found in one of 2 types of motor ganglia in the PNS:

- Chain or paravertebral
- **Collateral or prevertebral** (found only in abdomen or pelvis)

Table 6-1. Sympathetic = Thoracolumbar Outflow

Origin (Preganglionic)	Site of Synapse (Postganglionic)	Innervation (Target)
Spinal cord levels T1–L2	Sympathetic chain ganglia (paravertebral ganglia)	Smooth muscle, cardiac muscle and glands of **body wall** and **limbs** (T1–L2), **head** (T1–2) and **thoracic viscera** (T1–5).
Thoracic splanchnic nerves T5–T12	Prevertebral ganglia (collateral) (e.g., celiac, aorticorenal, superior mesenteric ganglia)	Smooth muscle and glands of the **foregut** and **midgut**
Lumbar splanchnic nerves L1–L2	Prevertebral ganglia (collateral) (e.g., inferior mesenteric and pelvic ganglia)	Smooth muscle and glands of the **pelvic viscera** and **hindgut**

Note

m = muscle

a = artery

Gray rami
* Rejoin branches of spinal nerve to body wall and limps

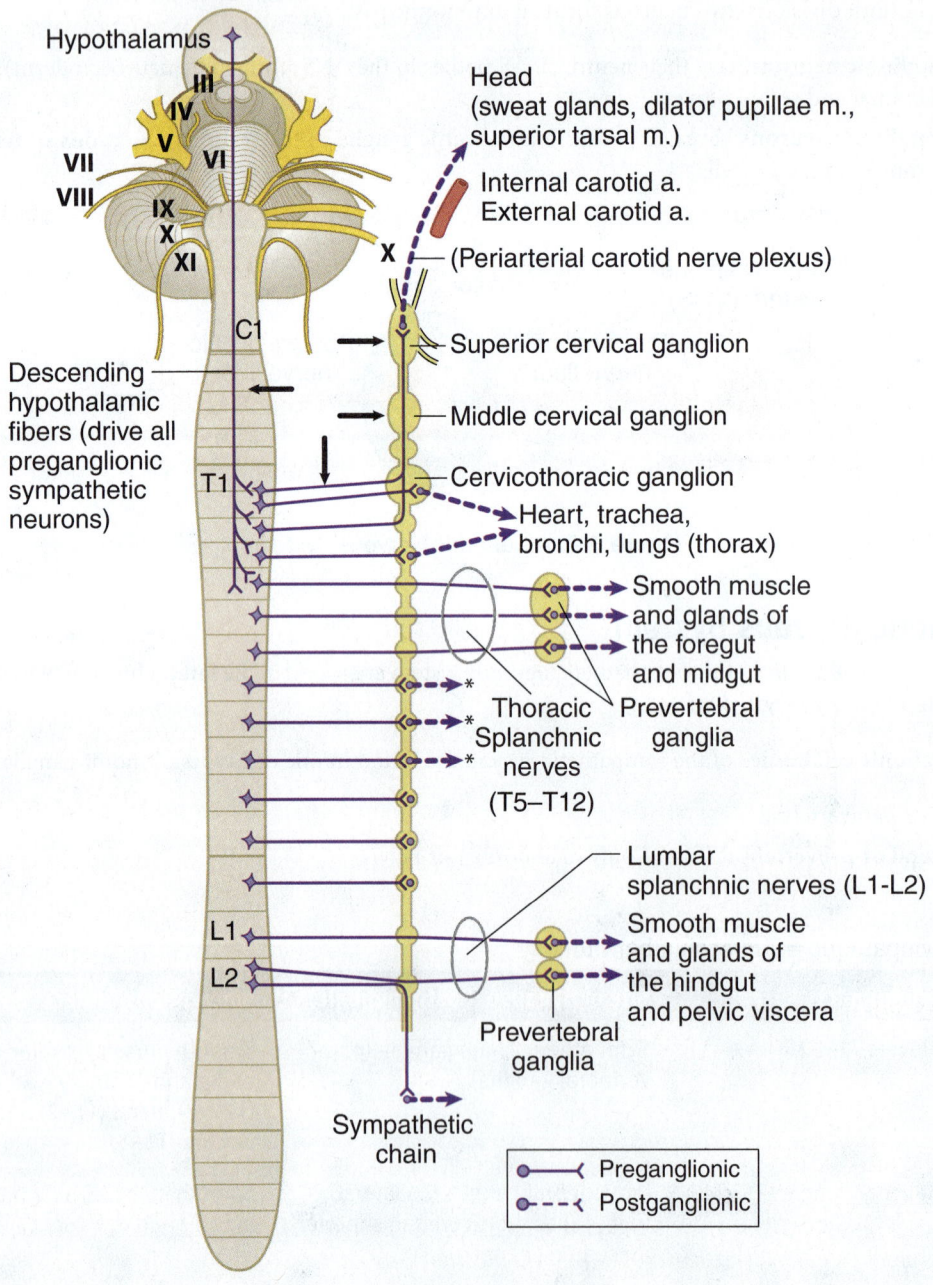

Figure 6-7. Overview of Sympathetic Outflow

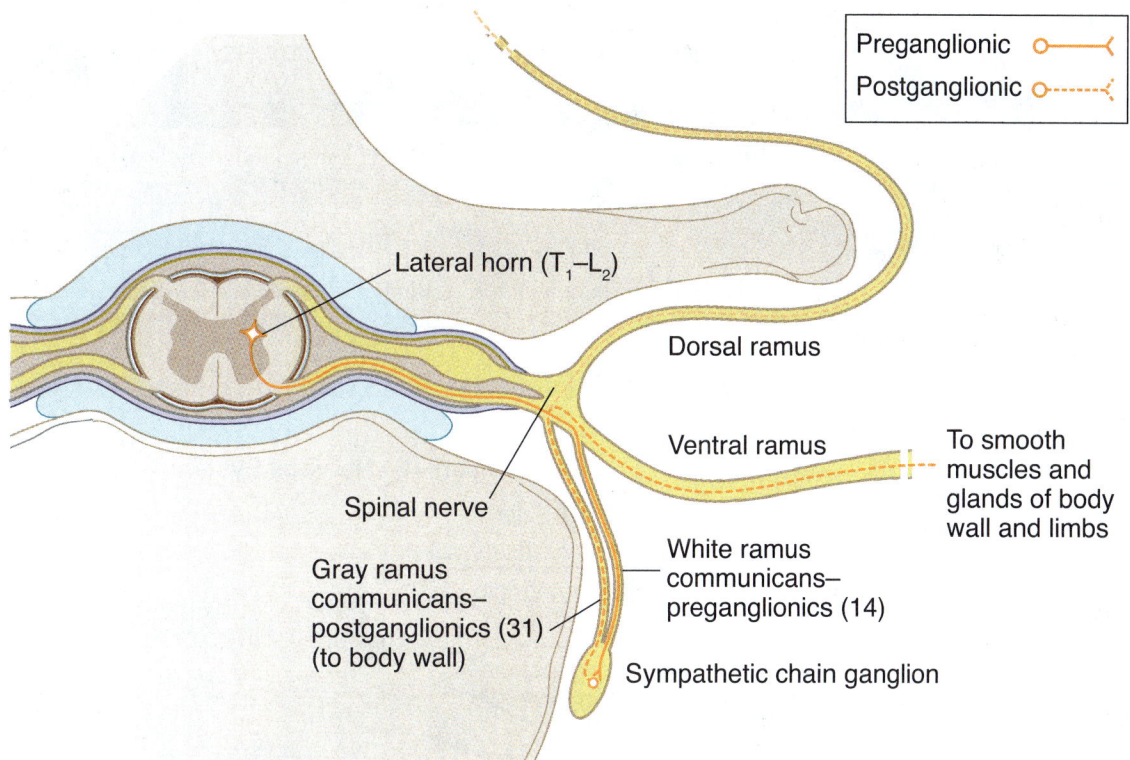

Preganglionic o——<
Postganglionic o----<

Lateral horn (T₁–L₂)

Dorsal ramus

Ventral ramus

To smooth muscles and glands of body wall and limbs

Spinal nerve

White ramus communicans– preganglionics (14)

Gray ramus communicans– postganglionics (31) (to body wall)

Sympathetic chain ganglion

Figure 6-8. Cross Section of Spinal Cord Showing Sympathetic Outflow

Note
White rami are preganglionic sympathetics that all enter the sympathetic trunk of ganglia. They may synapse with ganglion at point of entry or go up or down and synapse above or below point of entry. If a white ramus does not synapse, it passes through ganglion and becomes a root of a thoracic or lumbar splanchnic nerve.

Parasympathetic Nervous System

The **preganglionic cell bodies** of the parasympathetic nervous system are found in the **CNS** in one of 2 places:

- Gray matter of brain stem associated with **cranial nerves III, VII, IX, and X,** or
- Spinal cord gray in **sacral segments S2 3, and 4 (pelvic splanchnics)**

The **postganglionic cell bodies** of the parasympathetic nervous system are found in **terminal ganglia** in the PNS that are usually located near the organ innervated or in the wall of the organ.

Table 6-2. Parasympathetic = Craniosacral Outflow

Origin (Preganglionic)	Site of Synapse (Postganglionic)	Innervation (Target)
Cranial nerves III, VII, IX	4 cranial ganglia	Glands and smooth muscle of the **head**
Cranial nerve X	Terminal ganglia (in or near the walls of viscera)	Viscera of the neck, **thorax**, **foregut**, and **midgut**
Pelvic splanchnic nerves S 2, 3, 4	Terminal ganglia (in or near the walls of viscera)	**Hindgut** and **pelvic viscera** (including the bladder, rectum, and erectile tissue)

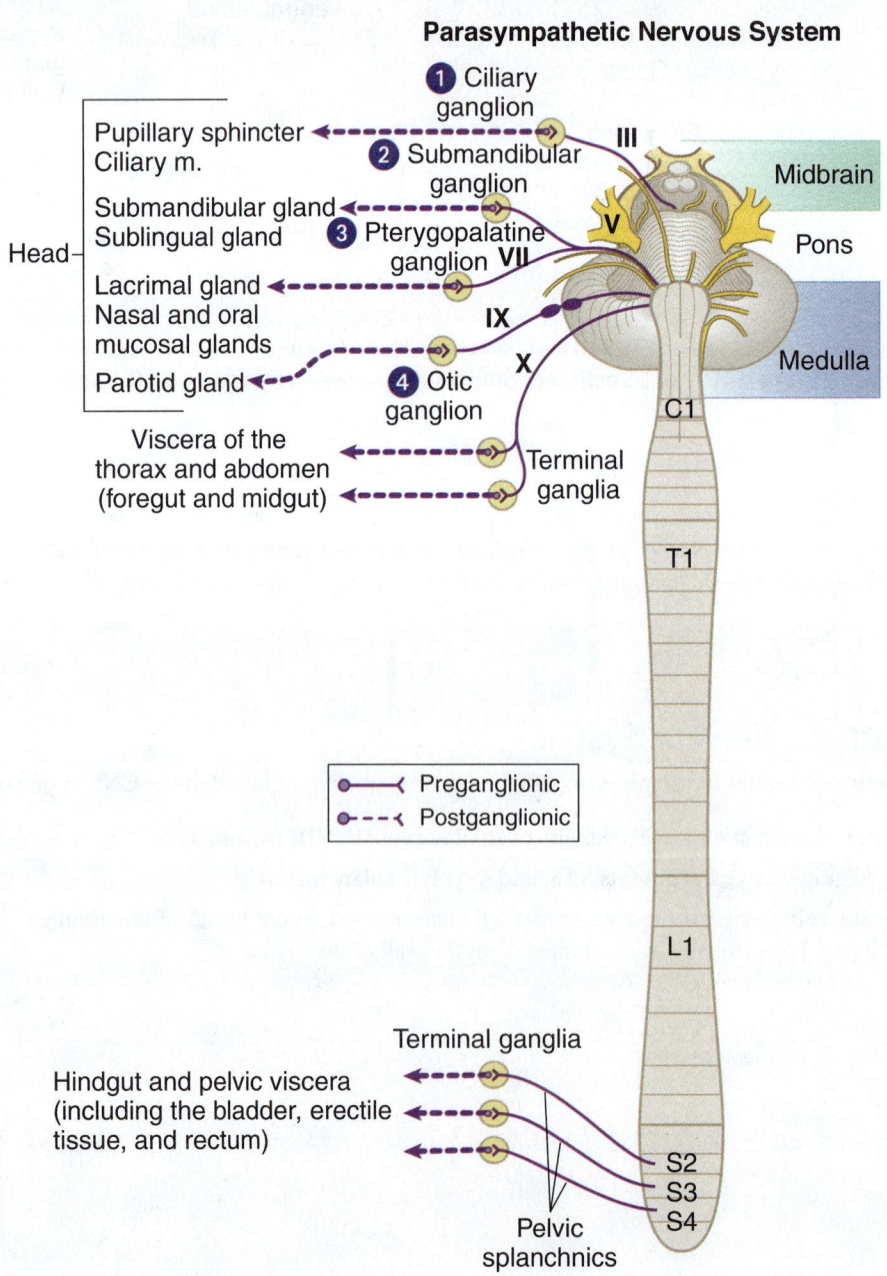

Figure 6-9. Overview of Parasympathetic Outflow

Learning Objectives

- ❏ Solve problems concerning the chest wall
- ❏ Use knowledge of pleura and pleural cavity
- ❏ Interpret scenarios on respiratory histology
- ❏ Solve problems concerning the mediastinum
- ❏ Interpret scenarios on heart histology

CHEST WALL

Breast

The breast (mammary gland) is a subcutaneous glandular organ of the superficial pectoral region. It is a modified sweat gland, specialized in women for the production and secretion of milk. A variable amount of fat surrounds the glandular tissue and duct system and is responsible for the shape and size of the female breast.

Cooper ligaments

Cooper ligaments are suspensory ligaments that attach the mammary gland to the skin and run from the skin to the deep fascia.

> **Clinical Correlate**
>
> The presence of a tumor within the breast can distort Cooper ligaments, which results in dimpling of the skin (orange-peel appearance).

Arterial supply

There is an extensive blood supply to the mammary tissues. The two prominent blood supplies are:

- **Internal thoracic artery (internal mammary)**, a branch of the subclavian artery which supplies the medial aspect of the gland.
- **Lateral thoracic artery**, a branch of the axillary artery which contributes to the blood supply to the lateral part of the gland. On the lateral aspect of the chest wall, the lateral thoracic artery courses with the **long thoracic nerve**, superficial to the serratus anterior muscle.

Lymphatic drainage

The lymphatic drainage of the breast is critical due to its important role in metastasis of breast cancer. The lymphatic drainage of the breast follows two primary routes:

1. Laterally, most of the lymphatic flow (75%) drains from the nipple and the superior, lateral, and inferior quadrants of the breast to the **axillary nodes**, initially to the **pectoral group**.

2. From the medial quadrant, most lymph drains to the **parasternal nodes**, which accompany the internal thoracic vessels. It is also through this medial route that cancer can spread to the **opposite breast**.

ADULT THORACIC CAVITY

The **thoracic cavity** is kidney-shaped on cross section and is bounded anterolaterally by the bony thorax (sternum, ribs, and intercostal spaces) and posteriorly by the thoracic vertebrae. Superiorly, the thoracic cavity communicates through the **thoracic inlet** with the base of the neck. Inferiorly, the **thoracic outlet** is closed by the diaphragm which separates the thoracic from the abdominal cavity.

The thoracic cavity is divided into two **lateral compartments** containing the lungs and their covering of serous membranes and a **central compartment** called the **mediastinum** (discussed later) which contains most of the viscera of the thorax (Figure 7-1B).

Intercostal Spaces

- There are 11 **intercostal spaces** within the thoracic wall (Figure 7-1A). The spaces are filled in by three layers of intercostal muscles and their related fasciae and are bounded superiorly and inferiorly by the adjacent ribs.

- The **costal groove** is located along the inferior border of each rib (upper aspect of the intercostal space) and provides protection for the intercostal nerve, artery, and vein which are located in the groove. The vein is most superior and the nerve is inferior in the groove (VAN).

- The intercostal arteries are contributed to anteriorly from branches of the internal thoracic artery (branch of the subclavian artery) and posteriorly from branches of the thoracic aorta. Thus, the intercostal arteries can provide a potential collateral circulation between the subclavian artery and the thoracic aorta.

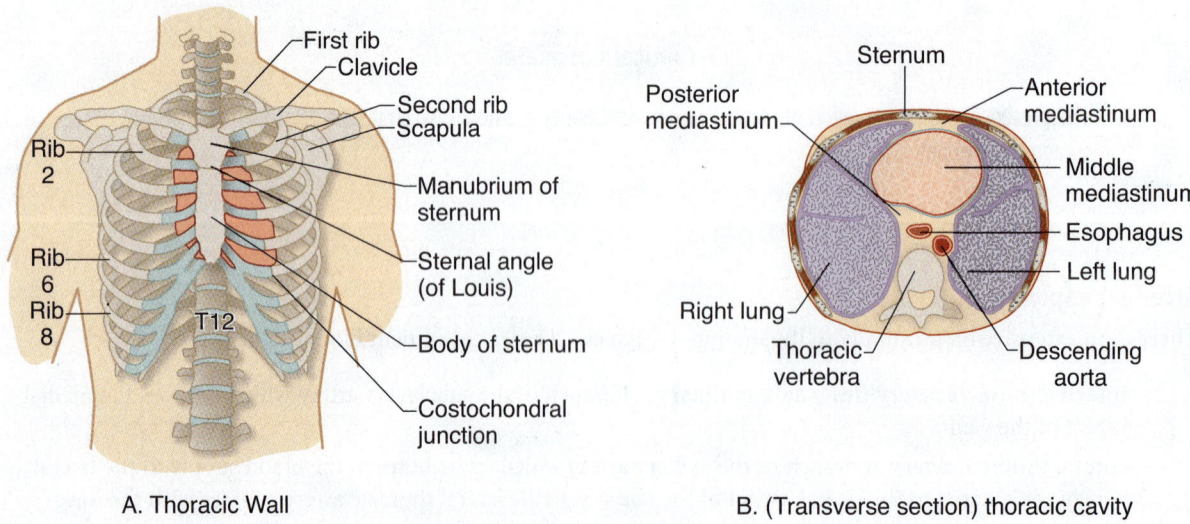

A. Thoracic Wall

B. (Transverse section) thoracic cavity

Figure 7-1. Thoracic Cavity

PLEURA AND PLEURAL CAVITY

Serous Membranes

Within the thoracic and abdominal cavities there are three serous mesodermal-derived membranes which form a covering for the lungs (**pleura**), heart (**pericardium**), and abdominal viscera (**peritoneum**).

Each of these double-layered membranes permits friction-reducing movements of the viscera against adjacent structures.

The outer layer of the serous membranes is referred to as the **parietal layer;** and the inner layer which is applied directly to the surface of the organ, is called the **visceral layer**. The two layers are continuous and there is a potential space (pleural cavity) between the parietal and visceral layers containing a thin layer of serous fluid.

Pleura

The **pleura** is the serous membrane that invests the lungs in the lateral compartments of the thoracic cavity. The external **parietal pleura** lines and attaches to the inner surfaces of the chest wall, diaphragm, and mediastinum. The innermost **visceral** layer reflects from the parietal layer at the hilum of the lungs and is firmly attached to and follows the contours of the lung. Visceral and parietal pleura are continuous at the root of the lung.

The **parietal pleura** is regionally named by its relationship to the thoracic wall and mediastinum:

- **Costal parietal pleura** is lateral and lines the inner surfaces of the ribs and intercostal spaces
- **Diaphragmatic parietal pleura** lines the thoracic surface of the diaphragm
- **Mediastinal parietal pleura** is medial and lines the mediastinum. The mediastinal pleura reflects and becomes continuous with the visceral pleura at the hilum.
- **Cervical parietal pleura** extends into the neck above the first rib where it covers the apex of the lung.

The **visceral pleura** tightly invests the surface of the lungs, following all of the fissures and lobes of the lung.

Clinical Correlate
Inflammation of the parietal pleural layers (**pleurisy**) produces sharp pain upon respiration.

Pleural Cavity

The **pleural cavity** is the potential space between the parietal and visceral layers of the pleura. It is a closed space which contains a small amount of serous fluid that lubricates the opposing parietal and visceral layers.

The introduction of air into the pleural cavity may cause the lung to collapse, resulting in a **pneumothorax** which causes shortness of breath and painful respiration. The lung collapses due to the loss of the negative pressure of the pleural cavity during a pneumothorax.

LUNGS

The lungs and the pleural membranes are located in the lateral compartment of the thoracic cavity. The lungs are separated from each other in the midline by the mediastinum. The **hilum** of the lung is on the medial surface and serves for passage of structures in the root of the lung: the pulmonary vessels, primary bronchi, nerves, and lymphatics.

Surfaces and Regions

Each of the lungs has three surfaces:

- The **costal surface** is smooth and convex and is related laterally to the ribs and tissues of the chest wall.
- The **mediastinal surface** is concave and is related medially to the middle mediastinum and the heart. The mediastinal surfaces contain the **root** of the lung and a deep **cardiac impression**, more pronounced on the left lung.
- The **diaphragmatic surface** (base) is concave and rests on the superior surface of the diaphragm. It is more superior on the right owing to the presence of the liver.
- The **apex** (cupola) of the lung projects superiorly into the root of the neck above the level of the first rib and is crossed anteriorly by the subclavian artery and vein.

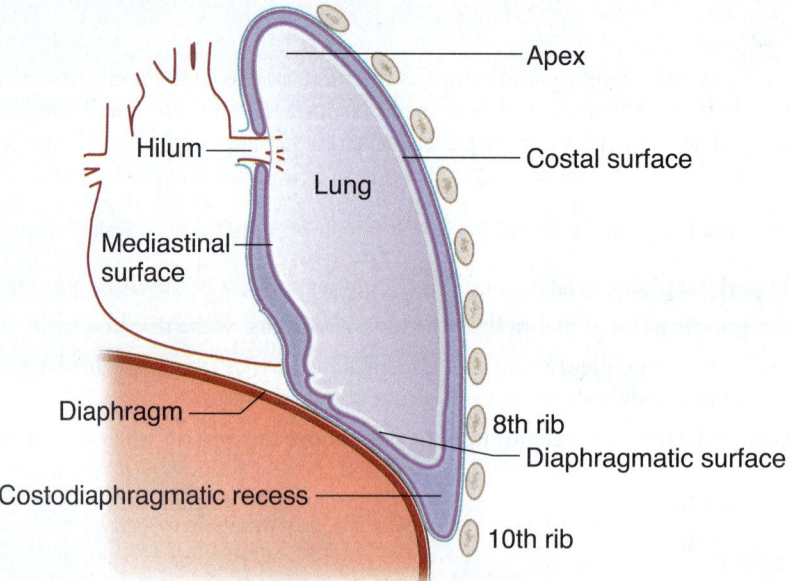

Figure 7-2. Surfaces of the Lung

Lobes and Fissures

- The **right lung** is divided into three lobes (**superior, middle, inferior**) separated by two fissures, the **oblique** and **horizontal fissures** (Figure 7-3). The horizontal fissure separates the superior from the middle lobe and the oblique fissure separates the middle from the inferior lobe.
- The **left lung** is divided into two lobes (**superior, inferior**) separated by an **oblique fissure** (Figure 7-3). The **lingula** of the upper lobe of the left lung corresponds to the middle lobe of the right lung.
- The **horizontal fissure** of the right lung follows the curvature of the **4th rib,** ending medially at the 4th costal cartilage.
- The **oblique fissure** of both lungs projects anteriorly at approximately the **5th intercostal space** in the midclavicular line, ending medially deep to the 6th costal cartilage.

Clinical Correlate

Aspiration of a foreign body will more often enter the **right primary bronchus**, which is shorter, wider, and more vertical than the left primary bronchus. When the individual is vertical, the foreign body usually falls into the **posterior basal segment** of the **right inferior lobe.**

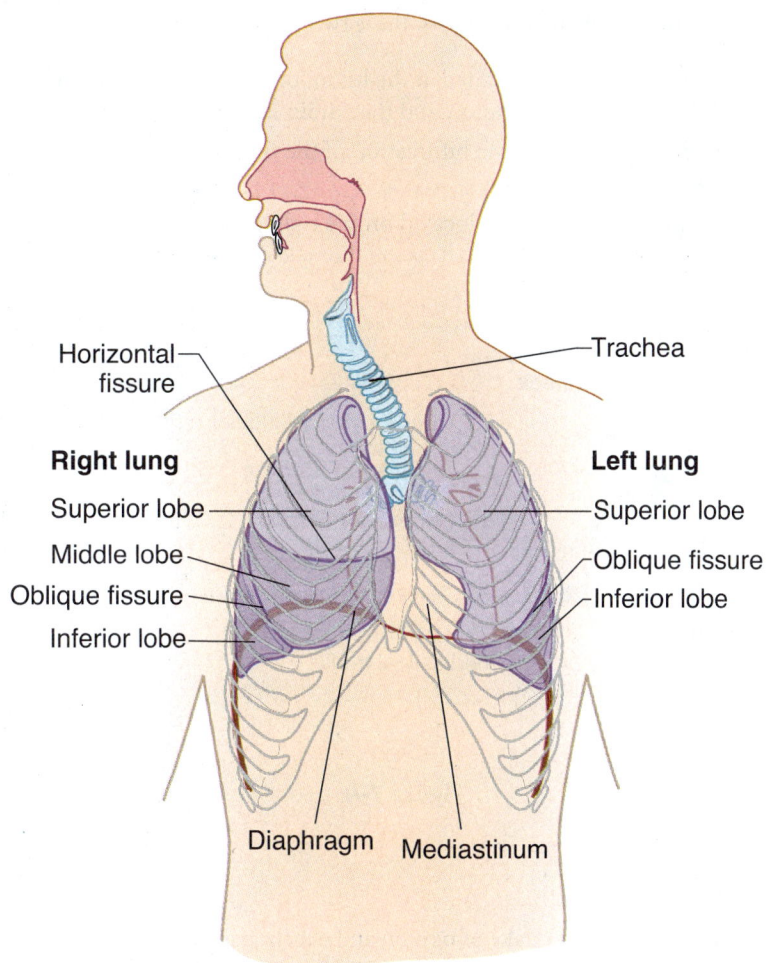

Figure 7-3. Lobes and Fissures of Lungs

Lymphatic System

The **lymphatic system** consists of an extensive network of lymph capillaries, vessels, and nodes that drain extracellular fluid from most of the body tissues and organs. The lymph flow will return to the blood venous system by two major lymphatic vessels, the **right lymphatic duct** and the **thoracic duct** on the left (Figure 7-4A). These two vessels drain into the junction of the internal jugular and the subclavian veins on their respective sides.

- The **thoracic duct** carries all lymphatic drainage from the body below the diaphragm and on the left side of the trunk and head above the diaphragm (Figure 7-4B).
- **The right lymphatic duct** drains lymph flow from the right head and neck and the right side of the trunk above the diaphragm.

Lymphatic Drainage

The lymphatic drainage of the lungs is extensive and drains by way of **superficial** and **deep** lymphatic plexuses. The superficial plexus is immediately deep to the visceral pleura. The deep plexus begins deeply in the lungs and drains through **pulmonary nodes** which follow the bronchial tree toward the hilum.

The major nodes involved in the lymphatic drainage of these two plexuses are:

- **Bronchopulmonary (hilar) nodes** are located at the hilum of the lungs. They receive lymph drainage from both superficial and deep lymphatic plexuses, and they drain into the tracheobronchial nodes.

- **Tracheobronchial nodes** are located at the bifurcation of the trachea, and they drain into the right and left bronchomediastinal nodes and trunk.

- **Bronchomediastinal nodes** and trunk are located on the right and left sides of the trachea, and they drain superiorly into either the right lymphatic duct or the thoracic duct on the left.

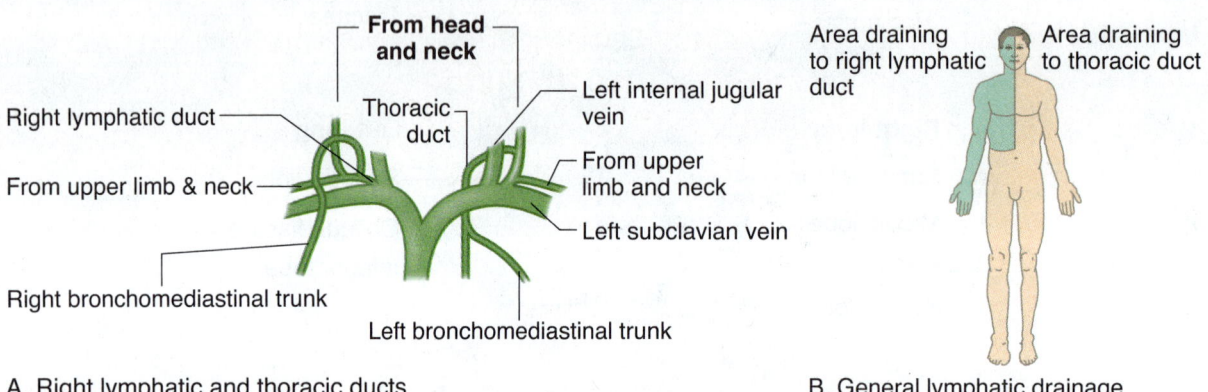

A. Right lymphatic and thoracic ducts

B. General lymphatic drainage

Figure 7-4.

RESPIRATORY HISTOLOGY

The lung is an organ that functions in the intake of oxygen and exhaling of CO_2. Approximately 14 times each minute, we take in about 500 mL of air per breath. Inspired air will be spread over 120 square meters of the surface area of the lungs. The air–blood barrier has to be thin enough for air to pass across but tough enough to keep the blood cells inside their capillaries.

Lungs are opened to the outside world so that they are susceptible to environmental insults in the form of pollution and infectious bacteria.

The lungs receive the entire cardiac output and are positioned to modify various blood components. The pulmonary endothelium plays an active role in the metabolic transformation of lipoproteins and prostaglandins. **The enzyme that converts angiotensin I to angiotensin II is produced by the lung endothelial cells.**

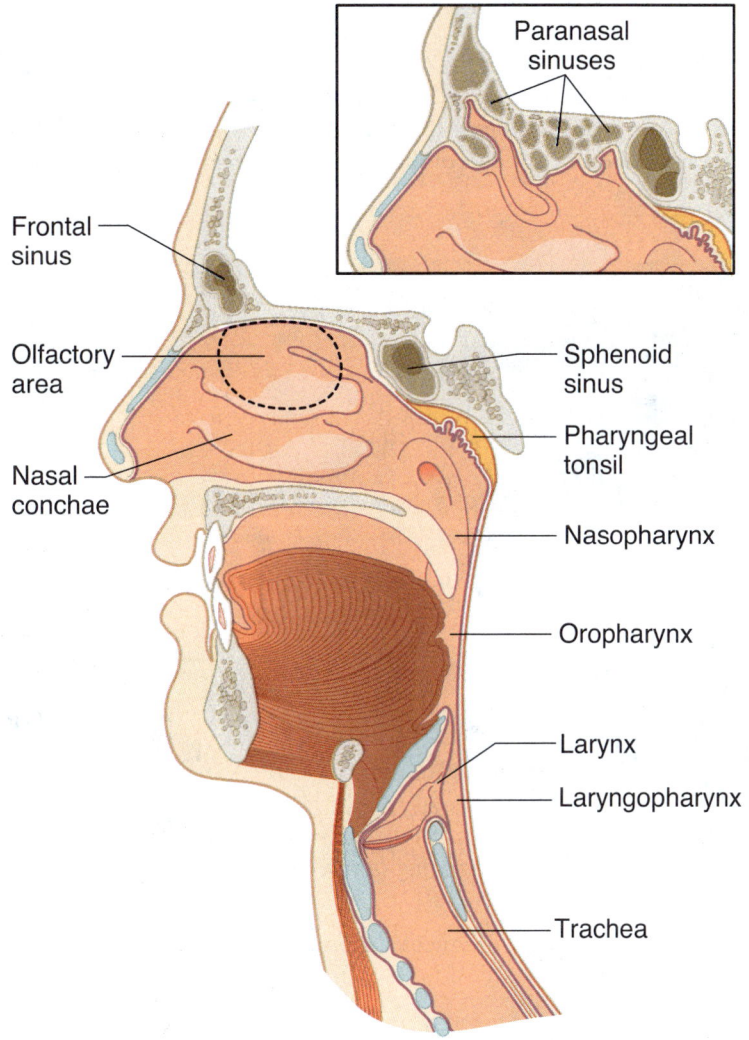

Figure 7-5. Respiratory Pathways

Table 7-1. Histologic Features of Trachea, Bronchi, and Bronchioles

	Trachea	Bronchi	Bronchioles
Epithelia	Pseudostratified ciliated columnar (PCC) cells, goblet cells	PCC to simple columnar cells	Ciliated, some goblet cells, Clara cells in terminal bronchioles
Cartilage	16–20 C-shaped cartilaginous rings	Irregular plates	None
Glands	Seromucous glands	Fewer seromucous glands	None
Smooth muscle	Between open ends of C-shaped cartilage	Prominent	Highest proportion of smooth muscle in the bronchial tree
Elastic fibers	Present	Abundant	Abundant

TRACHEA

The **trachea** is a hollow tube, about 10 cm in length (and about 2 cm in diameter), extending from the larynx to its bifurcation at the carina to form a primary bronchus for each lung. The most striking structures of the trachea are the C-shaped hyaline cartilage rings. In the human there are about 16 to 20 of them distributed along the length of the trachea. The rings overlap in the anterior part of the trachea. The free posterior ends of the C-shaped cartilages are interconnected by smooth-muscle cells.

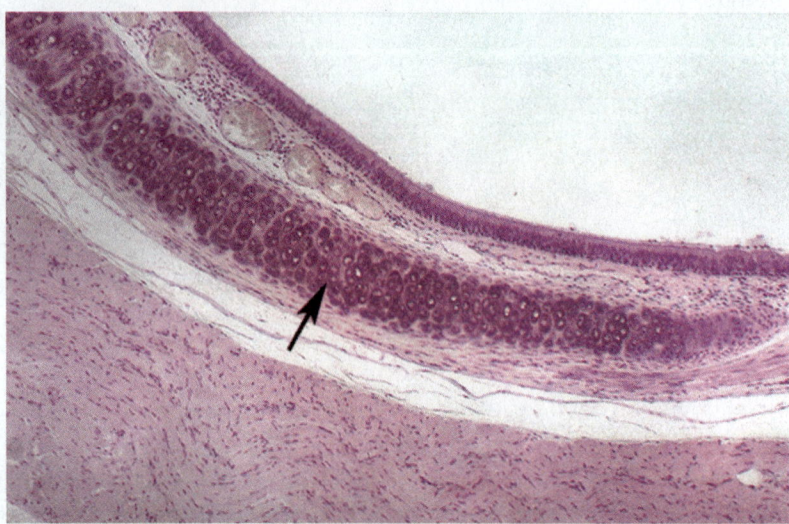

Copyright McGraw-Hill Companies. Used with permission.

Figure 7-6. Trachea with a hyaline cartilage ring (arrow) and pseudostratified columnar epithelium

The trachea is composed of concentric rings of mucosa, submucosa, an incomplete muscularis, and an complete adventitia.

- The mucosa has three components: a pseudostratified epithelium, an underlying vascularized loose connective tissue (lamina propria) that contains immune cells, and a thin layer of smooth-muscle cells (muscularis mucosa).
- The submucosa is a vascular service area containing large blood vessels. Collagen fibers, lymphatic vessels and nerves are also present in this layer.
- The outside covering of the trachea, the adventitia, is composed of several layers of loose connective tissue.

The epithelial lining of the trachea and bronchi is pseudostratified columnar in which all cells lie on the same basal membrane but only some reach the luminal surface. The only other place in the body with this epithelium is the male reproductive tract.

Clinical Correlate

If mucosal clearance is ineffective, or the mechanism overwhelmed, infection (pathogenic bacteria) or pneumoconiosis (dust-related disease) may follow.

In cystic fibrosis, the secreted mucus is thick or viscous and the cilia have a difficult time moving it toward the pharynx. Patients with this disease have frequent infections of the respiratory system.

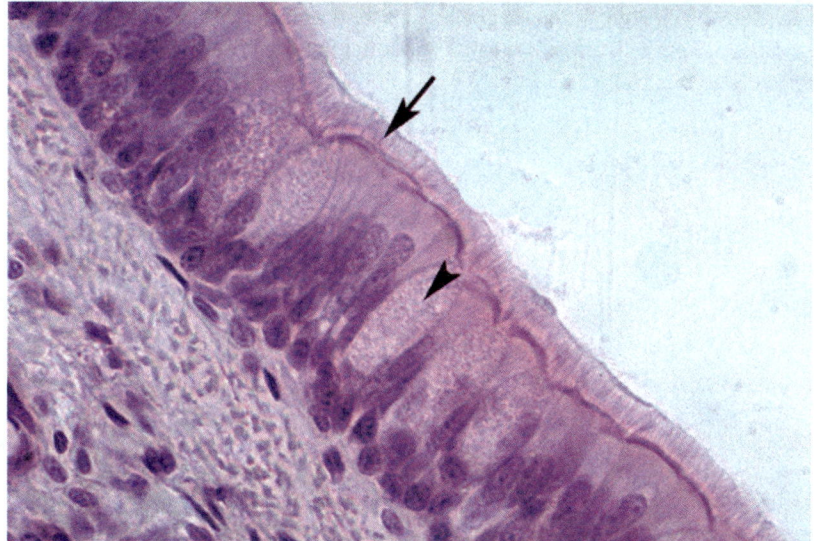

Figure 7-7. Pseudostratified columnar epithelium with goblet cells (arrowhead)
surrounded by ciliated cells (arrow)

Tracheal Epithelial Cell Types

Columnar cells extend from the basal membrane to the luminal surface. These cells contain approximately 200 to 300 apical cilia per cell that are intermingled with microvilli. The cilia are motile and beat to help move the secreted mucus layer over the lining of the trachea and out of the respiratory system.

Goblet cells secrete a polysaccharide mucous material into the lumen of trachea. Mucus production is supplemented by secretions of the submucosal mixed glands. The mucus layer of the respiratory system traps particulate substances (dust, bacteria, and viruses) and absorbs noxious water-soluble gases such as ozone and sulfur dioxide. The mucus sticky layer is moved by the beating cilia toward the pharynx where it is swallowed. This movement is known as the mucociliary escalator system. Most material (dust and bacteria) is trapped in the mucus layer, and is removed and digested.

Pulmonary neuroendocrine (PNE) cells are comparable to the endocrine cells in the gut. These epithelial neuroendocrine cells have been given various names:

- **APUD cells** (Amino-Precursor-Uptake-Decarboxylase), **DNES cells** (Diffuse NeuroEndocrine System) and **K** (Kulchitsky) **cells.** These cells occur in clusters and are often located at airway branch points.
- **Brush cells** may represent goblet cells that have secreted their products or intermediate stages in the formation of goblet or the tall ciliated cells. They have short microvilli on their apical surfaces. Some of these cells have synapses with intraepithelial nerves, suggesting that these cells may be sensory receptors.

Clinical Correlate

The columnar and goblet cells are sensitive to irritation. The ciliated cells become taller, and there is an increase in the number of goblet cells and submucosal glands.

Intensive irritation from smoking leads to a squamous metaplasia where the ciliated epithelium becomes a squamous epithelium. This process is reversible.

Basal cells are stem cells for the ciliated and goblet cells. The stem cells lie on the basal membrane but do not extend to the lumen of the trachea. These cells, along with the epithelial neuroendocrine cells, are responsible for the pseudostratified appearance of the trachea.

BRONCHI

The **bronchial tree** forms a branching airway from the trachea to the bronchioles. When the primary bronchi enter the lung, they give rise to 5 secondary or lobar bronchi—3 for the right lung and 2 for the left. The 5 lobes are further subdivided into 10 tertiary or segmental bronchi in each lung, which form bronchopulmonary segments.

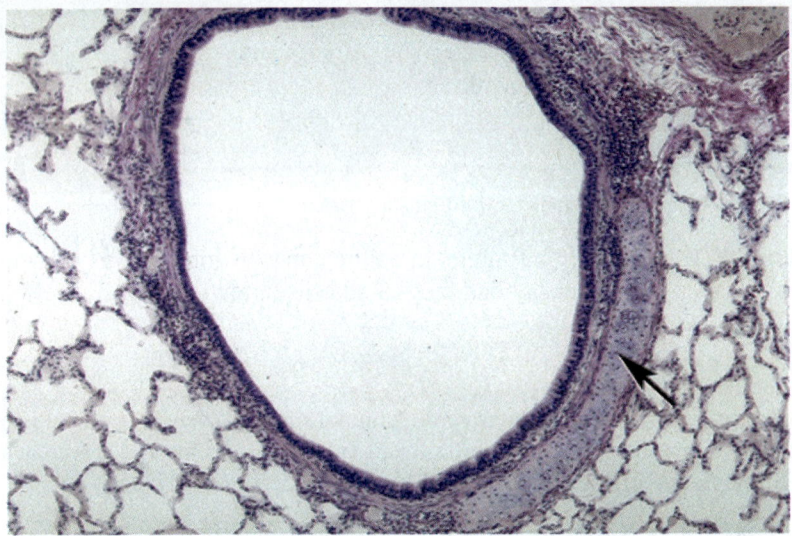

Figure 7-8. Bronchus with a plate of cartilage (arrow)

The epithelial lining of the bronchi is also pseudostratified. It consists of **ciliated columnar cells, basal cells, mucus cells, brush cells and neuroendocrine** (APUD, DNES, or K) **cells.** There are also seromucous glands in the submucosa that empty onto the epithelial surface via ducts. The walls of bronchi contain irregular plates of cartilage and circular smooth-muscle fascicles bound together by elastic fibers. The number of goblet cells and submucosa glands decreases from the trachea to the small bronchi.

Clinical Correlate

Cystic fibrosis that results in abnormally thick mucus is in part due to defective chloride transport by Clara cells.

BRONCHIOLES

The **wall of a bronchiole** does not contain cartilage or glands. The smooth-muscle fascicles are bound together by elastic fibers. The epithelium is still ciliated, but is a simple cuboidal or columnar epithelium rather than pseudostratified. The epithelial lining of the airway is composed of **ciliated cells** (goblet and basal cells are absent in the terminal bronchioles) and an additional type called the **Clara cell.**

Clara cells (also called bronchiolar secretory cells) are nonciliated and **secrete a serous solution similar to surfactant**. They aid in the **detoxification of airborne toxins**, and serve as a **stem cell for the ciliated cells** and for themselves. The number of Clara cells increases in response to increased levels of pollutants like cigarette smoke. **Clara cells are most abundant in the terminal bronchioles, where they make up about 80 % of the epithelial cell lining;** they are also involved with chloride ion transport into the lumens of the terminal bronchioles.

Clinical Correlate

Chronic obstructive pulmonary disease (COPD) affects the bronchioles and includes emphysema and asthma.

- Emphysema is caused by a loss of elastic fibers and results in chronic airflow obstruction.
- Asthma is a chronic process characterized by a reversible narrowing of airways.
- Asthma is reversible; emphysema is not.

Terminal Bronchioles

The **terminal bronchiole** is the last conducting bronchiole. This bronchiole is followed by **respiratory bronchioles** which are periodically interrupted by alveoli in their walls. The goblet cells are absent from the epithelial linings of the respiratory bronchioles, but are still lined with a sparse ciliated cuboidal epithelium that prevent the movement of mucous into the alveoli. After the last respiratory bronchiole, the wall of the airway disappears and air enters the alveoli.

ALVEOLAR DUCTS, ALVEOLAR SACS, AND THE ALVEOLI

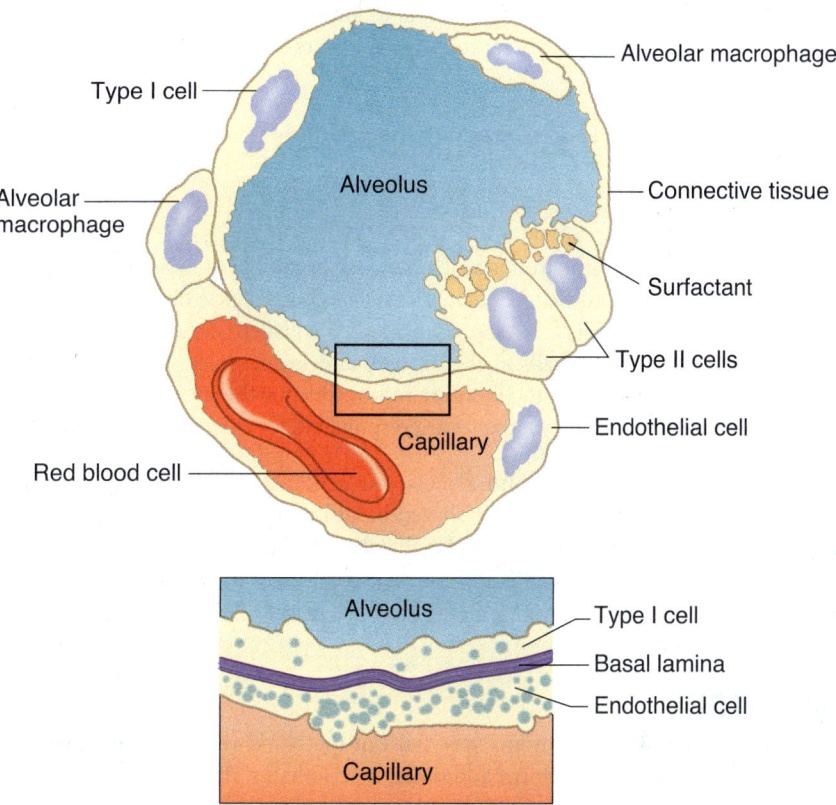

Figure 7-9. Alveolus and blood–air barrier

The **alveolar ducts and sacs** have little or no walls and consist almost entirely of alveoli. The alveoli constitute 80 to 85% of the volume of the normal lung. There are 300 million alveoli in the lungs. Each alveolus is approximately 200 microns in diameter. The cuboidal epithelium of the respiratory bronchioles and the alveolar ducts are continuous with the squamous cells lining the alveoli.

The **type I pneumocyte** is the major cell lining cell of the alveolar surfaces (also called small alveolar cell or alveolar type I cell).

- These cells represent only 40% of the alveolar lining cells, but are spread so thinly that they cover about 90 to 95% of the surface.
- Primarily involved in gas exchange.
- These cells are post-mitotic.

The **type II pneumocyte** is the other major alveolar cell (also called the great alveolar cell because of its size). Other names for this cell type include granular pneumocyte, septal cell, corner cell, niche cell, and alveolar type II.

- Though they constitute 60% of the cells lining the alveoli, they form only 5 to 10% of the surface.
- Produce and secrete surfactant
- They are large, round cells with "myelin figures" in their apical cytoplasm which represent the remnants of surfactant after histological processing.
- The type II cells serve as stem cells for themselves and the type I cell.

Surfactant

Surfactant is essential to maintain the normal respiratory mechanics of the alveoli. Production of surfactant in the fetus is essential for the survival of the neonate as it takes its first breath. Surfactant is composed of a mixture of phospholipids and surfactant proteins whose function is to aid in the spreading of the surfactant at the alveolar air–water interface. The phospholipids act as a detergent which lowers the surface tension of the alveoli and prevents alveolar collapse during expiration.

Most surfactant is recycled back to Type II cells for reutilization; some of it undergoes phagocytosis by macrophages.

Alveolar Wall

In the **alveolar wall** under the alveolar epithelium is a rich network of capillaries arising from pulmonary arteries. The alveolar wall contains a variety of cells and extracellular fibers. The cells include fibroblasts, macrophages, myofibroblasts, smooth-muscle cells, and occasional mast cells. Type I and II collagens, as well as elastic fibers, are in the septa. Type I collagen is present primarily in the walls of the bronchi and bronchioles. Twenty percent of the mass of the lung consists of collagen and elastic fibers. Elastic fibers are responsible for the stretching and recoiling activities of the alveoli during respiration. These microscopic elements are responsible for the recoil of the lungs during expiration.

Gas exchange occurs between capillary blood and alveolar air across the blood–gas barrier. This barrier consists of surfactant, the squamous Type I pneumocytes, a shared basal lamina, and capillary endothelium. The distance between the lumen of the capillary and the lumen of the alveolus can be as thin as 0.1 microns. There are openings in the wall of most alveoli that form the **pores of Kohn**. These pores are thought to be important in collateral ventilation. The diameter of these alveolar pores can be as large as 10 to 15 microns.

Alveolar Macrophages

The **alveolar macrophages** are derived from monocytes that exit the blood vessels in the lungs. The resident alveolar macrophages can undergo limited mitoses to form additional macrophages. These cells can reside in the interalveolar septa as well as in the alveoli. Alveolar macrophages that patrol the alveolar surfaces may pass through the pores of Kohn.

There are about 1 to 3 macrophages per alveolus. Alveolar macrophages vary in size from 15 to 40 microns in diameter. These macrophages represent the last defense mechanism of the lung. Macrophages can pass out of the alveoli to the bronchioles and enter the lymphatics or become trapped in the moving mucus layer and propelled toward the pharynx to be swallowed and digested.

Clinical Correlate

Alveolar macrophages have several other names: **dust cells** because they have phagocytosed dust or cigarette particles, and **heart failure cells** because they have phagocytosed blood cells that have escaped into the alveolar space during congestive heart failure.

EMBRYOLOGY OF THE HEART

Formation of Heart Tube

The heart begins to develop from splanchnic **mesoderm** in the latter half of the third week within the cardiogenic area of the cranial end of the embryo. **Neural crest cells m**igrate into the developing heart and play an important role in cardiac development. The cardiogenic cells condense to form a pair of primordial heart tubes which will fuse into a single **heart tube** during body folding.

- The heart tube undergoes dextral looping (bends to the right) and rotation.
- The upper truncus arteriosus (ventricular) end of the tube grows more rapidly and folds downward and **ventrally** and to the right.
- The atria and sinus venosus lower part of the tube fold upward and **dorsally** and to the left. These foldings begin to place the chambers of the heart in their postnatal anatomic positions.

Fetal Circulation

Venous systems associated with the fetal heart

There are three major venous systems that flow into the sinus venosus end of the heart tube.

- **Viteline (omphalomesenteric) veins** drain deoxygenated blood from the yolk stalk; they will coalesce and form the veins of the liver (sinusoids, hepatic portal vein, hepatic vein) and part of the inferior vena cava.
- **Umbilical vein** carries oxygenated blood from the placenta.
- **Cardinal veins** carry deoxygenated blood from the body of the embryo; they will coalesce and contribute to some of the major veins of the body (brachiocephalic, superior vena cava, inferior vena cava, azygos, renal).

Arterial systems associated with the fetal heart

During fetal circulation, oxygenated blood flood from the placenta to the fetus passes through the **umbilical vein**. Three **vascular shunts** develop in the fetal circulation to bypass blood flow around the liver and lungs (Figure 7-16).

1. The **ductus venosus** allows oxygenated blood in the umbilical vein to bypass the sinusoids of the liver into the inferior vena cava and to the right atrium. From the right atrium, oxygenated blood flows mostly through the foramen ovale into the left atrium then left ventricle and into the systemic circulation.
2. The **foramen ovale** develops during atrial septation to allow oxygenated blood to bypass the pulmonary circulation. Note that this is a **right-to-left** shunting of blood during fetal life.
3. During fetal circulation, the superior vena cava drains deoxygenated blood from the upper limbs and head into the right atrium. Most of this blood flow is directed into the right ventricle and into the pulmonary trunk. The **ductus arteriosus** opens into the underside of the aorta just **distal** to the origin of the left subclavian artery and shunts this deoxygenated blood from the pulmonary trunk to the aorta to bypass the pulmonary circulation.

The shunting of blood through the foramen ovale and through the ductus arteriosus (right to left) during fetal life occurs because of a **right-to-left pressure gradient**.

Pressure Gradients
Fetal
$\quad$ R → L
Postnatal
$\quad$ L → R

Postnatal circulation

Following birth, these three shunts will close because of changes in the pressure gradients and in oxygen tensions. The umbilical vein closes and reduces blood flow into the right atrium. The ductus venosus also closes. Lung expansion reduces pulmonary resistence and results in increased flow to the lungs and increased venous return to the left atrium.

- Closure of the foramen ovale occurs as a result of the increase in left atrial pressure and reduction in right atrial pressure.
- Closure of the ductus venosus and ductus arteriosus occurs over the next several hours as a result of the contraction of smooth muscles in its wall and increased oxygen tension.
- The release of bradykinin and the immediate drop of prostaglandin E at birth also facilitate the closure of the ductus arteriosus.

The changes which occur between pre- and postnatal circulation are summarized here

Table 7-2. Adult Vestiges Derived from the Fetal Circulatory System

Changes After Birth	Remnant in Adult
Closure of right and left umbilical arteries	Medial umbilical ligaments
Closure of the umbilical vein	Ligamentum teres of liver
Closure of ductus venosus	Ligamentum venosum
Closure of foramen ovale	Fossa ovalis
Closure of ductus arteriosus	Ligamentum arteriosum

Atrial Septal Defects

Atrial septal defect (ASD) is one of several congenital heart defects. It is more common in female births than in male. Postnatally, ASDs result **in left-to-right shunting** and are **non-cyanotic conditions**.

In a Nutshell

Postnatal Shunts

- **Right-to-left** shunts are **cyanotic conditions**.
- **Left-to-right** shunts are **non-cyanotic conditions**.

Two clinically important ASDs are the **secundum** and **primum** types.

1. **Secundum-type ASD** is the most common ASD. It is caused by either an excessive resorption of the SP or an underdevelopment and reduced size of the SS or both. This ASD results in variable openings between the right and left atria in the central part of the atrial septum above the limbus. If the ASD is small, clinical symptoms may be delayed as late as age 30.

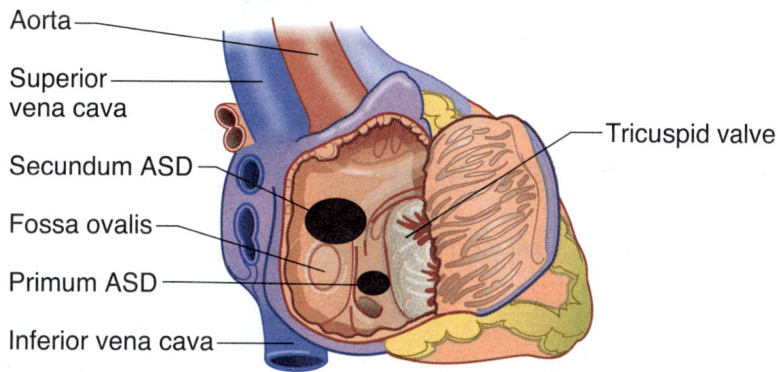

Figure 7-10. Secundum and Primum Atrial Septal Defect

2. **Primum type ASD** is less common than secundum ASD and results from a failure of the septum premium to fuse with the endocardial cushions, and may be combined with defects of the endocardial cushions. Primum ASDs occur in the lower aspect of the atrial wall, usually with a normal formed fossa ovalis. If the endocardial </ix>cushion is involved, a primum ASD can also be associated with a defect of the membranous interventricular septum and the atrioventricular valves.

Clinical Correlate

Ventricular septal defect (VSD) is the most common of the congenital heart defects, being more common in males than in females. The most common VSD is a **membranous ventricular septal defect**, associated with the failure of **neural crest** cells to migrate into the endocardial cushions.

A membranous VSD is caused by the failure of the membranous interventricular (IV) septum to develop, and it results in **left-to-right shunting** of blood through the IV foramen. Patients with left-to-right shunting complain of **excessive fatigue upon exertion**. Left-to-right shunting of blood is **noncyanotic** but causes increased blood flow and pressure to the lungs (pulmonary hypertension).

Patent Ductus Arteriosus

A **patent ductus arteriosus** (PDA) occurs when the ductus arteriosus (a connection between the pulmonary trunk and aorta) fails to close after birth. PDA is common in premature infants and in cases of maternal rubella infection.

- Postnatally, a PDA causes a **left-to-right** shunt (from aorta to pulmonary trunk) and is **non-cyanotic**. The newborn presents with a machine-like murmur.

- Normally, the ductus arteriosus closes within a few hours after birth via smooth-muscle contraction to form the **ligamentum arteriosum**. Prostaglandin E (PGE) and low oxygen tension sustain patency of the ductus arteriosus in the fetal period.

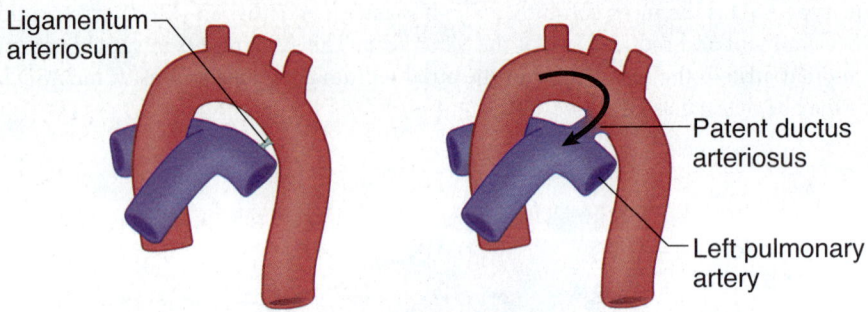

A. Normal obliterated ductus arteriosus   B. Patent ductus arteriosus

Figure 7-11. Ductus Arteriosus

Truncus arteriosus defects

Three classic **cyanotic congenital heart abnormalities** occur with defects in the development of the aorticopulmonary septum and are related to the failure of neural crest cells to migrate into the truncus arteriosus:

1. **Tetralogy of Fallot** (Figure 7-12) is the **most common** cyanotic congenital heart defect. Tetralogy occurs when the AP septum fails to align properly and shifts anteriorly to the right. This causes **right-to-left** shunting of blood with resultant **cyanosis** that is usually present sometime after birth. Imaging typically shows a boot-shaped heart due to the enlarged right ventricule.

   - There are four major defects in Tetralogy of Fallot:
     - Pulmonary stenosis (most important)
     - Overriding aorta (receives blood from both ventricles)
     - Membranous interventricular septal defect
     - Right ventricular hypertrophy (develops secondarily)

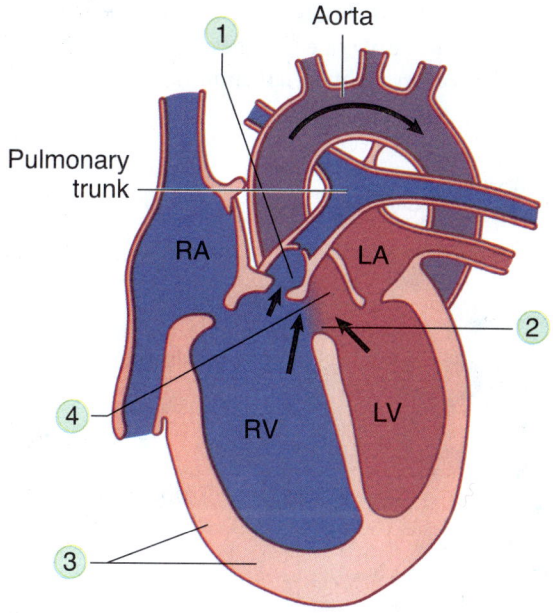

Figure 7-12. Tetralogy of Fallot

2. **Transposition of the great vessels** (Figure 7-13) occurs when the AP septum fails to develop in a spiral fashion and results in the aorta arising from the right ventricle and the pulmonary trunk arising from the left ventricle. This causes **right-to-left** shunting of blood with resultant **cyanosis**.

  • Transposition is the most common cause of severe cyanosis that persists immediately at birth. Transposition results in producing two closed circulation loops.

  • Infants born alive with this defect usually have other defects (PDA, VSD, ASD) that allow mixing of oxygenated and deoxygenated blood to sustain life.

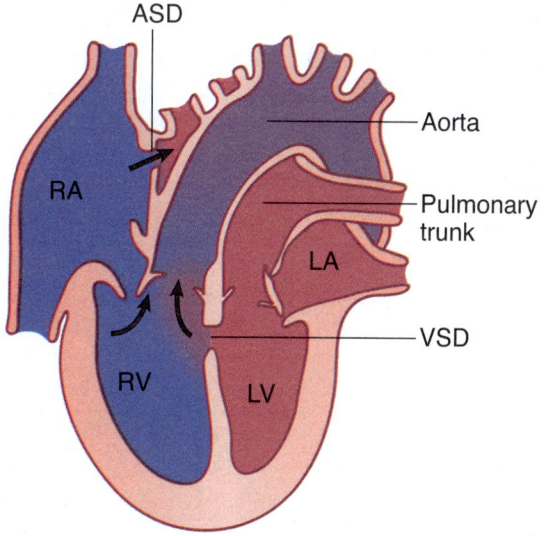

Figure 7-13. Transposition of the Great Vessels

3. **Persistent truncus arteriosus** (Figure 7-14) occurs when there is only partial development of the AP septum. This results in a condition where only one large vessel leaves the heart that receives blood from both the right and left ventricles. This causes **right-to-left** shunting of blood with resultant **cyanosis**. This defect is <u>always accompanied</u> by a membranous VSD.

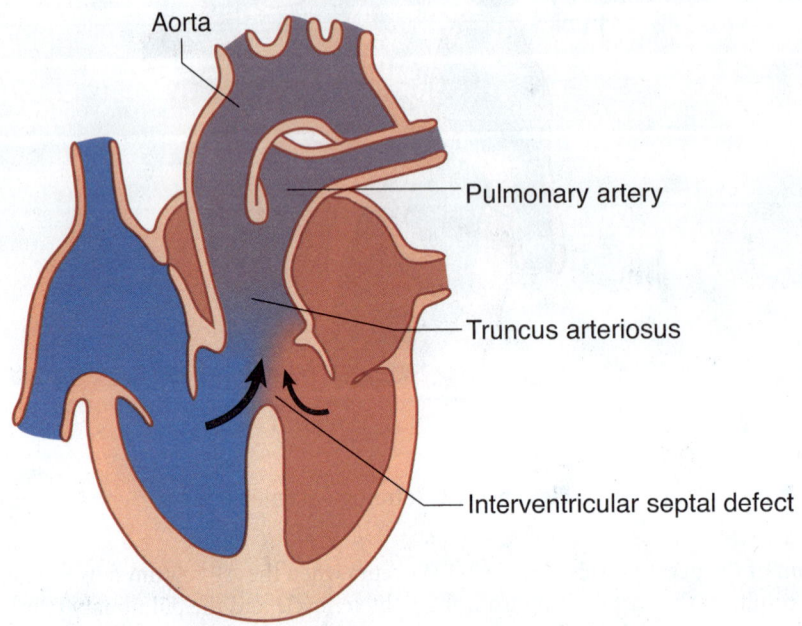

Figure 7-14. Persistent Truncus Arteriosus

In a Nutshell

Non-cyanotic congenital (left-to-right) heart defects at birth:

- Atrial septal defect
- Ventricular septal defects
- Patent ductus arteriosus

Cyanotic congenital (right-to-left) heart defects at birth

- Transposition of great vessels
- Tetralogy of Fallot
- Persistent truncus arteriosus

MEDIASTINUM

General Features

The **mediastinum** is the central, midline compartment of the thoracic cavity. It is bounded anteriorly by the sternum, posteriorly by the 12 thoracic vertebrae, and laterally by the pleural cavities.

- Superiorly, the mediastinum is continuous with the neck through the **thoracic inlet**; and inferiorly, is closed by the diaphragm. The mediastinum contains most of the viscera of the thoracic cavities except from the lungs (and pleura) and the sympathetic trunk.

- The sympathetic trunks are primarily located paravertebrally, just outside the posterior mediastinum. However, the greater, lesser, and least thoracic splanchnic nerves, which convey preganglionic sympathetic fibers to the collateral (prevertebral) ganglia below the diaphragm, enter the posterior mediastinum after leaving the sympathetic trunks.

- The mediastinum is divided into **superior** and **inferior** mediastina by a plane passing from the **sternal angle (of Louis)** anteriorly to the intervertebral disc between T4 and T5 posteriorly. The sternal angle and plane are **important clinical landmarks**. The inferior mediastinum is classically subdivided into **anterior, middle, and posterior** mediastina.

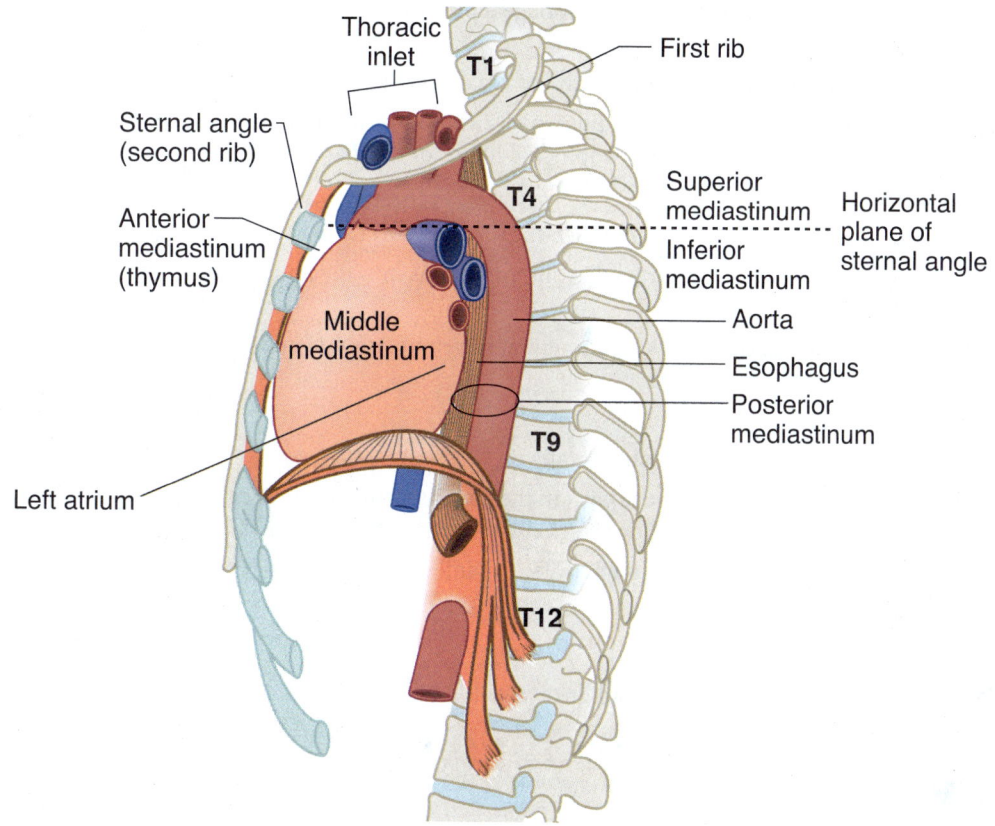

Figure 7-15. Divisions of the Mediastinum

Anterior Mediastinum

The anterior mediastinum is the small interval between the sternum and the anterior surface of the pericardium. It contains fat and areolar tissue and the inferior part of the **thymus gland**. A tumor of the thymus (**thymoma**) can develop in the anterior or superior mediastina

Posterior Mediastinum

The **posterior mediastinum** is located between the posterior surface of the pericardium and the T5-T12 thoracic vertebrae. Inferiorly, it is closed by the diaphragm.

There are four vertically oriented structures coursing within the posterior mediastinum:

- **Thoracic (descending) aorta**
  - Important branches are the **bronchial, esophageal,** and **posterior intercostal arteries**
  - Passes through the **aortic hiatus** (with the thoracic duct) at the T12 vertebral level to become the abdominal aorta
- **Esophagus**
  - Lies immediately posterior to the left primary bronchus and the **left atrium,** forming an important radiological relationship
  - Covered by the **anterior and posterior esophageal plexuses** which are derived from the left and right vagus nerves, respectively
  - Passes through the **esophageal hiatus** (with the vagal nerve trunks) at the T10 vertebral level
  - Is constricted (1) at its origin from the pharynx, (2) posterior to the arch of the aorta, (3) posterior to the left primary bronchus, and (4) at the esophageal hiatus of the diaphragm.
- **Thoracic duct**
  - Lies posterior to the esophagus and between the thoracic aorta and azygos vein
  - Ascends the posterior and superior mediastina and drains into the junction of the left subclavian and internal jugular veins
  - Arises from the cisterna chyli in the abdomen (at vertebral level L1) and enters the mediastinum through the **aortic hiatus** of the diaphragm
- **Azygos system of veins**
  - Drains the posterior and thoracic lateral wall
  - Communicates with the inferior vena cava in the abdomen and terminates by arching over the root of the right lung to empty into the **superior vena cava** above the pericardium
  - Forms a **collateral venous circulation** between the inferior and superior vena cava

Middle Mediastinum

The middle mediastinum contains the heart and great vessels and pericardium and will be discussed later.

Superior Mediastinum

The **superior mediastinum** is located between the manubrium of the sternum, anteriorly, and the thoracic vertebrae 1-4, posteriorly. As with all mediastina, the parietal pleura and the lungs form the lateral boundary. The thoracic inlet connects superiorly with the neck and the horizontal plane through the sternal angle forms the inferior boundary.

- The superior mediastinum contains the thymus, great arteries and veins associated with the upper aspect of the heart, trachea, and esophagus.
- The vagus and phrenic nerves and the thoracic duct also course through the mediastinum.
- Note that the pulmonary trunk and arteries are located completely in the middle mediastinum and are not found in the superior mediastinum.

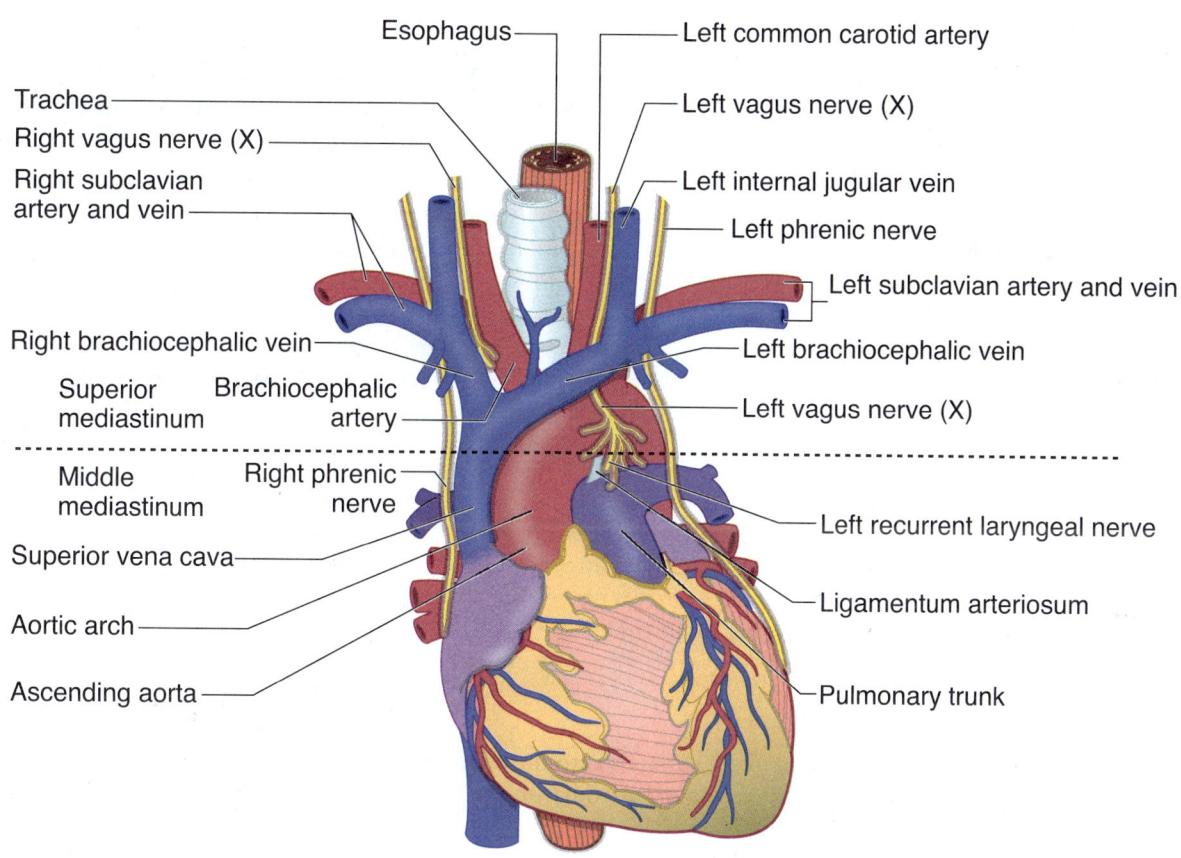

Figure 7-16. Structures of the Mediastinum

The relationships of these structures in the superior mediastinum are best visualized in **a ventral to dorsal** orientation between the sternum anteriorly and the vertebrae posteriorly:

- **Thymus**: Located posterior to the manubrium, usually atrophies in the adult and remains as fatty tissue
- **Right and left brachiocephalic veins**: Right vein descends almost vertically and the left vein obliquely crosses the superior mediastinum posterior to the thymic remnants.
  - The two veins join to form the **superior vena cava** posterior to the **right first costal cartilage**.
  - The superior vena cava descends and drains into the right atrium **deep to the right third costal cartilage.**
- **Aortic arch and its three branches**: Aortic arch begins and ends at the plane of the sternal angle and is located just **inferior** to the left brachiocephalic vein. As a very important radiological landmark, the origins of the three branches of the aortic arch (**brachiocephalic, left common carotid, and left subclavian**) are directly **posterior** to the left brachiocephalic vein.
- **Trachea**: Lies posterior to the aortic arch and bifurcates at the level of T4 vertebra to form the right and left primary bronchi. The **carina** is an internal projection of cartilage at the bifurcation.
- **Esophagus**: Lies posterior to the trachea and courses posterior to the left primary bronchus to enter the posterior mediastinum

In addition to these structures, the superior mediastinum also contains the **right and left vagus** and **phrenic nerves** and the superior end of the **thoracic duct.**

Vagus nerves

- Right and left vagus nerves contribute to the pulmonary and cardiac plexuses.
- In the neck, the right vagus nerve gives rise to the **right recurrent laryngeal nerve**, which passes under the right subclavian artery to ascend in the groove between the esophagus and the trachea to reach the larynx. **Note:** The right recurrent laryngeal nerve is not in the mediastinum.
- The left vagus nerve gives rise to the **left recurrent laryngeal nerve** in the superior mediastinum, which passes under the aortic arch and ligamentum arteriosum to ascend to the larynx.

Thoracic duct

The thoracic duct is the largest lymphatic channel in the body. It returns lymph to the venous circulation at the junction of the left internal jugular vein and the left subclavian vein.

Phrenic nerves

Phrenic nerves arise from the ventral rami of **cervical nerves 3, 4, and 5.** The nerves are the sole motor supply of the diaphragm and convey sensory information from the central portion of both the superior and inferior portions of the diaphragm and parietal pleura. Both phrenic nerves pass through the middle mediatstinum lateral between the fibrous pericardium and pleura, and anterior to the root of the lung.

Coarctation of the Aorta

Coarctation of the aorta is a narrowing of the aorta distal to the origin of the left subclavian artery. Two types are usually identified based on if the constriction is found proximal or distal to the opening of the ductus arteriosus (DA).

Middle Mediastinum

The middle mediastinum contains the pericardium, the heart, parts of the great vessels, and the phrenic nerves.

Pericardium

The pericardium is the serous sac covering the heart and is the only one of the three serous membranes that has three layers: an outer **fibrous layer** and a double-layered **parietal and visceral serous** layers.

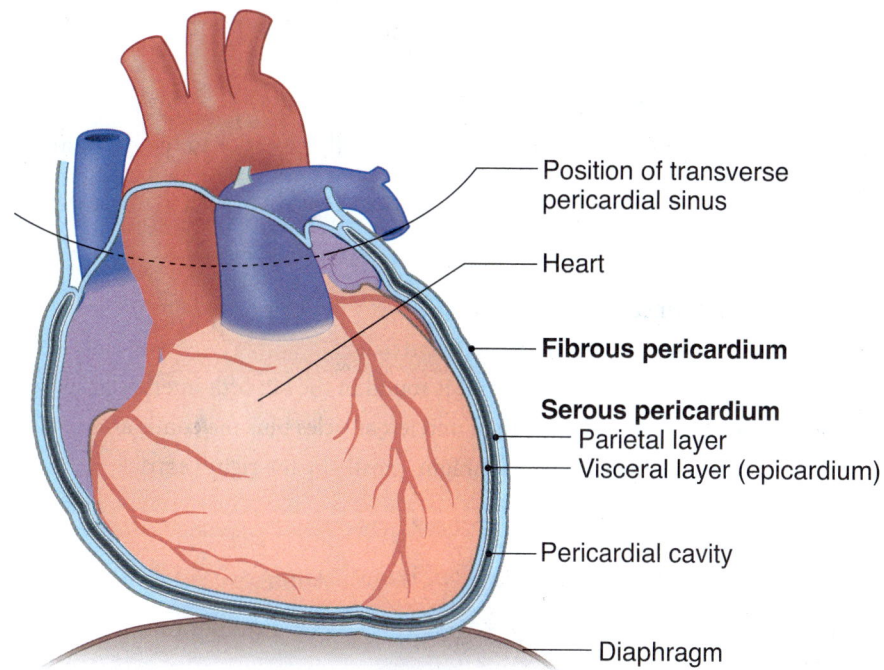

- Position of transverse pericardial sinus
- Heart
- **Fibrous pericardium**
- **Serous pericardium**
  - Parietal layer
  - Visceral layer (epicardium)
- Pericardial cavity
- Diaphragm

Figure 7-17. Layers of the Pericardium

The **fibrous pericardium** surrounds the entire heart and the great vessels at the upper aspect of the heart. It is firmly attached below to the central tendon of the diaphragm and superiorly to the adventitia of the great vessels at the plane of the sternal angle (level of the second rib). The fibrous pericardium is very strong and maintains the position of the heart within the middle mediastinum.

The **serous pericardium** is double-layered and formed by the outer **parietal layer** that lines the inner aspect of the fibrous pericardium and the inner **visceral layer** (epicardium) that covers the surface of the heart. The reflection between these two serous layers is at the base of the great vessels.

Clinical Correlate

Cardiac tamponade is the pathological accumulation of fluids (serous or blood) within the pericardial cavity. The fluid compresses the heart and restricts venous filling during diastole and reduces cardiac output.

The **pericardial cavity** is the potential space between the parietal and visceral layers containing a small amount of serous fluid that allows free movement of the beating heart. The pericardial cavity is expanded to form two sinuses:

- The **transverse pericardial sinus** is a space posterior to the ascending aorta and pulmonary trunk and anterior to the superior vena cava and pulmonary veins. Note that it separates the great arteries from the great veins. The transverse sinus is useful in cardiac surgery to allow isolation of the aorta and pulmonary trunk.
- The **oblique pericardial sinus** is the blind, inverted, U-shaped space posterior to the heart and bounded by reflection of serous pericardium around the four pulmonary veins and the inferior vena cava as they enter the heart.

HEART

External Features of the Heart

The heart lies obliquely within the middle mediastinum, mostly posterior to the sternum. Externally, the heart can be described by its **borders** and **surfaces.**

Borders of the heart

- The **right border** is formed by the **right atrium.**
- The **left border** is mainly formed by the **left ventricle.**
- The **apex** is the tip of the **left ventricle,** and is found in the left fifth intercostal space.
- The superior border is formed by the right and left auricles plus the conus arteriosus of the right ventricle.
- The inferior border is formed at the diaphragm, mostly by the right ventricle.

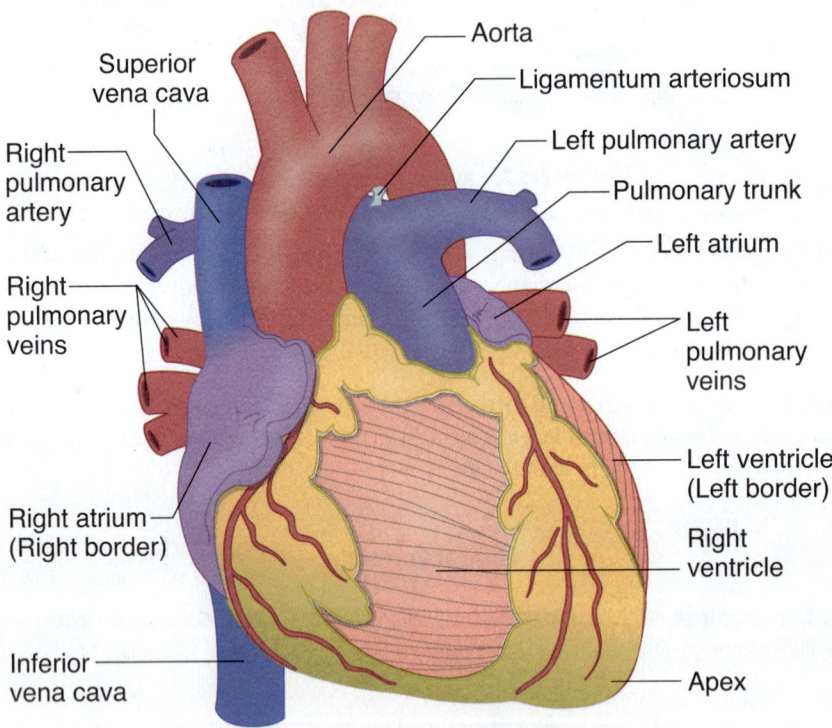

Figure 7-18. Sternocostal View of the Heart

Surfaces of the heart

- The **anterior (sternocostal) surface** is formed primarily by the **right ventricle.**
- The **posterior surface** is formed primarily by the **left atrium.**
- The **diaphragmatic surface** is formed primarily by the **left ventricle.**

Internal Features of the Heart

Chambers of the Heart

1. Right atrium

The right atrium receives venous blood from the entire body with the exception of blood from the pulmonary veins.

- **Auricle**

  The auricle is derived from the fetal atrium; it has rough myocardium known as pectinate muscles.

- **Sinus Venarum**

  The sinus venarum is the smooth-walled portion of the atrium, which receives blood from the superior and inferior venae cavae. It developed from the **sinus venosus**.

- **Crista Terminalis**

  The crista terminalis is the vertical ridge that separates the smooth from the rough portion (pectinate muscles) of the right atrium; it extends longitudinally from the superior vena cava to the inferior vena cava. The **SA node** is in the upper part of the crista terminalis.

- **Fossa Ovalis**

  The fossa ovalis is close to the foramen ovale, an opening in the interatrial septum which allows blood entering the right atrium from the inferior vena cava to pass directly to the left side of the heart.

- **Tricuspid Valve**

  The right AV (tricuspid) valve communicates with the right ventricle.

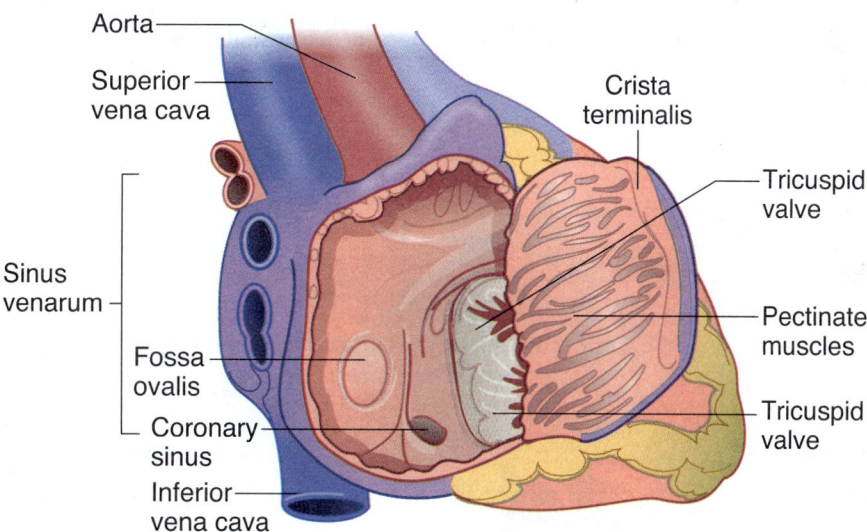

Figure 7-19. Inside the Right Atrium

2. Left atrium

The left atrium receives oxygenated blood from the lungs via the pulmonary veins. There are four openings: the upper right and left and the lower right and left pulmonary veins.

- **Bicuspid Valve**

  The left AV orifice is guarded by the mitral (bicuspid) valve; it allows oxygenated blood to pass from the left atrium to the left ventricle.

3. Right ventricle

The right ventricle (Figure 7-20) receives blood from the right atrium via the tricuspid valve; outflow is to the pulmonary trunk via the pulmonary semilunar valve.

- **Trabeculae Carneae**

  The trabeculae carneae are ridges of myocardium in the ventricular wall.

- **Papillary Muscles**

  The papillary muscles project into the cavity of the ventricle and attach to cusps of the AV valve by the strands of the chordae tendineae.

- **Chordae Tendineae**

  The chordae tendineae are fibrous cords between the papillary muscles and the valve leaflets that control closure of the valve during contraction of the ventricle.

- **Infundibulum**

  The infundibulum is the smooth area of the right ventricle leading to the pulmonary valve.

- **Septomarginal Trabecula (moderator band)**

  This is a band of cardiac muscle between the interventricular septum and the anterior papillary muscle that conducts part of the cardiac conduction system.

4. Left Ventricle

Blood enters from the left atrium through the mitral valve and is pumped out to the aorta through the aortic valve (Figure 7-20).

- **Trabeculae Carneae**

  The trabeculae carneae are ridges of myocardium in the ventricular wall, normally thicker than those of the right ventricle.

- **Papillary Muscles**

  The papillary muscles, usually two large ones, are attached by the chordae tendineae to the cusps of the bicuspid valve.

- **Chordae Tendinae**

  Same as right ventricle.

- **Aortic Vestibule**

  The aortic vestibule leads to the aortic semilunar valve and ascending aorta.

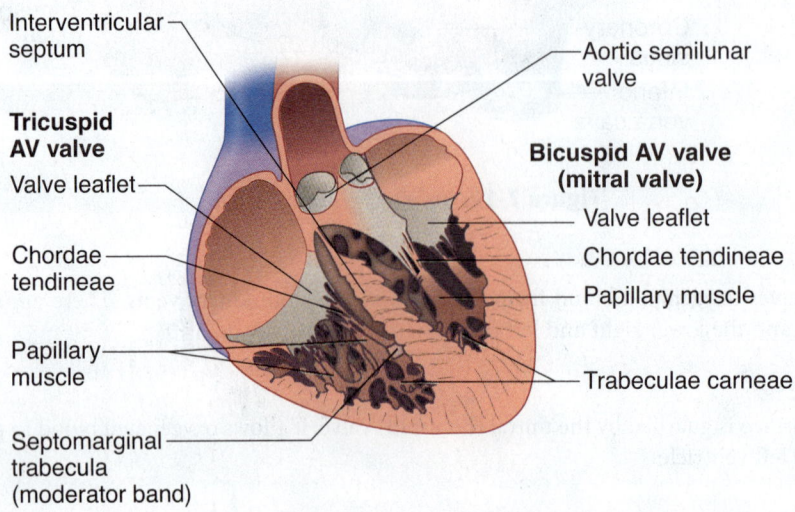

Figure 7-20. Right and Left Ventricles

HEART HISTOLOGY

Cardiac muscle is striated in the same manner as skeletal muscle, but it differs in being composed of smaller cells (fibers) with only one or two nuclei. The nuclei are located centrally, instead of peripherally.

Layers of the Heart Wall

The heart wall is composed of three distinct layers: an outer epicardium, a middle myocardium and an inner endocardium. The epicardium, or visceral layer of serous pericardium, consists of a simple squamous epithelium (mesothelium) and its underlying connective tissue. The connective tissue contains a large number of fat cells and the coronary vessels. The muscular wall of the heart is the myocardium and is composed mainly of cardiac muscle cells. The endocardium, which lines the chambers of the heart, is composed of a simple squamous epithelium, the endothelium, and a thin layer of connective tissue. Cardiac muscle is striated like skeletal muscle, but these cells are smaller, with centrally placed nuclei. Cardiac muscle has a similar but somewhat less well developed T-tubule system compared to skeletal muscle that is located at the Z-line.

Intercalated Discs

Intercalated discs are special junctional complexes that join myocardial cells. The intercalated discs appear as dark, transverse lines in the light microscope. These disks contain gap junctions and adhering junctions. These junctions permit the spread of electrical (gap) and mechanical (adhering) effects through the walls of the heart, synchronizing activity and for the pumping action of the heart chambers. While intercalated discs allow coordinated action of the myocardial cells, the squeezing and twisting movements of the heart chambers (particularly the left ventricle) during systole are due to the disposition of cardiac myocytes.

Purkinje cells are modified cardiac muscle cells with fewer contractile filaments. They are specialized for electrical impulse conduction rather than contraction. Purkinje cells are found in the conduction system of the heart.

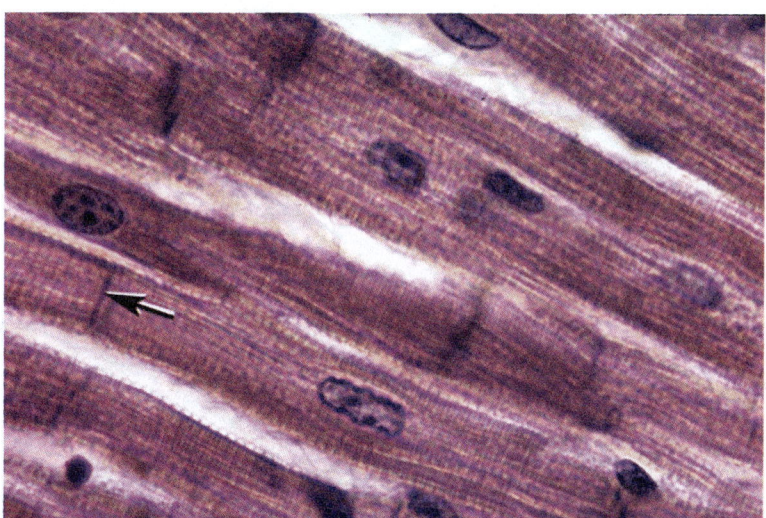

Figure 7-21. Cardiac muscle cells with centrally placed nuclei and intercalated disks (arrow)

Auscultation of Heart Valves

Points of auscultation of the **semilunar valves** (aortic and pulmonary) and the **atrioventricular valves** (tricuspid and mitral or bicuspid) are shown in Figure 7-22. The first heart sound occurs at the closure of the atrioventricular valves at the beginning of systole and the second heart sound occurs at the closure of the aortic and pulmonary semilunar valves at the end of systole.

Valves of the Heart

1. <u>Atrioventricular</u>
   Right Heart: Tricuspid
   Left Heart: Bicuspid

2. <u>Semilunar</u>
   Aortic (3 cusps)
   Pulmonary (3 cusps)

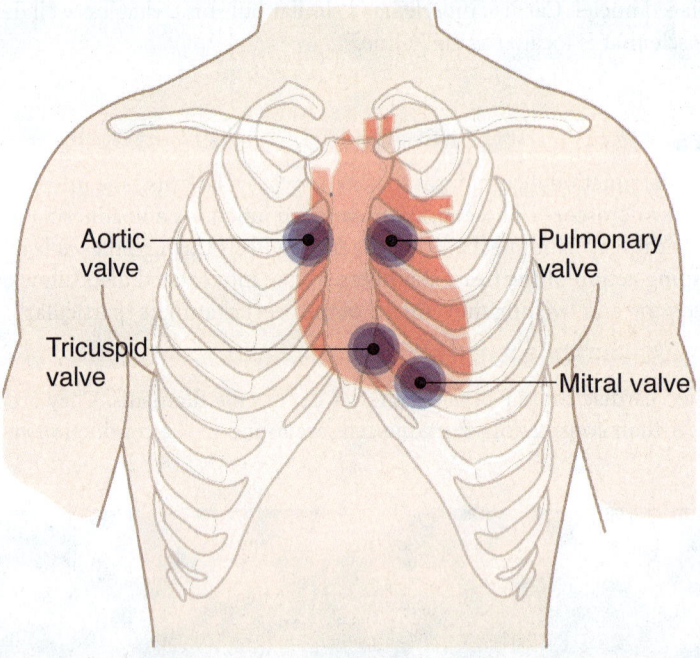

Figure 7-22. Surface Projections of the Heart

Heart Murmurs

Murmurs in valvular heart disease result when there is **valvular insufficiency or regurgitation** (the valves fail to close completely) or **stenosis** (narrowing of the valves). The **aortic and mitral valves** are more commonly </ix>involved in valvular heart disease.

For most of ventricular systole, the mitral valve should be closed and the aortic valve should be open, so that "common **systolic** valvular defects" include **mitral insufficiency** and **aortic stenosis**. For most of ventricular diastole, the mitral valve should be open and the aortic valve should be closed, so that "common **diastolic** valvular defects" include **mitral stenosis** and **aortic insufficiency**.

A heart murmur is heard downstream from the valve. Thus, stenosis is orthograde direction from valve and insufficiency is retrograde direction from valve.

Table 7-3. Heart Murmurs

	Stenosis	Insufficiency
A-V Valves	Diastolic Murmur	Systolic Murmur
Tricuspid (right)		
Mitral (left)		
Outflow Valves	Systolic Murmur	Diastolic Murmur
Pulmonic (right)		
Aortic (left)		

Arterial Supply of the Heart

The blood supply to the myocardium is provided by branches of the **right and left coronary arteries.** These two arteries are the only branches of the ascending aorta and arise from the **right and left aortic sinuses of the ascending aorta**, respectively. Blood flow enters the coronary arteries during diastole.

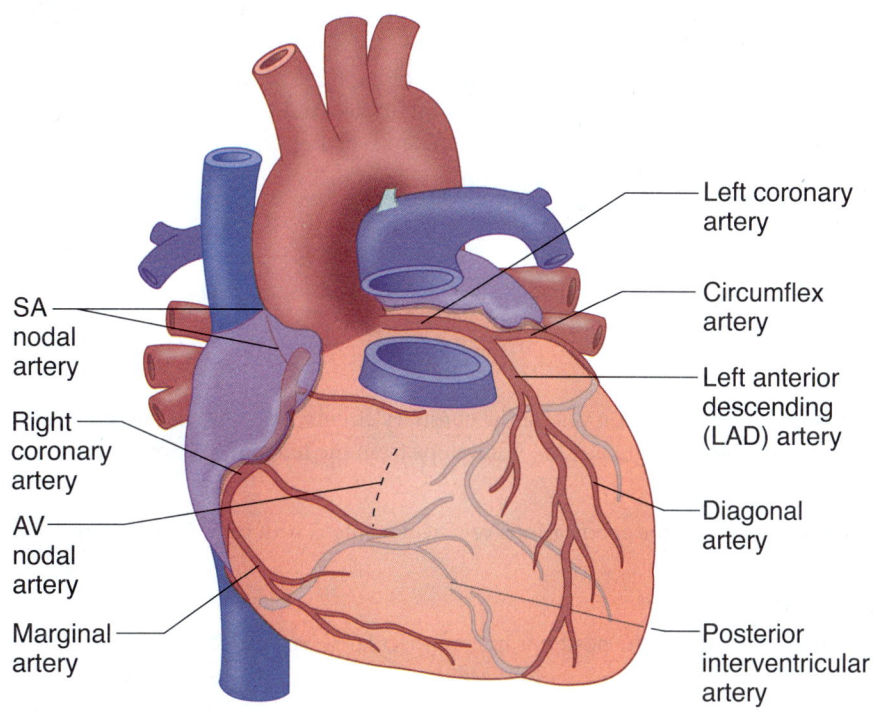

Figure 7-23. Arterial Supply to the Heart

Clinical Correlate

In myocardial infarction, the left anterior descending artery is obstructed in 50% of cases, the right coronary in 30%, and the circumflex artery in 20% of cases.

Right coronary artery

The **right coronary artery** courses in the coronary sulcus and supplies major parts of the right atrium and the right ventricle.

The branches of the right coronary include the following:

- **Sinoatrial (SA) nodal artery:** One of the first branches of the right coronary, it encircles the base of the superior vena cava to supply the **SA node.**
- **Atrioventricular (AV) nodal artery:** It arises from the distal end of the right coronary artery as it forms the posterior interventricular artery and penetrates the interatrial septum to supply the **AV node.**
- **Posterior interventricular artery:** It is the terminal distribution of the right coronary artery and courses in the posterior interventricular sulcus to supply parts of the right and left ventricles and, importantly, **the posterior third** of the interventricular septum.

Left coronary artery

The **left coronary artery** travels a short course between the left auricle and ventricle, and divides into two branches: **anterior interventricular or left anterior descending (LAD) artery** and **circumflex artery**.

- The **anterior interventricular artery** descends in the anterior interventricular sulcus and provides branches to the(1) **anterior left ventricle wall**, (2) **anterior two-thirds of the interventricular septum**,(3) **bundle of His**, and (4) **apex**. The LAD is the most common site of coronary occlusion.
- The **circumflex artery** courses around the left border of the heart in the coronary sulcus and supplies (1) the **left</ix> border of the heart** via the **marginal branch** and (2) ends on the posterior aspect of the left ventricle and supplies the **posterior-inferior** left ventricular wall.

Venous Drainage of the Heart

The major cardiac veins draining the heart course in the sulci and accompany the arteries but do not carry the same names. The major veins are the following:

- **Coronary sinus**

  The coronary sinus is the </ix>main vein of the coronary circulation; it lies in the posterior coronary sulcus. It drains to an opening in the right atrium. It develops from the **left sinus venosus**.

- **Great cardiac vein**

  The great cardiac vein lies in the anterior interventricular sulcus with the LAD artery. It is the main tributary of the coronary sinus.

- **Middle cardiac vein**

  The middle cardiac vein lies in the posterior interventricular sulcus with the posterior interventricular artery. It joins the coronary sinus.

- **Venae cordis minimae (the besian veins) and anterior cardiac veins**

  The venae cordis minimae and anterior cardiac veins open directly to the chambers of the heart.

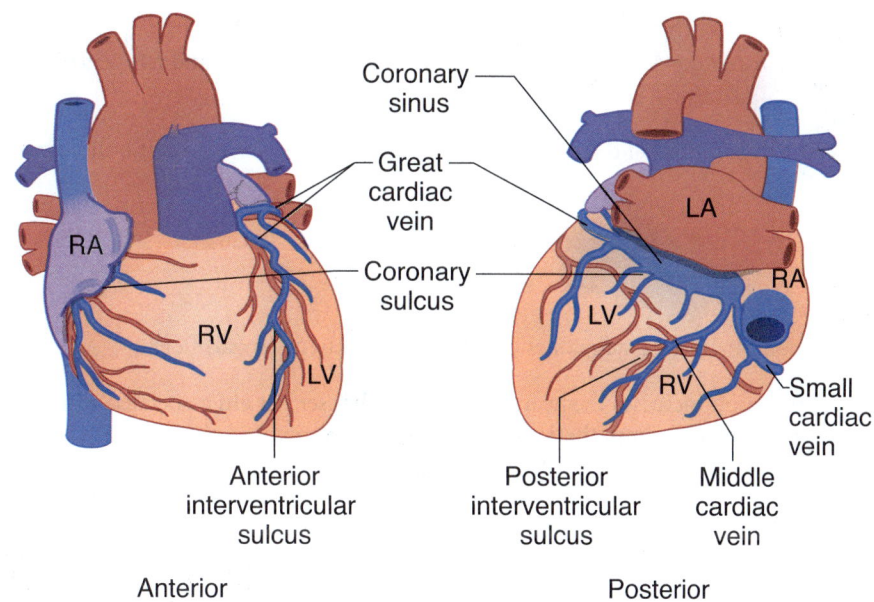

Figure 7-24. Venous Drainage of the Heart

Conducting System of the Heart

The **cardiac conduction system is** a specialized group of myocardial cells that initiates the periodic contractions of the heart due to their ability to depolarize at a faster rate than other cardiac myocytes. Electrical activity spreads through the walls of the atria from the SA node and is quickly passed by way of internodal fibers to the atrioventricular node. From the atrioventricular node, activity passes through the bundle of His and then down the right and left bundle branches in the interventricular septum. The bundle branches reach additional specialized cardiac muscle fibers known as Purkinje fibers in the ventricular walls.

- The Purkinje fibers run in several bundles along the endocardial surface and initiate ventricle activity starting at the apex of the ventricles.
- Purkinje fibers have a large cross section, a cytoplasm with few contractile fibrils and a large content of glycogen.

SA node

The SA node initiates the impulse for contraction of heart muscle (and is therefore termed the "pacemaker" of the heart). It is located at the superior end of the crista terminalis, where the superior vena cava enters the right atrium (Figure 7-25).

The SA node is supplied by the SA nodal branch of the **right coronary artery**.

Impulse production is speeded up by sympathetic nervous stimulation; it is slowed by parasympathetic (vagal) stimulation.

AV node

The AV node receives impulses from the SA node. The AV node is located in the interatrial septum near the opening of the coronary sinus. The AV node slows the impulse so that it reaches the ventricles after it has reached the atria.

The AV node is supplied by the **right coronary artery**.

Bundle of His

The **bundle of His** originates in the AV node. It conducts impulses to the right and left ventricles. It is supplied by the **LAD artery**.

In the right ventricle, the moderator band (septomarginal trabecula) contains the right bundle branch.

Impulses pass from the right and left bundle branches to the papillary muscles and ventricular myocardium.

Innervation

The cardiac plexus is a combination of sympathetic and parasympathetic (vagal) fibers.

- **Sympathetic** stimulation increases the heart rate. Nerves that sense **pain** associated with coronary artery ischemia (angina) follow the **sympathetic pathways** back into spinal cord segments T1–T5.

- **Parasympathetic** stimulation slows the heart rate. Sensory nerves that carry the afferent limb of cardiac **reflexes** travel with the **vagus nerve**.

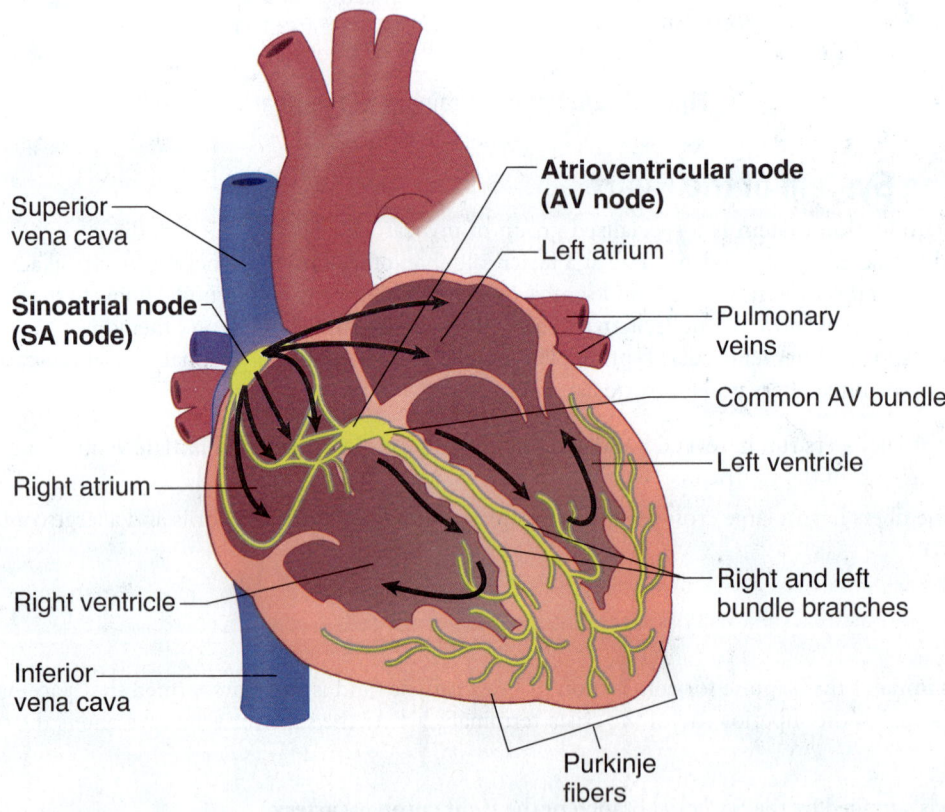

Figure 7-25. Cardiac Conduction System

DIAPHRAGM

Composition

The diaphragm is composed of a muscular portion and a central tendon. It is dome-shaped, and descends upon contraction of its muscular portion. It is innervated by the **phrenic nerves** that arise from spinal cord segments **C3 through C5**.

Apertures in the Diaphragm

Caval hiatus

Located to the right of the midline at the level of T8, within the central tendon (Figure 7-26)

Transmits the inferior vena cava and some branches of the right phrenic nerve

Esophageal hiatus

Located to the left of the midline at the level of T10, within the muscle of the right crus

Transmits the esophagus and the anterior and posterior vagus trunks

Aortic hiatus

Located in the midline at the level of T12, behind the two crura. Transmits the aorta and the thoracic duct.

Clinical Correlate

A **congenital diaphragmatic hernia** is a herniation of abdominal contents into the plural cavity due to the failure of the **pleuroperitoneal membranes** to develop properly.

An **esophageal hiatal hernia** is a herniation of the stomach into the pleural cavity due to an abnormally large esophageal hiatus to the diaphragm. This condition renders the esophagogastric sphincter incompetent so that contents reflux into the esophagus.

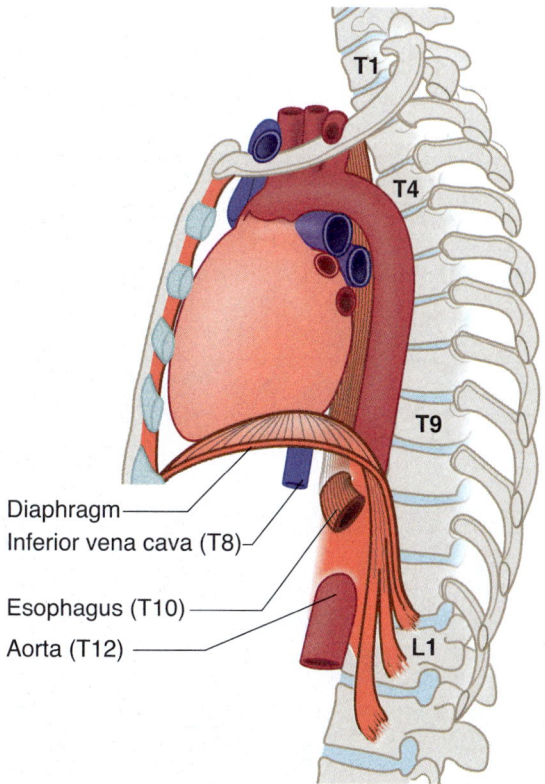

Figure 7-26. The Diaphragm

Learning Objectives

❏ Answer questions about embryology of the GI system

❏ Answer questions about GI histology, innervation, and immune functions

❏ Solve problems concerning arterial supply and venous drainage to abdominal viscera

❏ Explain information related to posterior abdominal body wall

❏ Answer questions about urinary histology and function

ANTERIOR ABDOMINAL WALL

Surface Anatomy

Linea Alba

The linea alba is a shallow groove that runs vertically in the median plane from the xiphoid to the pubis. It separates the right and left rectus abdominis muscles. The components of the rectus sheath intersect at the linea alba.

Linea Semilunaris

The linea semilunaris is a curved line defining the lateral border of the rectus abdominis, a bilateral feature.

MUSCLES AND FASCIAE OF ANTERIOR BODY WALL

The anterolateral abdominal body wall is a multilayer of fat, fasciae, and muscles (with their aponeuroses) that support and protect the abdominal contents. Three flat abdominal muscles are arranged in layers and the rectus abdominis is oriented vertically adjacent to the midline, extending between the costal margin and the pubis. Abdominal muscles are important in respiration, defecation, micturition, childbirth, etc. The layers of tissue that make up the abdominal wall are described superficial to deep.

In a Nutshell

Anterior Abdominal Wall Layers

- Skin
- Superficial fascia
  - Camper (fatty)
  - Scarpa (fibrous)
- External oblique
- Internal oblique
- Transversus abdominis
- Transversalis fascia
- Extraperitoneal connective tissue
- Parietal peritoneum

Layers of Anterior Abdominal Wall

Skin

Superficial fascia: The superficial fascia of the anterior abdominal wall below the umbilicus consists of two layers:

- **Camper** (fatty) fascia is the outer, subcutaneous layer of superficial fascia that is variable in thickness owing to the presence of fat.
- **Scarpa** (membranous) fascia is the deeper layer of superficial fascia devoid of fat. It is continuous into the perineum with various perineal fascial layers (Colles' fascia, dartos fascia of the scrotum, superficial fascia of the clitoris or penis).

Muscles

External abdominal oblique muscle and aponeurosis: This is the most superficial of the three flat muscles of the abdominal wall. Its contributions to the abdominal wall and inguinal region are the following:

- **Inguinal ligament** is the inferior rolled under aponeurotic fibers of the external oblique that extend between the anterior superior iliac spine and the pubic tubercle. Medially, the fibers of the inguinal ligament form a flattened, horizontal shelf called the **lacunar ligament** that attaches deeply to the pectineal line of the pubis and continues as the pectineal ligament. Lacunar ligament forms the medial border of a femoral hernia.
- **Superficial inguinal ring** is a vertical triangular cleft in the external oblique aponeurosis that represents the medial opening of the inguinal canal just superior and lateral to the pubic tubercle. It transmits the structures of the female and male inguinal canals.
- **External spermatic fascia** is the outer layer of the three coverings of the spermatic cord formed at the superficial inguinal ring in males.
- **Rectus sheath**: The external aponeuroses contribute to the anterior layer of the rectus sheath.

Internal abdominal oblique muscle and aponeurosis: This middle layer of the three flat muscles originates, in part, from the lateral two-thirds of the inguinal ligament. The internal oblique fibers course medially and arch over the inguinal canal in parallel with the arching fibers of the transversus abdominis muscle. The contributions of the internal abdominal oblique to the abdominal wall and inguinal region are the following:

> **Conjoint tendon** (**falx inguinalis**) is formed by the combined arching fibers of the internal oblique and the transversus abdominis muscles that insert on the pubic crest posterior to the superficial inguinal ring.

> **Rectus sheath:** The internal aponeuroses contribute to the layers of the rectus sheath.

> **Cremasteric muscle and fascia** represent the middle layer of the spermatic fascia covering the spermatic cord and testis in the male. It forms in the inguinal canal.

Transversus abdominis muscle and aponeurosis: This is the deepest of the flat muscles. The transversus muscle originates, in part, from the lateral one-third of the inguinal ligament and arches over the inguinal canal with the internal oblique fibers to contribute to the **conjoint tendon**. The aponeuroses of the transversus muscle also contribute to the layers of the rectus sheath. Note that it does not contribute to any of the layers of the spermatic fasciae.

Abdominopelvic Fasciae and Peritoneum

Transversalis fascia: This fascia forms a continuous lining of the entire abdominopelvic cavity. Its contributions to the inguinal region include the following:

- **Deep inguinal ring** is formed by an outpouching of the transversalis fascia immediately above the midpoint of the inguinal ligament and represents the lateral and deep opening of the inguinal canal. The **inferior epigastric vessels** are **medial** to the deep ring.

- **Internal spermatic fascia** is the deepest of the coverings of the spermatic cord formed at the deep ring in the male.

- **Femoral sheath** is an inferior extension of the transversalis fascia deep to the inguinal ligament into the thigh containing the femoral artery and vein and the femoral canal (site of femoral hernia).

- **Rectus sheath**: The transversalis fascia contributes to the posterior layer of the rectus sheath.

Extraperitoneal connective tissue: This is a thin layer of loose connective tissue and fat surrounding the abdominopelvic cavity, being most prominent around the kidneys. The **gonads** develop from the urogenital ridge within this layer.

Parietal peritoneum: This is the outer serous membrane that lines the abdominopelvic cavity.

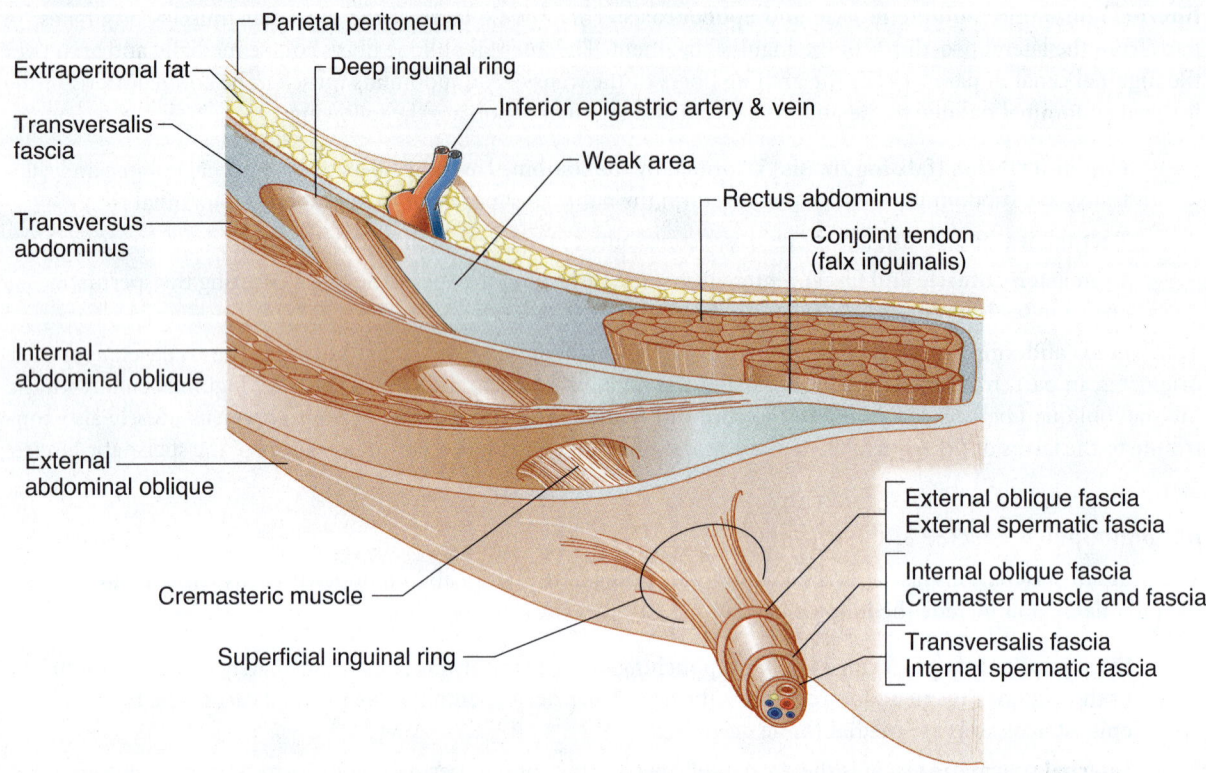

Figure 8-1. Layers of Anterolateral Abdominal Wall and Inguinal Canal

Nerves, Blood Vessels, and Lymphatics of Abdominal Wall

Innervation of the skin and musculature of the anterior abdominal wall is via branches of the ventral primary rami of the lower 6 thoracic spinal nerves (includes the subcostal nerve), plus the iliohypogastric and ilioinguinal branches of the ventral primary rami of L1.

The major **arterial blood supply** to the anterior wall is derived from the superior epigastric branch of the internal thoracic artery, as well as the inferior epigastric and the deep circumflex iliac branches of the external iliac artery.

Venous drainage from the anterior wall is to the superficial epigastric, the lateral thoracic veins superiorly and the great saphenous vein inferiorly.

Lymph drainage from tissues of the anterior wall is to axillary nodes superiorly and to superficial inguinal nodes inferiorly.

INGUINAL REGION AND CANAL

The **inguinal canal** is the oblique passage way (approximately 4 cm long) in the lower aspect of the anterior abdominal wall running parallel and superior to the medial half of the inguinal ligament. Clinically, the inguinal region is important because it is the area where inguinal hernias occur.

The entrance into the canal is the **deep inguinal ring**, located just lateral to the inferior epigastric vessels and immediately superior to the midpoint of the inguinal ligament.

The **superficial inguinal ring** is the medial opening of the canal superolateral to the pubic tubercle.

Contents of the Inguinal Canal

1. Female Inguinal Canal

Round ligament of the uterus: The round ligament extends between the uterus and the labia majora and is a remnant of the caudal genital ligament and the homologue of the gubernaculum testis of the male.

Ilioinguinal nerve (L1) is a branch of the lumbar plexus that exits the superficial ring to supply the skin of the anterior part of the mons pubis and labia majora.

2. Male Inguinal Canal

Ilioinguinal nerve (L1) is a branch of the lumbar plexus that exits the superficial ring to supply the skin of the lateral and anterior scrotum.

The spermatic cord is formed during descent of the testis and contains structures that are related to the testis. The cord begins at the deep ring and courses through the inguinal canal and exits the superficial ring to enter the scrotum. The spermatic cord is covered by three layers of spermatic fascia: external, middle, and internal. The cord contains the following:

- **Testicular artery:** A branch of the abdominal aorta that supplies the testis.
- **Pampiniform venous plexus:** An extensive network of veins draining the testis located within the scrotum and spermatic cord. The veins of the plexus coalesce to form the testicular vein at the deep ring. The venous plexus assists in the regulation of the temperature of the testis.
- **Vas deferens** (ductus deferens) and its artery
- **Autonomic nerves**
- **Lymphatics:** Lymphatic drainage of the testis will drain into the lumbar (aortic) nodes of the lumbar region and not to the superficial inguinal nodes which drain the rest of the male perineum.

EMBRYOLOGY OF THE GASTROINTESTINAL SYSTEM

Primitive Gut Tube

- The primitive gut tube is formed by incorporation of the **yolk sac** into the embryo during 2 body foldings: **head to tail (cranial-caudal)** and **lateral foldings** (Figure 8-3A).
- The epithelial lining of the mucosa of the primitive gut tube is derived from **endoderm**. The lamina propria, muscularis mucosae, submucosa, muscularis externa, and adventitia/serosa are derived from **mesoderm**.
- The primitive gut tube is divided into **the foregut, midgut, and hindgut**, each supplied by a specific artery and autonomic nerves.

Table 8-1. Adult Structures Derived from Each of the 3 Divisions of the Primitive Gut Tube

Foregut	Midgut	Hindgut
Artery: celiac	**Artery:** superior mesenteric	**Artery:** inferior mesenteric
Parasympathetic innervation: vagus nerves	**Parasympathetic innervation:** vagus nerves	**Parasympathetic innervation:** pelvic splanchnic nerves
Sympathetic innervation: • Preganglionics: thoracic splanchnic nerves, T5–T9 • Postganglionic cell bodies: celiac ganglion	**Sympathetic innervation:** • Preganglionics: thoracic splanchnic nerves, T9–T12 • Postganglionic cell bodies: superior mesenteric ganglion	**Sympathetic innervation:** • Preganglionics: lumbar splanchnic nerves, L1–L2 • Postganglionic cell bodies: inferior mesenteric ganglion
Referred Pain: Epigastrium	**Referred Pain:** Umbilical	**Referred Pain:** Hypogastrium
Foregut Derivatives	**Midgut Derivatives**	**Hindgut Derivatives**
Esophagus	Duodenum (second, third, and fourth parts)	Transverse colon (distal third—splenic flexure)
Stomach	Jejunum	Descending colon
Duodenum (first and second parts)	Ileum	Sigmoid colon
Liver	Cecum	Rectum
Pancreas	Appendix	Anal canal (above pectinate line)
Biliary apparatus	Ascending colon	
Gallbladder	Transverse colon (proximal two-thirds)	

In a Nutshell

The lower respiratory tract, liver and biliary system, and pancreas all develop from an **endodermal outgrowth of the foregut**.

PERITONEUM

Layers of Peritoneum

The peritoneum is the serous membrane related to the viscera of the abdominal cavity. It is divided into two layers: **parietal** and **visceral**.

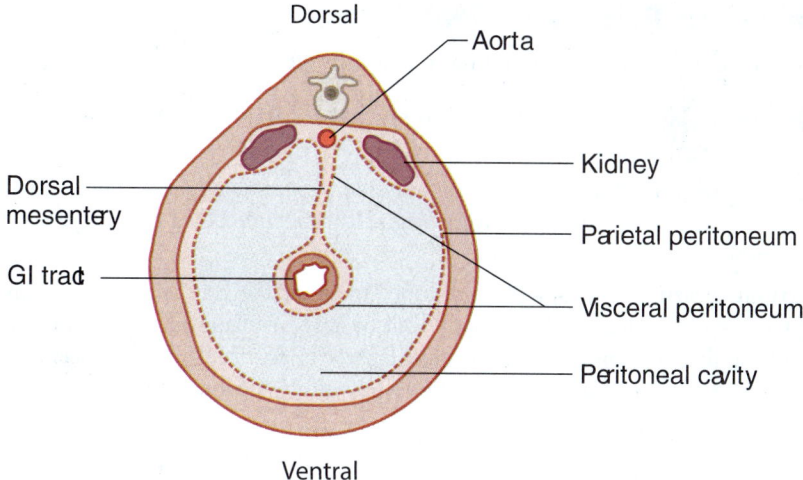

Figure 8-2. Peritoneum

Clinical Correlate

Inflammation of the parietal peritoneum (peritonitis) results in sharp pain that is localized over the area.

---

1. **Parietal Layer**

   The parietal layer lines the body wall and covers the retroperitoneal organs on one surface. Parietal peritoneum is very sensitive to somatic pain and is innervated by the lower intercostal nerves and the ilioinguinal and the iliohypogastric nerves of the lumbar plexus.

2. **Visceral Layer**

   The visceral layer encloses the surfaces of the intraperitoneal organs. The visceral peritoneum usually forms double-layered peritoneal membranes (mesenteries) that suspend parts of the GI tract from the body wall. The mesenteries allow for the passage of vessels, nerves, and lymphatics to reach the GI tract.

   Different terms describe the postnatal remnants of mesenteries in the abdomen and include the following:

   - **Omentum:** Lesser and greater omenta attach to the lesser or greater curvatures of the stomach, respectively.
   - **Mesocolon:** Transverse and sigmoid mesocolon attach to the transverse colon or the sigmoid colon, respectively.
   - **Ligaments:** Reflections of mesenteries between organs or the body wall, named according to their attachments

Peritoneal Cavity

The peritoneal cavity is the potential space located between the parietal and visceral peritoneal layers. The 90° rotation and the shift of the embryonic mesenteries divides the peritoneal cavity into two sacs.

- **The lesser sac (omental bursa)** is a cul-de-sac formed posterior to the stomach and the lesser omentum
- **The greater sac** is formed by the larger area of the remaining peritoneal cavity. The only communication between the lesser sac and the greater sac is the **epiploic foramen (of Winslow)**.

Intraperitoneal versus Retroperitoneal Organs

The abdominal viscera are classified according to their relationship to the peritoneum (Table 8-2).

- **Intraperitoneal organs** are suspended by a mesentery and are almost completely enclosed in visceral peritoneum. These organs are mobile.
- **Retroperitoneal organs** are partially covered on one side with parietal peritoneum and are immobile or fixed organs. Many retroperitoneal organs were originally suspended by a mesentery and become secondarily retroperitoneal.

Secondary Retroperitonealization: Parts of the gut tube (most of the duodenum, pancreas, ascending colon, descending colon, part of rectum) fuse with the body wall by way of fusion of visceral peritoneum with parietal peritoneum. This results in these organs becoming secondarily retroperitoneal and the visceral peritoneum covering the organ being renamed as the parietal peritoneum. The vessels within the mesentery of these gut structures become secondarily retroperitoneal.

Table 8-2. Intraperitoneal and Retroperitoneal Organs

Major Intraperitoneal Organs (suspended by a mesentery)	Major Secondary Retroperitoneal Organs (lost a mesentery during development)	Major Primary Retroperitoneal Organs (never had a mesentery)
Stomach	Duodenum, 2nd and 3rd parts	Kidneys
Liver and gallbladder	Head, neck, and body of pancreas	Adrenal glands
Spleen	Ascending colon	Ureters
Duodenum, 1st part	Descending colon	Aorta
Tail of pancreas	Upper rectum	Inferior vena cava
Jejunum		Lower rectum
Ileum		Anal canal
Appendix		
Transverse colon		
Sigmoid colon		

Epiploic Foramen (of Winslow)

The **epiploic foramen** is the opening between omental bursa and greater peritoneal sac. The boundaries of the epiploic foramen are the following:

- **Anteriorly:** Hepatoduodenal ligament and the hepatic portal vein
- **Posteriorly:** Inferior vena cava
- **Superiorly:** Caudate lobe of the liver
- **Inferiorly:** First part of the duodenum

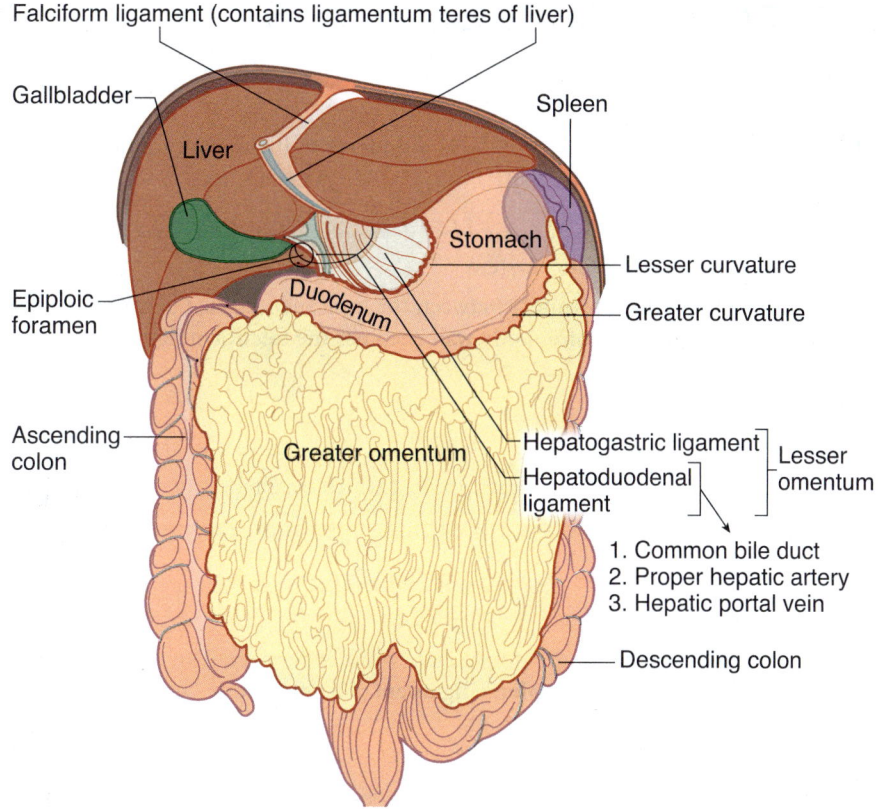

Figure 8-3. Peritoneal Membranes

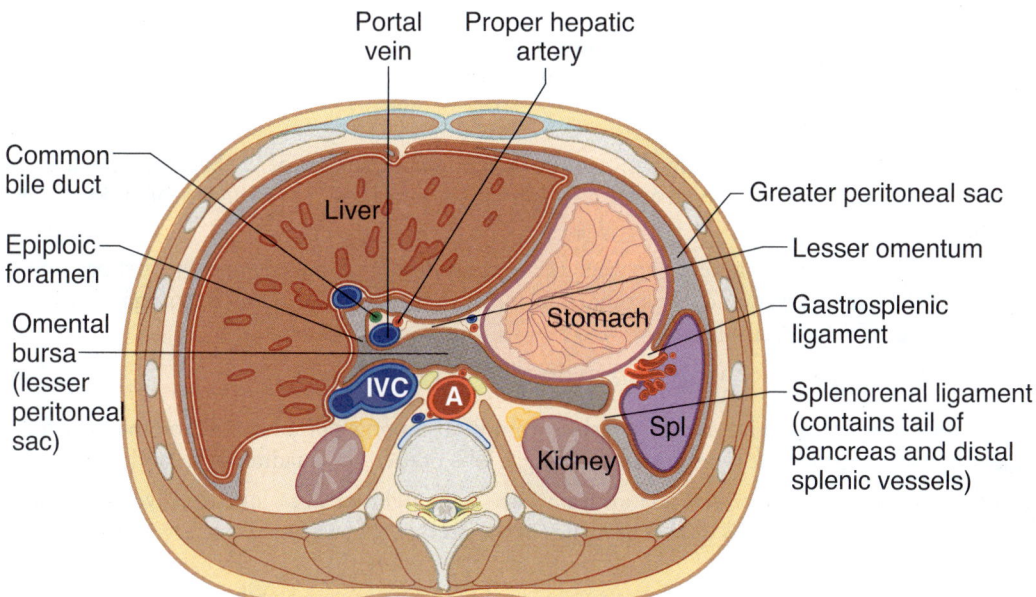

Figure 8-4. Greater and Lesser Peritoneal Sacs
IVC = inferior vena cava
A = aorta
Spl = spleen

DEVELOPMENT OF ABDOMINAL VISCERA

Liver

The hepatic diverticulum develops as an outgrowth of the **endoderm** of the foregut in the region of the duodenum near the border between the foregut and the midgut.

- This diverticulum enters the ventral embryonic mesentery and distally becomes the liver and gallbladder and proximately becomes the biliary duct system.
- The part of the ventral embryonic mesentery between the liver and gut tube becomes the **lesser omentum**, and the part between the liver and ventral body wall becomes the **falciform ligament**.

Pancreas

The pancreas develops from two pancreatic diverticula (buds), which evaginate from the **endodermal** lining of the foregut in the region of duodenum.

Spleen

The spleen develops from **mesoderm** within the dorsal embryonic mesentery. The embryonic mesentery between the spleen and the gut tube becomes the **gastrosplenic ligament**. The mesentery between the spleen and the dorsal body wall becomes the **splenorenal ligament**.

ABDOMINAL VISCERA

Liver

The liver has two surfaces: a superior or **diaphragmatic** surface and an inferior or a **visceral** surface (Figure 8-6). It lies mostly in the right aspect of the abdominal cavity and is protected by the rib cage. The liver is invested by visceral peritoneum:

- The reflection of visceral peritoneum between the diaphragmatic surface of the liver and the diaphragm forms the **falciform ligament**, which continues onto the liver as the coronary ligament and the right and left triangular ligaments.
- The extension of visceral peritoneum between the visceral surface of the liver and the first part of the duodenum and the lesser curvature of the stomach forms the **hepatoduodenal and hepatogastric ligaments** of the **lesser omentum**, respectively.

The liver is divided into two lobes of unequal size as described below.

- Fissures for the ligamentum teres and the ligamentum venosum, the porta hepatis, and the fossa for the gallbladder further subdivide the right lobe into the right lobe proper, the quadrate lobe, and the caudate lobe.
- The quadrate and caudate lobes are anatomically part of the right lobe but functionally part of the left. They receive their blood supply from the left branches of the portal vein and hepatic artery and secrete bile to the left hepatic duct.

The liver has a central hilus, or porta hepatis, which receives venous blood from the **portal vein** and arterial blood from the **hepatic artery**.

- The central hilus also transmits the common bile duct, which collects bile produced by the liver.
- These structures, known collectively as the portal triad, are located in the hepatoduodenal ligament, which is the right free border of the lesser omentum.

The **hepatic veins** drain the liver by collecting blood from the liver sinusoids and returning it to the inferior vena cava.

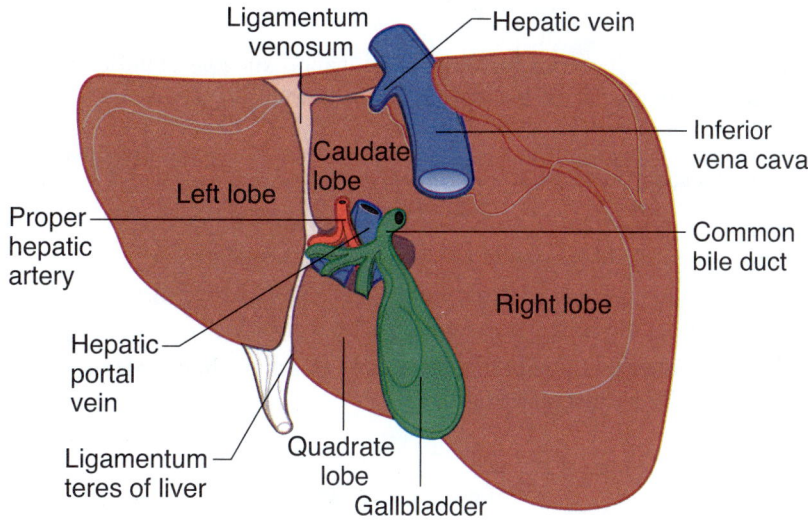

Figure 8-5. Visceral Surface of the Liver

Gallbladder

The gallbladder lies in a fossa on the visceral surface of the liver to the right of the quadrate lobe. It stores and concentrates bile, which enters and leaves through the cystic duct.

- The cystic duct joins the common hepatic duct to form the **common bile duct**.
- The common bile duct descends in the hepatoduodenal ligament, then passes posterior to the first part of the duodenum. The common bile duct penetrates the head of the pancreas where it joins the main pancreatic duct and forms the **hepatopancreatic ampulla,** which drains into the second part of the duodenum at the **major duodenal papilla**.

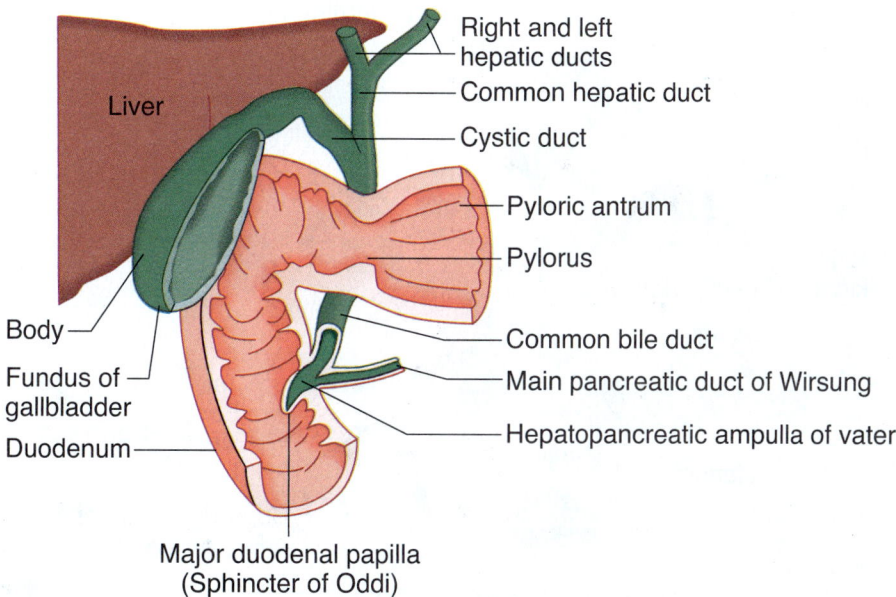

Figure 8-6. Biliary Ducts

Pancreas

The pancreas horizontally crosses the posterior abdominal wall at approximately at the level of the transpyloric plane (Figure 8-8). The gland consists of four parts: **head, neck, body, and tail**.

- The head of the pancreas rests within the C-shaped area formed by the duodenum and is traversed by the common bile duct. The head of the pancreas includes the **uncinate process** which is crossed by the superior mesenteric vessels.
- Posterior to the neck is the site of formation of the hepatic portal vein.
- The body passes to the left and passes anterior to the aorta and the left kidney. The splenic artery undulates along the superior border of the body of the pancreas with the splenic vein coursing posterior to the body.
- The tail of the pancreas enters the **splenorenal ligament** to reach the hilum of the spleen. The tail is the only part of the pancreas that is **intraperitoneal**.

Clinical Correlate
Carcinoma of the pancreas commonly occurs in the **head of the pancreas** and may constrict the main **pancreatic duct** and the **common bile duct**. Obstruction of the bile duct may result in **jaundice**.

The main **pancreatic duct** courses through the body and tail of the pancreas to reach the head of the pancreas, where it joins with the common bile duct to form the hepatopancreatic ampulla.

The head of the pancreas receives its blood supply from the **superior and inferior pancreaticoduodenal branches** of the gastroduodenal and superior mesenteric arteries, respectively. This region is important for **collateral circulation** because there are anastomoses between these branches of the celiac trunk and superior mesenteric artery.

The neck, body, and tail of the pancreas receive their blood supply from the **splenic artery**.

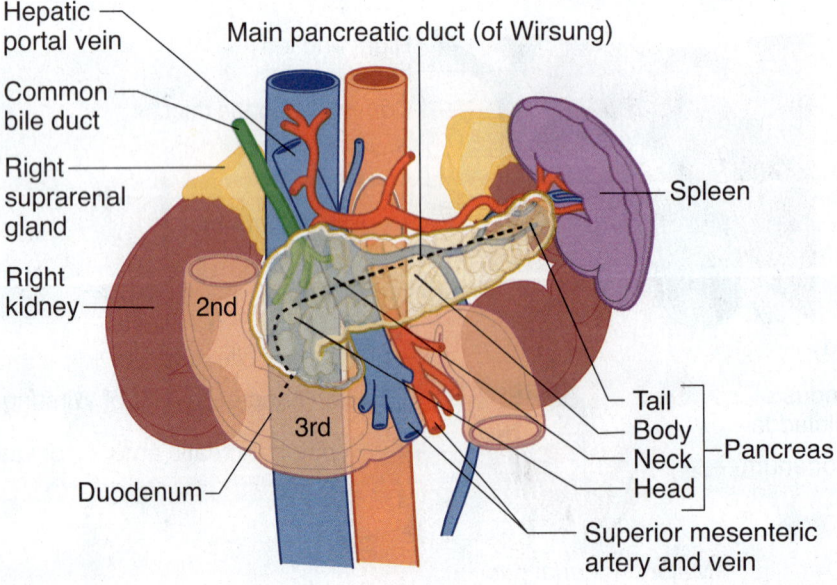

Figure 8-7. Adult Pancreas

Spleen

The spleen is a peritoneal organ in the upper left quadrant that is deep to the left 9th, 10th, and 11th ribs. The visceral surface of the spleen is in contact with the left colic flexure, stomach, and left kidney. Inasmuch as the spleen lies above the costal margin, a normal-sized spleen is not palpable.

The splenic artery and vein reach the hilus of the spleen by traversing the **splenorenal ligament**.

Stomach

The stomach has a right **lesser curvature**, which is connected to the porta hepatis of the liver by the lesser omentum (hepatogastric ligament), and a left **greater curvature** from which the greater omentum is suspended.

The cardiac region receives the esophagus; and the dome-shaped upper portion of the stomach, which is normally filled with air, is the fundus. The main central part of the stomach is the body. The pyloric portion of the stomach has a thick muscular wall and narrow lumen that empties into the duodenum approximately in the transpyloric plane (L1 vertebra).

Duodenum

The duodenum is C-shaped, has four parts, and is located retroperitoneal except for the first part.

- The first part is referred to as the duodenal cap (bulb). The gastroduodenal artery and the common bile duct descend posterior to the first part.
- The second part (descending) receives the **common bile duct** and main **pancreatic duct** at the hepatopancreatic ampulla (of Vater). Smooth muscle in the wall of the duodenal papilla is known as the sphincter of Oddi.
- Note that the foregut terminates at the point of entry of the common bile duct; the remainder of the duodenum is part of the midgut.

Jejunum and Ileum

The jejunum begins at the duodenojejunal junction and comprises 2/5 of the remaining small intestine. The beginning of the ileum is not clearly demarcated; it consists of the distal 3/5 of the small bowel.

The jejunoileum is suspended from the posterior body wall by the mesentery proper. Although the root of the mesentery is only 6 inches long, the mobile part of the small intestine is approximately 22 feet in length.

Colon

Cecum

The cecum is the first part of the colon, or large intestine, and begins at the ileocecal junction. It is a blind pouch, which often has a mesentery and gives rise to the vermiform appendix. The appendix has its own mesentery, the mesoappendix.

Ascending colon

The ascending colon lies retroperitoneally and lacks a mesentery. It is continuous with the transverse colon at the right (hepatic) flexure of colon.

Transverse colon

The transverse colon has its own mesentery called the **transverse mesocolon**. It becomes continuous with the descending colon at the left (splenic) flexure of colon. The midgut terminates at the junction of the proximal two-thirds and distal one-third of the transverse colon.

Descending colon

The descending colon lacks a mesentery. It joins the sigmoid colon where the large bowel crosses the pelvic brim.

Sigmoid colon

The sigmoid colon is suspended by the **sigmoid mesocolon**. It is the terminal portion of the large intestine and enters the pelvis to continue as the rectum.

Rectum

The superior one-third of the rectum is covered by peritoneum anteriorly and laterally. It is the fixed, terminal, straight portion of the hindgut.

Anal Canal

- The **anal canal** is about 1.5 inches long and opens distally at the anus. The anal canal is continuous with the rectum at the pelvic diaphragm where it makes a 90-degree posterior bend (anorectal flexure) below the rectum.
- The **puborectalis component** of the pelvic diaphragm pulls the flexure forward, helping to maintain fecal continence.
- The **internal anal sphincter** is circular smooth muscle that surrounds the anal canal. The **sympathetics** (lumbar splanchnics) **increase** the tone of the muscle and the **parasympathetics** (pelvic splanchnics) **relax** the muscle during defecation.
- The **external anal sphincter** is circular voluntary skeletal muscle surrounding the canal that is voluntarily controlled by the inferior rectal branch of the **pudendal nerve** and **relaxes** during defecation.
- The anal canal is divided in an upper and lower parts separated by the **pectinate line**, an elevation of the mucous membrane at the distal ends of the anal columns. A comparison of the features of the anal canal above and below the pectinate line is shown in the following table.

GASTROINTESTINAL HISTOLOGY

The alimentary or gastrointestinal (GI) tract is a muscular tube that runs from the oral cavity to the anal canal. The GI tract walls are composed of four layers: mucosa, submucosa, muscularis externa, and serosa.

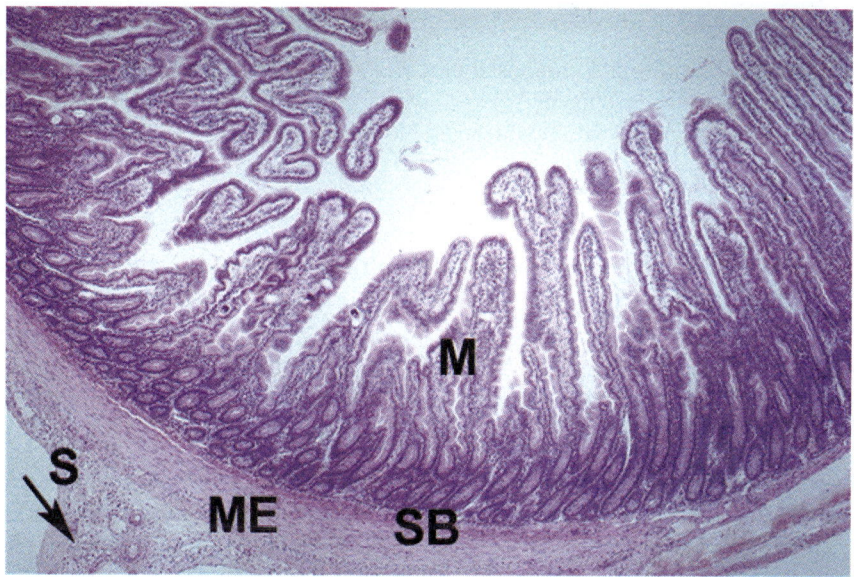

Copyright McGraw-Hill Companies. Used with permission.

Figure 8-8. Organization of the GI tract
Mucosa (M) submucosa (SB), muscularis externa (ME),
serosa or visceral peritoneum (S), mesentery (arrow)

Mucosa

The **mucosa** is the innermost layer and has three components.

- The **epithelium** lining the lumen varies in different regions depending on whether the function is primarily conductive and protective (stratified squamous; in the pharynx and esophagus), or secretory and absorptive (simple columnar; stomach and intestine).

- The **lamina propria** is a layer of areolar connective tissue that supports the epithelium and attaches it to the underlying muscularis mucosae. Numerous capillaries form extensive networks in the lamina propria (particularly in the small intestine).

  Within the lamina propria are blind-ended lymphatic vessels (lacteals) that carry out absorbed nutrients and white blood cells (particularly lymphocytes). The GALT (gut- associated lymphoid tissue), responsible for IgA production, is located within the lamina propria.

- The **muscularis mucosa** is a thin smooth-muscle layer that marks the innermost edge of the mucosa. The muscle confers some motility to the mucosa and facilitates discharge of secretions from glands. In the small intestine, a few strands of smooth muscle may run into the lamina propria and up to the tips of villi.

Submucosa

The **submucosa** is a layer of loose areolar connective tissue that attaches the mucosa to the muscularis externa and houses the larger blood vessels and mucus-secreting glands.

Muscularis Externa

The **muscularis externa** is usually comprised of two layers of muscle: an inner circular and an outer longitudinal. The muscularis externa controls the lumen size and is responsible for peristalsis. The muscle is striated in the upper third of the esophagus and smooth elsewhere.

Serosa

The **serosa** (or peritoneum of anatomy) is composed of a mesothelium (a thin epithelium lining the thoracic and abdominal cavities) and loose connective tissue. In the abdominal cavity, the serosa surrounds each intestinal loop and then doubles to form the mesentery within which run blood and lymphatic vessels.

INNERVATION

The GI tract has both intrinsic and extrinsic innervation. The intrinsic innervation is entirely located within the walls of the GI tract. The **intrinsic** system is capable of autonomous generation of peristalsis and glandular secretions. An interconnected network of ganglia and nerves located in the submucosa forms the Meissner's plexus and controls much of the intrinsic motility of the lining of the alimentary tract. Auerbach's plexus contains a second network of neuronal ganglia, and is located between the two muscle layers of the muscularis externa. All GI-tract smooth muscle is interconnected by gap junctions.

The **extrinsic** autonomic innervation to the GI tract is from the parasympathetic (stimulatory) and sympathetic (inhibitory) axons that modulate the activity of the intrinsic innervation. Sensory fibers accompany the parasympathetic nerves and mediate visceral reflexes and sensations, such as hunger and rectal fullness. Visceral pain fibers course back to the CNS with the sympathetic innervation. Pain results from excessive contraction and or distention of the smooth muscle. Visceral pain is referred to the body wall dermatomes that match the sympathetic innervation to that GI tract structure.

Clinical Correlate

Hirschsprung disease or aganglionic megacolon is a genetic disease present in approximately 1 out of 5,000 live births. It may result from mutations that affect the migration of neural crest cells into the gut. This results in a deficiency of terminal ganglion cells in Auerbach's plexus and affects of digestive tract motility, particularly in the rectum (peristalsis is not as effective and constipation results).

IMMUNE FUNCTIONS

The lumen of the GI tract is normally colonized by abundant bacterial flora. The majority of the bacteria in the body—comprising about 500 different species—are in our gut, where they enjoy a rich growth medium within a long, warm tube. Most of these bacteria are beneficial (vitamins B_{12} and K production, additional digestion, protection against pathogenic bacteria) but a few species of pathogenic microbes appear at times. Our gut has defense mechanisms to fight these pathogens (GALT and Paneth cells).

REGIONAL DIFFERENCES

Major differences lie in the general organization of the mucosa (glands, folds, villi, etc.) and in the types of cells comprising the epithelia and associated glands in the GI tract.

Table 8-3. Histology of Specific Regions

Region	Major Characteristics	Mucosal Cell Types at Surface	Function of Surface Mucosal Cells
Esophagus	• Nonkeratinized stratified squamous epithelium • Skeletal muscle in muscularis externa (upper 1/3) • Smooth muscle (lower 1/3)	—	—
Stomach (body and fundus)	*Rugae:* shallow pits; deep glands	Mucus cells	Secrete mucus; form protective layer against acid; tight junctions between these cells probably contribute to the acid barrier of the epithelium.
		Chief cells	Secrete pepsinogen and lipase precursor
		Parietal cells	Secrete HCl and intrinsic factor
		Enteroendocrine (EE) cells	Secrete a variety of peptide hormones
Pylorus	Deep pits; shallow, branched glands	Mucous cells	Same as above
		Parietal cells	Same as above
		EE cells	High concentration of gastrin
Small intestine	Villi, plicae, and crypts	Columnar absorptive cells	Contain numerous microvilli that greatly increase the luminal surface area, facilitating absorption
Duodenum	Brunner glands, which discharge alkaline secretion	Goblet cells	Secrete acid glycoproteins that protect mucosal linings
		Paneth cells	Contains granules that contain lysozyme. May play a role in regulating intestinal flora
		EE cells	High concentration of cells that secrete cholecystokinin and secretin
Jejunum	Villi, well developed plica, crypts	Same cell types as found in the duodenal epithelium	Same as above
Ileum	Aggregations of lymph nodules called Peyer's patches	M cells found over lymphatic nodules and Peyer's patches	Endocytose and transport antigen from the lumen to lymphoid cells
Large intestine	Lacks villi, crypts	Mainly mucus-secreting and absorptive cells	Transports Na^+ (actively) and water (passively) out of lumen

Oral Cavity

Note: details of oral tissue (mucosa, teeth, tongue, salivary glands, etc.) can be found in the Physiology and Dental Anatomy section.

The epithelium of the oral cavity is a stratified squamous epithelium. Mucous and serous secretions of the salivary glands lubricate food, rinse the oral cavity, moisten the food for swallowing and provide partial antibacterial protection. Secretions of IgA from plasma cells within the connective tissue are transported through the gland epithelia to help protect against microbial attachment and invasion.

Esophagus

The esophagus is also lined by a stratified squamous epithelium. In the lower part of the esophagus there is an abrupt transition to the simple columnar epithelium of the stomach. Langerhans cells—macrophage-like antigen-presenting cells—are present in the epithelial lining. The muscularis externa of the esophagus consists of striated muscle in the upper third, smooth muscle in the distal third, and a combination of both in the middle third.

Stomach

The stomach has three distinct histological areas: the cardia, body, and pyloric antrum. The mucosa of the stomach is thrown into folds (rugae) when empty, but disappears when the stomach is full. The surface is lined by a simple columnar epithelium. The stomach begins digestion by initiating the chemical and enzymatic breakdown of ingested food. Proteins are initially denatured by the acidic gastric juice before being hydrolyzed to polypeptide fragments by the enzyme pepsin. The chyme consists of denatured and partially broken-up food particles suspended in a semi-fluid, highly acidic medium.

Gastric pits form numerous deep tubular invaginations that line the inner surface of the stomach. The gastric pits are closely spaced; they penetrate into the thickness of the mucosa and extend into gastric glands. The transition between pits and glands is marked by the isthmus, where there is a narrowing of the lumen, and by a change in cellular composition of the epithelium. The glands are coiled in the cardiac and pyloric regions of the stomach and straight in the fundus and body regions. Glands in the body of the stomach deliver gastric juice (containing HCl and enzymes, rennin and lipase) to each pit, and from there to the stomach lumen. There are about 5 million glands in the stomach, secreting some 2 liters of fluid per day.

Mucus-secreting cells are located on the inner surface of the stomach, in the pit and in the neck, the transitional region between pits and glands. These cells produce a thick layer of mucus which covers and protects the stomach. The mucus falls into two categories: the surface mucus is composed of neutral glycoproteins, while the mucus secreted by the neck mucus cells is composed of acidic glycoproteins. In cardiac and pyloric regions, mucus cells are also the major cell type in the glands.

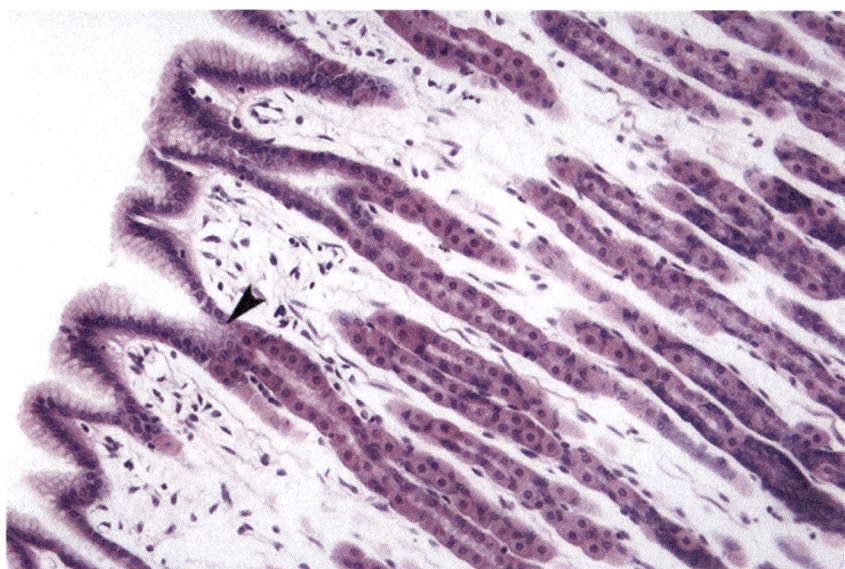

Copyright McGraw-Hill Companies. Used with permission.

Figure 8-9. Cardiac part of the stomach with gastric pits and coiled gastric glands. Stem cells that regenerate all stomach cells are located at the isthmus (arrowhead)

Clinical Correlate

Acetylcholine and gastrin increase HCL secretion by parietal cells. Histamine potentiates both by binding to the histamine H_2 receptor. Cimetidine and H_2 antagonists inhibit histamine.

Infection by *Helicobacter pylori* affects the gastric mucosal lining and allows pepsin, HCl, and proteases to erode the mucosa.

Oxyntic or parietal cells secrete 0.1N HCl into the stomach lumen and bicarbonate ions into the lamina propria (a byproduct of the acid production) in response to histamine, gastrin, and acetylcholine. These cells also secrete intrinsic factor (a glycoprotein necessary for absorption of vitamin B_{12}).

- Vitamin B_{12} is required for production of erythrocytes; deficiencies result in pernicious anemia and a disruption of peripheral and central nervous system myelin (see subacute combined degeneration in *Neuroscience* section).

Parietal cells, located in the upper regions of the gastric glands, have a broader base and narrower apex. Their structure varies greatly depending on their functional state.

Chief or **peptic cells** secrete pepsinogen, an enzyme precursor that is stored in secretory (zymogen) granules before its induced secretion. Pepsinogen is inactive and protects the peptic cells from autodigestion. Low pH, in the stomach lumen, converts pepsinogen to pepsin.

The **enteroendocrine cells** or APUD cells (amine precursor uptake and decarboxylation) are present throughout the GI tract and are also found in the respiratory tract. They constitute a diffuse neuroendocrine system that collectively accounts for more cells than all other endocrine organs in the body. Enteroendocrine cells are dispersed throughout the GI tract so that they can receive and transmit local signals.

The **stem cells** responsible for the regeneration of all types of cells in the stomach epithelium are **located in the isthmus**. Their mitotic rate can be influenced by the presence of gastrin and by damage (aspirin, alcohol, bile salt reflux). Renewal of many gastric epithelial cells occurs every 4–7 days.

Small Intestine

The small intestine is tubular in shape and has a total length of about 21 feet. The effective internal surface area of the small intestine is greatly increased by the plicae circulares, villi and microvilli.

Plicae circulares (circular folds or valves of Kerckring) are foldings of the inner surface that involve both mucosa and sub-mucosa. Plicae circulares increase the surface area by a factor of 3.

Villi arise above the muscularis mucosae and they include the lamina propria and epithelium of the mucosa. Villi increase the surface area by a factor of 10.

Microvilli of the absorptive epithelial cells increase the surface area by a factor of 20–30. The surface area of microvilli is increased even further by the presence surface membrane glycoproteins, constituting the glycocalyx to which enzymes are bound.

The luminal surface of the small intestine is perforated by the openings of numerous tubular invaginations (the crypts of Lieberkühn) analogous to the glands of the stomach. The crypts penetrate through the lamina propria and reach the muscularis mucosae.

The small intestine completes digestion, absorbs the digested food constituents (amino acids, monosaccharides, fatty acids) and transports it into blood and lymphatic vessels.

The **duodenum** is the proximal pyloric end of the small intestine. Distal to the duodenum is the **jejunum**, and then the **ileum**.

In the small intestine, the chyme from the stomach is **mixed** with mucosal cell secretions, exocrine pancreatic juice, and bile.

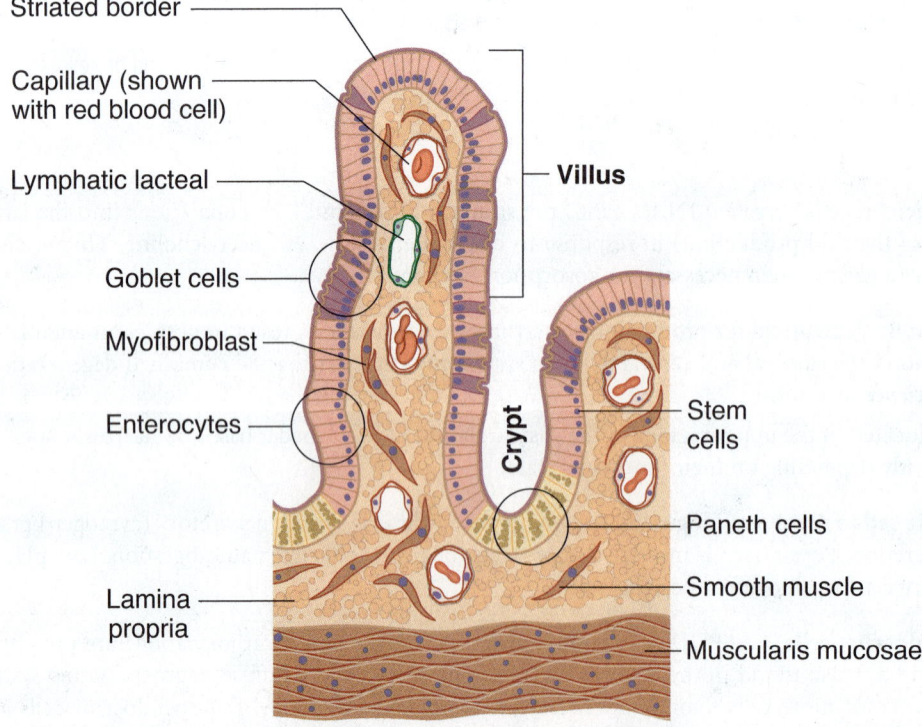

Figure 8-10. Small Intestine Mucosal Histology

Mucus production occurs in surface epithelial cells throughout the GI tract, by **Brunner glands** in the duodenum and **goblet cells** in the mucosa throughout the intestine.

> ### Clinical Correlate
>
> Any compromise of the mucous protection can lead to significant damage and irritation of the gastrointestinal tract, leading to gastritis, duodenitis, or even peptic ulcer disease.

Mucus functions include lubrication of the GI tract, binding bacteria, and trapping immunoglobulins where they have access to pathogens.

The **rate of mucus** secretion is increased by cholinergic stimulation, chemical irritation, and physical irritation.

In the **duodenum,** the acidic chyme from the stomach is neutralized by the neutral or alkaline mucus secretions of glands located in the submucosal or Brunner's glands. The duodenum also receives digestive enzymes and bicarbonate from the pancreas and bile from the liver (via gallbladder) through the bile duct, continuing the digestive process.

> ### Clinical Correlate
>
> Peristalsis is activated by the **parasympathetic system**. For those suffering from decreased intestinal motility manifesting as constipation (paralytic ileus, diabetic gastroparesis), dopaminergic and cholinergic agents are often used (e.g., metoclopramide).

In the **jejunum,** the digestion process continues via enterocyte-produced enzymes and absorbs food products. The plicae circulares are best developed here. In the **ileum,** a major site of immune reactivity, the mucosa is more heavily infiltrated with lymphocytes and the accompanying antigen-presenting cells than the duodenum and jejunum. Numerous primary and secondary lymphatic nodules (Peyer's patches) are always present in the ileum's mucosa, though their location is not fixed in time. In the infant, maternal IgGs that are ingested are recognized by the Fc receptors in microvilli and endocytosed to provide passive immunity. In the adult, only trace amounts of intact proteins are transferred from lumen to lamina propria, but IgAs produced in GALT in the ileum are transported in the opposite direction into the lumen.

> ### Note
>
> Histologically, the duodenum contains submucosal Brunner's glands, and the ileum contains Peyer's patches in the lamina propria. The jejunum can be easily recognized because it has neither Brunner's glands nor Peyer's patches.

Throughout the small intestine, the simple columnar intestinal epithelium has five types of differentiated cells, all derived from a common pool of stem cells.

1. **Goblet cells** secrete mucous that protects the surface of the intestine with a viscous fluid consisting of glycoproteins (20% peptides, 80% carbohydrates).
2. **Enterocytes** have two major functions. Enterocytes participate in the final digestion steps and they absorb the digested food (in the form of amino acids, monosaccharides, and emulsified fats) by transporting it from the lumen of the intestine to the lamina propria, where it is carried away by blood vessels and lymphatics.

3. **Paneth cells** are cells located at the base of the crypts, especially in the jejunum and ileum; they contain visible acidophilic secretory granules located in the apical region of the cells. These cells protect the body against pathogenic microorganisms by secreting lysozyme and defensins (or cryptins) that destroy bacteria. Their life span is about 20 days.

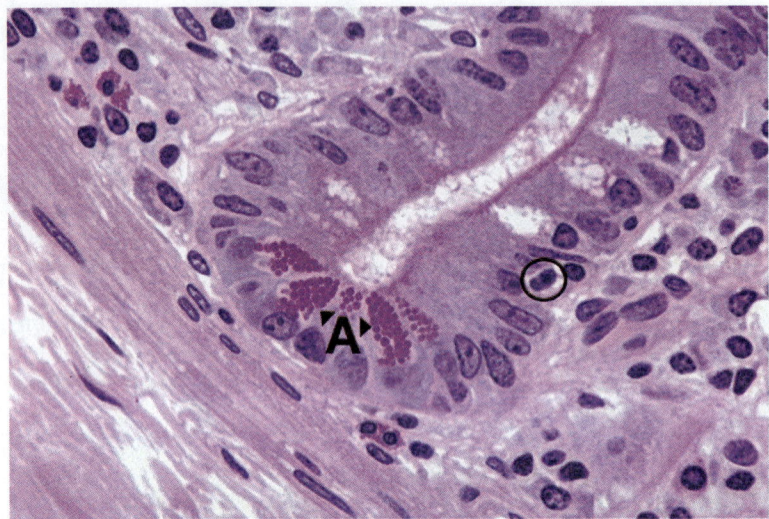

Copyright McGraw-Hill Companies. Used with permission.

Figure 8-11. Cells at the base of crypts of Lieberkühn include Paneth cells (A) with large apical granules of lysozyme, and an adjacent stem cell (circle) undergoing mitosis.

4. **Enteroendocrine cells** of the small and large intestine, like those of the stomach, secrete hormones that control the function of the GI tracts and associated organs. They are located in the lower half of the crypts and are detectable by silver-based stains.

5. **Stem cells** are located in the crypts, about one-third of the way up from the bottom. Their progeny differentiate into all the other cell types. **The epithelial lining of the small intestine, particularly that covering the villi, completely renews itself every 5 days (or longer, during starvation).** The newly created cells (goblet, enterocytes, and enteroendocrine cells) migrate up from the crypts, while the cells at the tips of microvilli undergo apoptosis and slough off. There is also a group of fibroblasts that accompany these epithelial cells as they move toward the tips of the villi. Other cells move to the base of the crypts, replenishing the population of Paneth and enteroendocrine cells.

Gut-associated lymphatic tissue (GALT): Throughout the intestine, the lamina propria is heavily infiltrated with macrophages and lymphocytes. Peyer's patches are patches of GALT that are prominent in the ileum. M cells in the epithelium transport luminal antigens to their base, where they are detected by B lymphocytes and taken up by antigen-presenting macrophages.

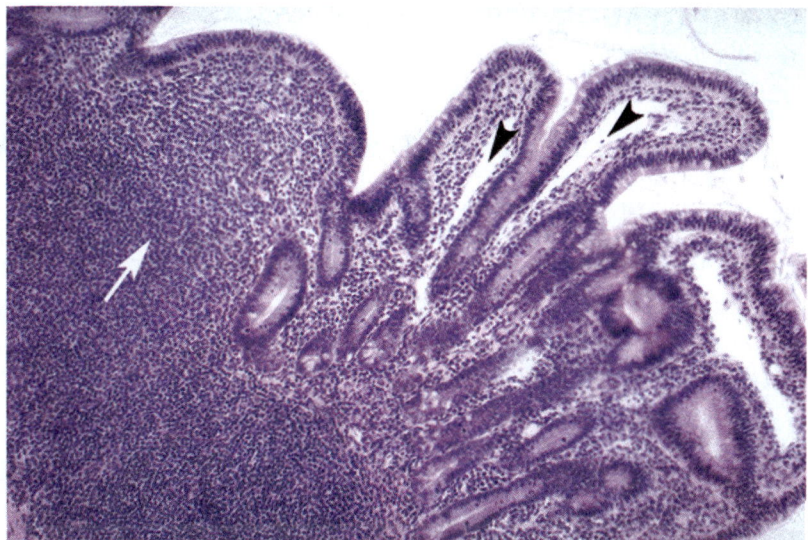

Copyright McGraw-Hill Companies. Used with permission.

Figure 8-12. Ileum with Payer's patches (arrow) and central lacteals (arrowheads) in the lamina propria of the villi

Large Intestine

The **large intestine** includes the cecum (with appendix), ascending, transverse, and descending colon, sigmoid colon, rectum, and anus. The large intestine has a wide lumen, strong musculature, and longitudinal muscle that is separated into three strands, the teniae coli. The inner surface has no plicae and no villi but consists of short crypts of Lieberkühn.

General features

- The colon is larger in diameter and shorter in length than is the small intestine. Fecal material moves from the **cecum**, through the colon (**ascending**, **transverse**, **descending**, and **sigmoid colons**), rectum, and anal canal.
- Three longitudinal bands of muscle, the **teniae coli**, constitute the outer layer. Because the colon is longer than these bands, pouching occurs, creating **haustra** between the teniae and giving the colon its characteristic "caterpillar" appearance.
- The mucosa has **no villi**, and mucus is secreted by short, inward-projecting colonic glands.
- Abundant lymphoid follicles are found in the cecum and appendix, and more sparsely elsewhere.
- The major functions of the colon are **reabsorption of fluid and electrolytes** and **temporary storage of feces**.

Defecation

Rectal distention with feces activates intrinsic and cord reflexes that cause relaxation of the internal anal sphincter (smooth muscle) and produce the urge to defecate. If the external anal sphincter (skeletal muscle innervated by the **pudendal nerve**) is then voluntarily relaxed, and intra-abdominal pressure is increased via the **Valsalva maneuver**, defecation occurs. If the external sphincter is held contracted, the urge to defecate temporarily diminishes.

Throughout the large intestine, the epithelium contains goblet, absorptive, and enteroendocrine cells. Unlike the small intestine, about half of the epithelial cells are mucus-secreting goblet cells, providing lubrication. The major function of the large intestine is fluid retrieval. Some digestion is still occurring, mainly the breakdown of cellulose by the permanent bacterial flora. Stem cells are in the lower part of the crypts.

GASTROINTESTINAL GLANDS

Salivary Glands

Note: more information concerning salivary glands can be found in the Dental Anatomy section.

The major salivary glands are all branched tubuloalveolar glands, with secretory **acini** that drain into **ducts**, which drain into the oral cavity. Acini contain **serous**, **mucous**, or both types of secretory cells, as well as **myoepithelial cells**, both surrounded by a basal lamina. Serous cells secrete various proteins and enzymes. Mucous cells secrete predominantly glycosylated mucins.

Table 8-4. Gastrointestinal Glands

Salivary glands
  Submandibular
  Parotid
  Sublingual
	• Produce approximately 1.5 L/day of saliva
	• Presence of food in the mouth; the taste, smell, sight, or thought of food; or the stimulation of vagal afferents at the distal end of the esophagus increase production of saliva	

Functions	• Initial triglyceride digestion (lingual lipase) • Initial starch digestion (α-amylase) • Lubrication	
Regulation	**Parasympathetic**	↑ synthesis and secretion of **watery** saliva via muscarinic receptor stimulation; (anti-cholinergics → dry mouth)
	Sympathetic	↑ synthesis and secretion of **viscous** saliva via β-adrenergic receptor stimulation

The ducts that drain the glands increase in size and are lined by an epithelium that transitions from cuboidal to columnar to pseudostratified to stratified columnar cells. The smallest ducts, **intercalated ducts**, have myoepithelial cells; the next larger ducts, **striated ducts**, have columnar cells with basal striations, caused by basal infolding of cell membranes between prominent mitochondria. These columnar cells make the saliva hypotonic by transporting Na and Cl ions out of saliva back into the blood. They also add bicarbonate to increase the pH of the saliva.

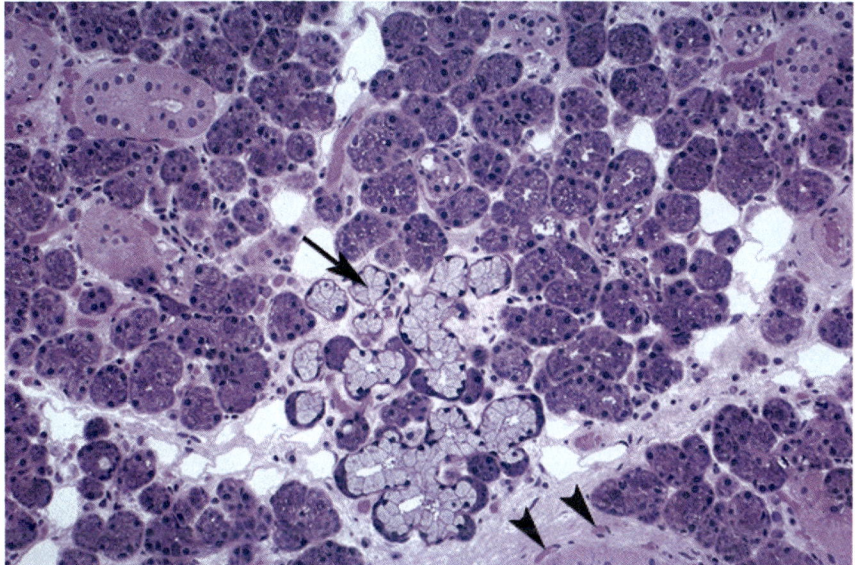

Figure 8-13. Submandibular with a mix of light-staining mucus acini (arrow) adjacent to dark-staining serous acini Small vessels (arrowheads)

Clinical Correlate

The parotid gland is the major site of the mumps and rabies viruses that are transmitted in saliva.

Benign tumors most frequently appear at the parotid gland; their removal is complicated by the facial nerve traversing the gland.

- The **parotid glands** lie on the surface of the masseter muscles in the lateral face, in front of each external auditory meatus. The parotids are **entirely serous** salivary glands that drain inside each cheek through **Stensen's ducts** which open above the second maxillary molar. The parotid glands contribute 25% of the volume of saliva.

- The **submandibular glands** lie inside the lower edge of the mandible, and are mixed serous/mucous glands with a **predominance of serous** cells. They drain in the floor of the mouth near the base of the tongue through **Wharton's ducts**. The submandibular glands contribute 70% of the volume of saliva.

- The **sublingual glands** lie at the base of the tongue, and are also mixed serous/mucous glands with a **predominance of mucous** cells. They drain into the mouth through multiple small ducts. They also send secretions through **Bartolin's duct** to connect to **Wharton's duct**, merging the secretions of both glands. The sublingual glands contribute 5% of the volume of saliva.

Exocrine Pancreas

The pancreas is a branched tubuloacinar exocrine gland with **acini**. The acini are composed of secretory cells that produce multiple digestive enzymes including proteases, lipases, and amylases. Acinar cells are functionally polarized, with basophilic RER at their basal ends below the nucleus, and membrane-bound, enzyme-containing eosinophilic **zymogen granules** toward their apex.

The endocrine-producing cells of the **islets of Langerhans** are embedded within the exocrine pancreas.

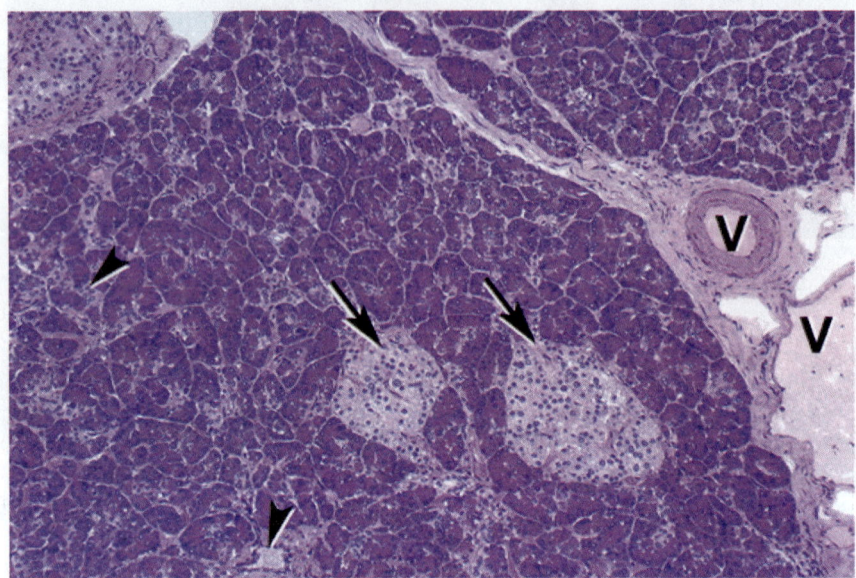

Figure 8-14. Pancreas with light-staining islets of Langerhans (arrows) surrounded by exocrine acini with ducts (arrowheads) and adjacent blood vessels (V)

Unlike salivary glands, the **pancreas lacks myoepithelial cells** in acini and **lacks striated ducts**. Also, unlike salivary glands, the cells of the intercalated ducts extend partially into the lumen of pancreatic acini as **centroacinar cells**. The pancreas does not usually have mucinous cells in acini, but may have mucinous cells in its ducts.

Pancreatic acini drain via progressively larger ducts into the duodenum. The main pancreatic **duct (of Wirsung)** is the distal portion of the dorsal pancreatic duct that joined the ventral pancreatic duct in the head of the pancreas. The main duct typically joins with the common bile duct and enters the duodenum through the **ampulla of Vater** (controlled by the **sphincter of Oddi**). Sometimes the pancreas has a persistent accessory duct with separate drainage into the duodenum, the **accessory duct of Santorini**, and a persisting remnant of the proximal part of the dorsal pancreatic duct.

Liver

The liver is the largest visceral organ and gland (both exocrine and endocrine) in the body. **Hepatocytes**, of endodermal epithelial origin, carry out both exocrine and endocrine functions. The liver has unusual capillaries, the hepatic **sinusoids**, that facilitate exchange (uptake and secretion) between hepatocytes and blood. The liver has **Kupffer cells**, specialized cells of the mononuclear phagocyte system (blood monocyte derived) which patrol the **space of Disse** between hepatocytes and blood.

The liver has epithelial lined exocrine (excretory) ducts, the **bile ducts**, lined by **biliary epithelium**, which drain hepatocyte products (bile) into the duodenum, ultimately through the common bile duct. Blood flow into the liver is dual (75% from **portal vein**, 25% from **hepatic artery**), while blood flow out is via **hepatic veins** into the inferior vena cava.

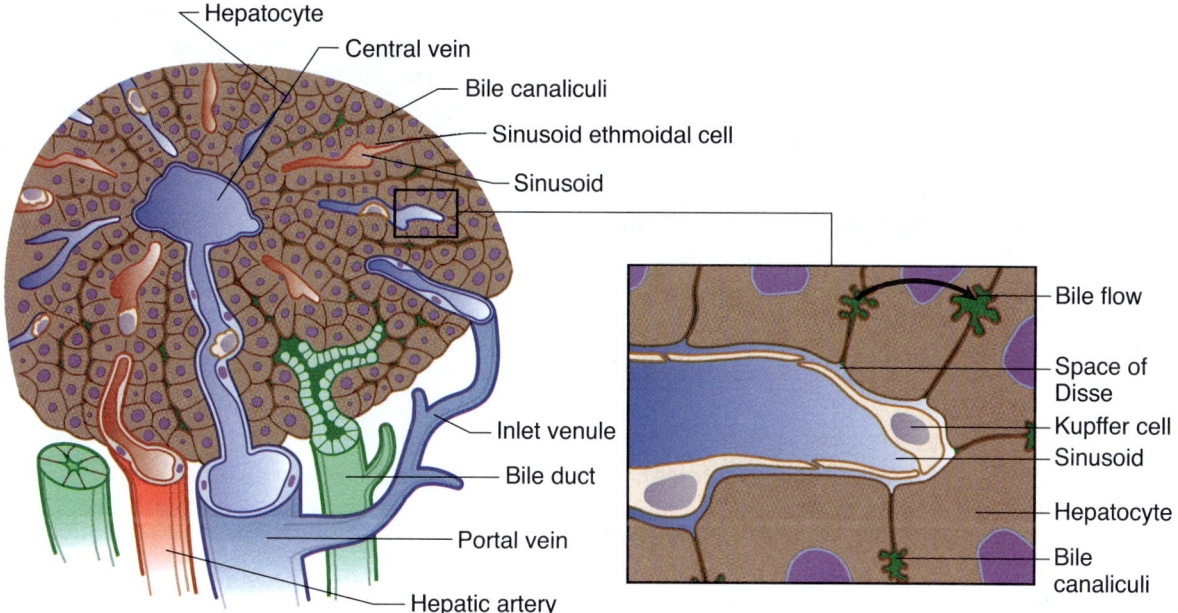

Figure 8-15. Organization of a Liver Lobule

Hepatocytes are functionally polarized, like many other epithelial cells, but rather than being polarized along a single axis, each hepatocyte has multiple "**basal**" and "**apical**" surfaces.

- Where 2 hepatocytes abut, their "apical" surfaces form bile **canaliculi**, extracellular grooved bile channels joined by tight and occluding junctions between adjacent hepatocytes. Bile is secreted into bile canaliculi, which drains into progressively larger bile ducts and empties into the duodenum.

- Where a hepatocyte abuts a sinusoid, its membrane has microvilli, representing a "basal" or basolateral surface. Exchange between blood and hepatocytes is facilitated by the surface microvilli. This exchange occurs in the space of Disse which is between the fenestrated endothelial cells of the sinusoid and the basal surface of hepatocytes.

The hepatic artery and portal vein enter and the common hepatic duct exits the liver in the hepatic **hilum**. Within the liver, branches of the hepatic artery, portal vein, and bile duct tend to run together in thin connective tissue bands. When seen in cross section, these three structures and their connective tissue are called a **portal triad or portal tract**. Blood from portal vein and hepatic artery branches both flow through and mix in hepatic sinusoids that run between cords or plates of hepatocytes. After passing by hepatocytes, the sinusoidal blood flows into hepatic venules, which form progressively larger branches draining into the right and left hepatic veins which drain into the inferior vena cava.

A **classic hepatic lobule** is a hexagonal structure with a portal tract at each corner of the hexagon and a central vein in the center of the hexagon. Blood flow is from the triads into the central vein and bile flow is opposite, from the central vein to the triads.

A **portal lobule** is a triangular structure with a central vein at each corner and a portal tract in the center. Bile flows from the periphery of the portal lobule into the central triad.

A **hepatic acinus** is based on blood flow from the hepatic artery branches to central veins. As hepatic arterial blood flow enters the sinusoids from side branches extending away from the center of the hepatic triad (rather than directly from the triad), the center of the acinus is conceived of as centered on such a branch extending out from a triad (or between 2 triads) and ending at 2 nearby central veins, resulting in a roughly elliptical structure with portal tracts at the 2 furthest poles and 2 central veins at the 2 closest edges.

In the acinus, the hepatocytes receiving the first blood flow (and the most oxygen and nutrients) are designated **zone 1**, while those receiving the last blood flow (and least oxygen and nutrients) are near the central veins and designated **zone 3**. **Zone 2** hepatocytes are in between zones 1 and 3. This model helps to explain the **differential effect on hepatocytes of changes in blood flow, oxygenation, etc**. Zone 3 is most susceptible to injury by decreased oxygenation of blood or decreased blood flow into the liver (as well as stagnation of blood drainage out of the liver due to congestive heart failure).

The metabolic activity of hepatocytes varies within the zones of the acinus. Zone 1 hepatocytes are most involved in glycogen synthesis and plasma protein synthesis (albumin, coagulation factors and complement components). Zone 3 cells are most concerned with lipid, drug, and alcohol metabolism and detoxification.

Clinical Correlate

When stimulated during liver injury, Ito cells may release type I collagen and other matrix components into the space of Disse, **contributing to scarring** of the liver in some diseases (cirrhosis due to ethanol). This may lead to the development of portal hypertension, portacaval anastomoses, and esophageal or rectal bleeding.

Ito cells (stellate cells) are mesenchymal cells that live in the space of Disse. They contain fat and are involved in **storage of fat-soluble vitamins, mainly vitamin A**.

Bile formation by hepatocytes serves both an exocrine and excretory function. Bile salts secreted into the duodenum aid in fat emulsification and absorption, as well as excretion of endogenous metabolites (bilirubin) and drug metabolites that cannot be excreted by the kidney.

Clinical Correlate

Disturbance of the balance in the components of bile can lead to precipitation of one or more of the bile components, resulting in stone (or **calculus**) formation or **lithiasis** in the gallbladder and/or bile ducts.

Gallbladder

The gallbladder is lined by a simple columnar epithelium with both absorptive and mucin secretory function, with underlying lamina propria. Unlike the gut tube, the gallbladder **lacks muscularis mucosae and submucosa,** and the muscularis externa is not organized into two distinct layers like the gut. The surface of the gallbladder is covered by peritoneal serosa (mesothelium). The gallbladder has a wide end, the **fundus**, and a narrowing **neck**, which empties into the **cystic duct** and which has spiral valves of Heister. The cystic duct joins the **common hepatic duct** to form the **common bile duct**, which joins the pancreatic duct at or just before the ampulla of Vater.

Note

Bile has three main functions:

1) Absorption of fats from intestinal lumen

2) Excretion

3) Transport of IgA

The gallbladder stores and concentrates bile by absorption of electrolytes and water. After a meal, entrance of lipid into the duodenum stimulates enteroendocrine cells of the duodenum to secrete cholecystokinin, which stimulates contraction and emptying of the gallbladder. At the same time, it relaxes the sphincter of Oddi in the ampulla of Vater. This delivers a bolus of bile into the duodenum.

ARTERIAL SUPPLY TO ABDOMINAL VISCERA

The blood supply to the abdominal viscera and the body wall is provided by branches of the abdominal aorta. The aorta enters the abdomen by passing through the aortic hiatus of the diaphragm at the **T12 vertebra**. It descends on the lumbar vertebra just to the left of the midline and bifurcates at the **L4 vertebral** level. During its short course in the abdomen, the aorta gives origin to three groups of branches: (a) **3 unpaired visceral branches**, (b) **3 paired visceral branches**, and (c) several **parietal branches** to the body wall.

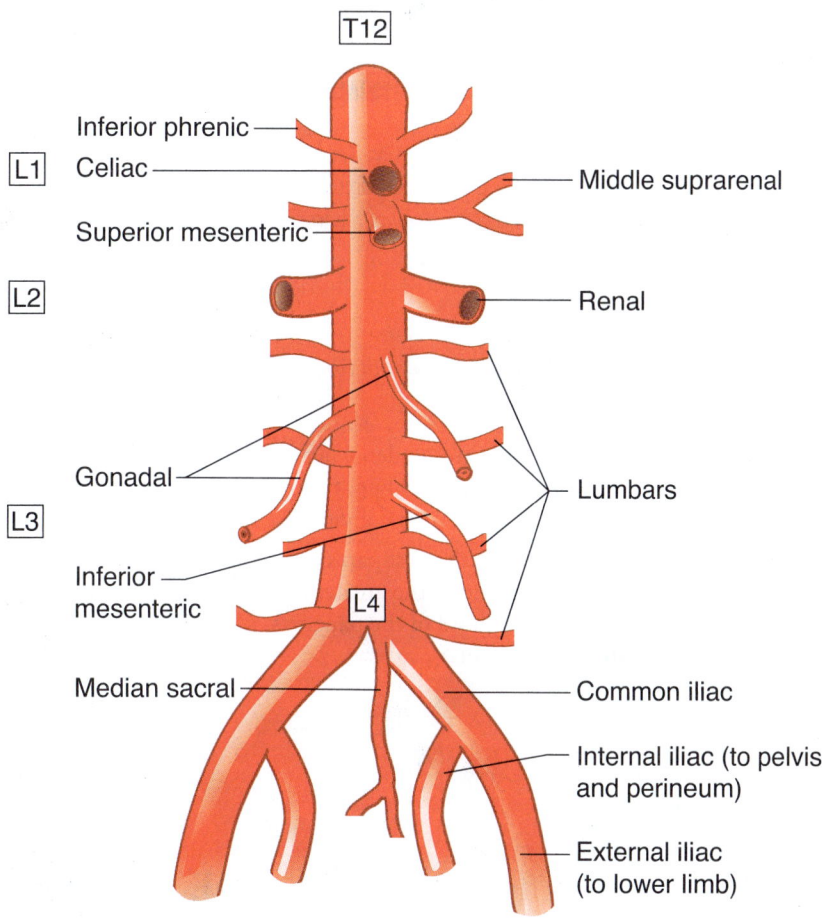

Figure 8-16. Visceral and Parietal Branches of the Abdominal Aorta

Three Unpaired Visceral Arteries

Celiac Artery (Trunk)

The **celiac artery** (Figure 8-17) is the blood supply to the structures derived from the foregut. The artery arises from the anterior surface of the aorta just inferior to the aortic hiatus at the level of T12–L1 vertebra. The celiac artery passes above the superior border of the pancreas and then divides into 3 retroperitoneal branches.

The **left gastric artery** courses superiorly and upward to the left to reach the **lesser curvature** of the stomach. The artery enters the lesser omentum and follows the lesser curvature distally to the pylorus. The distribution of the left gastric includes the following:

- **Esophageal branch** to the distal one inch of the esophagus in the abdomen
- **Most of the lesser curvature**

The **splenic artery** is the longest branch of the celiac trunk and runs a very tortuous course along the superior border of the pancreas. The artery is retroperitoneal until it reaches the tail of the pancreas, where it enters the splenorenal ligament to enter the hilum of the spleen. The distributions of the splenic artery include:

- **Direct branches to the spleen**
- **Direct branches to the neck, body, and tail of pancreas**
- **Left gastroepiploic artery** that supplies the left side of the **greater curvature** of the stomach
- **Short gastric** branches that supply to the **fundus** of the stomach

---

Clinical Correlate

The most common site for an abdominal aneurysm is in the area between the renal arteries and the bifurcation of the abdominal aorta. Signs include decreased circulation to the lower limbs and pain radiating down the back of the lower limbs. The most common site of atherosclerotic plaques is at the bifurcation of the abdominal aorta.

The **common hepatic artery** passes to the right to reach the superior surface of the first part of the duodenum, where it divides into its two terminal branches:

- **Proper hepatic artery** ascends within the hepatoduodenal ligament of the lesser omentum to reach the porta hepatis, where it divides into the **right and left hepatic arteries**. The right and left arteries enter the two lobes of the liver, with the right hepatic artery first giving rise to the **cystic artery** to the gallbladder.
- **Gastroduodenal artery** descends posterior to the first part of the duodenum and divides into the **right gastroepiploic artery** (supplies the pyloric end of the greater curvature of the stomach) and the **superior pancreaticoduodenal arteries** (supplies the head of the pancreas, where it anastomoses the inferior pancreaticoduodenal branches of the superior mesenteric artery).

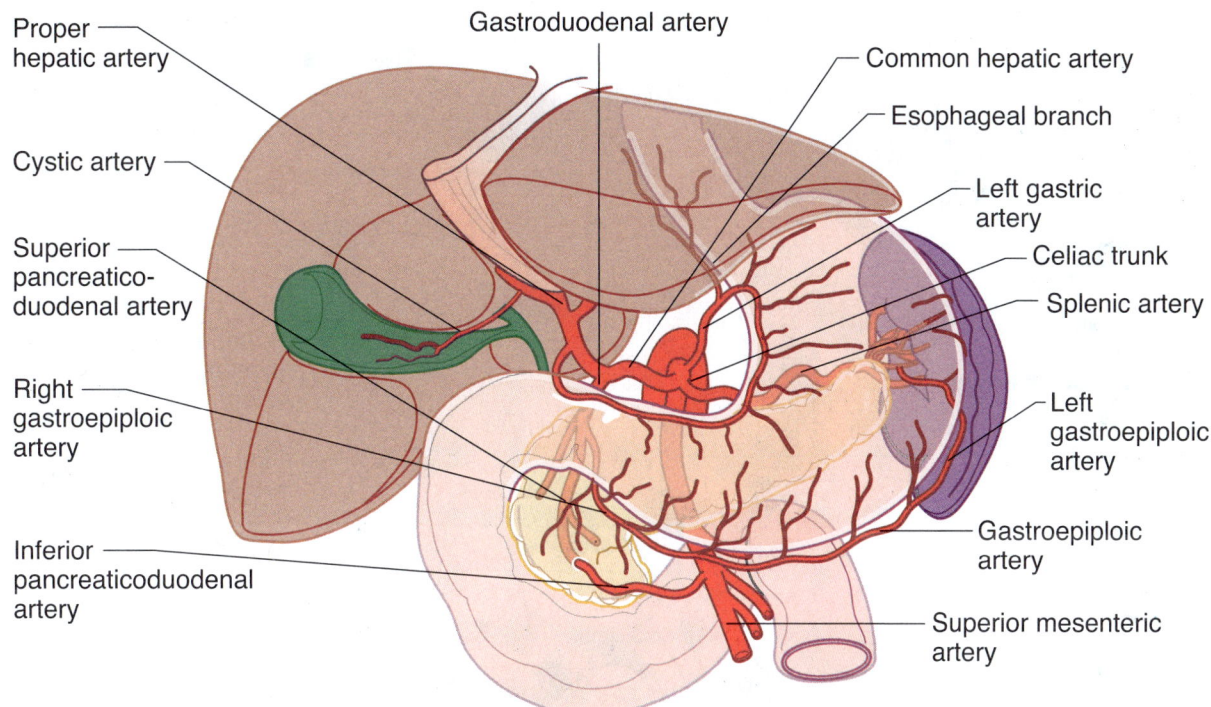

Figure 8-17. Celiac Artery

Superior Mesenteric Artery

The **superior mesenteric artery** (SMA) (Figure 8-18) supplies the viscera of the midgut. The SMA arises from the aorta deep to the neck of the pancreas just below the origin of the celiac artery at the L1 vertebral level. It then descends anterior to the uncinate process of the pancreas and the third part of the duodenum to enter the mesentery proper. The superior mesenteric vein is to the right of the artery. Branches of the SMA include:

1. **Inferior pancreaticoduodenal arteries** which anastomose with the superior pancreaticoduodenal branches of the gastroduodenal artery in the head of the pancreas

2. **Intestinal arteries** arise as 12–15 branches from the left side of the SMA and segmentally supply the jejunum and ileum. Distally, they form vascular arcades and vasa recta arteries at the wall of the gut.

3. **Ileocolic artery** is the most inferior branch which descends to the lower right quadrant to supply the distal ileum and cecum.

4. **Right colic artery** passes to the right to supply the ascending colon.

5. **Middle colic artery** ascends and enters the transverse mesocolon to supply the proximal two-thirds of the transverse colon.

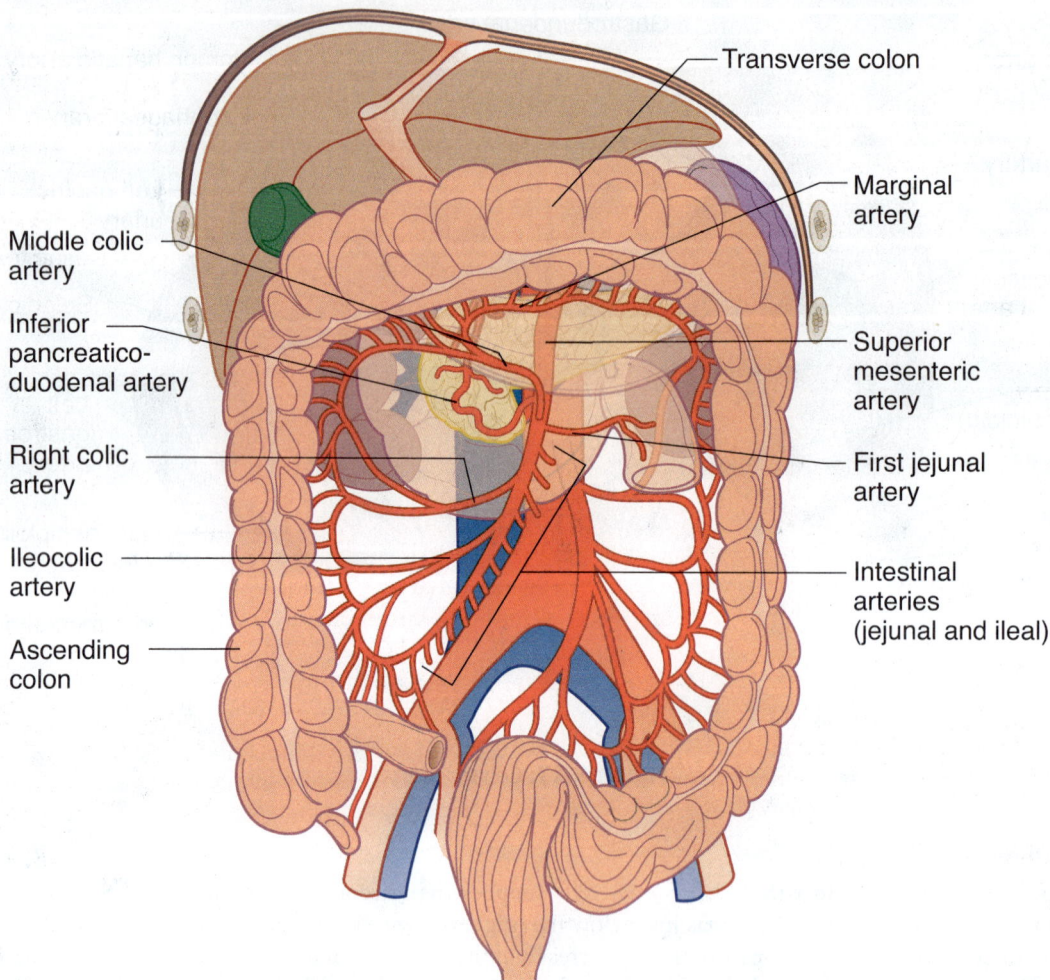

Figure 8-18. Distribution of Superior Mesenteric Artery

Inferior Mesenteric Artery

The inferior mesenteric artery (IMA) (Figure 8-19) is the third unpaired visceral branch of the aorta that supplies the hindgut (distal third of the transverse colon to the pectinate line). The IMA arises from the aorta just above its bifurcation at the level of the L3 vertebra. It descends retroperitoneally and inferiorly to the left and gives rise to three branches:

1. **Left colic artery** supplies the distal third of the transverse colon and the descending colon
2. **Sigmoid arteries** to the sigmoid colon
3. **Superior rectal artery** descends into the pelvis and supplies the superior aspect of the rectum and anal canal.

The branches of the SMA and IMA to the ascending, transverse and descending parts of the large intestines are interconnected by a continual arterial arch called the **marginal artery.** The marginal artery provides a collateral circulation between the parts of the large intestines if there is a vascular obstruction in some part of the SMA and IMA.

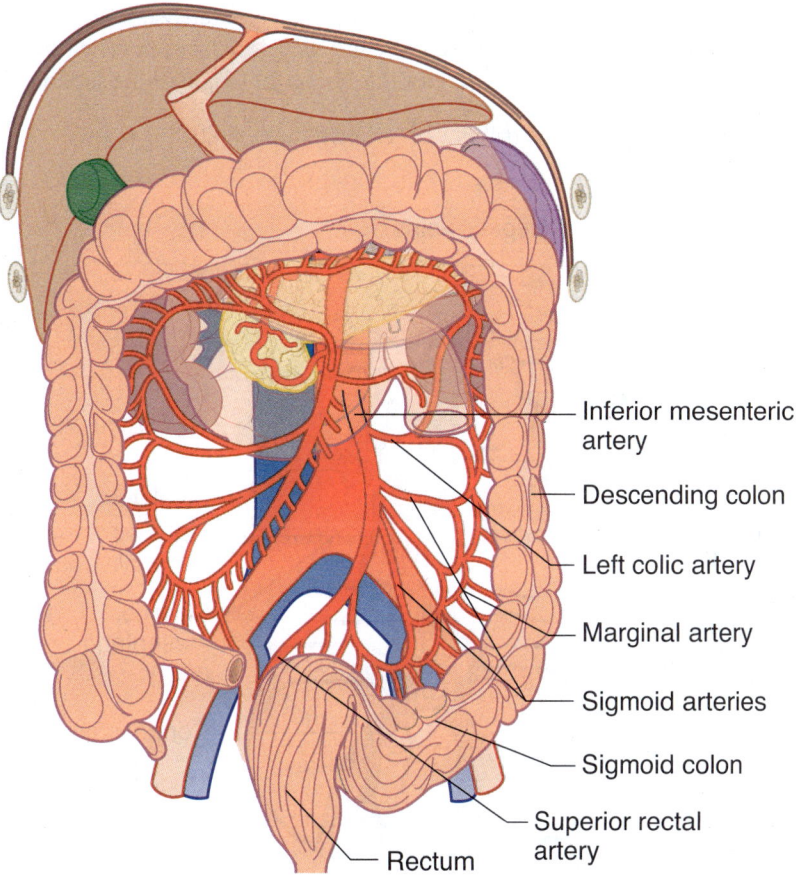

Figure 8-19. Distribution of Inferior Mesenteric Artery

Labels (top to bottom): Inferior mesenteric artery; Descending colon; Left colic artery; Marginal artery; Sigmoid arteries; Sigmoid colon; Superior rectal artery; Rectum

Three Paired Visceral Arteries

- **Middle suprarenal arteries** branch from the aorta above the renal arteries and supply the medial parts of the suprarenal gland.
- **Renal arteries** are large paired vessels that arise from the aorta at the upper border of the L2 vertebra. They course horizontally to the hila of the kidneys. The right renal artery is the longer than the left and passes posterior to the inferior vena cava.
- **Gonadal arteries** arise from the anterior surface of the aorta just inferior to the renal arteries. They descend retroperitoneally on the ventral surface of the psoas major muscle.

VENOUS DRAINAGE OF ABDOMINAL VISCERA

Inferior Vena Cava

The **inferior vena cava** forms to the right of the lumbar vertebrae and the abdominal aorta by the union of the two common iliac veins at the **L5 vertebral level** (Figure 8-20). The inferior vena cava ascends to the right of the midline and passes through the caval hiatus of the diaphragm at the **T8 vertebral level**. The inferior vena cava receives blood from the lower limbs, pelvis and perineum, paired abdominal viscera, and body wall. Note that the vena cava does not receive blood directly from the GI tract, except the lower rectum and anal canal.

Note that the **right tributaries** (right gonadal, right suprarenal) drain separately into the inferior vena cava. But on the left side, the left gonadal and left suprarenal veins drain into the left renal vein, which then drains into the vena cava. The left renal vein crosses anterior to the aorta, just inferior to the origin of the superior mesenteric artery.

The drainage of the inferior vena cava and its tributaries is shown in the following figure.

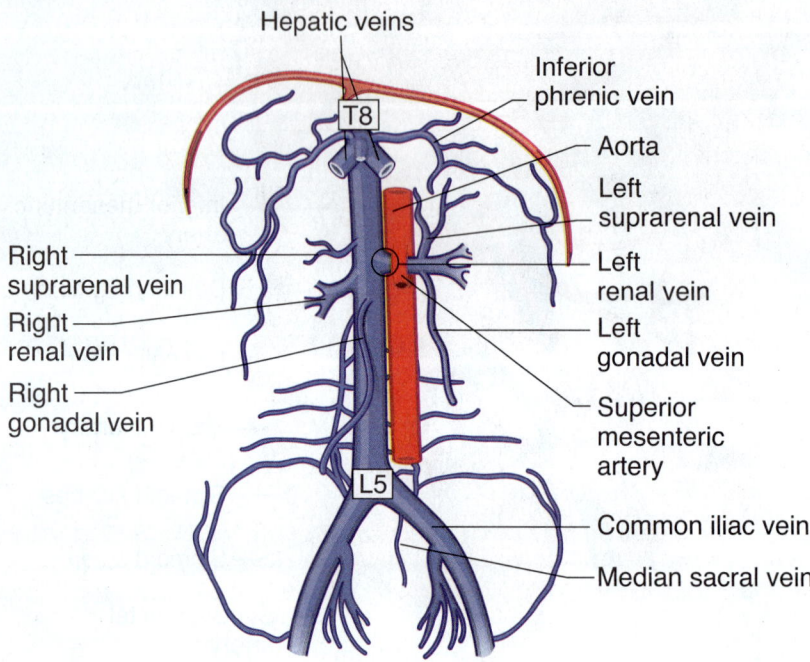

Figure 8-20. Inferior Vena Cava and Tributaries

Hepatic Portal System

The **hepatic portal system** is an extensive network of veins that receives the blood flow from the GI tract above the pectinate line. The venous flow is carried to the liver via the **hepatic portal vein** where it enters the liver sinusoids, which drain to the hepatic veins, which then drain into the inferior vena cava and ultimately into the right atrium.

The hepatic portal vein is formed by the union of the **superior mesenteric** (drains midgut) and **splenic** (drains foregut) veins posterior to the **neck of the pancreas. The inferior mesenteric vein** (drains hindgut) usually drains into splenic vein.

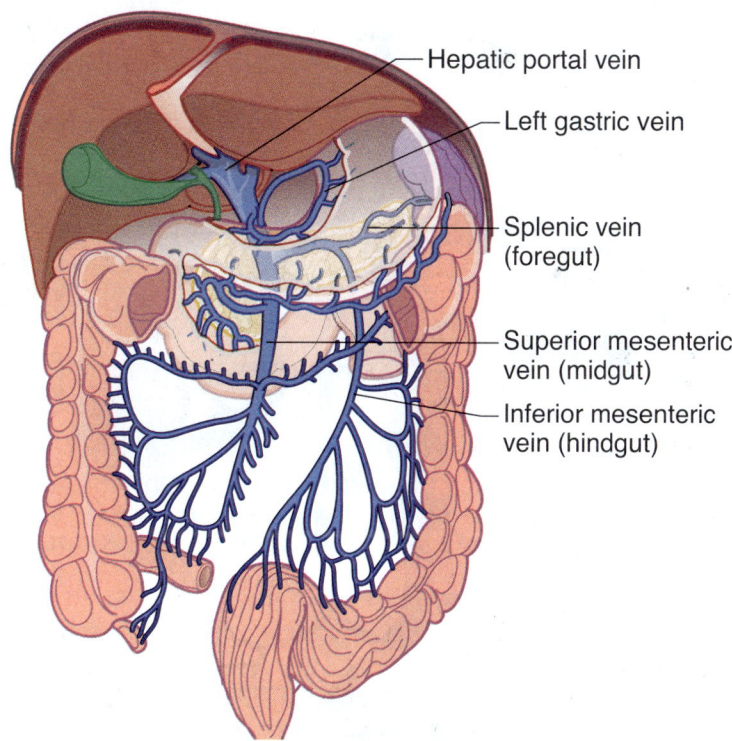

- Hepatic portal vein
- Left gastric vein
- Splenic vein (foregut)
- Superior mesenteric vein (midgut)
- Inferior mesenteric vein (hindgut)

Figure 8-21. Hepatic Portal System

Portalcaval (Systemic) Anastomoses

If there is an obstruction to flow through the portal system (portal hypertension), blood can flow in a retrograde direction (because of the absence of valves in the portal system) and pass through anastomoses to reach the caval system. Sites for these anastomoses include the **esophageal veins, rectal veins**, and **thoracoepigastric veins**. Enlargement of these veins may result in esophageal varices, hemorrhoids, and a caput medusae.

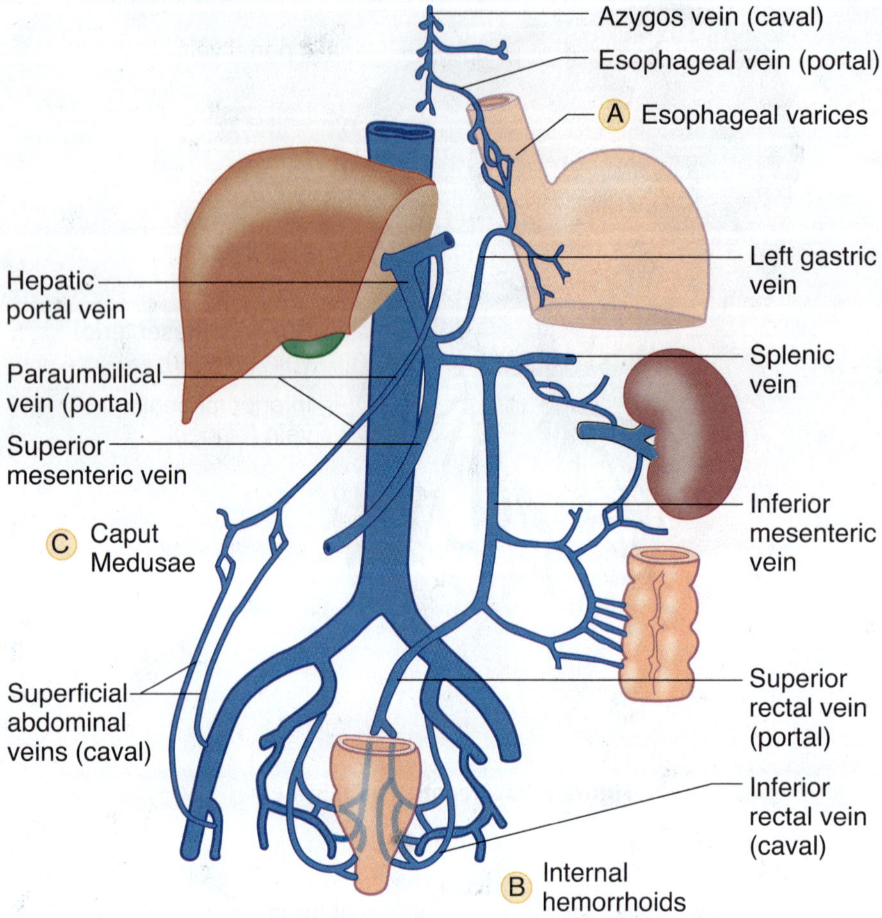
Azygos vein (caval)
Esophageal vein (portal)
A Esophageal varices
Hepatic portal vein
Left gastric vein
Splenic vein
Paraumbilical vein (portal)
Superior mesenteric vein
Inferior mesenteric vein
C Caput Medusae
Superficial abdominal veins (caval)
Superior rectal vein (portal)
Inferior rectal vein (caval)
B Internal hemorrhoids

Figure 8-22. Chief Portacaval Anastomoses

POSTERIOR ABDOMINAL BODY WALL

Embryology of Kidneys and Ureter

Renal development is characterized by 3 successive, slightly overlapping kidney systems: pronephros, mesonephros, and metanephros.

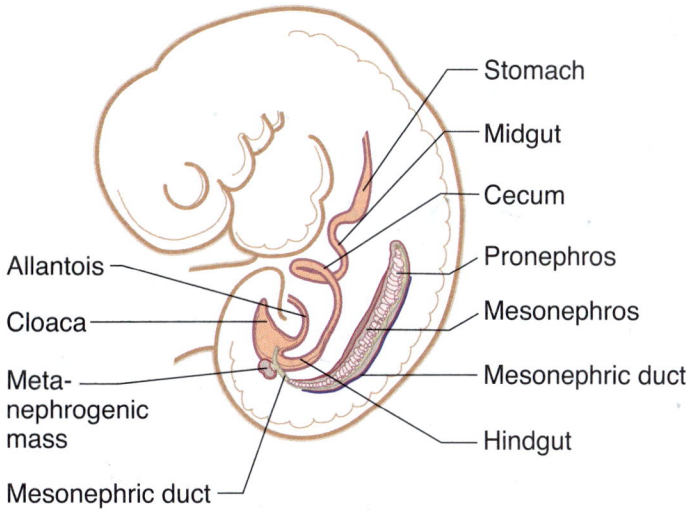

Figure 8-23. Pronephros, Mesonephros, and Metanephros

Pronephros

During week 4, segmented nephrotomes appear in the cervical intermediate mesoderm of the embryo. These structures grow laterally and canalize to form nephric tubules. The first tubules formed regress before the last ones are formed. By the end of week 4, the pronephros disappears and does not function.

Mesonephros

In week 5, the mesonephros appears as S-shaped tubules in the intermediate mesoderm of the thoracic and lumbar regions of the embryo.

- The medial end of each tubule enlarges to form a Bowman's capsule into which a tuft of capillaries, or glomerulus, invaginates.
- The lateral end of each tubule opens into the **mesonephric (Wolffian) duct**, an intermediate mesoderm derivative. The duct drains into the hindgut.
- Mesonephric tubules function temporarily and degenerate by the beginning of month 3. The mesonephric duct persists in the male as the ductus epididymidis, ductus deferens, and the ejaculatory duct. It disappears in the female.

Metanephros

During week 5, the metanephros, or permanent kidney, develops from two sources: the **ureteric bud**, a diverticulum of the mesonephric duct, and the **metanephric mass** (blastema), from intermediate mesoderm of the lumbar and sacral regions.

The **ureteric bud** penetrates the metanephric mass, which condenses around the diverticulum to form the metanephrogenic cap. The bud dilates to form the renal pelvis, which subsequently splits into the cranial and caudal major calyces. Each major calyx buds into the metanephric tissue to form the minor calyces. One to 3 million collecting tubules develop from the minor calyces, thus forming the renal pyramids. The ureteric bud forms the **drainage components** of the urinary system (calyces, pelvis, ureter).

Penetration of collecting tubules into the **metanephric mass** induces cells of the tissue cap to form **nephrons**, or excretory units.

- Lengthening of the excretory tubule gives rise to the proximal convoluted tubule, the loop of Henle, and the distal convoluted tubule.

Positional change of the kidneys

The kidneys develop in the pelvis but appear to ascend into the abdomen as a result of fetal growth of the lumbar and sacral regions. With their ascent, the ureters elongate, and the kidneys become vascularized by arteries which arise from the abdominal aorta.

Posterior Abdominal Wall and Pelvic Viscera

Kidneys

The kidneys are a pair of bean-shaped organs approximately 12 cm long. They extend from vertebral level T12 to L3 when the body is in the erect position. The right kidney is positioned slightly lower than the left because of the mass of the liver.

Ureters

Ureters are fibromuscular tubes that connect the kidneys to the urinary bladder in the pelvis. They run posterior to the ductus deferens in males and posterior to the uterine artery in females. They begin as continuations of the renal pelves and run retroperitoneally, crossing the external iliac arteries as they pass over the pelvic brim.

Urinary Bladder

- **Structure**
  - The urinary bladder is covered superiorly by peritoneum.
  - The body is a hollow muscular cavity.
  - The neck is continuous with the urethra.
  - The trigone is a smooth, triangular area of mucosa located internally at the base of the bladder.
  - The base of the triangle is superior and bounded by the two openings of the ureters. The apex of the trigone points inferiorly and is the opening for the urethra.
- **Blood Supply**
  - The bladder is supplied by vesicular branches of the internal iliac arteries and umbilical arteries.
  - The vesicular venous plexus drains to internal iliac veins.
- **Lymphatics**
  - Drain to the external and internal iliac nodes
- **Innervation**
  - Parasympathetic innervation is from sacral segments S2, S3, and S4. The preganglionic parasympathetic fibers travel in **pelvic splanchnic nerves** to reach the **detrusor muscle**.
  - Sympathetic innervation is through fibers derived from L1 through L2 (**lumbar splanchnics**). These fibers supply the **trigone muscle** and the **internal urethral sphincter**.

In a Nutshell

Parasympathetic fibers facilitate micturition and sympathetic fibers inhibit micturition.

Urethra

The male urethra is a muscular tube approximately 20 cm in length. The urethra in men extends from the neck of the bladder through the prostate gland (prostatic urethra) to the urogenital diaphragm of the perineum (membranous urethra), and then to the external opening of the glans (penile or spongy urethra).

The male urethra is anatomically divided into three portions: prostatic, membranous, and spongy (penile).

- The **distal spongy urethra** of the male is derived from the ectodermal cells of the glans penis.

The female urethra is approximately 4 cm in length and extends from the neck of the bladder to the external urethral orifice of the vulva.

URINARY HISTOLOGY AND FUNCTION

The urinary system consists of two kidneys, two ureters, the bladder, and the urethra.

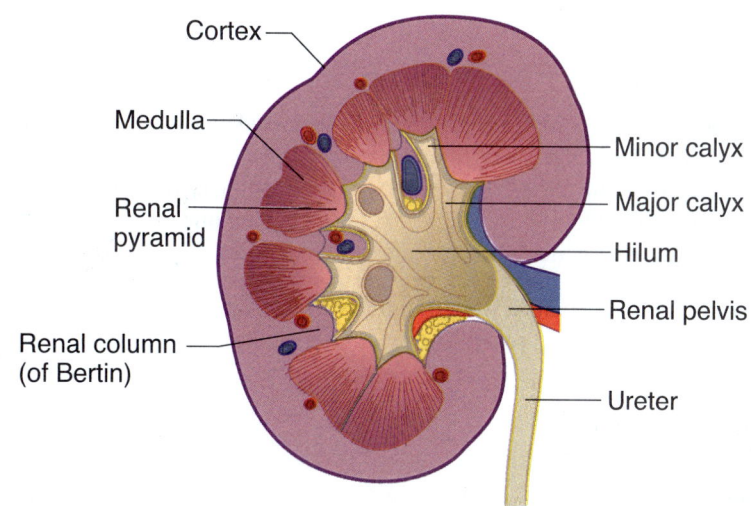

Figure 8-24. Organization of the Kidney

Urinary Functions

The urinary system functions in the removal of waste products from blood. The kidney also functions in fluid balance, salt balance, and acid-base balance. The kidney functions as an endocrine gland; it produces and releases renin, which leads to an increase in extracellular fluid volume; erythropoietin, which stimulates erythropoiesis; and prostaglandins, which act as vasodilators.

A sagittal section through the center of a kidney shows a capsule (connective tissue) surrounding and protecting the organ, a wide band of cortex showing radial striations and the presence of glomeruli, and a medulla in the shape of an inverted pyramid. The medulla in turn shows an outer and inner zone. The blunted tip of the pyramid, called the **papilla**, borders a space that is surrounded by calices of the ureter. The collecting ducts are invaginations of the papilla's epithelium and the urine drains from their open ends into the calices.

Table 8-5. Basic Functions of the Kidneys

Fluid balance	Maintain normal extracellular fluid (ECF) and intracellular fluid (ICF) volumes
Electrolytes	Balance excretion with intake to maintain normal plasma concentrations
Wastes	Excrete metabolic wastes (nitrogenous products, acids, toxins, etc.)
Fuels	Reabsorb metabolic fuels (glucose, lactate, amino acids, etc.)
Blood pressure	Regulate ECF volume for the long-term control of blood pressure
Acid–base	Regulate absorption and excretion of H^+ and HCO_3^- to control acid–base balance

Organization of the Kidney

The cortex is divided into lobules, and contains nephron elements mixed with vascular elements and stroma (a small amount of connective tissue). At the center of each lobule is a medullary ray, containing tubules that are parallel to each other and oriented radially in the cortex. The tubules in the medullary rays are continuous with those in the medulla. Along the two edges of each lobule are glomeruli, located along one or two rows. Radially oriented arterioles and venules with a large lumen are located at the edges of the lobules.

The medulla is comprised of radially arranged straight tubules which run from cortex to papilla, vascular elements, and stroma (a small amount of connective tissue). The medulla is divided into two zones. A wide strip in proximity to the cortex, the outer medulla contains profiles of tubules with different appearances. The inner medulla has fewer profiles of similar tubes.

Blood Circulation

The renal artery enters the kidney at the hilum, near the ureter. The artery branches into interlobar arteries, which travel to the medulla–cortex border remaining outside the medullary pyramids. The vessels branch into arcuate arteries (and veins) that follow the edge of the cortex. The arcuate arteries branch into interlobular arterioles that travel tangentially in the cortex at the edges of the lobules. Intralobular arterioles, feeding the glomeruli, branch off the interlobular arterioles at each renal corpuscle.

The kidneys receive 25% of total cardiac output, 1,700 liters in 24 hours. Each intralobular arteriole enters a renal corpuscle at the vascular pole as afferent arteriole and forms a convoluted tuft of capillaries (the glomerulus). A second arteriole (the efferent arteriole) exits the corpuscle. This is a unique situation due to the fact that the pressure remains high in the glomerulus in order to allow filtration.

The efferent arterioles carrying blood out of the glomeruli make a second capillary bed. This second capillary bed has lower blood pressure than the glomerulus and it connects to venules at its distal end. The arteriole-capillary-arteriole-capillary-vein sequence in the kidney is unique in the body. The efferent arterioles from glomeruli in the upper cortex divide into a complex capillary system in the cortex.

NEPHRON

The functional unit within the kidney is the nephron. Each kidney contains 1–1.3 million nephrons. Nephrons connect to collecting ducts, and collecting ducts receive urine from several nephrons and converge with each other before opening to and letting the urine flow out of the kidney. The nephron and the collecting duct form the uriniferous tubule.

The nephron is a tube about 55 mm in length in the human kidney. It starts at one end with Bowman's capsule, which is the enlarged end of the nephron. Bowman's capsule has been invaginated by a tuft of capillaries of the glomerulus so that it has two layers: the visceral layer is in direct contact with the capillary endothelium, and the parietal layer surrounds an approximately spherical urinary space. Bowman's capsule and glomerulus of capillaries form a renal corpuscle.

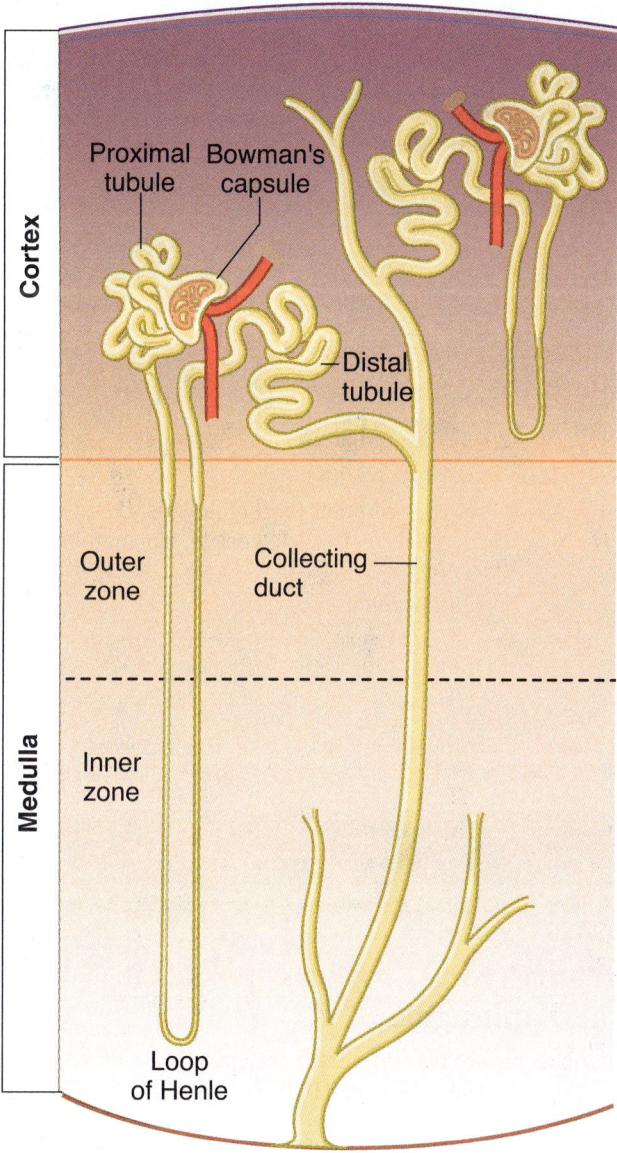

Figure 8-25. Nephron

PELVIS

Embryology of the Reproductive System

Table 8-6. Embryology of Reproductive System

Male and Female Development		
Adult Female and Male Reproductive Structures Derived From Precursors of the Indifferent Embryo		
Adult Female	**Indifferent Embryo**	**Adult Male**
Ovary, follicles, rete ovarii	Gonads $\xrightarrow[\text{TDF}]{+}$	Testes, seminiferous tubules, rete testes
Uterine tubes, uterus, cervix, and upper part of vagina ←	Paramesonephric ducts $\xrightarrow{\text{MIF}}$	Appendix of testes
Duct of Gartner	Mesonephric ducts $\xrightarrow[\text{Testosterone}]{+}$	Epididymis, ductus deferens, seminal vesicle, ejaculatory duct
Clitoris	Genital tubercle	Glans and body of penis
Labia minora	Urogenital folds	Ventral aspect of penis
Labia majora	Labioscrotal swellings	Scrotum

DHT (for penis rows)

Abbreviations: DHT, dihydrotestosterone; MIF, Müllerian-inhibiting factors; TDF, testes-determining factor

Pelvic and Urogenital Diaphragms

The **pelvic and urogenital diaphragms** are two important skeletal muscle diaphragms that provide support of the pelvic and perineal structures. They are each innervated by branches of the pudendal nerve.

- The **pelvic diaphragm** forms the muscular floor of the pelvis and separates the pelvic cavity from the perineum. The pelvic diaphragm is a strong support for the pelvic organs and transmits the distal parts of the genitourinary system and GI tract from the pelvis to the perineum.
  - The diaphragm is formed by two layers of fascia and the two muscles: the **levator ani** and coccygeus.
  - The **puborectalis** component of the levator ani muscle forms a muscular sling around the anorectal junction, marks the boundary between the rectum and anal canal and is important in fecal continence.

- The muscular **urogenital diaphragm** is located in the perineum inferior to the pelvic diaphragm. It is formed by two muscles (**sphincter urethrae** and deep transverse perineus muscles) which extend horizontally between the two ischiopubic rami.

  — The diaphragm is penetrated by the urethra in the male and the urethra and vagina in the female.

  — The sphincter urethrae muscle serves as an **external urethral sphincter** (voluntary muscle of micturition) which surrounds the membranous urethra and maintains urinary continence.

Male Pelvic Viscera

The position of organs and peritoneum in the male pelvis is illustrated here:

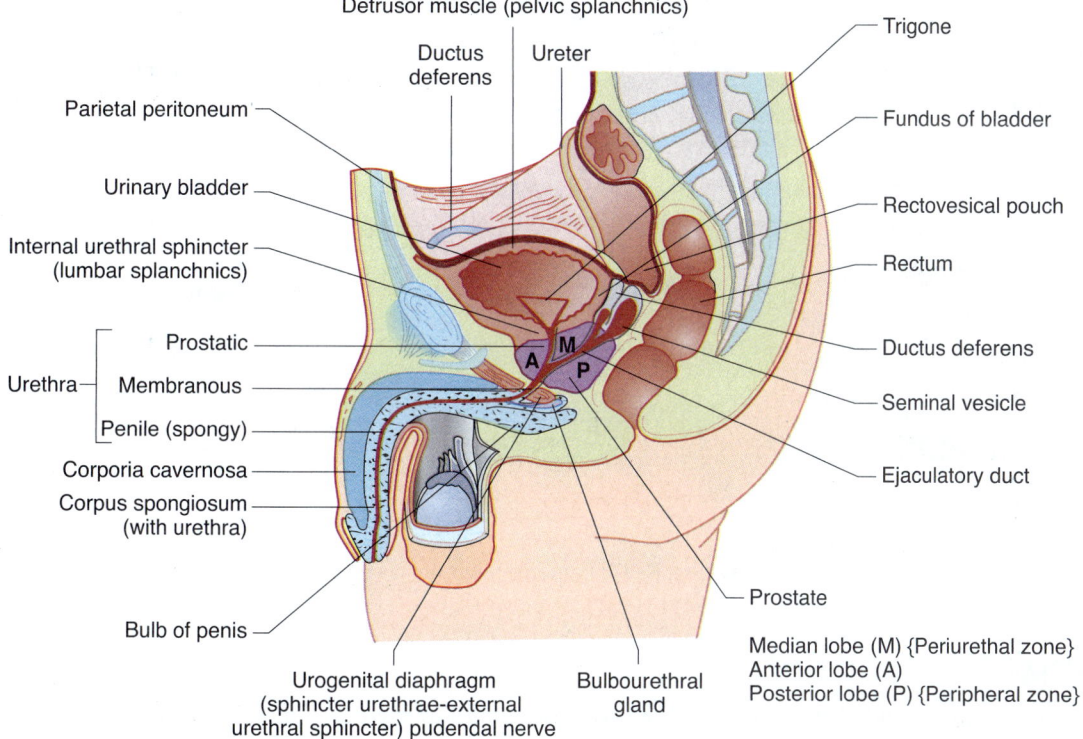

Figure 8-26. Male Pelvis

Clinical Correlate

Hyperplasia of the Prostate

An enlarged prostate gland will compress the urethra. The patient will complain of the urge to urinate often and has difficulty with starting urination.

Because the prostate gland is enclosed in a dense connective tissue capsule, hypertrophy will compress the prostatic portion of the urethra.

Female Pelvic Viscera

The position of organs and peritoneum in the female pelvis is illustrated here:

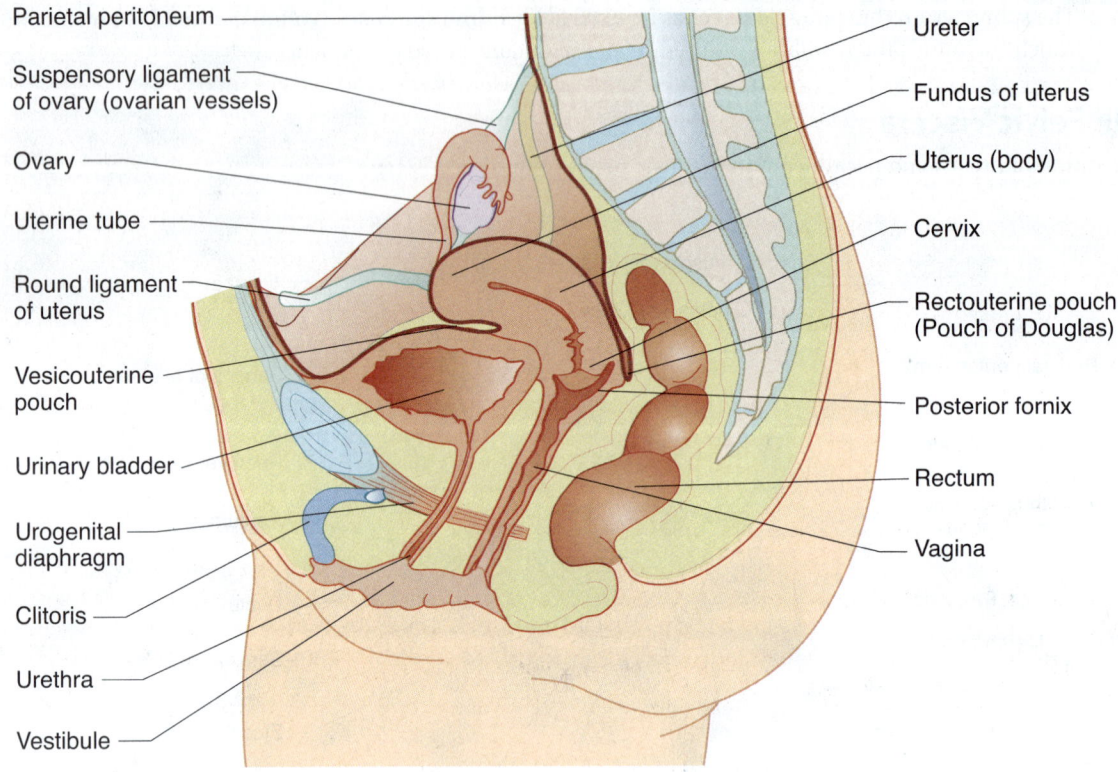

Parietal peritoneum

Suspensory ligament of ovary (ovarian vessels)

Ovary

Uterine tube

Round ligament of uterus

Vesicouterine pouch

Urinary bladder

Urogenital diaphragm

Clitoris

Urethra

Vestibule

Ureter

Fundus of uterus

Uterus (body)

Cervix

Rectouterine pouch (Pouch of Douglas)

Posterior fornix

Rectum

Vagina

Figure 8-27. Female Pelvis

PERINEUM

The **perineum** is the diamond-shaped outlet of the pelvis located below the pelvic diaphragm. The perineum is divided by a transverse line between the ischial tuberosities into the **anal** and **urogenital triangles** (Figure 8-42).

- The sensory and motor innervation to the perineum is provided by the **pudendal nerve** (S2, 3, 4) of the sacral plexus.
- The blood supply is provided by the **internal pudendal artery,** a branch of the internal iliac artery.
- The pudendal nerve and vessels cross the ischial spine posteriorly to enter the perineum.

Anal Triangle

The **anal triangle** is posterior and contains the **anal canal** surrounded by thefat-filled**ischioanal fossa.**

- The anal canal is guarded by a smooth-muscle **internal anal sphincter** innervated by the ANS and an **external anal sphincter** of skeletal muscle innervated by the pudendal nerve.
- The pudendal canal transmitting the pudendal nerve and internal pudendal vessels is found on the lateral aspect of the ischioanal fossa.

Urogenital Triangle

The **urogenital triangle** forms the anterior aspect of the perineum and contains the superficial and root structures of the external genitalia. The urogenital triangle is divided into **superficial** and **deep perineal spaces** (**pouches**).

Superficial Perineal Pouch (Space)

The superficial perineal pouch is located between the **perineal membrane** of the urogenital diaphragm and the **superficial perineal (Colles') fascia**.

It contains:

- Crura of penis or clitoris: erectile tissue
- Bulb of penis (in the male): erectile tissue; contains urethra
- Bulbs of vestibule (in the female): erectile tissue in lateral walls of vestibule
- Ischiocavernosus muscle: skeletal muscle that covers crura of penis or clitoris
- Bulbospongiosus muscle: skeletal muscle that covers bulb of penis or bulb of vestibule
- Greater vestibular (Bartholin) gland (in female only): homologous to Cowper gland

Deep Perineal Pouch (Space)

The deep perineal pouch is formed by the fasciae and muscles of the **urogenital diaphragm**. It contains:

- Sphincter urethrae muscle—serves as voluntary external sphincter of the urethra
- Deep transverse perineal muscle
- Bulbourethral (Cowper) gland (in the male only)—duct enters bulbar urethra

MALE REPRODUCTIVE HISTOLOGY

Testis

The testis is surrounded by a dense fibrous capsule called the **tunica albuginea**. The tunica albuginea is continuous with many of the interlobular septa that divide the testis into approximately 250 pyramidal compartments (testicular lobules).

Within each lobule are 1-4 tubes, **seminiferous tubules,** where spermatozoa are produced. Each tubule is a coiled, non-branching closed loop that is 150–200 μm in diameter and 30–70 cm in length. Both ends of each tubule converge on the rete testes. The seminiferous tubules contain spermatogenic cells, Sertoli cells, and a well-defined basal lamina.

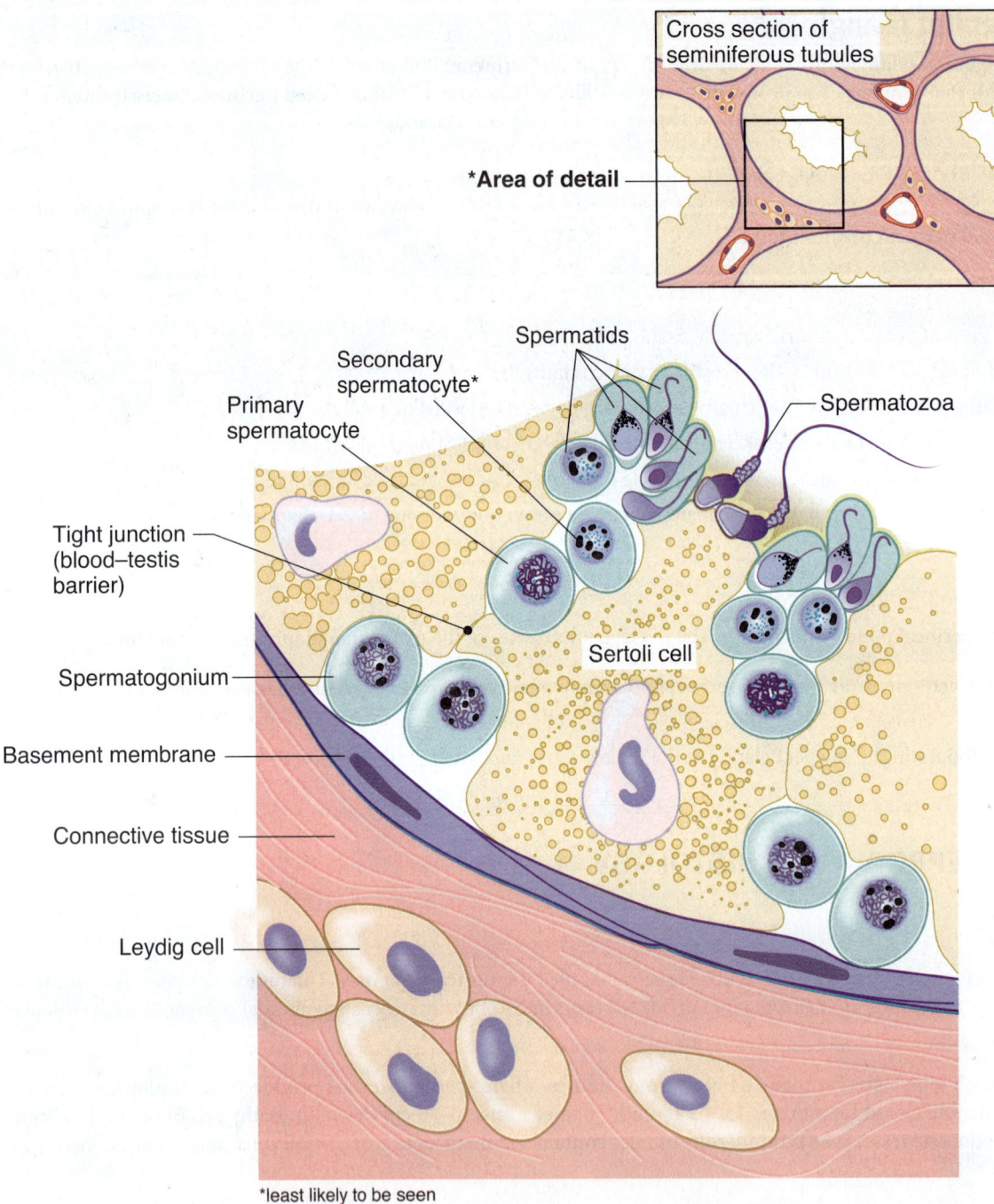

Cross section of seminiferous tubules

*Area of detail

Spermatids

Secondary spermatocyte*

Primary spermatocyte

Spermatozoa

Tight junction (blood–testis barrier)

Sertoli cell

Spermatogonium

Basement membrane

Connective tissue

Leydig cell

*least likely to be seen

Figure 8-28. Seminiferous tubule diagram

Spermatogenesis

The spermatogenic </ix>cells (germinal epithelium) are stacked in 4 to 8 layers that occupy the space between the basement membrane and the lumen of the seminiferous tubule. The stem cells (**spermatogonia**) are adjacent to the basement membrane. As the cells develop, they move from the basal to the luminal side of the tubule.

At puberty the stem cells resume mitosis, producing more stem cells as well as differentiated spermatogonia (type A and B) that are committed to meiosis. **Type B spermatogonia** differentiate into primary spermatocytes that enter meiosis. **Primary spermatocytes** (4n, diploid) pass through a long prophase (10 days to 2 weeks) and </ix>after the first meiotic division form 2 secondary spermatocytes (2n, haploid). The **secondary spermatocytes** rapidly undergo the second meiotic division in a matter of minutes (**and are rarely seen in histologic sections**) to produce the **spermatids** (1n, haploid).

The progeny of a single maturing spermatogonium remain connected to one another by cytoplasmic bridges throughout their differentiation into mature sperm.

Spermiogenesis

Spermiogenesis transforms haploid spermatids into spermatozoa. This process of differentiation involves formation of the acrosome, condensation, and elongation of the nucleus; development of the flagellum; and loss of much of the cytoplasm.

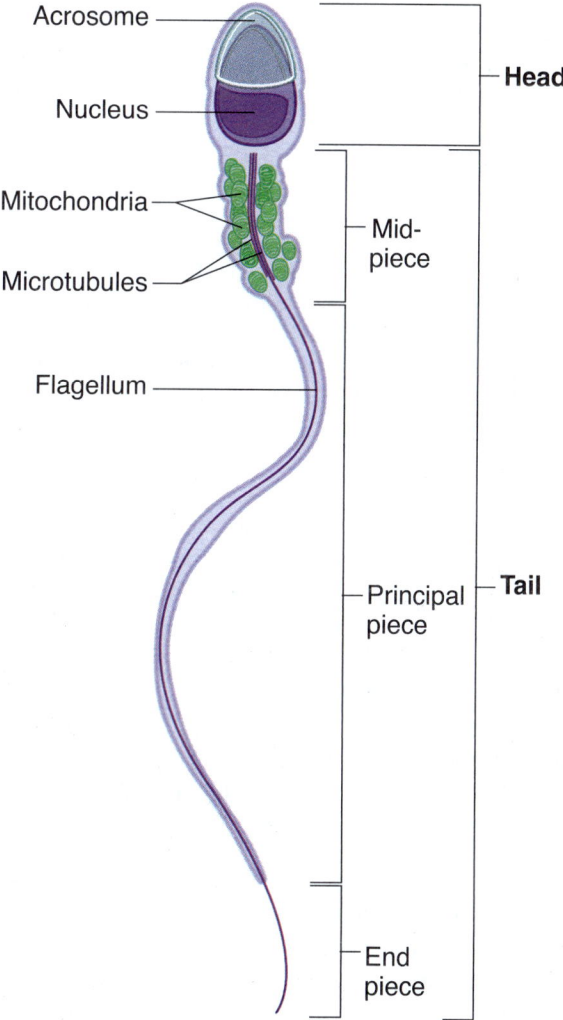

Figure 8-29. Spermatozoan

The acrosome, which is located over the anterior half of the nucleus, is derived from the Golgi complex of the spermatid and contains several hydrolytic enzymes such as hyaluronidase, neuraminidase, and acid phosphatase; these enzymes dissociate cells of the corona radiata and digest the zona pellucida of the recently produced secondary oocyte.

The basic structure of a flagellum is similar to that of a cilium. Movement is a result of the interaction among </ix>microtubules, ATP, and dynein.

Sertoli Cells and the Blood–Testis Barrier

Sertoli cells are tall columnar epithelial cells. These multifunctional cells are the predominant cells in the seminiferous tubule prior to puberty and in elderly men but comprise only 10% of the cells during times of maximal spermatogenesis.

- Irregular in shape; the base adheres to the basal lamina and the apical end extends to the lumen. The nucleus tends to be oval with the long axis oriented perpendicular to the basement membrane.
- The cytoplasmic extensions make contact with neighboring Sertoli cells via tight junctions, forming the **blood–testis barrier** by separating the seminiferous tubule into a basal and an adlumenal compartment.
- Do not divide during the reproductive period.
- Support, protect, and provide nutrition to the developing spermatozoa. During spermiogenesis, the excess spermatid cytoplasm is shed as residual bodies that are phagocytized by Sertoli cells. They also phagocytize germ cells that fail to mature.
- Secrete **androgen-binding protein** that binds testosterone and dihydrotestosterone. High concentrations of these hormones are essential for normal germ-cell maturation. The production of androgen-binding protein is stimulated by **follicle-stimulating hormone** (FSH receptors are on Sertoli cells).
- Secrete **inhibin**, which suppresses FSH synthesis.
- Produce anti-Müllerian hormone during fetal life that suppresses the development of female internal reproductive structures.

The blood–testis barrier is a network of Sertoli cells which divides the seminiferous tubule into a basal compartment (containing the spermatogonia and the earliest primary spermatocytes) and an adlumenal compartment (containing the remaining spermatocytes and spermatids). The basal compartment has free access to material found in blood, while the more advanced stages of spermatogenesis are protected from blood-borne products by the **barrier** formed by the tight junctions between the Sertoli cells. The primary spermatocytes traverse this barrier by a mechanism not yet understood.

Interstitial Tissues of the Testis

The interstitial tissue lying between the seminiferous tubules is a loose network of connective tissue composed of fibroblasts, collagen, blood and lymphatic vessels, and **Leydig cells** (also called interstitial cells). The Leydig cells synthesize testosterone.

Genital Ducts

The seminiferous tubules empty into the **rete testis** and then into 10–20 **ductuli efferentes**. The ductuli are lined by a single layer of epithelial cells, some of which are ciliated. The ciliary action propels the nonmotile spermatozoa. The non-ciliated cells reabsorb some of the fluid produced by the testis. A thin band of smooth muscle surrounds each ductus.

The spermatozoa pass from the ducti efferentes to the **epididymis**. The major function of this highly convoluted duct (approximately 5 m long) is the accumulation, storage, and maturation of spermatozoa. It is in the epididymis that the spermatozoa become motile. The epididymis is lined with a pseudostratified columnar epithelium which contains stereocilia (tall microvilli) on the luminal surface. This epithelium resorbs testicular fluid, phagocytizes residual bodies and poorly formed spermatozoa, and secretes substances thought to play a role in the maturation of spermatozoa.

The **ductus (vas) deferens** conducts spermatozoa from the epididymis to the ejaculatory duct and then into the prostatic **urethra**. The ductus (vas) deferens is a thick walled muscular tube consisting of an inner and outer layer of longitudinal smooth muscle and an intermediate circular layer. Vasectomy or the bilateral ligation of the vas deferens prevents movement of spermatozoa from the epididymis to the urethra.

Accessory Glands

Seminal Vesicles

The **seminal vesicles** are a pair of glands situated on the posterior and inferior surfaces of the bladder. These highly convoluted glands have a folded mucosa lined with pseudostratified columnar epithelium. The columnar epithelium is rich in secretory granules that displace the nuclei to the cell base.

The seminal vesicles produce a secretion that constitutes approximately 70% of human ejaculate and is rich in spermatozoa-activating substances such as fructose, citrate, prostaglandins, and several proteins. Fructose, which is a major nutrient for sperm, provides the energy for motility. The duct of each seminal vesicle joins a ductus deferens to form an ejaculatory duct. The ejaculatory duct traverses the prostate to empty into the prostatic urethra.

Prostate

The **prostate** is a collection of 30–50 branched tubuloalveolar glands whose ducts empty into the urethra. The prostate is surrounded by a fibroelastic capsule that is rich in smooth muscle. There are two types of glands in the prostate, periurethral submucosal glands and the main prostatic glands in the periphery. Glandular epithelium is pseudostratified columnar with pale, foamy cytoplasm and numerous secretory granules. The products of the secretory granules include acid phosphatase, citric acid, fibrinolysin, and other proteins.

Table 8-7. Male Reproductive Physiology

Penile Erection
Erection occurs in response to parasympathetic stimulation (pelvic splanchnic nerves). Nitric oxide is released, causing relaxation of the corpus cavernosum and corpus spongiosum, which allows blood to accumulate in the trabeculae of erectile tissue.
Ejaculation
• **Sympathetic** nervous system stimulation (lumbar splanchnic nerves) mediates movement of mature spermatozoa from the epididymis and vas deferens into the ejaculatory duct.   • Accessory glands such as the bulbourethral (Cowper) glands, prostate, and seminal vesicles secrete fluids that aid in sperm survival and fertility.   • **Somatic motor efferents** (pudendal nerve) that innervate the bulbospongiosus and ischiocavernous muscles at the base of the penis stimulate the rapid ejection of semen out the urethra during ejaculation. Peristaltic waves in the vas deferens aid in a more complete ejection of semen through the urethra.

FEMALE REPRODUCTIVE HISTOLOGY

Ovary

The paired **ovaries** have two major functions: to produce the female gametes and to produce the steroid hormones which prepare the endometrium for conception and maintain pregnancy should fertilization occur. The ovaries are 3 cm long, 1.5 cm wide, and 1 cm thick. They consist of a **medullary region**, which contains a rich vascular bed with a cellular loose connective tissue, and a **cortical region** where the ovarian follicles reside.

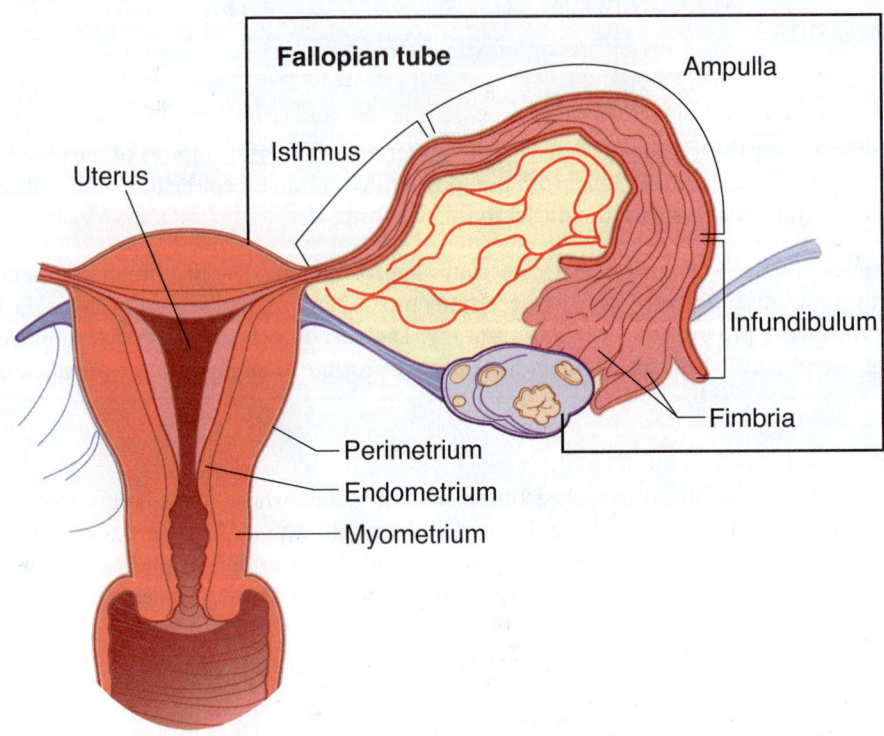

Figure 8-30. Female Reproductive System

Folliculogenesis and Ovulation

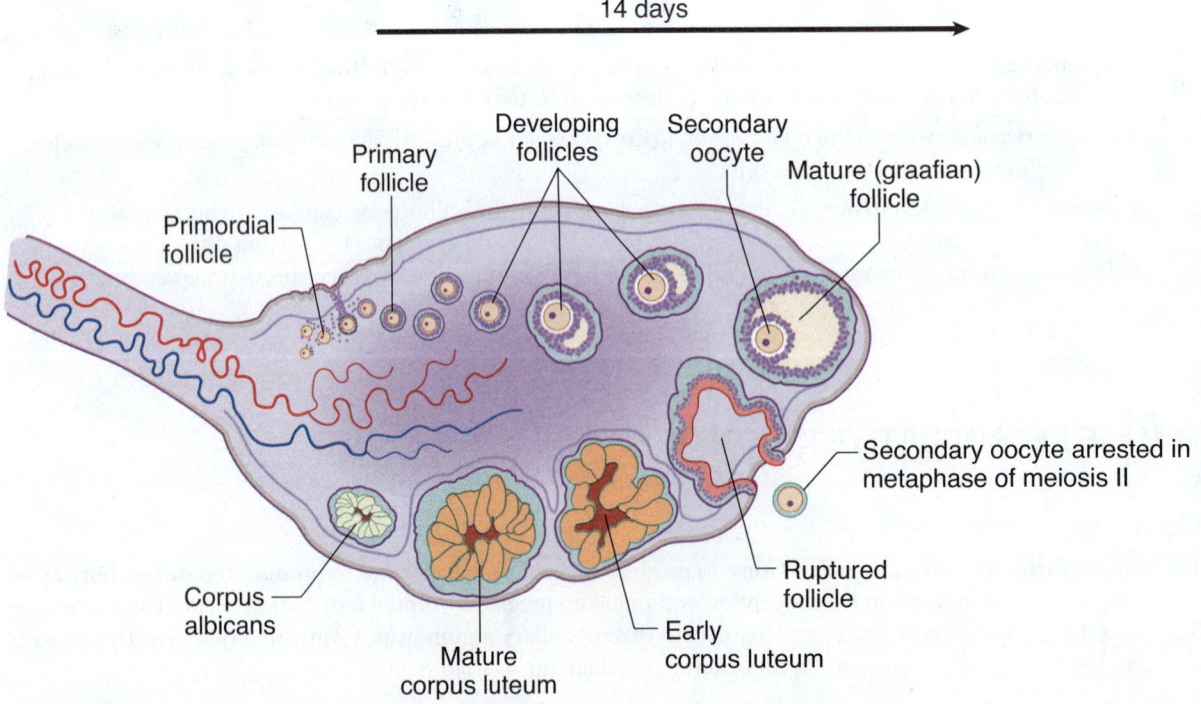

Figure 8-31. Follicular Development

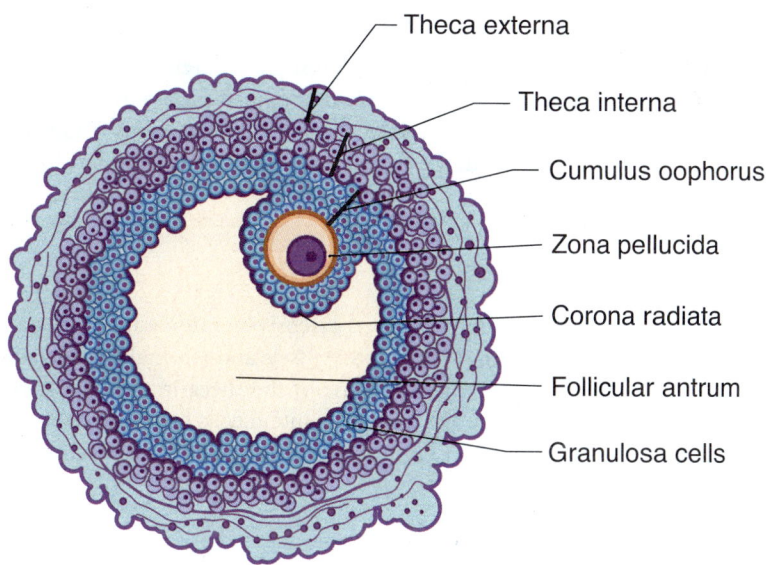

Figure 8-32. Graafian Follicle

Ovarian Follicles

An ovarian follicle consists of an oocyte surrounded by one or more layers of follicular cells, the **granulosa cells**. In utero, each ovary initially contains 3 million primordial germ cells. Many undergo atresia as the number of follicles in a normal young adult woman is estimated to be 400,000. A typical woman will ovulate only around 450 ova during her reproductive years. All other follicles (with their oocytes) will fail to mature and will undergo atresia.

Before birth, primordial germ cells differentiate into oogonia that proliferate by mitotic division until they number in the millions. They all enter prophase of the first meiotic division in utero and become arrested (they are now designated as **primordial follicles**). The primordial follicles consist of a primary oocyte surrounded by a single layer of squamous follicular cells, which are joined to one another by desmosomes.

Around the time of sexual maturity, the primordial follicles undergo further growth to become **primary follicles** in which the oocyte is surrounded by two or more layers of cuboidal cells. In each menstrual cycle after puberty, several primary follicles enter a phase of rapid growth. The oocyte enlarges and the surrounding follicular cells (now called granulosa cells) proliferate. Gap junctions form between the granulosa cells. A thick layer of glycoprotein called the **zona pellucida** is secreted (probably by both the oocyte and granulosa cells) in the space between the oocyte and granulosa cells. Cellular processes of the granulosa cells and microvilli of the oocyte penetrate the zona pellucida and make contact with one another via gap junctions. Around this time the stroma surrounding the follicle differentiates into a cellular layer called the **theca folliculi**. These cells are separated from the granulosa cells by a thick basement membrane. As development proceeds, 2 zones are apparent in the theca: the **theca interna** (richly vascularized) and the **theca externa** (mostly connective tissue). Cells of the theca interna synthesize androgenic steroids that diffuse into the follicle and are converted to estradiol by the granulosa cells.

As the follicle grows, follicular fluid, which contains mainly plasma, glycosaminoglycans and steroids accumulates between the cells. The cavities containing the fluid coalesce and form a larger cavity, the **antrum**. At this point, when the antrum is present, the follicles are called **secondary follicles**. The oocyte is at its full size and it is situated in a thickened area of the granulosa called the **cumulus oophorus**.

The mature follicle (**graafian follicle**) completes the first meiotic division (haploid, 2N amount of DNA) just prior to ovulation. The first polar body contains little cytoplasm and remains within the zona pellucida. The Graafian follicle rapidly commences the second meiotic division where it arrests in metaphase awaiting ovulation and fertilization. The second meiotic division is not completed unless fertilization occurs. The fluid filled antrum has greatly enlarged in the Graafian follicle and the cumulus oophorus diminishes leaving the oocyte surrounded by the corona radiata. After ovulation, the corona radiata remains around the ovum where it persists throughout fertilization and for some time during the passage of the ovum through the oviduct.

Ovulation

Ovulation occurs approximately mid-cycle and is stimulated by a surge of luteinizing hormone secreted by the anterior pituitary. Ovulation consists of rupture of the mature follicle and liberation of the secondary oocyte (ovum) that will be caught by the infundibulum, the dilated distal end of the oviduct. The ovum remains viable for a maximum of 24 hours. Fertilization most commonly occurs in the ampulla of the oviduct. If not fertilized, the ovum undergoes autolysis in the oviduct.

Corpus Luteum

After ovulation, the wall of the follicle collapses and becomes extensively infolded, forming a temporary endocrine gland called the **corpus luteum**. During this process the blood vessels and stromal cells invade the previously avascular layer of granulosa cells and the granulosa cells and those of the theca interna hypertrophy and form lutein cells (granulosa lutein cells and theca lutein cells). The granulosa lutein cells now secrete progesterone and estrogen and the theca lutein cells secrete androstenedione and progesterone. Progesterone prevents the development of new follicles, thereby preventing ovulation.

In the absence of pregnancy the corpus luteum lasts only 10–14 days. The lutein cells undergo apoptosis and are phagocytized by invading macrophages. The site of the corpus luteum is subsequently occupied by a scar of dense connective tissue, the **corpus albicans**.

When pregnancy does occur, human chorionic gonadotropin produced by the placenta will stimulate the corpus luteum for about 6 months and then decline. It continues to secrete progesterone until the end of pregnancy. The corpus luteum of pregnancy is large, sometimes reaching 5 cm in diameter.

Oviducts

The **oviduct** (Fallopian tube) is a muscular tube of about 12 cm in length. One end extends laterally into the wall of the uterus and the other end opens into the peritoneal cavity next to the ovary. The oviduct receives the ovum from the ovary, provides an appropriate environment for its fertilization, and transports it to the uterus. The **infundibulum** opens into the peritoneal cavity to receive the ovum. Finger-like projections (fimbriae) extend from the end of the tube and envelop the ovulation site to direct the ovum to the tube.

Adjacent to the infundibulum is the **ampulla**, where fertilization usually takes place. A slender portion of the oviduct called the **isthmus** is next to the ampulla. The **intramural segment** penetrates the wall of the uterus.

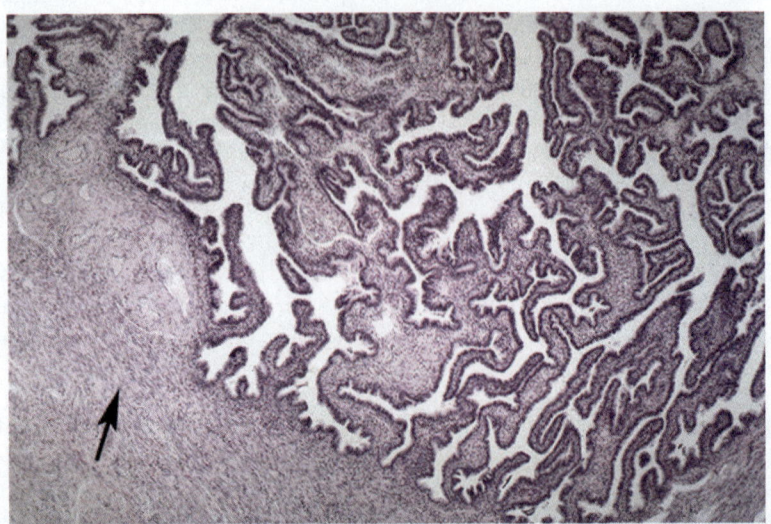

Figure 8-33. Oviduct with simple columnar epithelium and underlying layer of smooth muscle (arrow)

The wall of the oviduct has three layers: a mucosa, a muscularis, and a serosa composed of visceral peritoneum. The mucosa has longitudinal folds that are most numerous in the ampulla. The epithelium lining the mucosa is simple columnar. Some cells are ciliated and the other are secretory. The cilia beat toward the uterus, causing movement of the viscous liquid film (derived predominantly from the secretory cells) that covers the surface of the cells. The secretion has nutrient and protective functions for the ovum and promotes activation of spermatozoa. Movement of the liquid together with contraction of the muscle layer transports the ovum or fertilized egg (zygote) to the uterus.

Ciliary action is not essential, so women with **immotile cilia syndrome** (**Kartagener's syndrome**) will have a normal tubal transport of the ovum. The muscularis consists of smooth-muscle fibers in a inner circular layer and an outer longitudinal layer.

An **ectopic pregnancy** occurs when the fertilized ovum implants, most commonly in the wall of the ampulla of the oviduct. Partial development proceeds for a time but the tube is too thin and the embryo cannot survive. The vascular placental tissues that have penetrated the thin wall cause brisk bleeding into the lumen of the tube and peritoneal cavity when the tube bursts.

Uterus

The **uterus** is a pear-shaped organ that consists of a fundus, which lies above the entrance sties of the oviducts; a **body** (**corpus**), which lies below the entry point of the oviducts and the internal os; a narrowing of the uterine cavity; and a lower cylindrical structure, the **cervix**, which lies below the internal os. The wall of the uterus is relatively thick and has three layers. Depending upon the part of the uterus, there is either an outer serosa (connective tissue and mesothelium) or adventitia (connective tissue). The two other layers are the **myometrium** (smooth muscle) and the **endometrium** (the mucosa of the uterus).

The myometrium is composed of bundles of smooth-muscle fibers separated by connective tissue. During pregnancy, the myometrium goes through a period of growth as a result of hyperplasia and hypertrophy. The endometriumconsists of epithelium and lamina propria containing simple tubular glands that occasionally branch in their deeper portions. The epithelial cells are a mixture of ciliated and secretory simple columnar cells.

The endometrial layer can be divided into two zones. The **functionalis** is the part that is sloughed off at menstruation and replaced during each menstrual cycle, and the **basalis** is the portion retained after menstruation that subsequently proliferates and provides a new epithelium and lamina propria. The bases of the uterine glands, which lie deep in the basalis, are the source of the stem cells that divide and migrate to form the new epithelial lining.

Vagina

The wall of the **vagina** has no glands and consists of three layers: the mucosa, a muscular layer, and an adventitia. The mucus found in the vagina comes from the glands of the uterine cervix. The epithelium of the mucosa is stratified squamous. This thick layer of cells contains glycogen granules and may contain some keratohyalin. The muscular layer of the vagina is composed of longitudinal bundles of smooth muscle.

Mammary Glands

The mammary glands enlarge significantly during pregnancy as a result of proliferation of alveoli at the ends of the terminal ducts. Alveoli are spherical collections of epithelial cells that become the active milk-secreting structures during lactation. The milk accumulates in the lumen of the alveoli and in the lactiferous ducts. Lymphocytes and plasma cells are located in the connective tissue surrounding the alveoli. The plasma cell population increases significantly at the end of pregnancy and is responsible for the secretion of IgA that confers passive immunity on the newborn.

Learning Objectives

❏ Solve problems concerning brachial plexus

❏ Answer questions about muscle innervation

❏ Solve problems concerning sensory innervation and nerve injuries

❏ Use knowledge of arterial supply and major anastomoses

❏ Solve problems concerning carpal tunnel

BRACHIAL PLEXUS

The **brachial plexus** provides the motor and sensory innervation to the upper limb and is formed by the ventral rami of C5 through T1 spinal nerves.

Five major nerves arise from the brachial plexus:

• The **musculocutaneous, median,** and **ulnar** nerves contain **anterior division fibers** and innervate muscles in the anterior arm, anterior forearm, and palmer compartments that function mainly as flexors.

• The **axillary** and **radial** nerves contain **posterior division fibers** and innervate muscles in the posterior arm and posterior forearm compartments that function mainly as extensors.

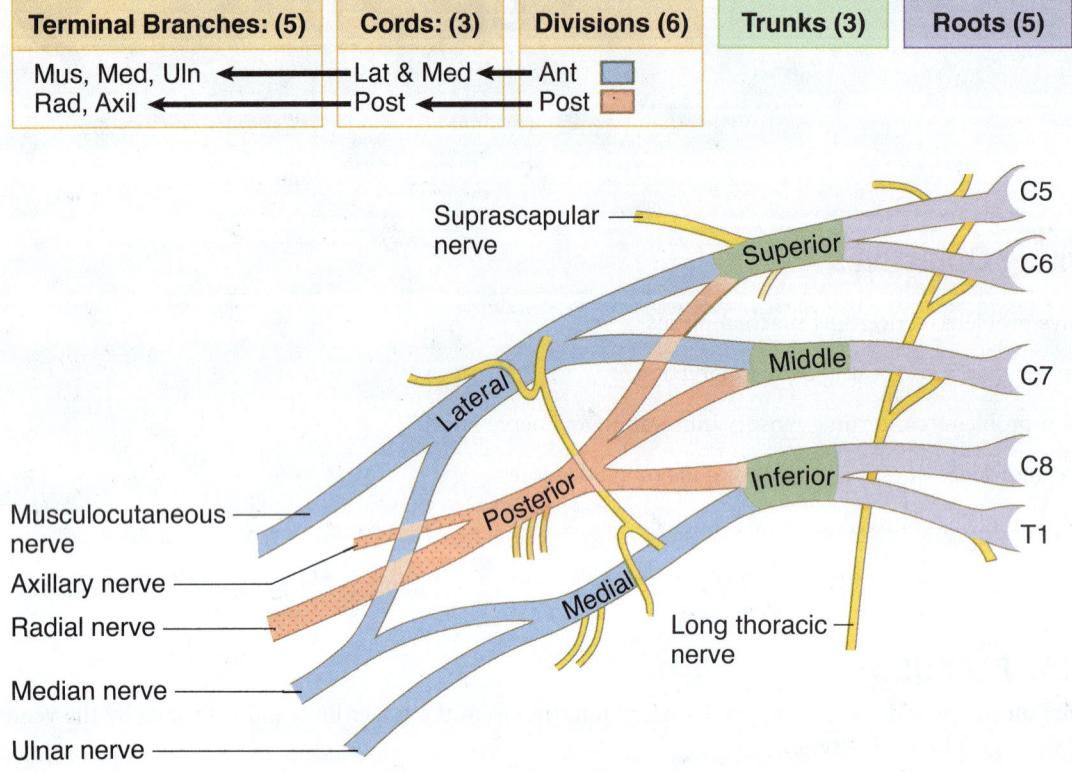

Terminal Branches: (5)	Cords: (3)	Divisions (6)	Trunks (3)	Roots (5)
Mus, Med, Uln ←	Lat & Med ←	Ant ▢		
Rad, Axil ←	Post ←	Post ▢		

Figure 9-1. Brachial Plexus

MUSCLE INNERVATION

Terminal Nerves of Upper Limbs

The motor innervation by the 5 terminal nerves of the arm muscles is summarized in the following table.

Table 9-1. Major Motor Innervations by the 5 Terminal Nerves

Terminal Nerve	Muscles Innervated	Primary Actions
Musculocutaneous nerve C5–6	All the muscles of the **anterior compartment** of the arm	Flex elbow Supination (biceps brachii)
Median nerve C5–T1	**A. Forearm** • **Anterior compartment** except 1.5 muscles by ulnar nerve (flexor carpi ulnaris and the ulnar half of the flexor digitorum profundus) **B. Hand** • **Thenar compartment** • **Central compartment** Lumbricals: Digits 2 and 3	Flex wrist and all digits Pronation Opposition of thumb Flex metacarpophalangeal (MP) and extend interphalangeal (PIP and DIP) joints of digits 2 and 3
Ulnar nerve C8–T1	**A. Forearm** Anterior Compartment: 1 [1/2] muscles not innervated by the median nerve **B. Hand** • Hypothenar compartment • **Central compartment** – Interossei muscles: Palmar and Dorsal • Lumbricals: Digits 4 & 5 • Adductor pollicis	Flex wrist (weak) and digits 4 and 5 Dorsal – Abduct digits 2-5 (DAB) Palmar – Adduct digits 2-5 (PAD) Assist Lumbricals in MP flexion and IP extension digits 2–5 Flex MP and extend PIP & DIP joints of digits 4 and 5 Adduct the thumb
Axillary nerve C5–6	Deltoid Teres minor	Abduct shoulder—15°–110° Lateral rotation of shoulder
Radial nerve C5–T1	**Posterior compartment** muscles of the arm and forearm	Extend MP, wrist, and elbow Supination (supinator muscle)

Collateral Nerves

In addition to the 5 terminal nerves, there are several collateral nerves that arise from the brachial plexus proximal to the terminal nerves (i.e., from the rami, trunks, or cords). These nerves innervate proximal limb muscles (shoulder girdle muscles). The following table summarizes the collateral nerves.

Table 9-2. The Collateral Nerves of the Brachial plexus

Collateral Nerve	Muscles or Skin Innervated
Dorsal scapular nerve	Rhomboids
Long thoracic nerve	Serratus anterior—protracts and rotates scapula superiorly
Suprascapular nerve C5–6	Supraspinatus—abduct shoulder 0–15°
	Infraspinatus—laterally rotate shoulder
Lateral pectoral nerve	Pectoralis major
Medial pectoral nerve	Pectoralis major and minor
Upper subscapular nerve	Subscapularis
Middle subscapular (thoracodorsal) nerve	Latissimus dorsi
Lower subscapular nerve	Subscapularis and teres major
Medial brachial cutaneous nerve	Skin of medial arm
Medial antebrachial cutaneous nerve	Skin of medial forearm

Segmental Innervation to Muscles of Upper Limbs

The **segmental innervation** to the muscles of the upper limbs has a **proximal–distal gradient**, i.e., the more proximal muscles are innervated by the higher segments (C5 and C6) and the more distal muscles are innervated by the lower segments (C8 and T1). Therefore, the intrinsic shoulder muscles are innervated by C5 and C6, the intrinsic hand muscles are innervated by C8 and T1, the distal arm and proximal forearm muscles are innervated by C6 and C7, and the more distal forearm muscles are innervated by C7 and C8.

SENSORY INNERVATION

The skin of the palm is supplied by the median and ulnar nerves. The **median** supplies the lateral 3½ digits and the adjacent area of the lateral palm and the thenar eminence. The **ulnar** supplies the medial 1½ digits and skin of the hypothenar eminence. The **radial** nerve supplies skin of the dorsum of the hand in the area of the first dorsal web space, including the skin over the anatomic snuffbox.

The sensory innervation of the hand is summarized in the following figure.

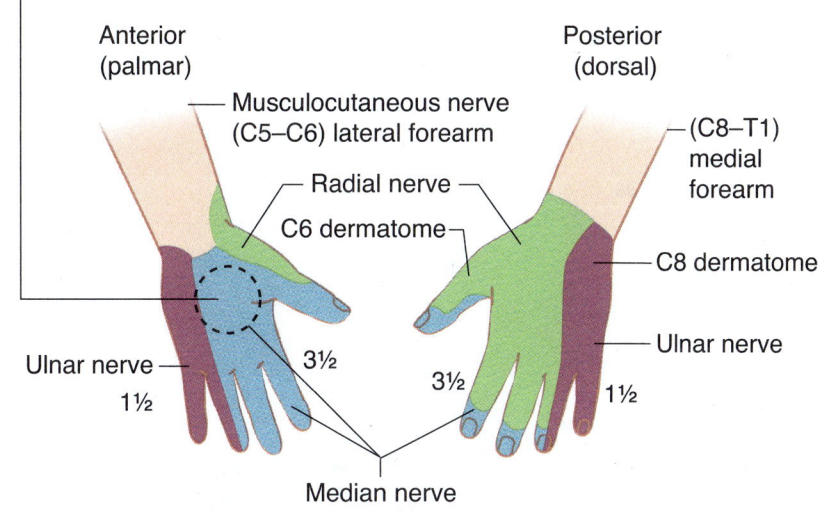

Figure 9-2. Sensory Innervation of the Hand and Forearm

Note
Palm sensation is not affected by carpal tunnel syndrome; the superficial palmar cutaneous branch of median nerve passes superficial to the carpal tunnel.

ARTERIAL SUPPLY AND MAJOR ANASTOMOSES

Arterial Supply to the Upper Limb

Subclavian artery
Branch of brachiocephalic trunk on the right and aortic arch on the left.

Axillary artery
- From the first rib to the posterior edge of the teres major muscle
- Three major branches:
  - Lateral thoracic artery—supplies mammary gland; runs with long thoracic nerve
  - Subscapular artery—collateral to shoulder with suprascapular branch of subclavian artery
  - Posterior humeral circumflex artery—at surgical neck with axillary nerve

Brachial artery
Profunda brachii artery with radial nerve in radial groove—at midshaft of humerus

Radial artery
Deep palmar arch

Ulnar artery

- Common interosseus artery
- Superficial palmar arch

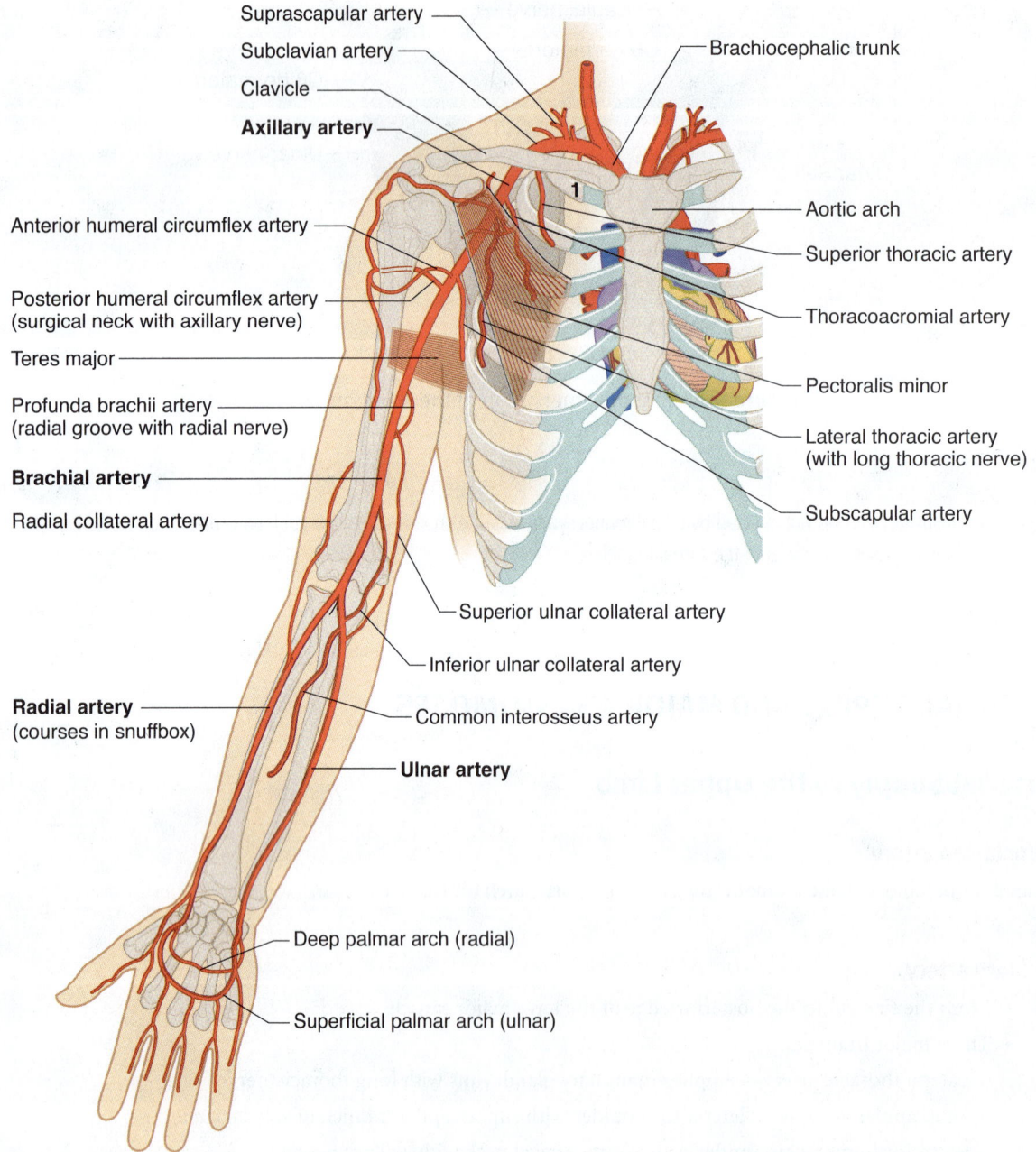

Suprascapular artery

Subclavian artery

Clavicle

Axillary artery

Anterior humeral circumflex artery

Posterior humeral circumflex artery
(surgical neck with axillary nerve)

Teres major

Profunda brachii artery
(radial groove with radial nerve)

Brachial artery

Radial collateral artery

Radial artery
(courses in snuffbox)

Brachiocephalic trunk

1

Aortic arch

Superior thoracic artery

Thoracoacromial artery

Pectoralis minor

Lateral thoracic artery
(with long thoracic nerve)

Subscapular artery

Superior ulnar collateral artery

Inferior ulnar collateral artery

Common interosseus artery

Ulnar artery

Deep palmar arch (radial)

Superficial palmar arch (ulnar)

Figure 9-3. Arterial Supply to the Upper Limb

Collateral Circulation

Shoulder

Subscapular branch of axillary and suprascapular branch of subclavian arteries

Hand

Superficial and deep palmar arches

CARPAL TUNNEL

The carpal tunnel is the fibro-osseous tunnel located on the ventral aspect of the wrist.

- The tunnel is bounded **anteriorly** by the **flexor retinaculum** and **posteriorly** by the proximal row of **carpal bones (lunate)**.
- The carpal tunnel transmits 9 tendons and the radial and ulnar bursae (4 tendons of the **flexor digitorum superficialis**, 4 tendons of the **flexor digitorum profundus**, and the tendon of the **flexor pollicis longus**) and the **median nerve.**
- There are **no** blood vessels or any branches of the radial or ulnar nerves in the carpal tunnel.

Carpal Tunnel Syndrome

Entrapment of the median nerve and other structures in the carpal tunnel due to any condition that reduces the space results in **carpal tunnel syndrome**. The median nerve is the only nerve affected and the patient will present withatrophy of the thenar compartment muscles and weakness of the thenar muscles (opposition of the thumb— **ape hand**).

There is also **sensory loss** and numbness on the palmar surfaces of the **lateral 3½ digits**. Note that the skin on the lateral side of the palm (thenar eminence) is spared because the **palmar cutaneous branch of the median nerve** which supplies the lateral palm enters the hand **superficial** to the flexor retinaculum and does not course through the carpal tunnel.

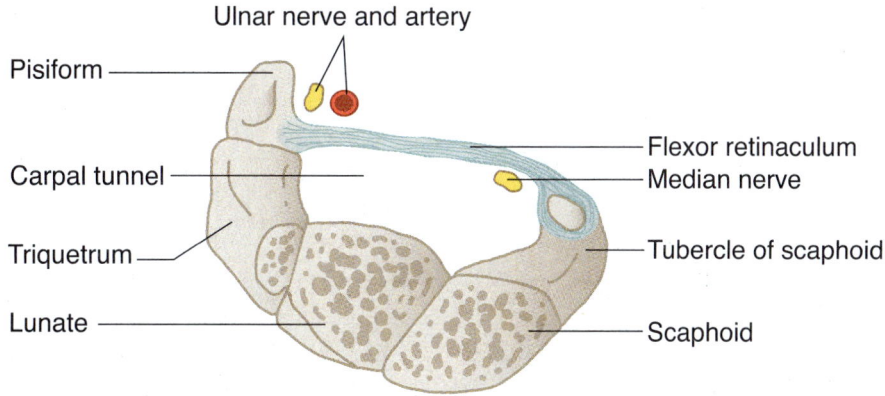

Figure 9-4. Carpal Tunnel at Proximal Row of Carpal Bones

ROTATOR CUFF

The tendons of rotator cuff muscles strengthen the glenohumeral joint and include the **supraspinatus, infraspinatus, teres minor**, and **subscapularis**(the **SITS**) muscles. The tendons of the muscles of the rotator cuff may become torn or inflamed.

The tendon of the **supraspinatus** is most commonly affected. Patients with rotator cuff tears experience pain anteriorly and superiorly to the glenohumeral joint during abduction.

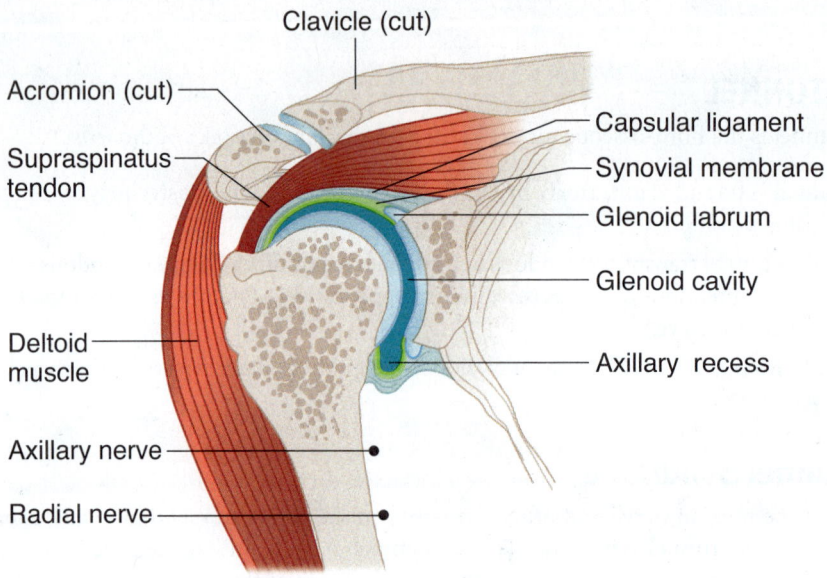

Figure 9-5. Rotator Cuff

Learning Objectives

❑ Answer questions about carotid and subclavian arteries

❑ Demonstrate understanding of embryology of the head and neck

❑ Demonstrate knowledge of major muscles and major bones of the head

❑ Answer questions about cranial meninges and dural venous sinuses

❑ Interpret scenarios on orbital muscles and their innervation

NECK

Thoracic Outlet

The thoracic outlet is the space bounded by the manubrium, the first rib, and T1 vertebra. The interval between the anterior and middle scalene muscles and the first rib (**scalene triangle**) transmits the structures coursing between the thorax, upper limb and lower neck.

- The triangle contains the **trunks of the brachial plexus** and the **subclavian artery**(Figure 10-1).
- Note that the subclavian vein and the phrenic nerve (C 3, 4, and 5) are on the anterior surface of the anterior scalene muscle and are not in the scalene triangle.

Thoracic Outlet Syndrome

Thoracic outlet syndrome results from the compression of the **trunks of the brachial plexus and the subclavian artery** within the scalene triangle. Compression of these structures can result from tumors of the neck (Pancoast on apex of lung), a cervical rib or hypertrophy of the scalene muscles. The lower trunk of the brachial plexus (C8, T1) is usually the first to be affected. Clinical symptoms include the following:

- Numbness and pain on the medial aspect of the forearm and hand
- Weakness of the muscles supplied by the ulnar nerve in the hand (claw hand)
- Decreased blood flow into the upper limb, indicated by a weakened radial pulse
- Compression can also affect the cervical sympathetic trunk (Horner's syndrome) and the recurrent laryngeal nerves (hoarseness).

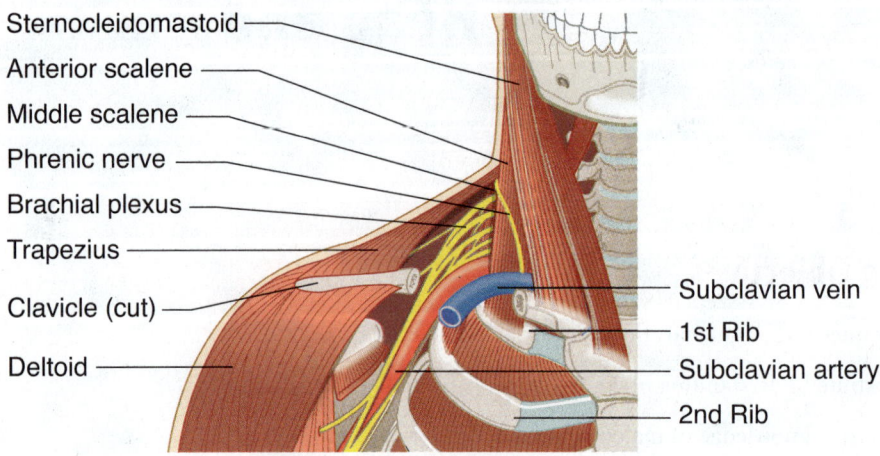

Figure 10-1. Scalene Triangle of the Neck

CAROTID AND SUBCLAVIAN ARTERIES

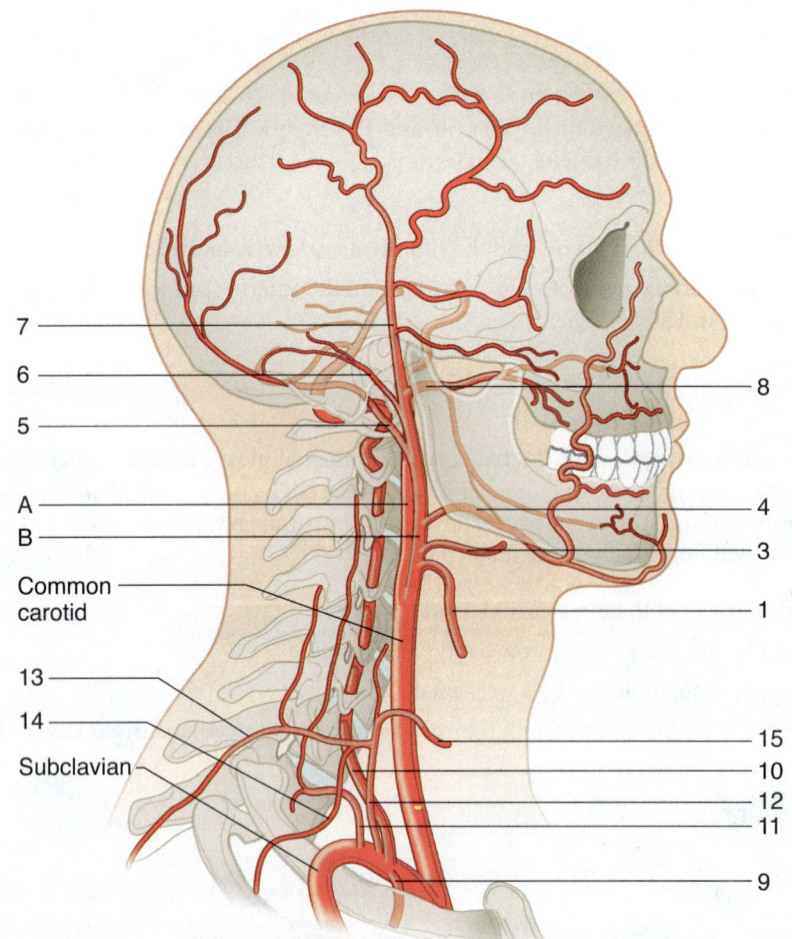

Common Carotid Artery
A. Internal carotid artery— opthalmic artery and brain
B. External carotid artery
1. Superior thyroid
2. Ascending pharyngeal (not shown)
3. Lingual
4. Facial
5. Occipital
6. Posterior auricular
7. Superficial temporal
8. Maxillary—deep face; middle meningeal artery

Subclavian Artery
9. Internal thoracic— cardiac bypass
10. Vertebral—brain
11. Costocervical
12. Thyrocervical
13. Transverse cervical
14. Suprascapular— collaterals to shoulder
15. Inferior thyroid

Figure 10-2. Arteries to the Head and Neck

EMBRYOLOGY OF THE HEAD AND NECK

Pharyngeal Apparatus

The pharyngeal apparatus consists of the following:

- **Pharyngeal arches** (1, 2, 3, 4, and 6) composed of **mesoderm and neural crest**
- **Pharyngeal pouches** (1, 2, 3, 4) lined with **endoderm**
- **Pharyngeal grooves or clefts** (1, 2, 3, and 4) lined **with ectoderm**

The anatomic associations relating to these structures in the fetus and adult are summarized in Figures 10-3 and 10-4.

Table 10-1 summarizes the relationships among the nerves, arteries, muscles, and skeletal elements derived from the pharyngeal arches.

Table 10-2 shows which adult structures are derived from the pharyngeal pouches.

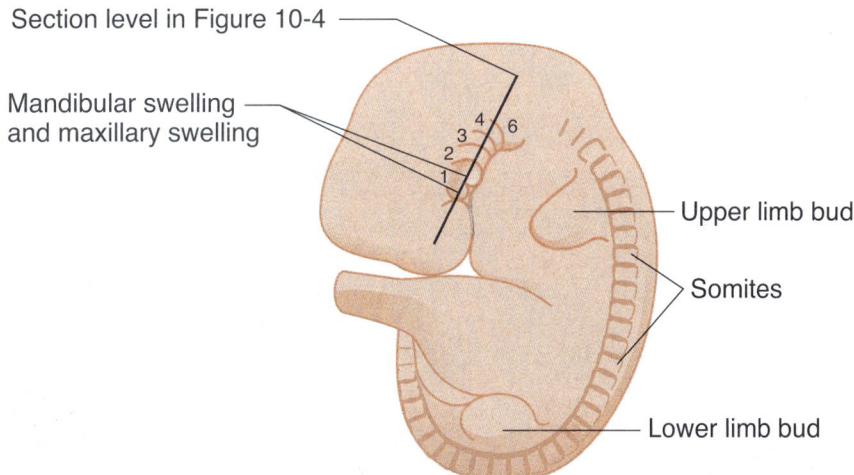

Figure 10-3. The Fetal Pharyngeal Apparatus

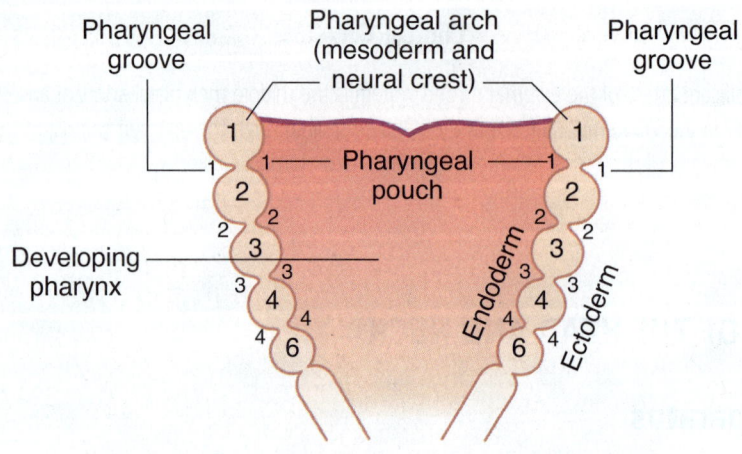

Figure 10-4. Section through the Developing Pharynx

Pharyngeal arches

The components of the pharyngeal arches are summarized in the following table.

Table 10-1. Components of the Pharyngeal Arches

Arch	Nerve* (Neural Ectoderm)	Artery (Aortic Arch Mesoderm)	Muscle (Mesoderm)	Skeletal/Cartilage (Neural Crest)
1	Trigeminal: mandibular nerve		Four muscles of mastication: — Masseter — Temporalis — Lateral pterygoid — Medial pterygoid Plus: — Digastric (anterior belly) — Mylohyoid — Tensor tympani — Tensor veli palatini	Maxilla Mandible Incus Malleus
2	VII		Muscles of facial expression: Plus: — Digastric (posterior belly) — Stylohyoid — Stapedius	Stapes Styloid process Lesser horn and upper body of hyoid bone

(Continue)

Arch	Nerve* (Neural Ectoderm)	Artery (Aortic Arch Mesoderm)	Muscle (Mesoderm)	Skeletal/Cartilage (Neural Crest)
3	IX	Right and left common carotid arteriesRight and left internal carotid arteries	Stylopharyngeus muscle	Greater horn and lower body of hyoid bone
4	X — Superior laryngeal nerve — Pharyngeal branches	Right subclavian artery (right arch) Arch of aorta (left arch)	Cricothyroid muscle Soft palate Pharynx (5 muscles)	Thyroid cartilage
6	X Recurrent laryngeal nerve	Right and left pulmonary arteries Ductus arteriosus (left arch)	Intrinsic muscles of larynx (except cricothyroid muscle)	All other laryngeal cartilages

*Nerves are not derived from pharyngeal arch; they grow into the arch.

Note: The **ocular muscles** (III, IV, VI) and the **tongue muscles** (XII) do not derive from pharyngeal arch mesoderm but from mesoderm of the occipital somites (somitomeres).

Pharyngeal pouches

The anatomic structures relating to the pharyngeal pouches are summarized in Figure 10-5 and Table 10-2.

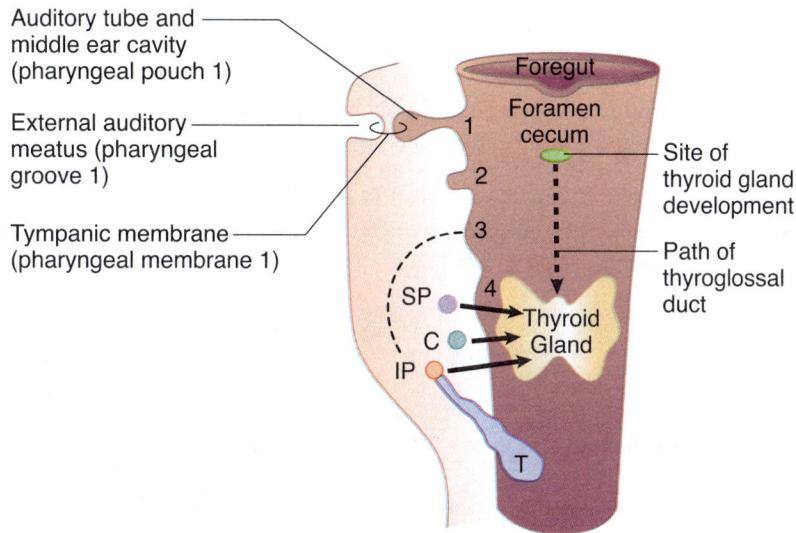

Figure 10-5. Fetal Pharyngeal Pouches
IP: Inferior parathyroid gland
SP: Superior parathyroid gland
T: Thymus
C: C-cells of thyroid

The adult structures derived from the fetal pharyngeal pouches are summarized in Table 10-2.

Table 10-2. Adult Structures Derived From the Fetal Pharyngeal Pouches

Pouch	Adult Derivatives
1	Epithelial lining of auditory tube and middle ear cavity
2	Epithelial lining of crypts of palatine tonsil
3	Inferior parathyroid (IP) gland Thymus (T)
4	Superior parathyroid (SP) gland C-cells of thyroid

*Neural crest cells migrate to form parafollicular C-cells of the thyroid.

Clinical Correlate

Normally, the second, third, and fourth pharyngeal grooves are obliterated by overgrowth of the second pharyngeal arch. Failure of a cleft to be completely obliterated results in a branchial cyst or **lateral cervical cyst.**

Pharyngeal grooves (clefts)

Pharyngeal groove 1 gives rise to the epithelial lining of **external auditory meatus.**

All other grooves are obliterated.

Thyroid Gland

The thyroid gland does not develop from a pharyngeal pouch. It develops from the **thyroid diverticulum,** which forms from the midline endoderm in the floor of the pharynx.

- The thyroid diverticulum migrates caudally to its adult anatomic position in the neck but remains connected to the foregut via the **thyroglossal duct,** which is later obliterated.
- The former site of the thyroglossal duct is indicated in the adult by the **foramen cecum** (Figures 10-5 and 10-6).

Tongue

Note: more information about the tongue can be found in the Dental Anatomy section.

The **anterior two-thirds of the tongue** is associated with **pharyngeal arches 1 and 2.** General sensation is carried by the lingual branch of the mandibular nerve (cranial nerve [CN] V). Taste sensation is carried by **chorda tympani of CN VII** (Figure 10-6).

The **posterior one third of the tongue** is associated with **pharyngeal arch 3.** General sensation and taste are carried by **CN IX.**

Most of the muscles of the tongue are innervated by CN XII.

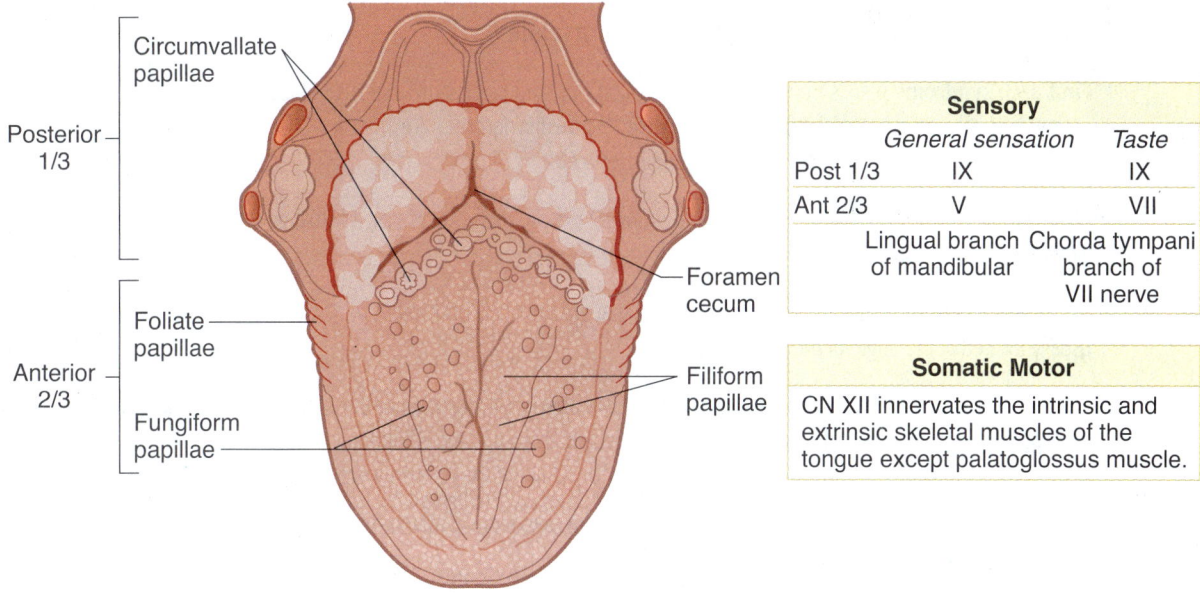

Posterior 1/3
- Circumvallate papillae
- Foramen cecum

Anterior 2/3
- Foliate papillae
- Fungiform papillae
- Filiform papillae

Sensory		
	General sensation	*Taste*
Post 1/3	IX	IX
Ant 2/3	V	VII
	Lingual branch of mandibular	Chorda tympani branch of VII nerve

Somatic Motor
CN XII innervates the intrinsic and extrinsic skeletal muscles of the tongue except palatoglossus muscle.

Figure 10-6. Tongue

Development of the Face and Palate

The **face** develops from 5 primordia of mesoderm (neural crest) of the first pharyngeal arch: a single frontonasal prominence, the pair of maxillary prominences, and the pair of mandibular prominences.

- The **intermaxillary segment** forms when the 2 medial nasal prominences of the frontonasal prominences fuse together at the midline and form the **philtrum of the lip** and the **primary palate**.
- The **secondary palate** forms from palatine shelves (maxillary prominence), which fuse in the midline, posterior to the incisive foramen.
- The primary and secondary palates fuse at the **incisive foramen** to form the definitive hard palate.

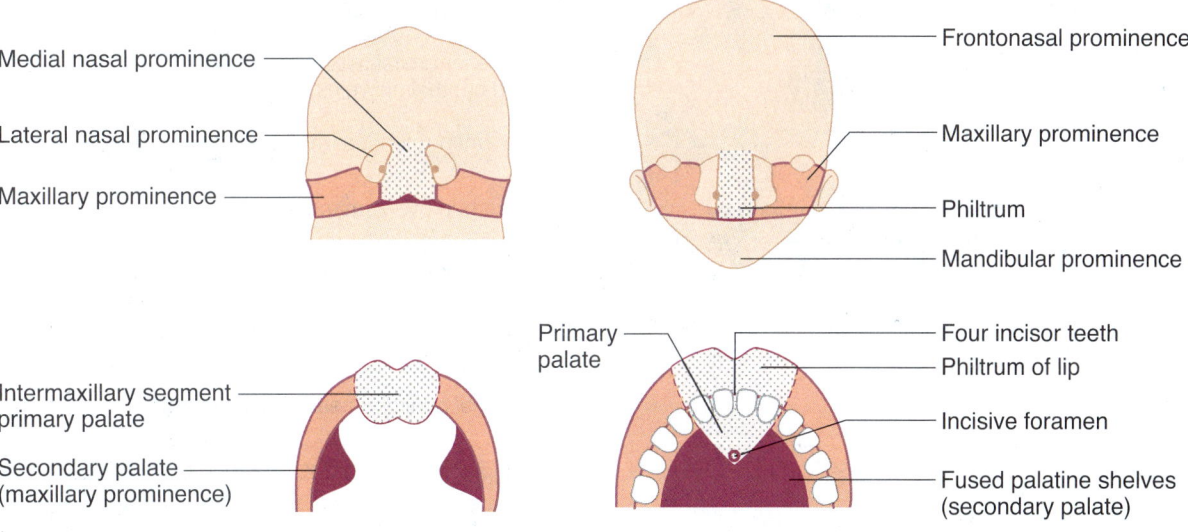

- Medial nasal prominence
- Lateral nasal prominence
- Maxillary prominence
- Frontonasal prominence
- Maxillary prominence
- Philtrum
- Mandibular prominence

- Intermaxillary segment primary palate
- Secondary palate (maxillary prominence)
- Primary palate
- Four incisor teeth
- Philtrum of lip
- Incisive foramen
- Fused palatine shelves (secondary palate)

Figure 10-7. Face and Palate Development

Clinical Correlate

First arch syndrome results from abnormal formation of pharyngeal arch 1 because of faulty migration of neural crest cells, causing facial anomalies. Two well-described syndromes are Treacher Collins syndrome and Pierre Robin sequence. Both defects involve neural crest cells.

Pharyngeal fistula occurs when pouch 2 and groove 2 persist, thereby forming a fistula generally found along the anterior border of the muscle.

Pharyngeal cyst occurs when pharyngeal grooves that are normally obliterated persist, forming a cyst usually located at the angle of the mandible.

Ectopic thyroid, parathyroid, or thymus results from abnormal migration of these glands from their embryonic position to their adult anatomic position. Ectopic thyroid tissue is found along the midline of the neck. Ectopic parathyroid or thymus tissue is generally found along the lateral aspect of the neck. May be an important issue during neck surgery.

Thyroglossal duct cyst or fistula occurs when parts of the thyroglossal duct persist, generally in the midline near the hyoid bone. The cyst may also be found at the base of the tongue (lingual cyst).

DiGeorge sequence occurs when pharyngeal pouches 3 and 4 fail to differentiate into the parathyroid glands and thymus. Neural crest cells are involved.

Cleft lip occurs when the maxillary prominence fails to fuse with the medial nasal prominence.

Cleft palate occurs when the palatine shelves fail to fuse with each other or the primary palate.

CRANIUM

Cranial Fossae

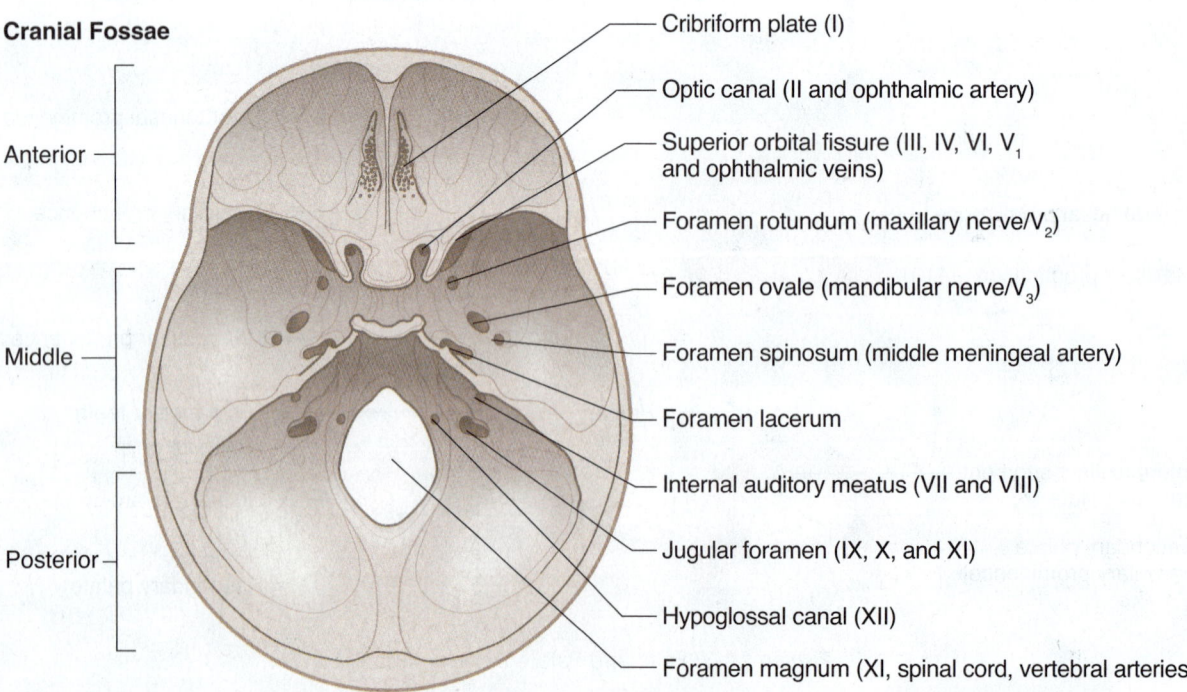

Anterior

Middle

Posterior

Cribriform plate (I)

Optic canal (II and ophthalmic artery)

Superior orbital fissure (III, IV, VI, V_1 and ophthalmic veins)

Foramen rotundum (maxillary nerve/V_2)

Foramen ovale (mandibular nerve/V_3)

Foramen spinosum (middle meningeal artery)

Foramen lacerum

Internal auditory meatus (VII and VIII)

Jugular foramen (IX, X, and XI)

Hypoglossal canal (XII)

Foramen magnum (XI, spinal cord, vertebral arteries)

Figure 10-8. Foramina: Cranial Fossae

Clinical Correlate

Jugular fobramen syndrome may be caused by a tumor pressing on CN IX, X, and XI. Patients present with hoarseness, dysphagia (CN IX and X), loss of sensation over the oropharynx and posterior third of the tongue (CN IX), and trapezius and sternocleidomastoid weakness (CN XI). The nearby CN XII may be involved producing tongue deviation to the lesioned side.

Bones

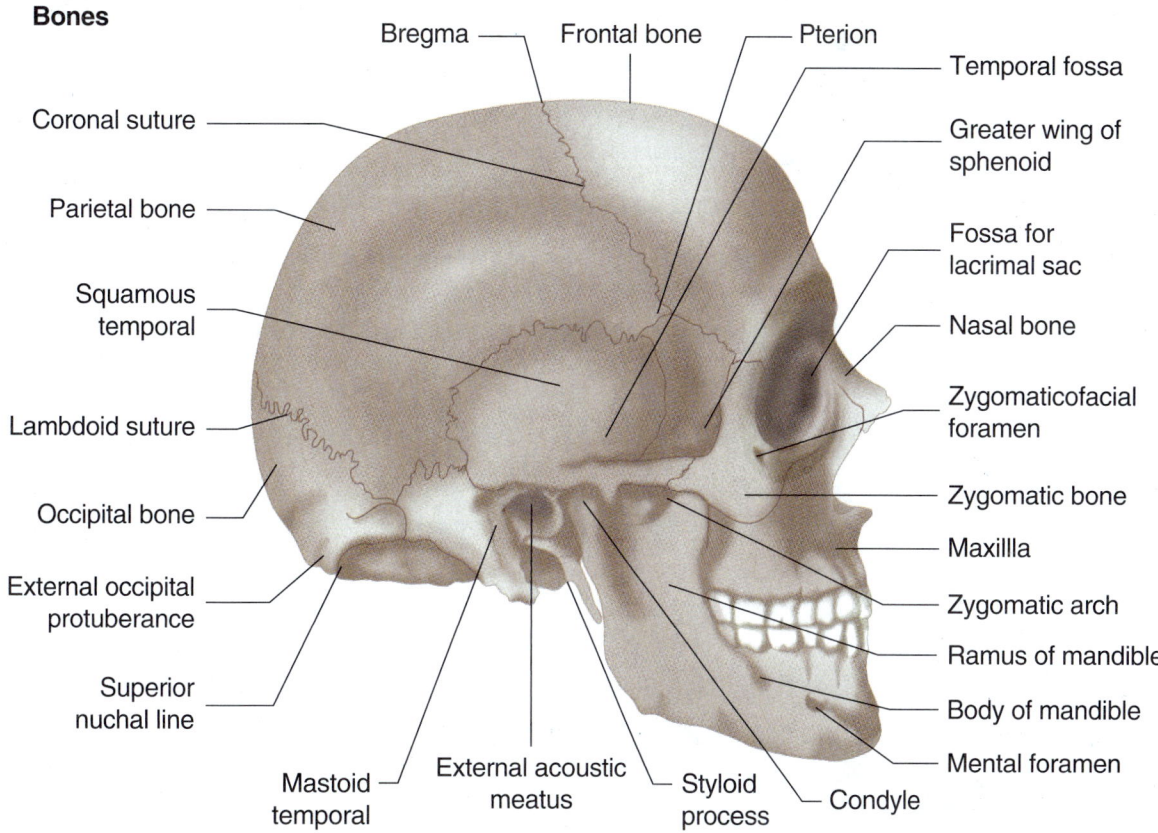

Figure 10-9. Lateral aspect of the skull

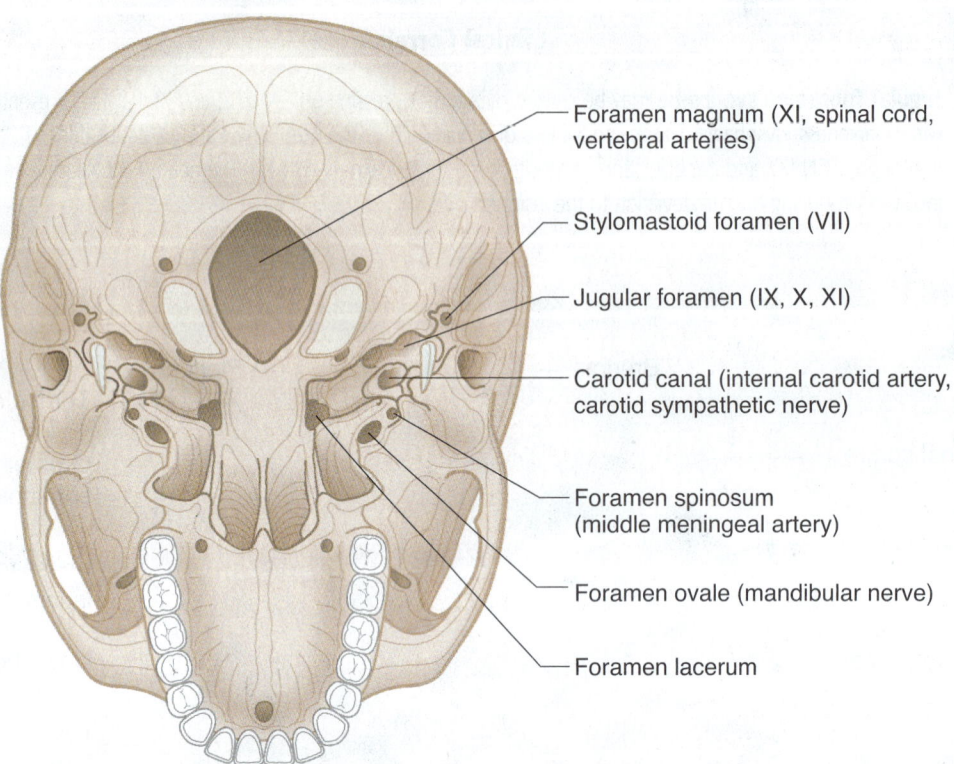

Figure 10-10. Foramina: Base of Skull

Foramen magnum (XI, spinal cord, vertebral arteries)

Stylomastoid foramen (VII)

Jugular foramen (IX, X, XI)

Carotid canal (internal carotid artery, carotid sympathetic nerve)

Foramen spinosum (middle meningeal artery)

Foramen ovale (mandibular nerve)

Foramen lacerum

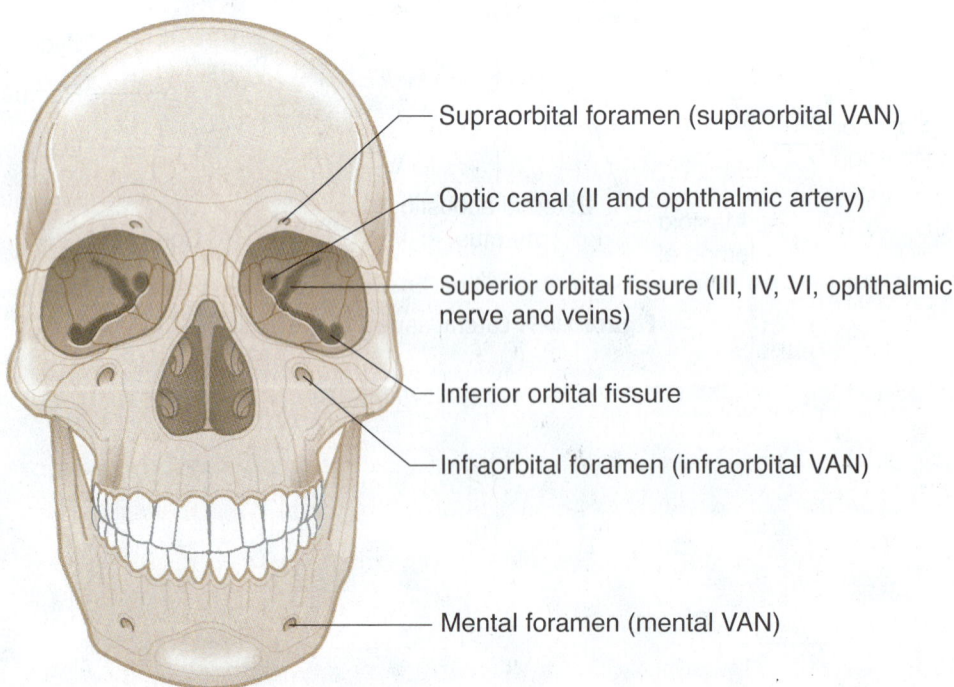

Figure 10-11. Foramina: Front of Skull

Supraorbital foramen (supraorbital VAN)

Optic canal (II and ophthalmic artery)

Superior orbital fissure (III, IV, VI, ophthalmic nerve and veins)

Inferior orbital fissure

Infraorbital foramen (infraorbital VAN)

Mental foramen (mental VAN)

CRANIAL MENINGES AND DURAL VENOUS SINUSES

Cranial Meninges

The brain is covered by 3 meninges that are continuous through the foramen magnum with the spinal meninges. There are several similarities and differences between spinal and cranial meninges (Figure 10-12).

- **Pia mater** tightly invests the surfaces of the brain and cannot be dissected away, having the same relationship with the brain as spinal pia mater.

- **Dura mater** is the thickest of the 3 meninges and, unlike the spinal dura, consists of 2 layers (**periosteal and meningeal**) that are fused together during most of their course in the cranial cavity.

  - **Periosteal layer**: This outer layer lines the inner surfaces of the flat bones and serves as their periosteum. The periosteal layer can easily be peeled away from the bones.

  - **Meningeal (true dura) layer**: This is the innermost layer that is mostly fused with the periosteal dura mater throughout the cranial cavity. At certain points in the cranium, the meningeal layer separates from the periosteal layer and forms the dural venous sinuses and connective tissue foldings or duplications: **falx cerebri, diaphragma sellae and tentorium cerebelli**. These duplications separate and support different parts of the CNS.

- **Arachnoid** is the thin, delicate membrane which lines and follows the inner surface of the meningeal dura.

  - Projections of arachnoid called **arachnoid granulations** penetrate through the dura mater and extend into the superior sagittal dural venous sinus. Arachnoid granulations are where CSF returns to the systemic venous circulation.

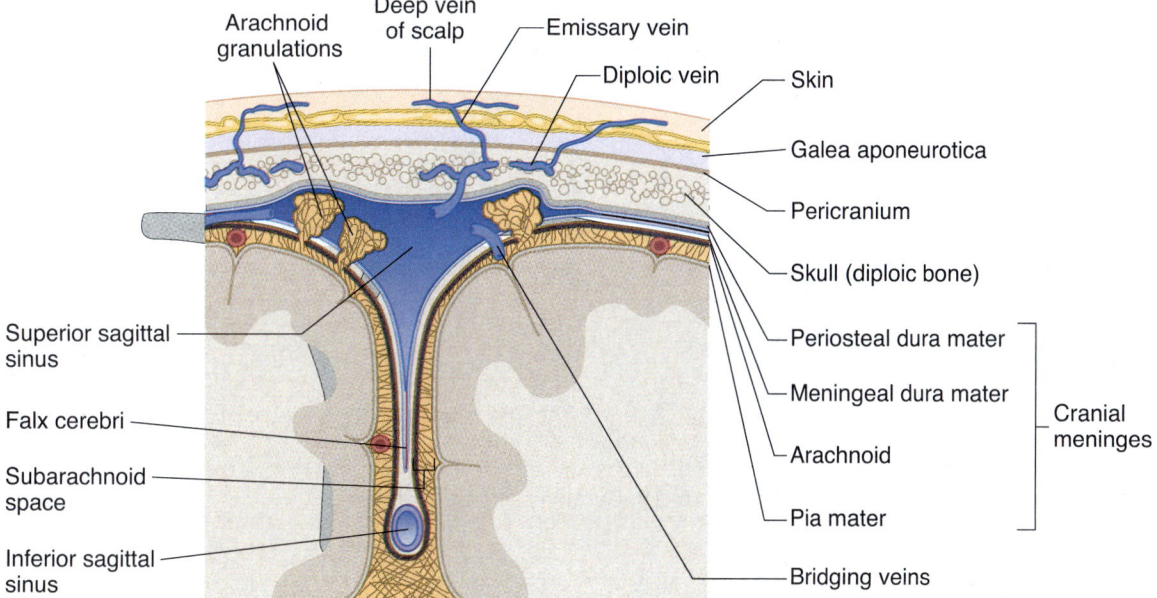

Figure 10-12. Coronal Section of the Dural Sinuses

Spaces related to the cranial meninges

- **Epidural space** is a potential space between the periosteal dura and the bones of the skull: site of epidural hematomas (described later).

- **Subdural space** is the potential space between the meningeal dura and the arachnoid membrane: site of subdural hematomas (described later).

- **Subarachnoid space** lies between the arachnoid and pia mater containing CSF: site of subarachnoid hemorrhage (described later).

Dural Venous Sinuses

Dural venous sinuses are formed at different points in the cranial cavity where the **periosteal** and **meningeal** dural layers separate to form endothelial lined venous channels called dural venous sinuses (Figures 10-12 and 10-13). The sinuses provide the major venous drainage from most structures within the cranial cavity. They drain mostly into the internal jugular vein, which exits the cranial floor at the jugular foramen. Most of the dural venous sinuses are located in the two largest duplications of meningeal dura mater (**falx cerebri** and the **tentorium cerebelli**).

The primary tributaries that flow into the sinuses are:

- **Cerebral** and **cerebelli veins** that form **bridging veins** which pass across the subdural space to drain into the sinuses
- **Emissary** veins are valveless channels that course through the bones of the skull and allow dural sinuses to communicate with extracranial veins.
- **Diploic veins** drain the spongy (diploe) core of the flat bones.
- **Arachnoid granulations** are where CSF returns to the venous circulation.
- **Meningeal veins** drain the meninges.

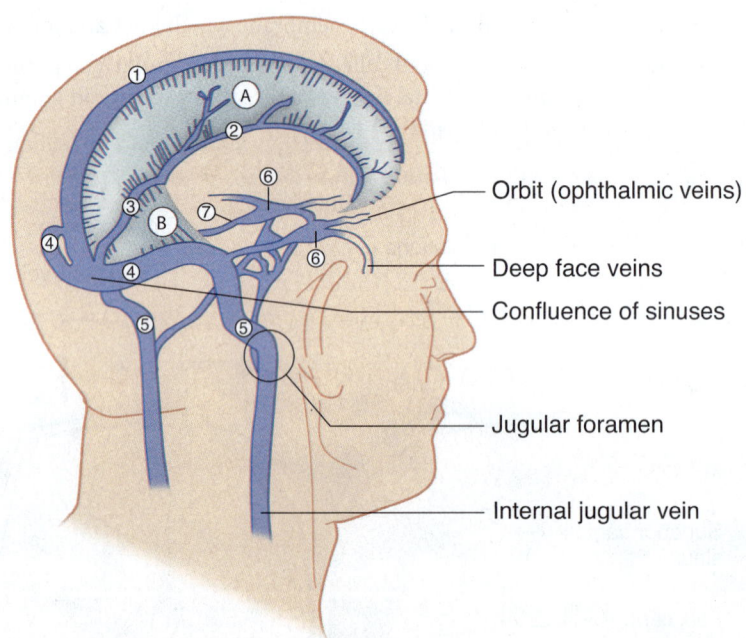

Names of the Major Dural Sinuses

1. Superior sagittal*
2. Inferior sagittal
3. Straight*
4. Transverse* (2)
5. Sigmoid (2)
6. Cavernous (2)
7. Superior petrosal (2)

* Drain into the confluence of sinuses located at the inion.

Folds (Duplications) of Dura Mater

A. Falx cerebri
B. Tentorium cerebelli

Orbit (ophthalmic veins)

Deep face veins

Confluence of sinuses

Jugular foramen

Internal jugular vein

Figure 10-13. Dural Venous Sinuses

Major dural venous sinuses

The major dural venous sinuses are:

- The **superior sagittal sinus** is located in the midsagittal plane along the superior aspect of the falx cerebri. It drains primarily into the confluence of the sinuses.

- The **inferior sagittal sinus** is located in the midsagittal plane near the inferior margin of the falx cerebri. It terminates by joining with the great cerebral vein (of Galen) to form the straight sinus at the junction of the falx cerebri and tentorium cerebelli.

- The **straight sinus** is formed by the union of the inferior sagittal sinus and the great cerebral vein. It usually terminates by draining into the confluens of sinuses (or into the transverse sinus).

- The **occipital sinus** is a small sinus found in the posterior border of the tentorium cerebelli. It drains into the confluens of sinuses.

- The **confluens of sinuses** is formed by the union of the superior sagittal, straight, and occipital sinuses posteriorly at the occipital bone. It drains laterally into the 2 transverse sinuses.

- The **transverse sinuses** are paired sinuses in the tentorium cerebelli and attached to the occipital bone that drain venous blood from the confluens of sinuses into the sigmoid sinuses.

- The **sigmoid sinuses** are paired and form a S-shaped channel in the floor of the posterior cranial fossa. The sigmoid sinus drains into the **internal jugular vein** at the **jugular foramen**.

- The paired **cavernous sinuses** are located on either side of the body of the sphenoid bone (Figure I-14).
  - Each sinus receives blood primarily from the **orbit (ophthalmic veins)** and via emissary veins from the **deep face**(pterygoid venous plexus). Superficial veins of the maxillary face drain into the medial angle of the eye, enter the ophthalmic veins, and drain into the cavernous sinus.

  - Each cavernous sinus 1 via the superior and inferior petrosal sinuses into the sigmoid sinus and internal jugular vein, respectively.

  - The cavernous sinuses are the **most clinically significant** dural sinuses because of their relationship to a number of cranial nerves. **CN III** and **IV** and the **ophthalmic and maxillary** divisions of the trigeminal nerve are located in lateral wall of the sinus. **CN VI** and **internal carotid artery** are located centrally in the sinus.

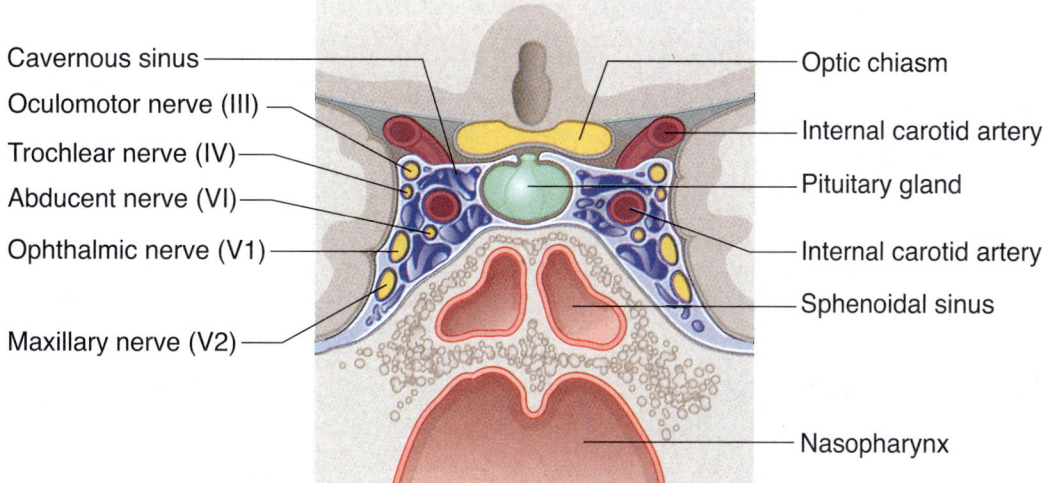

Figure 10-14. Coronal Section Through Pituitary Gland and Cavernous Sinuses

ORBITAL MUSCLES AND THEIR INNERVATION

In the orbit, there are 6 extraocular muscles that move the eyeball (Figure 10-15). A seventh muscle, the levator palpebrae superioris, elevates the upper eyelid.

- Four of the 6 extraocular muscles (the superior, inferior, and medial rectus, and the inferior oblique, plus the levator palpebrae superioris) are innervated by the oculomotor nerve (CN III).

- The superior oblique muscle is the only muscle innervated by the trochlear nerve (CN IV).

- The lateral rectus is the only muscle innervated by the abducens nerve (CN VI).

- The levator palpebrae superioris is composed of skeletal muscle innervated by the oculomotor nerve (CN III) and smooth muscle (the superior tarsal muscle) innervated by sympathetic fibers.

- Sympathetic fibers reach the orbit from a plexus on the internal carotid artery of postganglionic axons that originate from cell bodies in the superior cervical ganglion.

- The orbital muscles and their actions are illustrated in the following figure.

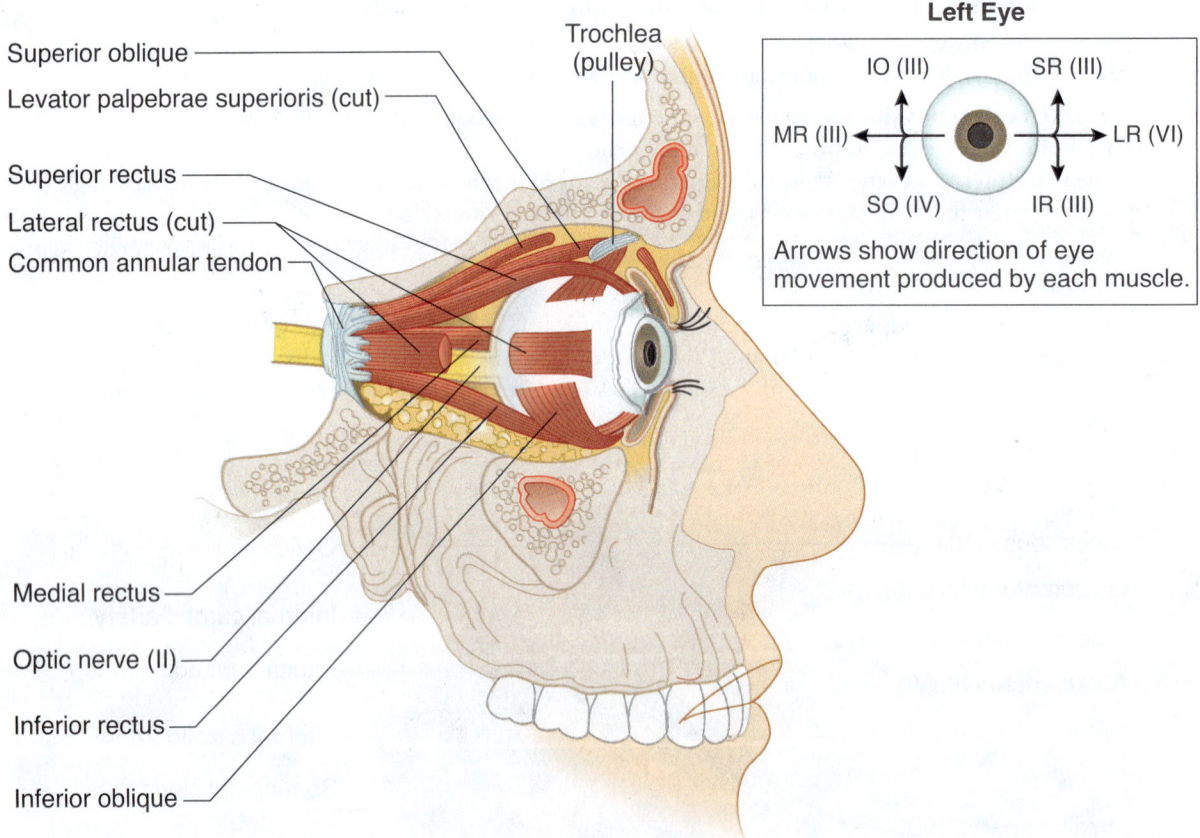

Figure 10-15. Muscles of the Eye

Nervous System Organization and Development

11

Learning Objectives

❑ Use knowledge of general organization and development of the nervous system

❑ Explain information related to autonomic nervous system

The central nervous system consists of the brain and spinal cord, which develop from the neural tube.

The peripheral nervous system (PNS) contains cranial and spinal nerves that consist of neurons that give rise to axons, which grow out of the **neural tube**, and neurons derived from **neural crest cells**. Skeletal motor neurons and axons of preganglionic autonomic neurons are derived from the neural tube.

Neural crest cells form sensory neurons and postganglionic autonomic neurons. The neuronal cell bodies of these neurons are found in ganglia. Therefore, all ganglia found in the PNS contain either sensory or postganglionic autonomic neurons and are derived from neural crest cells.

Chromaffin cells are neural crest cells, which migrate into the adrenal medulla to form postganglionic sympathetic neurons.

Development of the Nervous System

Neurulation

- **Neurulation** begins in the third week; both CNS and PNS derived from neuroectoderm.
- The **notochord** induces the overlying ectoderm to form the **neural plate (neuroectoderm)**.
- By end of the third week, **neural folds** grow over midline and fuse to form **neural tube**.
- During closure, **neural crest** cells also form from neuroectoderm.
- **Neural tube** 3 primary vesicles → 5 primary vesicles → brain and spinal cord
- Brain stem and spinal cord have an **alar** plate (**sensory**) and a **basal** plate (**motor**); plates are separated by the **sulcus limitans**.
- **Neural crest** → sensory and postganglionic autonomic neurons, and other non-neuronal cell types.
- **Peripheral NS (PNS):** cranial nerves (12 pairs) and spinal nerves (31 pairs)

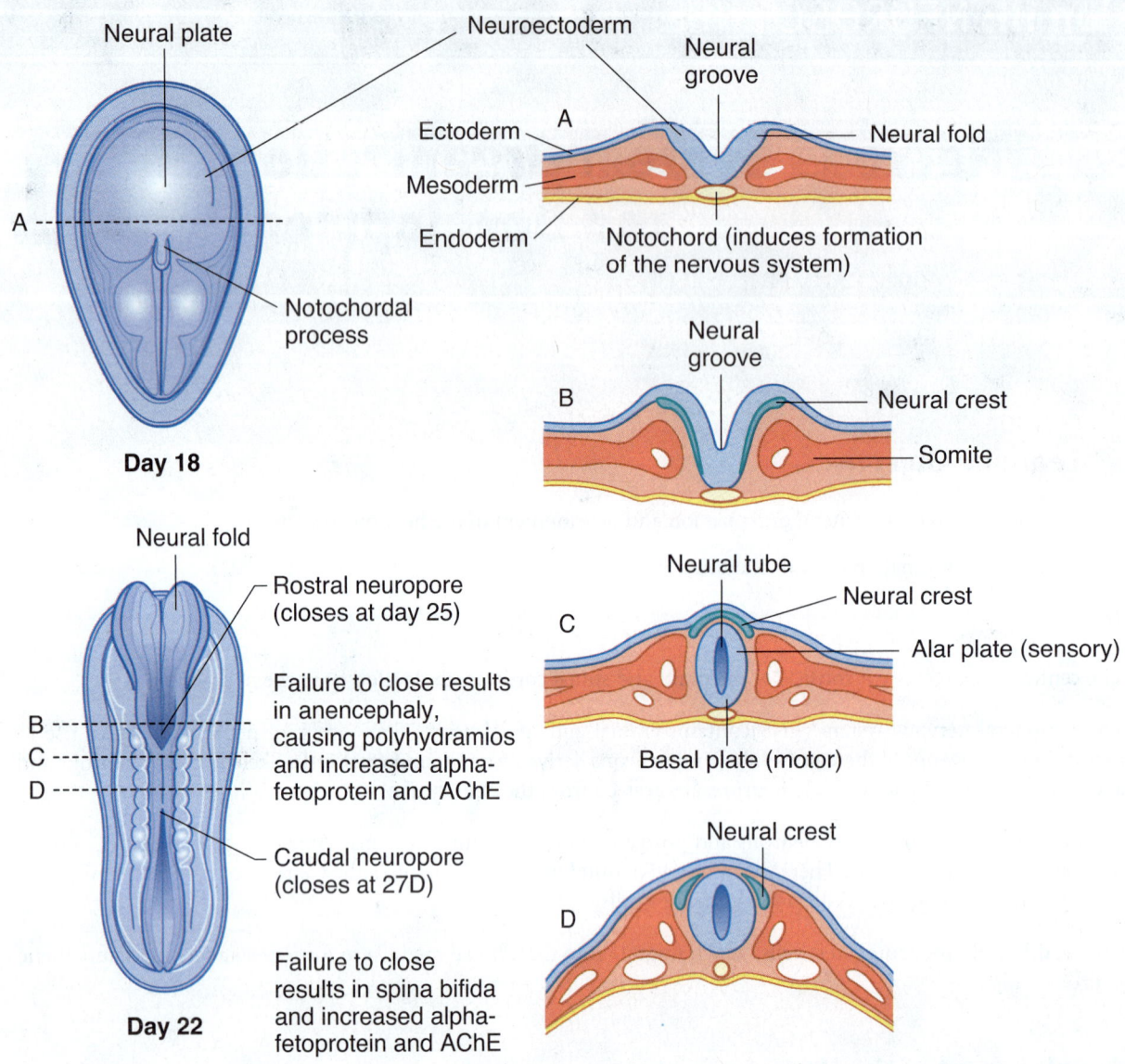

Figure 11-1. Development of Nervous System

Central Nervous System

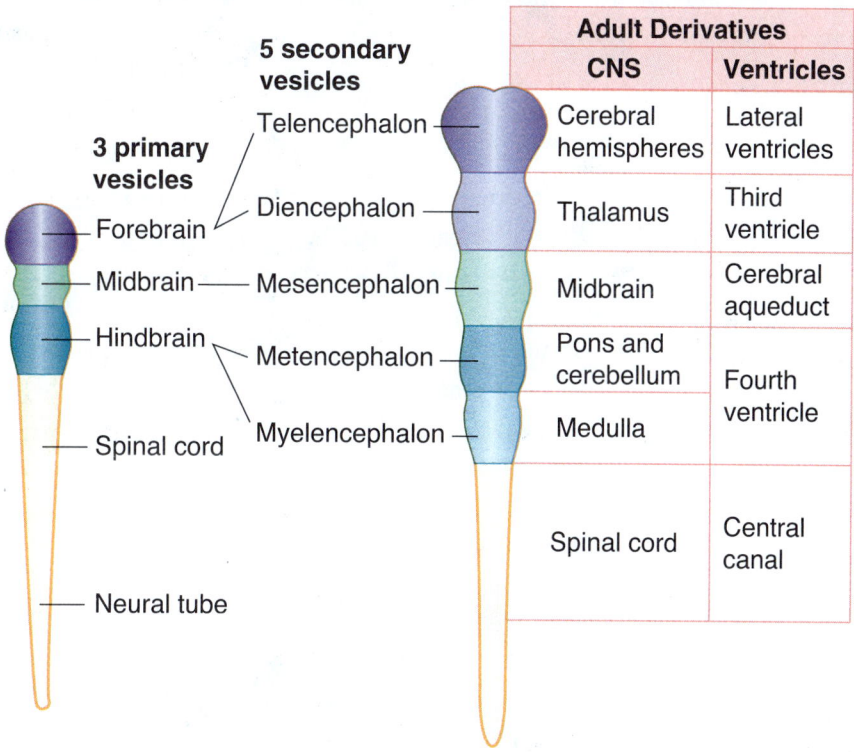

Figure 11-2. Adult Derivatives of Secondary Brain Vesicles

Table 11-1. Germ Layer Derivatives

Ectoderm	Mesoderm	Endoderm
Surface ectoderm	Muscle	**Forms epithelial parts of:**
Epidermis	Smooth	Tonsils
Hair	Cardiac	Thymus
Nails	Skeletal	Pharynx
Inner ear, external ear	Connective tissue	Larynx
Enamel of teeth	All serous membranes	Trachea
Lens of eye	Bone and cartilage	Bronchi
Anterior pituitary (Rathke's pouch)	Blood, lymph, cardiovascular organs	Lungs
Parotid gland	Adrenal cortex	Urinary bladder
Neuroectoderm	Gonads and internal reproductive organs	Urethra
Neural tube	Spleen	Tympanic cavity
Central nervous system	Kidney and ureter	Auditory tube
Retina and optic nerve	Dura mater	GI tract
Pineal gland		**Forms parenchyma of:**
Neurohypophysis		Liver
Astrocytes		Pancreas
Oligodendrocytes (CNS myelin)		Tonsils
Neural crest		Thyroid gland
Adrenal medulla		Parathyroid glands
Ganglia		Glands of the GI tract
Sensory (unipolar)		Submandibular gland
Autonomic (postganglionic)		Sublingual gland
Pigment cells (melanocytes)		
Schwann cells (PNS myelin)		
Meninges		
Pia and arachnoid mater		
Pharyngeal arch cartilage (First Arch Syndromes)		
Odontoblasts		
Parafollicular (C) cells		
Aorticopulmonary septum (Tetrology of Fallot)		
Endocardial cushions (Down Syndrome)		

Yolk sac derivatives:

Primordial germ cells

Early blood and blood vessels

AUTONOMIC NERVOUS SYSTEM: GENERAL ORGANIZATION

The autonomic nervous system (ANS) is responsible for the motor innervation of smooth muscle, cardiac muscle, and glands of the body. The ANS is composed of two divisions: sympathetic and parasympathetic.

In both divisions there are two neurons in the peripheral distribution of the motor innervation.

1. Preganglionic neuron with cell body in CNS
2. Postganglionic neuron with cell body in a ganglion in the PNS

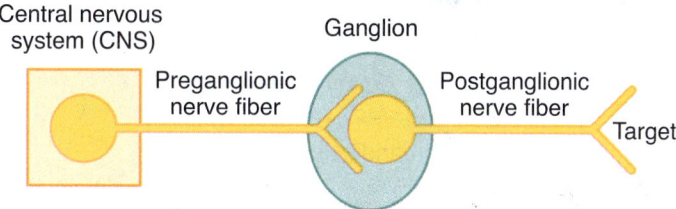

Figure 11-3. Autonomic Nervous System

Peripheral Nervous System

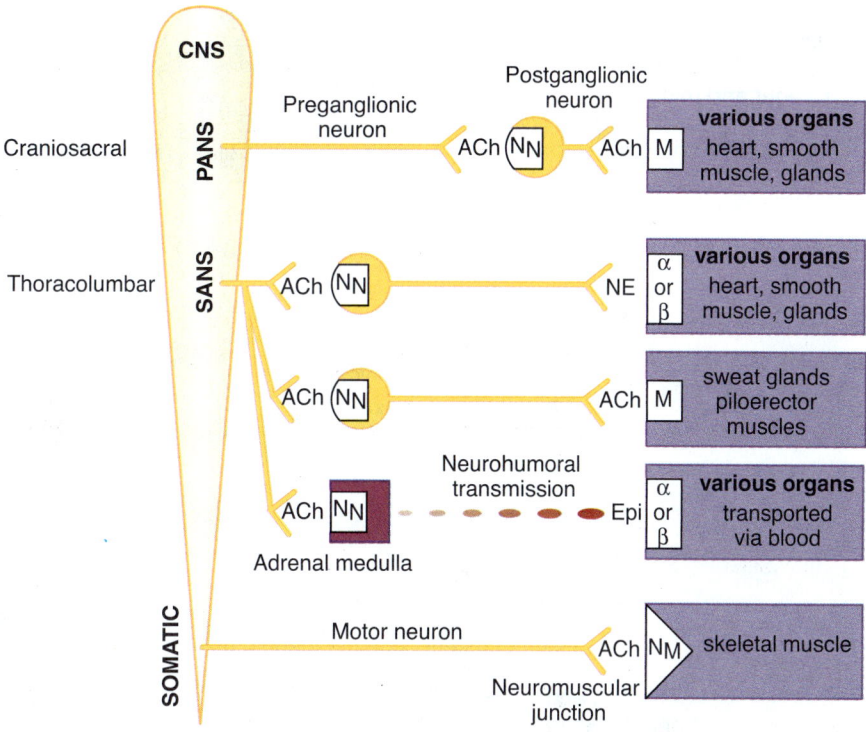

Figure 11-4. Autonomic and Somatic Nervous System Neurotransmitters/Receptors
N_N: neuronal nicotinic receptor
N_M: muscle nicotinic receptor
NE: norepinephrine
M: muscarinic receptor
ACh: acetylcholine

- **Somatic nervous system:** 1 neuron (from CNS → effector organ)
- **ANS:** 2 neurons (from CNS → effector organ)
  - **Preganglionic** neuron: cell body in CNS
  - **Postganglionic** neuron: cell body in ganglia in PNS
  - **Parasympathetic:** long preganglionic, short postganglionic
  - **Sympathetic:** short preganglionic, long postganglionic (except adrenal medulla)

Parasympathetic Nervous System

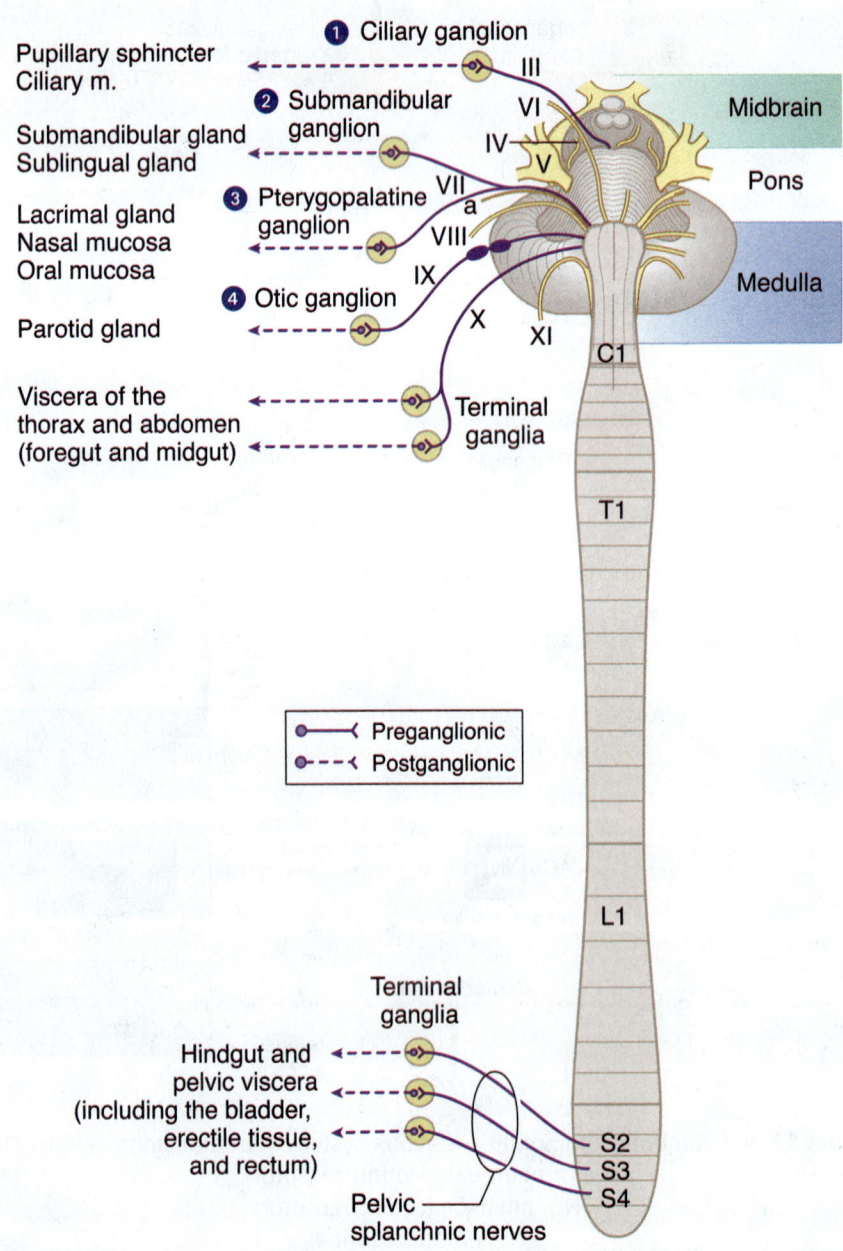

Figure 11-5. Overview of Parasympathetic Outflow

Table 11-2. Parasympathetic = Craniosacral Outflow

Origin	Site of Synapse	Innervation
Cranial nerves III, VII, IX	Four cranial ganglia	Glands and smooth muscle of the head
Cranial nerve X	Terminal ganglia (in or near the walls of viscera)	Viscera of the neck, thorax, foregut, and midgut
Pelvic splanchnic nerves (S2, S3, S4)	Terminal ganglia (in or near the walls of viscera)	Hindgut and pelvic viscera (including bladder and erectile tissue)

Sympathetic Nervous System

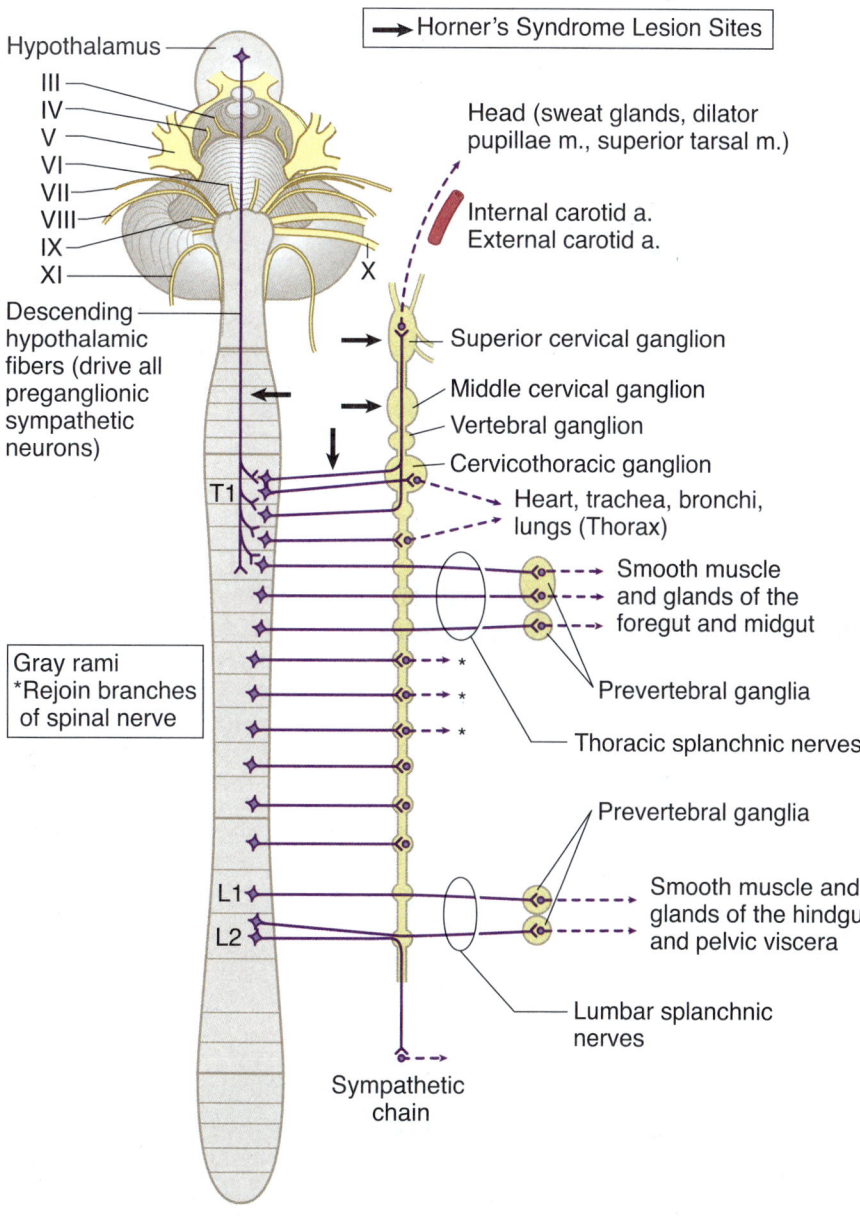

Figure 11-6. Overview of Sympathetic Outflow

Table 11-3. Sympathetic = Thoracolumbar Outflow

Origin	Site of Synapse	Innervation
Spinal cord levels T1–L2	Sympathetic chain ganglia (paravertebral ganglia)	Smooth muscle and glands of body wall and limbs; head and thoracic viscera
Thoracic splanchnic nerves T5–T12	Prevertebral ganglia (collateral; e.g., celiac, aorticorenal superior mesenteric ganglia)	Smooth muscle and glands of the foregut and midgut
Lumbar splanchnic nerves L1, L2	Prevertebral ganglia (collateral; e.g., inferior mesenteric and pelvic ganglia)	Smooth muscle and glands of the pelvic viscera and hindgut

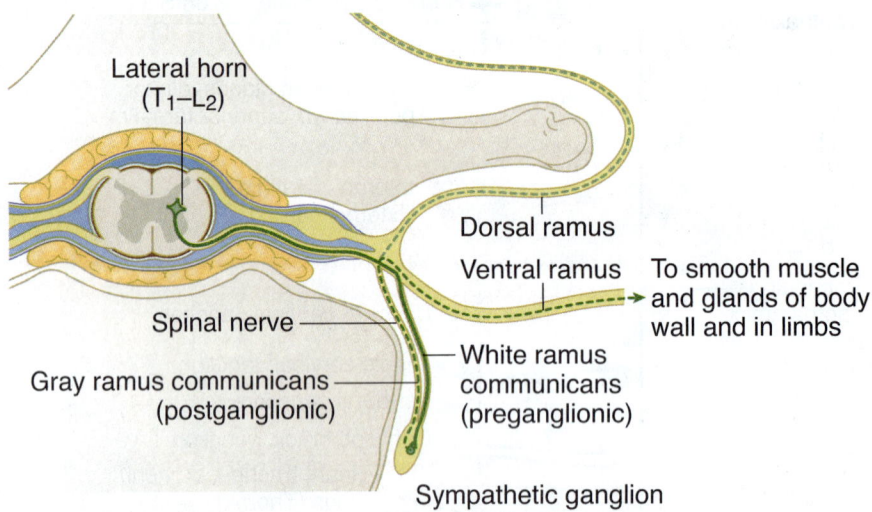

Figure 11-7. Cross Section of Spinal Cord Showing Sympathetic Outflow
Gray rami are postganglionics that rejoin spinal nerves to go to the body wall.

Histology of the Nervous System 12

Learning Objectives

❏ Explain information related to neurons

❏ Solve problems concerning disorders of myelination

NEURONS

Neurons are cells that are morphologically and functionally polarized so that information may pass from one end of the cell to the other.

Neurons may be classified by the form and number of their processes as bipolar, unipolar, or multipolar. The cell body of the neuron contains the nucleus and membrane-bound cytoplasmic organelles typical of a eukaryotic cell, including endoplasmic reticulum (ER), Golgi apparatus, mitochondria, and lysosomes. The nucleus and nucleolus are prominent in neurons.

The cytoplasm contains Nissl substance, clumps of rough ER with bound polysomes. The cytoplasm also contains free polysomes; free and bound polysomes in the Nissl substance are sites of protein synthesis.

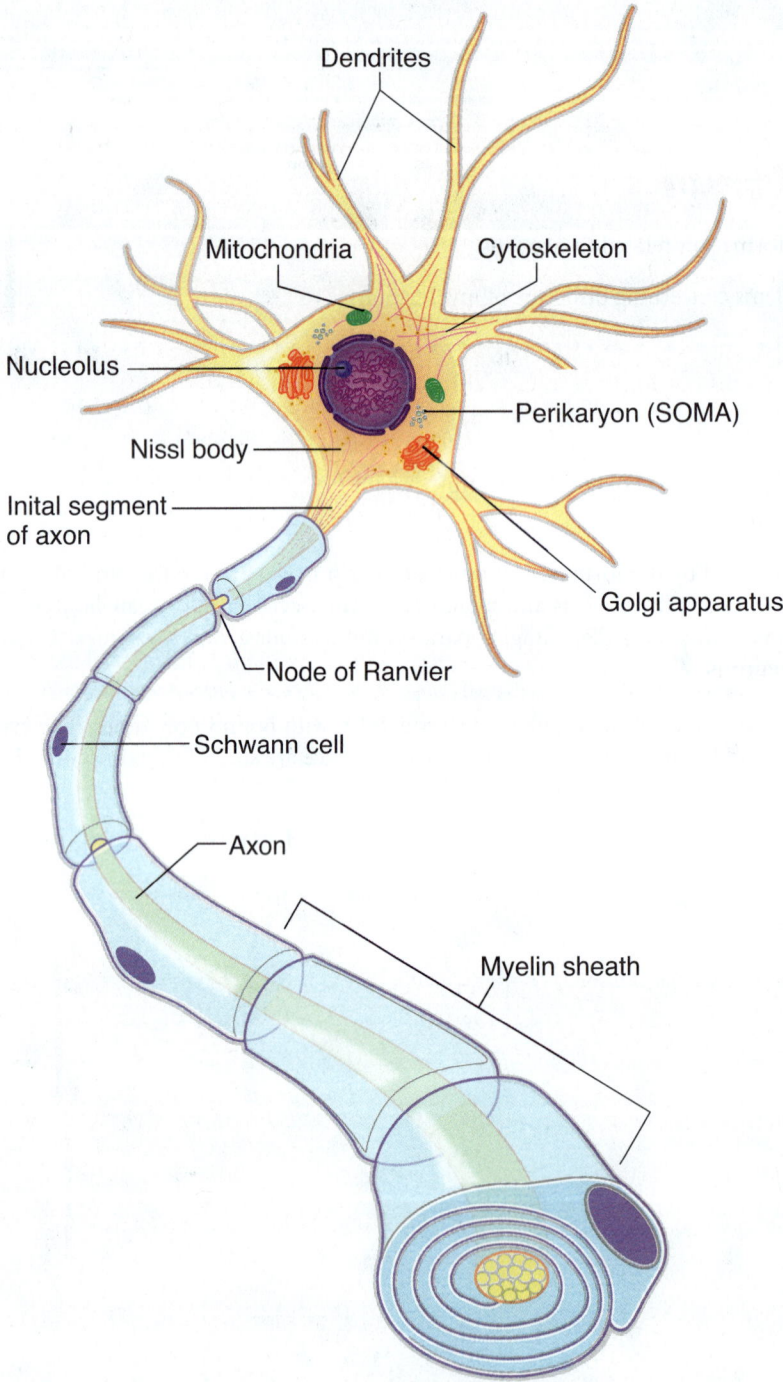

Figure 12-1. Neuron Structure

Cytoskeleton

The **cytoskeleton of the neuron** consists of microfilaments, neurofilaments, and microtubules.

Neurofilaments provide structural support for the neuron and are most numerous in the axon and the proximal parts of dendrites.

Microfilaments form a matrix near the periphery of the neuron. A microfilament matrix is prominent in growth cones of neuronal processes and functions to aid in the motility of growth cones during development. A microfilament matrix is prominent in dendrites and forms structural specializations at synaptic membranes. **Microtubules** are found in all parts of the neuron, and are the cytoplasmic organelles used in axonal transport.

Dendrites taper from the cell body and provide the major surface for synaptic contacts with axons of other neurons. **Dendrites may contain spines**, which are small cytoplasmic extensions that dramatically increase the surface area of dendrites. Dendrites may be highly branched; the branching pattern of dendrites may be used to define a particular neuronal cell type.

The **axon** has a **uniform diameter and may branch at right angles into collaterals** along the length of the axon, in particular near its distal end. The proximal part of the axon is usually marked by an **axon hillock**, a tapered extension of the cell body that lacks Nissl substance.

The initial segment is adjacent to the axon hillock. The membrane of the initial segment contains numerous voltage-sensitive sodium ion channels. The initial segment is the "trigger zone" of an axon where conduction of electrical activity as an action potential is initiated.

If the axon is myelinated, the myelin sheath begins at the initial segment. The cytoplasm of the entire axon lacks free polysomes, Nissl substance, and Golgi apparatus but contains mitochondria and smooth ER.

Anterograde axonal transport moves proteins and membranes that are synthesized in the cell body through the axon to the synaptic terminal. In **fast anterograde transport**, there is a rapid (100–400 mm/day) movement of materials from the cell body to the axon terminal.

Fast anterograde transport is dependent on **kinesin,** which acts as the motor molecule.

Fast anterograde transport delivers precursors of peptide neurotransmitters to synaptic terminals. In **slow anterograde transport**, there is a slow (1–2 mm/day) anterograde movement of soluble cytoplasmic components. Cytoskeletal proteins, enzymes, and precursors of small molecule neurotransmitters are transported to synaptic terminals by slow anterograde transport. Slow transport is not dependent on microtubules or ATPase motor molecules.

Retrograde axonal transport returns intracellular material from the synaptic terminal to the cell body to be recycled or digested by lysosomes.

Retrograde transport uses microtubules and is slower than anterograde transport (60–100 mm/day). It is dependent on dynein, an ATPase, which acts as the retrograde motor molecule. Retrograde transport also permits communication between the synaptic terminal and the cell body by transporting trophic factors emanating from the postsynaptic target or in the extracellular space.

Glial and Supporting Cells in the CNS and PNS

The supporting, or glial, cells of the CNS are small cells, which differ from neurons. Supporting cells have only one kind of process and do not form chemical synapses. Unlike neurons, supporting cells readily divide and proliferate; gliomas are the most common type of primary tumor of the CNS.

Astrocytes are the most numerous glial cells in the CNS and have large numbers of radiating processes. They provide the structural support or scaffolding for the CNS and contain large bundles of intermediate filaments that consist of **glial fibrillary acidic protein** (GFAP). Astrocytes have uptake systems that remove the neurotransmitter glutamate and K$^+$ ions from the extracellular space. Astrocytes have foot processes that contribute to the blood–brain barrier by forming a glial-limiting membrane. Astrocytes hypertrophy and proliferate after an injury to the CNS; they fill up the extracellular space left by degenerating neurons by forming an astroglial scar. **Radial glia** are precursors of astrocytes that guide neuroblast migration during CNS development.

Microglia cells are the smallest glial cells in the CNS. Unlike the rest of the CNS neurons and glia, which are derived from neuroectoderm, microglia are derived from bone marrow monocytes and enter the CNS after birth. Microglia provide a link between cells of the CNS and the immune system. Microglia proliferate and migrate to the site of a

CNS injury and phagocytose neuronal debris after injury. Pericytes are microglia that contribute to the blood–brain barrier.

Microglia determine the chances of survival of a CNS tissue graft and are the cells in the CNS that are targeted by the HIV-1 virus in patients with AIDS. The affected microglia may produce cytokines that are toxic to neurons.

CNS microglia that become phagocytic in response to neuronal tissue damage may secrete toxic free radicals. Accumulation of free radicals, such as superoxide, may lead to disruption of the calcium homeostasis of neurons.

Oligodendrocytes form myelin for axons in the CNS. Each of the processes of the oligodendrocyte can myelinate individual segments of many axons. Unmyelinated axons in the CNS are not ensheathed by oligodendrocyte cytoplasm.

Schwann cells are the supporting cells of the peripheral nervous system (PNS), and are derived from neural crest cells. Schwann cells form the myelin for axons and processes in the PNS. Each Schwann cell forms myelin for only a single internodal segment of a single axon. Unmyelinated axons in the PNS are enveloped by the cytoplasmic processes of a Schwann cell. Schwann cells act as phagocytes and remove neuronal debris in the PNS after injury. A **node of Ranvier** is the region between adjacent myelinated segments of axons in the CNS and the PNS.

In all myelinated axons, nodes of Ranvier are sites that permit action potentials to jump from node to node (saltatory conduction). Saltatory conduction dramatically increases the conduction velocity of impulses in myelinated axons.

Blood–Brain Barrier

- The blood–brain barrier restricts access of micro-organisms, proteins, cells, and drugs to the nervous system.
- The blood–brain barrier consists of capillary endothelial cells, an underlying basal lamina, astrocytes, and pericytes.
- Cerebral capillary endothelial cells and their intercellular tight junctions are the most important elements of the blood–brain barrier.
- Astrocytes and pericytes are found at the blood–brain barrier outside the basal lamina. Astrocytes have processes with "end feet" that cover more than 95% of the basal lamina adjacent to the capillary endothelial cells.

Substances cross the blood–brain barrier into the CNS by diffusion, by selective transport, and via ion channels. Oxygen and carbon dioxide are lipid-soluble gases that readily diffuse across the blood–brain barrier. Glucose, amino acids, and vitamins K and D are selectively transported across the blood–brain barrier. Sodium and potassium ions move across the blood–brain barrier through ion channels.

Response of Axons to Destructive Lesions (Severing an Axon or Axotomy) or Irritative Lesions (Compression of an Axon)

Anterograde or Wallerian degeneration distal to the cut occurs when an axon is severed in either the CNS or PNS. The closer the destructive lesion is to the neuronal cell body, the more likely the neuron is to die. In the PNS, anterograde degeneration of axons is rapid and complete after several weeks. In the PNS, the endoneurial Schwann cell sheath that envelops a degenerating axon does not degenerate and provides a scaffold for regeneration and remyelination of the axon.

Neurons with severed axons in the PNS are capable of complete axonal regeneration. Successful sprouts from the cut axon grow into and through endoneurial sheaths and are guided by Schwann cells back to their targets. Regeneration proceeds at the rate of 1–2 mm/day, which corresponds to the rate of slow anterograde transport.

Half of brain and spinal cord tumors are metastatic.

Learning Objectives

❏ Demonstrate understanding of ventricular system and venous drainage

❏ Explain information related to CSF distribution, secretion, and circulation

The brain and spinal cord float within a protective bath of cerebrospinal fluid (CSF), which is produced continuously by the choroid plexus within the ventricles of the brain.

Each part of the CNS contains a component of the ventricular system. There are four interconnected ventricles in the brain: two lateral ventricles, a third ventricle, and a fourth ventricle. A lateral ventricle is located deep within each cerebral hemisphere. Each lateral ventricle communicates with the third ventricle via an interventricular foramen (foramen of Monro). The third ventricle is found in the midline within the diencephalon and communicates with the fourth ventricle via the cerebral aqueduct (of Sylvius), which passes through the midbrain. The fourth ventricle is located between the dorsal surfaces of the pons and upper medulla and the ventral surface of the cerebellum. The fourth ventricle is continuous with the central canal of the lower medulla and spinal cord.

VENTRICULAR SYSTEM AND VENOUS DRAINAGE

The brain and spinal cord float within a protective bath of cerebrospinal fluid (CSF), which is produced by the lining of the ventricles, the choroid plexus. CSF circulation begins in the ventricles and then enters the subarachnoid space to surround the brain and spinal cord.

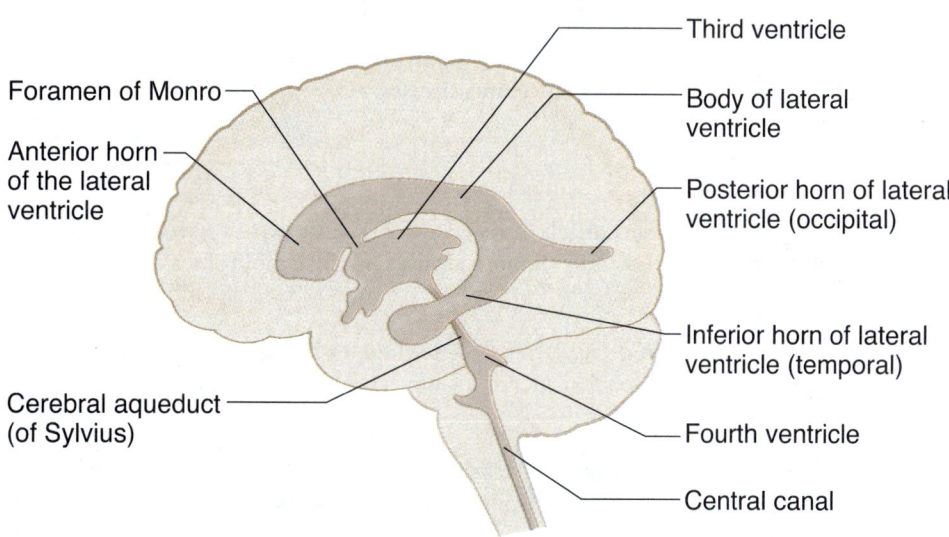

Figure 13-1. Ventricles and CSF Circulation

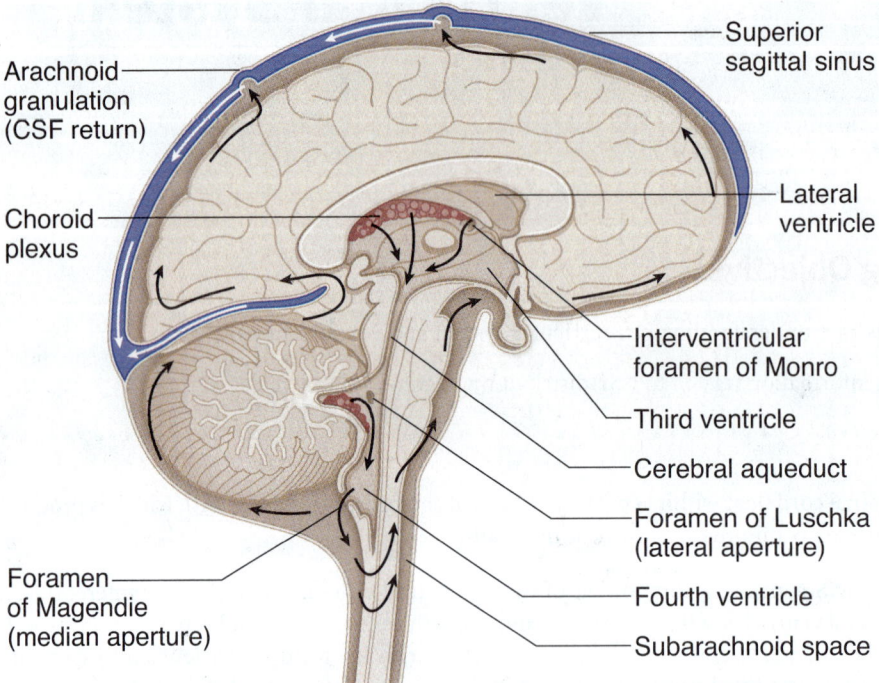

Figure 13-2. Sagittal Section of the Brain

interventricular foramen of Monro   cerebral aqueduct
Lateral ventricles ⌄→ third ventricle ⌄→ fourth ventricle –→ subarachnoid space
(via foramina of Luschka and foramen of Magendie)

CSF Production and Barriers

Choroid plexus—contains **choroid epithelial cells** and is in the lateral, third, and fourth ventricles. **Secretes CSF.** Tight junctions form **blood-CSF barrier**.

Blood-brain barrier—formed by capillary endothelium with tight junctions; astrocyte foot processes contribute.

Once CSF is in the subarachnoid space, it goes up over convexity of the brain and enters the venous circulation by passing through **arachnoid granulations** into **dural venous sinuses**.

Sinuses

Superior sagittal sinus (in superior margin of falx cerebri)—drains into two **transverse sinuses**. Each of these drains blood from the **confluence of sinuses** into **sigmoid sinuses**. Each sigmoid sinus exits the skull (via **jugular foramen**) as the **internal jugular veins**.

Inferior sagittal sinus (in inferior margin of falx cerebri)— terminates by joining with the great cerebral vein of Galen to form the **straight sinus** at the falx cerebri and tentorium cerebelli junction. This drains into the confluence of sinuses.

Cavernous sinus—a plexus of veins on either side of the **sella turcica**. Surrounds internal carotid artery and cranial nerves III, IV, V, and VI. It drains into the transverse sinus (via the **superior petrosal sinus**) and the internal jugular vein (via the **inferior petrosal sinus**).

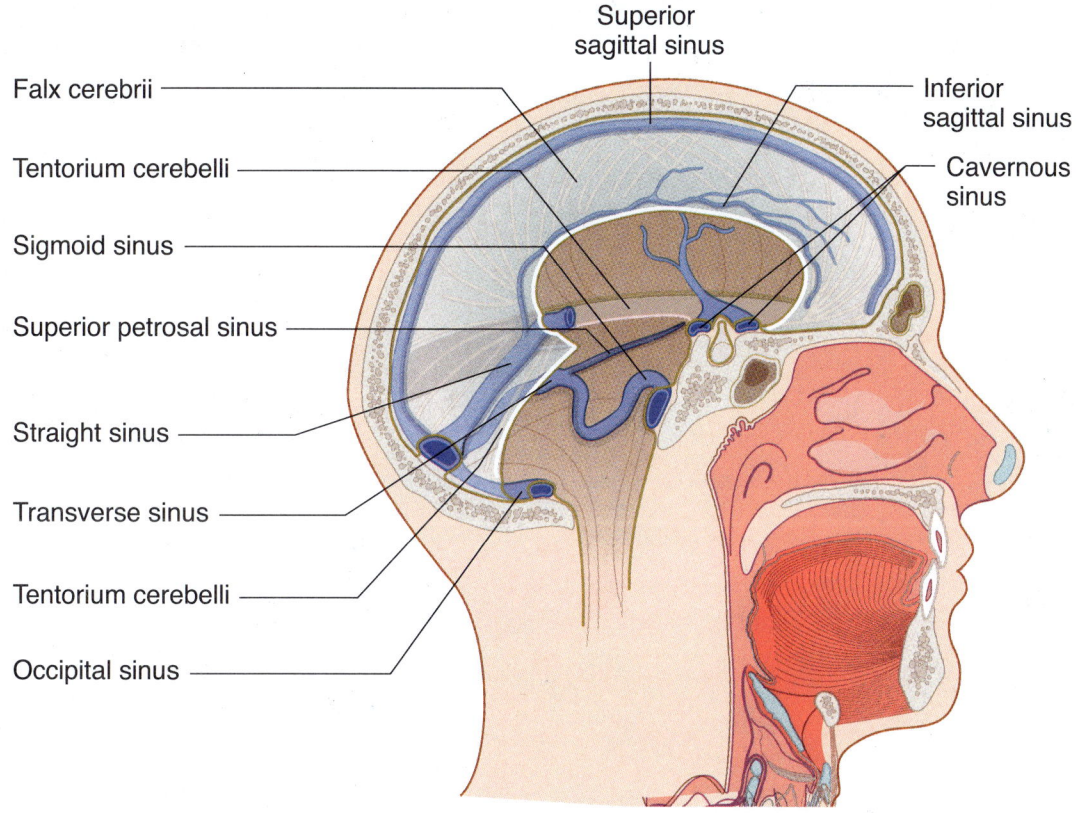

Figure 13-3. Dural Venous Sinuses

CSF DISTRIBUTION, SECRETION, AND CIRCULATION

CSF fills the subarachnoid space and the ventricles of the brain. The average adult has 90 to 150 mL of total CSF, although 400 to 500 mL is produced daily. Only 25 mL of CSF is found in the ventricles themselves.

Approximately 70% of the CSF is secreted by the choroid plexus, which consists of glomerular tufts of capillaries covered by ependymal cells that project into the ventricles (the remaining 30% represents metabolic water production). The choroid plexus is located in parts of each lateral ventricle, the third ventricle, and the fourth ventricle.

CSF from the lateral ventricles passes through the interventricular foramina of Monro into the third ventricle. From there, CSF flows through the aqueduct of Sylvius into the fourth ventricle. The only sites where CSF can leave the ventricles and enter the subarachnoid space outside the CNS arethrough three openings in the fourth ventricle, 2 lateral foramina of Luschka and the median foramen of Magendie.

Within the subarachnoid space, CSF also flows up over the convexity of the brain and around the spinal cord. Almost all CSF returns to the venous system by draining through arachnoid granulations into the superior sagittal dural venous sinus.

Normal CSF is a **clear** fluid, isotonic with serum (290–295 mOsm/L).

The Blood–CSF Barrier

The blood–CSF barrier is a mechanism that protects the chemical integrity of the brain. Tight junctions located along the epithelial cells of the choroid plexus form the blood–CSF barrier. Transport systems are similar but not identical to the those of blood–brain barrier. The ability of a substance (drug) to enter the CSF does not guarantee it will gain access to the brain.

The Spinal Cord

Learning Objectives

❏ Solve problems concerning general features

❏ Interpret scenarios on neural systems

GENERAL FEATURES

The spinal cord is housed in the vertebral canal. It is continuous with the medulla below the pyramidal decussation and terminates as the conus medullar is at the second lumbar vertebra of the adult. The roots of 31 pairs of spinal nerves arise segmentally from the spinal cord.

There are **8 cervical pairs** of spinal nerves (C1 through C8). The cervical enlargement (C5 through T1) gives rise to the rootlets that form the brachial plexus, which innervates the upper limbs.

There are **12 thoracic pairs** of spinal nerves (T1 through T12). Spinal nerves emanating from thoracic levels innervate most of the trunk.

There are **5 lumbar pairs** of spinal nerves (L1 through L5). The lumbar enlargement (L1 through S2) gives rise to rootlets that form the lumbar and sacral plexuses, which innervate the lower limbs.

There are **5 sacral pairs** of spinal nerves (S1 through S5). Spinal nerves at the sacral level innervate part of the lower limbs and the pelvis.

There is **1 coccygeal pair** of spinal nerves. The cauda equina consists of the dorsal and ventral roots of the lumbar, sacral, and coccygeal spinal nerves.

Inside the spinal cord, gray matter is centrally located and shaped like a butterfly. It contains neuronal cell bodies, their dendrites, and the proximal parts of axons. White matter surrounds the gray matter on all sides. White matter contains bundles of functionally similar axons called tracts or fasciculi, which ascend or descend in the spinal cord (Figures 14-1 and 14-2).

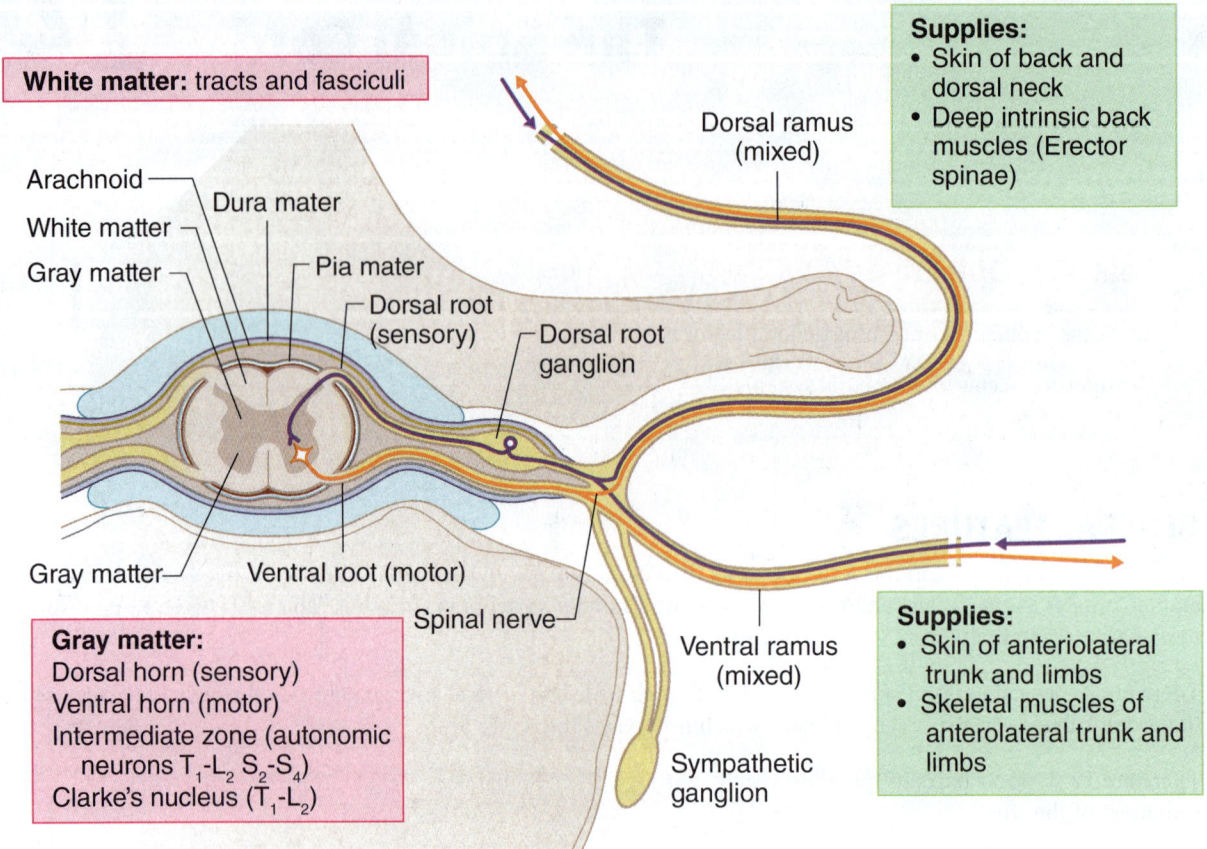

White matter: tracts and fasciculi

Supplies:
• Skin of back and dorsal neck
• Deep intrinsic back muscles (Erector spinae)

Dorsal ramus (mixed)

Arachnoid
Dura mater
White matter
Gray matter
Pia mater
Dorsal root (sensory)
Dorsal root ganglion

Gray matter
Ventral root (motor)
Spinal nerve
Ventral ramus (mixed)

Sympathetic ganglion

Supplies:
• Skin of anteriolateral trunk and limbs
• Skeletal muscles of anteriolateral trunk and limbs

Gray matter:
Dorsal horn (sensory)
Ventral horn (motor)
Intermediate zone (autonomic neurons T_1-L_2 S_2-S_4)
Clarke's nucleus (T_1-L_2)

Figure 14-1. Cross Section of Spinal Cord and Parts of Spinal Nerve

Table 14-1. General Spinal Cord Features

Conus medullaris	Caudal end of the spinal cord (S3–S5). In adult, ends at the L2 vertebra
Cauda equina	Nerve roots of the lumbar, sacral, and coccygeal spinal nerves
Filum terminale	Slender pial extension that tethers the spinal cord to the bottom of the vertebral column
Doral root ganglia	Cell bodies of primary sensory neurons
Dorsal and ventral roots	Each segment has a pair
Dorsal horn	**Sensory neurons**
Ventral horn	**Motor neurons**
Spinal nerve	Formed from dorsal and ventral roots (mixed nerve)
Cervical enlargement	(C5–T1) → branchial plexus → upper limbs
Lumbar enlargement	(L2–S3) → lumbar and sacral plexuses → lower limbs

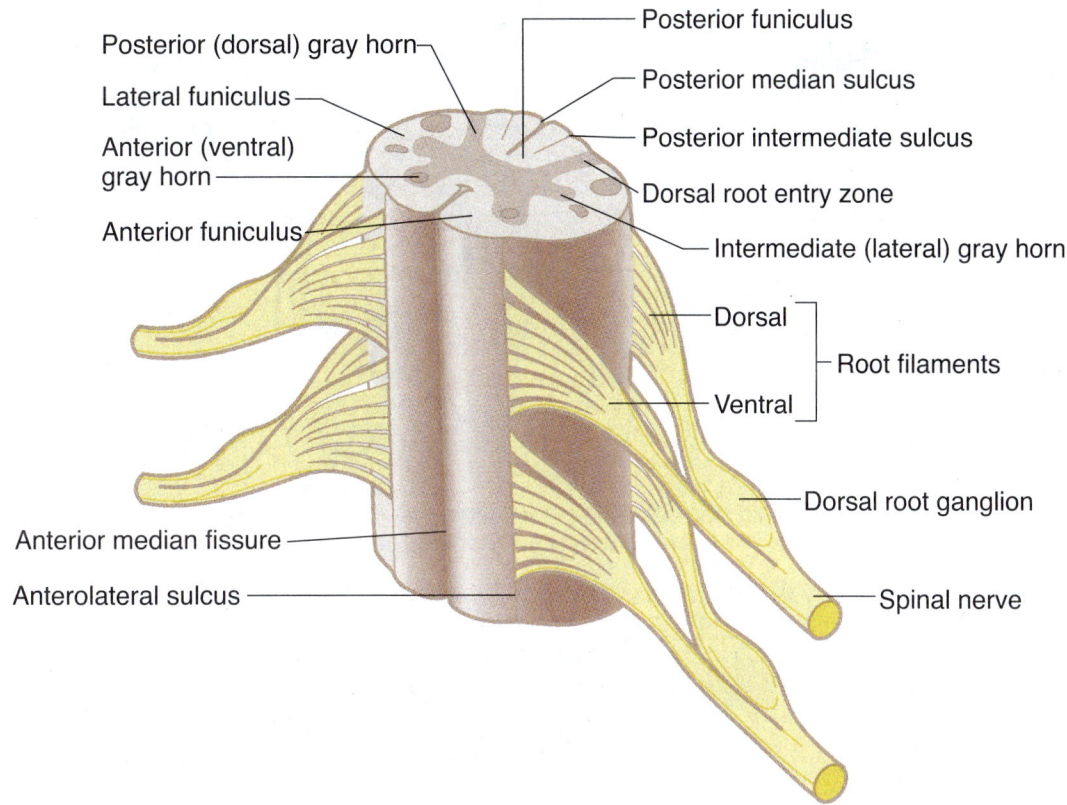

Posterior (dorsal) gray horn

Lateral funiculus

Anterior (ventral) gray horn

Anterior funiculus

Anterior median fissure

Anterolateral sulcus

Posterior funiculus

Posterior median sulcus

Posterior intermediate sulcus

Dorsal root entry zone

Intermediate (lateral) gray horn

Dorsal

Ventral

Root filaments

Dorsal root ganglion

Spinal nerve

Figure 14-2. General Spinal Cord Features

Dorsal Horn

The dorsal horn is dominated by neurons that respond to sensory stimulation. All incoming sensory fibers in spinal nerves enter the dorsolateral part of the cord adjacent to the dorsal horn in a dorsal root. Neurons in the dorsal horn project to higher levels of the CNS to carry sensations to the brain stem, cerebral cortex, or cerebellum. Other dorsal horn neurons participate in reflexes.

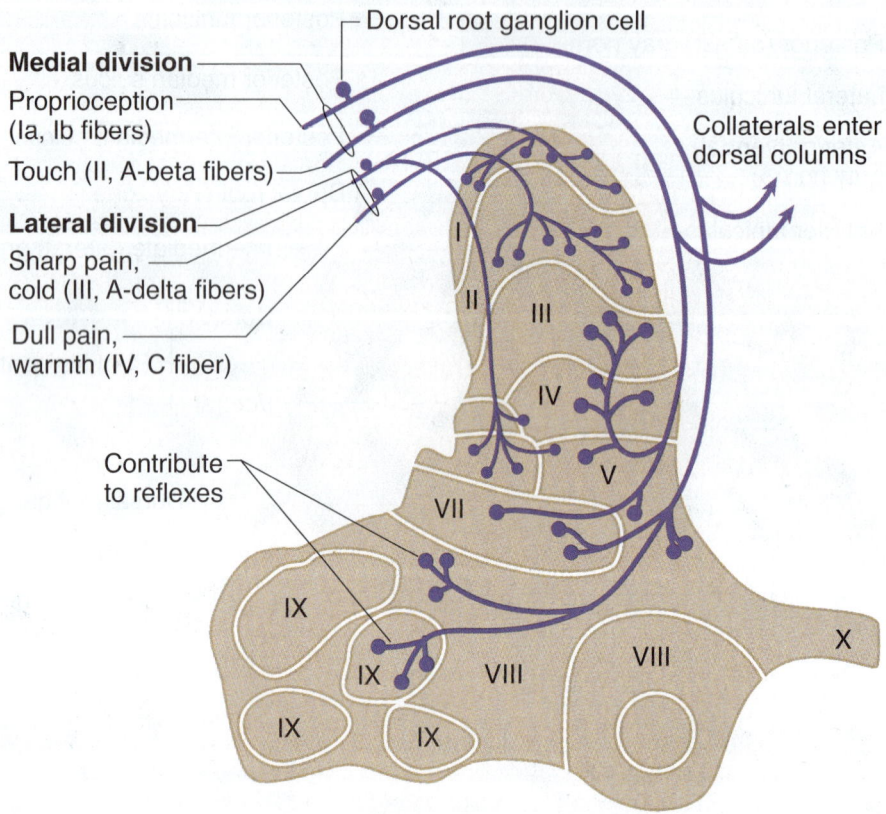

Figure 14-3. Fiber Types in Dorsal Roots and Sites of Termination in the Spinal Cord Gray Matter
Dorsal horn: rexed laminae I–VI
Ventral horn: rexed laminae VIII–IX
Intermediate zone: lamina VII

Ventral Horn

The ventral horn contains **alpha and gamma motoneurons**. The alpha motoneurons innervate skeletal muscle (extrafusal fibers) by way of a specialized synapse at a neuromuscular junction, and the gamma motoneurons innervate the contractile intrafusal muscle fibers of the muscle spindle. Within the ventral horn, alpha and gamma motoneurons that innervate flexors are dorsal to those that innervate extensors. Alpha and gamma motoneurons that innervate the proximal musculature are medial to those that innervate the distal musculature. Axons of alpha and gamma motoneurons and axons of preganglionic autonomic neurons leave the cord by way of a ventral root.

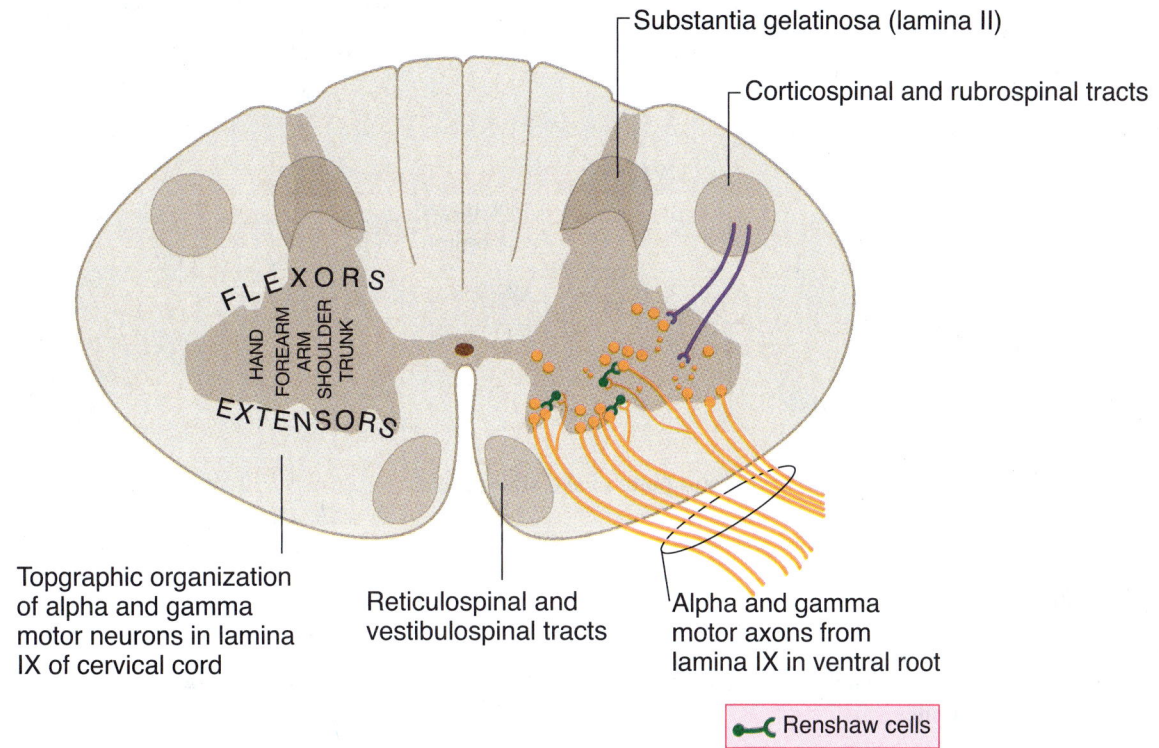

Figure 14-4. Topographic Organization of Alpha and Gamma Motoneurons (LMNs) in Lamina IX
C5–T1 and L2–S2 have large ventral horn.
Alpha motor neurons make skeletal muscles contract.
Gamma motor neurons make muscle spindles more sensitive to stretch.

Intermediate Zone

The intermediate zone of the spinal cord from T1 to L2 contains preganglionic sympathetic neuron cell bodies and Clarke nucleus, which sends unconscious proprioception to the cerebellum.

NEURAL SYSTEMS

There are three major neural systems in the spinal cord that use neurons in the gray matter and tracts or fasciculi of axons in the white matter. These neural systems have components that can be found at all levels of the CNS from the cerebral cortex to the tip of the spinal cord. An understanding of these three neural systems is essential to understanding the effects of lesions in the spinal cord and brain stem, and at higher levels of the CNS.

In a Nutshell

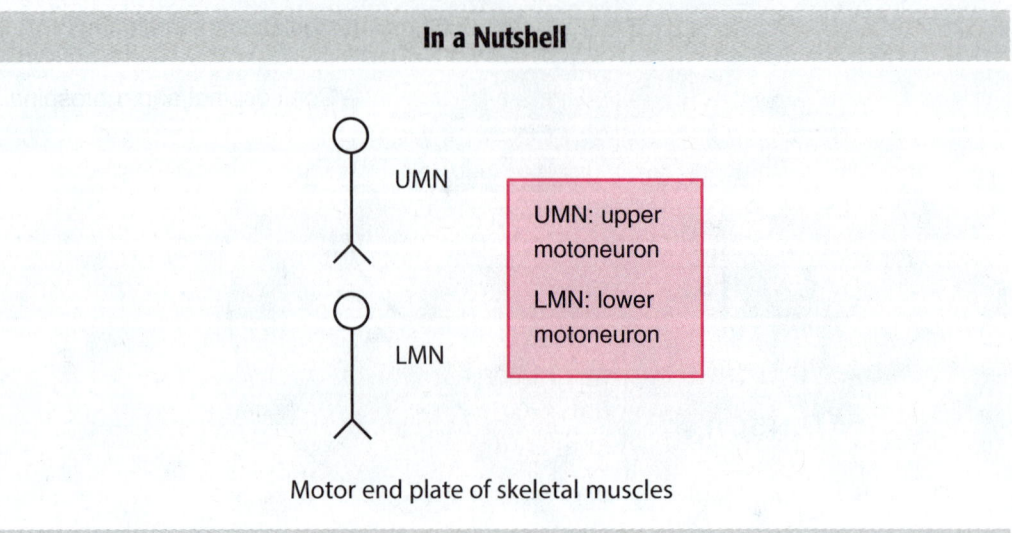

Motor end plate of skeletal muscles

Motor System

Voluntary innervation of skeletal muscle

Upper and Lower Motoneurons

Two motoneurons, an upper motoneuron and a lower motoneuron, together form the basic neural circuit involved in the voluntary contraction of skeletal muscle everywhere in the body. **The lower motoneurons are found in the ventral horn of the spinal cord** and in **cranial nerve nuclei in the brain stem**. Axons of lower motoneurons of spinal nerves exit in a ventral root, then join the spinal nerve to course in one of its branches to reach and synapse directly at a neuromuscular junction in skeletal muscle. Axons of lower motoneurons in the brain stem exit in a cranial nerve.

To initiate a voluntary contraction of skeletal muscle, a lower motoneuron must be innervated by an upper moto-neuron (Figure 14-5). The **cell bodies of upper motoneurons are found in the brain stem and cerebral cortex**, and their axons descend into the spinal cord in a tract to reach and synapse on lower motoneurons, or on interneurons, which then synapse on lower motoneurons. At a minimum, therefore, to initiate a voluntary contraction of skeletal muscle, two motoneurons, an upper and a lower, must be involved. The upper motoneuron innervates the lower motoneuron, and the lower motoneuron innervates the skeletal muscle.

The cell bodies of upper motoneurons are found in the red nucleus, reticular formation, and lateral vestibular nuclei of the brain stem, but the **most important location of upper motoneurons is in the cerebral cortex**. Axons of these cortical neurons course in the *corticospinal tract*.

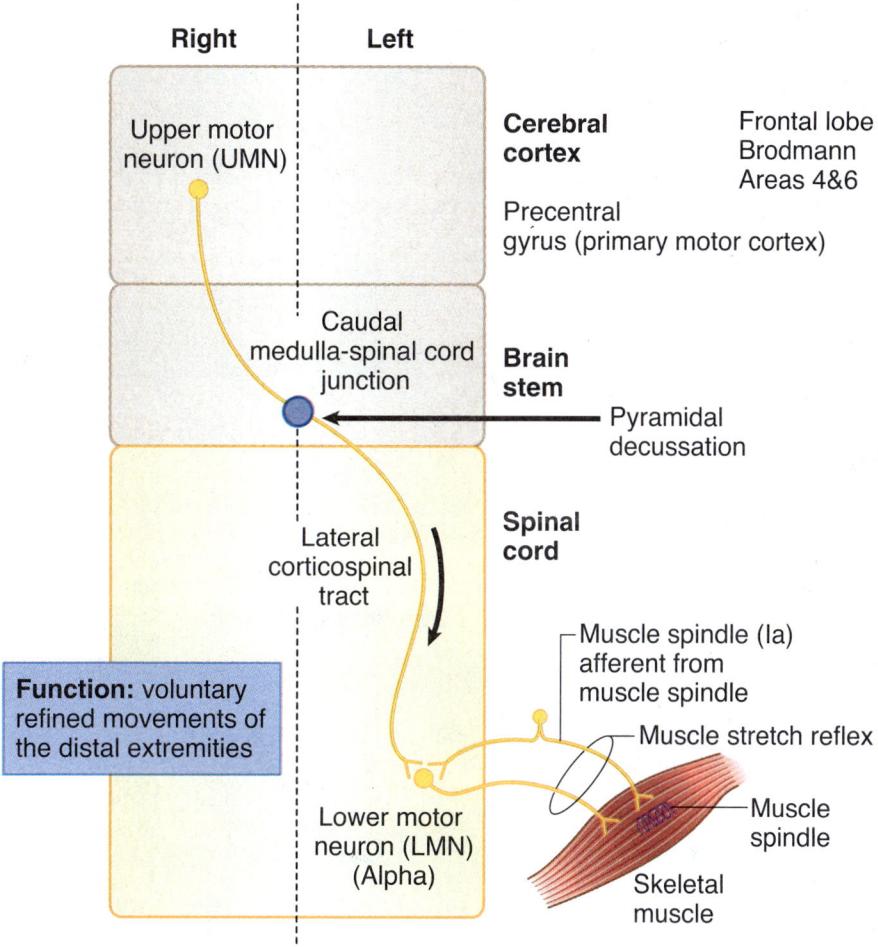

Figure 14-5. Voluntary Contraction of Skeletal Muscle: UMN and LMNs
UMNs have net inhibitory effect on muscle stretch reflexes.
Voluntary contraction: UMN → LMN
Reflect contraction: muscle sensory neuron → LMN

Corticospinal Tract

The primary motor cortex, located in the precentral gyrus of the frontal lobe, and the premotor area, located immediately anterior to the primary motor cortex, give rise to about 60% of the fibers of the corticospinal tract. Primary and secondary somatosensory cortical areas located in the parietal lobe give rise to about 40% of the fibers of the corticospinal tract.

Fibers in the corticospinal tract leave the cerebral cortex in the internal capsule, which carries all axons in and out of the cortex. Corticospinal fibers then descend through the length of the brain stem in the ventral portion of the midbrain, pons, and medulla.

In the lower medulla, 80 to 90% of corticospinal fibers cross at the decussation of the pyramids and continue in the contralateral spinal cord as the lateral corticospinal tract. The lateral corticospinal tract descends the full length of the cord in the lateral part of the white matter. As it descends, axons leave the tract and enter the gray matter of the ventral horn to synapse on lower motoneurons.

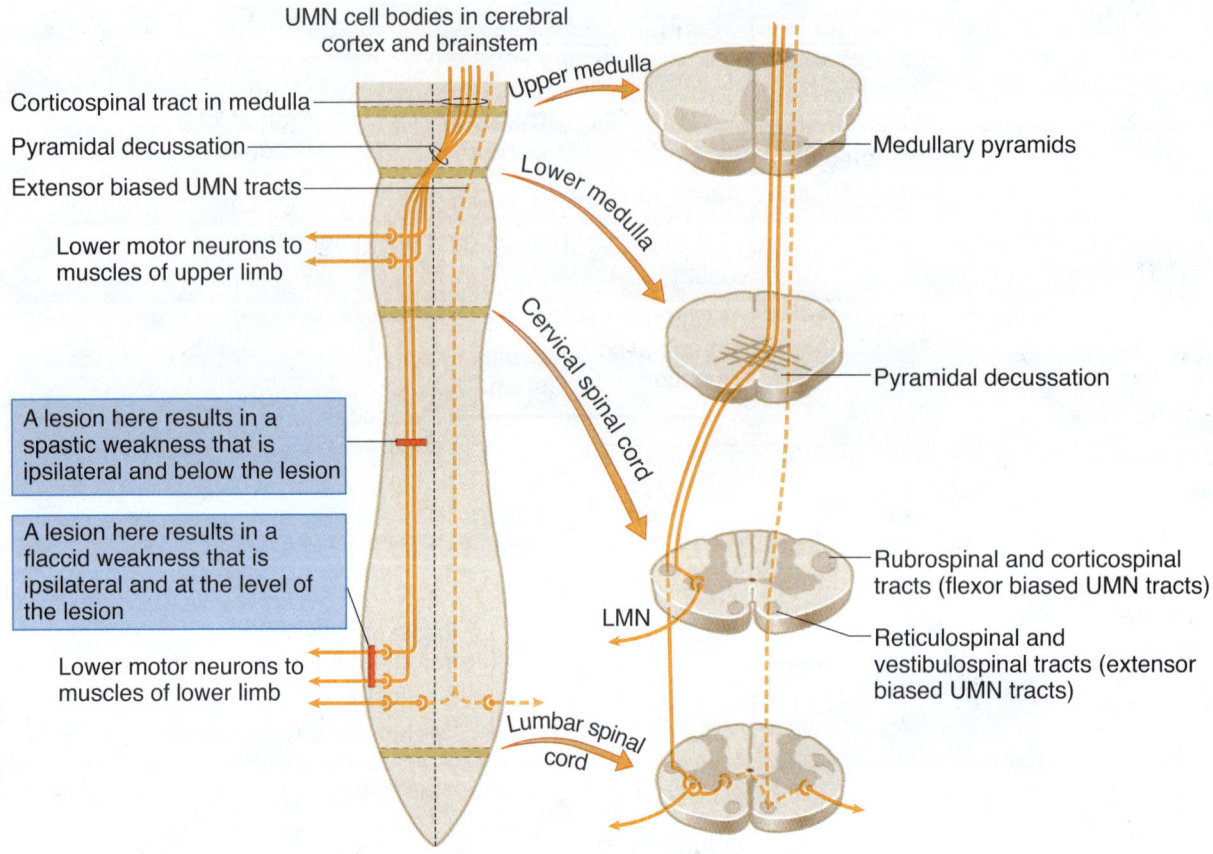

Figure 14-6. Course of Axons of Upper Motor Neurons in the Medulla and Spinal Cord with Representative Cross-Sections

Reflex innervation of skeletal muscle

A reflex is initiated by a stimulus of a sensory neuron, which in turn innervates a motoneuron and produces a motor response. In reflexes involving skeletal muscles, the sensory stimulus arises from receptors in the muscle, and the motor response is a contraction or relaxation of one or more skeletal muscles. In the spinal cord, lower motoneurons form the specific motor component of skeletal muscle reflexes. **Upper motoneurons provide descending control over the reflexes.**

Both alpha and gamma motoneurons are lower motoneurons that participate in reflexes.

- Alpha motoneurons are large cells in the ventral horn that innervate extrafusal muscle fibers. A single alpha motoneuron innervates a group of muscle fibers, which constitutes a motor unit, the basic unit for voluntary, postural, and reflex activity.

- Gamma motoneurons supply intrafusal muscle fibers, which are modified skeletal muscle fibers. The intrafusal muscle fibers form the muscle spindle, which acts as a sensory receptor in skeletal muscle stretch reflexes.

Both ends of the muscle spindle are connected in parallel with the extrafusal fibers, so these receptors monitor the length and rate of change in length of extrafusal fibers. Muscles involved with fine movements contain a greater density of spindles than those used in coarse movements.

Commonly tested muscle stretch reflexes

The **deep tendon (stretch, myotatic) reflex** is monosynaptic and ipsilateral. The **afferent limb** consists of a **muscle spindle, Ia sensory neuron,** and **efferent limb (lower motor neuron)**.These reflexes are useful in the clinical exam.

Reflex	Cord Segment Involved	Muscle Tested
Knee (patellar)	L2–L4 (femoral n.)	Quadriceps
Ankle	S1 (tibial n.)	Gastrocnemius
Elbow	C5–C6 (musculocutaneous n.)	Biceps
Elbow	C7–C8 (radial n.)	Triceps
Forearm	C5–C6 (radial n.)	Brachioradialis

Muscle stretch (myotatic) reflex

The muscle stretch (myotatic) reflex is the stereotyped contraction of a muscle in response to stretch of that muscle. **The stretch reflex is a basic reflex that occurs in all muscles and is the primary mechanism for regulating muscle tone.** Muscle tone is the tension present in all resting muscle. Tension is controlled by the stretch reflexes.

The best example of a muscle stretch or deep tendon reflex is the knee-jerk reflex. Tapping the patellar ligament stretches the quadriceps muscle and its muscle spindles. Stretch of the spindles activates sensory endings (Ia afferents), and afferent impulses are transmitted to the cord. Some impulses from stretch receptors carried by Ia fibers monosynaptically stimulate the alpha motoneurons that supply the quadriceps. This causes contraction of the muscle and a sudden extension of the leg at the knee. Afferent impulses simultaneously inhibit antagonist muscles through interneurons (in this case, hamstrings).

Inverse muscle stretch reflex

The inverse muscle stretch reflex monitors muscle tension. This reflex uses Golgi tendon organs (GTOs). These are encapsulated groups of nerve endings that terminate between collagenous tendon fibers at the junction of muscle and tendon. GTOs are oriented in series with the extrafusal fibers and respond to increases in force or tension generated in that muscle. Increases in force in a muscle increase the firing rate of Ib afferent neurons that innervate the GTOs, which, in turn, polysynaptically facilitate antagonists and inhibit agonist muscles.

Muscle tone and reflex activity can be influenced by **gamma motoneurons** and by upper motoneurons. Gamma motoneurons directly innervate the muscle spindles and regulate their sensitivity to stretch. Upper motoneurons innervate gamma motoneurons and also influence the sensitivity of muscle spindles to stretch. Stimulation of gamma motoneurons causes intrafusal muscle fibers located at the pole of each muscle spindle to contract, which activates alpha motoneurons, causing an increase in muscle tone.

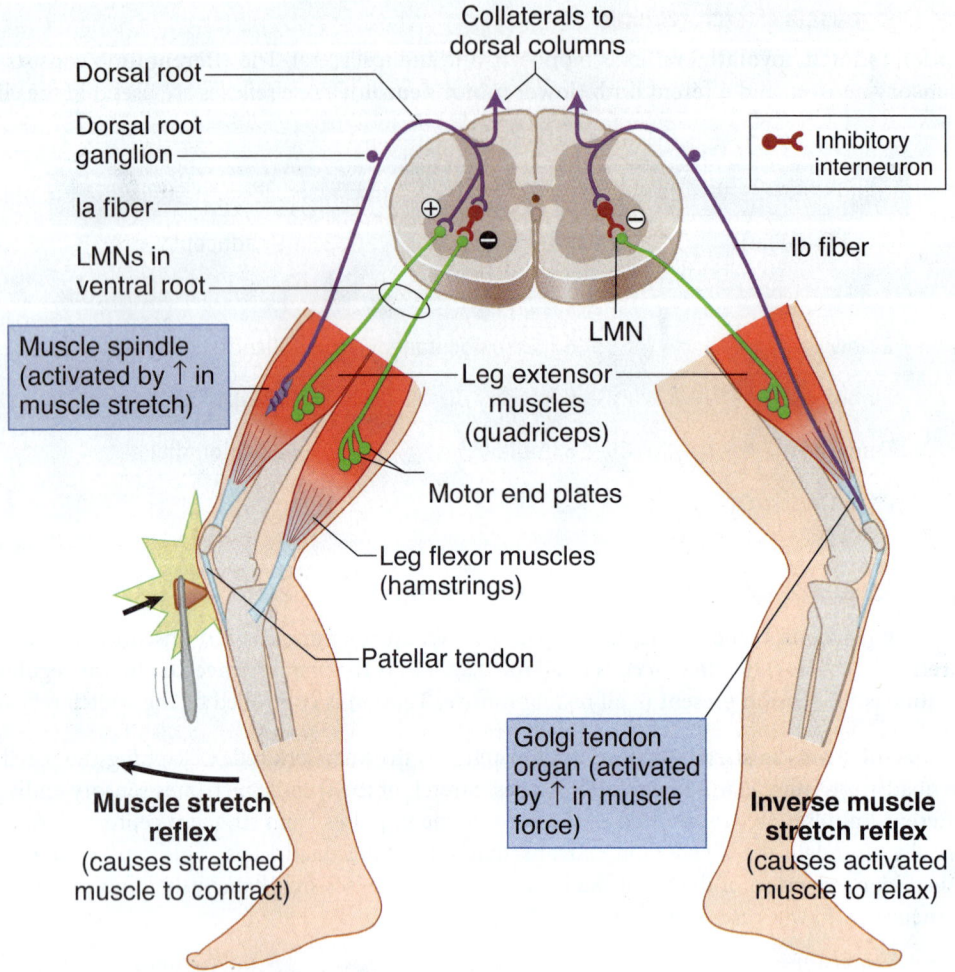

Figure 14-7. Muscle Stretch and Golgi Tendon Reflex Components

Flexor withdrawal reflex

The flexion withdrawal reflex is a protective reflex in which a stimulus (usually painful) causes withdrawal of the stimulated limb. This reflex may be accompanied by a crossed extension reflex in which the contralateral limb is extended to help support the body.

Sensory Systems

Two sensory systems, the dorsal column–medial lemniscal system and the anterolateral (spinothalamic) system, use three neurons to convey sensory information from peripheral sensory receptors to conscious levels of cerebral cortex. In both systems, the first sensory neuron that innervates a sensory receptor has a cell body in the dorsal root ganglion and carries the information into the spinal cord in the dorsal root of a spinal nerve. The first neuron synapses with a second neuron in the brain stem or the spinal cord, and the axon of the second neuron crosses the midline and is carried in a tract in the CNS. The axon of the second neuron then synapses on a third neuron that is in the thalamus. The axon of the third neuron projects to primary somatosensory cortex.

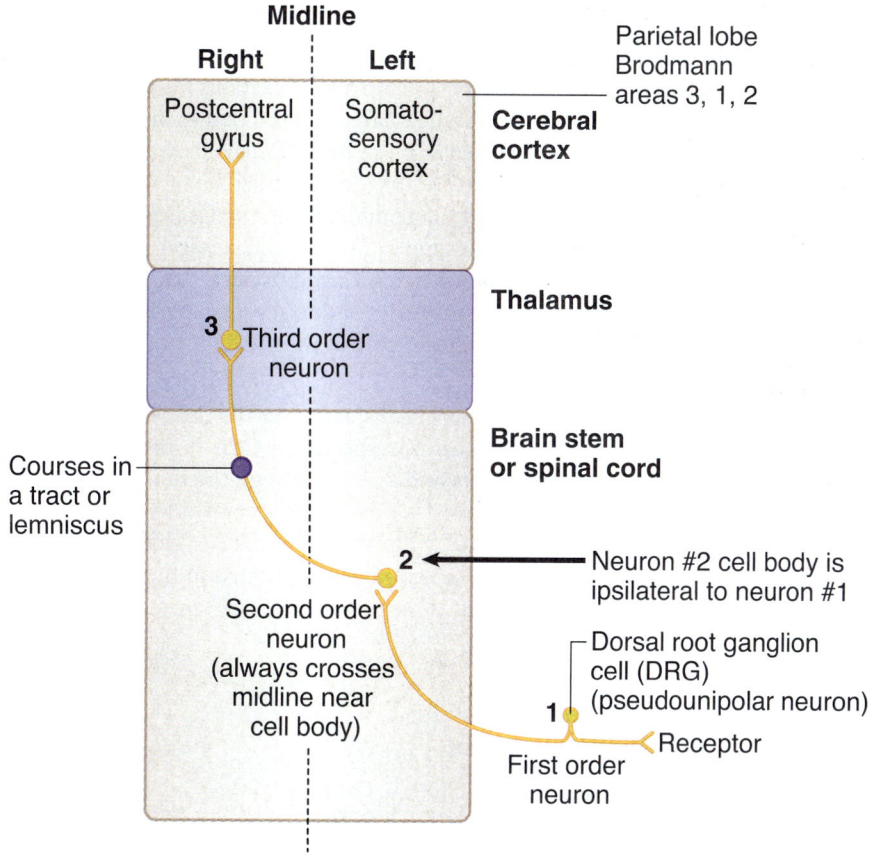

Figure 14-8. General Sensory Pathways
1: first-order neuron in sensory ganglion
2: second-order neuron in CNS (axon always crosses midline)
3: third-order neuron in thalamus

Ascending Pathways

The two most important ascending pathways use a 3-neuron system to convey sensory information to the cortex. Key general features are listed below.

Pathway	Function	Overview
Dorsal column–medial lemniscal system	Discriminative touch, conscious proprioception, vibration, pressure	**3-neuron system:** 1° neuron: cell body in **DRG**
Anterolateral system (spinothalamic)	Pain and temperature	2° neuron: **decussates** 3° neuron: **thalamus** **(VPL) → cortex**

Abbreviations: DRG, dorsal root ganglia; VPL, ventral posterolateral nucleus.

Dorsal column–medial lemniscal system

The dorsal column–medial lemniscal system carries sensory information for discriminative touch, joint position (kinesthetic or conscious proprioceptive) sense, vibratory, and pressure sensations from the trunk and limbs (Figures 14-9 and 14-10). The primary afferent neurons in this system have their cell bodies in the dorsal root ganglia, enter the cord via class II or A-beta dorsal root fibers, and then coalesce in the fasciculus gracilis or fasciculus cuneatus in the dorsal funiculus of the spinal cordfasciculus cuneatus in the dorsal funiculus of the spinal cord. The fasciculus gracilis, found at all spinal cord levels, is situated closest to the midline and carries input from the lower extremities and lower trunk. The fasciculus cuneatus, found only at upper thoracic and cervical spinal cord levels, is lateral to the fasciculus gracilis and carries input from the upper extremities and upper trunk. These two fasciculi form the dorsal columns of the spinal cord that carry the central processes of dorsal root ganglion cells and ascend the length of the spinal cord to reach their second neurons in the lower part of the medulla.

In the lower part of the medulla, fibers in the fasciculus gracilis and fasciculus cuneatus synapse with the second neurons found in the nucleus gracilis and nucleus cuneatus, respectively. Cells in these medullary nuclei give rise to fibers that cross the midline as internal arcuate fibers and ascend through the brain stem in the medial lemniscus ascend through the brain stem in the medial lemniscus. Fibers of the medial lemniscus terminate on cells of the ventral posterolateral (VPL) nucleus of the thalamus. From the VPL nucleus, thalamocortical fibers project to the primary somesthetic (somatosensory) area of the postcentral gyrus, located in the most anterior portion of the parietal lobe.

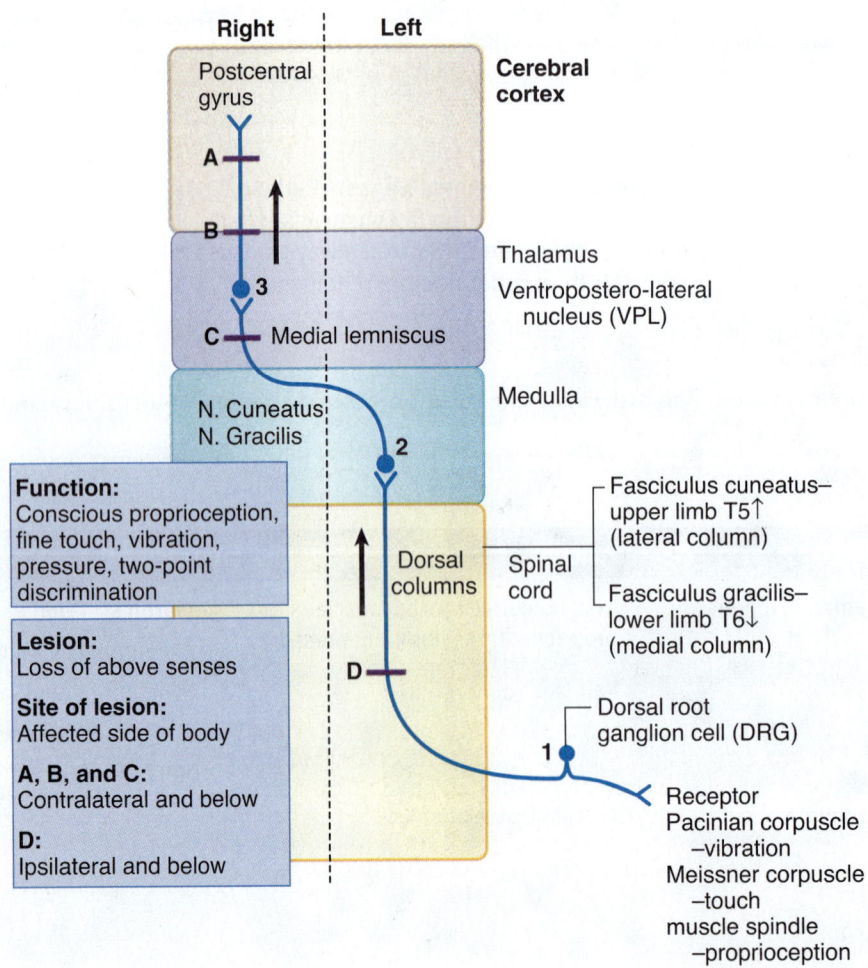

Figure 14-9. Dorsal Column Pathway–Medial Lemniscal System

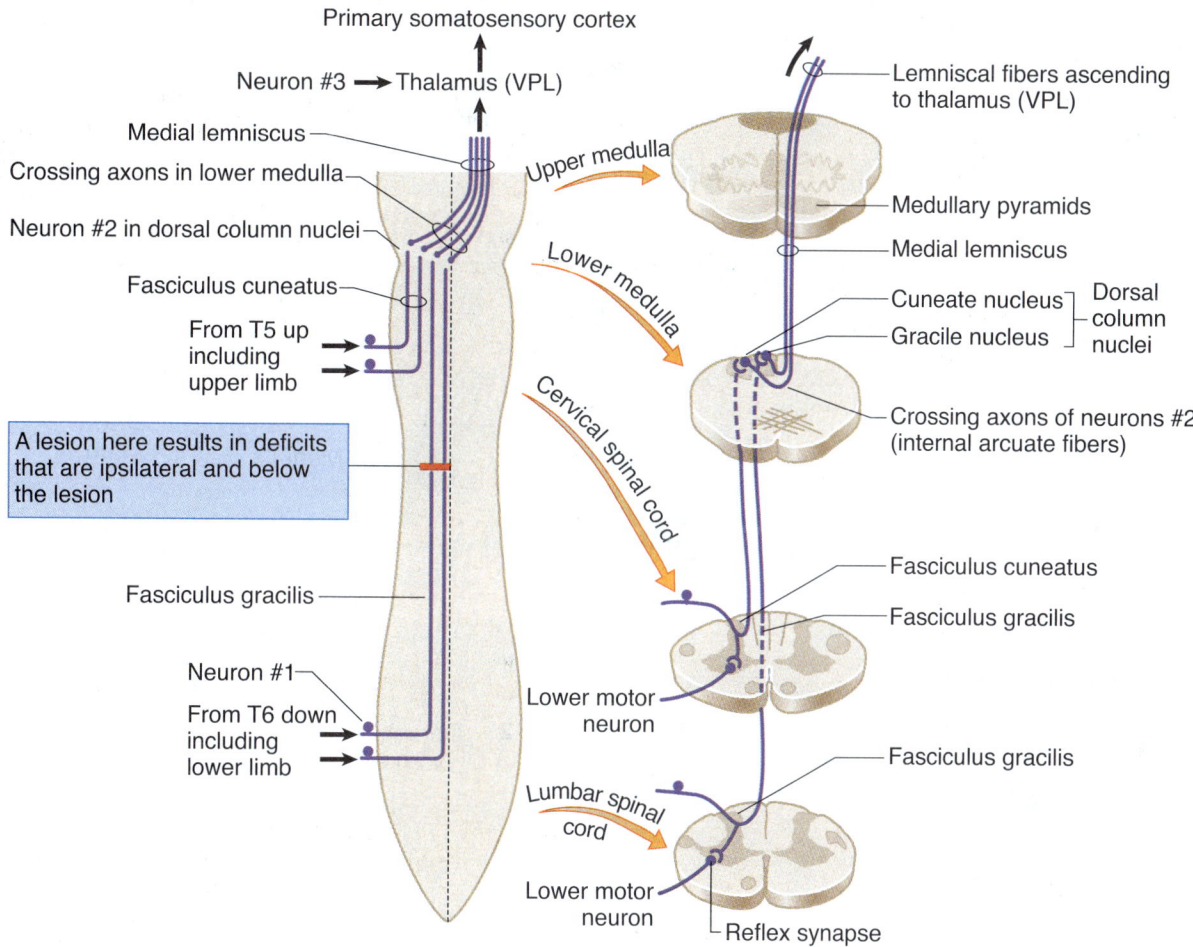

Figure 14-10. Dorsal Column/Medial Lemniscal System in the Spinal Cord and Medulla

Anterolateral (spinothalamic tract) system

The anterolateral system carries pain, temperature, and crude touch sensations from the extremities and trunk.

Pain and temperature fibers have cell bodies in the dorsal root ganglia and enter the spinal cord via A-delta and C or class III and class IV dorsal root fibers (Figure 14-11). Their fibers ascend or descend a couple of segments in the dorsolateral tract of Lissauer before entering and synapsing in the dorsal horn. The second neuron cell bodies are located in the dorsal horn gray matter. Axons from these cells cross in the ventral white commissure just below the central canal of the spinal cord and coalesce to form the spinothalamic tract in the ventral part of the lateral funiculus. The spinothalamic tract courses through the entire length of the spinal cord and the brain stem to terminate in the VPL nucleus of the thalamus. Cells in the VPL nucleus send pain and temperature information to the primary somatosensory cortex in the postcentral gyrus.

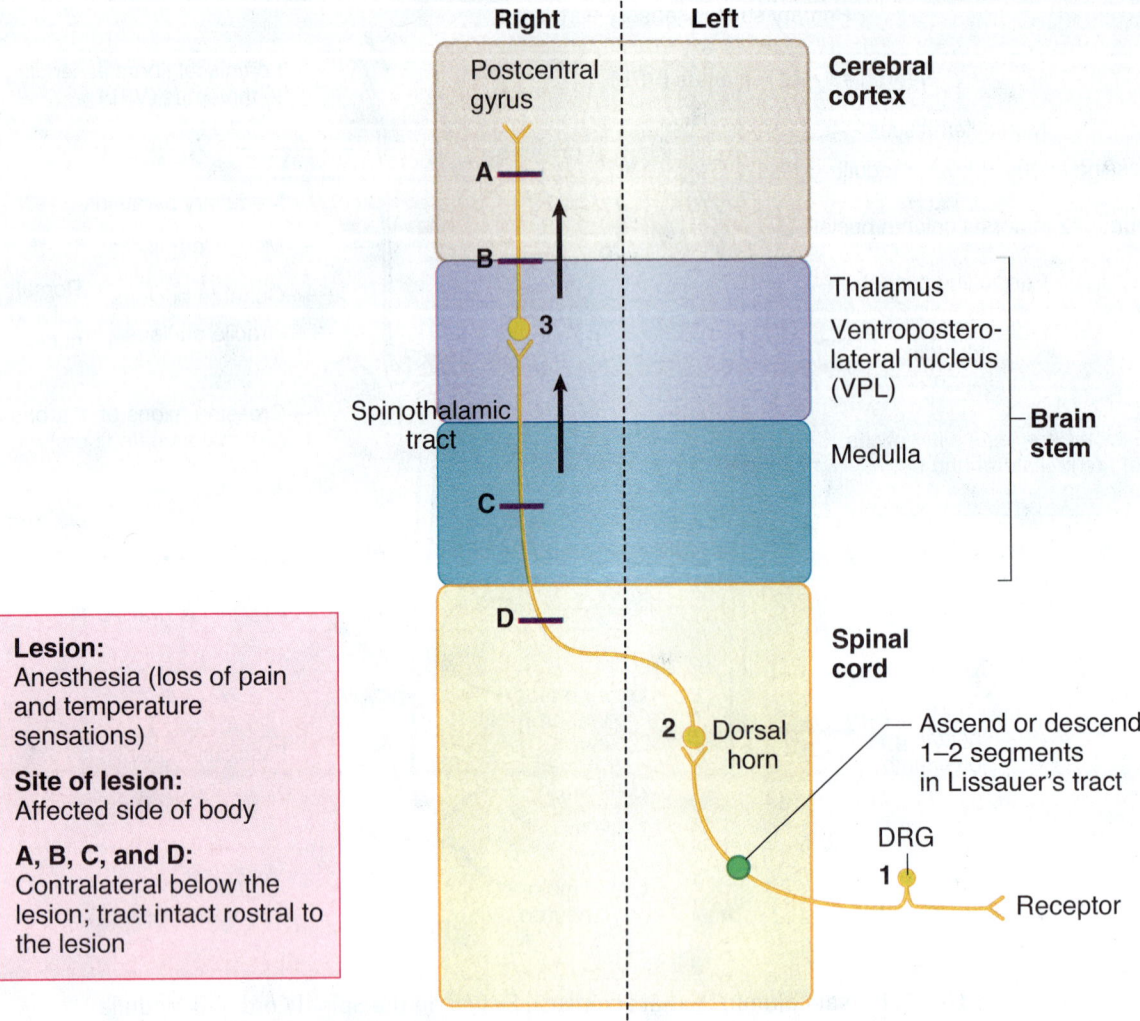

Figure 14-11. Spinothalamic Tract (Anterolateral System)

Lesion:
Anesthesia (loss of pain and temperature sensations)

Site of lesion:
Affected side of body

A, B, C, and D:
Contralateral below the lesion; tract intact rostral to the lesion

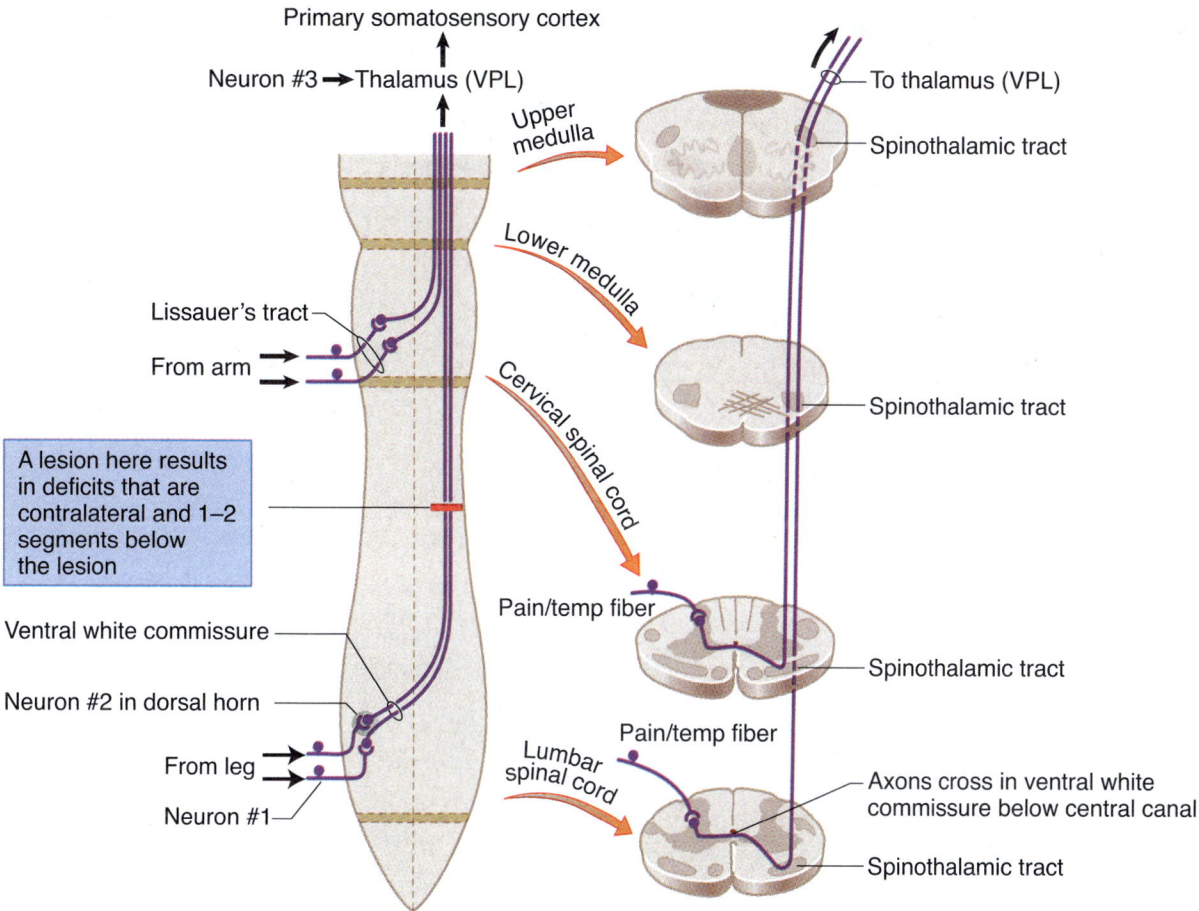

Figure 14-12. Anterolateral System in the Spinal Cord and Medulla

Spinocerebellar pathways

The spinocerebellar tracts mainly carry unconscious proprioceptive input from muscle spindles and GTOs to the cerebellum, where this information is used to help monitor and modulate movements. There are two major spino-cerebellar pathways:

- Dorsal spinocerebellar tract—carries input from the lower extremities and lower trunk.
- Cuneocerebellar tract—carries proprioceptive input to the cerebellum from the upper extremities and upper trunk.

The cell bodies of the dorsal spinocerebellar tract are found in Clarke's nucleus, which is situated in the spinal cord from T1 to L2. The cell bodies of the cuneocerebellar tract are found in the medulla in the external cuneate nucleus.

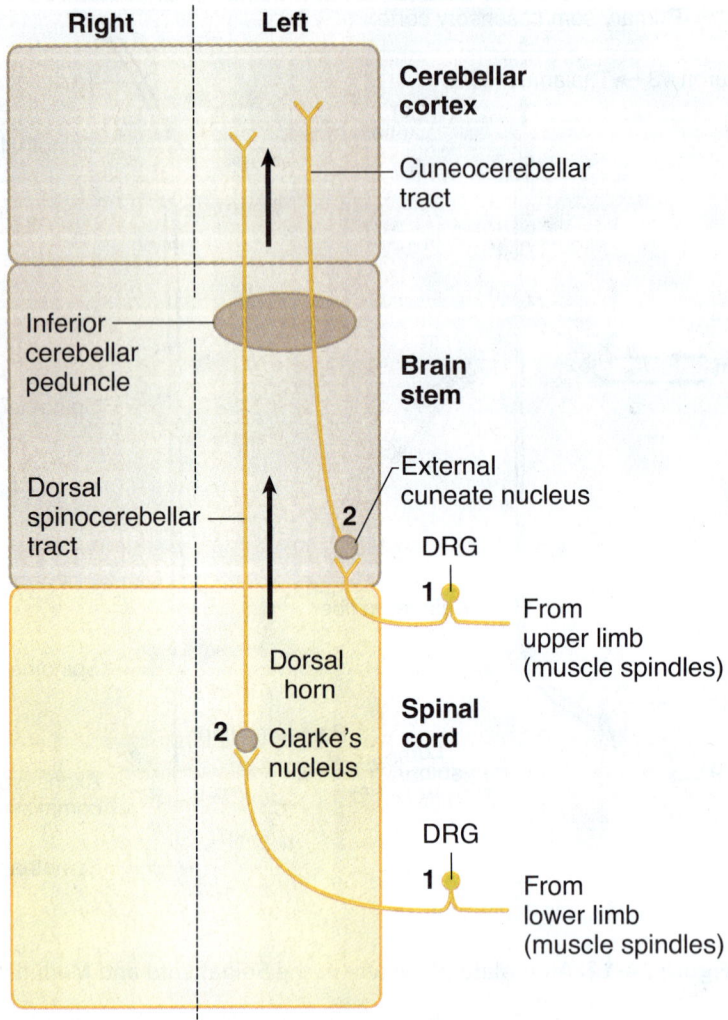

Figure 14-13. Spinocerebellar Tracts

The Brain Stem 15

Learning Objectives

❏ Answer questions about sensory and motor neural systems

❏ Interpret scenarios on midbrain

❏ Interpret scenarios on components of the ear, auditory, and vestibular systems

❏ Solve problems concerning blood supply to the brain stem

❏ Interpret scenarios on brain-stem lesions and reticular formation

The brain stem is divisible into three continuous parts: the midbrain, the pons, and the medulla. The midbrain is most rostral and begins just below the diencephalon. The pons is in the middle and is overlain by the cerebellum.

The medulla is caudal to the pons and is continuous with the spinal cord.

The brain stem is the home of the origins or sites of termination of fibers in 9 of the 12 cranial nerves (CNs).

CRANIAL NERVES

Two cranial nerves, the oculomotor and trochlear (CN III and IV), arise from the midbrain.

Four cranial nerves—the trigeminal, abducens, facial, and vestibulocochlear nerves (CN V, VI, VII, and VIII)—enter or exit from the pons.

Three cranial nerves—the glossopharyngeal, vagus, and hypoglossal nerves (CN IX, X, and XII)— enter or exit from the medulla. Fibers of the accessory nerve arise from the cervical spinal cord.

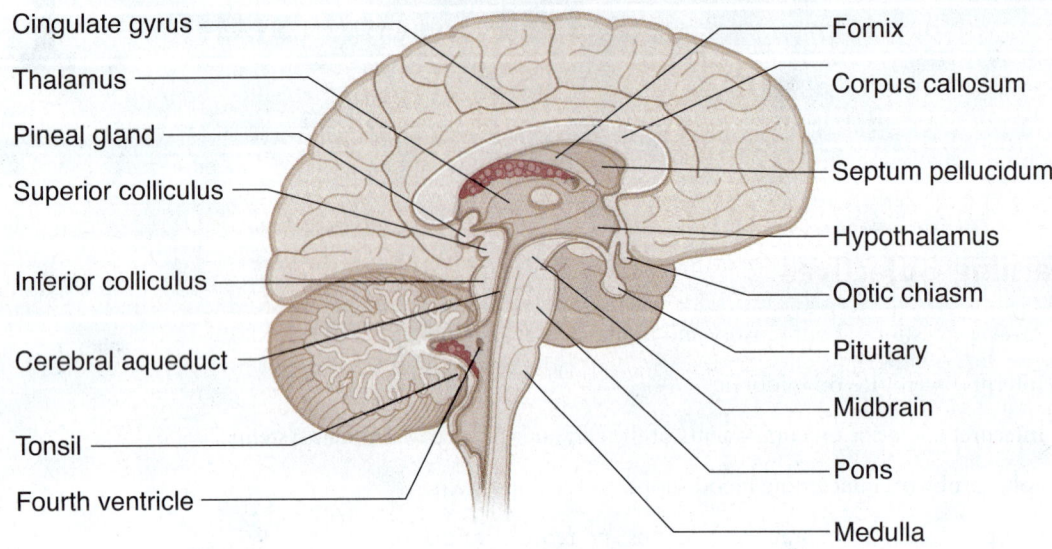

Figure 15-1. Brain: Mid-Sagittal Section

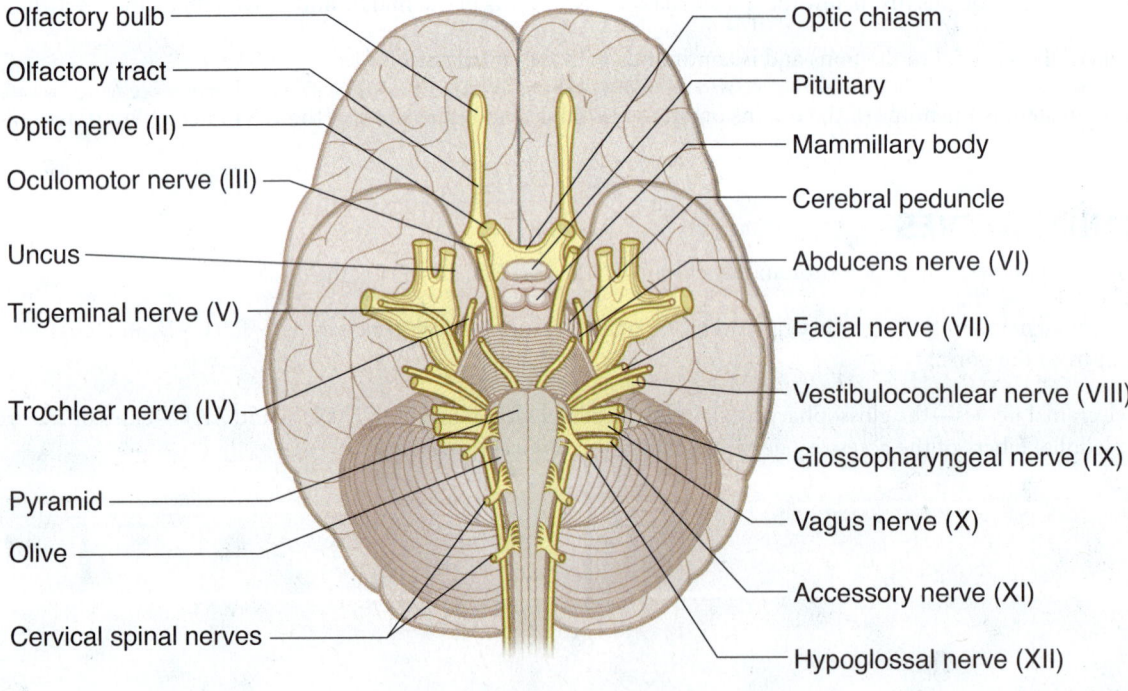

Figure 15-2. Brain: Inferior View

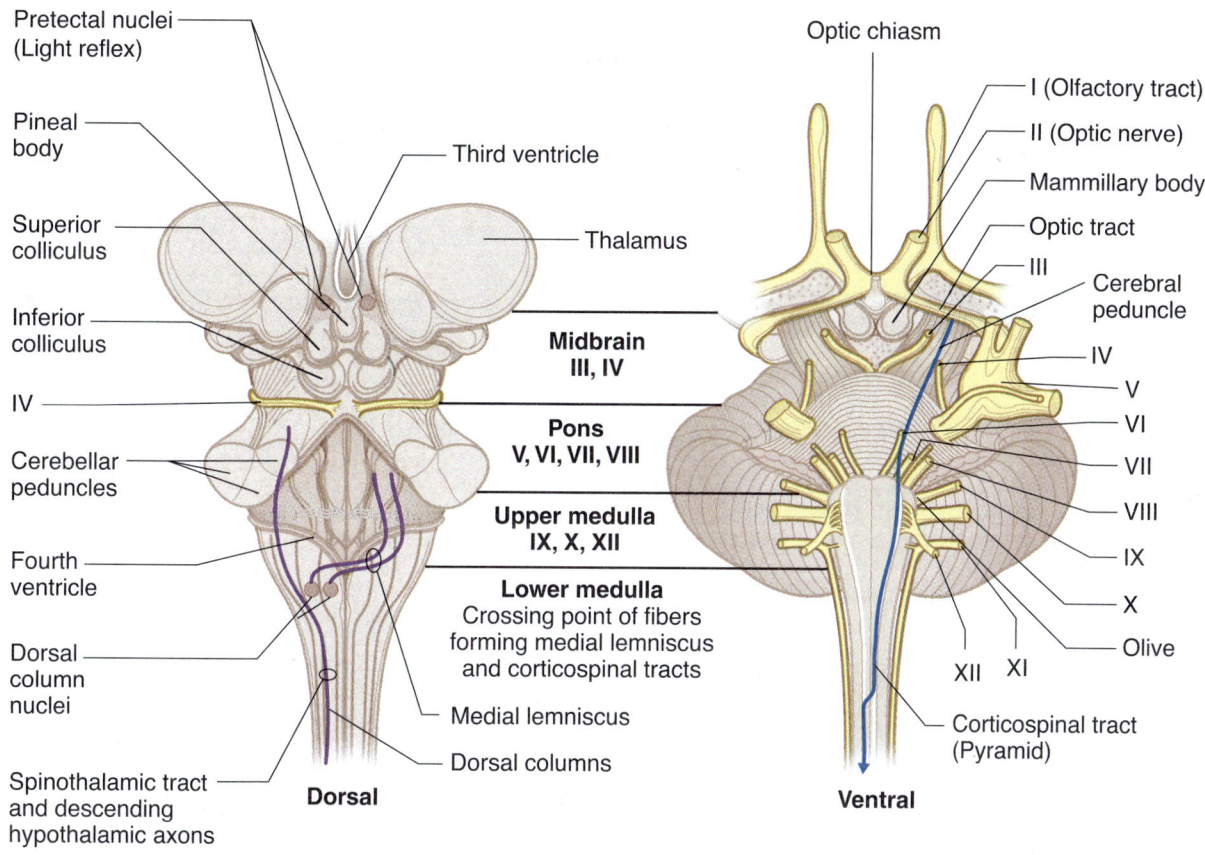

Figure 15-3. Brain Stem and Cranial Nerve: Surface Anatomy

Afferent fibers of cranial nerves enter the central nervous system (CNS) and terminate in relation to aggregates of neurons in sensory nuclei. Motor or efferent components of cranial nerves arise from motor nuclei. All motor and sensory nuclei that contribute fibers to cranial nerves are organized in a series of discontinuous columns according to the functional component that they contain. Motor nuclei are situated medially, closest to the midline, and sensory nuclei are situated lateral to the motor nuclei. A cranial nerve nucleus or nerve will be found at virtually every transverse sectional level of the brain stem.

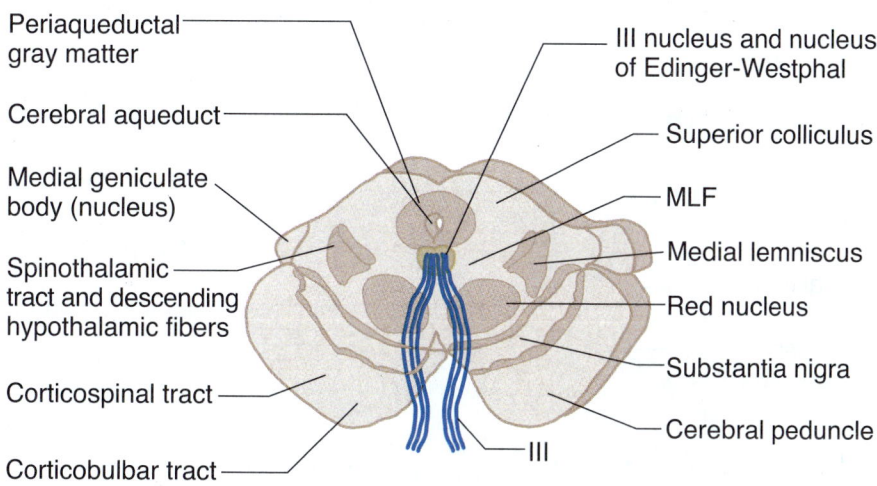

Figure 15-4A. Upper Midbrain; Level of Nerve III

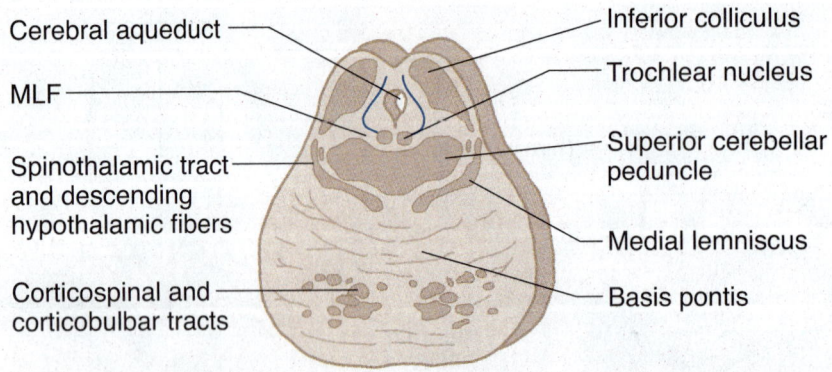

Figure 15-4B. Lower Midbrain; Level of Nucleus CN IV

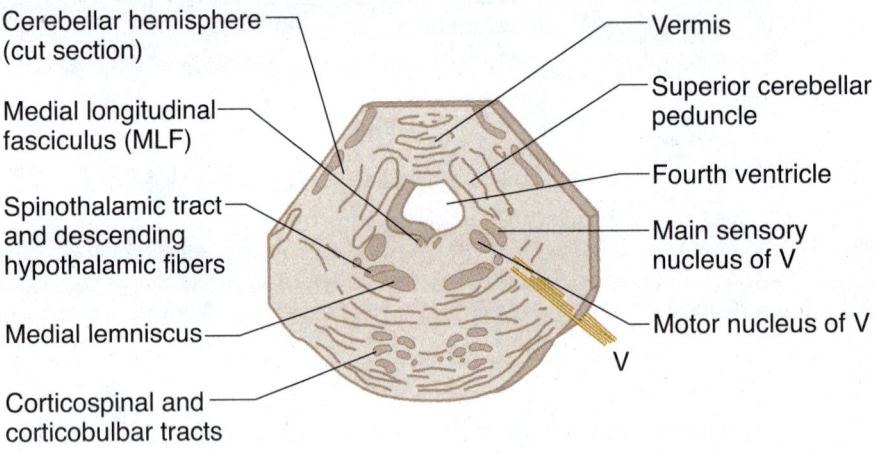

Figure 15-4C. Middle Pons; Level of Nerve V

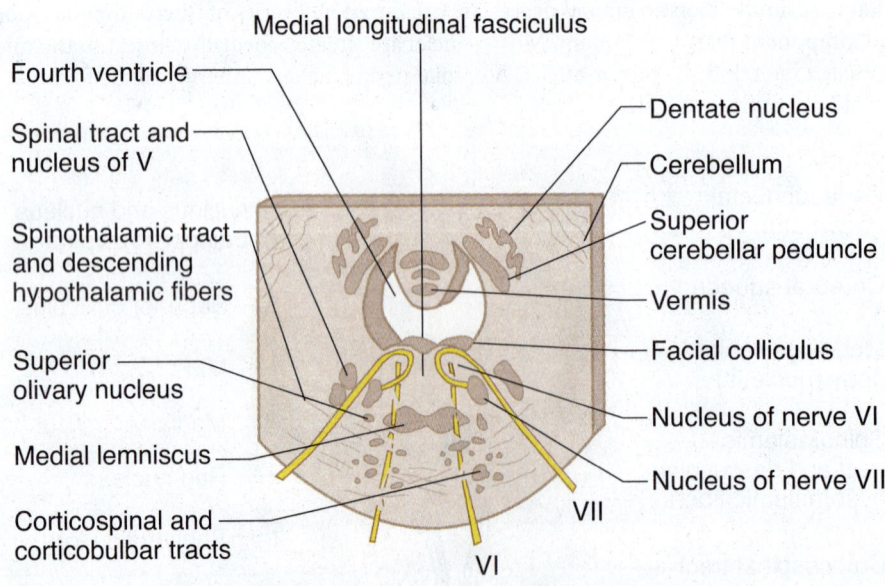

Figure 15-4D. Lower Pons; Level of Nerves VI and VII

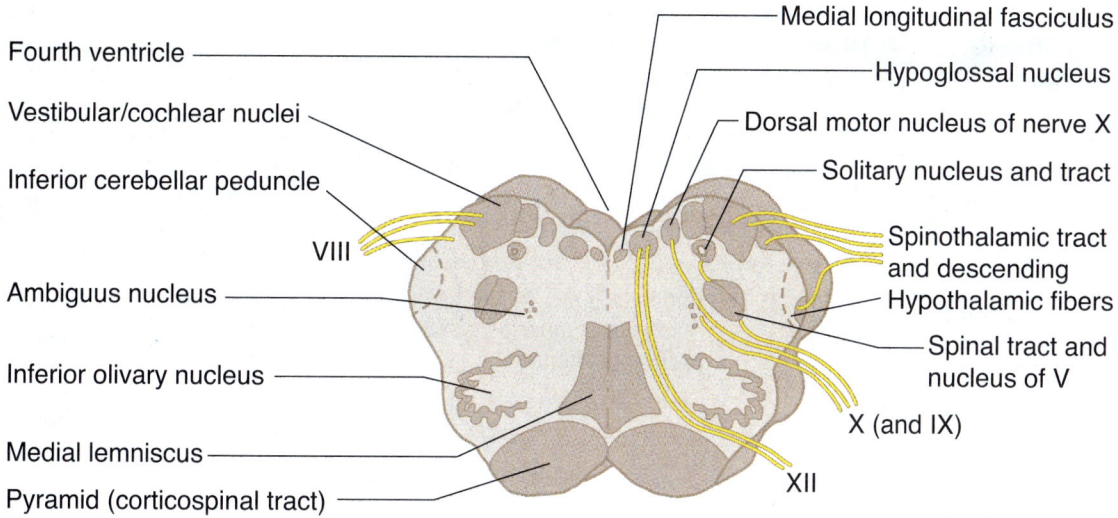

Figure 15-4E. Open Medulla

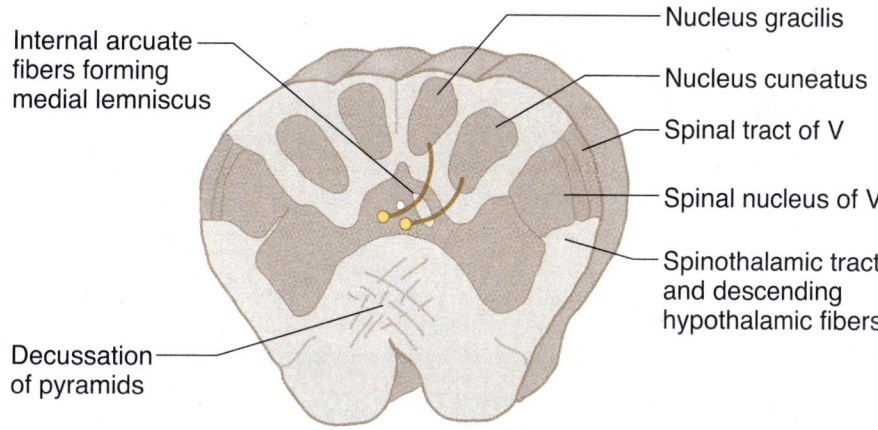

Figure 15-4F. Closed Medulla

Table 15-1. Cranial Nerves: Functional Features

CN	Name	Type	Function	Results of Lesions
I	Olfactory	Sensory	Smells	Anosmia
II	Optic	Sensory	Sees	Visual field deficits (anopsia)
				Loss of light reflex with III
				Only nerve to be affected by MS
III	Oculomotor	Motor	Innervates SR, IR, MR, IO extraocular muscles: adduction (MR) most important action	Diplopia, external strabismus
			Raises eyelid (levator palpebrae superioris)	Loss of parallel gaze
				Ptosis
			Constricts pupil (sphincter pupillae)	Dilated pupil, loss of light reflex with II
			Accommodates (ciliary muscle)	Loss of near response
IV	Trochlear	Motor	Superior oblique—depresses and abducts eyeball (makes eyeball look down and out)	Weakness looking down with adducted eye
			Intorts	Trouble going down stairs
				Head tilts away from lesioned side
V	Trigeminal Ophthalmic (V1) Maxillary (V2) Mandibular (V3)	Mixed	General sensation (touch, pain, temperature) of forehead/scalp/cornea	V1—loss of general sensation in skin of forehead/scalp
			General sensation of palate, nasal cavity, maxillary face, maxillary teeth	Loss of blink reflex with VII
				V2—loss of general sensation in skin over maxilla, maxillary teeth
			General sensation of anterior two-thirds of tongue, mandibular face, mandibular teeth	V3—loss of general sensation in skin over mandible, mandibular teeth, tongue, weakness in chewing
			Motor to muscles of mastication (temporalis, masseter, medial and lateral pterygoids) and anterior belly of digastric, mylohyoid, tensor tympani, tensor palati	Jaw deviation toward weak side
				Trigeminal neuralgia—intractable pain in V2 or V3 territory
VI	Abducens	Motor	Lateral rectus—abducts eyeball	Diplopia, internal strabismus
				Loss of parallel gaze, "pseudoptosis"

(Continue)

CN	Name	Type	Function	Results of Lesions
VII	Facial	Mixed	To muscles of facial expression, posterior belly of digastric, stylohyoid, stapedius	Corner of mouth droops, cannot close eye, cannot wrinkle forehead, loss of blink reflex, hyperacusis; Bell palsy—lesion of nerve in facial canal
			Salivation (submandibular, sublingual glands)	
			Skin behind ear	Pain behind ear
			Taste in anterior 2/3 of tongue/palate	Alteration or loss of taste (ageusia)
			Tears (lacrimal gland)	Eye dry and red
VIII	Vestibulocochlear	Sensory	Hearing	Sensorineural hearing loss
			Angular acceleration (head turning)	Loss of balance, nystagmus
			Linear acceleration (gravity)	
IX	Glossopharyngeal	Mixed	Oropharynx sensation, carotid sinus/body	Loss of gag reflex with X
			Salivation (parotid gland)	
			All sensation of posterior one-third of tongue	
			Motor to one muscle—stylopharyngeus	
X	Vagus	Mixed	To muscles of palate and pharynx for swallowing except tensor palati (V) and stylopharyngeus (IX)	Nasal speech, nasal regurgitation
				Dysphagia, palate droop
				Uvula pointing away from affected side
			To all muscles of larynx (phonates)	Hoarseness/fixed vocal cord
			Sensory of larynx and laryngopharynx	Loss of gag reflex with IX
			Sensory of GI tract	Loss of cough reflex
			To GI tract smooth muscle and glands in foregut and midgut	
XI	Accessory	Motor	Head rotation to opposite side (sternocleidomastoid)	Weakness turning chin to opposite side
			Elevates and rotates scapula (trapezius)	Shoulder droop
XII	Hypoglossal	Motor	Tongue movement (styloglossus, hyoglossus, genioglossus, and intrinsic tongue muscles—palatoglossus is by X)	Tongue pointing toward same (affected) side on protrusion

CN, cranial nerve; IO, inferior oblique; IR, inferior rectus; MR, medial rectus; MS, multiple sclerosis; SR, superior rectus

SENSORY AND MOTOR NEURAL SYSTEMS

Each of the following five ascending or descending neural tracts, fibers, or fasciculi courses through the brain stem and will be found at every transverse sectional level.

Medial Lemniscus

The medial lemniscus (ML) contains the axons from cell bodies found in the dorsal column nuclei (gracilis and cuneatus) in the caudal medulla and represents the second neuron in the pathway to the thalamus and cortex for discriminative touch, vibration, pressure, and conscious proprioception. The axons in the ML cross the midline of the medulla immediately after emerging from the dorsal column nuclei. Lesions in the ML, in any part of the brain stem, result in a loss of discriminative touch, vibration, pressure, and conscious proprioception from the **contralateral** side of the body.

Spinothalamic Tract (Part of Anterolateral System)

The spinothalamic tract has its cells of origin in the spinal cord and represents the crossed axons of the second neuron in the pathway conveying pain and temperature to the thalamus and cortex. Lesions of the spinothalamic tract, in any part of the brain stem, results in a loss of pain and temperature sensations from the **contralateral** side of the body.

Corticospinal Tract

The corticospinal tract controls the activity of lower motoneurons, and interneuron pools for lower motoneurons course through the brain stem on their way to the spinal cord. Lesions of this tract produce a spastic paresis in skeletal muscles of the body **contralateral** to the lesion site in the brain stem.

Descending Hypothalamic Fibers

The descending hypothalamic fibers arise in the hypothalamus and course without crossing through the brain stem to terminate on preganglionic sympathetic neurons in the spinal cord. Lesions of this pathway produce an ipsilateral **Horner syndrome.** Horner syndrome consists of miosis (pupillary constriction), ptosis (drooping eyelid), and anhidrosis (lack of sweating) in the face ipsilateral to the side of the lesion.

Descending hypothalamic fibers course with the spinothalamic fibers in the lateral part of the brain stem. Therefore, brain stem lesions producing Horner syndrome may also result in a contralateral loss of pain and temperature sensations from the limbs and body.

Medial Longitudinal Fasciculus

The medial longitudinal fasciculus is a fiber bundle interconnecting centers for horizontal gaze, the vestibular nuclei, and the nerve nuclei of CN III, IV, and VI, which innervate skeletal muscles that move the eyeball. This fiber bundle courses close to the dorsal midline of the brain stem and also contains vestibulospinal fibers, which course through the medulla to the spinal cord. Lesions of the fasciculus produce **internuclear ophthalmoplegia** and disrupt the vestibulo-ocular reflex.

MEDULLA

In the caudal medulla, two of the neural systems—the corticospinal and dorsal column–medial lemniscal pathways—send axons across the midline. The nucleus gracilis and nucleus cuneatus give rise to axons that decussate in the caudal medulla (the crossing axons are the internal arcuate fibers), which then form and ascend in the medial lemniscus.

The corticospinal (pyramidal) tracts, which are contained in the pyramids, course ventromedially through the medulla. Most of these fibers decussate in the caudal medulla just below the crossing of axons from the dorsal column nuclei, and then travel down the spinal cord as the (lateral) corticospinal tract.

The olives are located lateral to the pyramids in the rostral two-thirds of the medulla. The olives contain the convoluted inferior olivary nuclei. The olivary nuclei send climbing (olivocerebellar) fibers into the cerebellum through the inferior cerebellar peduncle. The olives are a key distinguishing feature of the medulla.

The spinothalamic tract and the descending hypothalamic fibers course together in the lateral part of the medulla below the inferior cerebellar peduncle and near the spinal nucleus and tract of CN V.

Cranial Nerve Nuclei

Spinal nucleus of V

The spinal nucleus of the trigeminal nerve (CN V) is located in a position analogous to the dorsal horn of the spinal cord. The spinal tract of the trigeminal nerve lies just lateral to this nucleus and extends from the upper cervical cord (C2) to the point of entry of the fifth cranial nerve in the pons. Central processes from cells in the trigeminal ganglion conveying pain and temperature sensations from the face enter the brain stem in the rostral pons but descend in the spinal tract of CN V and synapse on cells in the spinal nucleus.

Solitary nucleus

The solitary nucleus receives the axons of all general and special visceral afferent fibers carried into the CNS by CN VII, IX, and X. These include taste, cardiorespiratory, and gastrointestinal sensations carried by these cranial nerves. Taste and visceral sensory neurons all have their cell bodies in ganglia associated with CN VII, IX, and X outside the CNS.

Nucleus ambiguus

The nucleus ambiguus is a column of large motoneurons situated dorsal to the inferior olive. Axons arising from cells in this nucleus course in the ninth and tenth cranial nerves. The component to the ninth nerve is insignificant. In the tenth nerve, these fibers supply muscles of the soft palate, larynx, pharynx, and upper esophagus. A unilateral lesion will produce ipsilateral paralysis of the soft palate causing the uvula to deviate away from the lesioned nerve and nasal regurgitation of liquids, weakness of laryngeal muscles causing hoarseness, and pharyngeal weakness resulting in difficulty in swallowing.

Dorsal motor nucleus of CN X

These visceral motoneurons of CN X are located lateral to the hypoglossal nucleus in the floor of the fourth ventricle. This is a major parasympathetic nucleus of the brain stem, and it supplies preganglionic fibers innervating terminal ganglia in the thorax and the foregut and midgut parts of the gastrointestinal tract.

Hypoglossal nucleus

The hypoglossal nucleus is situated near the midline just beneath the central canal and fourth ventricle. This nucleus sends axons into the hypoglossal nerve to innervate all of the tongue muscles except the palatoglossus.

The accessory nucleus

The accessory nucleus is found in the cervical spinal cord. The axons of the spinal accessory nerve arise from the accessory nucleus, pass through the foramen magnum to enter the cranial cavity, and join the fibers of the vagus to exit the cranial cavity through the jugular foramen. As a result, intramedullary lesions do not affect fibers of the spinal accessory nerve. The spinal accessory nerve supplies the sternocleidomastoid and trapezius muscles.

The rootlets of the glossopharyngeal (CN IX) and vagus (CN X) nerves exit between the olive and the fibers of the inferior cerebellar peduncle. The hypoglossal nerve (CN XII) exits more medially between the olive and the medullary pyramid.

PONS

The pons is located between the medulla (caudally) and the midbrain (rostrally). The cerebellum overlies the pons. It is connected to the brain stem by three pairs of cerebellar peduncles. The fourth ventricle is found between the dorsal surface of the pons and the cerebellum. The ventral surface of the pons is dominated by fibers, which form a large ventral enlargement that carries fibers from pontine nuclei to the cerebellum in the middle cerebellar peduncle. This ventral enlargement is the key distinguishing feature of the pons.

The corticospinal tracts are more diffuse in the pons than in the medulla and are embedded in the transversely coursing fibers that enter the cerebellum in the middle cerebellar peduncle.

The medial lemniscus is still situated near the midline but is now separated from the corticospinal tracts by the fibers forming the middle cerebellar peduncle. The medial lemniscus has changed from a dorsoventral orientation in the medulla to a more horizontal orientation in the pons.

The spinothalamic tract and the descending hypothalamic fibers continue to course together in the lateral pons.

The lateral lemniscus, an ascending auditory pathway, is lateral and just dorsal to the medial lemniscus. The lateral lemniscus carries the bulk of ascending auditory fibers from both cochlear nuclei to the inferior colliculus of the midbrain.

The medial longitudinal fasciculus (MLF) is located near the midline just beneath the fourth ventricle.

Cranial Nerve Nuclei

Abducens nucleus

The abducens nucleus is found near the midline in the floor of the fourth ventricle just lateral to the MLF.

Facial motor nucleus

The facial motor nucleus is located ventrolateral to the abducens nucleus. Fibers from the facial nucleus curve around the posterior side of the abducens nucleus (the curve forms the internal genu of the facial nerve), then pass ventrolaterally to exit the brain stem at the pontomedullary junction.

Superior olivary nucleus

The superior olivary nucleus lies immediately ventral to the nucleus of CN VII and receives auditory impulses from both ears by way of the cochlear nuclei. The cochlear nuclei are found at the pontomedullary junction just lateral to the inferior cerebellar peduncle.

Vestibular nuclei

The vestibular nuclei are located near the posterior surface of the pons lateral to the abducens nucleus, and extend into the medulla.

Cochlear nuclei

The dorsal and ventral cochlear nuclei are found at the pontomedullary junction. All of the fibers of the cochlear part of CN VIII terminate here.

Trigeminal nuclei

Motor Nucleus—Pons

The motor nucleus of CN V is located in the pons just medial to the main sensory nucleus of the trigeminal and adjacent to the point of exit or entry of the trigeminal nerve fibers. These motor fibers supply the muscles of mastication (masseter, temporalis, and medial and lateral pterygoid.

Main Sensory Nucleus—Pons

The main sensory nucleus is located just lateral to the motor nucleus.

The main sensory nucleus receives tactile and pressure sensations from the face, scalp, oral cavity, nasal cavity, and dura.

Spinal Trigeminal Nucleus—Spinal cord to pons

The spinal trigeminal nucleus is a caudal continuation of the main sensory nucleus, extending from the mid pons through the medulla to the cervical cord. Central processes from cells in the trigeminal ganglion conveying pain and temperature sensations from the face descend in the spinal tract of V and synapse on cells in the spinal nucleus.

Mesencephalic Nucleus—Midbrain

The mesencephalic nucleus of CN V is located at the point of entry of the fifth nerve and extends into the midbrain. It receives proprioceptive input from joints, muscles of mastication, extraocular muscles, teeth, and the periodontium. Some of these fibers synapse monosynaptically on the motoneurons, forming the sensory limb of the jaw jerk reflex.

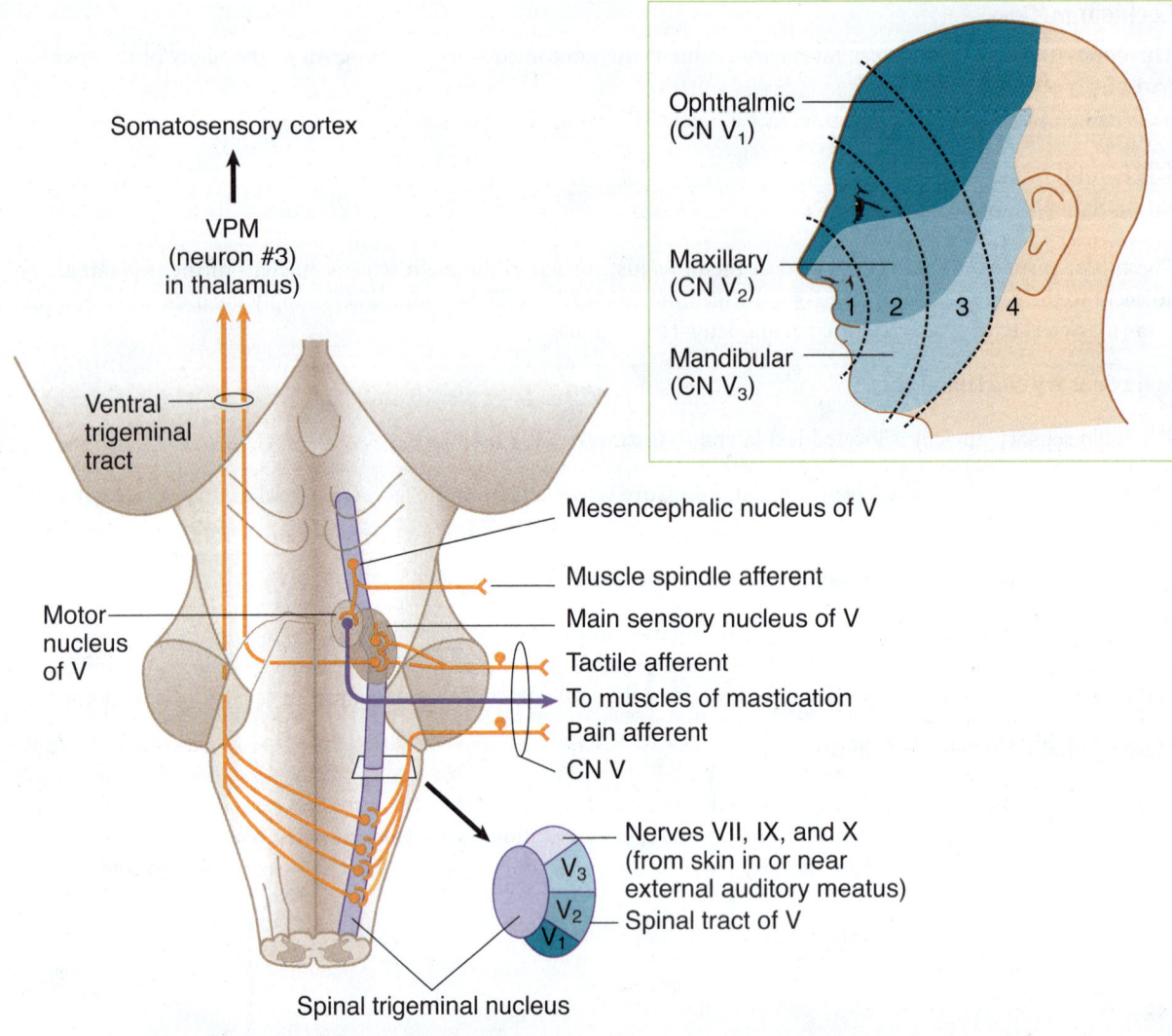

Figure 15-5. Shaded areas indicate regions of face and scalp innervated by branches of the 3 divisions of CN V. Dotted lines indicate concentric numbered "onion-skin" regions emanating posteriorly from nose and mouth that have a rostral to caudal representation in the spinal nucleus of V in the brain stem.

Note

VPM relays touch, pain, temperature (CN V) and taste (CN VII, IX) sensations to cortex.

Cranial Nerves V, VI, VII, and VIII

Four cranial nerves emerge from the pons. Cranial nerves VI, VII, and VIII emerge from the pontomedullary junction. The facial nerve is located medial to the vestibulocochlear nerve. The abducens nerve (CN VI) emerges near the midline lateral to the corticospinal tract. The trigeminal nerve (CN V) emerges from the middle of the pons.

MIDBRAIN

The midbrain (mesencephalon) is located between the pons and diencephalon. The cerebral aqueduct, a narrow channel that connects the third and fourth ventricles, passes through the midbrain. The inferior colliculi and superior colliculi are found on the dorsal aspect of the midbrain above the cerebral aqueduct. The inferior colliculus processes auditory information received bilaterally from the cochlear nuclei by axon fibers of the lateral lemniscus. The superior colliculi help direct movements of both eyes in gaze. The pretectal region is located just beneath the superior colliculi and in front of the oculomotor complex. This area contains interneurons involved in the pupillary light reflex. The massive cerebral peduncles extend ventrally from the midbrain. The cerebral peduncles contain corticospinal and corticobulbar fibers. The interpeduncular fossa is the space between the cerebral peduncles.

The substantia nigra is the largest nucleus of the midbrain. It appears black to dark brown in the freshly cut brain because nigral cells contain melanin pigments. Neurons in the substantia nigra utilize Dopamine and GABA as neurotransmitters.

The medial lemniscus and spinothalamic tract and descending hypothalamic fibers course together ventrolateral to the periaqueductal gray.

The MLF continues to be located near the midline, just beneath the cerebral aqueduct.

The mesencephalic nuclei of the trigeminal nerve are located on either side of the central gray.

Cranial Nerve Nuclei

The trochlear nucleus is located just beneath the periaqueductal gray near the midline between the superior and inferior colliculi. The oculomotor nucleus and the nucleus of Edinger-Westphal are found just beneath the periaqueductal gray near the midline at the level of the superior colliculi.

Two cranial nerves emerge from the midbrain: the oculomotor (CN III) and the trochlear (CN IV) nerves.

The **oculomotor nerve** arises from the oculomotor nucleus and exits ventrally from the midbrain in the interpeduncular fossa. CN III also contains preganglionic parasympathetic axons that arise from the nucleus of Edinger-Westphal, which lies adjacent to the oculomotor nucleus.

Axons of the **trochlear nerve** decussate in the superior medullary velum and exit the brain stem near the posterior midline just inferior to the inferior colliculi.

Corticobulbar (Corticonuclear) Innervation of Cranial Nerve Nuclei

Corticobulbar fibers serve as the source of upper motoneuron innervation of lower motoneurons in cranial nerve nuclei (Figure 15-6). Corticobulbar fibers arise in the motor cortex and influence lower motoneurons in all brain stem nuclei that innervate skeletal muscles. This includes:

- Muscles of mastication (CN V)
- Muscles of facial expression (CN VII) – (partially bilateral)
- Palate, pharynx, and larynx (CN X)
- Tongue (CN XII)
- Sternocleidomastoid and trapezius muscles (CN XI)

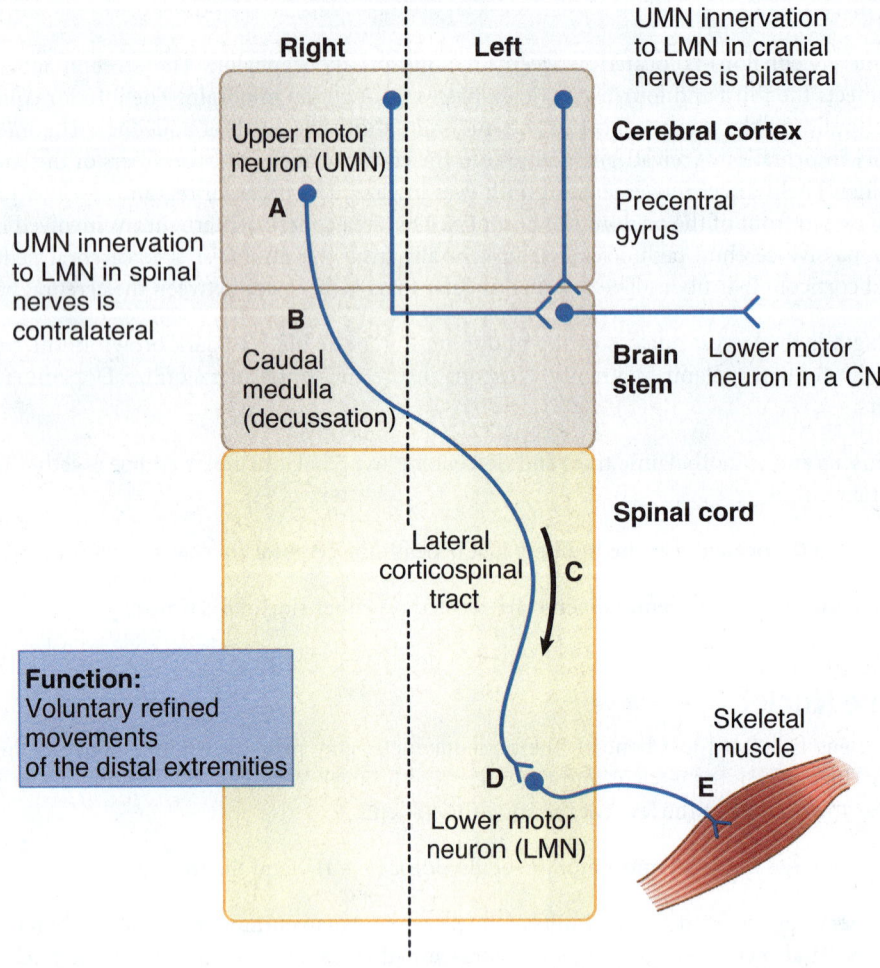

Figure 15-6. Upper Motor Neuron Innervation of Spinal Nerves and Cranial Nerves

The corticobulbar innervation of cranial nerve lower motoneurons is predominantly bilateral, in that each lower motoneuron in a cranial nerve nucleus receives input from corticobulbar axons arising from both the right and the left cerebral cortex. The major exception is that only some of the LMNs of the facial nerve (CN VII) receive a contralateral innervation.

Clinical Correlates

Facial Paralysis

The upper motoneuron innervation of lower motoneurons in the facial motor nucleus is different and clinically significant. Like most cranial nerve lower motoneurons, the corticobulbar innervation of facial motoneurons to muscles of the upper face (which wrinkle the forehead and shut the eyes) is bilateral. The corticobulbar innervation of facial motoneurons to muscles of the mouth, however, is contralateral only. Clinically, this means that one can differentiate between a lesion of the seventh nerve and a lesion of the corticobulbar fibers to the facial motor nucleus.

A facial nerve lesion (as in **Bell Palsy**) will result in a complete ipsilateral paralysis of muscles of facial expression, including an inability to wrinkle the forehead or shut the eyes and a drooping of the corner of the mouth. A corticobulbar lesion will result in only a drooping of the corner of the mouth on the contralateral side of the face and no other facial motor deficits. Generally, no other cranial deficits will be seen with corticobulbar lesions because virtually every other cranial nerve nucleus is bilaterally innervated. In some individuals, the hypoglossal nucleus may receive mainly contralateral corticobulbar innervation. If these corticobulbar fibers are lesioned, the tongue muscles undergo transient weakness without atrophy or fasciculations and may deviate away from the injured corticobulbar fibers. If, for example, the lesion is in corticobulbar fibers on the left, there is transient weakness of the right tongue muscles, causing a deviation of the tongue toward the right side upon protrusion.

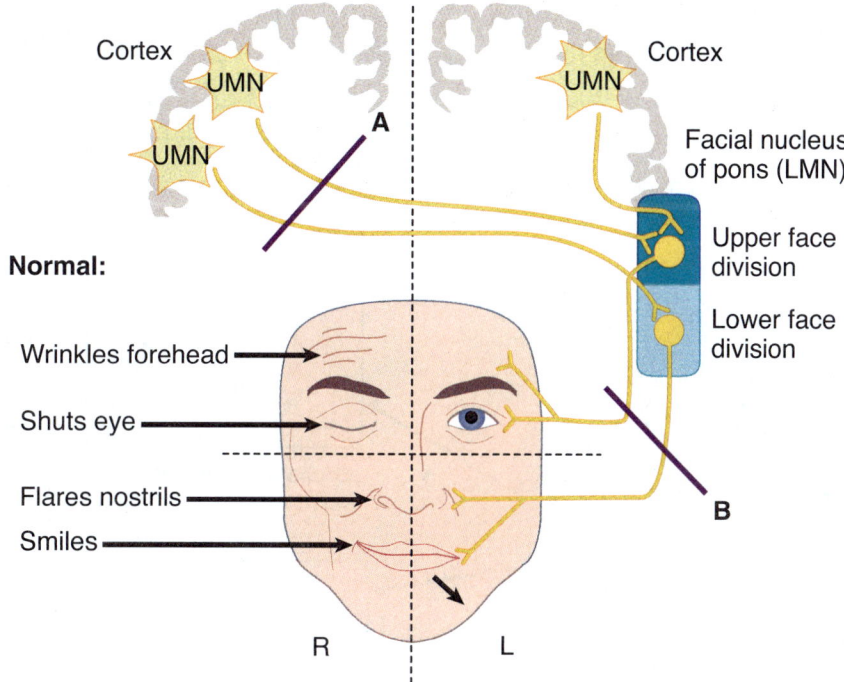

Figure 15-7. Corticobulbar Innervation of the Facial Motor Nucleus
Lesion A: left lower face weakness
Lesion B: complete left face weakness
UMN = upper motoneuron
LMN = lower motoneuron

COMPONENTS OF THE EAR, AUDITORY, AND VESTIBULAR SYSTEMS

Each ear consists of three components: two air-filled spaces, the external ear and the middle ear; and the fluid-filled spaces of the inner ear (Figures 15-8 and 15-9).

The external ear includes the pinna and the external auditory meatus, which extends to the tympanic membrane. Sound waves travel through the external auditory canal and cause the tympanic membrane (eardrum) to vibrate. Movement of the eardrum causes vibrations of the ossicles in the middle ear (i.e., the malleus, incus, and stapes). Vibrations of the ossicles are transferred through the oval window and into the inner ear.

The middle earlies in the temporal bone, where the chain of 3 ossicles connect the tympanic membrane to the oval window. These auditory ossicles amplify the vibrations received by the tympanic membrane and transmit them to the fluid of the inner ear with minimal energy loss. The malleus is inserted in the tympanic membrane, and the stapes is inserted into the membrane of the oval window. Two small skeletal muscles, the tensor tympani and the stapedius, contract to prevent damage to the inner ear when the ear is exposed to loud sounds. The middle-ear cavity communicates with the nasopharynx via the eustachian tube, which allows air pressure to be equalized on both sides of the tympanic membrane.

The inner ear consists of a labyrinth (osseous and membranous) of interconnected sacs (utricle and saccule) and channels (semicircular ducts and the cochlear duct) that contain patches of receptor or hair cells that respond to airborne vibrations or movements of the head. Both the cochlear duct and the sacs and channels of the vestibular labyrinth are filled with endolymph, which bathes the hairs of the hair cells. Endolymph is unique because it has the inorganic ionic composition of an intracellular fluid but it lies in an extracellular space. The intracellular ionic composition of endolymph is important for the function of hair cells. Perilymph, ionically like a typical extracellular fluid, lies outside the endolymph-filled labyrinth.

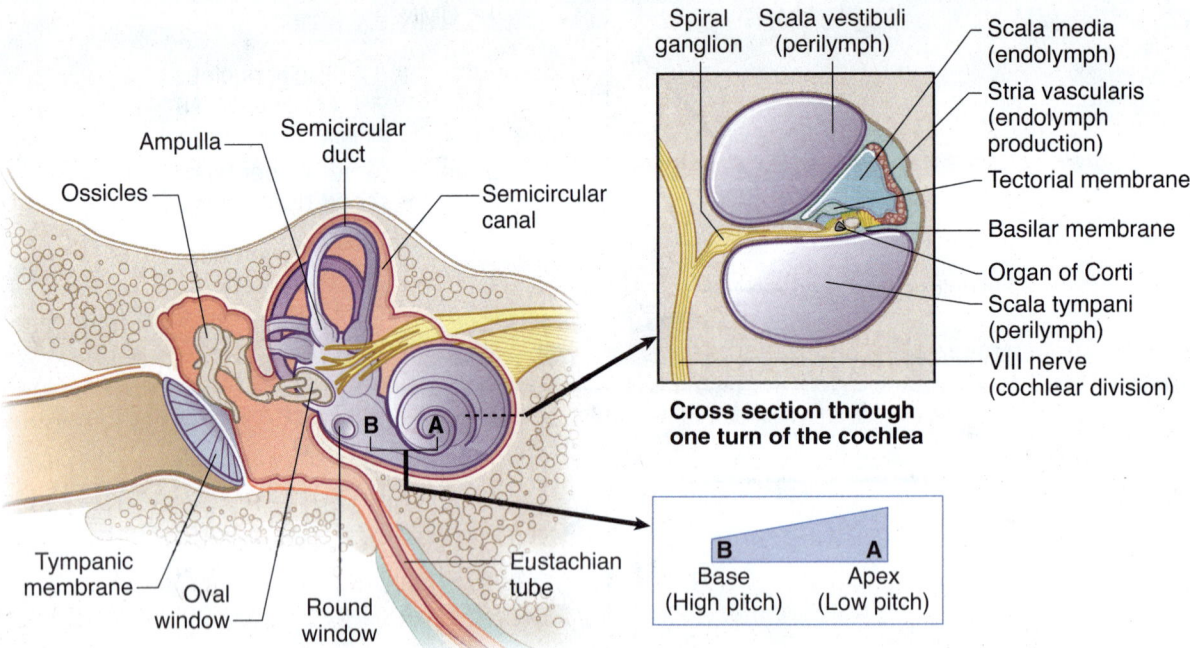

Figure 15-8. Structures of the Inner Ear

Auditory System

Cochlear duct

The cochlear duct is the auditory receptor of the inner ear. It contains hair cells, which respond to airborne vibrations transmitted by the ossicles to the oval window. The cochlear duct coils 2 and a quarter turns within the bony cochlea and contains hair cells situated on an elongated, highly flexible, basilar membrane. High-frequency sound waves cause maximum displacement of the basilar membrane and stimulation of hair cells at the base of the cochlea, whereas low-frequency sounds maximally stimulate hair cells at the apex of the cochlea.

Spiral ganglion

The spiral ganglion contains cell bodies whose peripheral axons innervate auditory hair cells of the organ of Corti. The central axons from these bipolar cells form the cochlear part of the eighth cranial nerve. All of the axons in the cochlear part of the eighth nerve enter the pontomedullary junction and synapse in the ventral and dorsal cochlear nuclei. Axons of cells in the ventral cochlear nuclei bilaterally innervate the superior olivary nuclei in the pons. The superior olivary nuclei are the first auditory nuclei to receive binaural input and use the binaural input to localize sound sources. The lateral lemniscus carries auditory input from the cochlear nuclei and the superior olivary nuclei to the inferior colliculus in the midbrain. Each lateral lemniscus carries information derived from both ears; however, input from the contralateral ear predominates.

Inferior colliculus

The inferior colliculus sends auditory information to the medial geniculate body (MGB) of the thalamus. From the MGB, the auditory radiation projects to the primary auditory cortex located on the posterior portion of the transverse temporal gyrus (Heschl's gyrus; Brodmann areas 41 and 42). The adjacent auditory association area makes connections with other parts of the cortex, including Wernicke's area, the cortical area for the comprehension of language.

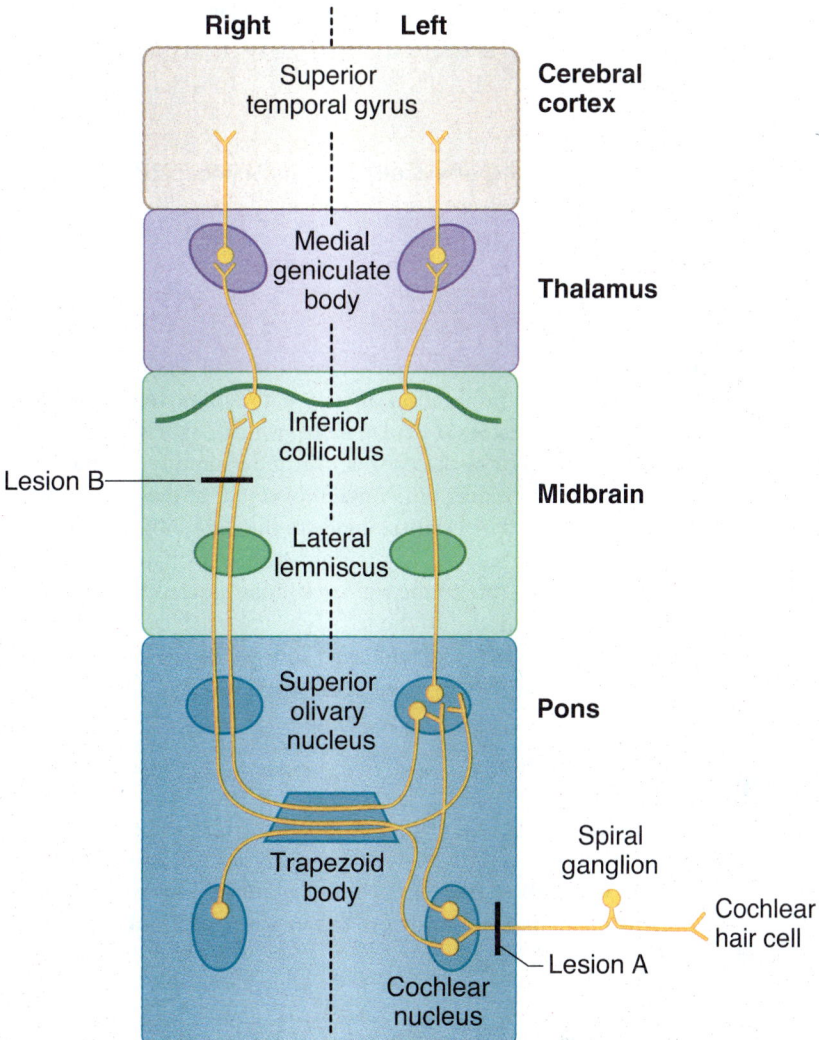

Figure 15-9. Auditory System

Hearing Loss

Conductive: passage of sound waves through external or middle ear is interrupted. Causes: obstruction, otosclerosis, otitis media

Sensorineural: damage to cochlea, CN VIII, or central auditory connections

Vestibular System

Sensory receptors

The vestibular system contains two kinds of sensory receptors, one kind in the utricle and the saccule and the other in the semicircular ducts.

The utricle and the saccule are two large sacs, each containing a patch of hair cells in a macula. Each macula responds to linear acceleration and detects positional changes in the head relative to gravity. There are three semicircular ducts in the inner ear, each lying in a bony semicircular canal. Each semicircular duct contains an ampullary crest of hair cells that detect changes in angular acceleration resulting from circular movements of the head. The three semicircular ducts—anterior, posterior, and horizontal—are oriented such that they lie in the three planes of space. Circular movements of the head in any plane will depolarize hair cells in a semicircular duct in one labyrinth and hyperpolarize hair cells in the corresponding duct in the opposite labyrinth.

Vestibular nuclei

There are four vestibular nuclei located in the rostral medulla and caudal pons. The vestibular nuclei receive afferents from the vestibular nerve, which innervates receptors located in the semicircular ducts, utricle, and saccule. Primary vestibular fibers terminate in the vestibular nuclei and the flocculonodular lobe of the cerebellum.

Vestibular fibers

Secondary vestibular fibers, originating in the vestibular nuclei, join the MLF and supply the motor nuclei of CN III, IV, and VI. These fibers are involved in the production of conjugate eye movements. These compensatory eye movements represent the efferent limb of the vestibulo-ocular reflex, which enables the eye to remain focused on a stationary target during movement of the head or neck. Most of our understanding of the vestibulo-ocular reflex is based on horizontal head turning and a corresponding horizontal movement of the eyes in the direction opposite to that of head turning. For example, when the head turns horizontally to the right, both eyes will move to the left using the following vestibulo-ocular structures. Head turning to the right stimulates hairs cells in the right semicircular ducts. The right eighth nerve increases its firing rate to the right vestibular nuclei. These nuclei then send axons by way of the MLF to the right oculomotor nucleus and to the left abducens nucleus. The right oculomotor nerve to the right medial rectus adducts the right eye, and the left abducens nerve to the left lateral rectus abducts the left eye. The net effect of stimulating these nuclei is that both eyes will look to the left.

Vestibular System (VIII)

Three semicircular ducts respond to **angular acceleration and deceleration** of the head. The **utricle** and **saccule** respond to **linear acceleration** and the pull of **gravity**. There are four **vestibular nuclei** in the medulla and pons, which receive information from CN VIII. Fibers from the vestibular nuclei join the MLF and supply the motor nuclei of CNs III, IV, and VI, thereby regulating conjugate eye movements. Vestibular nuclei also receive and send information to the **flocculonodular lobe** of the cerebellum.

In a Nutshell
Vestibular Functions:
Equilibrium
Posture
Vor

Vestibulo-Ocular Reflex

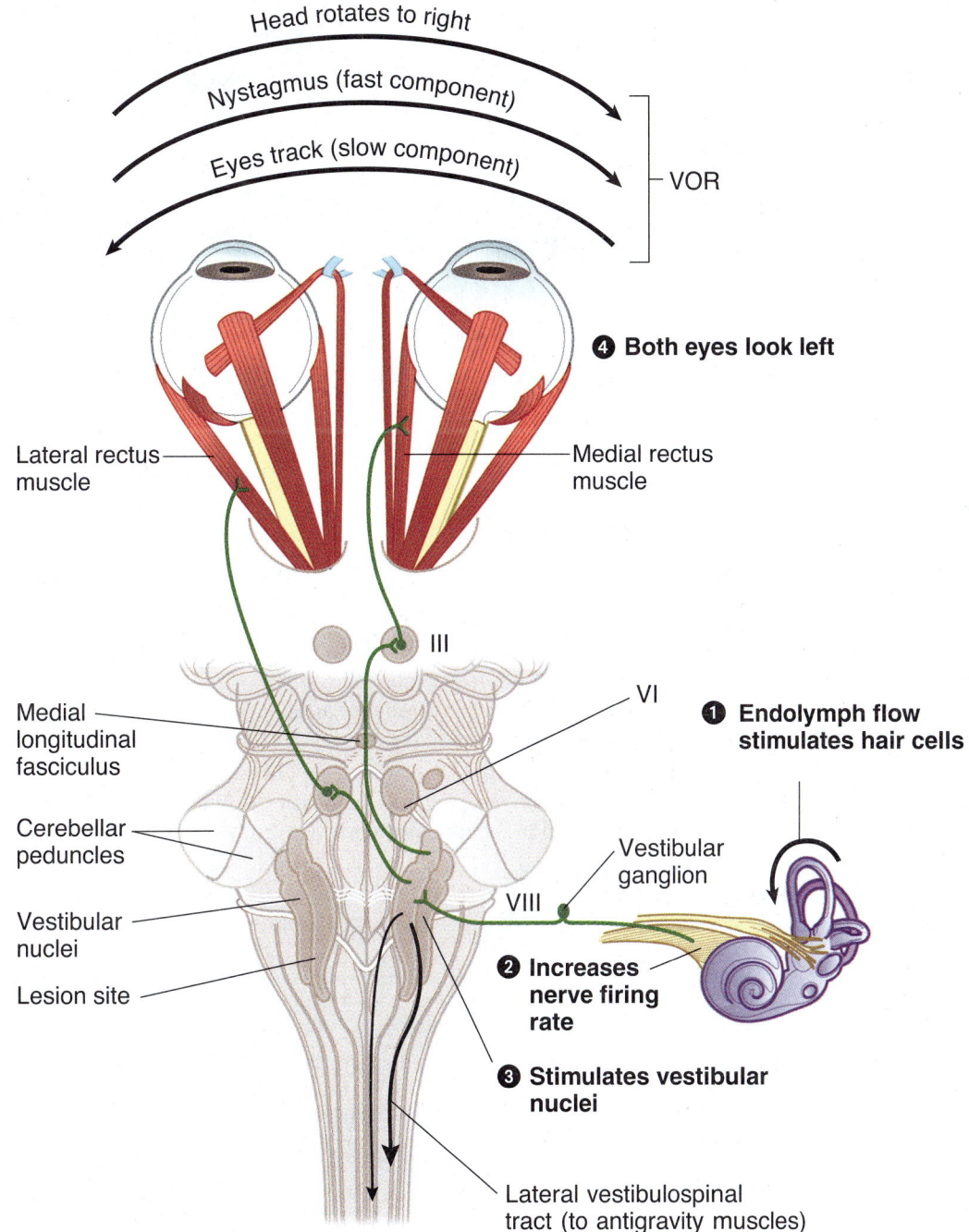

Figure 15-10. Vestibulo-Ocular Reflex (VOR)

BLOOD SUPPLY TO THE BRAIN STEM

Vertebral Artery

This artery is a branch of the subclavian that ascends through the foramina of the transverse processes of the upper 6 cervical vertebrae. It enters the posterior fossa by passing through the foramen magnum. The vertebral arteries continue up the ventral surface of the medulla and, at the caudal border of the pons, join to form the basilar artery.

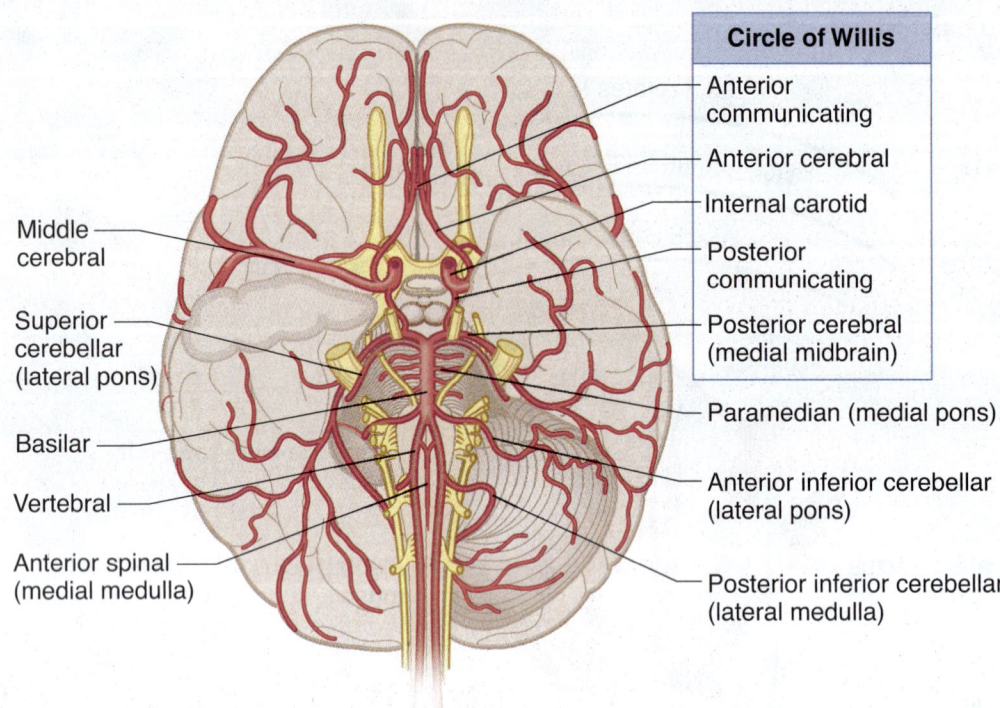

Figure 15-11. Arterial Supply of the Brain
AICA: anterior inferior cerebellar artery
PICA: posterior inferior cerebellar artery

Branches of the vertebral artery include: the anterior spinal artery, which supplies the ventrolateral two-thirds of the cervical spinal cord and the ventromedial part of the medulla; and the posterior inferior cerebellar artery (PICA), which supplies the cerebellum and the dorsolateral part of the medulla.

In a Nutshell

Brain stem:

Vertebral Artery:

1. ASA
2. PICA

Basilar:

1. AICA
2. Paramedian
3. Superior cerebellar
4. Posterior cerebral

Basilar Artery

The basilar artery is formed by the joining of the 2 vertebral arteries at the pontomedullary junction. It ascends along the ventral midline of the pons and terminates near the rostral border of the pons by dividing into the 2 posterior cerebral arteries. Branches include the anterior inferior cerebellar arteries (AICA) and the paramedian arteries.

Branches of the basilar artery include: the labyrinthine artery, which follows the course of the eighth cranial nerve and supplies the inner ear; the anterior inferior cerebellar artery, which supplies part of the pons and the anterior and inferior regions of the cerebellum; the superior cerebellar artery, which supplies part of the rostral pons and the superior region of the cerebellum; and pontine branches, which supply much of the pons via paramedian and circumferential vessels.

At the rostral end of the midbrain, the basilar artery divides into a pair of posterior cerebral arteries. Paramedian and circumferential branches of the posterior cerebral artery supply the midbrain.

BRAIN-STEM LESIONS

There are two keys to localizing brain-stem lesions. First, it is uncommon to injure parts of the brain stem without involving one or more cranial nerves. The cranial nerve signs will localize the lesion to the midbrain (CN III or IV), upper pons (CN V), lower pons (CN VI, VII, or VIII), or upper medulla (CN IX, X, or XII). Second, if the lesion is in the brain stem, the cranial nerve deficits will be seen with a lesion to one or more of the descending or ascending long tracts (corticospinal, medial lemniscus, spinothalamic, descending hypothalamic fibers). Lesions in the brain stem to any of the long tracts except for the descending hypothalamic fibers will result in a contralateral deficit. A unilateral lesion to the descending hypothalamic fibers that results in Horner syndrome is always seen ipsilateral to the side of the lesion.

RETICULAR FORMATION

The reticular formation is located in the brain stem and functions to coordinate and integrate the actions of different parts of the CNS. It plays an important role in the regulation of muscle and reflex activity and control of respiration, cardiovascular responses, behavioral arousal, and sleep.

Reticular Nuclei

Raphe nuclei

The raphe nuclei are a narrow column of cells in the midline of the brain stem, extending from the medulla to the midbrain. Cells in some of the raphe nuclei (e.g., the dorsal raphe nucleus) synthesize serotonin (5-hydroxytryptamine [5-HT]) from l-tryptophan and project to vast areas of the CNS. They play a role in mood, aggression, and the induction of non–rapid eye movement (non-REM) sleep.

Locus caeruleus

Cells in the locus caeruleus synthesize norepinephrine and send projections to most brain areas involved in the control of cortical activation (arousal). Decreased levels of norepinephrine are evident in REM (paradoxic) sleep.

Periaqueductal gray

The periaqueductal (central) gray is a collection of nuclei surrounding the cerebral aqueduct in the midbrain. Opioid receptors are present on many periaqueductal gray cells, the projections from which descend to modulate pain at the level of the dorsal horn of the spinal cord.

The Cerebellum 16

Learning Objectives

❏ Use knowledge of general features

❏ Use knowledge of cerebellar cytoarchitecture

❏ Solve problems concerning circuitry

GENERAL FEATURES

The cerebellum is derived from the metencephalon and is located dorsal to the pons and the medulla. The fourth ventricle is found between the cerebellum and the dorsal aspect of the pons. The cerebellum functions in the planning and fine-tuning of skeletal muscle contractions. It performs these tasks by comparing an intended with an actual performance.

The cerebellum consists of a midline vermis and 2 lateral cerebellar hemispheres. The cerebellar cortex consists of multiple parallel folds that are referred to as folia. The cerebellar cortex contains several maps of the skeletal muscles in the body.

The topographic arrangement of these maps indicates that the vermis controls the axial and proximal musculature of the limbs, the intermediate part of the hemisphere controls distal musculature, and the lateral part of the hemisphere is involved in motor planning.

The flocculonodular lobe is involved in control of balance and eye movements.

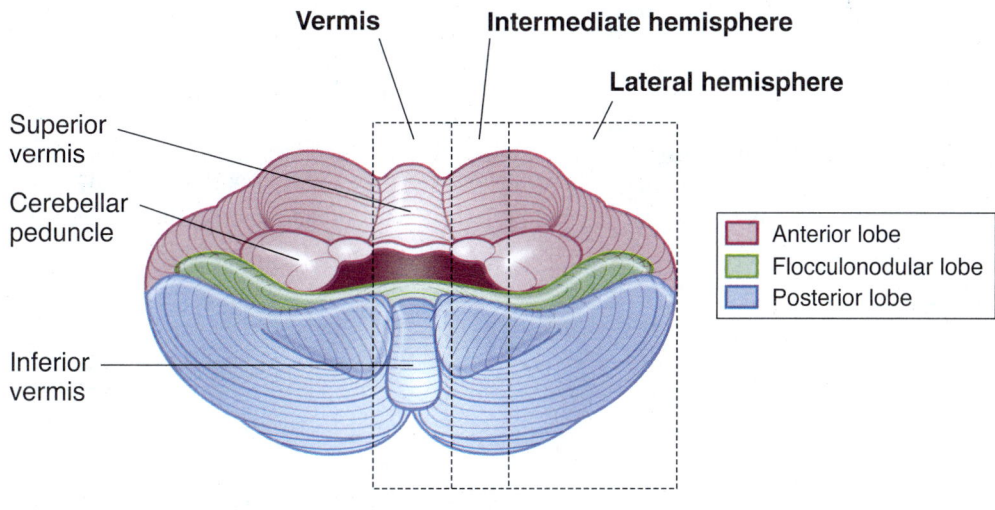

Figure 16-1. Cerebellum

Table 16-1. Cerebellum

Region	Function	Principle Input
Vermis and intermediate zones	Ongoing motor execution	Spinal cord
Hemisphere (lateral)	Planning/coordination	Cerebral cortex and inferior olivary nucleus
Flocculonodular lobe	Balance and eye movements	Vestibular nuclei (VIII)

Major input to the cerebellum travels in the inferior cerebellar peduncle (ICP) (restiform body) and middle cerebellar peduncle (MCP). Major outflow from the cerebellum travels in the superior cerebellar peduncle (SCP).

Table 16-2. Major Afferents to the Cerebellum

Name	Tract	Enter Cerebellum Via	Target and Function
Mossy fibers	Vestibulocerebellar	ICP	Excitatory terminals on granule cells (glutamate)
	Spinocerebellar (Cortico) pontocerebellar	ICP and SCP MCP (decussate)	
Climbing fibers	Olivocerebellar	ICP (decussate)	Excitatory terminals on Purkinje cells

Abbreviations: ICP, inferior cerebellar peduncle; MCP, middle cerebellar peduncle; SCP, superior cerebellar peduncle

CEREBELLAR CYTOARCHITECTURE

All afferent and efferent projections of the cerebellum traverse the ICP, MCP, or SCP. Most afferent input enters the cerebellum in the ICP and MCP; most efferent outflow leaves in the SCP (Figure 16-2 and Table 16-2).

Internally, the cerebellum consists of an outer cortex and an internal white matter (medullary substance).

The three cell layers of the cortex are the molecular layer, the Purkinje layer, and the granule cell layer.

The **molecular layer** is the outer layer and is made up of basket and stellate cells as well as parallel fibers, which are the axons of the granule cells. The extensive dendritic tree of the Purkinje cell extends into the molecular layer.

The **Purkinje layer** is the middle and most important layer of the cerebellar cortex. All of the inputs to the cerebellum are directed toward influencing the firing of Purkinje cells, and only axons of Purkinje cells leave the cerebellar cortex. A single axon exits from each Purkinje cell and projects to one of the deep cerebellar nuclei or to vestibular nuclei of the brain stem.

The **granule cell layer** is the innermost layer of cerebellar cortex and contains Golgi cells, granule cells, and glomeruli. Each glomerulus is surrounded by a glial capsule and contains a granule cell and axons of Golgi cells, which synapse with granule cells. The granule cell is the only excitatory neuron within the cerebellar cortex. All other neurons in the cerebellar cortex, including Purkinje, Golgi, basket, and stellate cells, are inhibitory.

Table 16-3. Cerebellum: Cell Types

Name	Target (Axon Termination)	Transmitter	Function
Purkinje cell	Deep cerebellar nuclei	GABA	Inhibitory*
Granule cell	Purkinje cell	Glutamate	Excitatory
Stellate cell	Purkinje cell	GABA	Inhibitory
Basket cell	Purkinje cell	GABA	Inhibitory
Golgi cell	Granule cell	GABA	Inhibitory

*Purkinje cells are the only outflow from the cerebellar cortex.

The internal white matter contains the deep cerebellar nuclei.

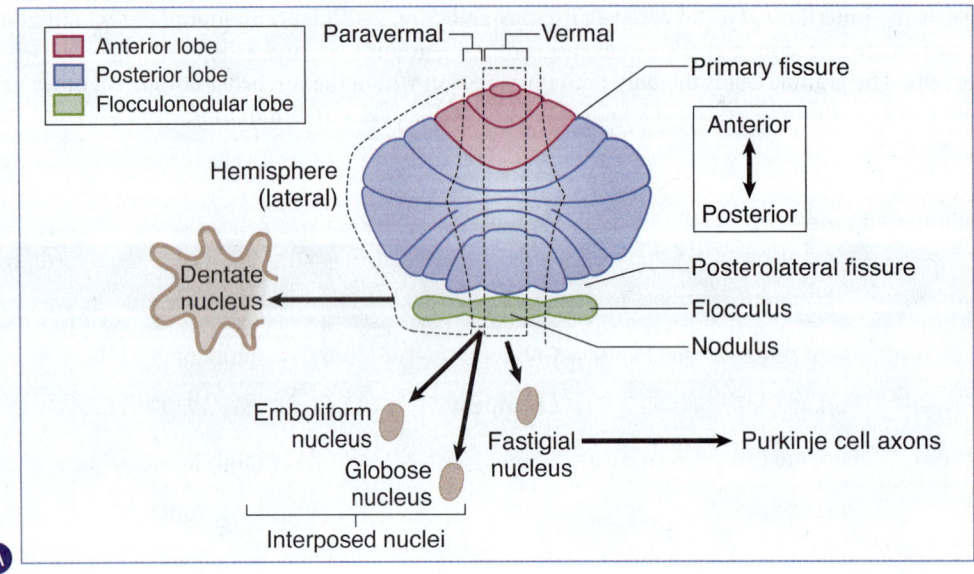

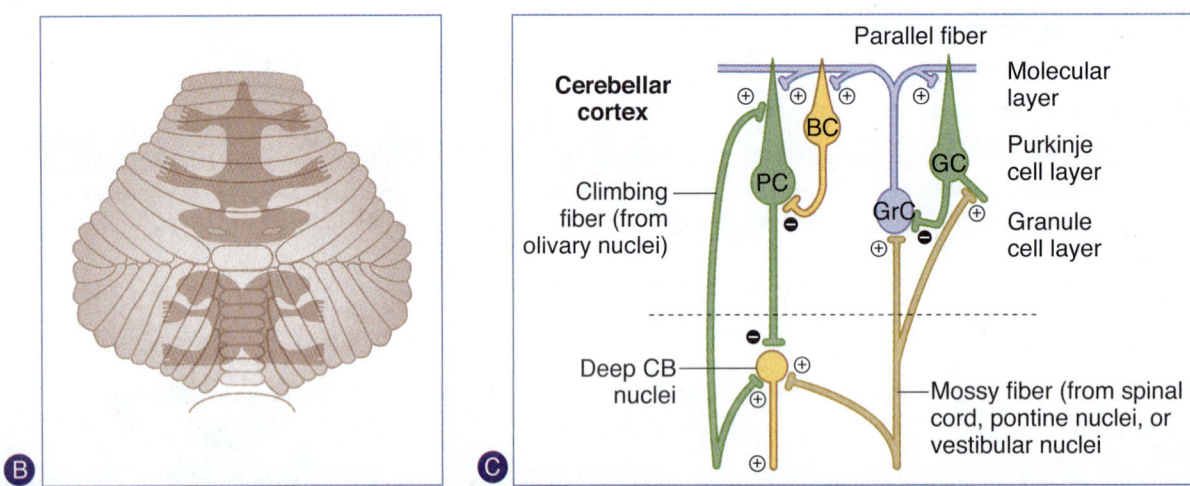

Figure 16-2. Cerebellar Organization (A) Parts of the cerebellar cortex and the deep cerebellar nuclei linked together by Purkinje cells (B) Topographic arrangement of skeletal muscles controlled by parts of the cerebellum (C) Cytology of the cerebellar cortex

GC: Golgi cell
BC: Basket cell
GrC: Granule cell

From medial to lateral, the deep cerebellar nuclei in the internal white matter are the fastigial nucleus, interposed nuclei, and dentate nucleus.

Two kinds of excitatory input enter the cerebellum in the form of climbing fibers and mossy fibers. Both types influence the firing of deep cerebellar nuclei by axon collaterals.

Climbing fibers originate exclusively from the inferior olivary complex of nuclei on the contralateral side of the medulla. Climbing fibers provide a direct powerful monosynaptic excitatory input to Purkinje cells.

Mossy fibers represent the axons from all other sources of cerebellar input. Mossy fibers provide an indirect, more diffuse excitatory input to Purkinje cells.

All mossy fibers exert an excitatory effect on **granule cells**. Each granule cell sends its axon into the molecular layer, where it gives off collaterals at a 90-degree angle that run parallel to the cortical surface (i.e., parallel fibers). These granule cell axons stimulate the apical dendrites of the Purkinje cells. Golgi cells receive excitatory input from mossy fibers and from the parallel fibers of the granule cells. The Golgi cell in turn inhibits the granule cell, which activated it in the first place.

The **basket** and **stellate cells**, which also receive excitatory input from parallel fibers of granule cells, inhibit Purkinje cells.

CIRCUITRY

The basic cerebellar circuits begin with Purkinje cells that receive excitatory input directly from climbing fibers and from parallel fibers of granule cells.

Purkinje cell axons project to and inhibit the deep cerebellar nuclei or the vestibular nuclei in an orderly fashion (Figure 16-3).

- Purkinje cells in the flocculonodular lobe project to the lateral vestibular nucleus.
- Purkinje cells in the vermis project to the fastigial nuclei.
- Purkinje cells in the intermediate hemisphere primarily project to the interposed (globose and emboliform) nuclei.
- Purkinje cells in the lateral cerebellar hemisphere project to the dentate nucleus.

Dysfunction

- **Hemisphere lesions** → ipsilateral symptoms: **intention** tremor, dysmetria, dysdiadochokinesia, scanning dysarthria, nystagmus, hypotonia
- **Vermal lesions** → truncal ataxia

Major Pathway

Purkinje cells → deep cerebellar nucleus; dentate nucleus → contralateral VL → first-degree motor cortex → pontine nuclei → contralateral cerebellar cortex

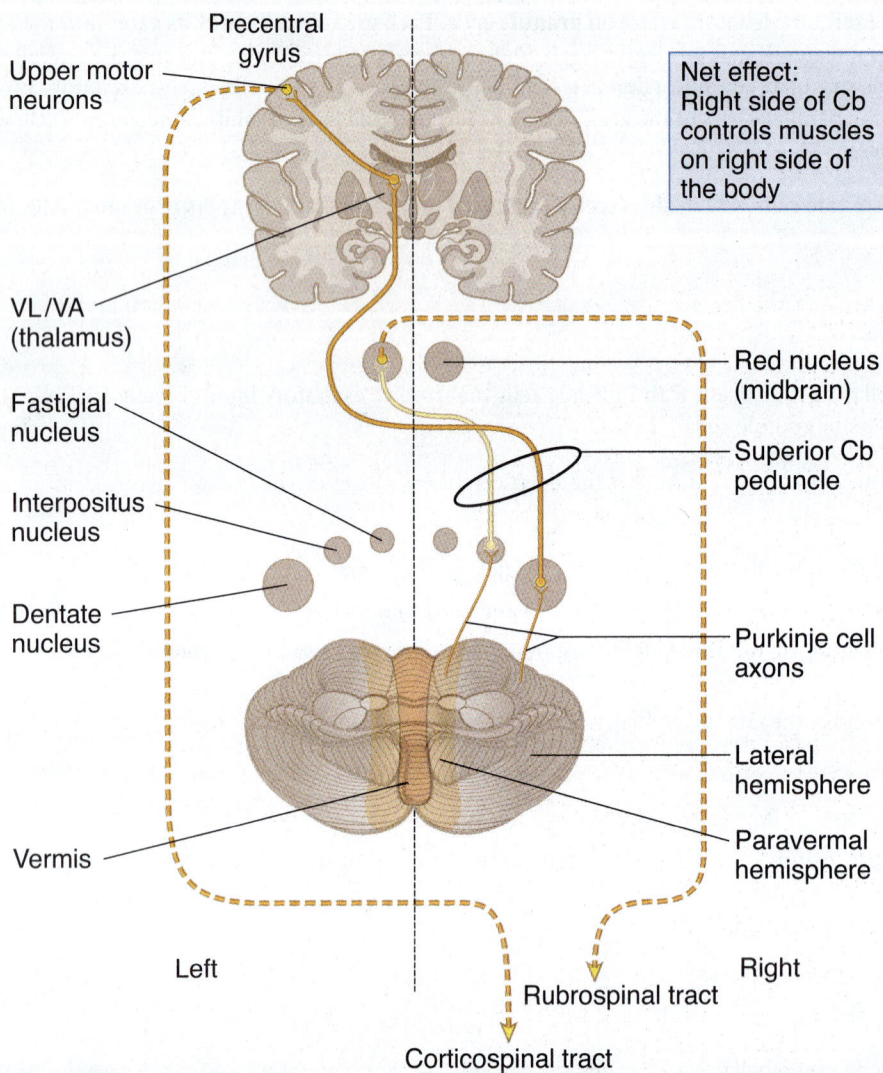

Figure 16-3. Cerebellar Efferents

Table 16-4. Major Efferents From the Cerebellum

Cerebellar Areas	Deep Cerebellar Nucleus	Efferents to:	Function
Vestibulocerebellum (flocculonodular lobe)	Fastigial nucleus	Vestibular nucleus	Elicit positional changes of eyes and trunk in response to movement of the head
Spinocerebellum (intermediate hemisphere)	Interpositus nucleus	Red nucleus Reticular formation	Influence LMNs via the reticulospinal and rubrospinal tracts to adjust posture and effect movement
Pontocerebellum (lateral hemispheres)	Dentate nucleus	Thalamus (VA, VL) then cortex	Influence on LMNs via the corticospinal tract, which effect voluntary movements, especially sequence and precision

Efferents from the deep cerebellar nuclei leave mainly through the SCP and influence all upper motoneurons. In particular, axons from the dentate and interposed nuclei leave through the SCP, cross the midline, and terminate in the ventrolateral (VL) nucleus of the thalamus.

The VL nucleus of the thalamus projects to primary motor cortex and influences the firing of corticospinal and corticobulbar neurons.

Axons from other deep cerebellar nuclei influence upper motoneurons in the red nucleus and in the reticular formation and vestibular nuclei.

Learning Objectives

❏ Solve problems concerning general features of the basal ganglia

GENERAL FEATURES

The basal ganglia initiate and provide gross control over skeletal muscle movements. The major components of the basal ganglia include:

- Striatum, which consists of the caudate nucleus and the putamen (telencephalon)
- External and internal segments of the globus pallidus (telencephalon)
- Substantia nigra (in midbrain)
- Subthalamic nucleus (in diencephalon)

Together with the cerebral cortex and the ventrolateral (VL) nucleus of the thalamus, these structures are interconnected to form two parallel but antagonistic circuits known as the direct and indirect basal ganglia pathways (Figures 17-1 and 17-2). Both pathways are driven by extensive inputs from large areas of cerebral cortex, and both project back to the motor cortex after a relay in the VL nucleus of the thalamus. Both pathways use a process known as "disinhibition" to mediate their effects, whereby one population of inhibitory neurons inhibits a second population of inhibitory neurons.

Direct Basal Ganglia Pathway

In the direct pathway, excitatory input from the cerebral cortex projects to striatal neurons in the caudate nucleus and putamen. Through disinhibition, activated inhibitory neurons in the striatum, which use γ-aminobutyric acid (GABA) as their neurotransmitter, project to and inhibit additional GABA neurons in the internal segment of the globus pallidus.

The GABA axons of the internal segment of the globus pallidus project to the thalamus (VL). Because their input to the thalamus is disinhibited, the thalamic input excites the motor cortex. The net effect of the disinhibition in the direct pathway results in an **increased** level of cortical excitation and the promotion of movement.

Indirect Basal Ganglia Pathway

In the indirect pathway, excitatory input from the cerebral cortex also projects to striatal neurons in the caudate nucleus and putamen. These inhibitory neurons in the striatum, which also use GABA as their neurotransmitter, project to and inhibit additional GABA neurons in the external segment of the globus pallidus.

The GABA axons of the external segment of the globus pallidus project to the subthalamic nucleus. Through disinhibition, the subthalamic nucleus excites inhibitory GABA neurons in the internal segment of the globus pallidus, which inhibits the thalamus. This decreases the level of cortical excitation, inhibiting movement. The net effect of the disinhibition in the indirect pathway results in a **decreased** level of cortical excitation, and a suppression of unwanted movement.

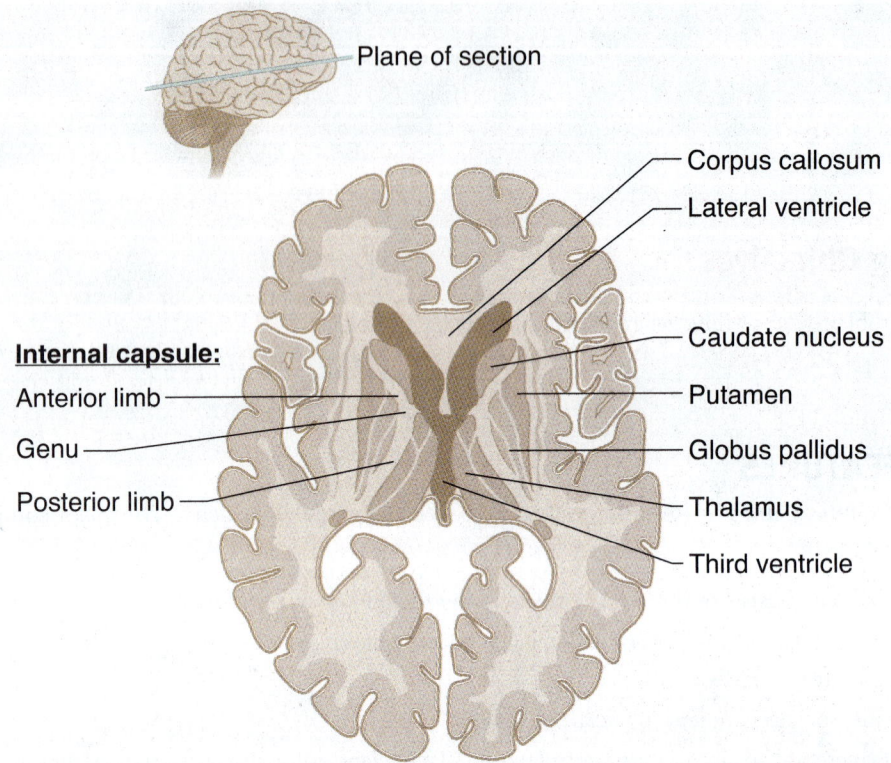

Plane of section

Internal capsule:

Anterior limb

Genu

Posterior limb

Corpus callosum

Lateral ventricle

Caudate nucleus

Putamen

Globus pallidus

Thalamus

Third ventricle

Figure 17-1.

Both basal ganglia pathways utilize 2 GABA neurons in series, and a "disinhibition."
Dopamine drives the direct pathway; acetylcholine (ACh) drives the indirect pathway.

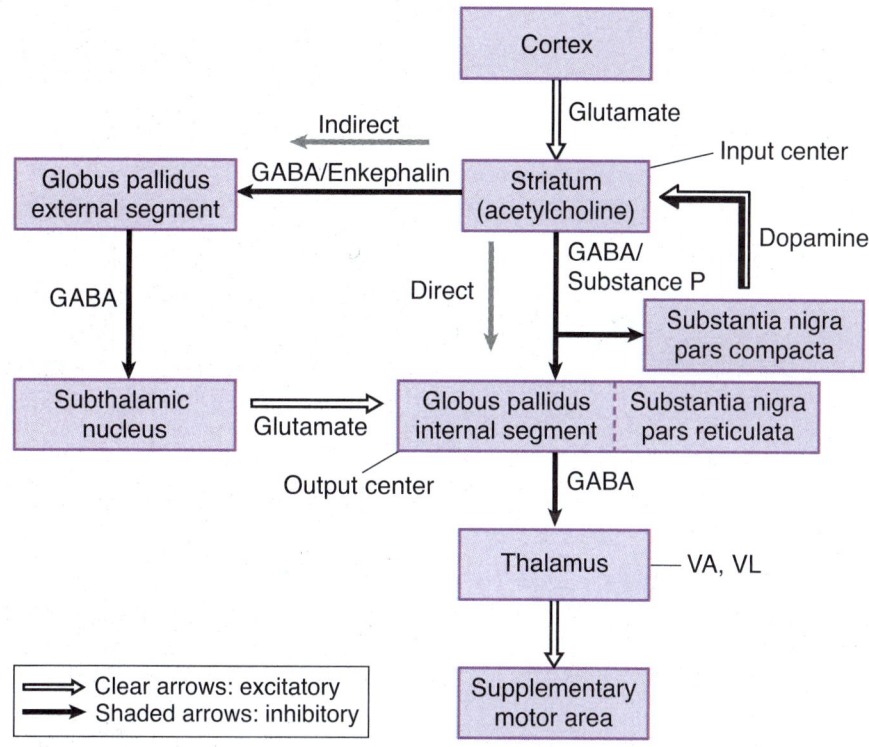

Figure 17-2.
VA/VL: ventral anterior/ventral lateral thalamic nuclei

Dopamine and cholinergic effects

In addition to the GABA neurons, two other sources of chemically significant neurons enhance the effects of the direct or indirect pathways.

Dopaminergic neurons in the substantia nigra in the midbrain project to the striatum. The effect of dopamine excites or drives the direct pathway, increasing cortical excitation. Dopamine excites the direct pathway through D_1 receptors and inhibits the indirect pathway through D_2 receptors.

Cholinergic neurons found within the striatum have the opposite effect. Acetylcholine (Ach) drives the indirect pathway, decreasing cortical excitation.

Visual Pathways 18

Learning Objectives

❏ Use knowledge of eyeball and optic nerve

❏ Solve problems concerning visual reflexes

EYEBALL AND OPTIC NERVE

Light must pass through the cornea, aqueous humor, pupil, lens, and vitreous humor before reaching the retina (Figure 18-1). It must then pass through the layers of the retina to reach the photoreceptive layer of rods and cones. The outer segments of rods and cones transduce light energy from photons into membrane potentials. Photopigments in rods and cones absorb photons, and this causes a conformational change in the molecular structure of these pigments. This molecular alteration causes sodium channels to close, a hyperpolarization of the membranes of the rods and cones, and a reduction in the amount of neurotransmitter released. Thus, rods and cones release less neurotransmitter in the light and more neurotransmitter in the dark.

Rods and cones have synaptic contacts on bipolar cells that project to ganglion cells. Axons from the ganglion cells converge at the optic disc to form the optic nerve, which enters the cranial cavity through the optic foramen. At the optic disc, these axons acquire a myelin sheath from the oligodendrocytes of the central nervous system (CNS).

Clinical Correlate

Vitamin A, necessary for retinal transduction, cannot be synthesized by humans. Dietary deficiency of vitamin A causes visual impairment resulting in night blindness.

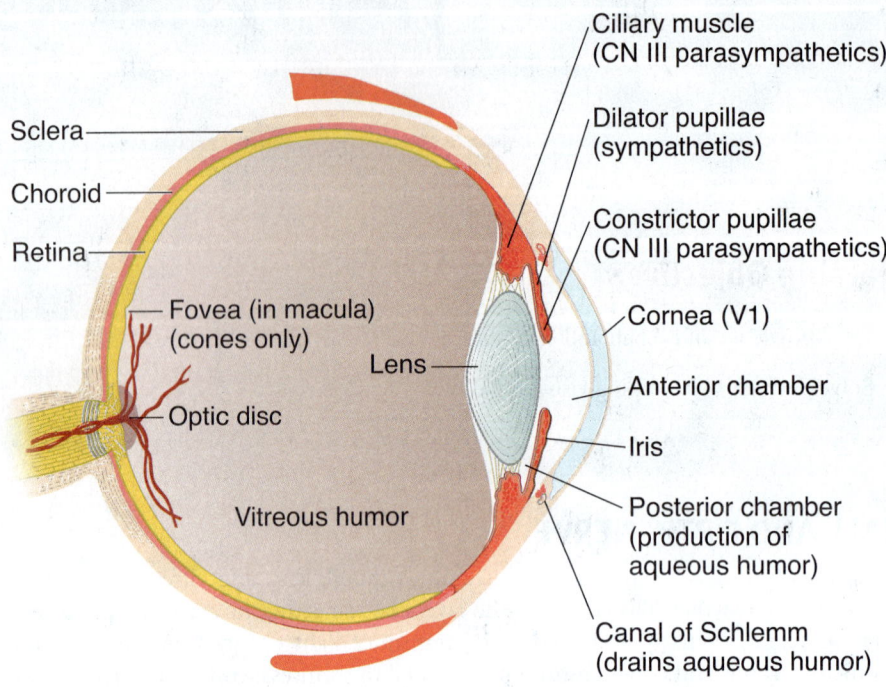

Figure 18-1. The Eyeball

Clinical Correlate

Decreased drainage into the canal of Schlemm is the most common cause of open-angle glaucoma.

Open-Angle Glaucoma

A chronic condition (often with increased intraocular pressure [IOP]) due to decreased reabsorption of aqueous humor, leading to progressive (painless) visual loss and, if left untreated, blindness. IOP is a balance between fluid formation and its drainage from the globe.

Narrow-Angle Glaucoma

An acute (painful) or chronic (genetic) condition with increased IOP due to blockade of the canal of Schlemm. Emergency treatment prior to surgery often involves cholinomimetics, carbonic anhydrase inhibitors, and/or mannitol.

VISUAL REFLEXES

Pupillary Light Reflex

When light is directed into an eye, it stimulates retinal photoreceptors and results in impulses carried in the optic nerve to the pretectal area. Cells in the pretectal area send axons to the Edinger-Westphal nuclei on both sides.

The Edinger-Westphal nucleus is the parasympathetic nucleus of the oculomotor nerve and gives rise to preganglionic parasympathetic fibers that pass in the third cranial nerve to the ciliary ganglion. Because cells in the pretectal area supply both Edinger-Westphal nuclei, shining light into one eye results in constriction of both the ipsilateral pupil (direct light reflex) and contralateral pupil (consensual light reflex).

Accommodation-Convergence Reaction

This reaction occurs when an individual attempts to focus on a nearby object after looking at a distant object. The oculomotor nerve carries the efferent fibers from the accommodation–convergence reaction, which consists of three components: accommodation, convergence, and pupillary constriction.

Accommodation refers to the reflex that increases the curvature of the lens needed for near vision. Preganglionic parasympathetic fibers arise in the Edinger-Westphal nucleus and pass via the oculomotor nerve to the ciliary ganglion. Postganglionic parasympathetic fibers from the ciliary ganglion supply the ciliary muscle. Contraction of this muscle relaxes the suspensory ligaments and allows the lens to increase its convexity (become more round). This increases the refractive index of the lens, permitting the image of a nearby object to focus on the retina.

Convergence results from contraction of both medial rectus muscles, which pull the eyes to look toward the nose. This allows the image of the near object to focus on the same part of the retina in each eye.

Pupillary constriction (miosis) results from contraction of the constrictor muscle of the iris. A smaller aperture gives the optic apparatus a greater depth of field. With Argyll Robertson pupils, both direct and consensual light reflexes are lost, but the accommodation–convergence reaction remains intact. This type of pupil is often seen in cases of neurosyphilis; however, it is sometimes seen in patients with multiple sclerosis, pineal tumors, or tabes dorsalis. The lesion site is believed to occur near the pretectal nuclei just rostral to the superior colliculi.

Table 18-1. Pupillary Light Reflex Pathway

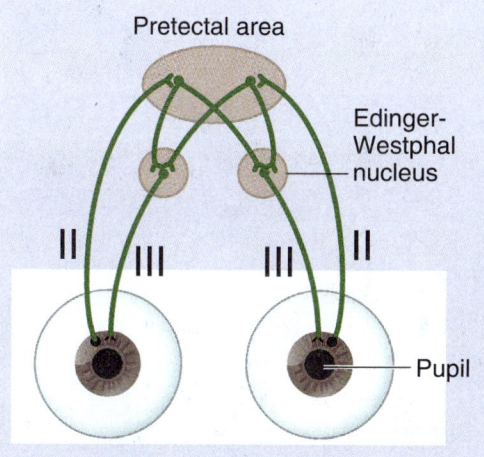

	Afferent Limb: CN II
Pretectal area	Light stimulates ganglion retinal cells → impulses travel up **CNII** which projects **bilaterally** to the **pretectal nuclei** (midbrain)
Edinger-Westphal nucleus	The pretectal nucleus projects **bilaterally** → **Edinger-Westphal nuclei (CN III)**
	Efferent Limb: CN III
Pupil	Edinger-Westphal nucleus (preganglionic parasympathetic) → **ciliary ganglion** (postganglionic parasympathetic) → **pupillary sphincter muscle** → **miosis**

Because cells in the pretectal area supply the Edinger-Westphal nuclei bilaterally, shining light in one eye → constriction in the ipsilateral pupil (direct light reflex) and the contralateral pupil (consensual light reflex).

Because this reflex does not involve the visual cortex, a person who is cortically blind can still have this reflex.

This is a simplified diagram; the ciliary ganglion is not shown.

Table 18-2. Accommodation-Convergence Reaction

When an individual focuses on a nearby object after looking at a distant object, 3 events occur:

1. **Accommodation**
2. **Convergence**
3. **Pupillary constriction (miosis)**

In general, stimuli from light → visual cortex → superior colliculus and pretectal nucleus → Edinger-Westphal nucleus (1, 3) and oculomotor nucleus (2).

Accommodation: Parasympathetic fibers contract the ciliary muscle, which relaxes suspensory ligaments, allowing the lens to increase its convexity (become more round). This increases the refractive index of the lens, thereby focusing a nearby object on the retina.

Convergence: Both medial rectus muscles contract, adducting both eyes.

Pupillary constriction: Parasympathetic fibers contract the pupillary sphincter muscle → miosis.

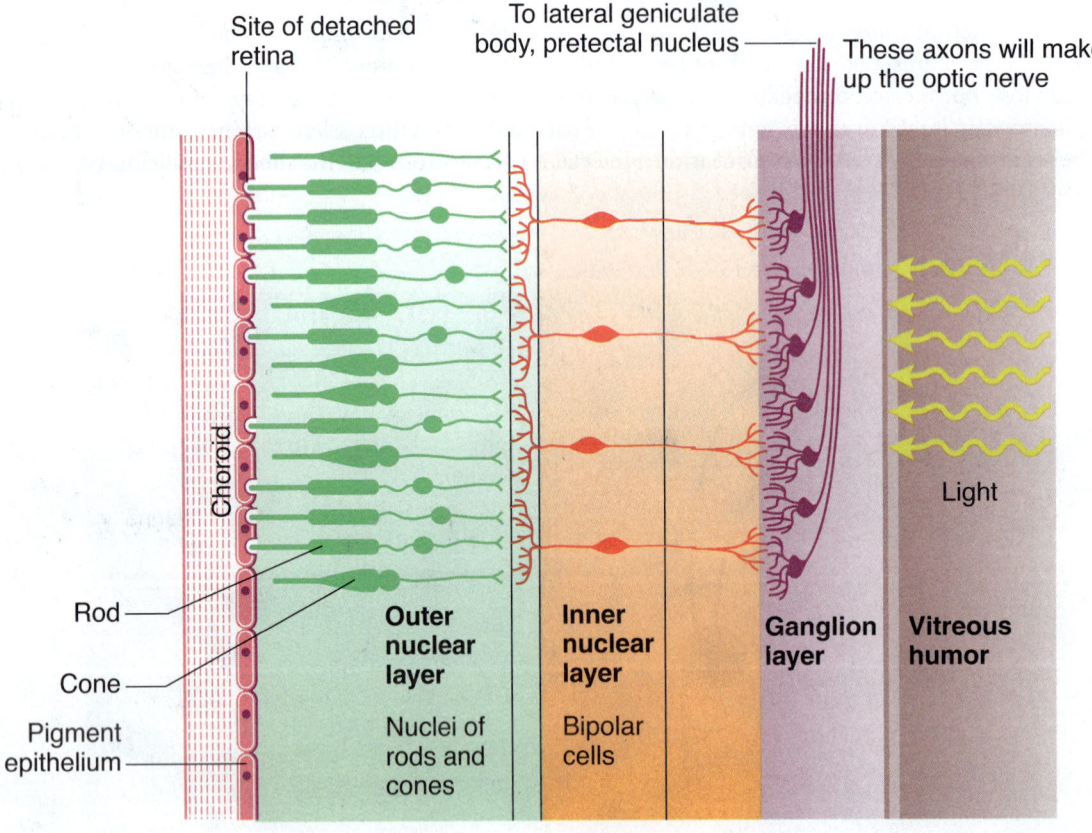

Figure 18-2. Retina

Notes

Photoreceptor Rods: one kind

- Achromatic
- Low-light sensitive
- Night vision, motion

Cones: 3 kinds

- Red, green, blue
- Chromatic
- Bright light sensitive
- Object recognition

At the optic chiasm, 60% of the optic nerve fibers from the nasal half of each retina cross and project into the contralateral optic tract (Figure 18-3). Fibers from the temporal retina do not cross at the chiasm and instead pass into the ipsilateral optic tract. The optic tract contains remixed optic nerve fibers from the temporal part of the ipsilateral retina and fibers from the nasal part of the contralateral retina. Because the eye inverts images like a camera, in reality each nasal retina receives information from a temporal hemifield, and each temporal retina receives information from a nasal hemifield. Most fibers in the optic tract project to the lateral geniculate nucleus. Optic tract fibers also project to the superior colliculi for reflex gaze, to the pretectal area for the light reflex, and to the suprachiasmatic nucleus of the hypothalamus for circadian rhythms.

Visual Field Defects

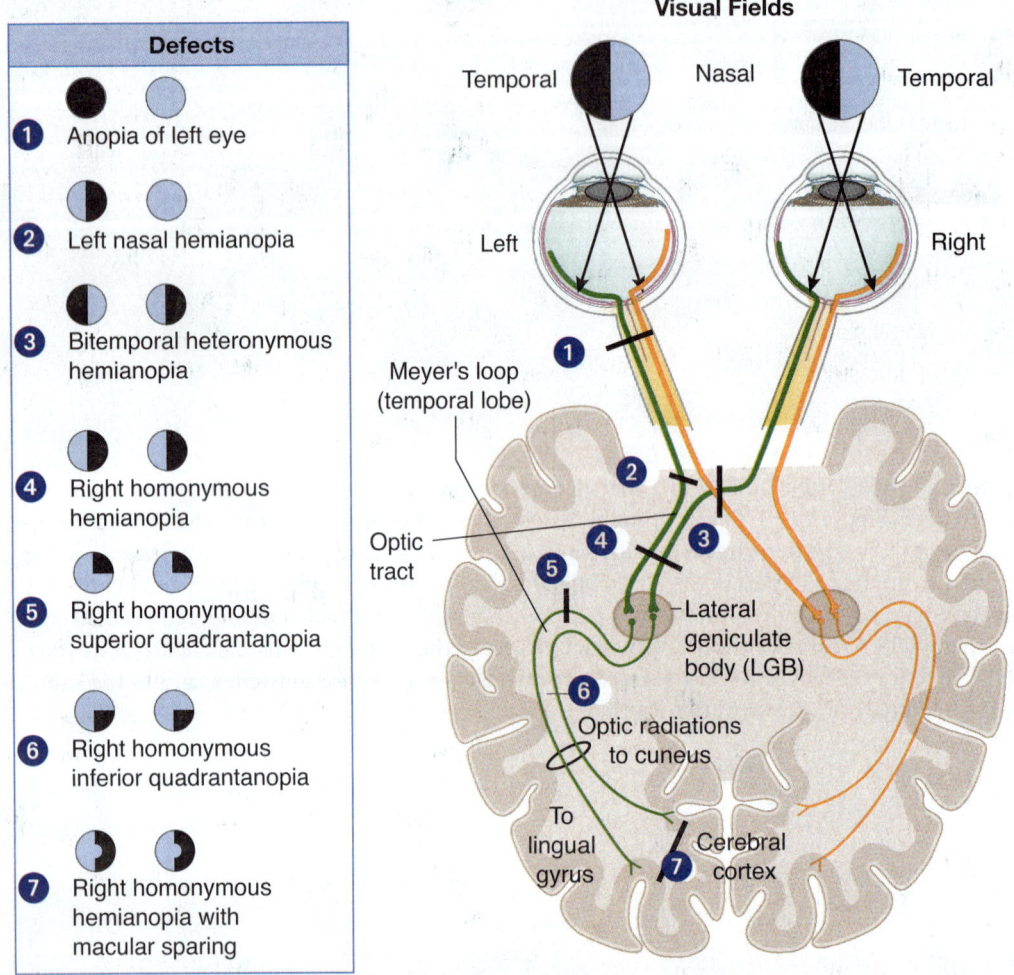

Figure 18-3. Visual Pathways 1, 2 Optic nerve, 3 Chiasm, 4 Tract

Visual information from **lower** retina courses in **lateral** fibers forming Meyer's **loop**, which projects to the lingual gyrus.

Notes

Like a camera, the lens inverts the image of the visual field, so the nasal retina receives information from the temporal visual field, and the temporal retina receives information from the nasal visual field.

At the **optic chiasm**, optic nerve fibers from the nasal half of each retina cross and project to the contralateral optic tract.

Most fibers from the **optic tract** project to the **lateral geniculate body (LGB)**; some also project to the pretectal area (light reflex), the superior colliculi (reflex gaze), and the suprachiasmatic nuclei (circadian rhythm). The LGB projects to the **primary visual cortex** (striate cortex, Brodmann area 17) of the occipital lobe via the optic radiations.

- Visual information from the lower retina (upper contralateral visual field) → temporal lobe (**Meyer loop**) → **lingual gyrus**
- Visual information from the upper retina (lower contralateral visual field) → parietal lobe → **cuneus gyrus**

The lateral geniculate body (LGB) is a laminated structure that receives input from the optic tract and gives rise to axons that terminate on cells in the primary visual cortex (striate cortex, Brodmann area 17) of the occipital lobe. The LGB laminae maintain a segregation of inputs from the ipsilateral and contralateral retina.

The axons from the LGB that project to the striate cortex are known as optic radiations, visual radiations, or the geniculocalcarine tract. The calcarine sulcus divides the striate cortex (primary visual cortex or Brodmann area 17) into the cuneus and the lingual gyri. The cuneus gyrus, which lies on the superior bank of the calcarine cortex, receives the medial fibers of the visual radiations. The lingual gyrus, which lies on the inferior bank of the calcarine cortex, receives the lateral fibers of the visual radiation. The medial fibers coursing in the visual radiations, which carry input from the upper retina (i.e., the lower contralateral visual field), pass from the LGB directly through the parietal lobe to reach the cuneus gyrus. Significantly, the lateral fibers coursing in the visual radiations, which carry input from the lower retina (i.e., the upper contralateral visual field), take a circuitous route from the LGB through Meyer loop anteriorly into the temporal lobe. The fibers of Meyer loop then turn posteriorly and course through the parietal lobe to reach the lingual gyrus in the striate cortex.

Learning Objectives

❏ Interpret scenarios on thalamus

❏ Demonstrate understanding of hypothalamus

❏ Use knowledge of epithalamus

The diencephalon can be divided into four parts: the thalamus, the hypothalamus, the epithalamus, and the subthalamus.

Diencephalon

Table 19-1. Thala cerebellum mus

Thalamus—serves as a major sensory relay for information that ultimately reaches the neocortex. Motor control areas (basal ganglia, cerebellum) also synapse in the thalamus before reaching the cortex. Other nuclei regulate states of consciousness.

Internal medullary lamina

Thalamic Nuclei	Input	Output
VPL	Sensory from **body and limbs**	Somatosensory cortex
VPM	Sensory from **face, taste**	Somatosensory cortex
VA/VL	**Motor** info from BG, cerebellum	Motor cortices
LGB	**Visual** from optic tract	First-degree visual cortex
MGB	**Auditory** from inferior colliculus	First-degree auditory cortex
AN	Mamillary nucleus (via mamillothalamic tract)	Cingulate gyrus (part of **Papez** circuit)
MD	(Dorsomedial nucleus). Involved in **memory** Damaged in **Wernicke-Korsakoff** syndrome	
Pulvinar	Helps integrate somesthetic, visual, and auditory input	
Midline/intralaminar	Involved in **arousal**	

Abbreviations: AN, anterior nuclear group; BG, basal ganglia; LGB, lateral geniculate body; MD, mediodorsal nucleus; MGB, medial geniculate body; VA, ventral anterior nucleus; VL, ventral lateral nucleus; VPL, ventroposterolateral nucleus; VPM, ventroposteromedial nucleus

THALAMUS

The thalamus serves as the major sensory relay for the ascending tactile, visual, auditory, and gustatory information that ultimately reaches the neocortex. Motor control areas such as the basal ganglia and cerebellum also synapse in thalamic nuclei before they reach their cortical destinations. Other nuclei participate in the regulation of states of consciousness.

Clinical Correlate

Thiamine deficiency in alcoholics results in degeneration of the dorsomedial nucleus of thalamus and the mammillary bodies, hippocampus, and vermis of the cerebellum (see chapter 20).

Major Thalamic Nuclei and Their Inputs and Outputs

Anterior nuclear group (part of the Papez circuit of limbic system)

Input is from the mammillary bodies via the mammillothalamic tract and from the cingulate gyrus; output is to the cingulate gyrus via the anterior limb of the internal capsule.

Medial nuclear group (part of limbic system)

Input is from the amygdala, prefrontal cortex, and temporal lobe; output is to the prefrontal cortex and cingulate gyrus. The most important nucleus is the dorsomedial nucleus.

Ventral nuclear group

Motor Nuclei

Ventral anterior nucleus (VA): Input to VA is from the globus pallidus, substantia nigra. Output is to the premotor and primary motor cortex.

Ventral lateral nucleus (VL): Input to VL is mainly from the globus pallidus and the dentate nucleus of the cerebellum. Output is to the primary motor cortex (Brodmann area 4).

Sensory Nuclei

Ventral posterolateral (VPL) nucleus: Input to VPL conveying somatosensory and nociceptive information ascends in the medial lemniscus and spinothalamic tract. Output is to primary somatosensory cortex (Brodmann areas 3, 1, and 2) of the parietal lobe.

Ventral posteromedial (VPM) nucleus: Input to VPM is from the ascending trigeminal and taste pathways. Output is to primary somatosensory cortex (Brodmann areas 3, 1, and 2) of the parietal lobe.

Medial geniculate body (nucleus): Input is from auditory information that ascends from the inferior colliculus. Output is to primary auditory cortex.

Lateral geniculate body (nucleus): Input is from the optic tract. Output is in the form of the geniculocalcarine or visual radiations that project to the primary visual (striate) cortex in the occipital lobe.

Midline and Intralaminar Nuclei

Midline and intralaminar nuclei receive input from the brain-stem reticular formation, and from the spinothalamic tract. Intralaminar nuclei send pain information to the cingulate gyrus.

These nuclei appear to be important in mediating desynchronization of the electroencephalogram (EEG) during behavioral arousal.

HYPOTHALAMUS

The hypothalamus is composed of numerous nuclei that have afferent and efferent connections with widespread regions of the nervous system, including the pituitary gland, the autonomic system, and the limbic system (Figure 19-1).

Table 19-2. Hypothalamus, Epithalamus, Subthalamus

Hypothalamus—helps maintain homeostasis; has roles in the autonomic, endocrine, and limbic systems	
Hypothalamic Nuclei	Functions and Lesions
Lateral hypothalamic	**Feeding center;** lesion → starvation
Ventromedial	**Satiety center;** lesion → hyperphagia, obesity, savage behavior
Suprachiasmatic	Regulates circadian rhythms, receives direct retinal input
Supraoptic and paraventricular	Synthesizes **ADH** and **oxytocin; regulates water balance** Lesion → **diabetes insipidus,** characterized by polydipsia and polyuria
Mamillary body	Input from hippocampus; damaged in Wernicke encephalopathy
Arcuate	Produces hypothalamic releasing and inhibiting factors and gives rise to tuberohypophysial tract Has neurons that produce dopamine (prolactin-inhibiting factor)
Anterior region	**Temperature regulation;** lesion → hyperthermia Stimulates the parasympathetic nervous system
Posterior region	**Temperature regulation;** lesion → poikilothermia (inability to thermoregulate) Stimulates sympathetic nervous system
Preoptic area	Regulates release of gonotrophic hormones; contains sexually dimorphic nucleus Lesion before puberty → arrested sexual development; lesion after puberty → amenorrhea or impotence
Dorsomedial	Stimulation → savage behavior
Epithalamus—Consists of pineal body and habenular nuclei. The **pineal body** secretes melatonin with a **circadian rhythm.**	
Subthalamus—The **subthalamic nucleus** is involved in **basal ganglia** circuitry. Lesion → **hemiballismus** (contralateral flinging movements of one or both extremities)	

Abbreviation: ADH, antidiuretic hormone

Major Hypothalamic Regions or Zones, and Their Nuclei

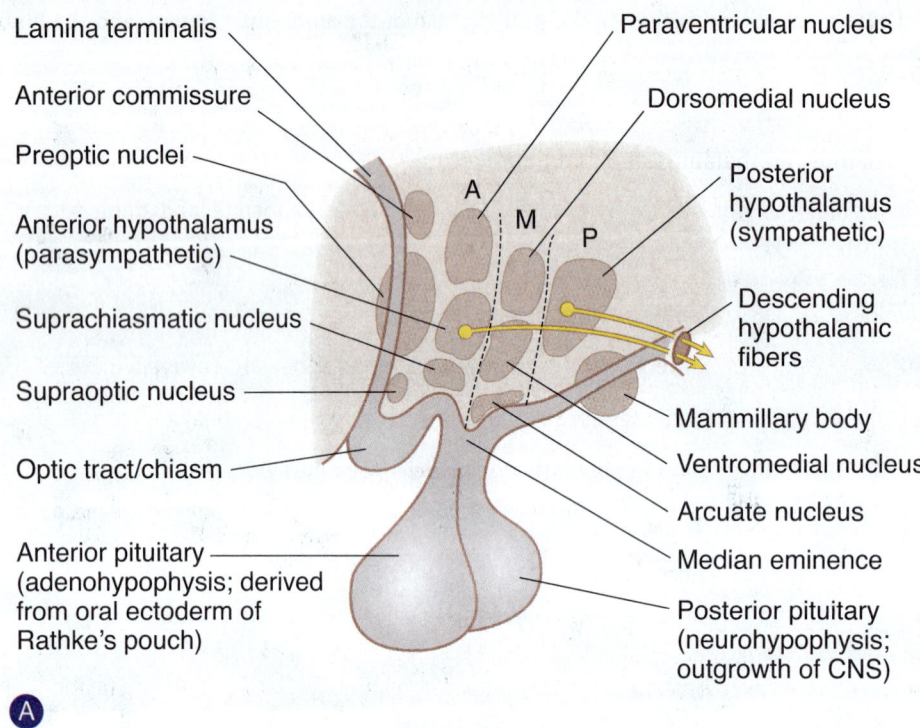

Lamina terminalis

Anterior commissure

Preoptic nuclei

Anterior hypothalamus
(parasympathetic)

Suprachiasmatic nucleus

Supraoptic nucleus

Optic tract/chiasm

Anterior pituitary
(adenohypophysis; derived
from oral ectoderm of
Rathke's pouch)

Paraventricular nucleus

Dorsomedial nucleus

Posterior
hypothalamus
(sympathetic)

Descending
hypothalamic
fibers

Mammillary body

Ventromedial nucleus

Arcuate nucleus

Median eminence

Posterior pituitary
(neurohypophysis;
outgrowth of CNS)

A

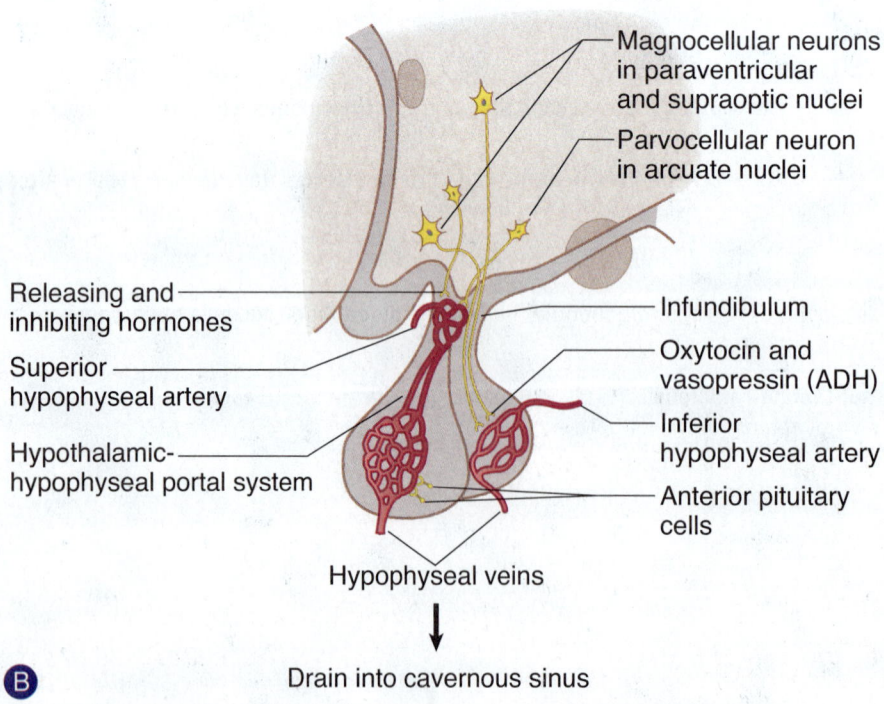

Magnocellular neurons
in paraventricular
and supraoptic nuclei

Parvocellular neuron
in arcuate nuclei

Releasing and
inhibiting hormones

Superior
hypophyseal artery

Hypothalamic-
hypophyseal portal system

Infundibulum

Oxytocin and
vasopressin (ADH)

Inferior
hypophyseal artery

Anterior pituitary
cells

Hypophyseal veins

Drain into cavernous sinus

B

Figure 19-1. (A) Organization of the Hypothalamus (Sagittal Section)
(B) Secretory Mechanisms of the Adeno- and Neuro-Hypophysis

Anterior region

Paraventricular and Supraoptic Nuclei

These nuclei synthesize the neuropeptides antidiuretic hormone (ADH) and oxytocin. Axons arising from these nuclei leave the hypothalamus and course in the supraopticohypophysial tract, which carries neurosecretory granules to the posterior pituitary gland, where they are released into capillaries. Lesions of the supraoptic nuclei lead to diabetes insipidus, which is characterized by polydipsia (excess water consumption) and polyuria (excess urination).

Suprachiasmatic Nucleus

Visual input from the retina by way of the optic tract terminates in the suprachiasmatic nucleus. This information helps set certain body rhythms to the 24-hour light-dark cycle (circadian rhythms).

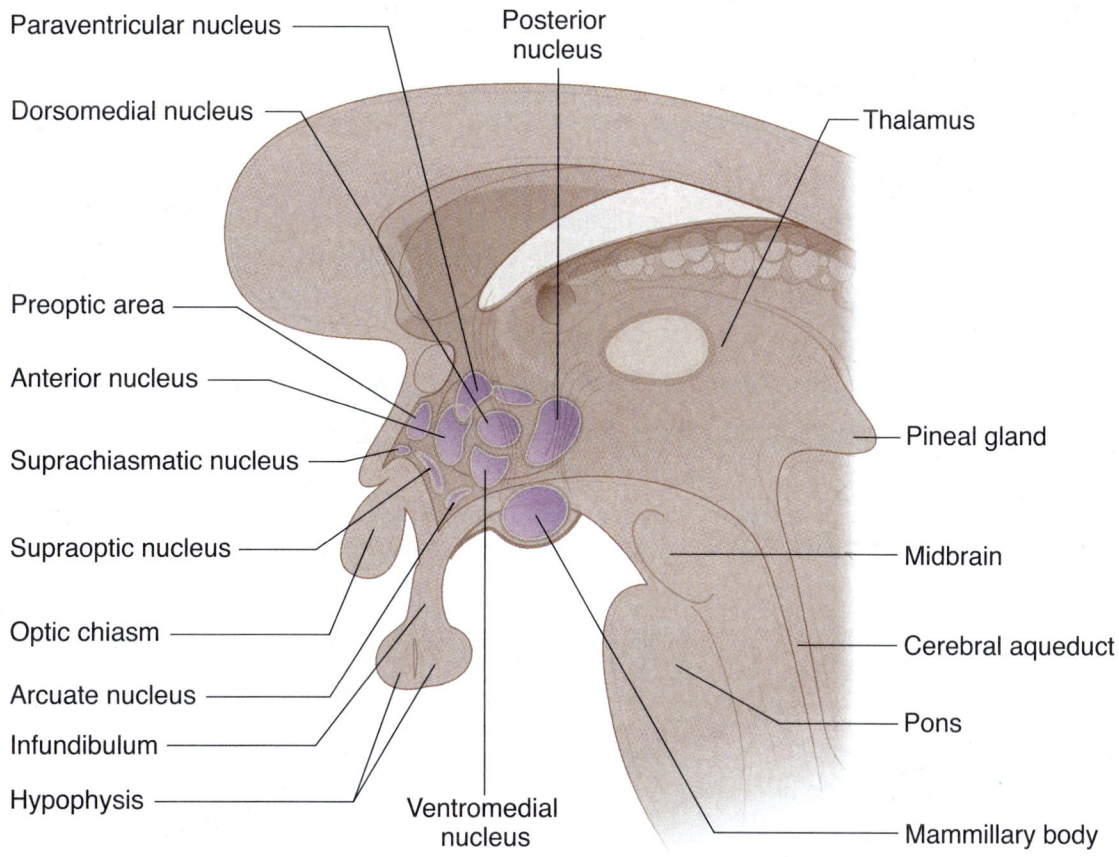

Figure 19-2. The Hypothalamic Nuclei

Tuberal region

Arcuate Nucleus

Cells in the arcuate nucleus produce releasing hormones and inhibitory factors, which enter capillaries in the tuberoinfundibular tract and pass through the hypophyseal-portal veins to reach the secondary capillary plexus in the anterior pituitary gland. Releasing hormones and inhibitory factors influence the secretory activity of the acidophils and basophils in the anterior pituitary. (See Histology section.)

Ventromedial Nucleus

The ventromedial hypothalamus is a satiety center and regulates food intake. Lesions of the ventromedial hypothalamus result in obesity.

Posterior region

Mammillary Bodies

The mammillary nuclei are located in the mammillary bodies and are part of the limbic system. The mammillothalamic tract originates in the mammillary nuclei and terminates in the anterior nuclear group of the thalamus.

Anterior hypothalamic zone

The anterior hypothalamic zone senses an elevation of body temperature and mediates the response to dissipate heat. Lesions of the anterior hypothalamus lead to hyperthermia.

Posterior hypothalamic zone

The posterior hypothalamic zone senses a decrease of body temperature and mediates the conservation of heat. Lesions of the posterior hypothalamus lead to poikilothermy (i.e., cold-blooded organisms). An individual with a lesion of the posterior hypothalamus has a body temperature that varies with the environmental temperature.

Lateral hypothalamic zone

The lateral hypothalamic zone is a feeding center; lesions of the lateral hypothalamus produce severe aphagia.

Preoptic area

The preoptic area is sensitive to androgens and estrogens, whereas other areas influence the production of sex hormones through their regulation of the anterior pituitary. Before puberty, hypothalamic lesions here may arrest sexual development.

After puberty, hypothalamic lesions in this area may result in amenorrhea or impotence.

EPITHALAMUS

The epithalamus is the part of the diencephalon located in the region of the posterior commissure that consists of the pineal body and the habenular nuclei.

The pineal body is a small, highly vascularized structure situated above the posterior commissure and attached by a stalk to the roof of the third ventricle.

The pineal body contains pinealocytes and glial cells but no neurons. Pinealocytes synthesize melatonin, serotonin, and cholecystokinin.

The pineal gland plays a role in growth, development, and the regulation of circadian rhythms.

Environmental light regulates the activity of the pineal gland through a retinal–suprachiasmatic– pineal pathway.

The subthalamus is reviewed with the basal ganglia.

Learning Objectives

❏ Answer questions about general features

❏ Solve problems concerning language and the dominant hemisphere

❏ Solve problems concerning blood supply

GENERAL FEATURES

The surface of the cerebral cortex is highly convoluted with the bulges or eminences, referred to as gyri; and the spaces separating the gyri, called sulci (Figures 20-1 and 20-2). Lobes of the cerebrum are divided according to prominent gyri and sulci that are fairly constant in humans.

Two prominent sulci on the lateral surface are key to understanding the divisions of the hemispheres. The lateral fissure (of Sylvius) separates the frontal and temporal lobes rostrally; further posteriorly, it partially separates the parietal and the temporal lobes. The central sulcus (of Rolando) is situated roughly perpendicular to the lateral fissure. The central sulcus separates the frontal and the parietal lobes. The occipital lobe extends posteriorly from the temporal and parietal lobes, but its boundaries on the lateral aspect of the hemisphere are indistinct. On the medial aspect of the hemisphere, the frontal and parietal lobes are separated by a cingulate sulcus from the cingulate gyrus. The cingulate is part of an artificial limbic lobe. Posteriorly, the parieto-occipital sulcus separates the parietal lobe from the occipital lobe. The calcarine sulcus divides the occipital lobe horizontally into a superior cuneus and an inferior lingual gyrus.

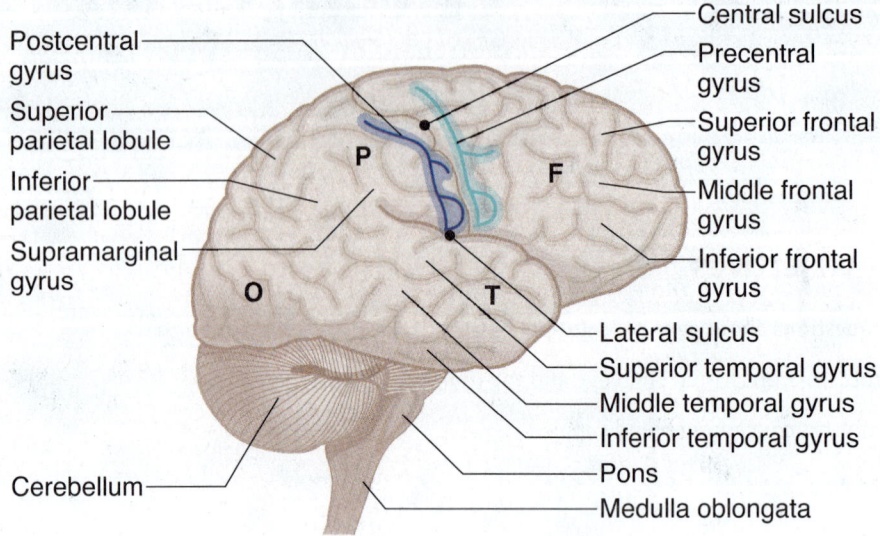

Figure 20-1. Lateral View of the Right Cerebral Hemisphere
F: frontal lobe
P: parietal lobe
T: temporal lobe
O: occipital lobe

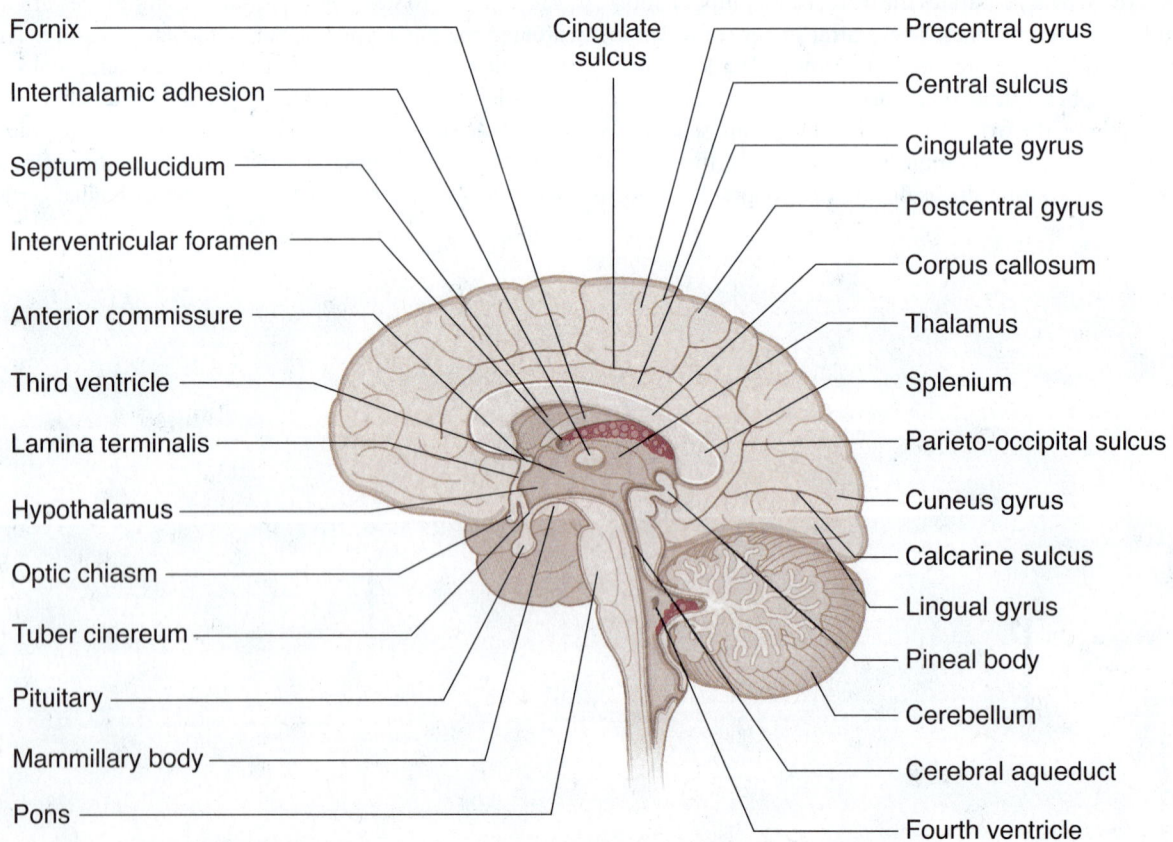

Figure 20-2. Medial View of the Right Cerebral Hemisphere

About 90% of the cortex is composed of six layers, which form the neocortex (Figure 20-5). The olfactory cortex and hippocampal formation are three-layered structures and together comprise the allocortex. All of the neocortex contains a six-layer cellular arrangement, but the actual structure varies considerably between different locations. On the basis of these variations in the cytoarchitecture, Brodmann divided the cortex into 47 areas, but only a few Brodmann numbers are used synonymously with functionally specific cortical areas.

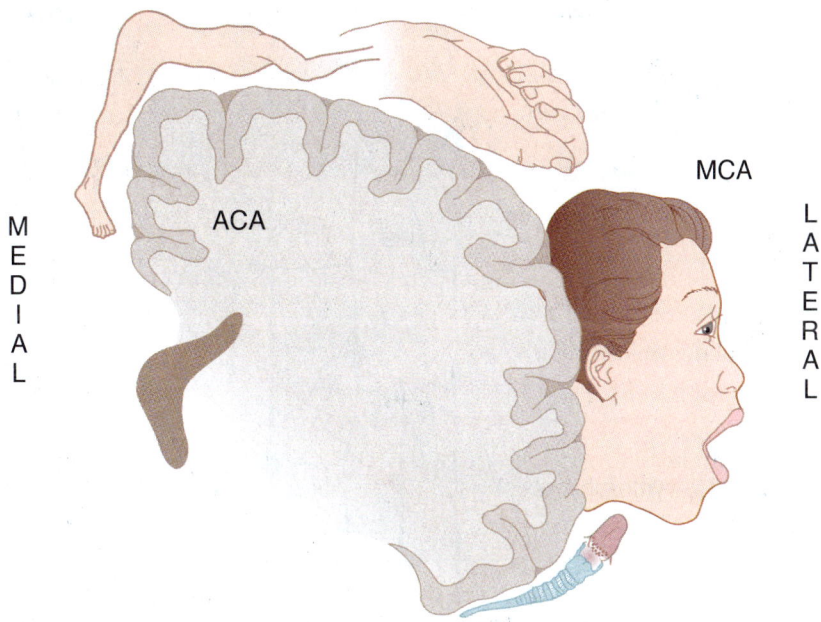

Figure 20-3. Motor Homunculus in Precentral Gyrus (Area 4)
Frontal Lobe (Coronal Section)

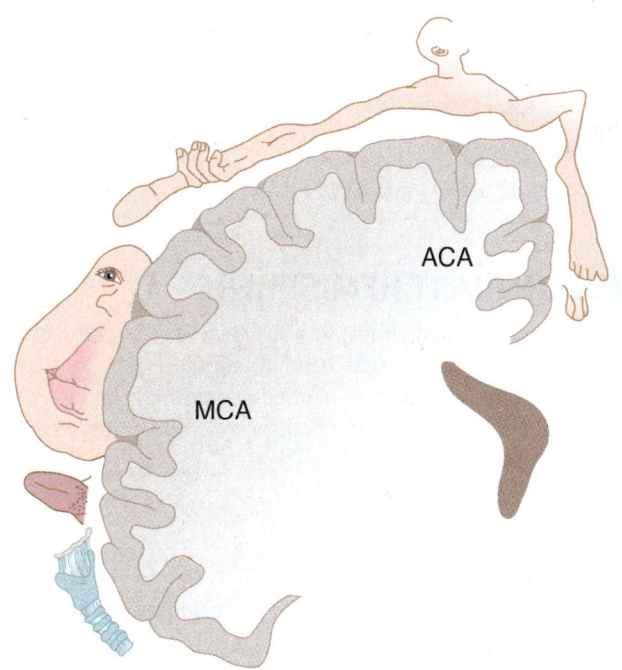

Figure 20-4. Sensory Homunculus in Postcentral Gyrus (Areas 3, 1, 2)
Parietal Lobe (Coronal Section)

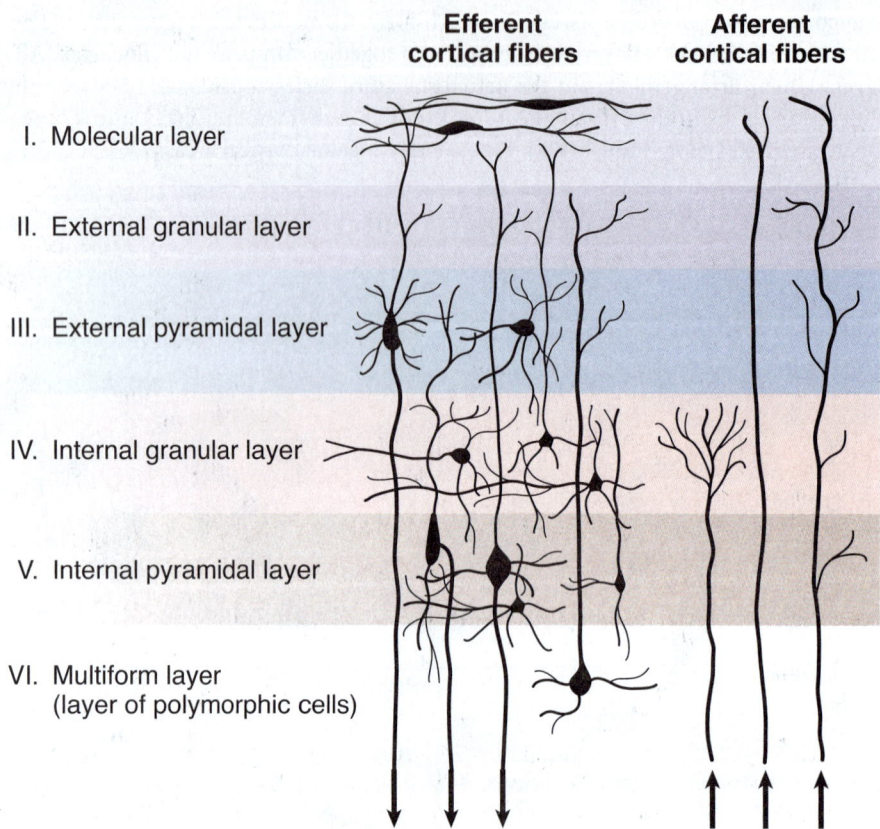

Efferent cortical fibers

Afferent cortical fibers

I. Molecular layer

II. External granular layer

III. External pyramidal layer

IV. Internal granular layer

V. Internal pyramidal layer

VI. Multiform layer
(layer of polymorphic cells)

Figure 20-5. The Six-Layered Neocortex

Note

The internal granular layer is the site of termination of the thalamocortical projections. In primary visual cortex, these fibers form a distinct Line of Gennari. The internal pyramidal layer gives rise to axons that form the corticospinal and corticobulbar tracts.

LANGUAGE AND THE DOMINANT HEMISPHERE

Most people (about 80%) are right-handed, which implies that the left side of the brain has more highly developed hand-controlling circuits. In the vast majority of right-handed people, speech and language functions are also predominantly organized in the left hemisphere. Most left-handed people show language functions bilaterally, although a few, with strong left-handed preferences, show right-sided speech and language functions.

BLOOD SUPPLY

The cortex is supplied by the 2 internal carotid arteries and the 2 vertebral arteries (Figures 20-6 and 20-7). On the base (or inferior surface) of the brain, branches of the internal carotid arteries and the basilar artery anastomose to form the circle of Willis. The anterior part of the circle lies in front of the optic chiasm, whereas the posterior part is situated just below the mammillary bodies. The circle of Willis is formed by the terminal part of the internal carotid arteries; the proximal parts of the anterior and posterior cerebral arteries and the anterior and posterior communicating arteries. The middle, anterior, and posterior cerebral arteries, which arise from the circle of Willis, supply all of the cerebral cortex, basal ganglia, and diencephalon.

The internal carotid artery arises from the bifurcation of the common carotid and enters the skull through the carotid canal. It enters the subarachnoid space and terminates by dividing into the anterior and middle cerebral arteries.

Just before splitting into the middle and anterior cerebral arteries, the internal carotid artery gives rise to the ophthalmic artery. The ophthalmic artery enters the orbit through the optic canal and supplies the eye, including the retina and optic nerve.

The middle cerebral artery is the larger terminal branch of the internal carotid artery. It supplies the bulk of the lateral surface of the hemisphere. Exceptions are the superior inch of the frontal and parietal lobes, which are supplied by the anterior cerebral artery, and the inferior part of the temporal lobe and the occipital pole, which are supplied by the posterior cerebral artery. The middle cerebral artery also supplies the genu and posterior limb of the internal capsule and the basal ganglia.

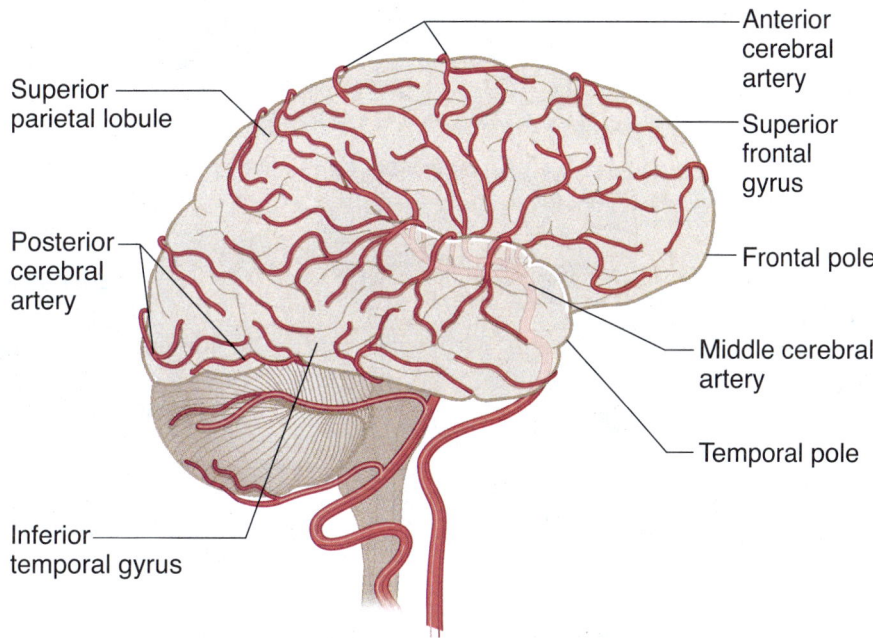

Figure 20-6. The Distributions of the Cerebral Arteries: Part 1

Note

The middle cerebral artery (MCA) supplies:

- the lateral surface of the frontal, parietal, and upper temporal lobes
- the posterior limb and genu of the internal capsule
- most of the basal ganglia

The anterior cerebral artery is the smaller terminal branch of the internal carotid artery. It is connected to the opposite anterior cerebral artery by the anterior communicating artery, completing the anterior part of the circle of Willis. The anterior cerebral artery supplies the medial surface of the frontal and parietal lobes, which include motor and sensory cortical areas for the pelvis and lower limbs. The anterior cerebral artery also supplies the anterior four-fifths of the corpus callosum and approximately 1 inch of the frontal and parietal cortex on the superior aspect of the lateral aspect of the hemisphere.

Occlusion of the anterior cerebral artery results in spastic paresis of the contralateral lower limb and anesthesia of the contralateral lower limb. Urinary incontinence may be present, but this usually occurs only with bilateral damage. A transcortical apraxia of the left limbs may result from involvement of the anterior portion of the corpus callosum. A transcortical apraxia occurs because the left hemisphere (language dominant) has been disconnected from the motor cortex of the right hemisphere. The anterior cerebral artery also supplies the anterior limb of the internal capsule.

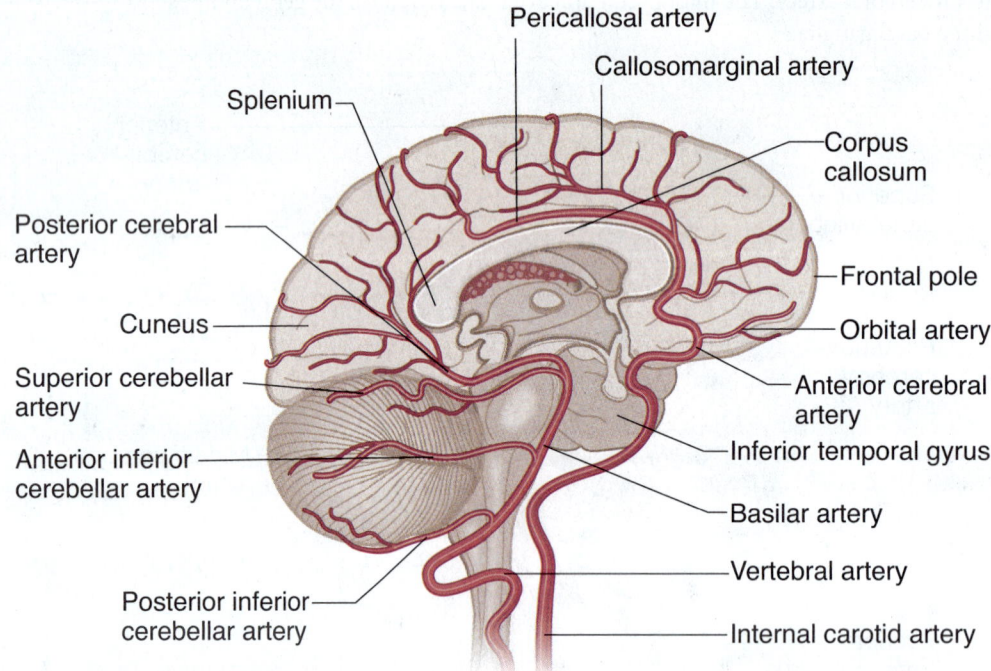

Figure 20-7. The Distributions of the Cerebral Arteries: Part 2

Notes

The anterior cerebral artery (ACA) Supplies:

1. Medial surface of frontal and parietal lobes
2. Anterior four-fifths of corpus callosum
3. Anterior limb of internal capsule

The posterior cerebral artery (PCA) Supplies:

1. Occipital lobe
2. Lower temporal lobe
3. Splenium
4. Midbrain

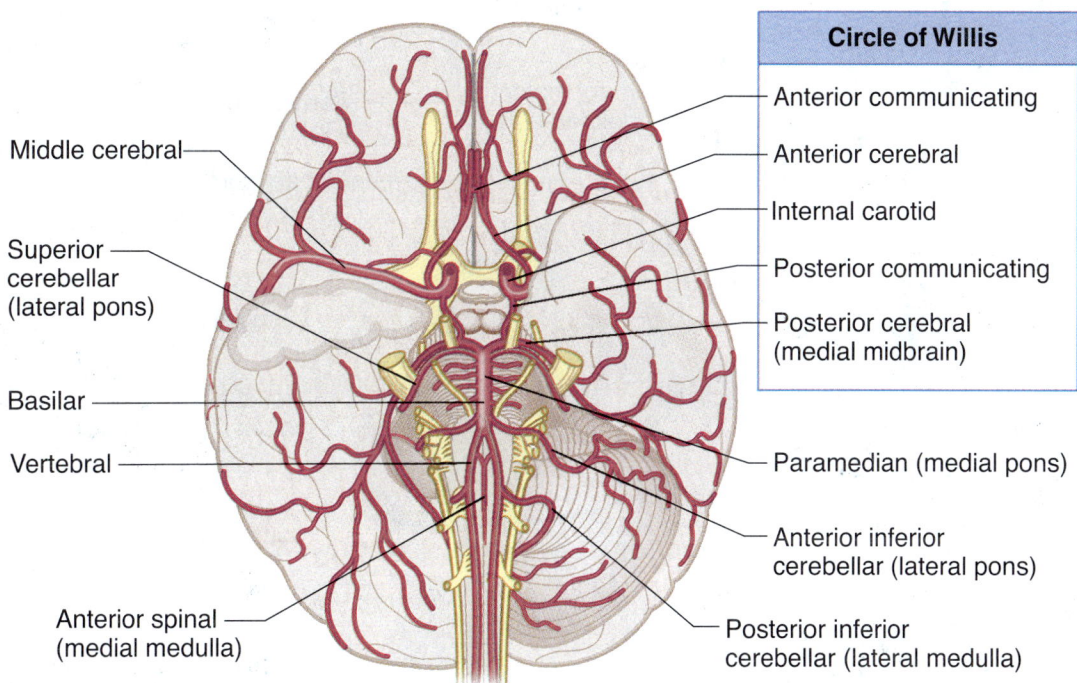

Middle cerebral

Superior cerebellar (lateral pons)

Basilar

Vertebral

Anterior spinal (medial medulla)

Circle of Willis

Anterior communicating

Anterior cerebral

Internal carotid

Posterior communicating

Posterior cerebral (medial midbrain)

Paramedian (medial pons)

Anterior inferior cerebellar (lateral pons)

Posterior inferior cerebellar (lateral medulla)

Figure 20-8. Arterial Supply of the Brain

Clinical Correlate

The most common aneurysm site in the circle of Willis is where the anterior communicating artery joins an anterior cerebral artery.

The posterior cerebral artery is formed by the terminal bifurcation of the basilar artery. The posterior communicating artery arises near the termination of the internal carotid artery and passes posteriorly to join the posterior cerebral artery. The posterior communicating arteries complete the circle of Willis by joining the vertebrobasilar and carotid circulations. The posterior cerebral artery supplies the occipital and temporal cortex on the inferior and lateral surfaces of the hemisphere, the occipital lobe and posterior two-thirds of the temporal lobe on the medial surface of the hemisphere, and the thalamus and subthalamic nucleus.

Occlusion of the posterior cerebral artery results in a homonymous hemianopia of the contralateral visual field with macular sparing.

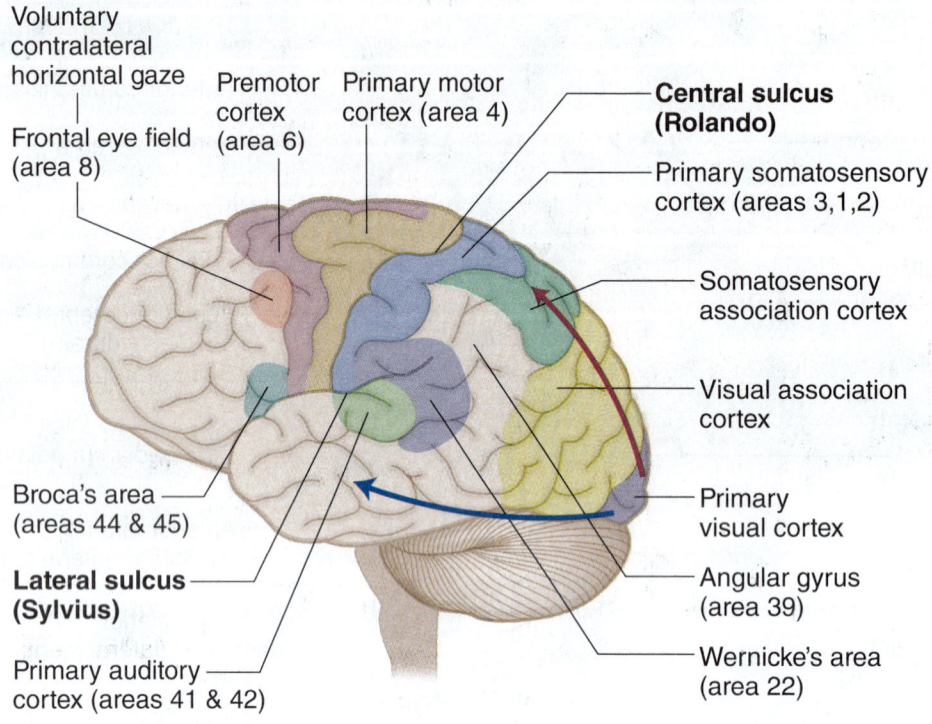

Figure 20-9. Cerebral Cortex: Functional Areas of Left (Dominant) Hemisphere

Frontal Lobe

A large part of the frontal cortex rostral to the central sulcus is related to the control of movements, primarily on the opposite side of the body. These areas include primary motor cortex (Brodmann area 4), premotor cortex (area 6), the frontal eye field (area 8), and the motor speech areas of Broca (area 44 and 45). Traditionally, area 4 is considered the primary motor cortex. It is in the precentral gyrus, immediately anterior to the central sulcus, and contains an orderly skeletal motor map of the contralateral side of the body.

The muscles of the head are represented most ventrally closest to the lateral fissure; then, proceeding dorsally, are the regions for the neck, upper limb, and trunk on the lateral aspect of the hemisphere. On the medial aspect of the hemisphere is the motor representation for the pelvis and lower limb.

Premotor cortex

Just anterior to area 4 is the premotor cortex (area 6). Neurons here are particularly active prior to the activation of area 4 neurons, so it is thought that the premotor cortex is involved in the planning of motor activities. Damage here results in an apraxia, a disruption of the patterning and execution of learned motor movements. Individual movements are intact, and there is no weakness, but the patient is unable to perform movements in the correct sequence.

Prefrontal cortex

The prefrontal cortex is located in front of the premotor area and represents about a quarter of the entire cerebral cortex in the human brain. This area is involved in organizing and planning the intellectual and emotional aspects of behavior, much as the adjacent premotor cortex is involved in planning its motor aspects.

Parietal Lobe

Primary somatosensory cortex

The parietal lobe begins just posterior to the central sulcus with the postcentral gyrus. The postcentral gyrus corresponds to Brodmann areas 3, 1, and 2 and contains primary somatosensory cortex. Like primary motor cortex, there is a similar somatotopic representation of the body here, with head, neck, upper limb, and trunk represented on the lateral aspect of the hemisphere, and pelvis and lower limb represented medially. These areas are concerned with discriminative touch, vibration, position sense, pain, and temperature. Lesions in somatosensory cortex result in impairment of all somatic sensations on the opposite side of the body, including the face and scalp.

Posterior parietal association cortex

Just posterior and ventral to the somatosensory areas is the posterior parietal association cortex, including Brodmann areas 5 and 7.

Wernicke area

The inferior part of the parietal lobe and adjacent part of the temporal lobe in the dominant (left) hemisphere, known as Wernicke area, are cortical regions that function in language comprehension. At a minimum, Wernicke area consists of area 22 in the temporal lobe but may also include areas 39 and 40 in the parietal lobe. Areas 39 (the angular gyrus) and 40 (the supramarginal gyrus) are regions of convergence of visual, auditory, and somatosensory information.

Occipital Lobe

The occipital lobe is essential for the reception and recognition of visual stimuli and contains primary visual and visual association cortex.

Visual cortex

The visual cortex is divided into striate (area 17) and extrastriate (areas 18 and 19). Area 17, also referred to as the primary visual cortex, lies on the medial portion of the occipital lobe on either side of the calcarine sulcus. Its major thalamic input is from the lateral geniculate nucleus. Some input fibers are gathered in a thick bundle that can be visible on the cut surface of the gross brain, called the line of Gennari. The retinal surface (and therefore the visual field) is represented in an orderly manner on the surface of area 17, such that damage to a discrete part of area 17 will produce a scotoma (i.e., a blind spot) in the corresponding portion of the visual field. A unilateral lesion inside area 17 results in a contralateral homonymous hemianopsia with macular sparing, usually caused by an infarct of a branch of the posterior cerebral artery. The area of the macula of the retina containing the fovea is spared because of a dual blood supply from both the posterior and middle cerebral arteries. The actual cortical area serving the macula is represented in the most posterior part of the occipital lobe. Blows to the back of the head or a blockage in occipital branches of the middle cerebral artery that supply this area may produce loss of macular representation of the visual fields. Bilateral visual cortex lesions result in cortical blindness; the patient cannot see, but pupillary reflexes are intact.

Visual association cortex

Anterior to the primary visual or striate cortex are extensive areas of visual association cortex. Visual association cortex is distributed throughout the entire occipital lobe and in the posterior parts of the parietal and temporal lobes. These regions receive fibers from the striate cortex and integrate complex visual input from both hemispheres. From the retina to the visual association cortex, information about form and color, versus motion, depth and spatial information are processed separately. Form and color information is processed by the parvocellular-blob system. This "cone stream" originates mainly in the central part of the retina, relays through separate layers of the lateral geniculate, and projects to blob zones of primary visual cortex. Blob zones project to the inferior part of the temporal lobe in areas 20 and 21. Unilateral lesions here result in achromatopsia, a complete loss of color vision in the contralateral hemifields. Patients see everything in shades of gray. Additionally, these patients may also present with prosopagnosia, an inability to recognize faces.

Motion and depth are processed by the magnocellular system. This "rod stream" originates in the peripheral part of the retina, relays through separate layers of the lateral geniculate, and projects to thick stripe zones of primary visual cortex. Striped areas project through the middle temporal lobe to the parietal lobe in areas 18 and 19. Lesions here result in a deficit in perceiving visual motion; visual fields, color vision, and reading are unaffected.

Temporal Lobe

Primary auditory cortex

On its superior and lateral aspect, the temporal lobe contains the primary auditory cortex. Auditory cortex (areas 41 and 42) is located on the 2 transverse gyri of Heschl, which cross the superior temporal lobe deep within the lateral sulcus. Much of the remaining superior temporal gyrus is occupied by area 22 (auditory association cortex), which receives a considerable projection from both areas 41 and 42 and projects widely to both parietal and occipital cortices.

Patients with unilateral damage to the primary auditory cortex show little loss of auditory sensitivity but have some difficulty in localizing sounds in the contralateral sound field. Area 22 is a component of Wernicke area in the dominant hemisphere, and lesions here produce a Wernicke aphasia.

Learning Objectives

❏ Solve problems concerning general features

❏ Solve problems concerning olfactory system

❏ Demonstrate understanding of limbic system

GENERAL FEATURES

The limbic system is involved in emotion, memory, attention, feeding, and mating behaviors. It consists of a core of cortical and diencephalic structures found on the medial aspect of the hemisphere. A prominent structure in the limbic system is the hippocampal formation on the medial aspect of the temporal lobe. The hippocampal formation extends along the floor of the inferior horn of the lateral ventricle in the temporal lobe and includes the hippocampus, the dentate gyrus, the subiculum, and adjacent entorhinal cortex. The hippocampus is characterized by a 3-layered cerebral cortex. Other limbic-related structures include the amygdala, which is located deep in the medial part of the anterior temporal lobe rostral to the hippocampus, and the septal nuclei, located medially between the anterior horns of the lateral ventricle. The limbic system is interconnected with thalamic and hypothalamic structures, including the anterior and dorsomedial nuclei of the thalamus and the mammillary bodies of the hypothalamus. The cingulate gyrus is the main limbic cortical area. The cingulate gyrus is located on the medial surface of each hemisphere above the corpus callosum. Limbic-related structures also project to wide areas of the prefrontal cortex.

In a Nutshell

Functions of the Limbic System

- Visceral–smell
- Sex drive
- Memory/Learning
- Behavior and emotions

OLFACTORY SYSTEM

Central projections of olfactory structures reach parts of the temporal lobe without a thalamic relay and the amygdala. The olfactory nerve consists of numerous fascicles of the central processes of bipolar neurons, which reach the anterior cranial fossa from the nasal cavity through openings in the cribriform plate of the ethmoid bone. These primary olfactory neurons differ from other primary sensory neurons in two ways. First, the cell bodies of these neurons, which lie scattered in the olfactory mucosa, are not collected together in a sensory ganglion, and second, primary olfactory neurons are continuously replaced. The life span of these cells ranges from 30 to 120 days in mammals.

Within the mucosa of the nasal cavity, the peripheral process of the primary olfactory neuron ramifies to reach the surface of the mucous membrane. The central processes of primary olfactory neurons terminate by synapsing with neurons found in the olfactory bulb. The bulb is a 6-layered outgrowth of the brain that rests on the cribriform plate. Olfactory information entering the olfactory bulb undergoes a great deal of convergence before the olfactory tract carries axons from the bulb to parts of the temporal lobe and amygdala.

Clinical Correlate

Olfactory deficits may be incomplete (hyposmia), distorted (dysosmia), or complete (anosmia). Olfactory deficits are caused by transport problems or by damage to the primary olfactory neurons or to neurons in the olfactory pathway to the central nervous system (CNS). Head injuries that fracture the cribriform plate can tear the central processes of olfactory nerve fibers as they pass through the plate to terminate in the olfactory bulb, or they may injure the bulb itself. Because the olfactory bulb is an outgrowth of the CNS covered by meninges, separation of the bulb from the plate may tear the meninges, resulting in cerebrospinal fluid (CSF) leaking through the cribriform plate into the nasal cavity.

LIMBIC SYSTEM

The limbic system is involved in emotion, memory, attention, feeding, and mating behaviors. It consists of a core of cortical and diencephalic structures found on the medial aspect of the hemisphere. The limbic system modulates feelings, such as fear, anxiety, sadness, happiness, sexual pleasure, and familiarity.

The Papez Circuit

A summary of the simplified connections of the limbic system is expressed by the Papez circuit. The Papez circuit oversimplifies the role of the limbic system in modulating feelings, such as fear, anxiety, sadness, happiness, sexual pleasure, and familiarity; yet, it provides a useful starting point for understanding the system. Arbitrarily, the Papez circuit begins and ends in the hippocampus. Axons of hippocampal pyramidal cells converge to form the fimbria and, finally, the fornix. The fornix projects mainly to the mammillary bodies in the hypothalamus. The mammillary bodies, in turn, project to the anterior nucleus of the thalamus by way of the mammillothalamic tract. The anterior nuclei project to the cingulate gyrus through the anterior limb of the internal capsule, and the cingulate gyrus communicates with the hippocampus through the cingulum and entorhinal cortex.

The amygdala functions to attach an emotional significance to a stimulus and helps imprint the emotional response in memory.

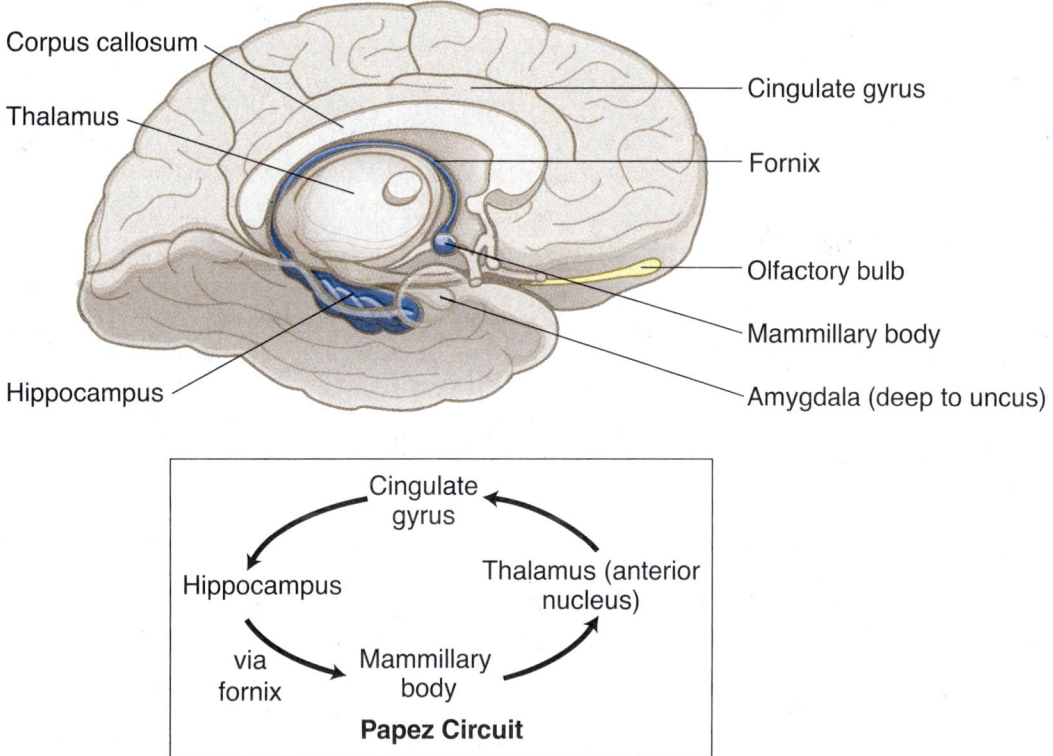

Figure 21-1. The Limbic System and Papez Circuit

Limbic Structures and Function

- Hippocampal formation (hippocampus, dentate gyrus, the subiculum, and entorhinal cortex)
- Amygdala
- Septal nuclei
- The hippocampus is important in learning and memory. The amygdala attaches an emotional significance to a stimulus and helps imprint the emotional response in memory.

Limbic Connections

- The limbic system is interconnected with anterior and dorsomedial nuclei of the thalamus and the mammillary bodies.
- The cingulate gyrus is the main limbic cortical area.
- Limbic-related structures also project to wide areas of the prefrontal cortex.
- Central projections of olfactory structures reach parts of the temporal lobe and the amygdala.

Papez Circuit

Axons of hippocampal pyramidal cells converge to form the fimbria and, finally, the fornix. The fornix projects mainly to the mammillary bodies in the hypothalamus. The mammillary bodies project to the anterior nucleus of the thalamus (mammillothalamic tract). The anterior nuclei project to the cingulate gyrus, and the cingulate gyrus projects to the entorhinal cortex (via the cingulum). The entorhinal cortex projects to the hippocampus (via the perforant pathway).

Microbiology

General Microbiology

1

Learning Objectives

❏ Answer questions about infectious disease epidemiology, pathogenicity, and major mechanisms of infectivity and toxicity

❏ Demonstrate knowledge about bacterial toxins

EPIDEMIOLOGY

Normal Flora

- Is found on body surfaces contiguous with the outside environment
- Is semi-permanent, varying with major life changes
- Can cause infection
  - if misplaced, e.g., fecal flora to urinary tract or abdominal cavity, or skin flora to catheter
  - or, if person becomes compromised, normal flora may overgrow (oral thrush)
- Contributes to health
  - protective host defense by maintaining conditions such as pH so other organisms may not grow
  - serves nutritional function by synthesizing: K and B vitamins
  - competition for space

In a Nutshell

Definitions:

Carrier: person colonized by a potential pathogen without overt disease.

Bacteremia: bacteria in bloodstream without overt clinical signs.

Septicemia: bacteria in bloodstream (multiplying) with clinical symptoms.

Table 1-1. Important Normal Flora

Site	Common or Medically Important Organisms	Less Common but Notable Organisms
Blood, internal organs	None, generally sterile	
Cutaneous surfaces including urethra and outer ear	*Staphylococcus epidermidis*	*Staphylococcus aureus*, Corynebacteria (diphtheroids), streptococci, anaerobes, e.g., peptostreptococci, yeasts (*Candida* spp.)
Nose	*Staphylococcus aureus*	*S. epidermidis*, diphtheroids, assorted streptococci
Oropharynx	**Viridans streptococci** including *Strep. mutans*[1]	Assorted streptococci, **nonpathogenic** *Neisseria*, **nontypeable**[2] *Haemophilus influenzae*, **Candida albicans**
Gingival crevices	Anaerobes: *Bacteroides, Prevotella, Fusobacterium, Streptococcus, Actinomyces*	
Stomach	None	
Colon (microaerophilic/anaerobic)	Babies; breast-fed only: *Bifidobacterium*	*Lactobacillus*, streptococci
	Adult: **Bacteroides**/*Prevotella* (Predominant organism) *Escherichia Bifidobacterium*	*Eubacterium, Fusobacterium, Lactobacillus*, assorted Gram-negative anaerobic rods, *Enterococcus faecalis* and other streptococci
Vagina	**Lactobacillus**[3]	Assorted streptococci, gram-negative rods, diphtheroids, yeasts, *Veillonella*

[1]**S. mutans** secretes a biofilm that glues it and other oral flora to teeth, producing **dental plaque**.

[2]Nontypeable for *Haemophilus* means no capsule.

[3]Group B streptococci colonize vagina of 15–20% of women and may infect the infant during labor or delivery, causing septicemia and/or meningitis (as may *E. coli* from fecal flora).

PATHOGENICITY (INFECTIVITY AND TOXICITY) MAJOR MECHANISMS

Colonization

(Important unless organism is traumatically implanted.)

Adherence to cell surfaces involves

- **Pili/fimbriae:** primary mechanism in most gram-negative cells.
- **Teichoic acids:** primary mechanism of gram-positive cells.
- **Adhesins:** colonizing factor adhesins, pertussis toxin, and hemagglutinins.
- **IgA proteases:** make it easier for pathogens to colonize.

Partial adherence to inert materials, **biofilms**: *Staph. epidermidis, Streptococcus mutans, Pseudomonas aeruginosa*

Avoiding Immediate Destruction by Host Defense System:

- **Anti-phagocytic surface components** (inhibit phagocytic uptake):
  - **Capsules**/slime layers:

    Streptococcus pyogenes M protein
    Streptococcus pneumoniae capsule
    Neisseria gonorrhoeae pili
    Staphylococcus aureus A protein
- **IgA proteases,** destruction of mucosal IgA: *Neisseria, Haemophilus, S. pneumoniae*

Note

Mnemonic

Streptococcus pneumoniae

Klebsiella pneumoniae

Haemophilus influenzae

Pseudomonas aeruginosa

Neisseria meningitidis

Cryptococcus neoformans

(**S**ome **K**illers **H**ave **P**retty **N**ice **C**apsules)

"Hunting and Gathering" Needed Nutrients:

- **Siderophores** steal (chelate) and import iron.

Antigenic Variation

- Changing surface antigens to avoid immune destruction
- *N. gonorrhoeae*—pili and outer membrane proteins
- *Trypanosoma brucei rhodesiense* and *T. b. gambiense*—phase variation
- Enterobacteriaceae: capsular and flagellar antigens may or may not be expressed
- HIV, influenza—antigenic drift

Ability to Survive Intracellularly

- **Evading intracellular killing by professional phagocytic cells** allows intracellular growth:

  — *M. tuberculosis* survives by inhibiting phagosome-lysosome fusion.

  — *Listeria* quickly escapes the phagosome into the cytoplasm **before** phagosome-lysosome fusion.

- **Invasins**: surface proteins that allow an organism to bind to and invade normally non-phagocytic human cells, escaping the immune system. Best studied invasin is on *Yersinia pseudotuberculosis* (an organism causing diarrhea).

- Damage from viruses is largely from intracellular replication, which either kills cells, transforms them or, in the case of latent viruses, may do no noticeable damage.

Type III Secretion Systems

- Tunnel from the bacteria to the host cell (macrophage) that delivers bacterial toxins directly to the host cell

- Have been demonstrated in many pathogens: *E. coli, Salmonella* species, *Yersinia* species, *P. aeruginosa*, and *Chlamydia*

Inflammation or Immune-Mediated Damage

Examples

- **Cross-reaction of bacteria-induced antibodies with tissue antigens** causes disease. Rheumatic fever (RF) is one example.

- **Delayed hypersensitivity and the granulomatous response** stimulated by the presence of intracellular bacteria is responsible for neurological damage in leprosy, cavitation in tuberculosis, and fallopian tube blockage resulting in infertility from *Chlamydia* PID (pelvic inflammatory disease).

- **Immune complexes** damage the kidney in post streptococcal acute glomerulonephritis (PSG).

- **Peptidoglycan-teichoic acid** (large fragments) of gram-positive cells:

  — Serves as a structural toxin released when cells die.

  — Chemotactic for neutrophils.

Physical Damage

- Swelling from infection in a fixed space damages tissues; examples: meningitis and cysticercosis.

- Large physical size of organism may cause problems; example: *Ascaris lumbricoides* blocking bile duct.

- Aggressive tissue invasion from *Entamoeba histolytica* causes intestinal ulceration and releases intestinal bacteria, compounding problems.

TOXINS

Toxins may aid in invasiveness, damage cells, inhibit cellular processes, or trigger immune response and damage.

Structural Toxins

- **Endotoxin** (Lipopolysaccharide = LPS)
  - LPS is part of the **gram-negative outer membrane.**
  - **Toxic portion is lipid A**: generally not released (and toxic) until death of cell. Exception: *N. meningitidis*, which over-produces outer membrane fragments.
  - **LPS is heat stable** and not strongly immunogenic so it **cannot be converted to a toxoid.**
  - Mechanism
    - **LPS activates macrophages,** leading to release of TNF-alpha, IL-1, and IL-6.
    - IL-1 is a major mediator of fever.
    - Macrophage activation and products lead to tissue damage.
    - Damage to the endothelium from **bradykinin-induced vasodilation leads to shock.**
    - **Coagulation** (DIC) is mediated through the **activation of Hageman factor**.
- **Peptidoglycan, Teichoic Acids**

Exotoxins

- Are **protein toxins,** generally **quite toxic** and **secreted by** bacterial **cells** (somegram +, some gram –)
- **Can be modified** by chemicals or heat to produce a **toxoid** that still is **immunogenic, but no longer toxic** so can be used as a vaccine
- **A-B** (or "two") **component** protein toxins
  - **B** component **binds** to specific cell receptors to facilitate the internalization of A.
  - **A** component is the **active (toxic) component** (often an enzyme such as an ADP ribosyl transferase).
  - Exotoxins may be subclassed as enterotoxins, neurotoxins, or cytotoxins.
- **Cytolysins**: lyse cells from outside by damaging membrane.
  - *C. perfringens* **alpha toxin** is a **lecithinase.**
  - *Staphylococcus aureus*alpha **toxin** inserts itself to form **pores** in the membrane.

Table 1-2. Major Exotoxins

	Organism (Gram)	Toxin	Mode of Action	Role in Disease
Inhibitors of Protein Synthesis	*Corynebacterium diphtheriae* (+)	Diphtheria toxin	ADP ribosyl transferase; inactivates eEF-2; 1′ targets: heart/nerves/epithelium	Inhibits eukaryotic cell protein synthesis
	Pseudomonas aeruginosa (−)	Exotoxin A	ADP ribosyl transferase; inactivates eEF-2; 1′ target: liver.	Inhibits eukaryotic cell protein synthesis
	Shigella dysenteriae (−)	Shiga toxin	Interferes with 60S ribosomal subunit	Inhibits protein synthesis in eukaryotic cells. Enterotoxic, cytotoxic, and neurotoxic
	Enterohemorrhagic *E. coli* (EHEC) (−)	Verotoxin (a shiga-like toxin)	Interferes with 60S ribosomal subunit	Inhibits protein synthesis in eukaryotic cells
Neurotoxins	*Clostridium tetani* (+)	Tetanus toxin	Blocks release of the inhibitory transmitters glycine and GABA	Inhibits neurotransmission in inhibitory synapses
	Clostridium botulinum (+)	Botulinum toxin	Blocks release of acetylcholine	Inhibits cholinergic synapses
Super-antigens	*Staphylococcus aureus* (+)	TSST-1	Superantigen	Fever, increased susceptibility to LPS, rash, shock, capillary leakage
	Streptococcus pyogenes (+)	Exotoxin A, a.k.a.: erythrogenic orpyrogenic toxin	Similar to TSST-1	Fever, increased susceptibility to LPS, rash, shock, capillary leakage, cardiotoxicity
cAMP Inducers	Enterotoxigenic *Escherichia coli* (−)	Heat labile toxin (LT)	LT stimulates an adenylate cyclase by ADP ribosylation of GTP binding protein	Both LT and ST promote secretion of fluid and electrolytes from intestinal epithelium
	Vibrio cholerae (−)	Cholera toxin	Similar to *E. coli* LT	Profuse, watery diarrhea
	Bacillus anthracis (+)	Anthrax toxin (3 proteins make 2 toxins)	EF = edema factor = adenylate cyclase LF = lethal factor PA = protective antigen(B component for both)	Decreases phagocytosis; causes edema, kills cells
	Bordetella pertussis (−)	Pertussis toxin	ADP ribosylates G_i, the negative regulator of adenylate cyclase → increased cAMP	Histamine-sensitizing Lymphocytosis promoting Islet activating
Cytolysins	*Clostridium perfringens* (+)	Alpha toxin	Lecithinase	Damages cell membranes; myonecrosis
	Staphylococcus aureus (+)	Alpha toxin	Toxin intercalates forming pores	Cell membrane becomes leaky

Medically Important Bacteria

2

Learning Objectives

❏ Answer questions about endospores, bacterial growth and death

❏ Demonstrate understanding of microorganism cultures, strains, and gram stain techniques

❏ Answer questions about distinguishing features, transmission, pathogenesis, diagnosis, treatment, and prevention of gram-positive cocci, gram-positive rods, gram-negative cocci, gram-negative bacilli, spirochetes, and unusual bacteria

❏ Differentiate organisms in the *Chlamydophila*, *Rickettsia*, and *Ehrlichia* genuses

❏ Answer questions about dental related microbiology, including streptococci, periodontal anaerobes, sterilization, and disinfection

Note

Nomenclature

Latin bacterial **family** names have "**-aceae**," e.g., Enterobacteriaceae.

Genus and species names are **italicized** and **abbreviated**, e.g., *Enterobacter aerogenes = E. aerogenes*.

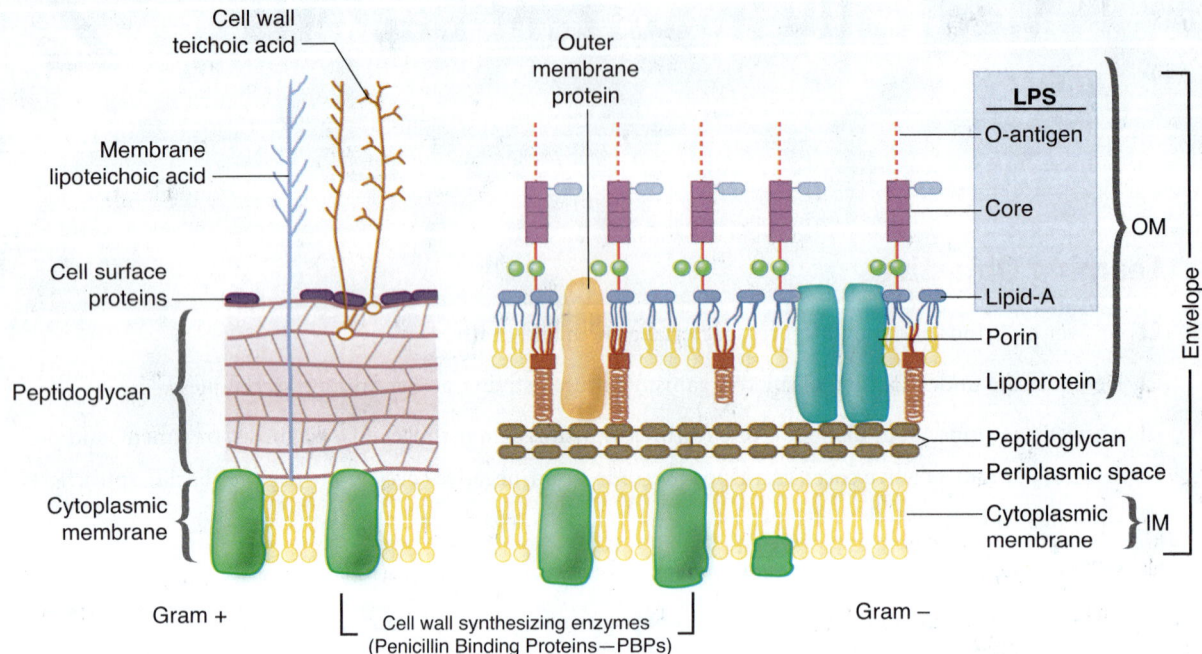

Figure 2-1. The Bacterial Cell Envelope

ENDOSPORES

Organisms: *Bacillus* and *Clostridium*

Function

- Survival not reproductive (1 bacterium → 1 spore)
- Resistance to chemicals, dessiccation, radiation, freezing, and heat
- Note that spore's resistance to heat is the basis for their use in autoclave spore tests. The tests use *Geobacillus* (formerly Bacillus) *stearothermophilus* to check sterilization of instruments.

Mechanism of resistance

- New enzymes (i.e., dipicolinic acid synthetase, heat-resistant catalase)
- Increases or decreases in other enzymes
- Dehydration: calcium dipicolinate in core
- Keratin spore coat

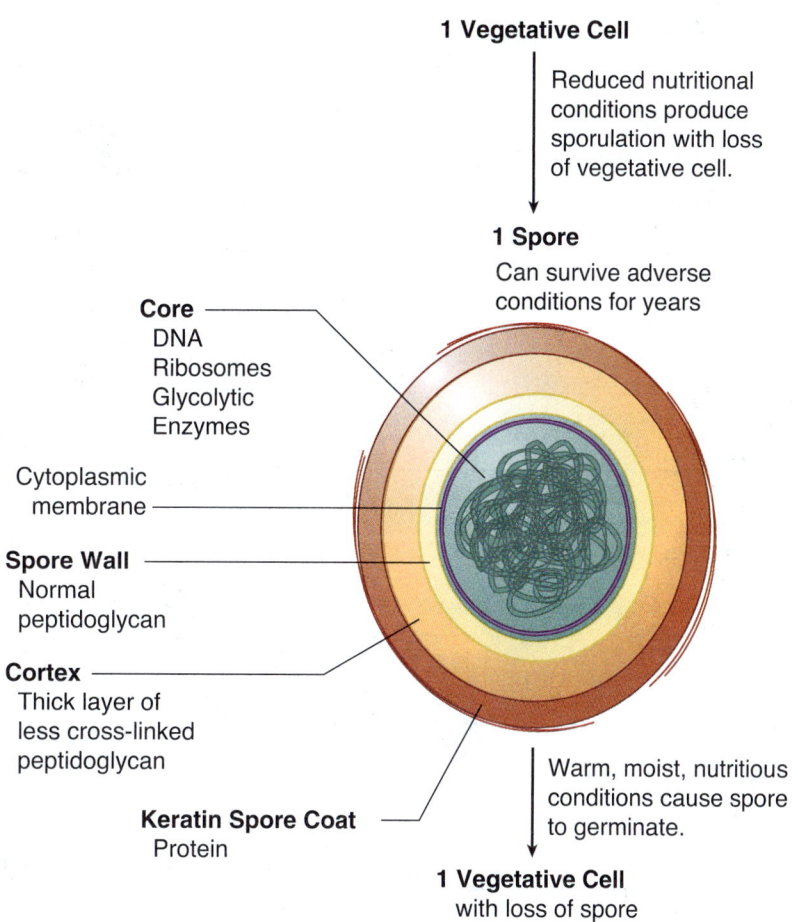

1 Vegetative Cell

Reduced nutritional
conditions produce
sporulation with loss
of vegetative cell.

1 Spore

Can survive adverse
conditions for years

Core
DNA
Ribosomes
Glycolytic
Enzymes

Cytoplasmic
membrane

Spore Wall
Normal
peptidoglycan

Cortex
Thick layer of
less cross-linked
peptidoglycan

Keratin Spore Coat
Protein

Warm, moist, nutritious
conditions cause spore
to germinate.

1 Vegetative Cell
with loss of spore

Figure 2-2. Endospore

Notes

Spores of fungi have a reproductive role.

The spore-forming genera are *Bacillus* and *Clostridium*.

BACTERIAL GROWTH AND DEATH

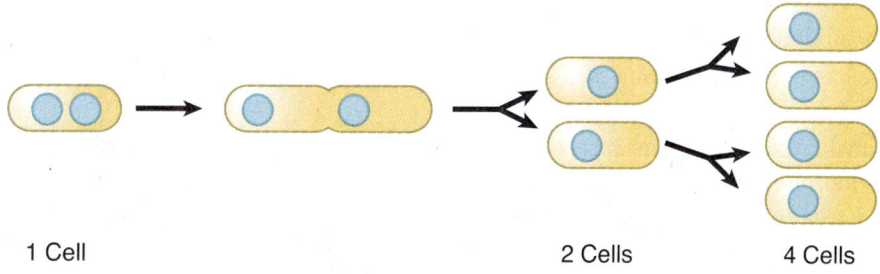

1 Cell   2 Cells   4 Cells

Figure 2-3. Exponential Growth by Binary Fission

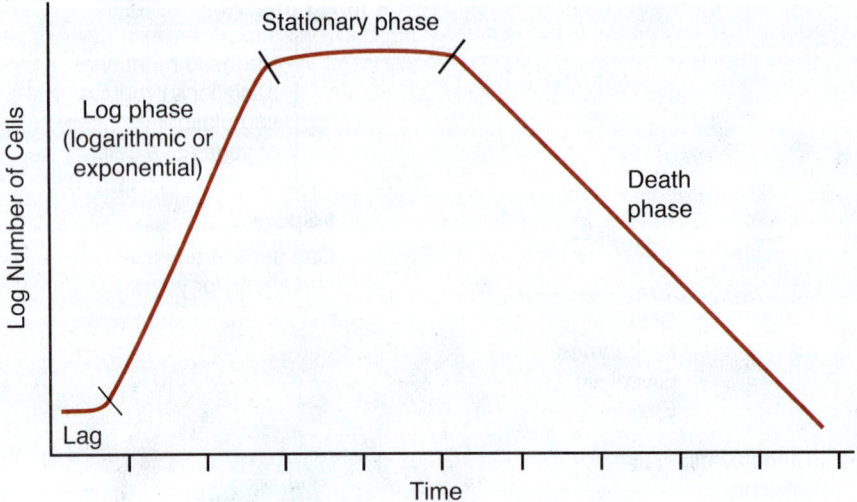

Figure 2-4. Bacterial Growth Curve

In a Nutshell

Lag Phase

- Initial Phase (only 1 lag phase)
- Detoxifying medium
- Turning on enzymes to utilize medium
- For exam, number of cells at beginning equals number of cells at end of lag phase.

Log Phase

- Rapid exponential growth
- Generation time = time it takes one cell to divide into two. This is determined during log phase.

Stationary Phase

- Nutrients used up
- Toxic products like acids and alkali begin to accumulate.
- Number of new cells equals the number of dying cells.

CULTURE OF MICROORGANISMS

- Obligate intracellular pathogens (viruses, rickettsias, chlamydias, etc.): Tissue cultures (cell cultures), eggs, animals, or not at all
- Facultative intracellular or extracellular organisms: Inert lab media (broths and agars)
  - Selective medium (S): A medium that selects for certain bacteria by inclusion of special nutrients and/or antibiotics.
  - Differential medium (D): A medium on which different bacteria can be distinguished by differences in colonial morphology or color.

Table 2-1. Oxygen Requirements and Toxicity

Classification	Characteristics	Important Genera
Obligate aerobes	Require oxygen Have no fermentative pathways Generally produce superoxide dismutase	*Mycobacterium* *Pseudomonas* (*Bacillus*)
Microaerophilic	Require low but not full oxygen tension	*Campylobacter* *Helicobacter*
Facultative anaerobes	Will respire aerobically until oxygen is depleted and then ferment	Most bacteria, e.g., *Enterobacteriaceae* *Streptococcus*
Obligate anaerobes	• Lack superoxide dismutase • Generally lack catalase • Are fermenters • Cannot use O_2 as terminal electron acceptor	*Actinomyces** *Bacteroides* *Clostridium* *Many periodontal disease organisms*

*ABCs of anaerobiosis = *Actinomyces*, *Bacteroides*, and *Clostridium*.

STAINS

Table 2-2. Gram Stain

Reagent	Gram-Positive	Gram-Negative
Crystal Violet (a very intense purple, small dye molecule)	Purple/Blue	Purple/Blue
Gram's Iodine	Purple/Blue (a large dye complex)	Purple/Blue (a large dye complex)
Acetone or Alcohol	Purple/Blue	Colorless
Safranin (a pale dye)	Purple/Blue	Red/Pink

All cocci are gram-positive except *Neisseria*, *Moraxella* and *Veillonella*.

All spore formers are gram-positive.

Background in stain modified for tissues will be pale red.

Table 2-3. Ziehl-Neelsen Acid Fast Stain (or Kinyoun)

Reagent	Acid Fast	Non-Acid Fast*
Carbol Fuchsin with heat**	Red (Hot Pink)	Red (Hot Pink)
Acid Alcohol	Red	Colorless
Methylene Blue***	Red	Blue

* *Mycobacterium* is acid fast. *Nocardia* is partially acid fast. All other bacteria are non-acid fast. Two protozoan parasites (*Cryptosporidium* and *Isospora*) have acid fast oocysts.

** Without the heat, the dye would not go in the mycobacterial cells.

*** Sputa and human cells will be blue.

GRAM-STAINING REACTIONS

(†Marked organisms have high numbers of questions on the Boards.)

Table 2-4. Gram-Positive Bacteria

Cocci		
	Staphylococcus†	
	Streptococcus†	
Rods		
	Aerobic or facultative anaerobic	
	Bacillus	
	Listeria	
	Corynebacterium†	
	Nocardia	
	Mycobacterium†	
	Anaerobic	
	Clostridium†	
	Actinomyces	
	Eubacterium	
	Propionibacterium	
	Lactobacillus	

Note: Spore formers are *Bacillus* and *Clostridium*.

Table 2-5. Non-Gram–staining Bacteria*

Mycoplasmataceae
Mycoplasma†
Ureaplasma

*Note:

Poorly visible on traditional Gram stain: ***Mycobacterium*** does not stain well with the Gram stain due to its waxy cell wall. It is considered gram-positive.

Most **spirochetes, chlamydiae,** and **rickettsias** are so thin that the color of the Gram stain cannot be seen. All have gram-negative cell walls.

Legionella (gram-negative) also does not stain well with the traditional Gram stain unless counterstain time is increased.

Table 2-6. Gram-Negative Bacteria

Aerobic		
Cocci	*Neisseria*†	
	Moraxella	
Rods		
	Pseudomonas	*Eikenella*
	Legionella	*Kingella*
	Brucella	
	Bordetella†	
	Francisella	
Helical or curved (and microaerophilic)		
	Campylobacter	
	Helicobacter	
Facultative anaerobic rods		
Enterobacteriaceae†		**Also:**
	Escherichia†	*Capnocytophaga*
	Shigella	*Actinobacillus*
	Salmonella†	*Cardiobacterium*
	Citrobacter	*Gardnerella*
	Klebsiella	
	Enterobacter	
	Serratia	
	Proteus	
	Yersinia†	
Vibrionaceae		
	Vibrio	

(*Continue*)

Pasteurellaceae	
	Pasteurella
	Haemophilus[†]
Anaerobic straight to helical rods	
	Bacteroides/Prevotella
	Fusobacterium
Spirochetes	
	Treponema[†]
	Borrelia
	Leptospira
Rickettsiaceae and relatives	*Rickettsia*[†]
	Bartonella
	Ehrlichia
Chlamydiaceae	
	Chlamydia[†]
	Chlamydophila

GRAM-POSITIVE COCCI

- *Staphylococcus*
- *Streptococcus*

Table 2-7. Major Species of Staphylococcus and Streptococcus and Identifying Features*

	Catalase	Coagulase	Hemolysis[†]	Distinguishing Features	Disease Presentations
			***Staphylococcus* Species**		
S. aureus	+	+	β	Ferments mannitol	Infective endocarditis (acute)
				Salt tolerant	Abscesses
					Toxic shock syndrome
					Gastroenteritis
					Suppurative lesions, pyoderma, impetigo
					Osteomyelitis

(Continue)

	Catalase	Coagulase	Hemolysis[†]	Distinguishing Features	Disease Presentations
S. epidermidis	+	−	γ	Novobiocin[S] Biofilm producer	Endocarditis in IV drug users Catheter and prosthetic device infections
S. saprophyticus	+	−	γ	Novobiocin[R]	UTIs in newly sexually active females
Streptococcus Species (Grouped by analysis of C carbohydrate)					
S. pyogenes (Group A)	−	−	β	Bacitracin[S] PYR[†]	Pharyngitis Scarlet fever Pyoderma/impetigo Suppurative lesions Rheumatic fever Acute glomerulonephritis
S. agalactiae (Group B)	−	−	β	Bacitracin[R] CAMP[+]	Neonatal septicemia and meningitis
S. pneumoniae (not groupable)	−	−	α	Optochin[S]	Pneumonia (community acquired) Adult meningitis Otitis media and sinusitis in children
Viridans group (not groupable)	−	−	α	Optochin[R]	Infective endocarditis Dental caries
Enterococcus sp. (Group D)	−	−	α, β, or γ	PYR[†] Esculin agar	Infective endocarditis Urinary and biliary infections
S. bovis	−	−	γ	Bile esculin[†]	Endocarditis, especially in patients with colon cancer

[†] β hemolysis = clear; α hemolysis = partial; γ hemolysis = no hemolysis

Definition of abbreviations: PYR, pyrrolidonyl arylamidase; [S], sensitive; [R], resistant

*Many of the diseases caused by *Staphylococcus* and *Streptococcus* are similar (i.e., skin infections, endocarditis). Therefore, laboratory tests are extremely important in differentiating between these organisms.

GENUS: *STAPHYLOCOCCUS*

Genus Features

- Gram-positive cocci in clusters
- **Catalase positive (streptococci are catalase negative)**

Species of Medical Importance

- *S. aureus*
- *S. epidermidis*
- *S. saprophyticus*

Staphylococcus aureus

Distinguishing Features

- Small, yellow colonies on blood agar
- **β-hemolytic**
- **Coagulase positive** (all other *Staphylococcus* species are negative)
- **Ferments mannitol** on mannitol salt agar

Reservoir

- Normal flora
  - Nasal mucosa (25% of population are carriers)
  - Skin

Transmission

- Hands
- Sneezing
- Surgical wounds
- Contaminated food
  - Custard pastries
  - Potato salad
  - Canned meats

Predisposing Factors for Infection

- Surgery/wounds
- Foreign body (tampons, surgical packing, sutures)
- Severe neutropenia (<500/μL)
- Intravenous drug abuse
- Chronic granulomatous disease
- Cystic fibrosis

Pathogenesis

- Protein A binds Fc component of IgG, inhibits phagocytosis
- **Enterotoxins:** fast acting, heat stable
- **Toxic shock syndrome toxin-1 (TSST-1):** superantigen (see chapter 6 of Immunology for further explanation of a superantigen)

- Coagulase: converts fibrinogen to fibrin clot
- Cytolytic toxin (α toxin): pore-forming toxin, Panton-Valentine leukocidin (PVL), forms pores in infected cells and is acquired by bacteriophage; associated with increased virulence, MRSA strains
- Exfolatins: skin-exfoliating toxins (involved in scalded skin syndrome [SSS]) and bullous impetigo

Diseases

Table 2-8. Staphylococcus aureus

Diseases	Clinical Symptoms	Pathogenicity Factors
Gastroenteritis (food poisoning)—toxin ingested preformed in food	**2–6 hours** after ingesting toxin: nausea, abdominal pain, vomiting, followed by diarrhea	Enterotoxins A–E preformed in food
Infective endocarditis (acute)	Fever, malaise, leukocytosis, heart murmur (may be absent initially)	Fibrin-platelet mesh, cytolytic toxins
Abscesses and mastitis	Subcutaneous tenderness, redness and swelling; hot	Coagulase, cytolysins
Toxic shock syndrome	Fever, hypotension, **scarlatiniform rash that desquamates (particularly on palms and soles)**, multiorgan failure	TSST-1
Impetigo	Erythematous papules to **bullae**	Coagulase, exfoliatins
Scalded skin syndrome	Diffuse epidermal peeling	Coagulase, exfoliatins
Pneumonia	Productive pneumonia with rapid onset, high rate of necrosis, and high fatality; nosocomial, ventilator, postinfluenza, IV drug abuse, CF, CGD, etc. Salmon-colored sputum	Coagulase, cytolysins
Surgical infections	Fever with cellulitis and/or abscesses	Coagulase, exfoliatins, ‡TSSTs
Osteomyelitis (most common cause)	Bone pain, fever, ± tissue swelling, redness; lytic bone lesions on imaging	Cytolysins, coagulase

Definition of abbreviations: CF, cystic fibrosis; CGD, chronic granulomatous disease.

Treatment

- Gastroenteritis is self-limiting.
- Nafcillin/oxacillin are drugs of choice because of widespread antibiotic resistance.
- For methicillin-resistant *Staphylococcus aureus* (MRSA): vancomycin
- For vancomycin-resistant *Staphylococcus aureus* (VRSA) or vancomycin-intermediate *S. aureus* (VISA): quinupristin/dalfopristin
- Note: Increasing importance of MRSA, MDRO, and related resistant organisms.

GENUS:*STREPTOCOCCUS*

Genus Features

- Gram-positive cocci in chains
- **Catalase negative**
- Serogrouped using known antibodies to the cell wall carbohydrates (Lancefield groups A–O)
  - *S. pneumoniae* serotyped via capsule
  - *S. pyogenes* serotyped via M protein

Species of Medical Importance

- *S. pyogenes*
- *S. agalactiae* (group B streptococci; GBS)
- *S. pneumoniae*
- Viridans streptococci
- *Enterococcus faecalis/Enterococcus faecium*
- *Streptococcus bovis*

Streptococcus pyogenes (Group A Streptococcus; GAS)

Distinguishing Features

- β **hemolytic**
- **Bacitracin sensitive**

Reservoir

- Human throat
- Skin

Transmission

- Direct contact
- Respiratory droplets

Pathogenesis

- **Hyaluronic acid: is non-immunogenic**
- **M-protein: antiphagocytic, M12 strains** associated with **acute glomerulonephritis**
- Streptolysin O: immunogenic, hemolysin/cytolysin
- Streptolysin S: not immunogenic, hemolysin/cytolysin

Spreading Factors

- Streptokinase: breaks down fibrin clot
- Streptococcal DNAse: liquefies pus, extension of lesion
- Hyaluronidase: hydrolyzes the ground substances of the connective tissues
- Exotoxins A–C (pyrogenic or erythrogenic exotoxins)
  - Phage-coded (i.e., the cells are lysogenized by a phage.)
  - Cause **fever and rash** of scarlet fever
    - ○ **Superantigens**

Diseases

Table 2-9. Acute Suppurative Group A Streptococcal Infections*

Diseases	Symptoms
Pharyngitis	Abrupt onset of sore throat, fever, malaise, and headache; tonsillar abscesses and tender anterior cervical lymph nodes
Scarlet fever	Above followed by a blanching **"sandpaper" rash** (palms and soles are usually spared), circumoral pallor, **strawberry tongue**, and nausea/vomiting
Pyoderma/impetigo	Pyogenic skin infection (honey-crusted lesions)

*Also, cellulitis/necrotizing fasciitis, puerperal fever, lymphangitis, erysipelas

Table 2-10. Nonsuppurative Sequelae to Group A Streptococcal Infections

Disease	Sequelae of	Mechanisms/Symptoms
Rheumatic fever	Pharyngitis with group A strep	Antibodies to heart tissue/2 weeks post pharyngitis, fever, joint inflammation, carditis, erythema marginatum (chorea later)type II hypersensitivity
Acute glomerulonephritis (M12 serotype)	Pharyngitis or skin infection	Immune complexes bound to glomeruli/pulmonary edema and hypertension, "smoky" urine (type III hypersensitivity)

Treatment
- Beta lactam drugs
- Macrolides are used in the case of penicillin allergy.

Prevention
- Prophylactic antibiotics should be considered in patients for at least 5 year post acute rheumatic fever.
- Beta lactams and macrolides

Streptococcus agalactiae (Group B Streptococci; GBS)

Distinguishing Features
- β **hemolytic**
- **Bacitracin resistant**

Reservoir
- Human vagina (15—20% of women)
- Gastrointestinal tract

Transmission—newborn infected during birth (increased risk with **prolonged labor after rupture of membranes**)

Pathogenesis

- Capsule
- β hemolysin and CAMP factor (polypeptide)

Diseases—neonatal septicemia and meningitis; most common causal agent

Treatment—ampicillin with an aminoglycoside or a cephalosporin

Prevention

- Prophylaxis during delivery in women with a positive vaginal or rectal culture of GBS, a history of recent infection with GBS, or prolonged labors after membrane rupture
- Ampicillin or penicillin drugs of choice
- Clindamycin or erythromycin for penicillin allergies

Streptococcus pneumoniae

Distinguishing Features

- **α hemolytic**
- **Optochin sensitive**
- **Lancet-shaped diplococci**
- **Lysed by bile**

Reservoir—human upper respiratory tract

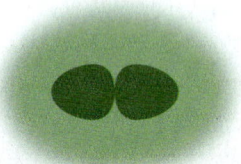

Figure 2-5. *Streptococcus pneumoniae*

Transmission

- Respiratory droplets
  - Not considered highly communicable
  - Often colonizes the nasopharynx without causing disease

In a Nutshell

Typical Pneumonia

Bacterial pneumonia such as *Streptococcus pneumoniae* elicits neutrophils; arachidonic acid metabolites (acute inflammatory mediators) cause pain and fever. *Pneumococcus* produces a lobar pneumonia with a productive cough, grows on blood agar, and usually responds well to penicillin treatment.

Predisposing Factors

- Antecedent influenza or measles infection
- Chronic obstructive pulmonary disease (COPD)
- Congestive heart failure (CHF)
- Alcoholism
- Asplenia predisposes to septicemia

Pathogenesis

- **Polysaccharide capsule** is the major virulence factor: anti- phagocytic
- IgA protease
- Teichoic acid
- Pneumolysin O: hemolysin/cytolysin
  - Damages respiratory epithelium
  - Inhibits leukocyte respiratory burst and inhibits classical complement fixation

Diseases

- Typical pneumonia
  - **Most common cause** (especially in sixth decade of life)
  - Shaking chills, high fever, lobar consolidation, **blood-tinged, "rusty" sputum**
- Adult meningitis
  - **Most common cause**
  - Peptidoglycan and teichoic acids are highly inflammatory in the CNS.
  - CSF reveals high WBCs (neutrophils) and low glucose, high protein
- Otitis media and sinusitis in children **most common cause**

Laboratory Diagnosis

- Gram stain of CSF
- PCR of CSF
- Quellung reaction: positive (swelling of the capsule with the addition of type-specific antiserum, no longer used but still tested!)
- Latex particle agglutination: test for capsular antigen in CSF

Treatment

- Bacterial pneumonia—macrolides
- Adult meningitis—Ceftriaxone or cefotaxime. Vancomycin may be added.
- Otitis media and sinusitis in children—amoxicillin, erythromycin for allergic individuals

Prevention

- Antibody to the capsule (over 80 different capsular serotypes) provides type-specific immunity
- Vaccine
  - Pediatric (PCV, pneumococcal conjugate vaccine)
    ○ Thirteen of the most common serotypes
    ○ Prevents invasive disease
- Adult (PPV, pneumococcal polysaccharide vaccine)
    ○ 23 of the most common capsular serotypes
    ○ Recommended for all adults ≥65 years of age and any at-risk individuals

Viridans Streptococci (*S. sanguis, S. mutans, S. salivarius, S. mitis, S. sanguinis, others*)

Distinguishing Features

- **α hemolytic**
- **Optochin resistant**

Reservoir—human oropharynx (normal flora)

Transmission—endogenous

Pathogenesis—dextran (biofilm)–mediated adherence onto tooth enamel or damaged heart valve and to each other (vegetation); growth in vegetation protects organism from immune system.

Diseases

- Dental caries—*S. mutans* dextran–mediated adherence glues oral flora onto teeth, forming plaque and causing dental caries.
- Caries initiated by *S. mutans,* but later deeper lesions will contain *Lactobacillus. Actinomyces* also said to be involved in root caries formation.
- Enamel caries initiated by lactic acid secretion (from fermentation). Demineralization occurs at pH 5 and below.
- Infective endocarditis (subacute)
  - Malaise, fatigue, anorexia, night sweats, weight loss, splinter hemorrhages
  - Predisposing conditions: damaged (or prosthetic) heart valve, cynanotic congenital conditions, previous endocarditis, *and* bacteremia-producing dental work without prophylactic antibiotics. ***See section below.***

Treatment—penicillin G with aminoglycosides for endocarditis

Prevention—prophylactic antibiotics prior to dental work for individuals with damaged heart valve

Details of Subacute Bacterial Endocarditis prevention for NBDE Part 1

General: SBE infection from a dental procedure depends on the combination of a susceptible cardiac condition and a bacteremia-inducing dental procedure.

DETAILS OF SBE DENTAL PROPHYLAXIS

SBE (sub-acute bacterial endocarditis) infection from a dental procedure depends on the combination of a susceptible cardiac condition and a bacteremia-inducing dental procedure. Conditions, procedures, and preventive antibiotics are reviewed periodically by the American Heart Association, dentists, microbiologists, and epidemiologists.

Their findings are then published and become the current guidelines. Current guidelines as of this writing are from 2007. Changes in the future may significantly alter the guidelines, and students will need to monitor future updates.

Susceptible Conditions

The number of susceptible cardiac conditions have been reduced over time, and currently include previous endocarditis, valvular damage, valvular surgery, cyanotic congenital conditions, and recent or incomplete repairs of these conditions. Note: many conditions previously requiring antibiotic prophylaxis no longer do, including mitral valve prolapse and rheumatic fever history. Many cardiac conditions **never** required prophylaxis, including pacemakers, coronary bypass surgery, angina, previous myocardial infarction, and others.

Table 2-11. Cardiac Conditions Associated With the Highest Risk of Adverse Outcome From Endocarditis for Which Prophylaxis Is Reasonable

Prosthetic cardiac valve or prosthetic material used for cardiac valve repair
Previous infectious endocarditis
Congenital heart disease (CHD)* as listed below: • Unrepaired cyanotic CHD, including palliative shunts and conduits • Completely repaired congenital heart defect with prosthetic material or device, whether placed by surgery or by catheter intervention, during the first 6 months after the procedure† • Repaired CHD with residual defects at the site or adjacent to the site of a prosthetic patch or prosthetic device (which inhibit endothelialization)
Cardiac transplantation recipients who develop cardiac valvulopathy

*Except for the conditions listed above, antibiotic prophylaxis is no longer recommended for any other form of CHD.

†Prophylaxis is reasonable because endothelialization of prosthetic material occurs within 6 months after the procedure.

Dental Procedures Requiring Premedication

Past versions of the AHA recommendations listed specific procedures to medicate or not medicate. The 2007 recommendations are for procedures that manipulate gingival or apical tissue or tear oral mucosa. Briefly: extractions, scaling, curettage, placement of matrix bands, endodontics, and prophylaxis normally require premedication, while X-ray films, denture adjustments, sealants, routine injections through uninfected tissue, orthodontic bracket placement, etc. do not. The general guideline is bleeding (ability to produce a bacteremia). AHA guidelines state that procedures which manipulate gingival or apical tissue or perforate oral mucosa will require premedication for susceptible individuals.

Antibiotic Regimens

There have been many changes to these regimens over time. Follow the table below precisely. Note that 2 grams amoxicillin 30-60 minutes before procedure is the standard regimen for non allergic, pill-swallowing patients. Note that there are many choices for the penicillin allergic patient (such as azithromycin, clarithromycin, clindamycin). Also note that children's doses are calculated by weight, and should never exceed the adult dose.

In terms of changes from prior years, note that there is only a pre-dose and no post-dose. Penicillin V, erythromycin, and vancomycin are not listed. Timing for all premedication is 30-60 minutes prior to procedure.

Table 2-12. Regimen for a Dental Procedure

Situation	Agent	Adults	Children
Oral	Amoxicillin	2 g	50mg/kg
Unable to take oral medication	Ampicillin OR	2 g IM or IV	50mg/kg IM or IV
	1 g IM or IV		
	Cefazolin/ceftriaxone		50mg/kg IM or IV
Allergic to penicillins or ampicillin—oral	Cephalexin*† OR	2 g	50mg/kg
	Clindamycin OR	600mg	20mg/kg
	Azithromycin/clarithromycin	500mg	15mg/kg
Allergic to penicillins or ampicillin and unable to take oral medication	Cefazolin or ceftriaxone† OR	1g IM or IV	50mg/kg IM or IV
	Clindamycin	600mg IM or IV	20mg/kg IM or IV

*Or other first- or second-generation oral cephalosporin in equivalent adult or pediatric dosage. †Cephalosporins should not be used in an individual with a history of anaphylaxis, angioedema, or urticaria with penicillins or ampicillin.

IM indicates intramuscular; IV, intravenous.

DENTAL CLINICAL MICROBIOLOGY

Clinical microbiology involves areas of infection control, preventing disease spread from patient to provider, provider to patient, and patient to patient through instruments, etc.

General Guidelines

- **Autoclave** is quickest and simplest and is used if there is no reason not to (i.e., tends to dull and corrode sharp edges, especially carbide steel).
- **Ethylene oxide** or **glutaraldehyde** (see below) is used for heat-sensitive materials.
- **Dri-Clave** or **ethylene oxide** is used when **sharp edges** are important to maintain. The main problem of Dri-Clave or ethylene oxide is turnaround time.
- Boiling can disinfect but never sterilize.
- Spores are not killed by long disinfectant soaking, unless extremely long periods are used, i.e., glutaraldehyde 8-12 hours. Otherwise, disinfectant soaking is not sterilization, merely high-level disinfection.
- Alcohols are generally good soaking but poor surface disinfectants because they evaporate easily.

Sterilization Versus Disinfection

Critical and Semi-critical instruments

By medical classification (Spaulding classification), critical instruments pierce skin or mucosa, or enter sterile area of the body. They must be single-use sterile disposable or sterilized. Semi-critical instruments touch (but do not pierce) mucus membranes. They are single-use sterile disposable, sterilized, or high-level disinfected.

Note that although an instrument like a dental mirror is *technically* semi-critical, ALL dental instruments are routinely sterilized.

Sterilization

- Absence of all life forms
- Kills spores of spore-forming bacteria (*Bacillus* and *Clostridium*)
- Can be tested by biological monitor (spore test) using *Geobacillus* spores

Disinfection

- Reduction of numbers of microorganisms to low level; elimination of pathogens to the point that the instrument or material is safe (biologically, but not legally). Routine dental instruments must be sterilized.
- Will not kill bacterial spores
- Instruments not considered "sterile"

Disinfection Methods

- Alcohols, phenols (also heat)—kill by protein denaturation
- Hypochlorites (bleach), iodines, silver compounds, mercury compounds, peroxides—kill by oxidation of sulfhydryl bonds
- Glutaraldehyde, ethylene oxide, and formaldehyde—kill by DNA alkylation
- Note that plain (non-disinfectant) soaps do not kill microorganisms directly. As emulsifying agents, they make it easier for bacteria to separate from skin surfaces and wash away.
- Mycobacterium is the "benchmark" (gold standard) for the effectiveness of disinfectants. They are extremely difficult to kill due to their fatty, waxy cell walls.
- Enveloped viruses (HIV) are easier to kill than non-enveloped viruses (Hepatitis A) when disinfectants are used on surfaces.

Sterilization Methods

- **Autoclave** (steam heat, pressure)—121 C, 20−30 min, 15 psi
- **Dry Heat** (Dri-Clave)—160 C, 1−2 hours
- **Ethylene oxide** (non heat chemical vapor)—8−12 hours (plus extra time to air out residue)
- **Combined heat/chemical** (chemiclave)—Formaldehyde and alcohol, 132 C, 20−40 psi, 20 minutes. Uncommon but tested.
- **Chemical soaking** (glutaraldehyde)—Must be long-term (8+ hours) otherwise considered disinfection

Preparation of Instruments

All instruments prior to sterilization must be clean and free of debris. In particular, bloody or proteinaceous debris is especially dangerous. It can shield microorganisms from the sterilizing effects of heat.

Failure to Sterilize

- Autoclave was overpacked.
- Time was insufficient; wrong cycle was used (wrapped instruments take more time than unwrapped, etc.).
- Autoclave cycle was interrupted (power problem or shut-off).
- Tissue/protein was left on the instrument

Sterilization Monitoring

Sterilization must be checked periodically to ensure that the process is completed adequately. Two basic methods exist:

- **Process indicators:** these show that adequate physical conditions were met to kill organisms (usually show sufficient temperature). They do NOT directly show that organisms were killed. They are often color change spots or squares on the instrument bag. Process indicators must be present on each bag of each load. While useful, for example, in clearly separating processed from unprocessed instruments, they are insufficient in legal and regulatory terms. A biological indicator must be used.

- **Biological indicators:** these strips or capsules contain Geobacillus spores. They are placed in the autoclave and then are cultured. If the autoclave is working correctly, the spores should not grow (negative growth). Usually, another capsule or strip is used as a control. It is not autoclaved, and is cultured. It should grow (positive growth). The control strip or capsule ensures that the spores were alive to begin with.

Spore tests must be run (minimally) weekly on each autoclave. This is the legal requirement for autoclave testing.

Geobacillus spores are the "benchmark" (gold standard) for sterilization.

GENUS: *ENTEROCOCCUS*

Genus Features

- **Catalase negative**
- **PYR+**

Species of Medical Importance

- *Enterococcus faecalis*
- *Enterococcus faecium*

Enterococcus faecalis/faecium

Distinguishing Features

- **Group D gram-positive cocci in chains**
- Catalase-negative, varied hemolysis

Reservoir—human colon, urethra ± and female genital tract

Transmission—endogenous

Pathogenesis

- Bile/salt tolerance allows survival in bowel and gall bladder.
- During medical procedures on GI or GU tract: *E. faecalis* → **bloodstream** → **previously damaged heart valves** → **endocarditis**

Diseases

- Urinary and biliary tract infections
- Infective (subacute) endocarditis in persons (often elderly) with damaged heart valves

Diagnosis

- Culture on blood agar
- Antibiotic sensitivities

Treatment

- All strains carry some drug resistance.

- Some **vancomycin-resistant strains of** *Enterococcus faecium* or *E. faecalis* (VRE) have no reliably effective treatment. In general for low-level resistance, use ampicillin, gentamicin, or streptomycin.

Prevention—prophylactic use of penicillin and gentamicin in patients with damaged heart valves prior to intestinal or urinary tract manipulations

GRAM-POSITIVE RODS

Table 2-13. Summary of Gram-Positive Rods

Genus	Spore	Aerobic Growth	Exotoxin	Facul-tative Intracel-lular	IC Hosts*	Acid Fast	Branch-ing Rods
Bacillus	+	+	+	−	−	−	−
Clostridium	+	−	+	−	−	−	−
Listeria	−	+	+	+	+	−	−
Corynebacterium	−	+	+	−	−	−	−
Actinomyces	−	−	−	−	−	−	+
Nocardia	−	+	−	−	+	+[†]	+
Mycobacterium	−	+	−	+	+	+	−

Definition of abbreviation: IC, immunocompromised.

*Column defines whether the organism a significant problem in IC hosts.

[†]*Nocardia* is considered partially acid fast.

GENUS: *BACILLUS*

Genus Features

- Gram-positive rods
- **Spore forming**
- **Aerobic**

Species of Medical Importance

- *Bacillus anthracis*
- *Bacillus cereus*

Bacillus anthracis

Distinguishing Features

- **Large,** boxcar-like, gram-positive, **spore-forming rods**
- **Capsule is polypeptide**
- **Potential biowarfare agent**

Reservoir—animals, skins, soils

Transmission—contact with infected animals or inhalation of spores (bioterrorism)

Pathogenesis

- Capsulepolypeptide, antiphagocytic, immunogenic
- **Anthrax toxin** includes three protein components

Diseases

- Cutaneous anthrax—papule → papule with vesicles (malignant pustules) → central necrosis (eschar) with erythematous border often with painful regional lymphadenopathy; fever in 50%
- Pulmonary (wool sorter's disease)
  - Life-threatening **pneumonia**; cough, fever, malaise, and ultimately facial edema, dyspnea, diaphoresis, cyanosis, and shock with **mediastinal hemorrhagic lymphadenitis**
- Gastrointestinal anthrax
  - Rare

Diagnosis

- Gram stain and culture of blood, respiratory secretions or lesions
- Serology
- PCR

Treatment—ciprofloxacin or doxycycline due to resistance to penicillin and doxycycline.

Prevention

- Toxoid vaccine (AVA, acellular vaccine adsorbed)
- Given to individuals in high risk occupations (military)

Bacillus cereus

Distinguishing Feature—spores

Reservoir—found in nature

Transmission

- Foodborne, intoxication
- Major association with fried rice from Chinese restaurants
- Associated with food kept warm, not hot (buffets)

Pathogenesis—two possible toxins:

- **Emetic toxin: preformed fast (1–6 hours)**, similar to *S. aureus* with vomiting and diarrhea; associated with **fried rice**
- Diarrheal toxin produced in vivo (meats, sauces): 18 hours, similar to *E. coli*

Diseases

- Gastroenteritis
  - Nonbloody
  - ± Vomiting

Diagnosis

- Clinical grounds
- Culture and Gram stain of implicated food

Treatment—self-limiting

- *Bacillus (Geobacillus stearothermophilus)*

Note: This nonpathogenic species is used for autoclave (sterility) spore testing. See "Dental Clinic Microbiology."

GENUS: *CLOSTRIDIUM*

Genus Features

- **Gram-positive rods**
- **Spore forming**
- **Anaerobic**

Species of Medical Importance

- *Clostridium tetani*
- *Clostridium botulinum*
- *Clostridium perfringens*
- *Clostridium difficile*

Clostridium tetani

Distinguishing Features

- **Large gram-positive, spore-forming rods**
- Anaerobes
- Produces tetanus toxin

Reservoir—soil

Transmission

- Puncture wounds/trauma (human bites)
- Requires low tissue oxygenation (E_h)

Pathogenesis

- Spores germinate in the tissues, producing **tetanus toxin** (an exotoxin also called **tetanospasmin).**
- Carried intra-axonally to CNS
- Excitatory neurons are unopposed → extreme muscle spasm
- One of the most toxic substances known

Disease—tetanus

- Risus sardonicus (facial spasm)
- Opisthotonus (hyperextension of spine)
- Extreme muscle spasms

Diagnosis—primarily a clinical diagnosis; organism is rarely isolated.

Treatment of Actual Tetanus

- **Hyperimmune human globulin (TIG) to neutralize toxin plus metronidazole or penicillin**

Prevention

- Toxoid is formaldehyde-inactivated toxin.
- Important because disinfectants have poor sporicidal action
- Care of wounds: proper wound cleansing and care plus treatment

Clostridium botulinum

Distinguishing Features

- **Anaerobic**
- **Gram-positive spore-forming rods**

Reservoir—soil/dust

Transmission—foodborne/traumatic implantation (commonly home-canned vegetables)

Pathogenesis

- **Spores** survive in soil and dust; **germinate** in moist, warm, nutritious but **nonacidic and anaerobic conditions**
- **Botulinum toxin**
  - **A-B polypeptide neurotoxin** (actually a series of 7 antigenically different; type A and B most common)
  - **Coded for by a prophage** (lysogenized *Clostridium botulinum).*
  - Highly toxic
  - **Heat labile** (unlike staph), 10 minutes 60.0°C
  - **Mechanism of action**
    - **Absorbed by gut** and carried by blood to peripheral nerve synapses
    - **Blocks release of acetylcholine** at the myoneuronal junction resulting in a reversible **flaccid paralysis** Disease(s)

Table 2-14. Forms of Botulism

Disease	Adult	Infant
Acquisition	**Preformed toxin ingested (toxicosis)** Poorly canned alkaline vegetables (green beans), smoked fish	**Spores ingested: household dust, honey** Toxin produced in gut (toxi-infection)
Prevention	**Proper canning; heat all canned foods**	**No honey first year**

Clostridium perfringens

Distinguishing Features

- Large **gram-positive, spore-forming** rods (spores rare in tissue), nonmotile

Reservoir—soil and human colon

Transmission—foodborne and traumatic implantation

Pathogenesis

- **Spores** germinate under anaerobic conditions in tissue.
- Vegetative cells produce:
  - **Alpha toxin** (phospholipase C) is a **lecithinase.** It disrupts membranes, damaging RBCs, platelets, WBCs, endothelial cells → massive hemolysis, tissue destruction, hepatic toxicity.
- Twelve other toxins damage tissues.
- **Enterotoxin** produced in intestines in food poisoning: disrupts ion transport → watery diarrhea, cramps.

Disease(s)

- Gas gangrene (myonecrosis)
  - Contamination of **wound with soil or feces**
  - **Tense tissue** (edema, gas) and exudate
  - Systemic symptoms include **fever** and **tachycardia** (disproportionate to fever), diaphoresis, pallor, etc.
  - **Rapid, high mortality**
- Food poisoning
  - **Reheated meat dishes,** organism grows to high numbers; 8–24 hour incubation
  - **Enterotoxin** production in gut; self-limiting noninflammatory, watery diarrhea

Diagnosis—clinical

Treatment

- Gangrene
  - Debridement, delayed closure, clindamycin and penicillin, hyperbaric chamber
- Food poisoning
  - Self-limiting

Clostridium difficile

Reservoir—human colon/gastrointestinal tract

Transmission—endogenous

Pathogenesis

- **Toxin A: enterotoxin damaging mucosa leading to fluid increase; granulocyte attractant**
- **Toxin B: cytotoxin: cytopathic**

Disease(s)—antibiotic-associated (clindamycin, cephalosporins, amoxicillin, ampicillin) **diarrhea, colitis, or pseudomembranous colitis** (yellow plaques on colon)

Diagnosis

- Culture is not diagnostic because organism is part of normal flora
- Stool exam for toxin production

Treatment

- Severe disease—**metronidazole**: use vancomycin only if no other drug available; to avoid selecting for vancomycin-resistant normal flora
- Mild disease—discontinue other antibiotic therapy

Prevention

- Caution in overprescribing broad-spectrum antibiotics (limited-spectrum drugs should be considered first)

GENUS: *LISTERIA*

Genus Features

- **Gram-positive, non–spore forming rods**
- **Facultative intracellular**
- **Tumbling motility**

Species of Medical Importance—*Listeria monocytogenes*

Listeria monocytogenes

Distinguishing Features

- Small gram-positive rods
- Beta hemolytic, nonspore-forming rod on blood agar, CAMP positive
- **Tumbling motility** in broth; actin jet motility in cells
- **Facultative intracellular parasite**
- **Cold growth**

Reservoir

- Widespread: animals (gastrointestinal and genital tracts), **unpasteurized milk products**, plants, and soil
- Cold growth: soft cheeses, deli meats, cabbages (coleslaw), hotdogs

Transmission—foodborne, vertical, or across the placenta

Pathogenesis

- **Listeriolysin O, a β-hemolysin:** facilitates rapid egress from phagosome into cytoplasm

Disease(s)

- Listeriosis (human, peaks in summer)
  - Healthy adults and children: generally asymptomatic or diarrhea with low % carriage
  - Pregnant women: symptomatic carriage, septicemia characterized by fever and chills; can cross the placenta in septicemia.
- Neonatal disease
  - **Early-onset:** in utero transmission; sepsis with high mortality
  - **Late-onset:** 2–3 weeks after birth from fecal exposure; meningitis with septicemia
- In immunocompromised patients
  - **Septicemia and meningitis** (most common clinical presentation)

Diagnosis

- Blood or CSF culture
- CSF wet mount or Gram stain

Treatment—ampicillin with gentamicin added for immunocompromised patients

Prevention—pregnant women or immunocompromised patients should not eat cold deli foods

GENUS: CORYNEBACTERIUM

Genus Features

- Gram-positive rods
- Non—spore forming
- Aerobic

Species of Medical Importance

- *Corynebacterium diphtheriae*
- Diphtheroids (normal flora)

Corynebacterium diphtheriae

Distinguishing Features

- Gray-to-black colonies of **club-shaped** gram-positive rods arranged in V or L shapes on **Gram stain**
- Aerobic, non—spore forming
- **Toxin-producing strains have β-prophage** carrying genes for the toxin (**lysogeny, β-corynephage**). The phage from one patient with diphtheria can infect the normal nontoxigenic diphtheroid of another person and cause diphtheria.

Reservoir—throat and nasopharynx

Transmission—bacterium or phage via respiratory droplets

Pathogenesis

- Organism **not invasive**; colonizes epithelium of oropharynx or skin in cutaneous diphtheria
- **Diphtheria toxin (A-B component)—inhibits protein synthesis**
- Effect on oropharynx: **Dirty gray pseudomembrane** (made up of dead cells and fibrin exudate, bacterial pigment)
- **Extension into larynx/trachea → obstruction**
- Effect of systemic circulation → **heart** and **nerve** damage

Disease—diphtheria (sore throat with **pseudomembrane, bull neck**, potential respiratory obstruction, **myocarditis**, cardiac dysfunction, **recurrent laryngeal nerve palsy**, and lower limb polyneuritis)

Treatment

- Erythromycin and antitoxin
- For endocarditis, intravenous penicillin and aminoglycosides for 4–6 weeks

Prevention— toxoid vaccine (formaldehyde-modified toxin is still immunogenic but with reduced toxicity), part of DTaP, DTP, or Td, boosters 10-year intervals

GENUS: *ACTINOMYCES*

Genus Characteristics

- **Anaerobic**
- Gram-positive **branching** rods
- **Non–acid fast**
- "Fungus-like" in appearance

Species of Medical Importance—*Actinomyces israelii*

Actinomyces israelii

Distinguishing Features

- Anaerobic
- Branching rods
- Non–acid fast

Reservoir—human; normal flora of **gingival crevices** and **female genital tract**

Transmission—endogenous

Pathogenesis—invasive growth in tissues with compromised oxygen supply

Disease—actinomycosis

- Generally not painful but **very invasive**, penetrating all tissues, including bone
- Tissue swelling → **draining abscesses** (sinus tracts) with **"sulfur" granules** (hard yellow microcolonies) in exudate that can be used for microscopy or culture
- Only in tissues with low oxygenation (E_h)
  - **Cervicofacial (lumpy jaw): dental trauma or poor oral hygiene**
  - **Pelvic: from thoracic or sometimes IUDs**
  - Abdominal: surgery or bowel trauma
  - Thoracic: aspiration with contiguous spread
  - CNS: **solitary brain abscess** (*Nocardia* will produce multiple foci)

Diagnosis

- Identify gram-positive branching bacilli in "sulfur granules"
- Colonies resemble molar tooth shape

Treatment—ampicillin or penicillin G and surgical drainage

GENUS: *NOCARDIA*

Genus Features

- **Gram-positive filaments breaking up into rods**
- **Aerobic**
- **Partially acid fast (some areas of smear will be blue and some red)**
- Note that *Mycobacteria* are the other acid-fast genus.

Species of Medical Importance

- *N. asteroides*
- *N. brasiliensis*

Nocardia asteroides and *Nocardia brasiliensis*

Distinguishing Features

- **Aerobic**
- **Gram-positive branching rods**
- **Partially acid fast**

Reservoir—soil and dust

Transmission—airborne or traumatic transplantation

Pathogenesis

- No toxins or virulence factors known
- **Immunosuppression and cancer predispose** to pulmonary infection

Disease(s)

- Nocardiosis
  - **Cavitary bronchopulmonary nocardiosis**
  - Symptoms: cough, fever, dyspnea, localized or diffuse pneumonia with cavitation
  - May spread hematogenously to brain (**brain abscesses**)
- Cutaneous/subcutaneous nocardiosis
  - Starts with traumatic implantation
  - Symptoms: **cellulitis** with swelling → **draining subcutaneous abscesses** with **granules** (mycetoma)

Diagnosis—culture of sputum or pus from cutaneous lesion

Treatment—sulfonamides (high dose) or trimethoprim/sulfamethoxazole (TMP-SMX)

GENUS: *MYCOBACTERIUM*

Genus Features

- **Acid fast rods** with a waxy cell wall
- **Obligate aerobe**
- Cell wall
  - Unique: **high concentration of lipids** containing long chain fatty acids called mycolic acids
  - Wall makes **mycobacteria highly resistant to:**
    - Desiccation
    - **Many chemicals** (including NaOH used to kill other bacteria in sputa before neutralizing and culturing)
- **Sensitive to UV**
- **Slow growth**

Species of Medical Importance

- *M. tuberculosis*
- *M. leprae*
- *M. avium-intracellulare*
- *M. kansasii*
- *M. scrofulaceum*
- *M. marinum*

Mycobacterium tuberculosis

Distinguishing Features

- **Auramine-rhodamine staining bacilli** (fluorescent apple green); no antibody involved (sensitive but not specific)
- **Acid fast**
- **Aerobic, slow growing**

Reservoir—human lungs

Transmission—respiratory droplets

Pathogenesis

- **Facultative intracellular organism** (most important)
- **Sulfatides**
  - **Inhibit phagosome-lysosome fusion,** allowing intracellular survival
- **Cord factor (trehalose dimycolate)**
  - Causes **serpentine growth** in vitro
  - **Inhibits leukocyte migration; disrupts mitochondrial respiration and oxidative phosphorylation**
- **Tuberculin** (surface protein) along with mycolic acid → delayed hypersensitivity and **cell-mediated immunity** (CMI)
  - Granulomas and caseation mediated by CMI
  - No exotoxins or endotoxin; damage done by immune system

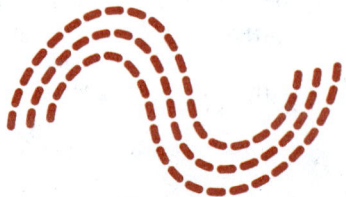

Figure 2-6. Cord Factor

Disease(s)

- Primary pulmonary tuberculosis
  - Organisms replicate in naive alveolar macrophages, killing the macrophages until CMI is set up (Ghon focus)
  - Macrophages transport the bacilli to the regional lymph node (**Ghon complex**) and most people heal without disease; Ghon complex calcifies
  - Organisms that are walled off within the Ghon complex remain viable unless treated
- Reactivational tuberculosis
  - Erosion of granulomas into airways (high oxygen) later in life under conditions of reduced T-cell immunity leads to mycobacterial replication and disease symptoms
  - Complex disease with the potential of infecting any organ system
  - May disseminate (miliary TB) through lymph or blood

Diagnosis

- Microscopy of sputum: screen with auramine-rhodamine stain
- **PPD skin test** (Mantoux): measure **zone of induration at 48–72 hours; positive if:**
  - ≥5 mm in HIV+ or anyone with recent TB exposure; AIDS patients have reduced ability to mount skin test.

- ≥10 mm in high-risk population: IV drug abusers, people living in poverty, or immigrants from high TB area
- ≥15 mm in low-risk population
- **Positive skin test indicates** only **exposure but not necessarily active disease.**
- Quantiferon-TB Gold Test: measures interferon-gamma production when leukocytes exposed to TB antigens
- Slow-growing (3–6 weeks) colonies in lab
- **No serodiagnosis**

Treatment

- **Multiple drugs critical** to treat infection
- Standard observed short-term therapy for uncomplicated pulmonary TB (rate where acquired resistance <4%):
  - First two months: rifampin + isoniazid + pyrazinamide + ethambutol (RIPE)
  - Next four months: rifampin and isoniazid
- Ethambutol or streptomycin added for possible drug-resistant cases
- Drug regimens may change over time

Prevention

- **Isoniazid** taken for nine months can prevent TB in persons with infection but no clinical symptoms.
- Bacille Calmette-Guérin (BCG) **vaccine** containing live, attenuated organisms may prevent disseminated disease; not used in U.S.
- BCG may cause long-term positive PPD reaction, making the test less useful.
- UV lights or HEPA filters used to treat potentially contaminated air.

Mycobacteria Other than Tuberculosis (MOTTS)

Distinguishing Features

- Atypical mycobacteria
- **Noncontagious**
- Found in surface waters, soil, cigarettes
- Commonly found in southeastern U.S.
- *M. avium* is an AIDS-defining infection

Mycobacterium leprae

Distinguishing Features

- **Acid fast rods (seen in punch biopsy)**
- **Obligate intracellular parasite** (cannot be cultured in vitro)
- Optimal growth at less than body temperature

Reservoir

- **Human** mucosa, skin, and nerves are only significant reservoirs
- Some infected armadillos in Texas and Louisiana

Transmission—nasal discharge from untreated lepromatous leprosy patients

Pathogenesis

- **Obligate intracellular parasite**
- Cooler parts of body, e.g., skin, mucous membranes, and peripheral nerves

Disease(s)—leprosy: a continuum of disease, which usually starts out with an indeterminate stage called "borderline." Two advanced forms are tuberculosis and lepromatous.

Diagnosis

- **Punch biopsy or nasal scrapings; acid fast stain**
- **Lepromin skin test** is positive in the tuberculoid but not in the lepromatous form
- No cultures

Treatment—multiple-drug therapy with dapsone and rifampin, with clofazimine added for lepromatous

Prevention—dapsone for close family contacts

GRAM-NEGATIVE COCCI

GENUS: *NEISSERIA*

Genus Features

- Gram negative
- Diplococci with flattened sides
- Oxidase positive

Species of Medical Importance

Table 2-15. Medically Important Neisseria Species

Organism	Capsule	Vaccine	Portal of Entry	Glucose Fermentation	Maltose Fermentation	β-Lactamase Production
N. meningitidis	Yes	Yes	Respiratory	Yes	Yes	Rare
N. gonorrhoeae	No	No	Genital	Yes	No	Common

Neisseria meningitidis

Distinguishing Features

- Gram-negative, kidney bean–shaped diplococci
- Large capsule

Reservoir—human nasopharynx (5–10% carriers)

Transmission

- Respiratory droplets; oropharyngeal colonization, spreads to the meninges via the bloodstream
- Disease occurs in only small percentage of colonized individuals.

Pathogenesis

- Important virulence factors
  - Polysaccharide **capsule:** antiphagocytic, antigenic
  - **IgA protease** allows oropharynx colonization.
  - **Endotoxin** (lipo**oligo**saccharide): fever, septic shock in meningococcemia, **overproduction of outer membrane**
  - Pili and outer membrane proteins important in ability to colonize and invade
  - Deficiency in late complement components (C5–C9) predisposes to bacteremia

Disease(s)

- Meningitis and meningococcemia
  - **Abrupt onset with fever, chills, malaise, prostration, and a rash that is generally petechial;** rapid decline
  - Fulminant cases: ecchymoses, DIC, shock, coma, and death (Waterhouse-Friderichsen syndrome)

Diagnosis

- Gram stain of the CSF
- Polymerase chain reaction (PCR)
- Latex agglutination (for capsular antigens in CSF)

Treatment

- Neonates/infants: ampicillin and cefotaxime
- Older infants, children, and adults: cefotaxime or ceftriaxone with or without vancomycin

Prevention

- **Vaccine:** capsular polysaccharide of strains **Y, W-135, C, and A**
  - Type B (50% of the cases in U.S.) capsule not a good immunogen
- Prophylaxis of close contacts: **rifampin** (or ciprofloxacin)

Neisseria gonorrhoeae

Distinguishing Features

- **Gram-negative**, kidney bean–shaped **diplococci**

Reservoir—human genital tract

Transmission

- Sexual contact, birth
- Sensitive to drying and cold

Pathogenesis

- **Pili**
  - **Attachment** to mucosal surfaces
  - **Inhibit phagocytic uptake**
  - **Antigenic** (immunogenic) **variation:** >1 million variants
- **Outer membrane proteins**
  - **IgA protease:** aids in colonization and cellular uptake
- **Organism invades mucosal surfaces and causes inflammation.**

Disease—gonorrhea

- Male: **urethritis,** proctitis
- Female: **endocervicitis,** PID (contiguous spread), arthritis, proctitis
- Infants: **ophthalmia**(rapidly leads to **blindness if untreated**)

Diagnosis

- Intracellular **gram-negative diplococci in PMNs** from urethral smear from symptomatic male.
- Commonly: diagnosis by **genetic probes** with amplification
- Culture

Treatment

- Ceftriaxone
- Test for *C. trachomatis* or treat with a doxycycline
- Penicillin-binding protein mutations led to gradual increases in penicillin resistance.
- Plasmid-mediated β-**lactamase** produces **high-level penicillin resistance.**

Prevention

- Adult forms: no vaccine; condoms
- Neonatal: silver nitrate or erythromycin ointment in eyes at birth

Moraxella catarrhalis

Distinguishing Features

- Gram-negative diplococcus
- Close relative of *Neisseria*

Reservoir— normal upper respiratory tract flora

Transmission—respiratory droplets

Pathogenesis—endotoxin may play role in disease

Disease(s)

- Otitis media
- Sinusitis
- Bronchitis and bronchopneumonia in elderly patients with COPD

Treatment

- Drug resistance is a problem; most strains produce a β-lactamase.
- Amoxicillin + clavulanate, second or third generation cephalosporin or TMP-SMX

GRAM-NEGATIVE BACILLI

GENUS: *PSEUDOMONAS*

Genus Features

- **Gram-negative rod**
- **Oxidase-positive**
- **Aerobic (nonfermenting)**

Species of Medical Importance—*Pseudomonas aeruginosa*

Pseudomonas aeruginosa

Distinguishing Features

- **Oxidase-positive, Gram-negative rods, nonfermenting**
- **Pigments: pyocyanin (blue-green)** and fluorescein
- **Grape-like odor**
- **Slime layer**
- **Biofilm**

Reservoir—ubiquitous in water

Transmission—water aerosols, raw vegetables, flowers

Pathogenesis

- **Endotoxin** causes inflammation in tissues and gram-negative shock in septicemia.
- *Pseudomonas* **exotoxin A** inhibiting protein synthesis (like diphtheria toxin)
- **Liver is the primary target.**
- **Capsule/slime layer:** antiphagocytic

Disease(s)

- Healthy people
  - Transient gastrointestinal tract colonization: loose stools (10% population)
  - Hot tub folliculitis
  - Eye ulcers: trauma, coma, or prolonged contact wear
- Burn patients
  - Gastrointestinal tract colonization → skin → colonization of eschar → **cellulitis (blue-green pus)** → **septicemia**
- Neutropenic patients
  - **Pneumonia** and **septicemias**—often **superinfections**
- Chronic granulomatous disease (CGD)
  - Pneumonias, septicemias (*Pseudomonas* is catalase positive)
- Otitis externa
  - Swimmers, diabetics, those with pierced ears
- Septicemias
  - Fever, shock ± skin lesions

- Catheterized patients
  - Urinary tract infections (UTIs)
- Cystic fibrosis
  - Early pulmonary colonization, recurrent pneumonias; **always** high **slime-producing strains**

Diagnosis—Gram stain and culture

Note

Drug Resistance in P. aeruginosa

Susceptibilities important.

Drug resistance very common:

Intrinsic resistance (missing high affinity porin some drugs enter through); Plasmid-mediated β-lactamases and acetylating enzymes.

Treatment—antipseudomonal penicillin and an aminoglycoside

Prevention

- Pasteurization or disinfection of water-related equipment, hand washing; prompt removal of catheters
- No flowers or raw vegetables in burn units

GENUS: *LEGIONELLA*

Genus Features

- **Weakly gram-negative**
- **Pleomorphic rods requiring cysteine and iron**
- **Water organisms**

Species of Medical Importance—*Legionella pneumophila*

Legionella pneumophila

Distinguishing Features

- **Stain poorly** with standard Gram stain; **gram-negative**
- **Fastidious** requiring increased **iron and cysteine** for laboratory culture (CYE, charcoal yeast extract)
- **Facultative intracellular**

Reservoir—rivers/streams/amebae; air-conditioning water cooling tanks

Transmission

- Aerosols from contaminated **air-conditioning**
- **No human-to-human transmission**

Predisposing Factors

- **Smokers over 55 years with high alcohol intake**
- **Immunosuppressed patients, e.g.,** renal transplant patients

Pathogenesis

- **Facultative intracellular** pathogen
- **Endotoxin**

Disease(s)

- Legionnaires disease ("atypical pneumonia")
    - Associated with air-conditioning systems, now routinely decontaminated
    - Pneumonia
    - Hyponatremia
    - Mental confusion
    - Diarrhea (no *Legionella* in gastrointestinal tract)
- Pontiac fever
    - Pneumonitis
    - No fatalities

Treatment

- Fluoroquinolone or azithromycin or erythromycin with rifampin for immunocompromised patients
- Drug must penetrate human cells.

Prevention—routine decontamination of air-conditioner cooling tanks

GENUS: *FRANCISELLA*

Genus Features

- **Gram-negative small rods**
- **Facultative intracellular pathogen**

Species of Medical Importance—*Francisella tularensis*

Francisella tularensis

Distinguishing Features

- Small gram-negative rod
- **Potential biowarfare agent**
- **Zoonosis**

Reservoir—many species of wild **animals**, especially rabbits, deer, and rodents

Transmission

- **Tick bite** *(Dermacentor)* → **ulceroglandular** disease, characterized by **fever**, ulcer at bite site, and regional lymph node enlargement and necrosis
- **Traumatic implantation** while skinning rabbits → ulceroglandular disease
- Aerosols (skinning rabbits) → pneumonia
- Ingestion (of undercooked, infected meat or contaminated water) produces typhoidal tularemia.

Pathogenesis

- **Facultative intracellular pathogen (localizes in reticuloendothelial cells)**
- Granulomatous response

Disease

- Tularemia
  - Endemic in every state of the U.S.

Treatment—streptomycin

Prevention

- Protect against tick bites, gloves while butchering rabbits

GENUS: *BORDETELLA*

Genus Features

- **Gram-negative small rods**
- **Strict aerobes**

Species of Medical Importance—*Bordetella pertussis*

Bordetella pertussis

Distinguishing Features

- Small **gram-negative,** aerobic **rods**
- Encapsulated organism

Reservoir—human (vaccinated)

Transmission— respiratory droplets

Pathogenesis

- *B. pertussis* **is a mucosal surface pathogen.**
- **Attachment** to nasopharyngeal ciliated epithelial cells is via:
  - Filamentous hemagglutinin
  - Pertussis toxin (on outer membrane) aids in attachment.
- **Toxins** damage respiratory epithelium.
  - **Adenylate cyclase toxin:** impairs leukocyte chemotaxis → inhibits phagocytosis and causes local edema
  - **Tracheal cytotoxin:** interferes with ciliary action; kills ciliated cells
  - Endotoxin
  - **Pertussis toxin** (A and B component, OM protein toxin): **ADP ribosylation of G$_i$** (inhibiting negative regulator of adenylate cyclase) interferes with transfer of signals from cell surface to intracellular mediator system.

Treatment

- Supportive care; hospitalization if <6 months old, erythromycin for 14 days including all household contacts
- Macrolides can also be given.

Prevention

- Vaccine: DTaP (acellular pertussis: filamentous hemagglutin plus pertussis toxoid); immunity wanes 5–7 years
- Babies are born with little or no immunity (IgA) from mother.

GENUS: *BRUCELLA*

Genus Features

- Gram-negative rods, aerobic
- **Zoonosis**
- Facultative intracellular pathogen
- **Potential biowarfare agent**

Species of Medical Importance

- *Brucella abortus*: cattle
- *Brucella melitensis:* goats
- *Brucella suis:* pigs

Brucella Species

Distinguishing Features

- Small **gram-negative** rods, aerobic
- Facultative intracellular
- Potential biowarfare agent

Reservoir—domestic livestock

Transmission

- **Unpasteurized dairy products**
- **Direct contact with the animal,** work in slaughterhouse

Pathogenesis

- **Endotoxin**
- **Facultative intracellular parasite** (localizes in cells of the RES, reticuloendothelial system) → **septicemia**
- **Granulomatous response** with central necrosis

Disease

- Brucellosis (undulant fever)
  - Acute septicemias
  - Fever 100–104°F (often in evening)
  - Influenza-like symptoms, including arthralgias, anorexia, myalgia, back pain
  - Sweating (profuse)
  - Hepatomegaly

Treatment

- Adults: rifampin and doxycycline

Prevention

- Vaccinate cattle.
- Pasteurize milk, especially goat milk.

GENUS: *CAMPYLOBACTER*

Genus Features

- Gram-negative curved rods with polar flagella ("gulls' wings")
- Oxidase-positive

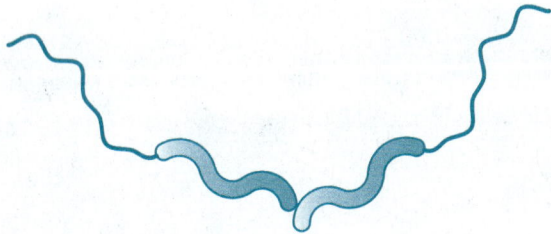

Figure 2-7. Campylobacter

Species of Medical Importance—*Campylobacter jejuni*

Campylobacter jejuni

Distinguishing Features—**microaerophilic**

Reservoir—intestinal tracts of humans, cattle, sheep, dogs, cats, **poultry**

Transmission—fecal-oral, primarily from **poultry**

Pathogenesis

- **Low infectious dose (as few as 500)**
- **Invades** mucosa of the colon, destroying mucosal surfaces; blood and **pus** in stools (inflammatory diarrhea)
- Rarely penetrates to cause septicemia

Disease

- Gastroenteritis
  - Common cause of infectious diarrhea worldwide
  - In U.S., *Campylobacter* enteritis > (*Salmonella* plus *Shigella*)
  - **Ten or more stools/day, may be frankly bloody**
  - Abdominal pain, fever, malaise, nausea, and vomiting
  - Generally **self-limiting in 3–5 days** but may last longer
  - Complications
    - **Guillain-Barré syndrome (GBS)**→ 30% of the GBS in the U.S.
    - Reactive arthritis

Treatment

- Mostly supportive via fluid and electrolyte replacement
- Erythromycin, fluoroquinolones, penicillin resistant

GENUS: *HELICOBACTER*

Genus Features

- Gram-negative spiral gastric bacilli with flagella
- **Microaerophilic**

Species of Medical Importance—*Helicobacter pylori*

Helicobacter pylori

Distinguishing Feature—urease positive

Reservoir—humans

Transmission

- Fecal-oral
- Oral-oral

Pathogenesis

- **Motile**
- **Urease-positive:** ammonium cloud neutralizes stomach acid, allowing survival in stomach acid during transit to border.
- **Mucinase** aids in penetration of mucous layer
- **Invasive** into stomach lining where pH is neutral
- Inflammation is prominent.

Diseases

- Chronic gastritis and duodenal ulcers
  - Associated with several forms of **stomach cancer**
  - Now classed by WHO as **type I carcinogen**

Treatment

- Myriad of regimens
  - Omeprazole + amoxicillin + clarithromycin is one example of triple therapy.

GENUS: *VIBRIO*

Genus Features

- **Gram-negative curved rod with polar flagella**

Species of Medical Importance

- *Vibrio cholerae*
- *Vibrio parahaemolyticus*
- *Vibrio vulnificus*

Vibrio cholerae

Reservoir

- Human colon; **no vertebrate animal carriers** (copepods or shellfish may be contaminated by water contamination)
- Human carriage may persist after untreated infection for months after infection; permanent carrier state is rare.

Transmission

- Fecal-oral spread; sensitive to stomach acid
- Requires high dose ($>10^7$ organisms), if stomach acid is normal

Pathogenesis

- Motility, mucinase, and toxin coregulated pili (TCP) aid in attachment to the intestinal mucosa.
- Cholera enterotoxin (choleragen) similar to *E. coli* LT

Disease

- Cholera
  - Rice water stools, **tremendous fluid loss**
  - Hypovolemic shock if not treated

Treatment

- **Fluid and electrolyte replacement**
- Doxycycline or ciprofloxacin shorten disease and reduce carriage

Prevention—proper sanitation; new vaccine

FAMILY: ENTEROBACTERIACEAE

Family Features

- **Gram-negative rods**
- **Facultative anaerobes**
- Catalase positive

Family Pathogenesis

- **Endotoxin**
- Some also produce **exotoxins.**
- **Antigens**
  - O= cell envelope or O antigen
  - H= flagellar (motile cells only) antigen
  - K = capsular polysaccharide antigen
  - Vi (virulence) = *Salmonella* capsular antigen

GENUS: *ESCHERICHIA*

Genus Features

- **Gram-negative rods**
- **Enterobacteriaceae**

Species of Medical Importance—*Escherichia coli*

Escherichia coli

Distinguishing Features

- **Gram-negative rod**
- **Facultative anaerobic, oxidase negative**

Reservoir

- **Human colon**; may colonize vagina or urethra
- Contaminated crops where human fecal fertilizer is used
- **Enterohemorrhagic strains: bovine feces**

Transmission

- Endogenous
- Fecal-oral
- Maternal fecal flora
- Enterohemorrhagic strains: bovine fecal contamination (raw or undercooked beef, milk, apple juice from fallen apples)

Disease Syndromes Caused by *Escherichia coli*

- UTI (most common cause)
- Neonatal septicemia/meningitis (second most common cause)
- Septicemia
- Gastroenteritis

GENUS: *KLEBSIELLA*

Genus Features

- **Gram-negative rods**
- **Enterobacteriaceae**
- **Major capsule**

Species of Medical Importance

- *Klebsiella pneumoniae*

Klebsiella pneumoniae

Distinguishing Features

- **Gram-negative rods** with **large** polysaccharide **capsule**

Reservoir—human colon and upper respiratory tract

Transmission—endogenous

Pathogenesis

- **Capsule:** impedes phagocytosis
- **Endotoxin:** causes fever, inflammation, and shock (septicemia)

Disease(s)

- Pneumonia
  - Community-acquired, most often in older males; most commonly in **patients with either chronic lung disease, alcoholism, or diabetes** (but this is not the most common cause of pneumonia in alcoholics; *S. pneumoniae* is.)
- Endogenous; assumed to reach lungs by inhalation of respiratory droplets from upper respiratory tract
- Frequent **abscesses** make it hard to treat; fatality rate high

- **Sputum is generally thick and bloody (currant jelly)** but not foul smelling as in anaerobic aspiration pneumonia.
- Urinary tract infections—**catheter-related**
- Septicemia—in immunocompromised patients, may originate from bowel defects or invasion of IV lines

Treatment

- Third-generation cephalosporin with or without an aminoglycoside

Prevention—good catheter care, limit use

In a Nutshell

Comparative Microbiology:

Major encapsulated organisms

Some **K**illers **H**ave **P**retty **N**ice **C**apsules:

Strep pneumoniae

Klebsiella pneumoniae

Haemophilus influenzae Type b (a-d)

Pseudomonas aeruginosa

Neisseria meningitidis

Cryptococcus neoformans (the yeast)

(Not a complete list, just the big ones.)

GENUS: *SHIGELLA*

Genus Features

- **Gram-negative rod**
- **Enterobacteriaceae**
- **Nonmotile**

Species of Medical Importance

- *Shigella sonnei* (**most common in U.S.**)
- *Shigella flexneri*
- *Shigella dysenteriae* (**most severe disease**)
- *Shigella boydii*

Shigella Species

Distinguishing Features

- **Gram-negative rods,** nonmotile

Reservoir—human colon only (no animal carriers)

Transmission—fecal-oral spread, person to person

Pathogenesis

- **Endotoxin** triggers inflammation.
- Shigellae **invade M cells** (membrane ruffling and macropinocytosis), get into the cytoplasm, replicate, and then **polymerize actin jet trails to go laterally** without going back out into the extracellular milieu. This produces **very shallow ulcers** and rarely causes invasion of blood vessels.
- **Shiga toxin:**

  – Produced by *S. dysenteriae*, type 1
  – Three activities: **neurotoxic, cytotoxic, enterotoxic**

Disease(s)

- Enterocolitis/shigellosis(most severe form is dysentery)
  – Few organisms required to start infection (1–10) (extremely acid resistant)
  – Organisms invade, producing bloody diarrhea.
  – **Fever (generally >101.0°F); lower abdominal cramps; tenesmus; diarrhea; shallow ulcers**

Treatment

- Mild cases: fluid and electrolyte replacement only
- Severe cases: antibiotics
- Resistance is mediated by plasmid-encoded enzymes.
- Many strains are ampicillin resistant.

Prevention—proper sanitation (sewage, clean drinking water, hand washing)

GENUS: *YERSINIA*

Genus Features

- **Gram-negative rods**
- **Enterobacteriaceae**

Species of Medical Importance

- *Yersinia pestis*
- *Yersinia enterocolitica*

Key Question Clues

Yersinia pestis

- Patient with high fever, buboes, conjunctivitis, pneumonia
- Exposure to small rodents, desert Southwest

Yersinia pestis

Distinguishing Features

- Small **gram-negative** rods with **bipolar staining**
- **Facultative intracellular parasite**

Reservoir

- **Zoonosis**
- **U.S. desert southwest: rodents** (e.g.,prairie dogs, chipmunks, squirrels)
- **Potential biowarfare agent**

Transmission

- Wild rodents **flea bite** → sylvatic plague
- Human-to-human transmission by **respiratory droplets**

Pathogenesis

- **Coagulase**-contaminated mouth parts of flea
- **Endotoxin** and exotoxin
- **Envelope antigen inhibits phagocytosis.**
- Type III secretion system suppresses cytokine production and resists phagocytic killing

Disease(s)

- Bubonic plague
  - Flea bites infected animal and then later uninfected human
  - Symptoms
    - **Rapidly increasing fever**
    - **Regional buboes**
    - **Conjunctivitis**
    - Leads to septicemia and death if untreated
- Pneumonic plague
  - Arises from septic pulmonary emboli in bubonic plague or **inhalation of organisms from infected individual**
  - **Highly contagious!**

Treatment—aminoglycosides

Prevention

- Animal control; avoid sick and dead animals.
- **Killed vaccine** (military)

GENUS: *PROTEUS*

Genus Features

- **Gram-negative rod**
- **Enterobacteriaceae**
- **Peritrichous flagella/** highly motile/"swarming motility"
- **Facultative anaerobe (Enterobacteriaceae), oxidase negative**

Species of Medical Importance

- *Proteus mirabilis* (90% of infections)
- *Proteus vulgaris*

Reservoir—human colon and environment (water and soil)

Transmission—endogenous

Pathogenesis

- **Urease raises urine pH to cause kidney stones** (staghorn renal calculi).
- **Motility** may aid entry into bladder.
- Endotoxin causes fever and shock when septicemia occurs.

Disease(s)

- Urinary tract infections
- Septicemia

Treatment

- Fluoroquinolones, TMP-SMX, or third-generation cephalosporin
- Remove stones, if present.

Prevention—promptly remove urinary tract catheters.

GENUS: *SALMONELLA*

Genus Features

- **Gram-negative rods (Enterobacteriaceae)**
- **Non–lactose fermenters**
- **Motile**

Species of Medical Importance

- *S. typhi*
- *S. enteritidis*
- *S. typhimurium*
- *S. choleraesuis*
- *S. paratyphi*
- *S. dublin*

Salmonella typhi

Distinguishing Features

- **Gram-negative rods,** highly motile with the **Vi capsule**
- Facultative anaerobe
- **Produces H_2S**
- **Sensitive to acid**

Reservoir

- **Humans only; no animal reservoirs**

Transmission

- **Fecal-oral** route from **human carriers (gall bladder)**
- **Decreased stomach acid or** impairment of mononuclear cells such as in **sickle cell disease predisposes** to *Salmonella* infections

Pathogenesis and Disease

- Typhoid fever (enteric fever), **S. typhi** (milder form: paratyphoid fever; *S. paratyphi*)
  - Organism ingested (requires large number if stomach acid is normal)
  - **Infection begins in ileocecal region**; constipation common
  - Host cell membranes "ruffle" from *Salmonella* contact.
  - *Salmonella* reach basolateral side of M cells, then **mesenteric lymph nodes and blood**
  - **Liver and spleen** are infected with additional release of bacteria to bloodstream → signs of **septicemia** (mainly fever).
  - *S. typhi* survives intracellularly and replicates in macrophages; **resistant to macrophage killing**
  - **Biliary system** (liver, gallbladder) is infected, organisms enter intestinal tract in bile.
  - Symptoms: **fever,** headache, abdominal pain, constipation more common than diarrhea
  - Complications if untreated: **necrosis of Peyer patches** with perforation, thrombophlebitis, cholecystitis, pneumonia, abscess formation, etc.

Treatment—fluoroquinolones or third-generation cephalosporins

Prevention

- Sanitation
- Three vaccine types, oral and parental

GENUS: *HAEMOPHILUS*

Genus Features

- **Gram-negative, pleomorphic rod**

Species of Medical Importance

- *Haemophilus influenzae*
- *Haemophilus ducreyi*

Haemophilus influenzae

Distinguishing Features

- Encapsulated, **gram-negative rod; 95%** of invasive disease caused by capsular type b

Reservoir—human nasopharynx

Transmission—respiratory droplets, shared toys

Pathogenesis

- **Polysaccharide capsule**
- Capsule important in diagnosis
- **IgA protease** is a mucosal colonizing factor.

Diseases

- Meningitis
  - **Epidemic in unvaccinated children ages 3 months to 2 years**
  - After maternal antibody has waned and before the immune response of the child is adequate
  - *H. influenzae* **was** most common cause of meningitis in 1- to 5-year-old children up to 1990.
  - Still a problem if child is <2 years and is not vaccinated

- Otitis media
- Bronchitis
- Pneumonia
- Epiglottitis

Treatment—cefotaxime or ceftriaxone for empirical therapy of meningitis

Prevention

- **Conjugate capsular polysaccharide-protein vaccine**
- Rifampin reduces oropharynx colonization and prevents meningitis in unvaccinated, close contacts <2 years of age.

Haemophilus ducreyi

Reservoir— human genitals

Transmission— sexual transmission and direct contact

Diseases

- Chancroid
- Genital ulcers: **soft, painful chancre** ("You do cry with ducreyi.")
- **Slow to heal without treatment**
- **Open lesions increase transmission of HIV.**

Treatment—azithromycin, ceftriaxone, or ciprofloxacin

GENUS: *BACTEROIDES*

Genus Features

- **Gram-negative rod**
- **Anaerobic**
- Modified LPS with reduced activity

Species of Medical Importance—*Bacteroides fragilis*

Bacteroides fragilis

Reservoir—human **colon; the genus** *Bacteroides* **is the predominant anaerobe.**

Transmission—**endogenous** from bowel defects

Pathogenesis

- Modified LPS has reduced endotoxin activity.
- Capsule is antiphagocytic.

Diseases—**septicemia, peritonitis (often mixed infections), and abdominal abscess**

Treatment

- Metronidazole, clindamycin, or cefoxitin; **abscesses should be surgically drained.**
- **Antibiotic resistance** is common

Prevention—prophylactic antibiotics for gastrointestinal or biliary tract surgery

ANAEROBIC BACTERIA AND PERIODONTAL DISEASE

For NBDE Part 1, only the basics of periodontal microbiology will be covered. Characteristics of the major periodontal disease entities are tested.

Periodontal disease organisms are usually gram-negative, strictly anaerobic, or both. Some are capnophilic (thrive in a high carbon dioxide environment). This is in contrast to most supragingival flora (Streptococcus, etc.).

Chronic Adult Periodontitis

Usually considered to be a microbial infection combined with an overly aggressive protective response to the bacteria. Collagen loss and alveolar bone loss result. The flora constitute a mixed infection, with participation by *Prevotella, Bacteroides, Porphyromonas, Eichenella, Veillonella, Capnocytophaga, Actinobacillus Fusobacteria, Spriochetes,* and others.

It is NOT caused by one specific organism or a few (as in dental caries).

Adult Necrotizing Ulcerative Gingivitis (ANUG); Trenchmouth

Also considered to be a mixed infection, with spirochetes, *Fusobacteria* and *Prevotella* predominating. It is marked by gray, sloughing papillae; foul odor; and significant pain. It is a different disease entity from chronic adult periodontitis.

Juvenile Periodontitis, Aggressive Periodontitis

Another distinct disease entity. Compared to adult chronic periodontal disease, it is characterized by younger age, specific sites (first molars, incisors), faster progression, lack of noticeable plaque and calculus, and a specific causal organism (*Actinobacillus actinomycetemcomitans*).

SPIROCHETES

Genus: *Treponema*

Genus Features

- **Spirochetes: spiral with axial filament (endoflagellum)**
- **Poorly visible on Gram stain but gram-negative envelope**

Species of Medical Importance—*Treponema pallidum*

Treponema pallidum

Distinguishing Features

- **Thin spirochete,** not reliably seen on Gram stain
- Basically a gram-negative cell envelope
- Outer membrane has endotoxin-like lipids.
- Axial filaments = endoflagella = periplasmic flagella
- Cannot culture in clinical lab; serodiagnosis
- Is an **obligate pathogen (but not intracellular)**

Reservoir—human genital tract

Transmission—transmitted **sexually** or **across the placenta**

Pathogenesis

- Disease characterized by **endarteritis resulting in lesions.**
- Strong tendency to chronicity

Table 2-16. Stages of Syphilis

Stage	Clinical	Diagnosis
Primary (10 d to 3 mo after exposure)	Nontender chancre; clean, indurated edge; contagious; heals spontaneously 3—6 weeks	**Dark-field or fluorescent microscopy of lesion** 50% of patients will be negative by nonspecific serology
Secondary (1 to 3 mo later)	Maculopapular (copper-colored) rash, diffuse, includes palms and soles, patchy alopecia Condylomata lata: flat, wartlike perianal and mucous membrane lesions; highly infectious	**Serology nonspecific and specific;** both positive
Latent	None	Positive serology
Tertiary (30% of untreated, years later)	Gummas (syphilitic granulomas), aortitis, CNS inflammation	**Serology: specific tests** Nonspecific may be negative
Congenital (babies of IV drug—using)	Stillbirth, keratitis, 8th nerve damage, notched teeth; most born asymptomatic or with rhinitis → widespread desquamating maculopapular rash	Serology: should revert to negative within 3 mo of birth if uninfected

Diagnosis

- **Visualize organisms by immunofluorescence or dark-field microscopy.**
- **Serology** important—two types of antibody:
  1. **Nontreponemal antibody (= reagin) screening tests**

     – **Examples:**
       o Venereal disease research lab (VDRL)
       o Rapid plasma reagin (RPR)
  2. **Specific tests for treponemal antibody (more expensive)**

     – **Earliest** antibodies; **bind to spirochetes**
       o These tests are more specific and positive earlier

Treatment

- **Benzathine penicillin** (long-acting form) for primary and secondary syphilis (no resistance to penicillin); penicillin G for congenital and late syphilis

Prevention—benzathine penicillin is given to contacts; no vaccine is available.

GENUS: *BORRELIA*

Genus Features

- **Larger spirochetes**
- **Gram negative**
- **Microaerophilic**
- **Difficult to culture**

Species of Medical Importance—*Borrelia burgdorferi* (10 species responsible for human disease)

Borrelia burgdorferi

Reservoirs—white-footed mice (nymphs) and **white-tailed deer (adult ticks)**

Transmission

- By *Ixodes* (deer) ticks and nymphs; worldwide but in 3 main areas in the U.S.:
  - *Ixodes scapularis* *(I. dammini)* in Northeast (e.g., Connecticut), Midwest (e.g., Wisconsin)
  - *Ixodes pacificus* on West Coast (e.g., California)
  - Late spring/early summer incidence

Pathogenesis

- *B. burgdorferi* **invades skin and spreads via the bloodstream to involve primarily the heart, joints, and central nervous system.**
- Arthritis is caused by immune complexes.

Disease

- Lyme disease (#1 tick-borne disease in the U.S.)

Stage 1: Early localized (3 days to 1 month)	Target rash
Stage 2: Early disseminated (days to weeks later) Organism spreads hematogenously	Fatigue
	Chills and fever
	Headache
	Muscle and joint pain
	Swollen lymph nodes
	Secondary annular skin lesions
Stage 3: Late persistent (months to years)	Bell palsy, headache, meningitis, extreme fatigue, conjunctivitis, palpitations, arrhythmias, myocarditis, pericarditis
	Arthritis, most common in knees, immune complex-mediated

Treatment

- Doxycycline, amoxicillin, or azithromycin/clarithromycin (primary)
- Ceftriaxone for secondary
- Doxycycline or ceftriaxone for arthritis

Prevention
- DEET; avoid tick bites
- Vaccine (OspA flagellar antigen) not used in the U.S.

GENUS: *LEPTOSPIRA*

Genus Features
- **Spirochetes: thin, with hooks**
- **Too thin to visualize, but gram-negative cell envelope**

Species of Medical Importance—*Leptospira interrogans*

UNUSUAL BACTERIA

Table 2-17. Comparison of the Chlamydiaceae, Rickettsiaceae, and Mycoplasmataceae with Typical Bacteria

	Typical Bacteria (*S. aureus*)	Chlamydiaceae	Rickettsiaceae	Mycoplasmataceae
Obligate intracellular parasite?	Mostly no	Yes	Yes	No
Make ATP?	Normal ATP	No ATP	Limited ATP	Normal ATP
Peptidoglycan layer in cell envelope?	Normal peptidoglycan	Modified* peptidoglycan	Normal peptidoglycan	No peptidoglycan

*Chlamydial peptidoglycan lacks muramic acid and is considered by some as modified, by others as absent.

FAMILY: CHLAMYDIACEAE

Family Features
- **Obligate intracellular bacteria**
- **Elementary body/reticulate body**
- **Not seen on Gram stain**
- **Cannot make ATP**
- **Cell wall lacks muramic acid**

Genera of Medical Importance
- *Chlamydia trachomatis*
- *Chlamydophila pneumoniae* (formerly *Chlamydia pneumoniae*)
- *Chlamydophila psittaci* (formerly *Chlamydia psittaci*)

Chlamydia trachomatis

Reservoir—human genital tract and eyes

Transmission—sexual contact and **at birth;** trachoma is transmitted by **hand-to-eye contact** and flies.

Pathogenesis—infection of nonciliated columnar or cuboidal epithelial cells of mucosal surfaces leads to **granulomatous response and damage.**

Diseases

- STDs in U.S.
    - **Serotypes D-K** (This is the most common **bacterial** STD in the U.S., although overall, herpes and HPV are more common.)
    - **Nongonococcal urethritis, cervicitis, PID,** and major portion of infertility (no resistance to reinfection)
    - **Inclusion conjunctivitis**
- Lymphogranuloma venereum
    - This STD is prevalent in Africa, Asia, and South America.
    - Painless ulcer at the site of contact
    - Swollen lymph nodes leading to genital elephantiasis in late stage
    - Tertiary: ulcers, fistulas, genital elephantiasis
- Trachoma
    - Leading cause of preventable infectious blindness
    - **Follicular conjunctivitis** leading to **conjunctival scarring,** and **inturned eyelashes** leading to **corneal scarring** and **blindness**

Treatment—doxycycline or azithromycin

Prevention

- Erythromycin is effective in infected mothers to prevent neonatal disease.
- Treat neonatal conjunctivitis with systemic erythromycin to prevent pneumonia.

GENUS: *CHLAMYDOPHILA*

Table 2-18. Diseases Caused by Chlamydophila Species

Organism	*C. pneumoniae*	*C. psittaci*
Distinguishing characteristics	Potential association with atherosclerosis	No glycogen in inclusion bodies
Reservoir	Human respiratory tract	Birds, **parrots,** turkeys (major U.S. reservoir)
Transmission	Respiratory droplets	Dust of dried bird secretions and feces
Pathogenesis	Intracellular growth; infects smooth muscle, endothelial cells, or coronary artery and macrophages	Intracellular growth
Disease	Atypical "walking" pneumonia; single lobe; bronchitis; scant sputum, prominent dry cough	Psittacosis (ornithosis); atypical pneumonia with hepatitis
Treatment	Macrolides and tetracycline	Doxycycline
Prevention	None	Avoid birds

GENUS: *RICKETTSIA*

Table 2-19. Infections Caused by Rickettsiae and Close Relatives

Group Disease	Bacterium	Arthropod Vector	Reservoir Host
Rocky Mountain Spotted Fever	*R. rickettsii*	Ticks	Ticks, dogs, rodents
Epidemic Typhus	*R. prowazekii*	Human louse	Humans
Endemic Typhus	*R. typhi*	Fleas	Rodents

Genus Features
- **Aerobic, gram-negative bacilli (too small to stain well with Gram stain)**
- **Obligate intracellular bacteria (do not make sufficient ATP for independent life)**

Species of Medical Importance
- *Rickettsia rickettsii*
- *Rickettsia prowazekii*
- *Rickettsia typhi*

Rickettsia rickettsii

Reservoir—small wild rodents and larger wild and domestic animals (dogs)

Transmission—hard ticks: *Dermacentor*

Pathogenesis—invade endothelial cells lining capillaries, causing vasculitis in many organs

Disease
- Rocky Mountain spotted fever (RMSF)
  - **Headache, fever (102°F)**, malaise, myalgias, toxicity, vomiting, and confusion
  - **Rash** (maculopapular) → **on ankles and wrists** and then spreads to the trunk, **palms, soles, and face**
  - **Ankle and wrist swelling**

Diagnosis
- Clinical symptoms (above) and tick bite
- **Start treatment without laboratory confirmation.**

Treatment—doxycycline

Prevention—tick protection and prompt removal

GENUS: *EHRLICHIA*

Genus Features
- **Gram-negative bacilli**
- **Obligate intracellular bacteria of mononuclear or granulocytic phagocytes**

Species of Medical Importance

- *Ehrlichia chaffeensis*
- *Anaplasma phagocytophila*

Ehrlichia chaffeensis/Anaplasma phagocytophila

Table 2-20. Summary of Diseases Caused by Ehrlichia Species

Organism	Reservoir	Transmission	Pathogenesis	Disease	Treatment
E. chaffeensis	Ticks and deer	Lone star tick (*Amblyomma*)	Infects monocytes and macrophages	Ehrlichiosis (monocytic)	Doxycycline
A. phagocyto-phila	Ticks, deer, mice	*Ixodes* ticks Coinfection with *Borrelia*	Infects neutrophils	Ehrlichiosis (granulocytic)	Doxycycline

Disease

- Similar to Rocky Mountain spotted fever but generally without rash
- Leukopenia
- Thrombocytopenia
- Morulae—mulberry-like structures inside infected cells

Treatment—doxycycline (begin before laboratory confirmation)

Prevention—no vaccine, avoid ticks

FAMILY: MYCOPLASMATACEAE

Family Features

- **Smallest free-living (extracellular) bacteria**
- **Missing peptidoglycan (no cell wall)**
- **Sterols in membrane**

Genera of Medical Importance

- *Mycoplasma pneumoniae*
- *Ureaplasma urealyticum*

Mycoplasma pneumoniae

Reservoir—human respiratory tract

Transmission—respiratory droplets; close contact: families, military recruits, medical school classes, college dorms

Pathogenesis

- Surface parasite: not invasive
- **Attaches to respiratory epithelium**
- **Inhibits ciliary action**
- **Produces hydrogen peroxide, superoxide radicals, and cytolytic enzymes,** which damage the respiratory epithelium, leading to necrosis and a bad, hacking cough (walking pneumonia)
- *M. pneumoniae* functions as superantigen, elicits production of IL-1, IL-6, and TNF-α

Disease

- Walking pneumonia
  - **Pharyngitis**
  - **May develop into an atypical pneumonia**
  - **Most common atypical pneumonia (along with viruses) in young adults**

Treatment—erythromycin, azithromycin, clarithromycin; **no cephalosporins or penicillins**

Prevention—none

Ureaplasma urealyticum

Distinguishing Features

- Member of family Mycoplasmataceae

Pathogenesis

- Urease positive

Diseases

- Urethritis, prostatitis, renal calculi

Treatment

- Erythromycin or tetracyclineMicrobiology

Microbial Genetics/ Drug Resistance

Learning Objectives

❑ Explain information related to rearrangement of DNA within a bacterium

❑ Answer questions about bacterial gene transfer

❑ Solve problems concerning mechanisms of bacterial DNA exchange and conjugal crosses

❑ Demonstrate understanding of drug resistance

❑ Explain information related to antibiotic susceptibility testing

THE BACTERIAL GENETIC MATERIAL

Three different types of DNA may be found in a bacterial cell: bacterial chromosomal DNA, plasmid DNA, or bacteriophage DNA.

Bacterial Chromosome (Genome)

- Most bacteria have only **one chromosome but often multiple copies** of it in the cell.
- Most bacterial chromosomes are a **large, covalently closed, circular DNA molecule**.
- The chromosome is **organized into loops** around a proteinaceous center. A single-stranded topoisomerase (1 nick) will relax only the nicked loop, allowing DNA synthesis or transcription.
- All **essential genes** are on the bacterial chromosome.

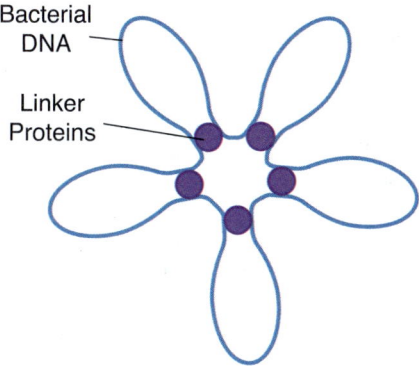

Figure 3-1. The Bacterial Chromosome

Plasmids

- Are **extrachromosomal genetic elements** found in bacteria (and eukaryotes)
- Are generally covalently closed, **circular DNA**
- Are **small** (1.5–400 kB)
- Can **replicate autonomously** in bacterial cells
- One subclass of plasmids, called **episomes**, may be integrated into the bacterial DNA. Episomes have insertion sequences matching those on the bacterial chromosome.
- Plasmids carry the genetic material for a variety of genes, e.g., the **fertility genes** directing conjugation (*tra* operon), many of the genes for **antibiotic resistance**, and most **bacterial exotoxins**.
- They contain genes that are **nonessential** for bacterial life.

Bacteriophage (= Phage = Bacterial Virus) Genome

- **Stable pieces of bacteriophage DNA** may be present in the bacterial cell.
- These are **generally repressed temperate phage (called prophage)** inserted into the bacterial chromosome.
- Besides the repressor protein, prophage DNA may also direct synthesis of other proteins. Most notable are gene products that make bacteria more pathogenic. This enhanced virulence is called **lysogenic conversion.**

REARRANGEMENT OF DNA WITHIN A BACTERIUM

Homologous Recombination

- Homologous recombination is a gene exchange process that may **stabilize genes** introduced into a cell by transformation, conjugation, or transduction.
- Imported bacterial DNA (transferred into a cell by transformation, conjugation, or transduction) is on short linear pieces of DNA called **exogenotes**. Most linear DNA is not stable in cells because it is broken down by exonucleases.
- Homologous recombination produces an **"exchange"** of DNA between the linear exogenote of DNA and a homologous region on the stable (circular) bacterial chromosome.
- Homologous recombination requires:
  - Several genes worth of **homology or near homology** between the DNA strands.
  - A series of recombination **enzymes**/factors coded for by the recombination genes

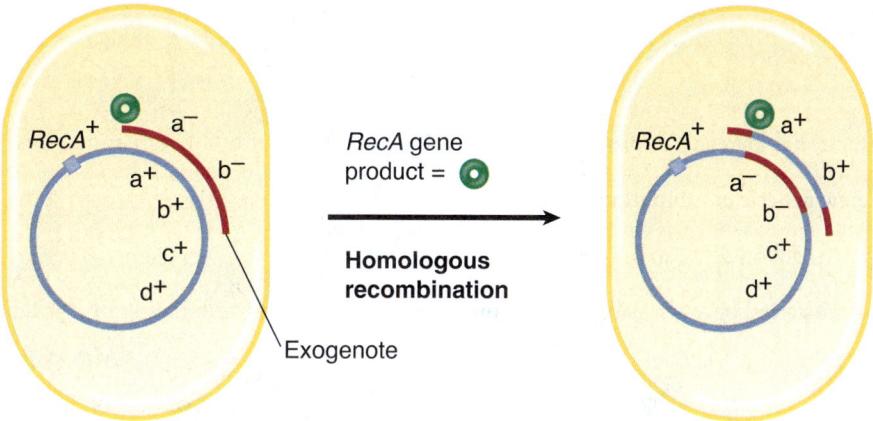

Genes ending up on the linear piece of DNA are lost. Those on the circular molecule become part of the cell's permanent genetic make up.

Figure 3-2. Homologous Recombination

Site-Specific Recombination

Site-specific recombination is the integration of one DNA molecule into another DNA molecule with which it has **no homology** except for a small site on each DNA (called an **attachment, integration, or insertion site**).

- Requires **restriction endonucleases** and restriction endonuclease sites on each DNA
- Because this process **integrates** rather than exchanges pieces of DNA, the end result is a molecule the **sum of the two original molecules**.

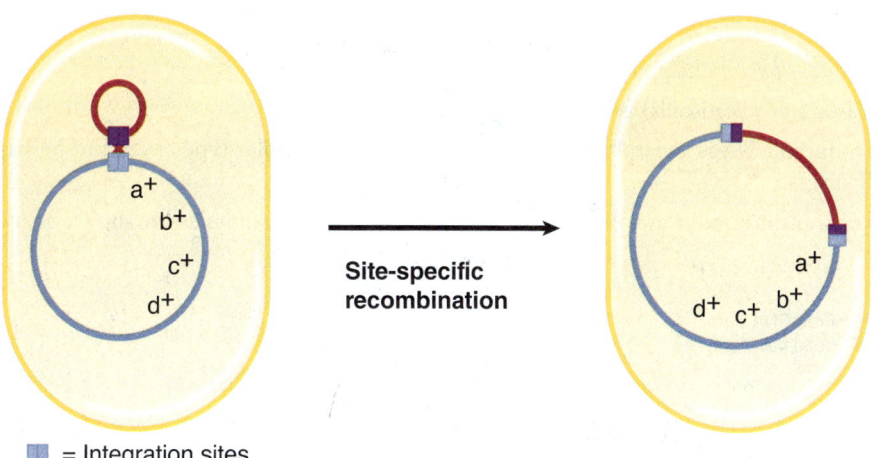

Figure 3-3. Site-Specific Recombination

Three major roles of site-specific integration

- Integration of a **fertility factor** to make an Hfr cell
- Integration of **temperate phage** DNA into a bacterial chromosome to create a prophage
- Movement and insertion of **transposons** (transposition is the name of site-specific integration of transposons)

GENE TRANSFER

Overview

Bacterial reproduction is asexual, so progeny are identical to parent cell with only rare mutations.

How do you get new genetic combinations in bacteria?

Answer: Gene transfer followed by stabilization of genes (recombination)

Any DNA that is transferred between bacterial cells must be stabilized by recombination or it will be lost.

In a Nutshell
DNA can be transferred from bacterium to bacterium by: • Conjugation   • Transformation   • Transduction

MECHANISMS OF DNA EXCHANGE

Transformation

Transformation is the uptake of naked DNA from the environment by competent cells.

- Cells become **competent (able to bind short pieces of DNA to the envelope and import them into the cell)** under certain environmental conditions.
- Some bacteria are capable of **natural transformation** (they are naturally competent): *Haemophilus influenzae*, *Streptococcus pneumoniae*, *Bacillus* species, and *Neisseria* species.
- DNA (released from dead cells) is taken up.
- Newly introduced DNA is generally linear, homologous DNA a similar type of cell but perhaps one that is genetically diverse.
- The steps of transformation of a nonencapsulated *Streptococcus pneumoniae* are shown below.

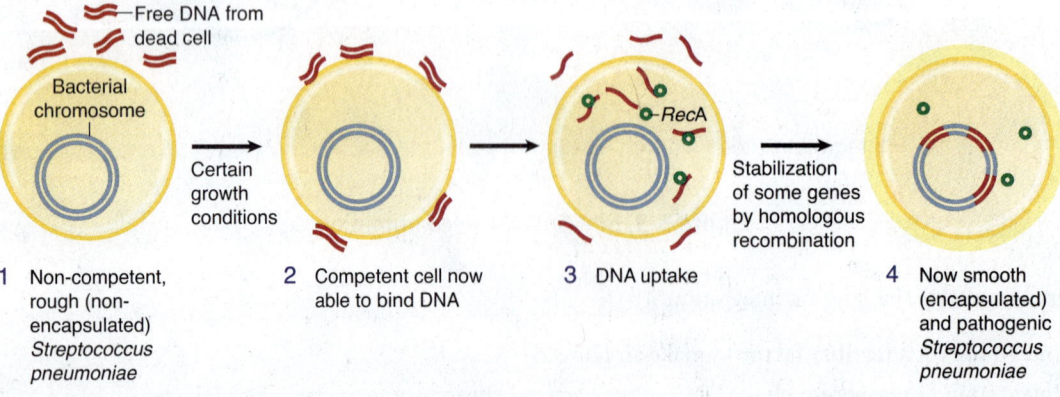

Figure 3-4. Transformation

Conjugation

Conjugation is gene transfer from one bacterial cell to another involving direct cell-to-cell contact.

- **Fertility factors control** conjugation.
- **Sex pili** (genes on F factor) play a role in establishing cell-to-cell contact.
- A **single strand** (or a portion thereof) of the double helix of DNA is transferred from the donor (or male) cell to the recipient or female cell.
- Chromosomal genes transferred in by conjugation have to be stabilized by **homologous recombination** (in an Hfr × F⁻ cross). Plasmid genes transferred by conjugation circularize and are stable without recombination (in an F⁺ × F⁻ cross).
- Conjugation with recombination may produce new genetic combinations.

Donor (male) cells

- All have fertility plasmids known as **F factors**. F factors have a series of important plasmid "fertility" genes called the transfer or ***tra* region**, which code for:
  - **Sex pili**
  - Genes whose products **stabilize mating pairs**
  - Genes that **direct conjugal DNA transfer**, and other genes.
- Have a region called ***oriT* (origin of transfer)** where a single strand break in the DNA will be made and then *oriT* begins the transfer of one strand of the double helix.
- Many have **insertion sequences** where the plasmid can be inserted into the bacterial chromosome combining to make one larger molecule of DNA.
- Donor cells in which the **fertility plasmid** is in its **free state** are called **F+ cells**.
- Donor cells in which the **fertility factor has inserted** itself into the bacterial chromosome are called **Hfr cells**. An integrated plasmid is called an episome.

Recipient (female) cells: F– cells

- Recipient cells **lack fertility factors**.
- In every cross, one cell must be an F-cell.

Mating types of bacterial cells

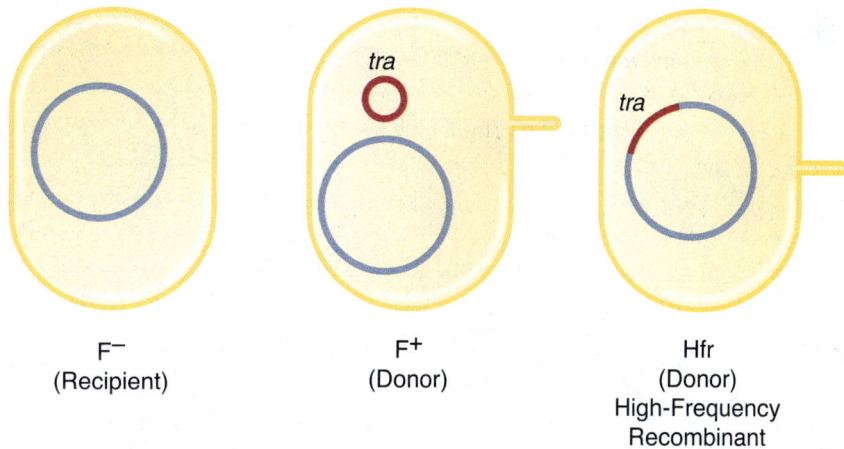

Figure 3-5. Mating Types of Bacteria

CONJUGAL CROSSES

There are two major types of crosses:

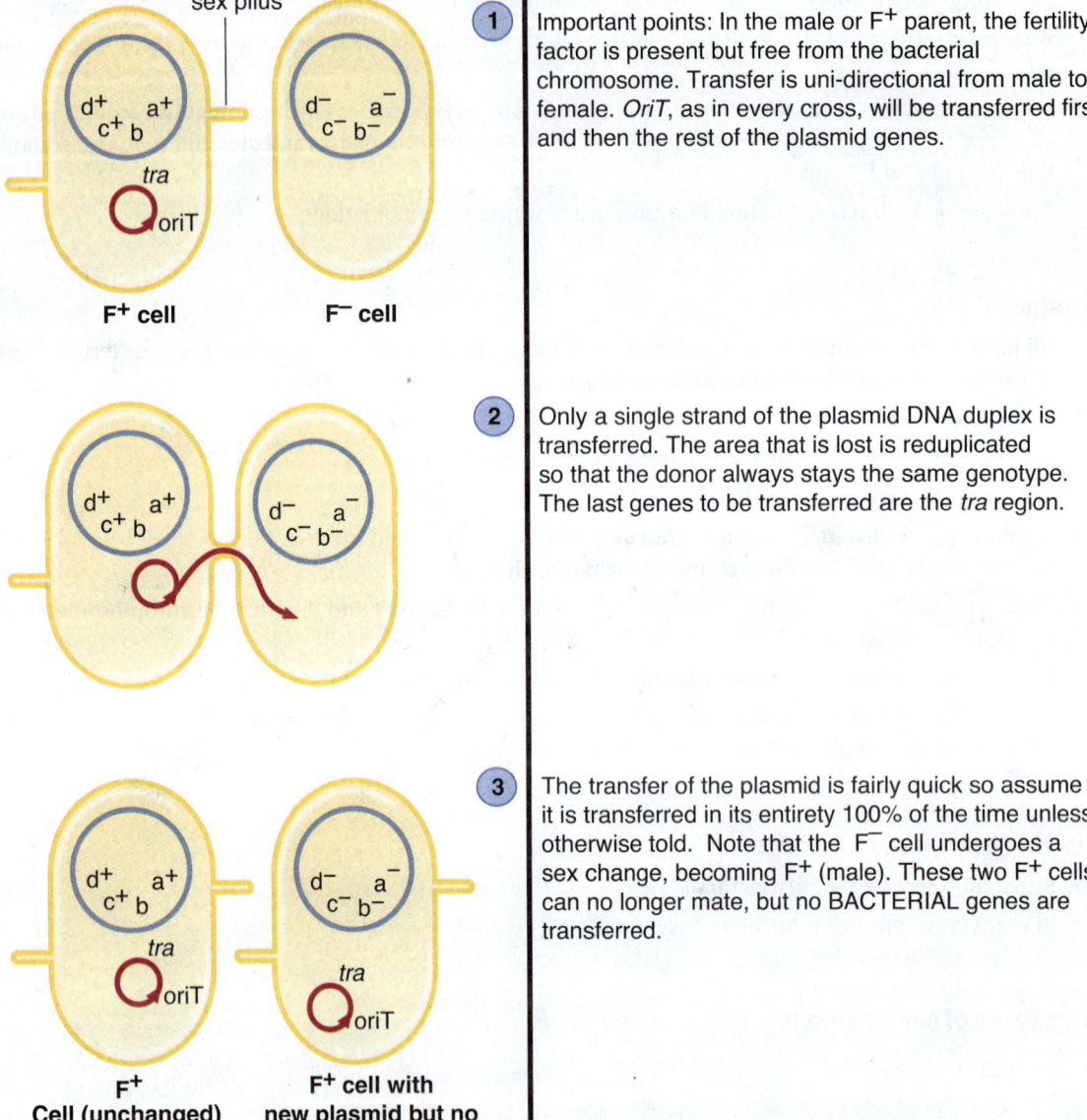

1. Important points: In the male or F⁺ parent, the fertility factor is present but free from the bacterial chromosome. Transfer is uni-directional from male to female. *OriT*, as in every cross, will be transferred first and then the rest of the plasmid genes.

2. Only a single strand of the plasmid DNA duplex is transferred. The area that is lost is reduplicated so that the donor always stays the same genotype. The last genes to be transferred are the *tra* region.

3. The transfer of the plasmid is fairly quick so assume it is transferred in its entirety 100% of the time unless otherwise told. Note that the F⁻ cell undergoes a sex change, becoming F⁺ (male). These two F⁺ cells can no longer mate, but no BACTERIAL genes are transferred.

Figure 3-6. The F+ by F− Conjugal Cross

Conjugation: 2nd type of cross Hfr × F⁻

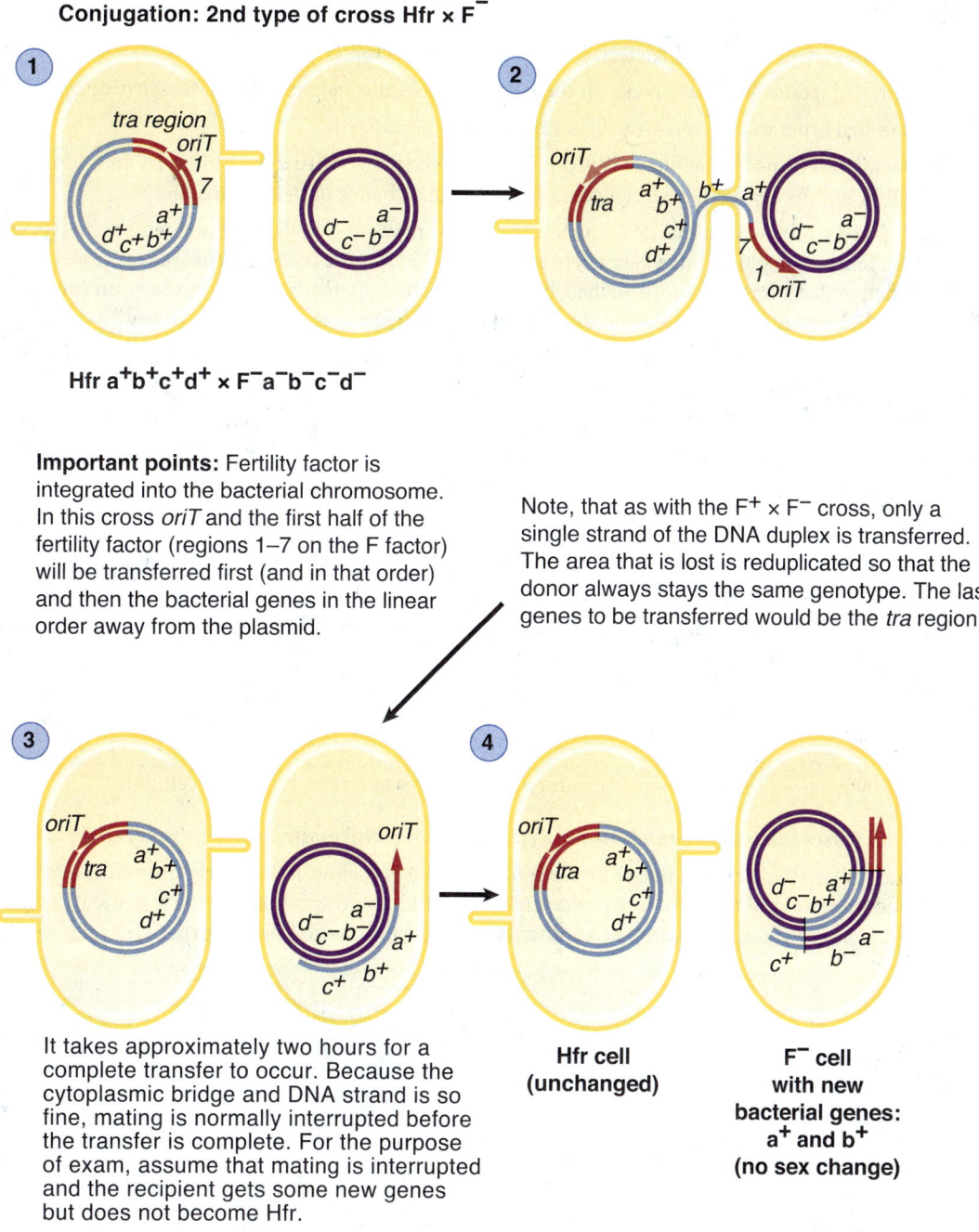

Hfr a⁺b⁺c⁺d⁺ × F⁻a⁻b⁻c⁻d⁻

Important points: Fertility factor is integrated into the bacterial chromosome. In this cross *oriT* and the first half of the fertility factor (regions 1–7 on the F factor) will be transferred first (and in that order) and then the bacterial genes in the linear order away from the plasmid.

Note, that as with the F⁺ × F⁻ cross, only a single strand of the DNA duplex is transferred. The area that is lost is reduplicated so that the donor always stays the same genotype. The last genes to be transferred would be the *tra* region.

It takes approximately two hours for a complete transfer to occur. Because the cytoplasmic bridge and DNA strand is so fine, mating is normally interrupted before the transfer is complete. For the purpose of exam, assume that mating is interrupted and the recipient gets some new genes but does not become Hfr.

Hfr cell (unchanged)

F⁻ cell with new bacterial genes: a⁺ and b⁺ (no sex change)

Figure 3-7. The Hfr by F⁻ Conjugal Cross

Transduction

- **Transduction** is the transfer of bacterial DNA by a phage vector.
- During transduction, the phage picks up the bacterial DNA through an error in phage production.
- There are **two types of transduction: generalized and specialized**.
  - A **generalized transducing phage** is produced when the phage **with a lytic life cycle** puts a piece of bacterial DNA into its head. All bacterial genes have an equal chance of being transduced.
  - **Specialized transduction** may occur when an error is made in the life cycle of a temperate (lysogenic) phage. **Temperate phage introduce their genomic DNA into the bacterial chromosome** at a specific site and then excise it later to complete their life cycle. If errors are made during the excision process, then bacterial chromosomal DNA can be carried along into the next generation of viruses.

To understand transduction, you need first to understand how a phage replicates normally so that you can understand how the errors are made.

Phage = bacteriophage = bacterial virus

Come in two major types:

- **Virulent phage** infect bacterial cells, always making more virus and lysing the cells (lytic replication).
- **Temperate phage** often infect without lysing the cells because they have the ability to repress active phage replication and to stably integrate their DNA into the bacterial chromosome. In the absence of functional repressor protein, they also may replicate lytically.

Lytic infection

Lytic infection, by phage or viruses, leads to production of viruses and their release by cell lysis.

- **Virulent viruses can only go into lytic life cycles and can accidentally carry out generalized transduction.**
- The lytic (or productive) life cycle of virulent phage is shown below. It is entirely normal except for a mistaken incorporation of bacterial DNA into one phage head, creating a transducing virus, shown at the bottom of the next page. Transduction of another bacterial cell is shown following that.

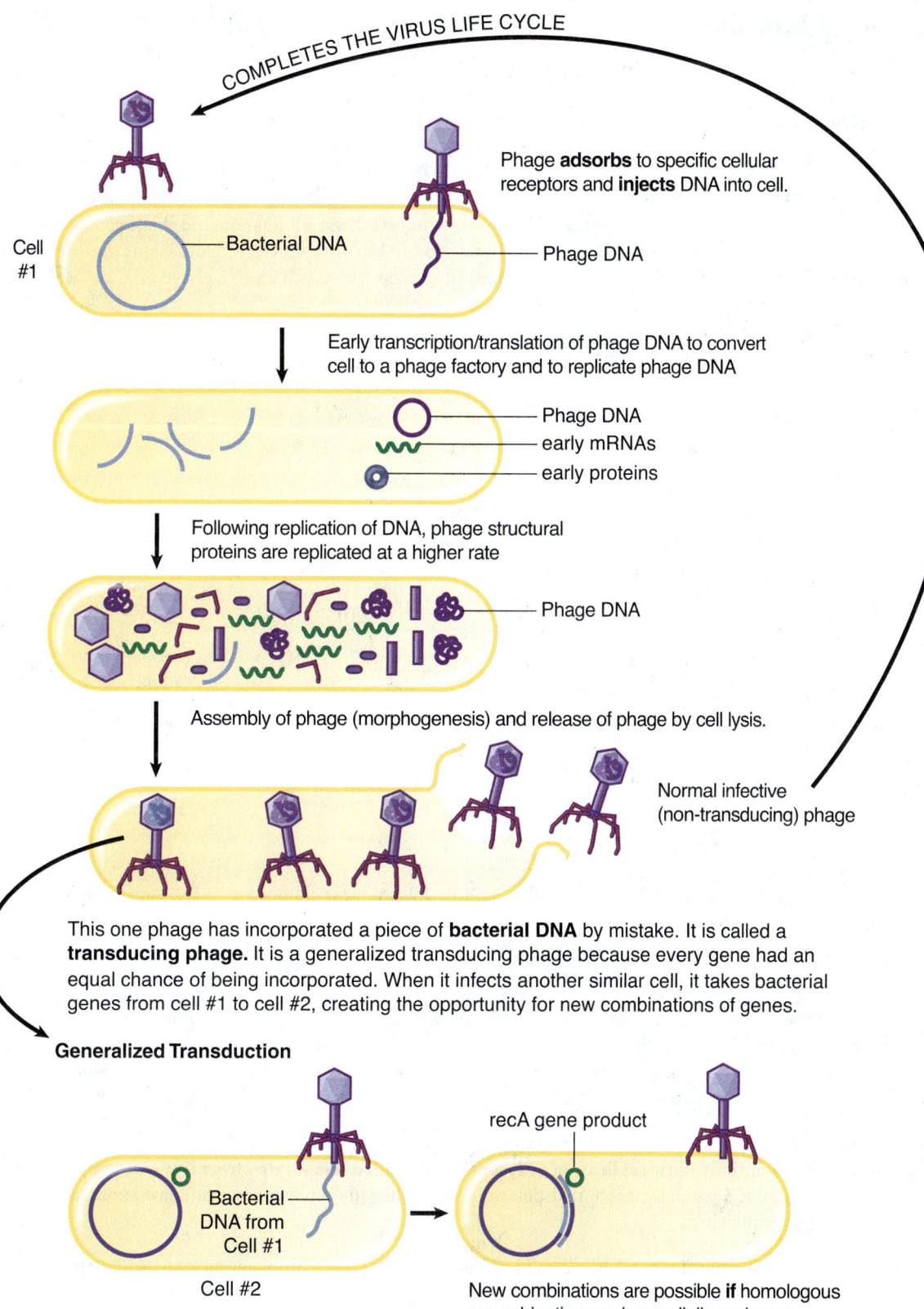

Figure 3-8. Generalized Transduction as an Accident of the Lytic Virus Life Cycle

Specialized Transduction as a Sequela to the Lysogenic Phage Life Cycle

Lysogeny

Temperate phage may become prophage (DNA stably integrated) or replicate lytically.

- When repressor is made, temperate phage insert their DNA into the bacterial chromosome where it stably stays as a **prophage**.

- If the repressor gene gets mutated or the repressor protein gets damaged then the prophage gets excised from the bacterial DNA and is induced into the lytic production of virus. On rare occasions these temperate phage can produce either specialized or generalized transducing viruses. Lambda phage of *E. coli* is the best studied. Most temperate phages have only a single insertion site.

- **Lambda inserts ONLY between *E. coli* genes *gal* and *bio* as shown below.**

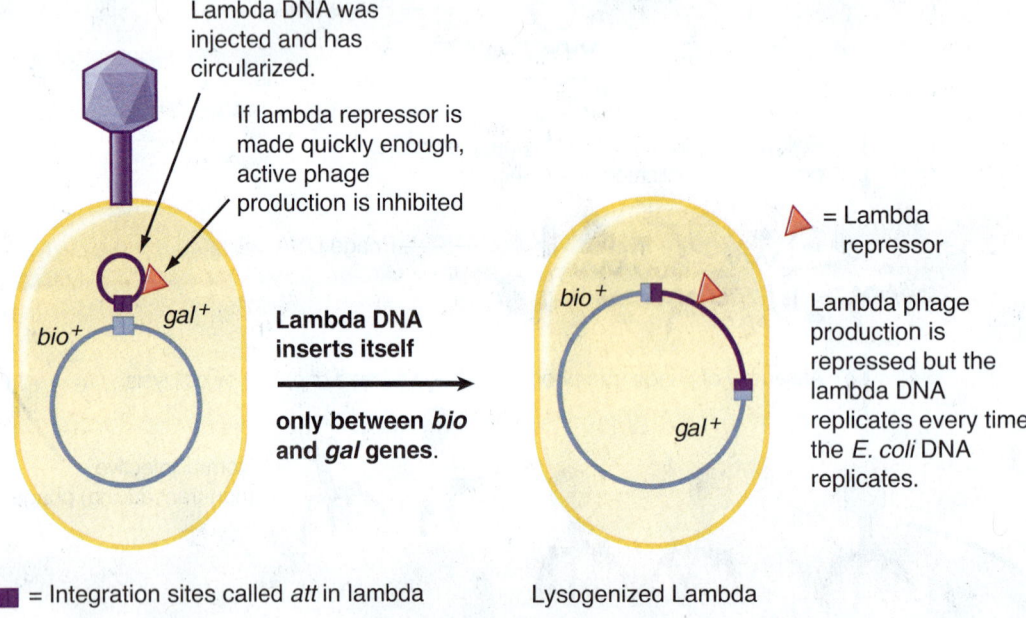

Figure 3-9. Lysogeny

Lysogeny is the state of a bacterial cell with a **stable phage DNA** (generally integrated into the bacterial DNA), **not undergoing lytic replication either because it is repressed or defective**. When the cell DNA replicates, the phage DNA also replicates and, as long as the repressor protein is not damaged, the lysogenic state continues ad infinitum. Defective phage (or defective viruses in the human equivalent) cannot go into an active replication unless a helper virus is present.

Phage that have both options (lytic replication or lysogeny) are called temperate phage. When a temperate phage first infects a cell there is a regulatory race that determines whether the repressor is made fast enough to prevent synthesis of phage components.

The lysogenized cell will replicate to produce two identical cells each with a prophage as long as the repressor gene product is present.

Lysogeny can confer new properties on a genus such as toxin production or antigens (**lysogenic conversion**):

C: Cholera toxin

O: Presence of specific prophage in *Salmonella* can affect **O** antigens.

B: Phage CE β or DE β cause *Clostridium botulinum* to produce **B**otulinum toxin.

E: **E**xotoxins A–C (erythrogenic or pyogenic) of *Streptococcus pyogenes*

D: Prophage beta causes *Corynebacterium diphtheriae* to make **D**iphtheria toxin.

S: **S**higa toxin

- (Mnemonic for phage-mediated pathogenic factors = COBEDS)
- Model for retrovirus provirus
- Allows specialized transduction

Induction

If the repressor is damaged (by UV, cold, or alkylating agents), then the prophage is excised and the cell goes into lytic replication phase. This process is called **induction**.

Most of the time this process is carried out **perfectly**, recreating the figure 8 of DNA that was the product of viral site-specific recombination, and normal (**nontransducing**) **phage** are produced.

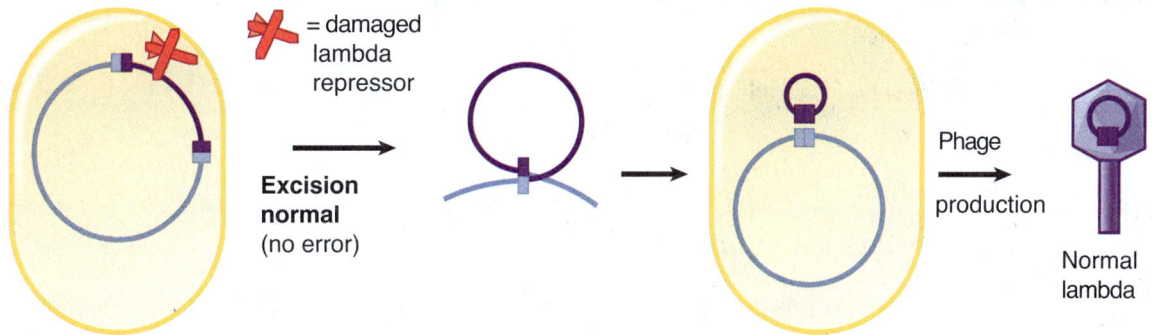

Figure 3-10. Normal Excision of a Lysogenic Phage

Rarely, in the excision process, an **excisional error** is made and **one of the bacterial genes next to the insertion site is removed attached to the lambda DNA, and a little bit of lambda DNA is left behind**. Only genes on one side *or* the other side of the virus insertion site can be incorporated by excisional error.

Because lambda has only one insertion site (between *gal* or *bio*), only *gal* <u>or</u> *bio* can be incorporated by excisional error.

Because all of the phage genes are still in the cell, phage are still made with the circular defective phage genome copied and put in each phage head. These are **specialized transducing phage** (only able to transduce *bio* or *gal*).

Specialized Transduction

Bacterial genes picked up by error in the excision process are transferred to another closely related but often genetically distinct cell. If any genes on the exogenote are stabilized by recombinational exchange, then new genetic combinations occur.

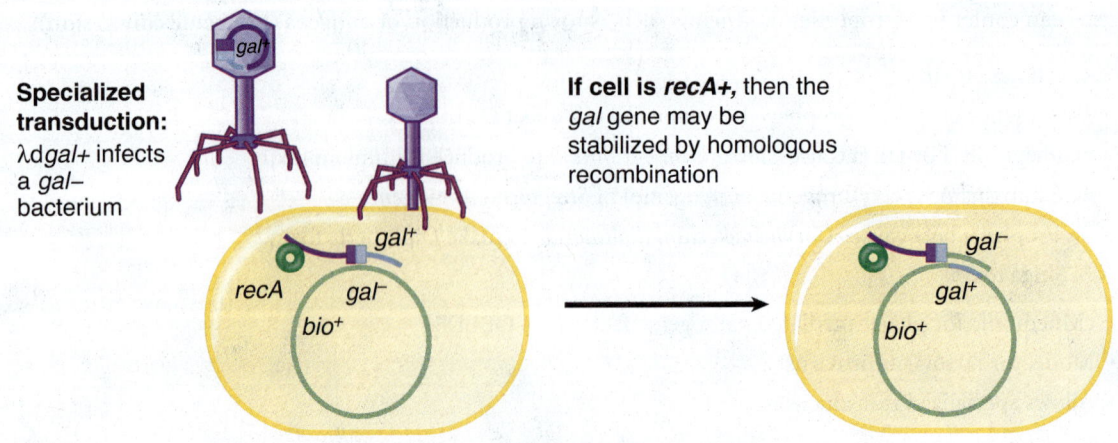

Figure 3-11. Specialized Transduction

Only those genes next to the phage insertion site can be transduced by specialized transduction.

Table 3-1. Comparison of Transformation, Conjugation, and Transduction

Requirement	Transformation	Conjugation	Transduction
Is cell-to-cell contact required?	No	Yes	No
Does it require an antecedent phage infection?	No	No	Yes
Is competency required?	Yes	No	No
Is naked (free) DNA involved?	Yes	No	No
Is recombination required to stabilize new genes?	Yes	No for F$^+$ × F$^-$ Yes for Hfr × F$^-$	Yes

Table 3-2. Comparison of Generalized and Specialized Transduction

	Generalized	Specialized
Mechanism	**Error in assembly**	**Error of excision** Requires stable insertion of prophage DNA (lysogeny)
What genes may be transferred?	**Any**	Only **genes next to the insertion site**

DRUG RESISTANCE

Overall Problem
- Drug resistance is becoming such a significant problem that there are
- bacteria for which most antibiotics no longer work. We are entering a "post-antibiotic era."
- Drug resistance can be transferred from one genus of bacteria to another, e.g., from normal flora to a pathogen.
- Three general types of antibiotic resistance exist: intrinsic, chromosome-mediated, and plasmid-mediated.

Intrinsic Drug Resistance
Bacteria are intrinsically resistant to an antibiotic if they lack the target molecule for the drug or if their normal anatomy and physiology makes them refractory to the drug's action.

- Bacteria that lack mycolic acids are intrinsically resistant to isoniazid.
- Bacteria such as *Mycoplasma* that lack peptidoglycan are intrinsically resistant to penicillin.

Chromosome-Mediated Antibiotic Resistance
The genes that determine this resistance are located on the bacterial chromosome.

- Most commonly these genes modify the **receptor for a drug** so that the drug can no longer bind (e.g., a mutation in a gene for a penicillin binding protein).
- In general, causes **low-level drug resistance** rather than high
- In methicillin-resistant *Staphylococcus aureus* a major penicillin-binding protein was mutated.
- Even low-level resistance may be clinically significant, e.g., in *Streptococcus pneumoniae* meningitis.

Plasmid-Mediated Drug Resistance
The genes that determine this resistance are located on plasmids.

- Plasmid-mediated resistance is created by a variety of mechanisms but often genes code for **enzymes that modify the drug.**
- R factors are conjugative plasmids carrying genes for drug resistance.
  - One section of the DNA (containing *oriT* and the *tra* gene region) mediates conjugation.
  - The other section (**R determinant**) carries genes for drug resistance. Multiple genes seem to have been inserted through **transpositional insertion** into a "hot spot."

How Do Multiple Drug-Resistance Plasmids Arise?
Gene cassettes/integrons/transposons:

- Are mobile genetic elements (DNA) that can move themselves or a copy from one molecule of DNA to another ("jumping genes")
- Are found in eukaryotic and bacterial cells and viruses
- Have at least one gene for a **transposase** (enzyme involved in the movement)
- Create additional **mutations** with their insertion into another totally unrelated gene

Table 3-3. Plasmid-Mediated Mechanisms of Bacterial Drug Resistance

Antimicrobial Agent	Mechanism
Penicillins and cephalosporins	Production of β-**lactamase**; cleavage of β-lactam rings
Aminoglycosides	Production of acetyltransferase, adenosyltransferase, or phosphotransferase; **inactivation of drug by acetylation**, adenosylation, or phosphorylation
Chloramphenicol	Production of acetyltransferase; **inactivation of drug by acetylation**
Tetracyclines	Increased **efflux** out of cell
Sulfonamides	Active **export** out of cell and lowered affinity of enzyme
Vancomycin	Ligase produces cell wall pentapeptides that terminate in d-alanine-d-lactate, which will not bind to drug

Transfer of Drug Resistance

Conjugation

Gram-negative bacilli

Plasmid mediated, transferred by conjugation.

Staphylococcus aureus (Methicillin Resistant = MRSA)

Resistance to methicillin is chromosomal, transferred by transduction. Most of the other antibiotic resistance is transferred by plasmids.

S. aureus recently acquired the genes for vancomycin resistance (van A and van B) from *Enterococcus faecalis* via a transposon on a multi-drug resistant conjugative plasmid. In *S. aureus*, the transposon moved from the *E. faecalis* plasmid to a multi-drug resistant plasmid in *S. aureus*. The new *S. aureus* super multi-drug resistant plasmid now contains resistance genes against β-lactams, vancomycin, aminoglycosides, trimethoprim, and some disinfectants and can be transferred to other strains via conjugation.

Enterococcus faecalis and ***faecium***

Resistance to vancomycin is carried on a multi-drug–resistant conjugative plasmid.

Neisseria gonorrhoeae

In ***Neisseria gonorrhoeae***, two plasmids are required to transfer drug resistances. In this bacterial species, drug resistance genes are located on **nonconjugative plasmids**. These are plasmids that have lost their *tra* operon but retained *oriT*. Nonconjugative plasmids may be transferred by conjugation as long as there is another fertility factor in the same cell with a functional *tra* operon. The process is referred to as **mobilization**.

Transformation

It is difficult to mark the movement of drug resistance genes through the process of transformation, but epidemiologic studies suggest that the spread of **penicillin-binding protein mutations of _Streptococcus pneumoniae_ occurs via transformation.**

Transduction

The high host cell specificity of bacteriophage limits transduction to a transfer mechanism between members of the same bacterial species. Nevertheless, in **_Staphylococcus aureus_ resistance to methicillin is chromosome mediated and transferred by transduction**. In _Pseudomonas aeruginosa_, imipenem resistance is transferred from one member of the species to another during transduction by wild-type bacteriophage.

ANTIBIOTIC SUSCEPTIBILITY TESTING

Sterilization, Disinfection, Pasteurization

Sterilization: complete removal or killing of all viable organisms.

Disinfection: the removal or killing of disease-causing organisms. Compounds for use on skin: antiseptics.

Pasteurization: the rapid heating and cooling of milk designed to kill milk-borne pathogens such as _Mycobacterium bovis_, _Brucella_, and _Listeria_.

Physical Methods of Control

Heat = saturated steam
- **Autoclaving (steam under pressure): 15 lbs pressure → 121°C 15–20 min** (sterilizing)

Radiation
- UV: formation of thymine–thymine pairs on adjacent DNA bases

Filtration
- HEPA (High Efficiency Particulate Air) filters for air
- Nitrocellulose or other known pore-size filters

Chemical Methods of Control

Agents damaging membranes
- **Detergents:** surface active compounds—most notable the quaternary ammonium compounds like benzalkonium chloride—interact with membrane through hydrophobic end disrupting membrane.
- **Alcohols:** disrupt membrane and denature proteins.
- **Phenols** and derivatives: damage membrane and denature proteins.

Agents modifying proteins
- **Chlorine:** oxidizing agent inactivating sulfhydryl-containing enzymes

- **Iodine and iodophors** (that have reduced toxicity): also oxidation of sulfhydryl-containing enzymes
- **Hydrogen peroxide:** oxidizing agent (sulfhydryl groups); catalase inactivates
- **Heavy metals:** (silver and mercury)—bind to sulfhydryl groups inhibiting enzyme activity
- **Ethylene oxide:** alkylating agent (sterilizing agent)
- **Formaldehyde** and glutaraldehyde: denatures protein and nucleic acids and alkylates amino and hydroxyl groups on both. Primarily an alkylator.

Modification of nucleic acids

- **Dyes:** like crystal violet and malachite green whose positively charged molecule binds to the negatively charged phosphate groups on the nucleic acids

Medically Important Viruses

Learning Objectives

❏ Demonstrate understanding of structure, morphology, and replication of medically important viruses

❏ Answer questions related to patterns of infection, resistance, and treatment of DNA viruses, positive-stranded RNA viruses, negative-stranded RNA viruses, double-stranded RNA viruses, onco-viruses, and prions

❏ Explain information related to viral hepatitis.

Bridge to Biochemistry

Positive-sense = coding strand

Negative-sense = template strand

STRUCTURE AND MORPHOLOGY

```
DNA              Structural
 or      +        proteins        =    Nucleocapsid    =    Naked capsid
RNA*            (capsomers, etc.)                            virus

Enzymes e.g., polymerase
```

```
Nucleocapsid    +    Host membrane with
                     viral-specified glycoproteins    =    Enveloped virus
                     (critical for infectiousness
                     of viral progeny)
```

Figure 4-1. The Basic Virion

*Positive-sense RNA = (+)RNA (can be used itself as mRNA)

ss = Single stranded

ds = Double stranded

*Negative-sense RNA = (−)RNA

- Complementary to mRNA

- Cannot be used as mRNA

- Requires virion-associated, RNA-dependent RNA polymerase (as part of the mature virus)

VIRAL STRUCTURE

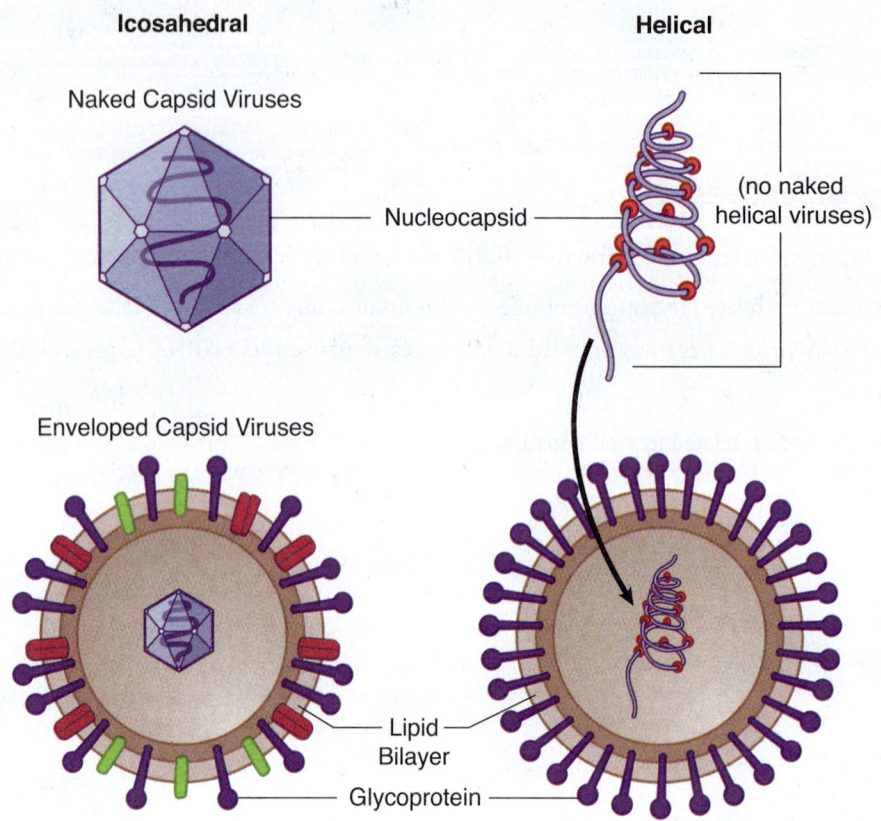

Figure 4-2. Morphology of Viruses

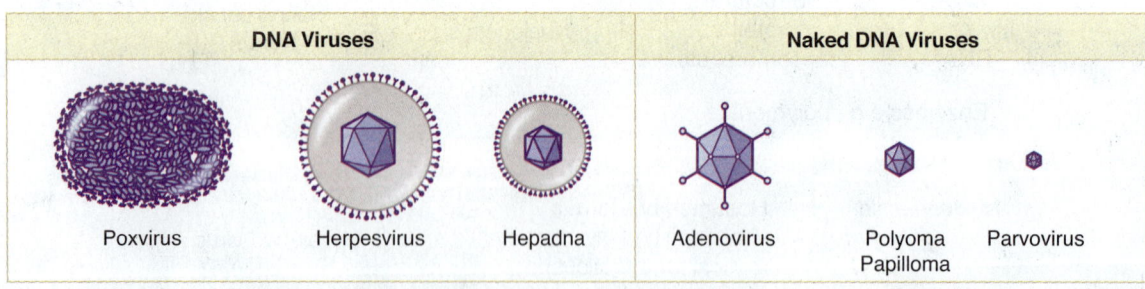

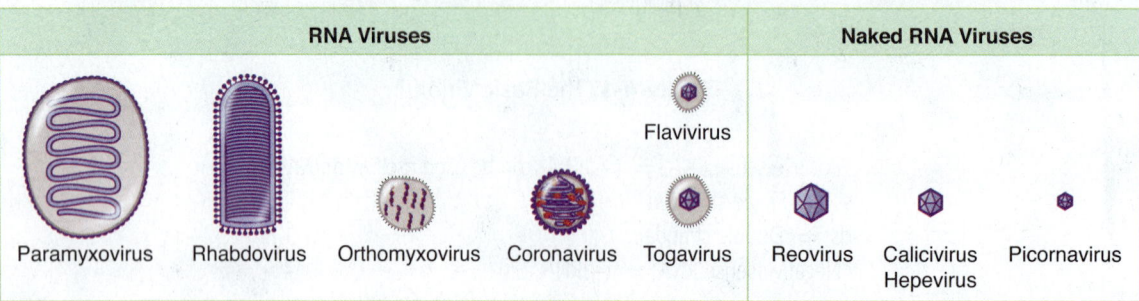

Figure 4-3. Relative Sizes and Shapes of Different Viruses

VIRAL REPLICATION

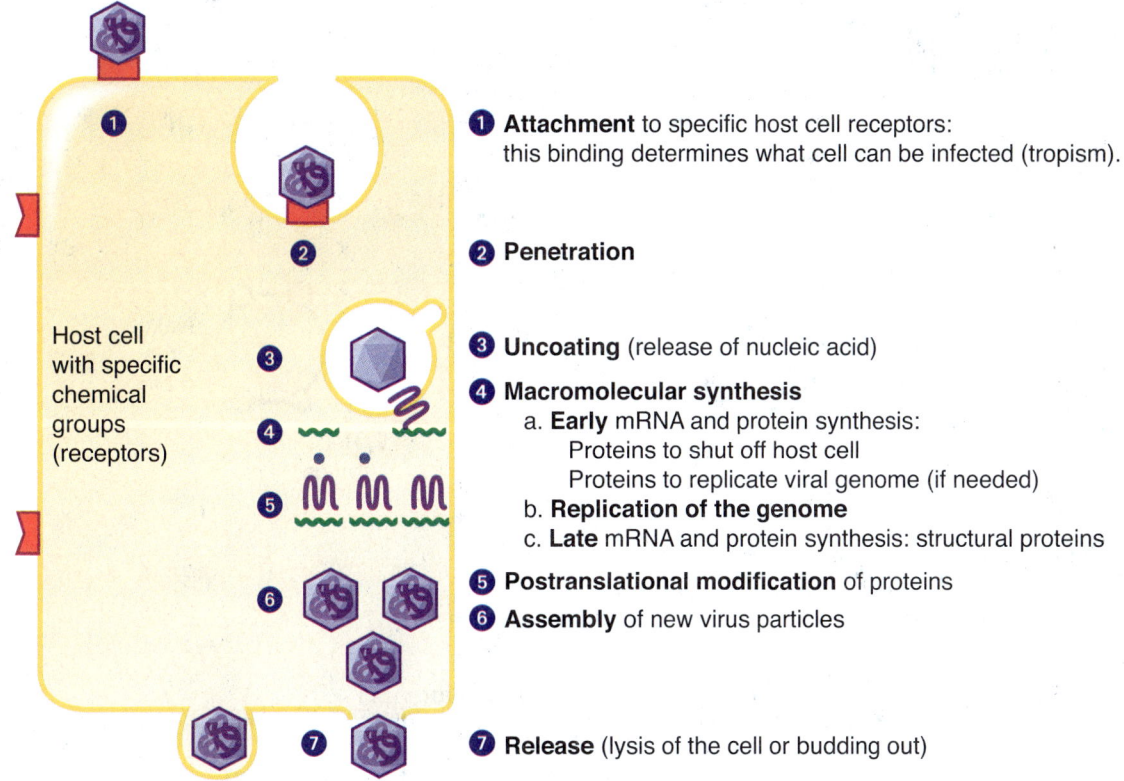

1. **Attachment** to specific host cell receptors: this binding determines what cell can be infected (tropism).

2. **Penetration**

3. **Uncoating** (release of nucleic acid)

4. **Macromolecular synthesis**
   a. **Early** mRNA and protein synthesis:
      Proteins to shut off host cell
      Proteins to replicate viral genome (if needed)
   b. **Replication of the genome**
   c. **Late** mRNA and protein synthesis: structural proteins

5. **Postranslational modification** of proteins

6. **Assembly** of new virus particles

7. **Release** (lysis of the cell or budding out)

Host cell with specific chemical groups (receptors)

Figure 4-4. Generalized Viral Replication Scheme

IMPORTANT STEPS IN VIRAL REPLICATION

Spread

Viruses are spread basically by the same mechanisms (e.g., respiratory droplets or sexually) as other pathogens.

Arthropod-borne viruses are referred to as **arboviruses**.

Most belong to three formal taxonomic groups

- Togavirus encephalitis viruses (a.k.a. alphaviruses)
- Flavivirus
- Bunyavirus

Vectors

- Mosquitoes are most common vectors.
- Ticks, biting midges, and sandflies are less common.

Attachment

Viruses bind through specific interaction with the host cell surface components <u>and</u>

- Specific **viral surface glycoproteins** of **enveloped viruses**, or
- Specific **viral surface proteins** of **naked viruses**.

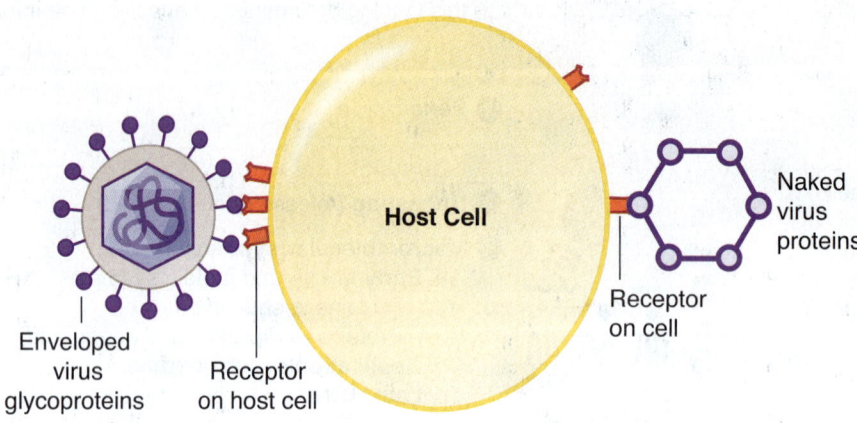

Figure 4-5. Attachment

These interactions (and the distribution of the receptors) **determine viral**

1. **Host range** (e.g., horses or humans)
2. **Tissue specificity** (e.g., liver versus heart; **tropism**)

Table 4-1. Specific Viral Receptors to Know

Virus	Target Cell	Receptor on Host Cell
HIV	Th cells, macrophages, microglia	CD4 plus CCR5 or CXCR4
EBV	B lymphocytes	CD21 = CR2
Rabies	Neurons	Acetylcholine receptor
Rhinovirus	Respiratory epithelial cells	ICAM-1

Table 4-2. Difference Between Naked and Enveloped Viruses

	Naked	Enveloped
Inactivated by heat, detergents, acid and organic solvents like ether and alcohols?	No	Yes, since the lipid envelope holds the glycoproteins essential for attachment. Dissolving the envelope inhibits attachment and therefore uptake.

Viral Entry Into Host Cell

Viral entry is by

- Receptor-mediated endocytosis
- Uptake via coated pits
- Or for those enveloped viruses with fusion proteins via fusion of the cell membrane with the viral envelope

Macromolecular Synthesis

How do the various viruses make their mRNA? mRNA production is diagrammed below.

- The major types of viral genomes are shown on the right.
- The replication intermediates necessary to make mRNA are shown in the gray area.

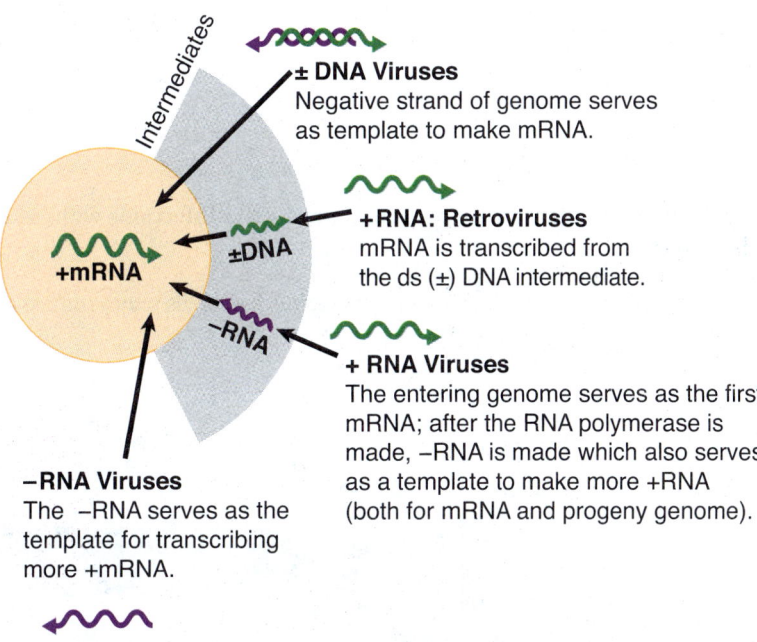

Figure 4-6. Production of Viral Messenger RNA

Replication of the Genomic Nucleic Acid (NA)

Progeny viruses have a nucleic acid sequence identical to the parent virus.

All single-stranded **RNA viruses replicate through a replicative intermediate**.

Going back to the Simplified Imaginary Teaching Viruses:

- If the parental genomic sequence is UUUUUUUUU, then the progeny must have the same sequence.
- (Poly AAA would make a polylysine capsid instead.)
- To make more poly UUU, a replicative intermediate of AAAAAAAAA would be required.
- The replicative intermediate is used to make new poly UUU.

Table 4-3. Strategy for Viral Genome Replication

Virus Type	Parental Genome	Intermediate Replicative Form	Progeny Genome
Most dsDNA viruses	dsDNA		dsDNA
Hepatitis B	dsDNA	ssRNA →	dsDNA
Most +ssRNA viruses	+ssRNA	−ssRNA	+ssRNA
Retroviruses	+ssRNA →	dsDNA	+ssRNA
−ssRNA viruses	−ssRNA	+ssRNA	−ssRNA

+ means an RNA which can serve as mRNA (or for the retroviruses has the same sequence.)

→ = RNA-dependent DNA polymerase

- Called reverse transcriptase for the retroviruses.
- Called the DNA polymerase for hepatitis B.
- Both actually make the first strand of the DNA using the RNA original and then break down the RNA and use the single strand of DNA as template to make the second strand.

Release of Viruses

Naked viruses lyse the host cells. Thus, there are **no persistent productive infections** with naked viruses (only cytolytic productive or latent infections).

Release of enveloped viruses: Budding leads to cell senescence (aging), but cells may produce a low level of virus for years as occurs in chronic hepatitis B.

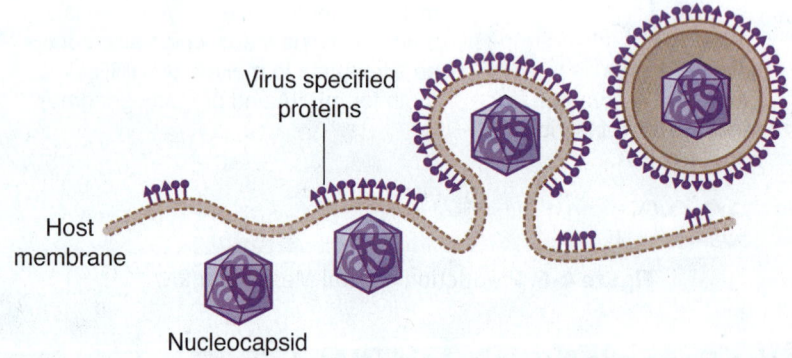

Figure 4-7. Release of Enveloped Virus

The glycoproteins on the enveloped viral surface are essential for viral infectivity.

PATTERNS OF VIRAL INFECTIONS

Table 4-4. Cellular Effects

Infection Type	Virus Production	Fate of Cell
Abortive	−	No effect: No virus is made nor is latency established; Virus is terminated
Cytolytic Naked viruses lyse host cells. Some enveloped viruses also are cytolytic, killing the cell in the process of replication.	+	Lysis of the host cell (death)
Persistent	+	Senescence (premature aging)
Productive (enveloped viruses)	−	No overt damage to host; no production of virus, but viral production may be turned on later.
Latent	±	
Transforming		Immortalization

HOST RESISTANCE TO VIRAL INFECTION

Primary Defenses

- Skin barrier (dead keratinized cells impervious to viruses)
- Skin has acids and other inhibitors produced by normal bacterial flora
- Mucociliary elevator

Immune Defense

Innate immune response

- Interferon
- Complement
- Natural killer cells

Adaptive immune response

- Antibody
- Cytotoxic T lymphocytes

Interferon Production

Interferons (IFNs) are a family of eukaryotic cell proteins classified according to the cell of origin. IFN-alpha and IFN-beta are produced by a variety of virus-infected cells. They:

- Act on target cells to **inhibit viral replication**.
- Do not act directly on the virus.
- Are **not virus-specific**.
- Are **species-specific** (e.g., mouse IFN versus human IFN).

Interferon inhibits viral protein synthesis

- Through activation of an RNA endonuclease, which digests viral RNA.
- By activation (by phosphorylation) of protein kinase that inactivates eIF2, inhibiting viral protein synthesis.

Exogenous human IFN (produced by recombinant DNA technology) may be used in antiviral therapy for chronic, active HBV and HCV infections.

Bridge to Biochemistry

Production of IFN and most immunologic cytokines is under the control of the transcription factor NFκB.

VIRAL HEPATITIS

Symptoms of Hepatitis

Fever, malaise, headache, anorexia, vomiting, dark urine, jaundice.

See more extensive coverage in chapter 19 of Pathology.

Table 4-5. Hepatitis Viruses (Hepatotropic)

	Hepatitis A	Hepatitis B	Hepatitis C	Hepatitis D	Hepatitis E
	"Infectious" (HAV)	"Serum" (HBV)	"Post-transfusion Non A, Non B" (HCV)	"Delta" (HDV)	"Enteric" (HEV)
Family	Picornavirus	Hepadnavirus	Flavivirus	Defective	Hepevirus
Features	RNA Naked Capsid	DNA Enveloped	RNA Enveloped	Circular RNA Enveloped	RNA Naked capsid
Transmission	Fecal-oral	Parenteral, sexual	Parenteral, sexual	Parenteral, sexual	Fecal-oral

(Continue)

	Hepatitis A	Hepatitis B	Hepatitis C	Hepatitis D	Hepatitis E
Disease presentation	Mild acute No chronic No sequellae	Acute; occasionally severe Chronic: 5–10% adults 90% infants Primary hepatocellular carcinoma, cirrhosis	Acute is usually subclinical 80% become chronic Primary hepatocellular carcinoma, cirrhosis	Co-infection with HBV: occasionally severe Superinfection with HBV: often severe Cirrhosis, fulminant hepatitis	Normal patients: mild Pregnant patients: severe No chronic
Mortality	<0.5%	1–2%	0.5–1%	High to very high	Normal patients 1–2% Third-trimester pregnant patients 25%
Diagnosis	IgM to HAV	HBsAg, IgM to HBcAg	Antibody to HCV, ELISA	Hepatitis D Ab, HBsAg	Antibody to HEV, ELISA

Note: Remember that hepatitis also may occur in other viral diseases (e.g., CMV and EBV infections, congenital rubella, and yellow fever).

Table 4-6. Hepatitis B Terminology and Markers

Abbreviation	Name and Description
HBV	Hepatitis B virus, a hepadnavirus (enveloped, partially double-stranded DNA virus); Dane particle = infectious HBV
HBsAg	Antigen found on surface of HBV; also found on spheres and filaments in patient's blood: positive during acute disease; continued presence indicates carrier state
HBsAb	Antibody to HBsAg; provides immunity to hepatitis B
HBcAg	Antigen associated with core of HBV
HBcAb	Antibody to HBcAg; positive during window phase; IgM HBcAb is an indicator of recent disease
HBeAg	A second, different antigenic determinant on the HBV core; important indicator of transmissibility
HBeAb	Antibody to e antigen; indicates low transmissibility
Delta agent	Small RNA virus with HBsAg envelope; defective virus that replicates only in HBV-infected cells
Window period	The period between the end of detection of HBsAg and the beginning of detection HBsAb

Table 4-7. Hepatitis B Serology

	HBsAg HBeAg* HBV-DNA	HBcAb IgM	HBcAb IgG	HBeAb	HBsAb
Acute infection	+	+	−	−	−
Window period	−	+/−	+	+	−
Prior infection	−	−	+	+	+
Immunization	−	−	−	−	+
Chronic infection	+	−	+	+/−	−

*HBeAg—Correlates with viral proliferation and infectivity.

DNA VIRUSES: CHARACTERISTICS

All DNA viruses:

- Are double-stranded, except parvovirus
- Are icosahedral, except poxviruses, which are a brick-shaped "complex"
- Replicate their DNA in the nucleus, except poxvirus

Table 4-8. DNA Viruses*

Virus Family	DNA type	Virion-Associated Polymerase	Envelope	DNA Replicates in:	Major Viruses
Parvovirus	ssDNA	No	Naked	Nucleus	B19
Papillomavirus Polyomavirus	dsDNA, circular	No	Naked	Nucleus	Papilloma, Polyoma
Adenovirus	dsDNA, linear	No	Naked	Nucleus	Adenoviruses
Hepadnavirus	Partially dsDNA, circular	Yes***	Enveloped	Nucleus, RNA intermediate	Hepatitis B
Herpes virus	dsDNA, linear	No	Enveloped (nuclear)	Nucleus; virus assembled in nucleus	HSV, Varicella-zoster, Epstein-Barr, Cytomegalovirus
Poxvirus	dsDNA, linear	Yes**	Enveloped	Cytoplasm	Variola, Vaccinia, Molluscum contagiosum

* Mnemonic: <u>P</u>ardon <u>P</u>apa <u>A</u>s <u>H</u>e <u>H</u>as <u>P</u>ox

** **Poxviruses** have a **virion-associated transcriptase** (DNA dependent RNA polymerase), so it can transcribe its own DNA in the cytoplasm and make all of the enzymes and factors necessary for replication of the poxvirus DNA in the cytoplasm.

*** Hepadnaviruses: DNA viruses that carry a DNA polymerase with reverse transcriptase activity to synthesize an RNA intermediate that is then used to make the genomic DNA. Hepatitis B is partially double-stranded with one complete strand.

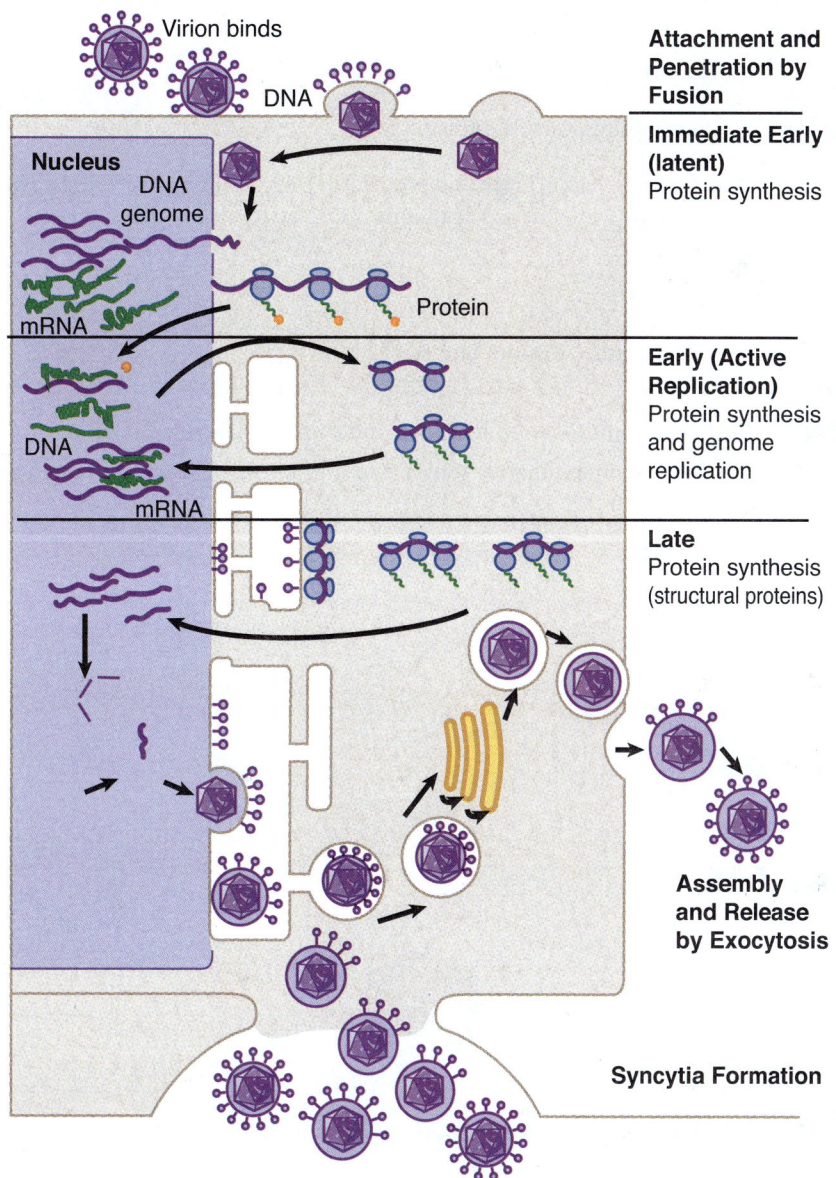

Figure 4-8. DNA Virus: Life Cycle of Herpes

PARVOVIRIDAE

Virus Characteristics

- ssDNA virus, linear
- Naked, icosahedral

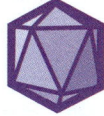

Figure 4-9. Parvovirus

Viruses of Medical Importance—B19

B19

Reservoir—human respiratory tract

Transmission—respiratory route, fomites, vertical transmission

Pathogenesis—B19 infects immature (cycling) erythroid progenitor cells, resulting in cell lysis. The resulting **anemia** is only clinically significant in patients with **sickle-cell anemia** and may result in **aplastic crisis**.

Diseases

- Children/adults
  - Fifth </ix>disease, erythema infectiosum, slapped cheek fever
  - 7–10 day incubation
  - Nonspecific "flu-like" symptoms followed by raised, indurated facial rash
  - Rash and arthralgias (adults predominantly) are due to immune complexes in the skin and joints
- Fetus
  - Severe anemia
  - Congestive heart failure
  - Hydrops fetalis
  - Spontaneous abortion

Diagnosis—serology and molecular analysis

Treatment—supportive care

PAPILLOMAVIRIDAE

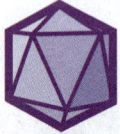

Figure 4-10. Papillomavirus

Virus Characteristics

- dsDNA virus, circular
- Naked, icosahedral

Viruses of Medical Importance

- Human papilloma virus (HPV)

Human Papilloma Virus (HPV)

Distinguishing Characteristics

- Over 75 serotypes
- Different serotypes are associated with different clinical presentations

Reservoir—human skin and genitals

Transmission—direct contact, fomites

Pathogenesis

- Virus infects basal layer of the skin and mucous membranes
- Hyperkeratosis leads to the formation of the "wart"
- Malignancy may result: **E6 and E7 inhibit tumor-suppressor genes p53 and Rb, respectively.**

Diseases

- Cutaneous warts
  - **Common warts** (serotypes 2 and 4) are predominantly found on the hands and fingers.
  - **Plantar warts** (serotype 1) are predominantly found on soles of feet and tend to be deeper and more painful.
- Anogenital warts (Condylomata acuminata)
  - Also cause laryngeal papillomas in infants and sexually active adults
  - **Over 90% of genital warts are serotypes 6 and 11 (benign)**
  - **Serotypes 16 and 18** (31 and 35) are preneoplastic (cervical intraepithelial neoplasia; CIN)
  - **95% of cases of CINs contain HPV DNA**
  - Viral genes E6 and E7 inactivate tumor-suppressor genes

Diagnosis

- Cutaneous—clinical grounds
- Genital—finding of koilocytic cells (cells with perinuclear cytoplasmic vacuolization and nuclear enlargement) in Pap smears
- In situ DNA probes and PCR can be used to confirm any diagnosis and type the HPV strain involved

Treatment

- Cryotherapy, electrocautery, or chemical means (salicylic acid)
- Imiquimod (induces proinflammatory cytokines), interferon-α, and virus-specific cidofovir

Prevention

- A vaccine composed of HPV capsid proteins produced by recombinant DNA technology
- Safe sex practices

POLYOMAVIRIDAE

Table 4-9. Summary of Polyomaviridae

Virus	Reservoir/ Transmission	Pathogenesis	Disease	Diagnosis	Treatment
BK	Respiratory	Latent infection in kidney	Renal disease in AIDS patients	ELISA, PCR	Supportive
JC	Respiratory	Infection in oligodendrocytes = demyelination	Progressive multifocal leukoencephalopathy (PML) in AIDS and transplant patients	ELISA, PCR	Supportive

ADENOVIRIDAE

Virus Characteristics

- dsDNA, nonenveloped
- Hexons, pentons, and fibers

Viruses of Medical Importance

- Adenovirus
- ~49 serotypes

Adenovirus

Reservoir—ubiquitous in humans and animals

Transmission—respiratory, fecal-oral, direct contact

Pathogenesis

- Penton fibers act as hemagglutinin.
- Purified penton fibers are toxic to cells.
- Virus is lytic in permissive cells and can be chronic or oncogenic in nonpermissive hosts. The adenoviruses are the standard example of a permissive host (where virus is produced) and nonpermissive host (where the virus is not produced, but transformed).

Disease

- Acute respiratory disease (ARD) and pneumonia
  - Spring and winter peak incidence
  - Children, young military recruits and college students serotypes 4, 7, and 21
- Pharyngoconjunctivitis
  - Swimming pool conjunctivitis, pink eye
  - Fever, sore throat, coryza, and red eyes
  - Nonpurulent
- Acute hemorrhagic cystitis
  - Boys ages 5 to 15 predominantly
  - Dysuria, hematuria
- Gastroenteritis
  - Daycare, not as common as rotavirus
  - Serotypes 40 and 41

Diagnosis—serology; ELISA

Treatment—supportive care

Prevention—live, nonattenuated vaccine

HERPESVIRIDAE

Virus Characteristics

- Large dsDNA
- Enveloped, icosahedral
- Derives envelope from nuclear membrane
- **Intranuclear inclusion bodies**
- **Establishes latency**

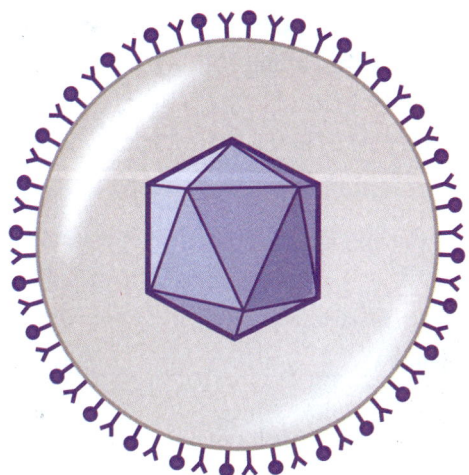

Figure 4-11. Herpesvirus

Viruses of Medical Importance

- Herpes simplex virus 1 and 2 (HSV)
- Varicella-zoster virus (VZV)
- Epstein-Barr virus (EBV)
- Cytomegalovirus (CMV)
- Human herpesvirus 6 (HHV-6)
- Human herpesvirus 8 (HHV-8)

HSV-1 and HSV-2

Reservoir—human mucosa and ganglia

Transmission—close personal contact (i.e., kissing, sexual contact)

Pathogenesis—HSV establishes infection in the mucosal epithelial cells and leads to the formation of vesicles. The virus travels up the ganglion to establish lifelong latent infection. Stress triggers reactivation of virus in nerve and recurrence of vesicles.

Diseases—The rule of thumb is that HSV-1 infections generally occur above the waist and HSV-2 infections generally occur below the waist.

HSV-1

- Gingivostomatitis and cold sores
  - Blister-like lesions on the oral mucosa
  - **Latent in trigeminal ganglion**
- Keratoconjunctivitis
  - Generally with lid swelling and vesicles
  - Dendritic ulcers may be seen
  - Untreated and repeat attacks may result in blindness
- Encephalitis
  - Fever, headache, and confusion
  - **Focal temporal lesions** and perivascular cuffing
  - If untreated, 70% mortality rate
  - Most common cause of viral encephalitis in the United States

HSV-2

- Genital infections
  - Painful genital vesicles
  - Systemic effects can include fever, malaise, and myalgia
  - **Latency in the sacral nerve ganglia**
- Neonatal herpes
  - Infection during passage through infected birth canal
  - Infections are usually severe:
    - Disseminated with liver involvement and high mortality
    - Encephalitis, high mortality
    - Skin, eyes, or mouth

Diagnosis

- Oral lesions—clinical
- Encephalitis
  - PCR on CSF
  - Large numbers of RBCs in CSF
- Genital infections—Tzank smear to show the formation of multinucleated giant cells and Cowdry type A intranuclear inclusions has been largely replaced by immunofluorescent staining, which can distinguish HSV-1 from HSV-2

Treatment—Acyclovir is a nucleoside analog that is only activated in cells infected with HSV-1, HSV-2 or VZV. This is because the virus thymidine kinase is required to activate the drug by placing the first phosphate on the drug, followed by the phosphorylation via cellular enzymes. Resistance to acyclovir occurs due to a mutation in the thymidine kinase. Famciclovir, valacyclovir, and penciclovir are alternatives if resistance develops.

Varicella Zoster Virus (VZV)

Reservoir—human mucosa and nerves

Transmission—respiratory droplets

Pathogenesis—VZV enters the respiratory tract → replicates in the local lymph nodes → primary viremia → spleen and liver → secondary viremia → skin (rash) → **latent in the dorsal root ganglia.** Reactivation of virus due to stress or immunocompromise causes vesicular lesions and severe nerve pain.

Diseases

- Chickenpox
  - Fever, pharyngitis, malaise, rhinitis
  - **Asynchronous rash**
  - One of the 5 "classic" childhood exanthems, less common due to vaccination
- Shingles
  - Zoster
  - Pain and vesicles restricted to one dermatome
  - Fifth or sixth decade of life
  - **Reactivation of latent infection**

Diagnosis

- Tzanck smear—Cowdry type A, intranuclear inclusions
- Antigen detection by PCR

Treatment

- Healthy adults with shingles—oral acyclovir
- Immunocompromised—IV acyclovir
- Aspirin contraindicated due to association with Reye syndrome

Prevention

- Live, attenuated vaccine, booster for 60-year-old to prevent shingles
- VZIG (varicella-zoster immunoglobulin) for postexposure prophylaxis of the immunocompromised

Epstein-Barr Virus (EBV)

Reservoir—humans

Transmission

- Saliva
- 90% of the adult population is seropositive

Pathogenesis

- Virus infects nasopharyngeal epithelial cells, salivary and lymphoid tissues → latent infection of B cells (EBV binds to CD21 and acts as a B-cell mitogen) → results in the production of atypical reactive T cells (Downey cells), which may constitute up to 70% of the WBC count
- Heterophile antibodies are produced (due to B cell mitogenesis)

Diseases

- Heterophile-positive mononucleosis, "kissing disease"
  - Fatigue, fever, sore throat, lymphadenopathy and splenomegaly
  - **Latency in B cells**

- Lymphoproliferative disease
  - Occurs in immunocompromised patients
  - T cells can't control the B-cell growth
- Hairy oral leukoplakia
  - Hyperproliferation of lingual epithelial cells
  - AIDS patients

Malignancies

- Burkitt lymphoma
  - Cancer of the maxilla, mandible, abdomen
  - Africa
  - Malaria cofactor
  - AIDS patients
  - Translocation juxtaposes c-myc oncogene to a very active promoter, such as an immunoglobulin gene promoter
- Nasopharyngeal carcinoma
  - Asia
  - Tumor cells of epithelial origin
- Hodgkin lymphoma

Diagnosis

- Heterophile-antibody positive (IgM antibodies that recognize the Paul-Bunnell antigen on sheep and bovine RBCs)

Treatment

- For uncomplicated mononucleosis, treatment is symptomatic

Cytomegalovirus (CMV)

Reservoir—humans

Transmission—saliva, sexual, parenteral, in utero

Pathogenesis

- CMV infects the salivary gland epithelial cells and establishes a persistent infection in fibroblasts, epithelial cells, and macrophages
- **Latency in mononuclear cells**

Disease

- Cytomegalic inclusion disease
  - Most common in utero infection in U.S.
  - Disease ranges from infected with no obvious defects to severe cytomegalic inclusion disease characterized by jaundice, hepatosplenomegaly, thrombocytic purpura ("blueberry muffin baby"), pneumonitis, and CNS damage to death
- Mononucleosis (children and adults)—heterophile-negative mononucleosis

- Interstitial pneumonitis to severe systemic infection—due to reactivation in a transplanted organ or in an AIDS patient
- CMV retinitis—common in AIDS patients

Diagnosis

- Owl-eye inclusion ("sight-o-megalo-virus") in biopsy material and urine
- Basophilic intranuclear inclusions
- Serology, DNA detection, virus culture

Treatment

- In healthy—supportive
- In immuncompromised (AIDS and transplant patients)—ganciclovir/foscarnet ± human immunoglobulin. Resistance to ganciclovir through hL97 gene.

Prevention

- Safe sex
- Screening of blood and organ donors

HHV-6

Reservoir—humans

Transmission—respiratory droplets

Pathogenesis—replicates in peripheral blood mononuclear cells

Disease

- Roseola (exanthema subitum)
- Fever for ~3–5 days followed by a lacy body rash

Diagnosis—clinical

Treatment—symptomatic

HHV-8

Reservoir—humans

Transmission—sexual contact, saliva, vertical, transplantation

Pathogenesis—HHV-8 has a gene that turns on vascular endothelial growth factor (VEGF), which plays a direct role in the development of Kaposi sarcoma

Disease—Kaposi sarcoma

Diagnosis

- Clinical
- Serology, PCR

Treatment—none

Table 4-10. Summary of Herpesvirus Infections

Virus	Site of Primary Infection	Clinical Presentation of Primary Infection	Site of Latency	Clinical Presentation of Recurrent Infection
HSV-1	Mucosa	Gingivostomatitis, keratoconjunctivitis, pharyngitis	Trigeminal ganglia	Cold sores
HSV-2	Mucosa	Genital herpes, neonatal herpes	Sacral ganglia	Genital herpes
VZV	Mucosa	Chickenpox	Dorsal root ganglia	Shingles (zoster)
EBV	Mucosal epithelial cells, B cells	Mononucleosis (heterophile ⊕)	B cells	Asymptomatic shedding of virus
CMV	Mononuclear cells, epithelial cells	Mononucleosis (heterophile –), cytomegalic inclusion disease	Mononuclear cells	Asymptomatic shedding of virus
HHV-6	Mononuclear cells	Roseola infantum	Mononuclear cells	Asymptomatic shedding of virus
HHV-8	Dermis	Kaposi sarcoma	?	?

POXVIRIDAE

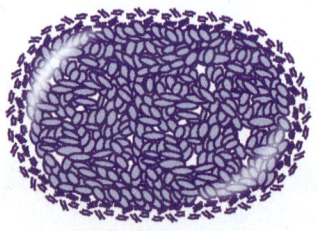

Figure 4-12. Poxvirus

Virus Characteristics

- Large dsDNA, enveloped
- Complex morphology
- Replicates in the cytoplasm
- Potential biowarfare agent

Viruses of Medical Importance

- Variola
- Vaccinia (vaccine strain)
- Molluscum contagiosum
- Orf
- Monkeypox

Variola/Smallpox

Reservoir

- Humans
- Variola has 1 serotype, which made eradication (1977) possible

Transmission—respiratory route

Pathogenesis

- Via inhalation, the virus enters the upper respiratory tract and disseminates via lymphatics → viremia
- After a secondary viremia, the virus infects all dermal tissues and internal organs
- Classic "pocks"

Disease

- 5–17 day incubation
- Prodrome of flu-like illness for 2–4 days
- Prodrome followed by rash, which begins in the mouth and spreads to the face, arms and legs, hands, and feet and can cover the entire body within 24 hours
- All vesicles are in the same stage of development (synchronous rash)

Diagnosis

- Clinical
- Guarnieri bodies found in infected cells (intracytoplasmic)

Treatment—supportive care

Prevention—live, attenuated vaccine

Molluscum contagiosum

Reservoir—humans

Transmission—direct contact (sexual) and fomites

Pathogenesis—replication in dermis

Disease

- Single or multiple (<20) benign, wart-like tumors
- Molluscum bodies in central caseous material (eosinophilic cytoplasmic inclusion bodies)

Diagnosis

- Clinical (warts are umbilicated)
- Eosinophilic cytoplasmic inclusion bodies

Treatment

- In healthy persons, self limiting
- Ritonavir, cidofovir in immunocompromised

RNA VIRUSES: CHARACTERISTICS

General Characteristics

- All RNA viruses are single stranded (ss), except Reovirus.
- ss(−)RNA viruses carry RNA-dependent RNA polymerase.
- A virion-associated polymerase is also carried by:
  - Reovirus
  - Arenavirus
  - Retrovirus (reverse transcriptase)
- Most are enveloped; the **only naked ones** are:
  - Picornavirus
  - Calicivirus and Hepevirus
  - Reovirus
- Some are segmented (different genes on different pieces of RNA)
  - **R**eovirus
  - **O**rthomyxovirus
  - **B**unyavirus
  - **A**renavirus

POSITIVE-STRANDED RNA VIRUSES

Table 4-11. Positive-Stranded RNA Viruses*

Virus Family	RNA Structure	Virion-Associated Polymerase	Envelope	Shape	Multiplies in	Major Viruses
Calicivirus	ss(+)RNA Linear Non-segmented	No polymerase	Naked	Icosahedral	Cytoplasm	Norwalk agent Noro-like virus
Hepevirus	↓	↓	↓	↓	↓	Hepatitis E
Picornavirus	ss(+)RNA Linear Non-segmented	No polymerase	Naked	Icosahedral	Cytoplasm	Polio** ECHO Enteroviruses Rhino Coxsackie Hepatitis A
Flavivirus	ss(+)RNA Linear Non-segmented	No polymerase	Enveloped	Icosahedral	Cytoplasm	Yellow fever Dengue St. Louis encephalitis Hepatitis C West Nile virus
Togavirus	ss(+)RNA Linear Non-segmented	No polymerase	Enveloped	Icosahedral	Cytoplasm	Rubella WEE, EEE Venezuelan encephalitis
Coronavirus	ss(+)RNA Linear Non-segmented	No polymerase	Enveloped	Helical	Cytoplasm	Coronaviruses SARS-CoV
Retrovirus	Diploid ss (+) RNA Linear Non-segmented	RNA dep. DNA polymerase	Enveloped	Icosahedral or truncated conical	Nucleus	HIV HTLV Sarcoma

*Mnemonic: (+)RNA Viruses: Call Henry Pico and Flo To Come Rightaway

**Mnemonic: Picornaviruses: PEE Co Rn A Viruses

Polio, Entero, Echo, Coxsackie, Rhino, Hep A

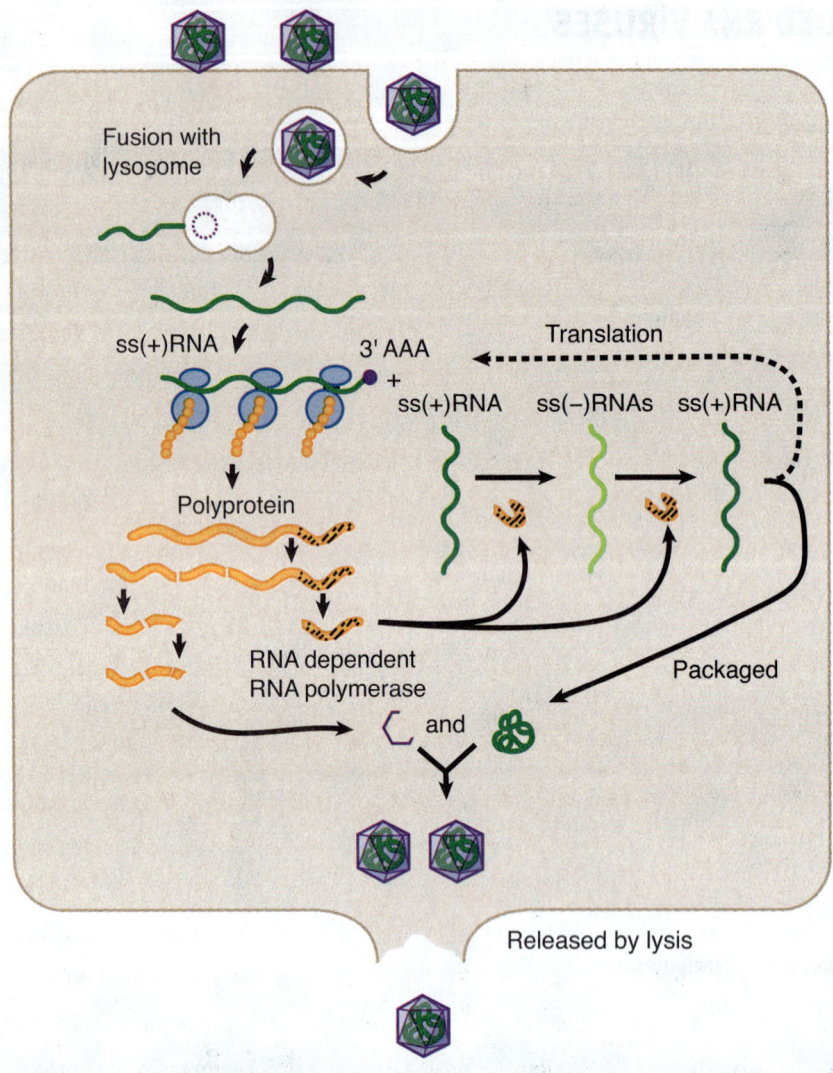

Figure 4-13. Positive-Sense RNA Virus Life Cycle

CALICIVIRIDAE

Family Characteristics

- Naked, icosahedral
- Positive-sense ssRNA

Viruses of Medical Importance

- Norwalk virus (Norovirus)
- Noro-like virus

Norwalk Virus

Reservoir—human gastrointestinal tract

Transmission—fecal-oral route, contaminated food and water

Disease—acute gastroenteritis

- Watery; no blood or pus in stools
- Nausea, vomiting, diarrhea
- 60% of all nonbacterial gastroenteritis in U.S.
- Outbreak of viral gastroenteritis in cruise ships attributed to Norovirus

Diagnosis—RIA, ELISA

Treatment

- No specific antiviral treatment
- Self-limiting

Prevention—handwashing

HEPEVIRIDAE

- Naked, icosahedral
- Positive-sense ssRNA

Hepatitis E Virus (previously discussed)

PICORNAVIRIDAE

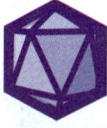

Figure 4-14. Picornavirus

Family Characteristics

- Small, naked, icosahedral
- Positive-sense ssRNA
- Summer/fall peak incidence
- Resistant to alcohol, detergents (naked capsid)
- Divided into genera:

  Enteroviruses:

  — Fecal-oral transmission, do *not* cause diarrhea

  — Peak age group <9 years

  — Stable at pH 3

Rhinoviruses:

 — Not stable under acidic conditions

 — Growth at 33°C

Heparnavirus

Viruses of Medical Importance

- Enteroviruses (acid stable)

  — Polio virus

  — Coxsackie virus A

  — Coxsackie virus B

  — Echoviruses

- Rhinoviruses (acid labile)

- Heparnaviruses—HAV

Table 4-12. Summary of Picornaviridae

Virus	Transmission	Pathogenesis	Diseases	Diagnosis	Treatment*/ Prevention
Enteroviruses					
Polio	Fecal-oral	Virus targets anterior horn motor neurons	Asymptomatic to FUO; aseptic meningitis; paralytic polio (flaccid asymmetric paralysis, no sensory loss)	Serology (virus absent from CSF)	No specific antiviral/ live vaccine (Sabin); killed vaccine (Salk)
		Neural fatigue (?)	Post-Polio Syndrome	Patient with polio decades earlier, progressive muscle atrophy	
Coxsackie A	Fecal-oral	Fecal-oral spread with potential for dissemination to other organs; often asymptomatic with viral shedding	Hand, foot, and mouth (A16); herpangina; aseptic meningitis; acute lymphoglandular pharyngitis; common cold	Virus isolation from throat, stool, or CSF	No specific treatment/ handwashing
Coxsackie B	Fecal-oral	As above	Bornholm disease (devil's grip); aseptic meningitis; severe systemic disease of newborns; **myocarditis**	As above	No specific/ handwashing
Echoviruses	Fecal-oral	As above	Fever and rash of unknown origin; aseptic meningitis	As above	No specific/ handwashing
Rhinovirus					
Rhinovirus	Respiratory	Acid labile; grows at 33°C; over 100 serotypes	Common cold; #1 cause, peak summer/fall	Clinical	No specific/ handwashing

(Continue)

Virus	Transmission	Pathogenesis	Diseases	Diagnosis	Treatment*/ Prevention
Heparnavirus					
HAV	Fecal-oral	Virus targets hepatocytes; liver function is impaired	Infectious hepatitis	IgM to HAV serology	No specific/ killed vaccine and hyperimmune serum

Definition of abbreviations: FUO, fever of unknown origin.

*Pleconaril (blocks uncoating by fitting into cleft in receptor-binding canyon of picornavirus capsid) is available on a limited basis. Must be administered early.

FLAVIVIRIDAE

Family Characteristics

- Enveloped, icosahedral
- Positive-sense ssRNA
- Arthropod-borne (arboviruses)

Viruses of Medical Importance

- St. Louis encephalitis virus (SLE)
- West Nile encephalitis virus (WNV)
- Dengue virus
- Yellow fever virus (YFV)
- Hepatitis C virus (HCV; discussed with the hepatitis viruses)

Table 4-13. Summary of Flaviviridae

Virus	Vector	Host(s)	Disease	Diagnosis	Prevention
SLE	Mosquito *(Culex)*	Birds	Encephalitis	Serology, hemagglutination inhibition, ELISA, latex particle agglutination	Vector control
WNV	Mosquito *(Culex)*	Birds (killed by virus)	Encephalitis	As above	Vector control
Dengue	Mosquito *(Aedes)*	Humans (monkeys)	Break bone fever (rash, muscle and joint pain), reinfection, can result in dengue hemorrhagic shock	As above	Vector control
YFV	Mosquito *(Aedes)*	Humans (monkeys)	Yellow fever: liver, kidney, heart, and GI (black vomit) damage	As above	Vector control/live, attenuated vaccine

Definition of abbreviations: FUO, fever of unknown origin; SLE, St. Louis encephalitis virus; WNV, West Nile encephalitis virus; YFV, yellow fever virus.

TOGAVIRIDAE

Family Characteristics

- Enveloped, icosahedral
- Positive-sense ssRNA

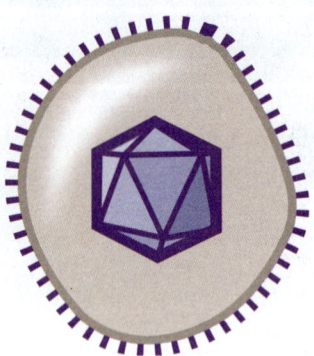

Figure 4-15. Togavirus

Viruses of Medical Importance

- **Alphaviruses (arboviruses)**
  - Eastern equine encephalitis virus (EEE)
  - Western equine encephalitis virus (WEE)
  - Venezuelan equine encephalitis virus (VEE)
- **Rubivirus**
  - Rubella

Table 4-14. Summary of Togaviridae

Virus	Vector	Host	Disease(s)	Diagnosis	Prevention
EEE, WEE, VEE	Mosquito	Birds, horses	Encephalitis	Cytopathology, immunofluorescence, RT-PCR, serology	Killed vaccines for EEE and WEE
Rubella	None	humans	German measles (erythematous rash begins on face, progresses to torso)	Serology	Live, attenuated vaccine
			CRS*		

Definition of abbreviations: CRS, congenital rubella syndrome; EEE, Eastern equine encephalitis virus; VEE, Venezuelan equine encephalitis virus; WEE, Western equine encephalitis virus.

*Congenital rubella syndrome—patent ductus arteriosis, pulmonary stenosis, cataracts, microcephaly, deafness. The effects are more serious if the maternal infection is acquired during the first 16 weeks' gestation.

CORONAVIRIDAE

Family Characteristics

- Enveloped, helical
- Positive-sense ssRNA
- Hemagglutinin molecules make up peplomers on virus surface, which give shape like sun with corona

Viruses of Medical Importance

- **Coronavirus**
- **Severe acute respiratory syndrome coronavirus (SARS-CoV)**

Coronavirus

- Second most common cause of the common cold
- Winter/spring peak incidence

SARS-CoV

Reservoir—birds and small mammals (civet cats)

Transmission

- Respiratory droplets
- Virus is also found in urine, sweat, and feces
- Original case is thought to have jumped from animal to human

Disease—severe acute respiratory syndrome (SARS)

- Atypical pneumonia
- Clinical case definition includes: fever of >100.4°F, flu-like illness, dry cough, dyspnea, and progressive hypoxia
- Chest x-ray may show patchy distribution of focal interstitial infiltrates

Diagnosis

- Includes clinical presentation and prior history of travel to endemic area or an association with someone who recently traveled to endemic area
- Lab tests: detection of antibodies to SARS-CoV, RT-PCR, and isolation of the virus in culture

Treatment

- Supportive
- Ribavirin and interferon are promising

RETROVIRIDAE

Family Characteristics

- Positive-sense ssRNA
- Virion-associated reverse transcriptase
- Enveloped

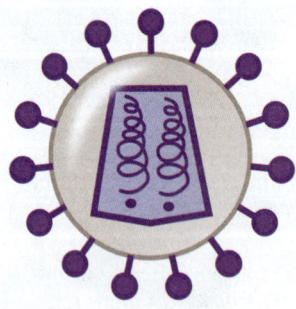

Figure 4-16. Retrovirus

Viruses of Medical Importance

- **Oncovirus group**
    - **Human T-cell leukemia/lymphotropic (HTLV)**
        - ○ Adult T-cell leukemia
        - ○ C-type particle (most oncoviruses, centrally located electron-dense nucleocapsid)
        - ○ Japan, Caribbean, southern U.S.
- **Lentivirus group—human immunodeficiency virus (HIV);** acquired immunodeficiency syndrome

Human Immunodeficiency Virus (HIV)

Distinguishing Characteristics

- The HIV virion contains:
    - Enveloped, truncated, conical capsid (type D retrovirus)
    - Two copies of the ss(+)RNA
    - RNA-dependent DNA polymerase (reverse transcriptase)
    - Integrase
    - Protease

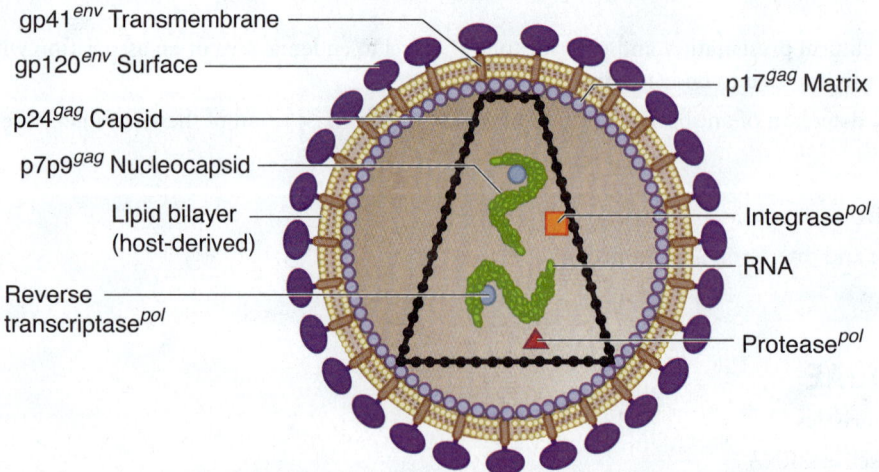

Figure 4-17. Structure and Genes of HIV

Table 4-15. Important HIV Genes and Their Functions

Gene	Product(s)	Function
Structural Genes		
Gag	Group-specific antigens	Structural proteins
	p24	Capsid protein
	p7p9	Core nucleocapsid proteins
	p17	Matrix protein
Pol	Reverse transcriptase	Produces dsDNA provirus (extremely error-prone, causes genetic drift of envelope glycoprotein
	Integrase	Viral DNA integration into host cell DNA
	Protease	Cleaves viral polyprotein
Env	gp120	Surface protein that binds to CD4 and coreceptors CCR5 (macrophages) and CXCR4 (T cells); tropism; genetic drift
	gp41	Transmembrane protein for viral fusion to host cell
Regulatory Genes		
LTR (U3, U5)	DNA, long terminal repeats	Integration and viral gene expression
Tat	Transactivator	Transactivator of transcription (upregulation); spliced gene
Rev	Regulatory protein	Upregulates transport of unspliced and spliced transcripts to the cell cytoplasm; a spliced gene
Nef	**Regulatory protein**	**Decreases CD4 and MHC I expression on host cells; manipulates T-cell activation pathways; required for progression to AIDS**

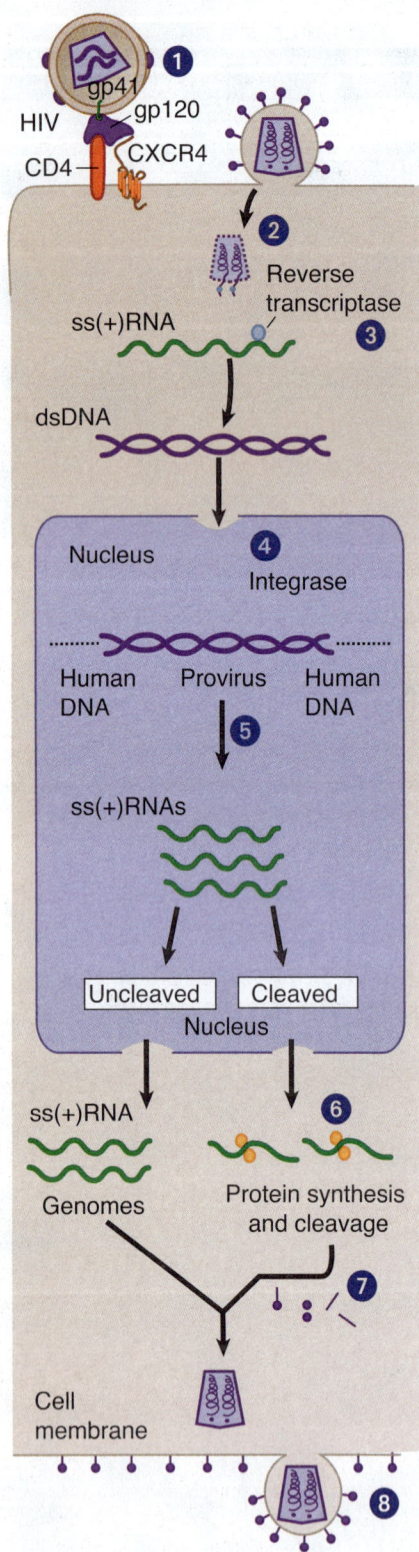

Figure 4-18. Retrovirus Life Cycle: HIV

1. Surface gp120 of HIV binds to CD4 of T-helper cells, macrophages, microglia, and coreceptors (*CCR5* and *CXCR4*) found on macrophages and Th cells, respectively.

2. HIV is taken into the cell, losing the envelope; the RNA is uncoated.

3. The RNA is copied using the virion-associated reverse transcriptase; ultimately dsDNA with long terminal repeats is made.

4. The DNA and integrase migrate to nucleus and the DNA is integrated into host DNA forming the **provirus**.

   The provirus remains in the host DNA.

   The rate of viral replication is regulated by the activity of the regulatory proteins (*tat/rev, nef*, etc).

   Tat upregulates transcription.

   Rev regulates transport of RNA to cytoplasm.

   Co-infections (e.g., mycobacterial) stimulate the HIV-infected cells to produce more virus.

5. Transcription produces ss(+)RNA, some cleaved and some remain intact.

   • Cleaved RNA will be used as mRNA.

   • Uncleaved RNA is used as genomic RNA.

6. Translation produces the proteins some of which are polyproteins that are cleaved by the HIV protease.

7. Assembly

8. Maturation/release of virus

Reservoir—human Th cells and macrophages

Transmission:

- Sexual contact
- Bloodborne (transfusions, dirty needles)
- CDC risk factors for needlesticks include depth of injury, width (bore) of needle, visible blood, and late stage AIDS diagnosis of source patient
- Vertical

Disease—acquired immunodeficiency syndrome (AIDS)

- Asymptomatic infection → persistent, generalized lymphadenopathy → symptomatic → AIDS-defining conditions
- Homozygous *CCR5* mutation → immune
- Heterozygous *CCR5* mutation → slow course
- The course of the illness follows the decline in CD4+ T cells (Figure II-4-19)
- Long-term survivors may result when virus lacks functional *nef* protein

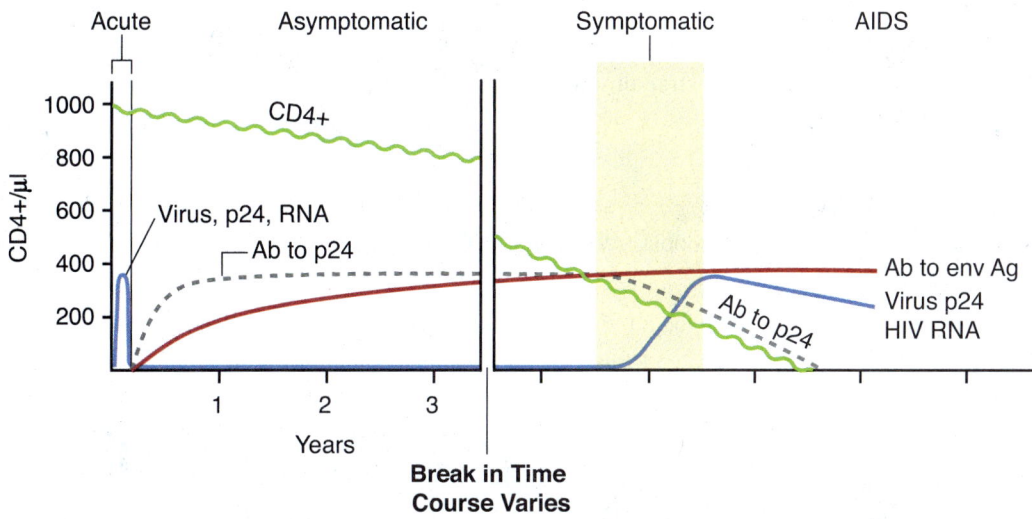

Figure 4-19. Clinical Stages of HIV Infection

Conditions of Early Symptomatic Period

- Bacillary angiomatosis (disseminated bartonellosis)
- Candidiasis (oral or persistent vulvovaginal)
- Cervical dysplasia or carcinoma in situ
- Constitutional symptoms (fever 38.5°C or diarrhea lasting >1 month)
- Hairy leukoplakia
- Idiopathic thrombocytopenic purpura
- Listeriosis
- Pelvic inflammatory disease (especially with abscess)
- Peripheral neuropathy

Conditions Associated with AIDS

- Encephalopathy, HIV-related
- Pneumonia, recurrent (leading cause of death)
- Fungal infections
- Candidiasis of esophagus, bronchi, trachea, or lungs
- Coccidioidomycosis, disseminated or extrapulmonary
- Cryptococcosis, extrapulmonary
- Histoplasmosis, disseminated or extrapulmonary
- *Pneumocystis jirovecii* pneumonia
- Malignancies
    - Invasive cervical carcinoma
    - Kaposi sarcoma; Burkitt, immunoblastic, or primary CNS lymphoma
- Viral infections
    - Cytomegalovirus retinitis (with loss of vision) or disease (other than liver, spleen, or nodes)
    - Herpes simplex: chronic ulcer(s) (>1 month); or bronchitis, pneumonitis, or esophagitis
    - Progressive multifocal leukoencephalopathy
    - Wasting syndrome due to HIV (TNF-α)
- Parasitic infections
    - Cryptosporidiosis, chronic intestinal (>1 month)
    - Isosporiasis, chronic intestinal (>1 month)
    - Toxoplasmosis of brain
- Bacterial infections
    - *Mycobacterium tuberculosis,* any site (pulmonary or extrapulmonary)
    - *Mycobacterium avium* complex or *M. kansasii* or other species or unidentified species, disseminated or extrapulmonary
    - *Salmonella* septicemia, recurrent

Table 4-16. Laboratory Analysis for HIV

Purpose	Test
Initial screening	Serologic: ELISA (HIV1 and HIV2 antibodies, p24 antigen)
Confirmation	Serologic: Western blot
Detection of virus in blood (evaluate **viral load**)	RT-PCR*
Detect HIV infection in newborns of HIV+ mother **(provirus)**	PCR*
Early marker of infection	p24 antigen
Evaluate progression of disease	CD4:CD8 T-cell ratio

*RT-PCR tests for circulating viral RNA and is used to monitor the efficacy of treatment. PCR detects integrated virus (provirus). Viral load has been demonstrated to be the best prognostic indicator during infection.

Table 4-17. Treatment

Mechanism	Name	Resistance
RT inhibitors Nuceloside or non-nucleoside analogs	End in "ine"	Common, leads to cross-resistance
Protease inhibitors	End in "inavir"	Common via protease mutations, leads to cross-resistance
HAART*	2 nucleoside analogs and 1 protease inhibitor	Increasing
Fusion inhibitors	Fuzeon, enfuvirtide	Not yet
CCR5 co-receptor antagonist	Maraviroc	Not yet
Integrase inhibitor	Raltegravir	Not yet

*HAART—highly active anti-retroviral therapy

Prevention

- Education/safe sex
- Blood/organ screening
- Infection control
- Vaccine development (currently none available)

NEGATIVE-STRANDED RNA VIRUSES

Table 4-18. Negative-Stranded RNA Viruses

Virus	RNA Structure	Virion-Associated Polymerase	Envelope	Shape	Multi-plies in	Major Viruses
Paramyxo-virus	ss(–)RNA Linear Non-segmented	Yes	Yes	Helical	Cytoplasm	Mumps Measles Respiratory syncytial Parainfluenza
Rhabdo-virus	ss(–)RNA Linear Non-segmented	Yes	Yes	Bullet-shaped helical	Cytoplasm	Rabies Vesicular stomatitis
Filovirus	ss(–)RNA Linear Non-segmented	Yes	Yes	Helical	Cytoplasm	Marburg Ebola
Orthomyxo-virus	ss(–) RNA Linear 8 segmented	Yes	Yes	Helical	Cytoplasm & nucleus	Influenza
Bunyavirus	ss(–)RNA Pseudocircular, 3 segments, 1 is ambisense	Yes	Yes	Helical	Cytoplasm	California encephalitis La Crosse encephalitis Hantavirus
Arenavirus	ss(–)RNA Circular 2 segments 1 (–)sense 1 ambisense	Yes	Yes	Helical	Cytoplasm	Lymphocytic choriomeningitis Lassa fever

Mnemonic for the ss(–)RNA viruses: <u>P</u>ain <u>R</u>esults <u>F</u>rom <u>O</u>ur <u>B</u>unions <u>A</u>lways. Gives them in order of size. You can remember these are the negative ones because pain is a negative thing. Another one: <u>B</u>ring <u>a</u>polymerase <u>o</u>r <u>f</u>ail <u>r</u>eplication.

Note that all are enveloped, all have virion-associated polymerase, and all have helical nucleocapsids. The oddballs are the last three:

- The orthomyxoviruses are linear (ortho) but with 8 (ortho/octo) segments, which is one of the reasons they can genetically "mix" it up. The orthomyxoviruses are also odd in that they replicate in both the nucleus and cytoplasm.
- The bunyaviruses are somewhat contortionists (circular): California playboy bunnies in a ménage à trois?
- The arenaviruses have one negative sense and one ambisense strand of RNA.

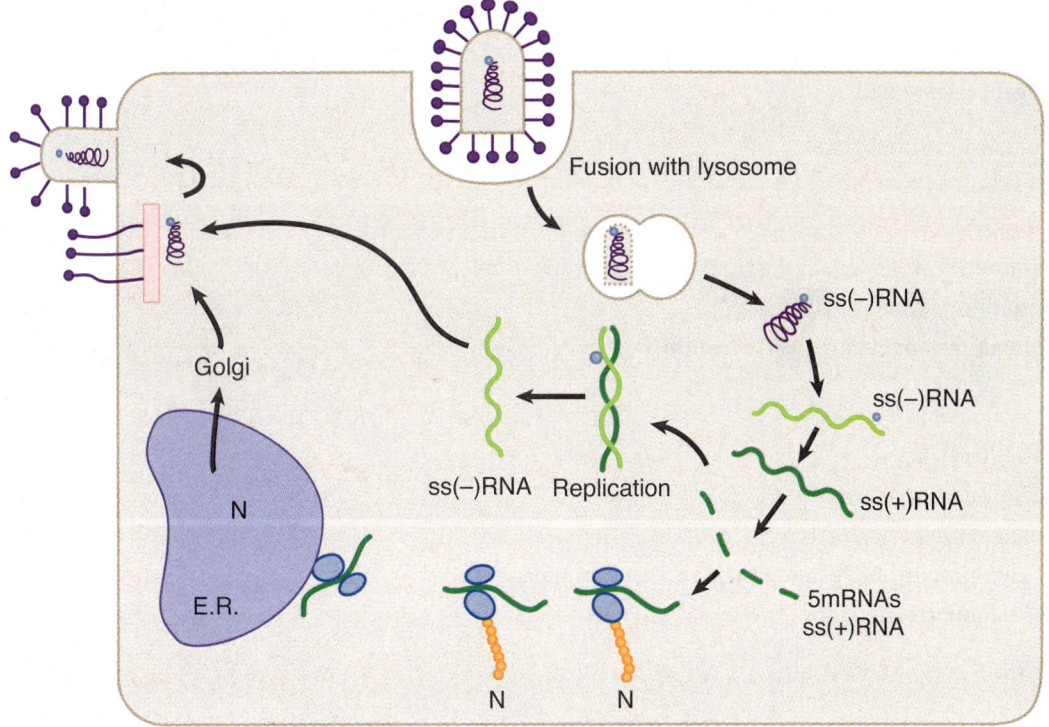

Figure 4-20. Negative-Sense RNA Virus Life Cycle

Abbreviations:

H = Hemagglutinin—surface glycoproteins that bind to sialic acid (N-acetylneuraminic acid) receptors

N = Neuraminidase—clips off sialic acids, thus aiding in release of virus

M = Matrix protein—membrane stabilizing protein underlying the viral envelope

F = Fusion protein—destabilizes host membrane

P = Polymerase associated with virion

PARAMYXOVIRIDAE

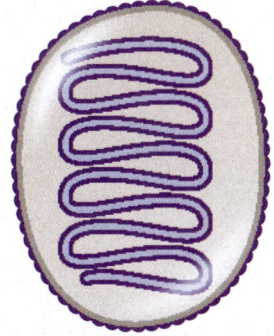

Figure 4-21. Paramyxovirus

Family Characteristics

- Enveloped, helical nucleocapsid
- Negative-sense ssRNA

Viruses of Medical Importance

- Measles
- Mumps
- Parainfluenza
- Respiratory syncytial virus (RSV)
- Human metapneumovirus (human MNV)

Measles Virus

Distinguishing Characteristics

- Single serotype
- H glycoprotein and fusion protein; no neuraminidase

Reservoir—human respiratory tract

Transmission—respiratory route

Pathogenesis

- Ability to cause cell:cell fusion → giant cells
- Virus can escape immune detection

Disease

- Measles
  - Presentation generally the 3 C's (cough, coryza, and conjunctivitis) with photophobia
  - Koplik spots → maculopapular rash from the ears down → giant cell pneumonia (Warthin-Finkeldey cells)
- Subacute sclerosing panencephalitis
  - Rare late complication
  - Defective measles virus persists in brain, acts as slow virus
  - Chronic CNS degeneration

Diagnosis—serology

Treatment

- Supportive
- Ribavirin (experimental)

Prevention—live, attenuated vaccine, MMR

Mumps Virus

Distinguishing Characteristics

- Negative-sense ssRNA
- Helical
- Enveloped
- Single HN glycoprotein, also F protein
- Single serotype

Reservoir—human respiratory tract

Transmission—person to person via respiratory droplets

Pathogenesis—lytic infection of epithelial cells of upper respiratory tract and parotid glands → spread throughout body.

Disease—mumps

- Asymptomatic to bilateral parotitis with fever, headache, and malaise
- Complications include pancreatitis, orchitis (leads to sterility in males), and meningoencephalitis

Diagnosis

- Clinical
- Serology; ELISA, IFA, hemagglutination inhibition

Treatment—supportive

Prevention—live, attenuated vaccine, M<u>M</u>R

Table 4-19. Summary of Additional Paramyxoviruses

Virus	Transmission	Disease(s)	Diagnosis	Treatment/Prevention
Parainfluenza	Respiratory	Older children and adults—subglottal swelling; hoarse, barking cough Infants—colds, bronchiolitis, pneumonia, **croup**	RT-PCR	Supportive/none
RSV	Respiratory	Adults—colds; infants/**preemies**—bronchiolitis and necrosis of bronchioles, atypical pneumonia (low fever, tachypnea, tachycardia, expiratory wheeze)	IFA, ELISA, RT-PCR	Ribavirin and anti-RSV Abs/none Palivizumab blocks fusion protein
Human MNV	Respiratory	Common cold (15% in kids), bronchiolitis, pneumonia	RT-PCR	Supportive/none

Definition of abbreviations: IFA, indirect fluorescent antibody; ELISA, enzyme-linked immunosorbent assay; RSV, respiratory syncytial virus; MNV, metapneumovirus; RT-PCR, reverse transcriptase-polymerase chain reaction.

RHABDOVIRIDAE
Family Characteristics
- Negative-sense ssRNA
- Bullet shaped
- Enveloped, helical

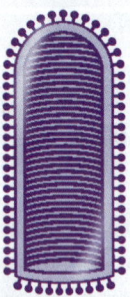

Figure 4-22. Rhabdovirus

Viruses of Medical Importance

- Rabies

Rabies Virus

Reservoir

- In the U.S., most cases sylvatic: bats, raccoons, foxes, and skunks
- Worldwide, dogs are primary reservoir

Transmission—bite or contact with a rabid animal

Pathogenesis

- After contact, virus binds to peripheral nerves by binding to nicotinic acetylcholine receptor *or* indirectly into the muscle at the site of inoculation
- Virus travels by **retrograde axoplasmic** transport to dorsal root ganglia and spinal cord
- Once virus gains access to spinal cord, brain becomes rapidly infected

Disease—rabies

- Nonspecific flu-like illness followed by neurologic symptoms of **hydrophobia**, seizures, disorientation, **hallucination**, coma, and death
- With rare exception, rabies fatal unless treated by immunoprophylaxis

Diagnosis

- Clinical
- Negri bodies, intracytoplasmic inclusion bodies (brain biopsy)
- DFA (impression smears of corneal epithelial cells), PCR (usually too late)

Treatment

- If symptoms are evident: *none*
- If suspect:
  - Postexposure prophylaxis
  - One dose of human rabies immunoglobulin (hRIG)
  - Five doses of rabies vaccine (day of, 3, 7, 14, 28)
  - Killed virus vaccine

Prevention

- Vaccine for high-risk individuals
- Vaccination program for domestic animals (U.S.)

FILOVIRIDAE

Family Characteristics

- Negative-sense ssRNA
- Enveloped, helical
- Filamentous

Viruses of Medical Importance

- Ebola virus
- Marburg virus

Table 4-20. Summary of Filoviruses

Virus	Reservoir	Transmission	Disease	Diagnosis	Treatment/ Prevention
Ebola, Marburg	Unknown	Direct contact (blood, secretions)	Fatal hemorrhagic fever	Level 4 isolation, ELISA, PCR	Supportive/ quarantine

ORTHOMYXOVIRIDAE

Family Characteristics

- Negative-sense ssRNA
- Enveloped
- Segmented (8 segments)
- Helical

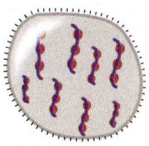

Figure 4-23. Orthomyxovirus

Viruses of Medical Importance

- Influenza A
- Influenza B

Influenza Virus

Distinguishing Features

- Envelope contains two glycoproteins, H and N
- Used to serotype virus

Reservoir

- Influenza A (birds, pigs, humans)
- Influenza B (humans only)

Transmission

- Direct contact
- Respiratory
- 1997 H5N1 strain jumped directly from birds to humans
- 2009 H1N1 strain—quadruple reassortment virus (North American swine, avian, human; Asian and European swine)

Pathogenesis

- Antigenic drift
  - Influenza A and B
  - Slight changes in antigenicity due to mutations in H and/or N
  - Causes epidemics
- Antigenic shift
  - *Influenza A only*
  - Rare genetic reassortment
  - Coinfection of cells with two different strains of influenza A (H5N1 and H3N2); reassortment of segments of genome
  - Production of a new agent to which population has no immunity
  - Responsible for pandemics

Disease—influenza

- Headache and malaise
- Fever, chills, myalgias, anorexia
- Bronchiolitis, croup, otitis media, vomiting (younger children)
- Pneumonia/secondary bacterial infections
- Can lead to Reye syndrome or Guillain-Barré syndrome

Diagnosis

- Rapid tests (serology)
- Clinical symptoms plus season

Treatment

- Amantadine/rimantadine (current isolates are commonly resistant)
  - Inhibit viral uncoating
  - Administer orally
- Zanamivir/oseltamivir
  - Neuraminidase inhibitors
  - Zanamivir is inhaled
  - Oseltamivir is given orally

Prevention

- Killed vaccine
  - Two strains of influenza A (H3N2, H1N1, for example) and one strain of influenza B are incorporated into the vaccine
- Live, attenuated vaccine
  - Intranasal administration
  - Similar composition
  - Currently recommended for ages 2–49

BUNYAVIRIDAE

Family Characteristics

- Negative-sense ssRNA
- Enveloped viruses
- Three segments, one ambisense
- Mostly arboviruses, except Hantavirus

Viruses of Medical Importance

- California encephalitis
- LaCrosse encephalitis
- Hantavirus (sin nombre)

Table 4-21. Summary of Bunyaviridae

Virus	Transmission	Disease	Diagnosis
California and La-Crosse encephalitis	Mosquito	Viral encephalitis	Serology
Hantavirus (sin nombre)	Rodent excrement, four-corners region, rainy season	Hantavirus pulmonary syndrome (cough, myalgia, dyspnea, tachycardia, pulmonary edema and effusion, and hypotension [mortality 50%])	RT-PCR

ARENAVIRIDAE

Family Characteristics

- Negative-sense ssRNA
- Pleomorphic, enveloped
- Virions have a sandy appearance (ribosomes in virion)
- Two segments, one ambisense

Viruses of Medical Importance

- Lymphocytic choriomeningitis virus (LCMV)
- Lassa fever virus

Table 4-22. Summary of Arenaviridae

Virus	Transmission	Disease	Diagnosis	Treatment
LCMV	Mice and pet hamsters (U.S.)	Influenza-like with meningeal signs	Serology, level 3 isolation	Supportive, ribavirin
Lassa fever	Rodents, human-to-human (West Africa)	Hemorrhagic fever with 50% fatality rate	Serology, level 4 isolation	Supportive, ribavirin

Definition of Abbreviations: LCMV, Lymphocytic choriomeningitis virus

DOUBLE-STRANDED RNA VIRUSES

Reoviridae

Table 4-23. Double-Stranded RNA Viruses

	RNA Structure	Polymerase	Envelope	Shape	Major Viruses
Reovirus	Linear dsRNA 10-11 segments	Yes	Naked	Icosahedral Double shelled	Reovirus Rotavirus Colorado Tick Fever Virus

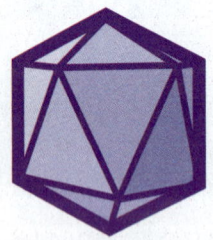

Figure 4-24. Reovirus

Table 4-24. Summary of Reoviridae

Virus	Transmission	Disease	Diagnosis	Treatment/Prevention
Reovirus	Fecal-oral, respiratory	Common cold, gastroenteritis	Serology	Self-limiting/none
Rotavirus	Fecal-oral	Gastroenteritis, no blood or pus	ELISA (stool)	Live, attenuated vaccine, oral

Definition of Abbreviations: ELISA, enzyme-linked immunosorbent assay.

ONCOGENIC VIRUSES

Definitions

Malignant transformation of cells

- Dedifferentiation
- Loss of growth control
- Immortalization
- Appearance of new surface antigens ("T" antigens)

Provirus

Viral DNA inserted into host DNA

Oncogenes

Genes with the potential to cause malignant transformation

Cellular oncogenes (abbreviated c-onc)

These are normal cellular genes whose products </ix>control regulation of cell growth and division (e.g., kinases, growth factors and their receptors, G proteins and nuclear regulatory proteins).

Viral oncogenes (abbreviated v-onc)

Genes carried by certain viruses causing cancer. Viral oncogenes are homologs of cellular oncogenes.

Tumor suppressor genes

These genes suppress, or constrain, cell growth and replication.

Major Concepts of Tumorigenesis

Mutation of a c-oncogene or tumor suppressor gene

- Mutation in one of these control genes may result in unregulated growth of cells.
- Example of mutated oncogene—*ras*
- Retinoblastoma (Rb) is an example of mutation in tumor suppressor gene.

Dosage effects

- Oncogenes in amplified DNA—increased number of copies results in overexpression of gene.
- **Translocation**, which links an oncogene with a more active enhancer and/or promoter, resulting in overexpression (Burkitt lymphoma)
- Provirus **insertional mutagenesis**—for example, a retrovirus with its very active transcriptional promoter/enhancer region, the LTR (long terminal repeat), may integrate (insert) near a cellular oncogene. This is one of the mechanisms by which retroviruses that do not have v-onc cause carcinoma.

- Infection with a virus carrying a v-onc: e.g., infection with a retrovirus carrying viral oncogenes such as *src*. The gene was probably picked up by a provirus inserted near a cellular oncogene picking up copies of c-onc. Viral progeny then contain the new oncogene now called v-onc. When a new cell is infected with the recombinant virus, the oncogene is now under the transcriptional control of the viral enhancer/promoter.

- Interaction between the products of oncogenes and tumor suppressor genes. Proteins E6 and E7 of the human papilloma virus combine with and inactivate the p53 and Rb, respectively.

Specific Viruses Associated with Human Cancers

EBV

- Burkitt lymphoma (BL) translocation t(8:14), nasopharyngeal, and thymic carcinoma
- BL occurs only in malarial regions; the plasmodia are thought to produce a slight immunosuppression.
- EBV stimulates B-cell replication and eventually, if a translocation of *c-myc* to the DNA region where genetic rearrangements involved in antibody synthesis occurs, BL develops.

Chronic HBV

Primary hepatocellular carcinoma

Chronic HCV

Primary hepatocellular carcinoma

HPV

- Cervical carcinoma
- Mechanism: inactivation of tumor suppressor gene

HTLV-1

- CD4+ T-cell leukemia/lymphomas
- Provirus insertion or capture

HTLV-2

- Hairy cell leukemia

PRION DISEASES

Table 4-25. Prion Diseases

Disease	Infectious agent	Host	Comments
Kuru	Prion	Human	Subacute spongiform encephalopathy (SSE); Fore Tribe, New Guinea; cannibalism
Creutzfeldt-Jakob disease (and variant)	Prion	Human	SSE Genetic predisposition; ingestion of infected cow brains
Gerstmann-Sträussler-Scheinker	Prion	Human	SSE
Fatal familial insomnia	Prion	Human	SSE
Scrapie	Prion	Sheep	SSE—scraping their wool off on fences

Table 4-26. Slow Conventional Viruses (Viruses)

Disease	Infectious agent	Host	Comments
Measles SSPE	Virus	Human having had measles	Subacute sclerosing panencephalitis
AIDS dementia	HIV	Human	Dementia
PML	JC virus	Human	Progressive multifocal leukoencephalopathy

VIRAL GENETICS

Genetic Reassortment = Genetic Shift

- Two different strains of a segmented RNA virus infect the same cell.
- Major new genetic combinations are produced through "shuffling," resulting in stable and dramatic changes.

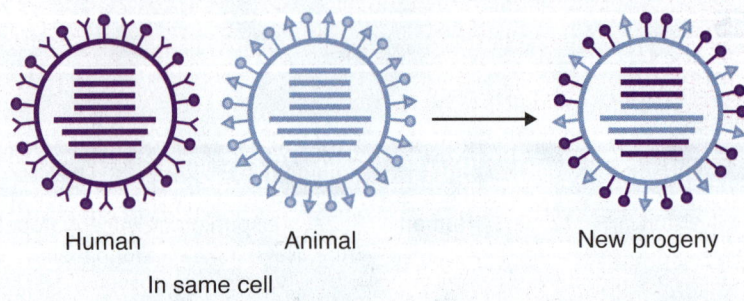

Figure 4-25. Genetic Reassortment in Influenza A

Genetic Drift

- Minor antigenic changes from mutation
- Occurs in many viruses, particularly RNA ones
- Most noted in HIV and influenza

Medically Important Fungi 5

Learning Objectives

❏ Demonstrate understanding of mycology and fungal morphology

❏ Differentiate between non-systemic fungal infections and deep fungal infections

❏ Answer questions concerning specific fungal infections, including those caused by *Candida*

MYCOLOGY

Mycology is the **study of fungi (molds, yeasts, and mushrooms).**

All fungi are

- **Eukaryotic** (e.g., true nucleus, 80S ribosomes, mitochondria, as are humans).
- **Complex carbohydrate cell walls: chitin, glucan, and mannan.**
- **Ergosterol** = Major membrane sterol

    Imidazole antifungals inhibit synthesis of ergosterol.
    Polyene antifungals bind more tightly to **ergosterol** than cholesterol.

FUNGAL MORPHOLOGY

Hyphae = filamentous cellular units of molds and mushrooms

Nonseptate Hyphae

- No cross walls
- Broad hyphae with **irregular width**
- **Broad angle of branching**

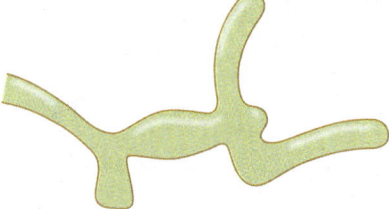

Figure 5-1. Nonseptate Hyphae

Septate Hyphae

- With **cross walls**
- Width is fairly regular (tube-like).

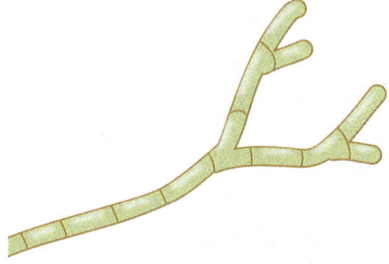

Figure 5-2. Septate Hyphae

Hyphal Coloration

- **Dematiaceous: dark colored** (gray, olive)
- **Hyaline: clear**

Mat of hyphae = mycelium

Yeasts = single celled (round to oval) fungi

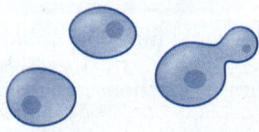

Figure 5-3. Yeasts

Dimorphic Fungi

- **Fungi able to convert from hyphal to yeast or yeast-like forms.**
- **Thermally dimorphic: in the "cold" are the mold form.**

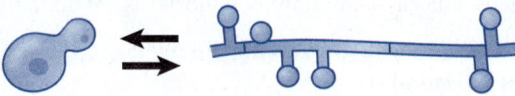

Figure 5-4. Dimorphic Fungi

Pseudohyphae (Candida albicans)

Hyphae with constrictions at each septum

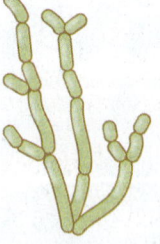

Figure 5-5. Candida Pseudohyphae

Spore types

Conidia

- **Asexual spores**
- Formed off of hyphae
- Common
- Airborne

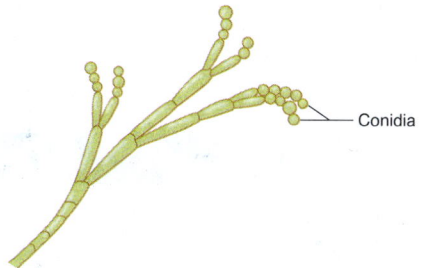

Figure 5-6. Conidia

Blastoconidia: "Buds" on yeasts (asexual budding daughter yeast cells)

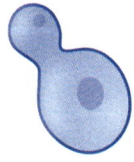

Figure 5-7. Blastoconidia

Arthroconidia: Asexual spores formed by a **"joint"**

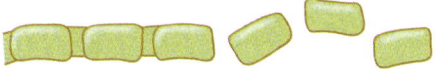

Figure 5-8. Arthroconidia

Spherules and Endospores *(Coccidioides)*: Spores inside the spherules in tissues

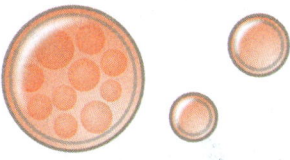

Figure 5-9. Endospores and Spherules

Diagnosis

Table 5-1. Microscopic Methods/Special Fungal Stains

Preparation	Fungal Color	Notes
KOH wet mount (KOH degrades human tissues leaving hyphae and yeasts visible)	Colorless (hyaline) refractive green or light olive to brown (dematiaceous) fungal elements	Heat gently; let sit 10 minutes; dissolves human cells
PAS	Hot pink	
Silver stain	Gray to black	*Pneumocystis*
Calcofluor white (can be done on wet mounts)	Bright blue-white on black	Scrapings or sections; fluorescent microscope needed
India ink wet mount of CSF sediment	Colorless cells with halos (capsule) on a black particulate background (*Cryptococcus neoformans*)	Only "rules in"; insensitive; misses 50% 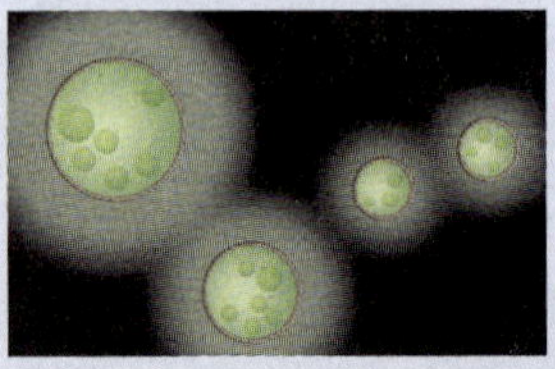

Figure 5-10. *Cryptococcus neoformans*

Culture

(May take several weeks.) Special fungal media: inhibitory mold agar is modification of Sabouraud with antibiotics.

- **Sabouraud agar**
- Blood agar
- Both of the above with antibiotics

Identification from cultures

- Fungal **morphology**
- PCR with nucleic acid probes

Serology

(E.g., antibody screen, complement fixation, etc.) Looking for patient antibody.

Fungal antigen detection: (CSF, serum)

Cryptococcal capsular polysaccharide detection by latex particle agglutination (LPA) or counter immunoelectrophoresis.

Skin tests

- Most useful for **epidemiology** or **demonstration of anergy** to an agent you know patient is infected with (grave prognosis)
- Otherwise, like tuberculosis, a skin test **only indicates exposure** to the agent.

NONSYSTEMIC FUNGAL INFECTIONS

Superficial Infections (Keratinized Tissues)

Malassezia furfur

Normal skin flora (lipophilic yeast)

Diseases

- **Pityriasis or tinea versicolor**
  - Superficial infection of keratinized cells
  - Moist, warm climates predispose
  - **Hypopigmented spots on the chest/back** (blotchy suntan)
  - KOH mount of skin scales: spaghetti and meatballs (bacon and eggs) **Yeast clusters & short curved septate hyphae**
  - Coppery-orange fluoresence under Wood lamp (UV)
  - Treatment is topical selenium sulfide; recurs.
- **Fungemia in premature infants** on intravenous lipid supplements

Cutaneous Fungal Infections (Without Systemic Disease)

Yeast or dermatophytic infections.

Yeast skin infections

- Commonly **cutaneous or mucocutaneous candidiasis**
- May disseminate in compromised patients
- Discussed with opportunistic fungi

Dermatophytes (group of fungi)

- **Filamentous** fungi (**monomorphic**)
- **Infect only skin and hair and/or nails** (do not disseminate)
- Three genera:

  Trichophyton—Infects skin, hair and nails

  Microsporum—Infects hair and skin

  Epidermophyton—Infects nails and skin

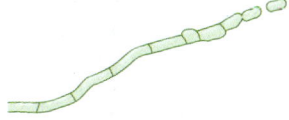

Figure 5-11. Dermatophyte

Diseases

- Dermatophytic Infections = **Tineas** (Ringworms)

  – Itching is the most common symptom of all tineas.

  – If **highly inflammatory**, generally from **animals** (zoophilic)

  – If **little inflammation**, generally from humans

  – Tinea capitis = ringworm of the scalp

  – The most serious of the tineas capiti is **favus** (tinea favosa), which causes **permanent hair loss** and is very contagious.

  – Tinea barbae = ringworm of the bearded region

  – Tinea corporis = dermatophytic infection of the glabrous skin

  – Tinea cruris = jock itch

  – Tinea pedis = athlete's foot

  – Tinea unguium = ringworm of the nails

Diagnosis

- *Microsporum* fluoresces a bright yellow-green (Wood lamp)
- **KOHmount** of nail or skin scrapings should show **arthroconidia and hyphae.**

Treatment

- Topical imidazoles or tolnaftate
- Oral imidazoles or griseofulvin where hairs are infected, or skin contact hurts
- **Keep areas dry.**

ID reaction

(Dermatophyt<u>id</u>) = Allergic response to circulating fungal antigens

Subcutaneous Mycoses

Sporothrix schenckii

Dimorphic Fungus

- **Environmental form:** on **plant material**, worldwide as **hyphae with rosettes and sleeves of conidia**
- **Traumatic implantation** (rose or plum tree thorns, wire/sphagnum moss)
- **Tissue form: cigar-shaped yeast** in tissue

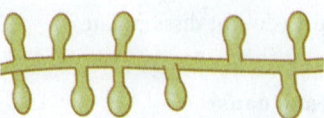

Figure 5-12. *Sporothrix* Hyphae

Diseases

- **Sporotrichosis (rose gardener disease): subcutaneous or lymphocutaneous lesions.** Treatment: itraconazole or **potassium iodide in milk**
- **Pulmonary** (acute or chronic) **sporotrichosis.** Urban alcoholics, particularly homeless (**alcoholic rose-garden-sleeper disease**)

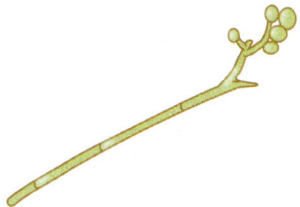

Figure 5-13. *Sporothrix*

Treatment: Itraconazole or amphotericin B

DEEP FUNGAL INFECTIONS

Classical Pathogens

Three important classical pathogens in the U.S.:

- *Histoplasma*
- *Coccidioides*
- *Blastomyces*

All three pathogens **cause**

- **Acute pulmonary** (asymptomatic or self-resolving in about **95%** of the cases)
- **Chronic** pulmonary, or
- **Disseminated** infections

Diagnosis

(Most people never see a doctor.)

- Sputum cytology (calcofluor white helpful)
- **Sputum cultures** on blood agar and **special fungal media** (inhibitory mold agar, Sabouraud)
- Peripheral blood cultures are useful for *Histoplasma* since it circulates in RES cells.

Histoplasma capsulatum

Dimorphic Fungus

- **Environmental form: hyphae** with **microconidia** and **tuberculate macroconidia**
  - Endemic region: **Eastern Great Lakes, Ohio, Mississippi, and Missouri River beds**
  - Found in **soil (dust) enriched with bird or bat feces**
  - Spelunking (cave exploring), cleaning chicken coops, or bulldozing starling roosts

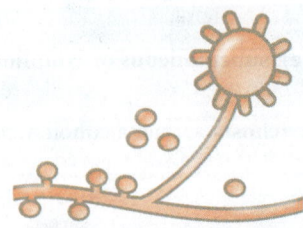

Figure 5-14. *Histoplasma* Environmental Form

- **Tissue form: small intracellular yeasts** with narrow neck on bud; **no capsule**
- **Facultative intracellular parasite** found in **reticuloendothelial (RES) cells** (tiny; can get 30 or so in a human cell)

Disease

Fungus flu (a pneumonia)

- Asymptomatic or acute (but self-resolving) pneumonia with flu-like symptomatology
- **Hepatosplenomegaly may be present** even in acute pulmonary infections (facultative intracellular RES)
- Very common in summer in endemic areas: children or newcomers (80% of adults are skin-test positive in some areas)
- Lesions have a tendency to **calcify as they heal**.
- Relapse potential increases with T cell immunosuppression.
- **Disseminated infections**: Mucocutaneous lesions are common; also common **in AIDS** patients in endemic area.

Treatment: Itraconazole for mild, amphotericin B for severe

Coccidioides immitis

Dimorphic Fungus

- **Environmental form: hyphae** breaking up into **arthroconidia** found **indesert sand**

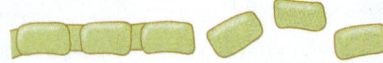

Figure 5-15. *Coccicioides immitis*

– Endemic region: **Southwestern United States**—Southern **California** (especially San Joaquin Valley), Arizona, New Mexico, Texas, Nevada
– Arthroconidia are inhaled, round up, and enlarged, becoming spherules inside which the cytoplasm walls off, forming endospores.
- **Tissue form: spherules with endospores**

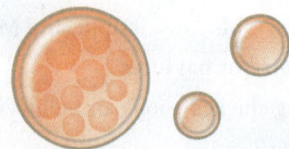

Figure 5-16. *Coccidioides immitis* Spherules

Disease: Valley fever (asymptomatic to **self-resolving pneumonia**)

- **Desert bumps** (erythema nodosum) and arthritis are generally good prognostic signs.
- Very common in endemic region
- **Pulmonary lesions have a tendency to calcify as they heal**.
- **Systemic infections are a problem in AIDS and immunocompromised patients** in endemic region (meningitis, mucocutaneous lesions).
- Tendency to **disseminate in third trimester of pregnancy**.

Treatment: Azoles for mild to moderate (itraconazole, etc.), amphotericin B for severe

Blastomyces dermatitidis

Dimorphic Fungus

Environmental form: hyphae with **nondescript conidia** (i.e., no fancy arrangements)

- Association not definitively known, **appears to be associated with rotting wood** such as beaver dams
- Endemic region: Upper Great Lakes, Ohio, Mississippi River beds, plus the southeastern seaboard of the U.S. and northern Minnesota into Canada

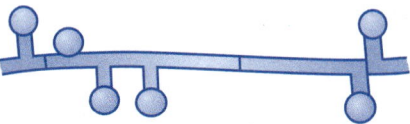

Figure 5-17. *Blastomyces dermatitidis* Hyphae with Conidia

Tissue form: broad-based budding yeasts and a double refractile cell wall (not capsule)

Disease: Blastomycosis

- Acute and chronic pulmonary disease
- Considered less likely to self-resolve than *Histoplasma* or *Coccidioides*, so many physicians will treat even acute infections.
- Disseminated disease

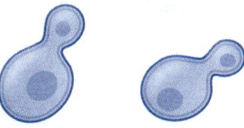

Figure 5-18. *Blastomyces dermatitidis* Broad-Based Budding Yeasts

Treatment: Itraconazole for mild, amphotericin B for severe

Opportunistic Fungi

Aspergillus fumigatus
Monomorphic filamentous fungus

- **Dichotomously branching**
- **Generally acute angles**
- **Frequent septate hyphae with 45° angles**
- One of our **major recyclers**: compost pits, moldy marijuana

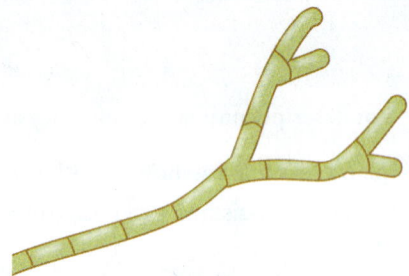

Figure 5-19. *Aspergillus* Showing Monomorphic Filamentous Fungus

Diseases/Predisposing Conditions

- **Allergic bronchopulmonary aspergillosis**/asthma, cystic fibrosis (growing in mucous plugs in the lung but not penetrating the lung tissue)
- **Fungus ball**: free in preformed lung cavities (surgical removal to reduce coughing, which may induce pulmonary hemorrhage)
- **Invasive aspergillosis**/severe neutropenia, CGD, CF, burns
  - Invades tissues causing infarcts and hemorrhage.
  - Nasal colonization → **pneumonia or meningitis**
  - **Cellulitis**/in burn patients; may also disseminate

Treatment: Voriconazole for invasive and aspergilloma, glucocorticoids + itraconazole for ABPA

Candida albicans (and other species of Candida)

- **Yeast** endogenous to our mucous membrane normal flora
- *C. albicans* yeasts form germ tubes at 37°C in serum.
- Forms **pseudohyphae** and **true hyphae** when it invades tissues (nonpathogenic *Candida* do not).

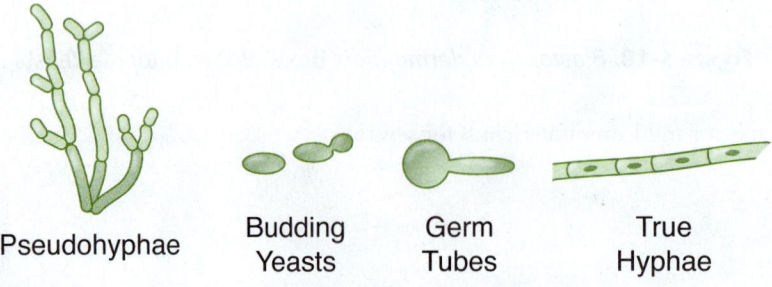

Pseudohyphae   Budding   Germ   True
                 Yeasts   Tubes   Hyphae

Figure 5-20. *Candida albicans*

Diseases/Predisposing Conditions

- **Perlèche**: crevices of mouth/malnutrition
- **Angular chelitis:** Growth at corners of the mouth
- **Inside of any dental appliance** (ex: complete denture) due to warmth, darkness, mositure in space between denture and tissue
- **Oral thrush**/prematurity, antibiotic use, immunocompromised (IC) host, AIDS
- **Esophagitis**/antibiotic use, IC host, AIDS
- **AIDS defining**: oral is not , but pharyngeal/espohageal is
- **Gastritis**/antibiotic use, IC host, AIDS
- **Septicemia** (with endophthalmitis and macronodular skin lesions)/immunocompromised, cancer, and intravenous (IV) patients
- **Endocarditis** (with transient septicemias)/**IV drug abusers**
- **Cutaneous infections**/obesity and infants; patients with rubber gloves
- **Yeast vaginitis**; particularly a problem in diabetic women
- Chronic mucocutaneous candidiasis/endocrine defects; anergy to *Candida*

Diagnosis

- KOH: pseudohyphae, true hyphae, budding yeasts
- Septicemia: culture lab identification: biochemical tests/formation of germ tubes
- Note that "psuedohyphae and chlamydospores" is classic description for NBDE 1

Treatment

- Topical imidazoles or oral imidazoles; nystatin
- Most common dental treatment—nystatin (Mycostatin) rinse or clotrimazole (Mycelex) troches (lozenges)
- Disseminated: Amphotericin B or fluconazole

Cryptococcus neoformans

Encapsulated Yeast (Monomorphic)

Environmental Source: Soil enriched with pigeon droppings

Diseases/Predisposing Conditions

- **Meningitis/Hodgkin, AIDS (the dominant meningitis)**
- **Acute pulmonary** (usually asymptomatic)/**pigeon breeders**

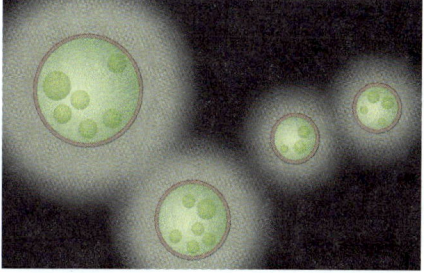

Cryptococcus neoformans

Diagnosis of Meningitis: CSF

- Detect capsular antigen in CSF (by latex particle agglutination or counter immunoelectrophoresis)
- India ink mount (misses 50%) of CSF sediment to find budding yeasts with capsular "halos"
- Cultures (urease positive yeast)

Treatment: AMB+5FC (flucytosine) until afebrile and culture negative (minimum of 10 weeks), then fluconazole

Mucor, Rhizopus, Absidia (Zygomycophyta)

Nonseptate filamentous fungi

Environmental Source: Soil; sporangiospores are inhaled

Disease

- **Rhinocerebral infection** caused by *Mucor* (or other zygomycophyta)
- (Old names: Mucormycosis = Phycomycosis = Zygomycosis)
- Characterized by paranasal swelling, necrotic tissues, hemorrhagic exudates from nose and eyes, and mental lethargy
- Occurs in **ketoacidotic diabetic patients and leukemic patients**
- These fungi penetrate without respect to anatomical barriers, progressing rapidly from sinuses into the brain tissue

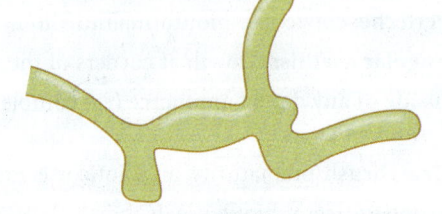

Figure 5-21. Nonseptate Hyphae with Broad Angles

Diagnosis: KOH of tissue; broad ribbon-like nonseptate hyphae with about 90° angles on branches.

Treatment

- Debride necrotic tissue and start Amphotericin B fast
- High fatality rate because of rapid growth and invasion

Pneumocystis jirovecii (formerly P. carinii)

Fungus (based on molecular techniques like **ribotyping**)

- **Obligate extracellular parasite**
- **Silver stained cysts in tissues**

Disease: Interstitial pneumonia

- Pneumonia in AIDS patients even with prophylaxis (mean CD4+/mm^3 of 26), malnourished babies, premature neonates, and some other IC adults and kids
- Symptoms: fever, cough, shortness of breath; sputum nonproductive except in smokers
- Serum leaks into alveoli, producing an exudate with a foamy or **honeycomb appearance on H & E stain.** (Silver stain reveals the holes in the exudate are actually the cysts and trophozoites, which do not stain with H & E.)
- X-ray: **patchy infiltrative** (ground glass appearance); the lower lobe periphery may be spared.

Diagnosis: Silver-staining cysts in bronchial alveolar lavage fluids or biopsy

Treatment: Trimethoprim/sulfamethoxazole for mild; dapsone for moderate to severe; pentamidine for treatment or prophylaxis

Emerging Drug Resistances in Fungi

- Fungi are developing drug resistances by mechanisms analogous to those seen in bacteria.
- Resistance to azoles (clotrimazole, miconazole, ketoconazole, fluconazole) becoming widespread
- *Aspergillus, Candida, Cryptococcus* Nonseptate Hyphae with Broad Angles

Medical Parasitology ⑥

Learning Objectives

❏ Demonstrate understanding of classification of parasites

❏ Use knowledge of important protozoan parasites

❏ Answer questions about important metazoan parasites

CLASSIFICATION OF PARASITES

Medical parasitology is the study of the invertebrate animals and the diseases they cause. Parasites are classified as protozoans or metazoans.

The most important organisms in the U.S. are identified in the following two tables in boldface type.

Table 6-1. Protozoans

Common Name	Amebae	Flagellates	Apicomplexa
Important Genera	***Entamoeba***	LUMINAL (GUT, UG)	BLOOD/TISSUE
	Naegleria	***Trichomonas***	***Plasmodium***
	Acanthamoeba	***Giardia***	***Toxoplasma***
		HEMOFLAGELLATES	*Babesia*
		Leishmania	INTESTINAL
		Trypanosoma	***Cryptosporidium***
			Isospora

Pneumocystis, which was formerly classified as a protozoan, has been determined to be a fungus through ribotyping and other molecular biologic techniques.

Table 6-2. Metazoans: Worms*

Phylum	Flat worms (Platyhelminthes)		Roundworms
Classes:	**Trematodes**	**Cestodes**	**Nematodes**
Common name:	(flukes)	(tapeworms)	(roundworms)
Genera:	*Fasciola*	*Diphyllobothrium*	<u>N</u>**ecator**
	Fasciolopsis	*Hymenolepis*	**Enterobius**
	Paragonimus	*Taenia*	⁀ⱳ uchereria/Brugia
	Clonorchis	*Echinococcus*	**Ascaris** and **Ancylostoma**
	Schistosoma		*Toxocara, Trichuris & Trichinella*
			Onchocerca
			Dracunculus
			Eye worm (Loa loa)
			Strongyloides

* Metazoans also include the Arthropoda, which serve mainly as intermediate hosts (the crustaceans) or as vectors of disease (the Arachnida and Insecta).

**Nematodes mnemonic.

Hosts

The infected host is classified as

- **Intermediate**—host in which **larval or asexual stages develop**.
- **Definitive** —host in which the **adult or sexual stages occur**.

Vectors

Vectors are **living transmitters** (e.g., a fly) of disease and may be

- **Mechanical,** which transport the parasite but there is no development of the parasite in the vector.
- **Biologic**, in which some stages of the life cycle occur.

IMPORTANT PROTOZOAN PARASITES

Table 6-3. Protozoan Parasites

Species	Disease/Organs Most Affected	Form/ Transmission	Diagnosis	Treatment
Entamoeba histolytica	***Amebiasis:*** dysentery **Inverted flask**-shaped lesions in large intestine with extension to peritoneum and liver, lungs, brain, and heart **Blood and pus** in stools **Liver abscesses**	Cysts Fecal-oral transmission—water, fresh fruits, and vegetables	Trophozoites: or cysts in stool: Serology: Nuclei have sharp central karyosome and fine chromatin "spokes."	Metronidazole followed by iodoquinol
Giardia lamblia	Giardiasis: Ventral sucking disk attaches to lining of duodenal wall, causing **a fatty, foul-smelling diarrhea** (diarrhea → *malabsorption* duodenum, jejunum)	Cysts Fecal (human, beaver, muskrat, etc.), oral transmission—water, food, day care, oral-anal sex	Trophozoites or cysts in stool or fecal antigen test (replaces "string" test) "Falling leaf" motility	Metronidazole
Cryptosporidium sp. *C. parvum*	Cryptosporidiosis: transient diarrhea in healthy, severe in immunocompromised hosts	Cysts Undercooked meat, water; not killed by chlorination	**Acid fast oocysts in stool:** Biopsy shows dots (cysts) in intestinal glands	Nothing is 100% effective; nitrazoxanide, puromycin, or azithromycin are the DOCs
Isospora belli	Transient diarrhea in AIDS patients; diarrhea mimics giardiasis malabsorption syndrome	Oocysts Ingestion Fecal-oral	**Acid-fast and elliptical oocysts in stool;** contain 2 sporocysts each with 4 sporozoites	TMP-SMX or pyrimethamine/ sulfadiazine

(Continue)

Species	Disease/Organs Most Affected	Form/ Transmission	Diagnosis	Treatment
Cyclospora cayetanensis	Self-limited diarrhea in immunocompetent; prolonged and severe **diarrhea in AIDS** patients	Oocysts, water	Fecal; **acid-fast and spherical oocysts**; contain 2 sporocysts each with 2 sporozoites; UV fluorescence	TMP-SMX
Microsporidia (6 genera)	Microsporidiosis: persistent, debilitating **diarrhea in AIDS** patients; other spp → neuro-logic, hepatitis, disseminated	Spores ingested	**Gram (+), acid-fast spores** in stool or biopsy material	None proven to be effective
Trichomonas vaginalis (urogenital)	Trichomoniasis: often as-ymptomatic or **frothy vaginal discharge**	Trophozoites **Sexual**	Motile trophozoites in methylene blue wet mount; **corkscrew motility**	**Metronidazole**

Free Living Amebae

- Occur in water or soil (*Naegleria, Acanthamoeba*)
- Occur in contact lens saline solutions (*Acanthamoeba*): cysts from dust contaminate

Table 6-4. Free Living Amoebae That Occasionally Infect Humans

Species	Disease / Locale	Form / Transmission	Diagnosis	Treatment
Naegleria	**Primary amebic meningoencephalitis** (PAM): severe **prefrontal headache**, nausea, high fever, **altered sense of smell**; often fatal	Free-living amebae picked up while swimming or **diving in very warm fresh water**	Motile trophozo-ites in CSF Culture on plates seeded with gram-negative bacteria; amebae will leave trails	Amphotericin B (rarely successful)
Acanthamoeba	**Keratitis; granuloma-tous amebic encepha-litis** (GAE) in immuno-compromised patients: insidious onset but progressive to death	Free living amebae in contaminated **contact lens solution (airborne cysts)** Not certain for GAE: inhala-tion or contact with con-taminated soil or water	Star-shaped cysts on biopsy; rarely seen in CSF Culture as above	Keratitis: topi-cal miconazole and propamidine isethionate GAE: ketoconazole, sul-famethazine (rarely successful)

Plasmodium Species

Each *Plasmodium* has two distinct hosts.

- A vertebrate such as the human where asexual phase (schizogony) takes place in the liver and red blood cells.
- An arthropod host (*Anopheles* mosquito) where gametogony (sexual phase) and sporogony take place.

Cause disease by a wide variety of mechanisms, including metabolism of hemoglobin and lysis of infected cells leading to anemia and to agglutination of infected RBC.

Cause paroxysms (chills, fever spike, and malarial rigors) when the infected RBC are lysed, liberating a new crop of merozoites.

Hemoflagellates (Trypanosomes and Leishmanias)

Hemoflagellates infect blood and tissues.

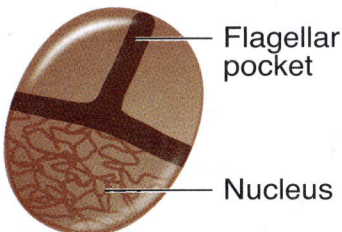

Flagellar pocket

Nucleus

Figure 6-1. Amastigote

Trypanosomes are found

- In human blood as trypomastigotes with flagellum and undulating membrane
- In tissues as **amastigotes(oval cells having neither the flagellum nor undulating membrane)**

Leishmania found always as amastigotes in macrophages.

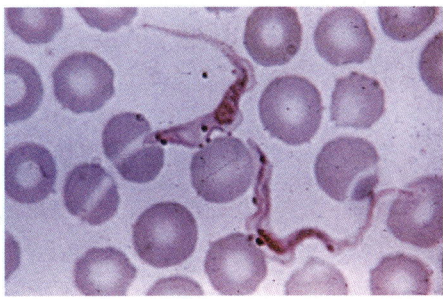

Trypomastigote in blood smear

Table 6-5. Hemoflagellates

Species	Disease	Vector/Form/ Transmission	Reservoirs	Diagnosis	Treatment
Trypanosoma cruzi*	**Chagas disease** (American trypanosomiasis) Latin America Swelling around eye: (**Romaña sign**) common early sign Cardiac muscle, liver, brain often involved	**Reduviid bug (kissing or cone bug**; genus *Triatoma*) passes trypomastigote (flagellated form) **in feces**; scratching implants in mucosa	Cats, dogs, armadillos, opossums Poverty housing	Blood films, **trypomastigotes**	Benzimidazole
Trypanosoma brucei gambiense Trypanosoma b. rhodesiense	**African sleeping sickness** (African trypanosomiasis) **Antigenic variation**	Trypomastigote in saliva of **tsetse fly** contaminates bite	Humans, some wild animals	Trypomastigotes in blood films, CSF High immuno-globulin levels in CSF	Acute: suramin Chronic: melarsoprol
Leishmania donovani** complex	**Visceral Leishmaniasis**	**Sandfly** bite	Urban: humans Rural: rodents and wild animals	**Amastigotes in macrophages** in bone marrow, liver, spleen	Stibogluco-nate sodium (from CDC)
Leishmania (About 15 different species)	Cutaneous Leishmaniasis (Oriental sore, etc.)	**Sandfly** bite	Urban: humans Rural: rodents and wild animals	**Amastigotes in macrophages** in cutaneous lesions	Stibogluco-nate sodium
Leishmania braziliensis complex	Mucocutaneous Leishmaniasis	**Sandfly** bite	Urban: humans Rural: rodents and wild animals	Same	Stibogluco-nate sodium

*T. cruzi: An estimated 1/2 million Americans are infected, creating some risk of transfusion transmission in U.S. In babies, acute infections often serious involving CNS.

In older children and adults, mild acute infections but may become chronic with the risk of development of cardiomyopathy and heart failure.

**Leishmania all: Intracellular, sandfly vector, stibogluconate.

Miscellaneous Apicomplexa Infecting Blood or Tissues

Table 6-6. Miscellaneous Apicomplexa Infecting Blood or Tissues

Species	Disease/Locale of Origin	Transmission	Diagnosis	Treatment
Babesia (primarily a disease of cattle) Humans: *Babesia microti*, WA1, & MO1 strains	Babesiosis (hemolytic, **malaria-like**) Same range as lyme: NE, N Central, California, and NW U.S.	***Ixodes* tick** **Co-infections with *Borrelia***	Giemsa stain of thin smear or hamster inoculation; small rings, maltese cross, tetrad in RBCs	Clindamycin + quinine
Toxoplasma gondii	See below	**Cat** is **essential definitive** host. Many other animals are intermediate host. Mode: 1) Raw meat in U.S. #1 = pork 2) Contact with cat feces	Serology High IgM or rising IgM acute infection	**Pyrimethamine + sulfadiazine**

Toxoplasmosis

Diseases

Healthy individuals

- *Toxoplasma* acquired after birth is most commonly asymptomatic or a mild, non-specific flu-like illness with lymphadenopathy and fever; heterophile-negative mononucleosis
- Once infected, as immunity develops, bradyzoites encyst, but generally remain viable as evidenced by a positive antibody titer.

Pregnant patients

- Women who acquire *Toxoplasma* as a primary infection during pregnancy present with flu-like illness/ heterophile-negative mononucleosis.
- If primary maternal infection occurs during pregnancy, the fetus may be infected.
- If *Toxoplasma* crosses the placenta early, severe congenital infections (intracerebral calcifications, chorioretinitis, hydro- or microcephaly or convulsions) may occur.
- If *Toxoplasma* crosses the placenta later, infection may be inapparent, but may lead to progressive blindness in the child later in life (teens).
- Maternal antibodies (secondary infection) protect the fetus during pregnancy, even if the mother is re-exposed during pregnancy.

AIDS patients

- Leading cause of focal CNS disease in AIDS patients
- Brain scan will describe ring-enhancing lesions.
- Unless prophylactic drugs are given, AIDS patients who are seropositive for *Toxoplasma* will have reactivational infections.

IMPORTANT METAZOAN PARASITES

Trematodes

- Are commonly called flukes.
- Are leaf-shaped worms, which are generally flat and fleshy.
- Are hermaphroditic except for *Schistosoma*, which has separate male and female.
- Have complicated life cycles occurring in two or more hosts.
- Have operculated eggs (except for *Schistosoma*), which contaminate water, perpetuating the life cycle, and which are also used to diagnose infections.
- **The first intermediate hosts are snails.**

Cestodes

- Are the tapeworms.
- Consist of three basic portions: the head or scolex; a "neck" section, which produces the proglottids; and the segments or proglottids, which mature as they move away from the scolex. (The combination of the neck and proglottids is called the strobila.)
- Are hermaphroditic, with each proglottid developing both male and female reproductive organs, and mature eggs developing in the most distal proglottids.
- Adhere to the mucosa via the scolex, which is knobby looking and has either suckers or a sucking groove.
- Have no gastrointestinal (GI) tract; they absorb nutrients from the host's GI tract.
- Are diagnosed by finding eggs or proglottids in the feces.
- Have for the most part complex life cycles involving extraintestinal larval forms in intermediate hosts. When humans are the intermediate host, these infections are generally more serious than the intestinal infections with adult tapeworms.
- Include *Taenia saginata* (beef tapeworm) and *Taenia solium* (pork tapeworm)

Nematodes

- Are the roundworms
- Cause a wide variety of diseases (pinworms, whipworms, hookworms, trichinosis, threadworms, filariasis, etc.)
- Have round unsegmented bodies
- Are transmitted by:
  - ingestion of eggs (*Enterobius, Ascaris,* or *Trichuris*);
  - direct invasion of skin by larval forms (*Necator, Ancylostoma,* or *Strongyloides*);
  - ingestion of meat containing larvae (*Trichinella*); or
  - infection involving insects transmitting the larvae with bites (*Wuchereria, Loa loa, Mansonella, Onchocerca,* and *Dracunculus*).

Comparative Microbiology

7

Learning Objectives

❏ Differentiate infectious organism that have clinically relevant and distinctive morphology, physiology, pathogenicity, epidemiology, transmission, pathology, lab diagnosis, treatment, or prevention

MORPHOLOGY/TAXONOMY

Spore-Forming Bacteria (Have Calcium Dipicolinate)

Bacillus

Clostridium

Non-motile Gram-Positive Rods

Corynebacterium diphtheriae

Nocardia

Clostridium perfringens (rest of the pathogenic *Clostridia* are motile)

Bacillus anthracis (most other *Bacillus* species are motile)

Acid Fast Organisms

Mycobacterium

Nocardia (partially acid fast)

Cryptosporidium oocysts

Isospora oocysts

Bacteria and Fungi That Characteristically Have Capsules

The "biggies" can be remembered by the mnemonic: **S**ome **K**illers **H**ave **P**retty **N**ice **C**apsules!

Streptococcus pneumoniae

Klebsiella pneumoniae

Haemophilus influenzae

Pseudomonas aeruginosa—slime producer especially in cystic fibrosis patients' lungs

Neisseria meningitidis

Cryptococcus neoformans (only encapsulated fungal pathogen)

Bordetella pertussis

Other Important Capsule Producers

E. coli meningeal strains have capsule, mostly K_1

Bacillus anthracis—poly D-glutamate capsule

Salmonella enterica subsp. *typhi*—(virulence; Vi) capsular antigen

Streptococcus pyogenes when first isolated; non-immunogenic (but anti-phagocytic) hyaluronic acid capsule

Biofilm Producers

Staphylococcus epidermidis (catheter-related infections)

Streptococcus mutans (dental plaque)

Pigment Production

Pseudomonas aeruginosa (blue-green)—pyocyanin, fluorescein

Serratia—red pigment

Staphylococcus aureus—yellow pigment

Photochromogenic and scotochromogenic *Mycobacteria*—Carotenoid pigments (yellow and orange)

Corynebacterium diphtheriae—black to gray

Unique Morphology/Staining

Metachromatic staining—*Corynebacterium*

Lancet-shaped diplococci—*Pneumococcus*

Kidney bean-shaped diplococci—*Neisseriae*

Bipolar staining—***Yersinia pestis***

Gulls wings—*Campylobacter*

Table 7-1. Viral Cytopathogenesis

Inclusion Bodies	Virus
Intracytoplasmic (Negri bodies)	Rabies
Intracytoplasmic acidophilic (Guarnieri)	Poxviruses
Intranuclear (Owl eye)	Cytomegalovirus
Intranuclear (Cowdry)	Herpes simplex virus
	Subacute sclerosing panencephalitis (measles) virus
Syncytia formation	**Virus**
	Herpes viruses
	Varicella-zoster
	Paramyxoviruses (measles, mumps, rubella and respiratory syncytial virus)
	HIV

PHYSIOLOGY

Table 7-2. Metabolism*

Aerobes	Anaerobes	Microaerophilic
Mycobacterium	*Actinomyces*	*Campylobacter*
Pseudomonas	*Bacteroides*	*Helicobacter*
Bacillus	*Clostridium*	
Nocardia	*Fusobacterium*	
Corynebacterium diphtheriae	*Prevotella*	
	Propionibacterium (aerotolerant)	
	Eubacterium	
	Lactobacillus (aerotolerant)	

*Most others are considered facultative anaerobes.

Enzymes

Oxidase

- **All Enterobacteriaceae are oxidase negative.**
- **All *Neisseria* are oxidase positive** (as are most other Gram-negative bacteria).

Urease Positive (mnemonic: PUNCH)

- All *Proteus* **species** produce urease; this leads to alkaline urine and may be associated with renal calculi.
- *Ureaplasma* (renal calculi)
- *Nocardia*
- *Cryptococcus* (the fungus)
- *Helicobacter*

Catalase

$$H_2O_2 \xrightarrow{\text{catalase}} H_2O + 1/2\ O_2$$

Staphylococci **have catalase,** *Streptococci* **do not.**

Most anaerobes lack catalase.

Catalase positive organisms are major problems in chronic granulomatous disease (CGD):

- All staphylococci
- *Pseudomonas aeruginosa*
- *Candida*
- *Aspergillus*
- Enterobacteriaceae

Coagulase positive

- *Staph. aureus*
- *Yersinia pestis*

DETERMINANTS OF PATHOGENICITY

Genetics

Genes encoding pathogenic factors reside on:

- The bacterial **chromosome**

    Endotoxin
- A **plasmid**

    Most toxins and multiple drug resistances
- A **bacteriophage genome** stably integrated into the host DNA as a prophage. Virulence modified by the stable presence of phage DNA in bacterial cell = lysogenic conversion.

Examples:

C = cholera toxin

O = *Salmonella* O antigen

B = Botulinum toxin (phage CEβ and DEβ)

E = Erythrogenic toxin of *Streptococcus pyogenes*

D = Diphtheria toxin (Corynephage β)

S = Shiga toxin

Mnemonic: **COBEDS** (when 2 people share a bed somebody gets a little pregnant [with phage])

Antigenic variation

> *Neisseria gonorrhoeae (pili)*
> *Borrelia recurrentis*
> *Trypanosoma brucei*
> HIV

Toxins

Table 7-3. Disease Due to Toxin Production

Bacterium	Disease	Activity of Toxin
Corynebacterium diphtheriae	**Diphtheria**	ADP ribosylation of eEF-2 results in inhibition of protein synthesis
Clostridium tetani	**Tetanus**	Binds to SV2 ganglioside protein receptor. SV2 enables internalization and cellular intoxication.
Clostridium botulinum	**Botulism**	Prevents release of acetylcholine
Vibrio cholerae	**Cholera**	Choleragen stimulates adenylate cyclase
E. coli (ETEC)	**Travelers' diarrhea**	LT stimulates adenylate cyclase
Clostridium difficile	Diarrhea	Toxin A and B inhibit protein synthesis and cause loss of intracellular K$^+$
Bordetella pertussis	Whooping cough	Hypoglycemia due to activation of islets Edema due to inhibition Gi Lymphocytosis due to inhibition of chemokine receptors Sensitivity to histamine

eEF-2 = eukaryotic elongation factor-2

Heat stable toxins

60°C

- *Staphylococcus aureus* enterotoxin
- ST toxin of *E. coli*
- *Yersinia enterocolitica* toxin

100°C

- Endotoxin

Toxins with ADP-ribosylating activity

Table 7-4. Toxins with A-B ADP-Ribosyl Transferase Activity

Toxin	ADP-Ribosylated Host Protein	Effect on Host Cell
Pseudomonas Exotoxin A	eEF-2	Inhibits translocation during protein synthesis
Exotoxin S	unknown	
Diphtheria toxin	eEF-2	Inhibits translocation during protein synthesis
E. coli heat-labile toxin (LT)	G-protein (G_S)	Increases cAMP in instestinal epithelium causing diarrhea
Cholera toxin	G-protein (G_S)	Increases cAMP in intestinal epithelium causing diarrhea
Pertussis toxin	G-protein (G_i)	Increases cAMP causing edema, lymphocytosis and increased insulin secretion

A is the ADP-ribosyl transferase.
B binds to cell receptor and translocates the A subunit into the cell.

Invasive factors

Table 7-5. Invasive Factors

Invasive Factor	Function	Bacteria
All capsules	Antiphagocytic	See earlier list with morphology
Slime layer (capsule or glycocalyx)	Antiphagocytic	*Pseudomonas*
M protein	Antiphagocytic	Group A Streptococci
A protein	Inhibits opsonization	*Staph. aureus*
Lipoteichoic acid	Attachment to host cells	All gram-positive bacteria
N. gonorrhoeae pili	Antiphagocytic	*N. gonorrhoeae*

Table 7-6. Extracellular Enzymes

Enzyme	Function	Bacteria
Hyaluronidase	Hydrolysis of ground substance	Group A Streptococci
Collagenase	Hydrolysis of collagen	*Clostridium perfringens* *Prevotella melaninogenica*
Kinases	Hydrolysis of fibrin	*Streptococcus* *Staphylococcus*
Lecithinase (alpha toxin)	Damage to membrane	*Clostridium perfringens*
Heparinase	May contribute to thrombophlebitis	*Bacteroides fragilis* *Prevotella melaninogenica*
IgA Proteases	Colonizing factor	*Neisseria* *Haemophilus* *Strep. pneumoniae*

Ability to Survive and Grow in Host Cell

Obligate Intracellular Parasites

Cannot be cultured on inert media. Virulence is due to the ability to survive and grow intracellularly where the organism is protected from many B-cell host defenses.

- Bacteria
    All Rickettsiae
    All Chlamydiaceae
    Mycobacterium leprae
- Viruses
    All are obligate intracellular parasites.
- Protozoa
    Plasmodium
    Toxoplasma gondii
    Babesia
    Leishmania
    Trypanosoma cruzi (amastigotes in cardiac muscle)
- Fungi
    None

Facultative intracellular parasites of humans

- Bacteria
    Francisella tularensis
    Listeria monocytogenes
    Mycobacterium tuberculosis
    Brucella species

Non-tuberculous *mycobacteria*

Salmonella enterica subsp. *typhi*

Legionella pneumophila

Yersinia pestis

Nocardia species

- Fungi

Histoplasma capsulatum

Obligate Parasites That Are Not Intracellular

(e.g., cannot be cultured on inert media but are found extracellularly in the body)

- *Treponema pallidum*
- *Pneumocystis jirovecii*

EPIDEMIOLOGY/TRANSMISSION

Bacteria That Have Humans as the Only Known Reservoir

Mycobacterium tuberculosis

M. leprae (armadillos in Texas)

Shigella species

Salmonella enterica subspecies **typhi**

Rickettsia prowazekii (epidemic typhus)

Group A β-hemolytic streptococcus

Neisseria meningitidis and *N. gonorrhoeae*

Corynebacterium diphtheriae

Streptococcus pneumoniae

Treponema pallidum

Chlamydia trachomatis

Zoonotic Organisms

(Diseases of animals transmissible to humans)

Bacillus anthracis

Salmonella enterica all subspecies except *typhi*

Leptospira

Borrelia

Listeria monocytogenes

Brucella species

Francisella tularensis

Pasteurella multocida (cat bites)

Vibrio parahaemolyticus (from fish)

Capnocytophaga canimorsus (dog bites)

Bartonella henselae (cat scratches)

Streptobacillus moniliformis (rat bite fever)

Mycobacterium marinum (fish tank granuloma)

Vibrio vulnificus (oysters)

Yersinia pestis, Y. enterocolitica, Y. pseudotuberculosis

Campylobacter fetus, C. jejuni

Most *Rickettsia*

Chlamydophila psittaci(birds)

Rabies virus

Arthropod Vectors in Human Disease: Insects

- Lice
    Epidemic or louse-borne typhus (*Pediculus h. humanus*)
    Epidemic relapsing fever
    Trench fever
- **True bugs**
    Chagas' disease (American trypanosomiasis)—kissing bugs (Reduviidae)
- Mosquitoes
    Malaria (*Anopheles* mosquito)
    Dengue (*Aedes*)
    Mosquito-borne encephalitides: WEE, EEE, VEE, SLE, WNV
    Yellow Fever (*Aedes*)
    Filariasis
- **Sandflies**
    Leishmaniasis
    Bartonellosis
- Midges
    Filariasis
- Blackflies
    Onchocerciasis
- Deerflies (*Chrysops*) and horse flies
    Loaloasis
    Tularemia

- Tsetse flies
    African trypanosomiasis
- Fleas
    Plague
    Endemic typhus

Arthropod Vectors That Are Not Insects

- Ticks
    Rocky Mountain spotted fever (*Dermacentor*)
    Colorado tick fever (*Dermacentor*)
    Lyme disease (*Ixodes*)
    Ehrlichia (Ixodes, Amblyomma)
    Babesiosis (*Ixodes*)
    Tularemia (*Dermacentor*)
    Recurrent fever or tick-borne relapsing fever (*Ornithodoros*, a soft tick)
- Mites
    Scrub typhus (*Leptotrombium*) (transovarial transmission in vector)
    Rickettsialpox

Parasitic Infections Transmitted by Ova

Enterobius vermicularis (pinworm)

Ascaris lumbricoides (roundworm)

Toxocara canis (visceral larva migrans)

Trichuris trichiura (whipworm)

Echinococcus granulosus/multilocularis

Taenia solium (cysticercosis)

All others are transmitted in larval stage.

Bacterial and Fungal Infections That Are Not Considered Contagious

(i.e., no human-to-human transmission)

Nontuberculous mycobacterial infections, e.g., ***Mycobacterium avium-intracellulare***

Non-spore forming anaerobes

Legionella pneumophila

All fungal infections except the dermatophytes

Infections That Cross the Placenta

(Mnemonic: TORCH)

*T*oxoplasma

Other (Syphilis)

Rubella

CMV

Herpes and **H**IV

<5% perinatal hepatitis B could possibly have been acquired by crossing placenta.

- Viruses
    - *Cytomegalovirus*
    - *Rubella*
    - HSV 2 (in primary infection)
    - Coxsackie B
    - Polio
    - HIV
    - B19
- Parasites
    - ***Toxoplasma gondii***
- Bacteria
    - ***Treponema pallidum***
    - ***Listeria monocytogenes***

Spread by Respiratory Droplet

Streptococcus pyogenes (Group A)

Streptococcus pneumoniae   Influenza

Neisseria meningitidis   Rubella

Mycobacterium tuberculosis   Measles

Bordetella pertussis   Chickenpox

Haemophilus influenzae   *Pneumocystis jirovecii*

Corynebacterium diphtheriae

Mycoplasma pneumoniae

Spread by Inhalation of Organisms from the Environment

Histoplasma

Coccidioides

Blastomyces

Nontuberculous mycobacteria, e.g., *M. avium-intracellulare* (*MAC*)

Legionella

Chlamydophila psittaci

Pseudomonas (also spread by ingestion and contact)

Spread by Oral/Fecal Route

(Infections may be spread by oral sex.)

Salmonella

Shigella

Campylobacter

Vibrio

Yersinia enterocolitica

Yersinia pseudotuberculosis

Bacillus cereus

Clostridium

Staphylococcus (also other routes commonly)

Enteroviruses, including poliovirus

Rotavirus

Norwalk agent

Hepatitis A

Toxoplasma—cat feces

Entamoeba

Giardia

All nematodes except filaria and *Trichinella*

All cestodes

Contact: (Person-to-Person) Nonsexual

Impetigo (*Strep* and *Staph*)

Staphylococcus

Herpes I

Epstein-Barr (kissing)

Hepatitis B (all body fluids)

Molluscum contagiosum (wrestling teams)

Contact: Sexual

Chlamydia	HPV	HBV
Neisseria	HIV	HCV
Treponema	HSV 2	
Trichomonas	CMV	

PATHOLOGY

Organisms that Produce Granulomas (most are intracellular, others have persistent antigen)

Fran Likes My Pal Bruce And His Blasted Cockerspaniel (in) Salt Lake City. (Mnemonic by M. Free.)

(ic) = intracellular organism

Francisella (ic)

Listeria (ic)

Mycobacterium (ic)

Treponema *pallidum*

Brucella (ic)

Actinomyces

Histoplasma (ic)

Blastomyces

Coccidioides

Schistosoma species

Lymphogranuloma venereum (ic)

Cat scratch fever

Infections Causing Intracerebral Calcifications

Toxoplasma

CMV

Cysticercosis

Cryptococcus neoformans

Tuberculous meningitis

LABORATORY DIAGNOSIS

Special Stains

- Silver stains

    Dieterle—*Legionella*

    Gomori methenamine—*Pneumocystis*, fungi

- Acid fast (Ziehl-Neelsen or Kinyoun)
    - *Mycobacterium, Nocardia*(partially AF), *Cryptosporidium, Isospora, Cyclospora*, and *Microsporidia* (oocysts in feces)
- India ink—*Cryptococcus* (if negative not a reliable diagnostic method)
- Calcofluor white—fungi
- Giemsa

    Blood protozoa (*Plasmodium, Babesia, Trypanosoma, Leishmania*)

    Histoplasma capsulatum in RES cells

Unusual Growth Requirements

Haemophilus (most species require one or both)

- **X factor** = protoporphyrin IX, the precursor of **hemin**
- **V factor** = NAD (nicotinamide dinucleotide) or NADP

Mycoplasma

- **Cholesterol**

Salt (halophilic organisms)

- *Staph aureus* will grow on high salt media.
- Group D enterococci will grow on 6.5% NaCl.
- *Vibrio* species requires NaCl to grow and grows at 6.5%.

Cysteine requirement for growth

- Four Sisters Ella of the Cysteine Chapel (mnemonic by M. Free)
- *Francisella, Legionella, Brucella*, and *Pasteurella*

Cultures that must be observed for a long time

- *Mycobacterium tuberculosis* and all non-tuberculous mycobacteria except rapid growers
- *Mycoplasma pneumoniae*
- Systemic fungal pathogens (*Blastomyces, Histoplasma*, and *Coccidioides* in U.S.)

TREATMENT/PREVENTION

Treat Prophylactically

- *Neisseria meningitidis* (household and day care contacts—vaccination also used in outbreaks)
- *Mycobacterium tuberculosis* with a recent skin test conversion or known household (i.e., significant) exposure; or persons under 35 with a positive skin test who have never been treated
- *Haemophilus influenzae* B (unvaccinated household contacts <6 years old)—also vaccinate
- *Neisseria gonorrhoeae* (sexual contacts)
- *Treponema pallidum* (sexual contacts)
- *Yersinia pestis*
- Neonatal eyes (*Neisseria gonorrhoeae, Chlamydia trachomatis, Treponema pallidum*)

Vaccines Available in the U.S.

Inactivated vaccines (RIP-A; Rest In Peace Always)

- Rabies
- Influenza virus
- Salk polio (killed)—all primary vaccinations in U.S., including IC patients
- Hepatitis A
- Japanese encephalitis and several other encephalitis vaccines
- *Vibrio cholerae*

Live, attenuated vaccines

- *Francisella tularensis*
- Measles (rubeola)
- Rubella
- Mumps (killed vaccine available for IC patients)
- Sabin polio (oral)
- Smallpox
- Yellow fever
- Varicella-Zoster
- Rotavirus

Live, Pathogenic Virus (in enteric-coated capsules)

- Adenovirus

Toxoid: Chemically Modified Toxin—-Vaccines

- Tetanus
- Diphtheria
- Pertussis toxoid (in DTaP)

Subunit Vaccines

- *Haemophilus*—purified capsular polysaccharide conjugated to protein
- *Neisseria meningitidis*—capsular polysaccharides, pediatric version is conjugated to protein
- Pneumococcal—capsular polysaccharide (7 and 23 serotypes) (pediatric version is conjugated to protein)

Recombinant Vaccines

- Hepatitis B—HBsAg (produced in yeast)
- Human papilloma virus vaccine, 4 capsid proteins

Antibacterial Agents

8

Learning Objectives

❏ Apply the principles of antimicrobial chemotherapy to select the best treatment

❏ Differentiate medications that inhibitor cell-wall synthesis, bacterial protein synthesis, and nucleic acid synthesis

❏ Answer questions about unclassified antibiotics

❏ Describe the differences between standard antibacterial agents and antitubercular drugs

PRINCIPLES OF ANTIMICROBIAL CHEMOTHERAPY

- Bactericidal
- Bacteriostatic
- Combinations:
  - Additive
  - Synergistic (penicillins plus aminoglycosides)
  - Antagonistic (penicillin plus tetracyclines)
- Mechanisms:

Table 8-1. Mechanism of Action of Antimicrobial Agents

Mechanism of Action	Antimicrobial Agents
Inhibition of bacterial cell-wall synthesis	Penicillins, cephalosporins, imipenem/meropenem, aztreonam, vancomycin
Inhibition of bacterial protein synthesis	Aminoglycosides, chloramphenicol, macrolides, tetracyclines, streptogramins, linezolid
Inhibition of nucleic synthesis	Fluoroquinolones, rifampin
Inhibition of folic acid synthesis	Sulfonamides, trimethoprim, pyrimethamine

• Resistance:

Table 8-2. Mechanisms of Resistance to Antimicrobial Agents

Antimicrobial Agents	Primary Mechanism(s) of Resistance
Penicillins and cephalosporins	Production of beta-lactamases, which cleave the beta-lactam ring structure; change in penicillin-binding proteins; change in porins
Aminoglycosides (gentamicin, streptomycin, amikacin, etc.)	Formation of enzymes that inactivate drugs via conjugation reactions that transfer acetyl, phosphoryl, or adenylyl groups
Macrolides (erythromycin, azithromycin, clarithromycin, etc.) and clindamycin	Formation of methyltransferases that alter drug binding sites on the 50S ribosomal subunit Active transport out of cells
Tetracyclines	Increased activity of transport systems that "pump" drugs out of the cell
Sulfonamides	Change in sensitivity to inhibition of target enzyme; increased formation of PABA; use of exogenous folic acid
Fluoroquinolones	Change in sensitivity to inhibition of target enzymes; increased activity of transport systems that promote drug efflux
Chloramphenicol	Formation of inactivating acetyltransferases

INHIBITORS OF CELL-WALL SYNTHESIS

• All cell-wall synthesis inhibitors are bactericidal.

Penicillins	Cephalosporins
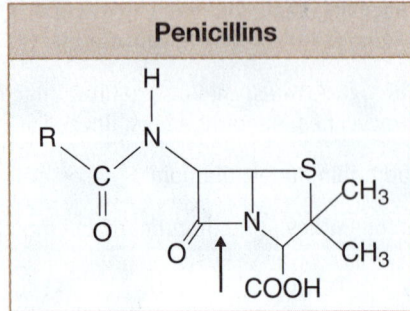	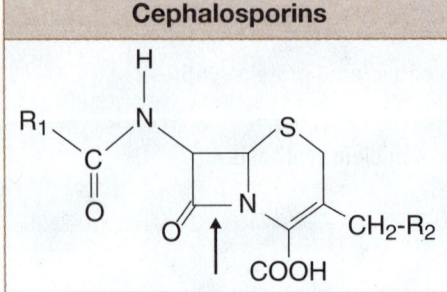

Figure 8-1. Beta-Lactam Antibiotics

Penicillins

- Mechanisms of action:
  - Bacterial cell wall is cross-linked polymer of polysaccharides and pentapeptides
  - Penicillins interact with cytoplasmic membrane-binding proteins (PBPs) to inhibit transpeptidation reactions involved in cross-linking, the final steps in cell-wall synthesis
- Mechanisms of resistance:
  - Penicillinases (beta-lactamases) break lactam ring structure (e.g., staphylococci)
  - Structural change in PBPs (e.g., methicillin-resistant *Staphylococcus aureus* [MRSA], penicillin-resistant pneumococci)
  - Change in porin structure (e.g., *Pseudomonas*)
- Subgroups and antimicrobial activity:
  - Narrow spectrum, beta-lactamase sensitive: penicillin G and penicillin V
    - Spectrum: streptococci, pneumococci, meningococci, *Treponema pallidum*
  - Very narrow spectrum, beta-lactamase resistant: nafcillin, methicillin, oxacillin
    - Spectrum: known or suspected staphylococci (not MRSA)
  - Broad spectrum, aminopenicillins, beta-lactamase sensitive: ampicillin and amoxicillin
    - Spectrum: gram-positive cocci (not staph), *E. coli, H. influenzae, Listeria monocytogenes* (ampicillin), *Borrelia burgdorferi* (amoxicillin), *H. pylori* (amoxicillin)
- Extended spectrum, antipseudomonal, beta-lactamase sensitive: ticarcillin, piperacillin
    - Spectrum: increased activity against gram-negative rods, including *Pseudomonas aeruginosa*
- General considerations:
  - Activity enhanced if used in combination with beta-lactamase inhibitors (clavulanic acid, sulbactam)
  - Synergy with aminoglycosides against pseudomonal and enterococcal species
- Pharmacokinetics:
  - Most are eliminated via active tubular secretion with secretion blocked by probenecid; dose reduction needed only in major renal dysfunction
  - Nafcillin and oxacillin eliminated largely in bile; ampicillin undergoes enterohepatic cycling, but excreted by the kidney
  - Benzathine penicillin G—repository form (half-life of 2 weeks)
- Side effects:
  - Hypersensitivity
- Incidence 5 to 7% with wide range of reactions (types I–IV). Urticarial skin rash common, but severe reactions, including anaphylaxis, are possible.
- Assume complete cross-allergenicity between individual penicillins
  - Other:
- GI distress (NVD), especially ampicillin
- Jarisch-Herxheimer reaction in treatment of syphilis

Cephalosporins

- Mechanisms of action and resistance: identical to penicillins
- Subgroups and antimicrobial activity:
  - First generation: cefazolin, cephalexin
    - Spectrum: gram-positive cocci (not MRSA), *E. coli,Klebsiella pneumoniae,* and some *Proteus* species
    - Common use in surgical prophylaxis
    - Pharmacokinetics: none enter CNS

— Second generation: cefotetan, cefaclor, cefuroxime

  o Spectrum: ↑ gram-negative coverage, including some anaerobes

  o Pharmacokinetics: no drugs enter the CNS, except cefuroxime

— Third generation: ceftriaxone (IM) and cefotaxime (parenteral), cefdinir and cefixime (oral)

  o Spectrum: gram-positive and gram-negative cocci (*Neisseria gonorrhea*), plus many gram-negative rods

  o Pharmacokinetics: most enter CNS; important in empiric management of meningitis and sepsis

— Fourth generation: cefepime (IV)

  o Even wider spectrum

  o Resistant to most beta-lactamases

  o Enters CNS

- Pharmacokinetics:

  o Renal clearance similar to penicillins, with active tubular secretion blocked by probenecid

  o Dose modification in renal dysfunction

  o Ceftriaxone is largely eliminated in the bile

- Side effects:

  o Hypersensitivity:

  Incidence: 2%
  Wide range, but rashes and drug fever most common
  Positive Coombs test, but rarely hemolysis
  Assume complete cross-allergenicity between individual cephalosporins and partial cross-allergenicity with penicillins (about 5%)
  Most authorities recommend avoiding cephalosporins in patients allergic to penicillins (for gram-positive organisms, consider macrolides; for gram-negative rods, consider aztreonam)

Clinical Correlate

Ceftaroline is an unclassified (fifth-generation) cephalosporin that can bind to the most often seen mutation of the PBP in MRSA.

Classic Clues

Organisms *not* covered by cephalosporins are "LAME":

Listeria monocytogenes

Atypicals (e.g., *Chlamydia*, *Mycoplasma*)

MRSA

Enterococci

Imipenem and Meropenem

- Mechanism of action:
  - Same as penicillins and cephalosporins
  - Resistant to beta-lactamases
- Spectrum:
  - Gram-positive cocci, gram-negative rods (e.g., *Enterobacter, Pseudomonas* spp.), and anaerobes
  - Important in-hospital agents for empiric use in severe life-threatening infections
- Side effects:
  - GI distress
  - Drug fever
  - CNS effects, including seizures

Vancomycin

- Mechanism of action:
  - Binding at the D-ala-D-ala muramyl pentapeptide to sterically hinder the transglycosylation reactions (and indirectly preventing transpeptidation) involved in elongation of peptidoglycan chains
  - Does not interfere with PBPs
- Spectrum:
  - MRSA
  - Enterococci
  - *Clostridium difficile* (backup drug)
- Resistance:
  - Vancomycin-resistant staphylococcal (VRSA) and enterococcal (VRE) strains emerging
  - Enterococcal resistance involves change in the muramyl pentapeptide "target," such that the terminal D-ala is replaced by D-lactate
- Pharmacokinetics:
  - Used IV and orally (not absorbed) in colitis
  - Enters most tissues (e.g., bone), but not CNS
  - Eliminated by renal filtration (important to decrease dose in renal dysfunction)
- Side effects:
  - "Red man syndrome" (histamine release)
  - Ototoxicity (usually permanent, additive with other drugs)
  - Nephrotoxicity (mild, but additive with other drugs)

INHIBITORS OF BACTERIAL PROTEIN SYNTHESIS

Table 8-3. Summary of Mechanisms of Protein Synthesis Inhibition

Event	Antibiotic(s) and Binding Site(s)	Mechanism(s)
1. Formation of initiation complex	Aminoglycosides (30S) Linezolid (50S)	Interfere with initiation codon functions—block association of 50S ribosomal subunit with mRNA-30S (static); misreading of code (aminoglycosides only)—incorporation of wrong amino acid (−cidal)
2. Amino-acid incorporation	Tetracyclines (30S) Dalfopristin/ quinupristin (50S)	Block the attachment of aminoacyl tRNA to acceptor site (−static)
3. Formation of peptide bond	Chloramphenicol (50S)	Inhibit the activity of peptidyltransferase (−static)
4. Translocation	Macrolides and clindamycin (50S)	Inhibit translocation of peptidyl-tRNA from acceptor to donor site (−static)

For mechanisms of resistance of antibiotics, see Table 9-2.

Aminoglycosides

- Activity and clinical uses:
  - Bactericidal, accumulated intracellularly in microorganisms via an O_2-dependent uptake → anaerobes are innately resistant
  - Useful spectrum includes gram-negative rods; **gentamicin**, **tobramycin**, and **amikacin** often used in combinations
  - Synergistic actions occur for infections caused by enterococci (with penicillin G or ampicillin) and *P. aeruginosa* (with an extended-spectrum penicillin or third-generation cephalosporin)
  - **Streptomycin** used in tuberculosis; is the DOC for bubonic plague and tularemia
- Pharmacokinetics:
  - Are polar compounds, not absorbed orally or widely distributed into tissues
- Side effects:
  - Nephrotoxicity
  - Ototoxicity
  - Neuromuscular blockade with ↓ release of ACh

Tetracyclines

- Activity and clinical uses:
  - Bacteriostatic drugs, actively taken up by susceptible bacteria
  - "Broad-spectrum" antibiotics, with good activity versus chlamydial and mycoplasmal species, *H. pylori* (GI ulcers), *Rickettsia, Borrelia burgdorferi, Brucella, Vibrio,* and *Treponema* (backup drug), use in periodontal disease treatment
- Specific drugs:
  - Tetracycline: commonly used in periodontal infections, tetracyclines concentrate in sulcular fluid
  - Doxycycline: more activity overall than tetracycline HCl and has particular usefulness in prostatitis because it reaches high levels in prostatic fluid, used for periodontal infections and decrease collagen resorption

- Doxycycline is used (high dose) as an antimicrobial and (low dose) as a collagen destruction preventive
- Minocycline: in saliva and tears at high concentrations and used in the meningococcal carrier state, used for periodontal infections
- Tigecycline: used in complicated skin, soft tissue, and intestinal infections due to resistant gram + (MRSA, VREF), gram –, and anaerobes

- Pharmacokinetics:
  - Kidney for most (↓ dose in renal dysfunction)
  - Liver for doxycycline
  - Chelators: tetracyclines bind divalent cations (Ca^{2+}, Mg^{2+}, Fe^{2+}), which ↓ their absorption

- Side effects:
  - Tooth enamel dysplasia and possible ↓ bone growth in children (avoid); cut-off age for children approximately age 8 (do not prescribe for children 8 and under or pregnant women)
  - Phototoxicity (demeclocycline, doxycycline)
  - GI distress (NVD), superinfections leading to candidiasis or colitis
  - Vestibular dysfunction (minocycline)
  - Have caused liver dysfunction during pregnancy at very high doses (contraindicated)

Clinical Correlate

Don't Use in Pregnancy

Aminoglycosides, fluoroquinolones, sulfonamides, tetracyclines

---

Classic Clues

Phototoxicity

- Tetracyclines
- Sulfonamides
- Quinolones

Chloramphenicol

- Activity and clinical uses:
  - Bacteriostatic with a wide spectrum of activity
  - Currently a backup drug for infections due to *Salmonella typhi*, *B. fragilis*, *Rickettsia*, and possibly in bacterial meningitis
- Pharmacokinetics:
  - Orally effective, with good tissue distribution, including CSF
  - Metabolized by hepatic glucuronidation
  - Inhibition of cytochrome P450
- Side effects:
  - Dose-dependent bone marrow suppression common; aplastic anemia rare (1 in 35,000)
  - "Gray baby" syndrome in neonates (↓ glucuronosyl transferase)

Macrolides

- Drugs: erythromycin, azithromycin, clarithromycin
- Activity and clinical uses:
  - Macrolides are wide-spectrum antibiotics
    - ○ Gram-positive cocci (not MRSA)
    - ○ Atypical organisms (*Chlamydia, Mycoplasma,* and *Ureaplasma* species)
    - ○ *Legionella pneumophila*
    - ○ *Campylobacter jejuni*
    - ○ *Mycobacterium avium-intracellulare (MAC)*
    - ○ *H. pylori*
- Pharmacokinetics:
  - They inhibit cytochrome P450s
- Side effects:
  - Macrolides stimulate motilin receptors and cause gastrointestinal distress (erythromycin, azithromycin > clarithromycin)
  - Macrolides cause reversible deafness at high doses
  - Increased QT interval
- Telithromycin: a ketolide active against macrolide-resistant *S. pneumonia*
- SBE Prophylaxis — both azithromycin and clarithromycin are used as premedication for subacute bacterial endocarditis

Clindamycin

- Not a macrolide, but has the same mechanisms of action and resistance
- Narrow spectrum: gram-positive cocci (including community-acquired MRSA) and anaerobes, including *B. fragilis* (backup drug)
- Concentration in bone has clinical value in osteomyelitis due to gram-positive cocci
- Side effect: pseudomembranous colitis (most likely cause)
- Special effectiveness vs. anaerobes — used in periodontal infections

Linezolid

- Mechanism of action:
  - Inhibits the formation of the initiation complex in bacterial translation systems by preventing formation of the N-formylmethionyl-tRNA-ribosome-mRNA ternary complex
- Spectrum:
  - Treatment of VRSA, VRE, and drug-resistant pneumococci
- Side effects: bone marrow suppression (platelets), MAO-A and B inhibitor

Quinupristin–Dalfopristin

- Mechanism of action:
  - Quinupristin and dalfopristinstreptogramins that act in concert via several mechanisms
  - Binding to sites on 50S ribosomal subunit, they prevent the interaction of amino-acyl-tRNA with acceptor site and stimulate its dissociation from ternary complex

– May also decrease the release of completed polypeptide by blocking its extrusion
- Spectrum:
    – Used parenterally in severe infections caused by vancomycin-resistant staphylococci (VRSA) and entero-cocci (VRE), as well as other drugresistant, gram-positive cocci
- Side effects:
    – Toxic potential remains to be established

INHIBITORS OF NUCLEIC ACID SYNTHESIS

Inhibitors of Folic Acid Synthesis
- Drugs: sulfonamides, trimethoprim, and pyrimethamine

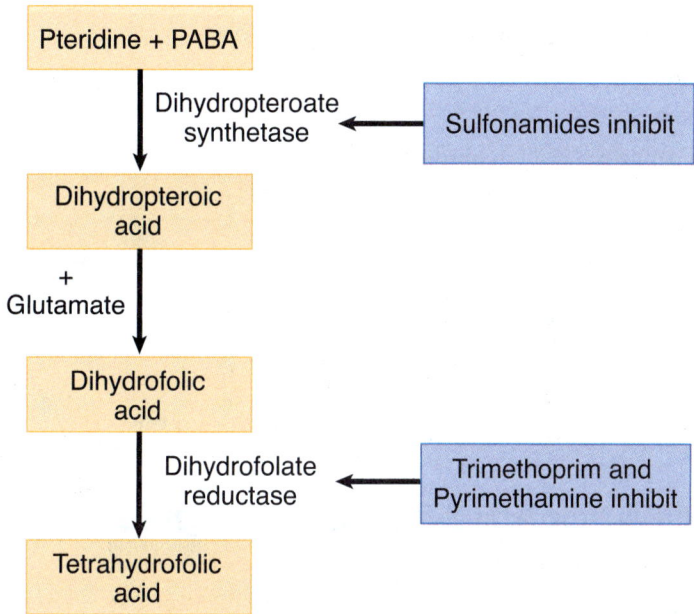

Figure 8-2. Inhibitors of Folic Acid Synthesis

Bridge to Biochemistry

Antimetabolites

Definition: a substance inhibiting cell growth by competing with, or substituting for, a natural substrate in an enzymatic process.

Sulfonamides and trimethoprim are antimetabolites, as are many antiviral agents and drugs used in cancer chemotherapy.

- Activity and clinical uses:
    – Sulfonamides alone are limited in use because of multiple resistance
    – Ag sulfadiazine used in burns

— Combination with dihydrofolate reductase inhibitors:

  ○ ↓ resistance

  ○ Synergy

— Uses of trimethoprim-sulfamethoxazole (cotrimoxazole):

  ○ Bacteria:

  DOC in *Nocardia*

  Listeria (backup)

  Gram-negative infections (*E. coli, Salmonella, Shigella, H. influenzae*)

  Gram-positive infections (*Staph.*, including community-acquired MRSA, *Strep.*)

  ○ Fungus: *Pneumocystis jiroveci* (back-up drugs are pentamidine and atovaquone)

  ○ Protozoa: *Toxoplasma gondii* (sulfadiazine + pyrimethamine)

- Pharmacokinetics:

— Sulfonamides are hepatically acetylated (conjugation)

— Renally excreted metabolites cause crystalluria (older drugs)

— High protein binding

  ○ Drug interaction

  ○ Kernicterus in neonates (avoid in third trimester)

- Side effects:

— Sulfonamides

  ○ Hypersensitivity (rashes, Stevens-Johnson syndrome)

  ○ Hemolysis in G6PD deficiency

  ○ Phototoxicity

— Trimethoprim or pyrimethamine

  ○ Bone marrow suppression (leukopenia)

Direct Inhibitors of Nucleic Acid Synthesis: Quinolones

- Drugs: ciprofloxacin, levofloxacin, and other "–floxacins"
- Mechanisms of action:

— Quinolones are bactericidal and interfere with DNA synthesis

— Inhibit topoisomerase II (DNA gyrase) and topoisomerase IV (responsible for separation of replicated DNA during cell division)

— Resistance is increasing

- Activity and clinical uses:

— Urinary tract infections (UTIs), particularly when resistant to cotrimoxazole

— Sexually transmitted diseases (STDs)/pelvic inflammatory diseases (PIDs): chlamydia, gonorrhea

— Skin, soft tissue, and bone infections by gram-negative organisms

— Diarrhea to *Shigella, Salmonella, E. coli, Campylobacter*

— Drug-resistant pneumococci (levofloxacin)

- Pharmacokinetics:
  - Iron, calcium limit their absorption
  - Eliminated mainly by kidney by filtration and active secretion (inhibited by probenecid)
- Side effects:
  - Tendonitis, tendon rupture
  - Phototoxicity, rashes
  - CNS effects (insomnia, dizziness, headache)
  - Contraindicated in pregnancy and in children (inhibition of chondrogenesis)

Note

The activity of quinolones includes *Bacillus anthracis*. Anthrax can also be treated with penicillins or tetracyclines.

UNCLASSIFIED ANTIBIOTIC: METRONIDAZOLE

- In anaerobes, converted to free radicals by ferredoxin, binds to DNA and other macromolecules, bactericidal
- Antiprotozoal: *Giardia, Trichomonas, Entamoeba*
- Antibacterial: strong activity against most anaerobic gram-negative *Bacteroides* species *Clostridium* species (DOC in pseudomembranous colitis), *Gardnerella*, and *H. pylori*
- Side effects:
  - Metallic taste
  - Disulfiram-like effect
- Mechanism unknown — note unusual spectrum of eukaryotes (protozoa) and prokaryotes (anaerobic bacteria)

ANTITUBERCULAR DRUGS

- Combination drug therapy is the rule to delay or prevent the emergence of resistance and to provide additive (possibly synergistic) effects against *Mycobacterium tuberculosis*.
- The primary drugs in combination regimens are isoniazid (INH), rifampin, ethambutol, and pyrazinamide. Regimens may include two to four of these drugs, but in the case of highly resistant organisms, other agents may also be required. Backup drugs include aminoglycosides (streptomycin, amikacin, kanamycin), fluoroquinolones, capreomycin (marked hearing loss), and cycloserine (neurotoxic).
- Prophylaxis: usually INH, but rifampin if intolerant. In suspected multidrug resistance, both drugs may be used in combination.
- Mechanisms of action, resistance, and side effects:

Table 8-4. Summary of the Actions, Resistance, and Side Effects of the Antitubercular Drugs

Drug	Mechanisms of Action and Resistance	Side Effects
Isoniazid (INH)	• Inhibits mycolic acid synthesis • Prodrug requiring conversion by catalase • High level resistance—deletions in *katG* gene (encodes catalase needed for INH bioactivation)	• Hepatitis (age-dependent) • Peripheral neuritis (use vitamin B_6) • Sideroblastic anemia (use vitamin B_6) • SLE in slow acetylators (rare)
Rifampin	• Inhibits DNA-dependent RNA polymerase (nucleic acid synthesis inhibitor)	• Hepatitis • Induction of P450 • Red-orange metabolites
Ethambutol	• Inhibits synthesis of arabinogalactan (cell-wall component)	• Dose-dependent retrobulbar neuritis $\rightarrow \downarrow$ visual acuity and red-green discrimination
Pyrazinamide		• Hepatitis • Hyperuricemia
Streptomycin	• Protein synthesis inhibition (*see* Aminoglycosides)	• Deafness • Vestibular dysfunction • Nephrotoxicity

---

Note

Mycobacterium avium-intracellulare (MAC)

- *Prophylaxis:* azithromycin (1 × week) or clarithromycin (daily)
- *Treatment:* clarithromycin + ethambutol ± rifabutin

Learning Objectives

❏ Demonstrate understanding of the use and side effects of polyenes (amphotericin B, nystatin), azoles (keto-conazole, fluconazole, itraconazole, voriconazole), and other antifungals

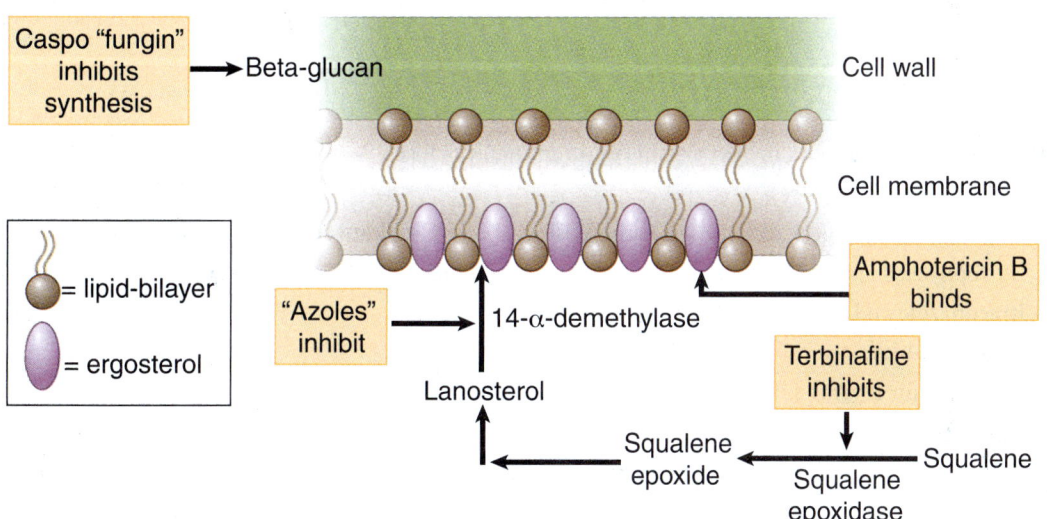

Figure 9-1. Mechanism of Action of Antifungal Drugs

POLYENES (AMPHOTERICIN B [AMP B], NYSTATIN)

- Mechanisms:
  - Amphoteric compounds with both polar and nonpolar structural components—interact with **ergosterol** in fungal membranes to form artificial "pores," which disrupt membrane permeability
  - Resistant fungal strains appear to have low ergosterol content in their cell membranes
- Activity and clinical uses:
  - Amphotericin B has wide fungicidal spectrum; remains the drug of choice (DOC) or co-DOC for severe infections caused by *Cryptococcus* and *Mucor*
  - Amphotericin B—synergistic with flucytosine in cryptococcoses
  - Nystatin (too toxic for systemic use)—used topically for localized infections (e.g., candidiasis)
- Pharmacokinetics:
  - Amphotericin B given by slow IV infusion—poor penetration into the CNS (intrathecal possible)
  - Slow clearance (half-life >2 weeks) via both metabolism and renal elimination

- Side effects:
  - Infusion-related
    - Fever, chills, muscle rigor, hypotension (histamine release) occur during IV infusion (a test dose is advisable)
  - Dose-dependent
    - Nephrotoxicity includes ↓ GFR, tubular acidosis, ↓ K^+ and Mg^{2+}, and anemia through ↓ erythropoietin

AZOLES (KETOCONAZOLE, FLUCONAZOLE, ITRACONAZOLE, VORICONAZOLE)

- Mechanism:
  - "Azoles" are fungicidal and interfere with the synthesis of ergosterol by inhibiting 14-a-demethylase, a fungal P450 enzyme, which converts lanosterol to ergosterol
  - Resistance occurs via decreased intracellular accumulation of azoles
- Activity and clinical uses:
  - Ketoconazole
    - Co-DOC for *Paracoccidioides* and backup for *Blastomyces* and *Histoplasma*
    - Oral use in mucocutaneous candidiasis or dermatophytoses
  - Fluconazole
    - DOC for esophageal and invasive candidiasis and coccidioidomycoses
    - Prophylaxis and suppression in cryptococcal meningitis
  - Itraconazole and Voriconazole
    - DOC in blastomycoses, sporotrichoses, aspergillosis
    - Backup for several other mycoses and candidiasis
  - Clotrimazole and miconazole
    - Used topically for candidal and dermatophytic infections, clotrimazole (Mycelex) "troche" is dissolved in mouth for topical contact with Candida
- Pharmacokinetics:
  - Effective orally
  - Absorption of ketoconazole ↓ by antacids
  - Absorption of itraconazole ↑ by food
  - Only fluconazole penetrates into the CSF and can be used in meningeal infection. Fluconazole is eliminated in the urine, largely in unchanged form.
  - Ketoconazole and itraconazole are metabolized by liver enzymes.
  - Inhibition of hepatic P450s
- Side effects:
  - ↓ synthesis of steroids, including cortisol and testosterone →↓ libido, gynecomastia, menstrual irregularities
  - ↑ liver function tests and rare hepatotoxicity

OTHER ANTIFUNGALS

- Flucytosine
  - Use in combination with amphotericin B in severe candidal and cryptococcal infections—enters CSF
  - Toxic to bone marrow
- Griseofulvin
  - Active only against dermatophytes (orally, not topically) by depositing in newly formed keratin and disrupting microtubule structure
  - Note unusual mechanism of microtubule inhibition
  - Side effects:
    - Disulfiram-like reaction
- Terbinafine
  - Active only against dermatophytes by inhibiting squalene epoxidase $\rightarrow\downarrow$ ergosterol
- Echinocandins (caspofungin and other "fungins")
  - Inhibit the synthesis of beta-1,2 glucan, a critical component of fungal cell walls
  - Back-up drugs given IV for disseminated and mucocutaneous *Candida* infections or invasive aspergillosis

Learning Objectives

❏ Answer questions about anti-herpetics and other antiviral agents

❏ Describe the appropriate treatment of HIV

❏ Solve problems concerning fusion inhibitors

Many antiviral drugs are antimetabolites that resemble the structure of naturally occurring purine and pyrimidine bases or their nucleoside forms. Antimetabolites are usually prodrugs requiring metabolic activation by host-cell or viral enzymes—commonly, such bioactivation involves phosphorylation reactions catalyzed by kinases.

Table 10-1. Mechanism of Action of Antiviral Drugs

Mechanism of Action	Major Drugs
Block viral penetration/uncoating	Amantadine, enfuvirtide, maraviroc
Inhibit viral DNA polymerases	Acyclovir, foscarnet, ganciclovir
Inhibit viral RNA polymerases	Foscarnet, ribavirin
Inhibit viral reverse transcriptase	Zidovudine, didanosine, zalcitabine, lamivudine, stavudine, nevirapine, efavirenz
Inhibit viral aspartate protease	Indinavir, ritonavir, saquinavir, nelfinavir
Inhibit viral neuraminidase	Zanamivir, oseltamivir

ANTIHERPETICS

Acyclovir

- Mechanisms of action:
  - Acyclovir-triphosphate is both a substrate for and inhibitor of viral DNA polymerase
  - When incorporated into the DNA molecule, acts as a chain terminator because it lacks the equivalent of a ribosyl 3′ hydroxyl group
- Activity and clinical uses:
  - Activity includes herpes simplex virus (HSV) and varicella-zoster virus (VZV)
  - There are topical, oral, and IV forms; has a short half-life
  - Reduces viral shedding in genital herpes; ↓ acute neuritis in shingles but has no effect on postherpetic neuralgia
  - Reduces symptoms if used early in chickenpox; prophylactic in immunocompromised patients

- Side effects:
  - Crystalluria and neurotoxicity
  - Is *not* hematotoxic
- Newer drugs—famciclovir and valacyclovir are approved for HSV infection and are similar to acyclovir in mechanism.

Ganciclovir

- Mechanisms of action:
  - Similar to that of acyclovir
  - Triphosphate form inhibits viral DNA polymerase and causes chain termination
- Activity and clinical uses:
  - HSV, VZV, and CMV
  - Mostly used in prophylaxis and treatment of CMV infections, including retinitis, in AIDS and transplant patients—relapses and retinal detachment occur
- Side effects:
  - Dose-limiting hematotoxicity, mucositis, fever, rash, and crystalluria

Foscarnet

- Mechanisms and clinical uses:
  - Not an antimetabolite, but still inhibits viral DNA and RNA polymerases
  - Uses identical to ganciclovir
- Side effects:
  - Dose-limiting nephrotoxicity

TREATMENT OF HIV

Reverse Transcriptase Inhibitors (RTIs)

- The original inhibitors of reverse transcriptases of HIV are nucleoside antimetabolites (e.g., zidovudine, the prototype) that are converted to active forms via phosphorylation reactions.
- **Nucleoside reverse transcriptase inhibitors (NRTIs):**
  - Are components of most combination drug regimens used in HIV infection
  - Are used together with a protease inhibitor (PI)
  - Highly active antiretroviral therapy (HAART) has often resulted in ↓ viral RNA, reversal of the decline in CD4 cells, and ↓ opportunistic infections
- **Nonnucleoside reverse transcriptase inhibitors (NNRTIs):**
  - RTIs that do not require metabolic activation: nevirapine, efavirenz
  - Are not myelosuppressant
  - Inhibit reverse transcriptase at a site different from the one NRTIs bind to
  - Additive or synergistic if used in combination with NRTIs and/or PIs

Zidovudine (Azidothymidine, ZDV, AZT)

- Mechanisms of action:
  - Phosphorylated nonspecifically to a triphosphate that can inhibit reverse transcriptase (RT) by competing with natural nucleotides and can also be incorporated into viral DNA to cause chain termination.
  - Resistance occurs by mutations (multiple) in the gene that codes for RT.
  - Originally used to prevent transfer of HIV from mother to newborn.
  - Used in most combination therapy after needlestick accidents (post-exposure prophylaxis).

Other NRTIs

- Mechanism of action identical to that of zidovudine
- Each requires metabolic activation to nucleotide forms that inhibit reverse transcriptase
- Resistance mechanisms are similar
- Not complete cross-resistance between NRTIs
- Drugs differ in their toxicity profiles and are less bone-marrow suppressing than AZT
- Examples: DDI, 3TC, FTC

Protease inhibitors (PI)

- Mechanisms of action:
  - Aspartate protease (*pol* gene encoded) is a viral enzyme that cleaves precursor polypeptides in HIV buds to form the proteins of the mature virus core.
  - The enzyme contains a dipeptide structure not seen in mammalian proteins. PIs bind to this dipeptide, inhibiting the enzyme.
- Clinical uses:
  - Ritonavir is the most commonly used protease inhibitor. Adverse effects of this group are discussed.
- Side effects:
  - Indinavir
    - Crystalluria (maintain hydration)
  - Ritonavir
    - Major drug interactions
  - General: syndrome of disordered lipid and CHO metabolism with central adiposity and insulin resistance

Clinical Correlate

HIV Prophylaxis

Usually a combination of NRTIs and PIs.
Exact combination changes over time.

Integrase Inhibitors

- Mechanism of action: prevents integration of viral genome in host cell DNA
  - Raltegravir

FUSION INHIBITORS

- Enfuvirtide and maraviroc block the entry of HIV into cells.

OTHER ANTIVIRALS

Amantadine, Rimantadine

Amantadine and rimantadine are no longer recommended as prophylaxis or treatment of influenza A viruses.

Zanamivir and Oseltamivir

- Mechanisms of action:
  - Inhibit neuraminidases of influenza A and B
  - Decreases the likelihood that the virus will penetrate uninfected cells
- Clinical uses: prophylaxis mainly, but may ↓ duration of flu symptoms by 2–3 days

Ribavirin

- Mechanisms:
  - Monophosphorylated form inhibits IMP dehydrogenase
  - Triphosphate inhibits viral RNA polymerase and end-capping of viral RNA
- Clinical uses:
  - Adjunct to alpha-interferons in hepatitis C
  - Management of respiratory syncytial virus
  - Lassa fever
  - Hantavirus
- Side effects:
  - Hematotoxic
  - Upper airway irritation
  - Teratogenic

Hepatitis C Treatment

- Sofosbuvir: nucleotide analog that inhibits RNA polymerase; combined with ribavirin or INT-α
- Simeprevir: hepatitis C protease inhibitor; combined with ribavirin or INT-α
- Note major increase in treatment effectiveness with these drugs as compared to interferon treatment

Antiprotozoal Agents

Learning Objectives

❏ Demonstrate understanding of drugs for malaria and helminthic infections

OVERVIEW

Table 11-1. Major Protozoal Infections and the Drugs of Choice

Infection	Drug of Choice	Comments
Amebiasis	Metronidazole	Diloxanide for noninvasive intestinal amebiasis
Giardiasis	Metronidazole	"Backpacker's diarrhea" from contaminated water or food
Trichomoniasis	Metronidazole	Treat both partners
Toxoplasmosis	Pyrimethamine + sulfadiazine	—
Leishmaniasis	Stibogluconate	—
Trypanosomiasis	Nifurtimox (Chagas disease) Arsenicals (African)	—

ANTIMALARIAL DRUGS

- Clinical uses:
  - Chloroquine-sensitive regions
    - Prophylaxis: chloroquine +/− primaquine
    - Backup drugs: hydroxychloroquine, primaquine, pyrimethamine-sulfadoxine
  - Chloroquine-resistant regions
    - Prophylaxis: mefloquine; backup drugs: doxycycline, atovaquone-proguanil
    - Treatment: quinine +/− either doxycycline or clindamycin or pyrimethamine
- Side effects:
  - Hemolytic anemia in G6PD deficiency (primaquine, quinine)
  - Cinchonism (quinine)

DRUGS FOR HELMINTHIC INFECTIONS

- Most intestinal nematodes (worms)
  - Albendazole
  - Pyrantel pamoate
- Most cestodes (tapeworms) and trematodes (flukes)
  - Praziquantel

Immunology

The Immune System

1

Learning Objectives

❏ Define and describe the components of the immune system

❏ Discriminate between innate and adaptive immunity

THE IMMUNE SYSTEM

The immune system is designed to recognize and respond to non-self antigen in a coordinated manner. Additionally, cells that are diseased, damaged, distressed or dying are recognized and eliminated by the immune system.

The immune system is divided into two complementary arms: the **innate** and the **adaptive** immune systems.

Innate Immunity

Innate immunity provides the body's first line of defense against infectious agents. It involves several defensive barriers:

- Anatomic and physical (skin, mucous membranes and normal flora)
- Physiologic (temperature, pH, anti-microbials and cytokines)
- Complement
- Cellular: phagocytes and granulocytes
- Inflammation

Innate immune defenses have the following characteristics in common:

- Are **present intrinsically** with or without previous stimulation
- Have **limited specificity** for shared microbe and cellular structures (pathogen-associated molecular patterns [PAMPs] and damage-associated molecular patterns [DAMPs])
- Have **limited diversity** as reflected by a limited number of pattern recognition receptors
- Are not enhanced in activity upon subsequent exposure—**no memory**

Adaptive Immunity

The components of the adaptive immune response are B and T lymphocytes and their effector cells.

Adaptive immune defenses have the following characteristics in common:

- Each B and T lymphocyte is **specific** for a particular antigen
- As a population, lymphocytes have extensive diversity
- Are enhanced with each repeat exposure—**immunologic memory**
- Are capable of **distinguishing self** from **non-self**
- Are **self-limiting**

The features of adaptive immunity are designed to give the individual the best possible defense against disease.

- **Specificity** is required, along with **immunologic memory,** to protect against persistent or recurrent challenge.
- **Diversity** is required to protect against the maximum number of potential pathogens.
- **Specialization** of effector function is necessary so that the most effective defense can be mounted against diverse challenges.
- The ability to **distinguish between self** (host cells) **and non-self** (pathogens) is vital in inhibiting an autoimmune response.
- **Self-limitation** allows the system to return to a basal resting state after a challenge to conserve energy and resources and to avoid uncontrolled cell proliferation resulting in leukemia or lymphoma.

Table 1-1. Innate versus Adaptive Immunity

Characteristics	Innate	Adaptive
Specificity	For pathogen-associated molecular patterns (PAMPs)	For specific antigens of microbial and nonmicrobial agents
Diversity	Limited	High
Memory	No	Yes
Self-reactivity	No	No
Components		
Anatomic and physiologic barriers	Skin, mucosa, normal flora, temperature, pH, antimicrobials, and cytokines	Lymph nodes, spleen, mucosal-associated lymphoid tissues
Blood proteins	Complement	Antibodies
Cells	Phagocytes, granulocytes and natural killer (NK) cells	B lymphocytes and T lymphocytes

Function

The innate and adaptive arms of the immune response work in collaboration to stop an infection. Once a pathogen has broken through the anatomic and physiologic barriers, the innate immune response is immediately activated, oftentimes it is able to contain and eliminate the infection.

When the innate immune response is unable to control the replication of a pathogen, the adaptive immune response is engaged and activated by the innate immune response in an antigen-specific manner. Typically, it takes 1-2 weeks after the primary infection for the adaptive immune response to begin clearance of the infection through the action of effector cells and antibodies.

Once an infection has been cleared, both the innate and adaptive immune responses cease. Antibodies and residual effector cells continue to provide protective immunity, while memory cells provide long-term immunologic protection from subsequent infection.

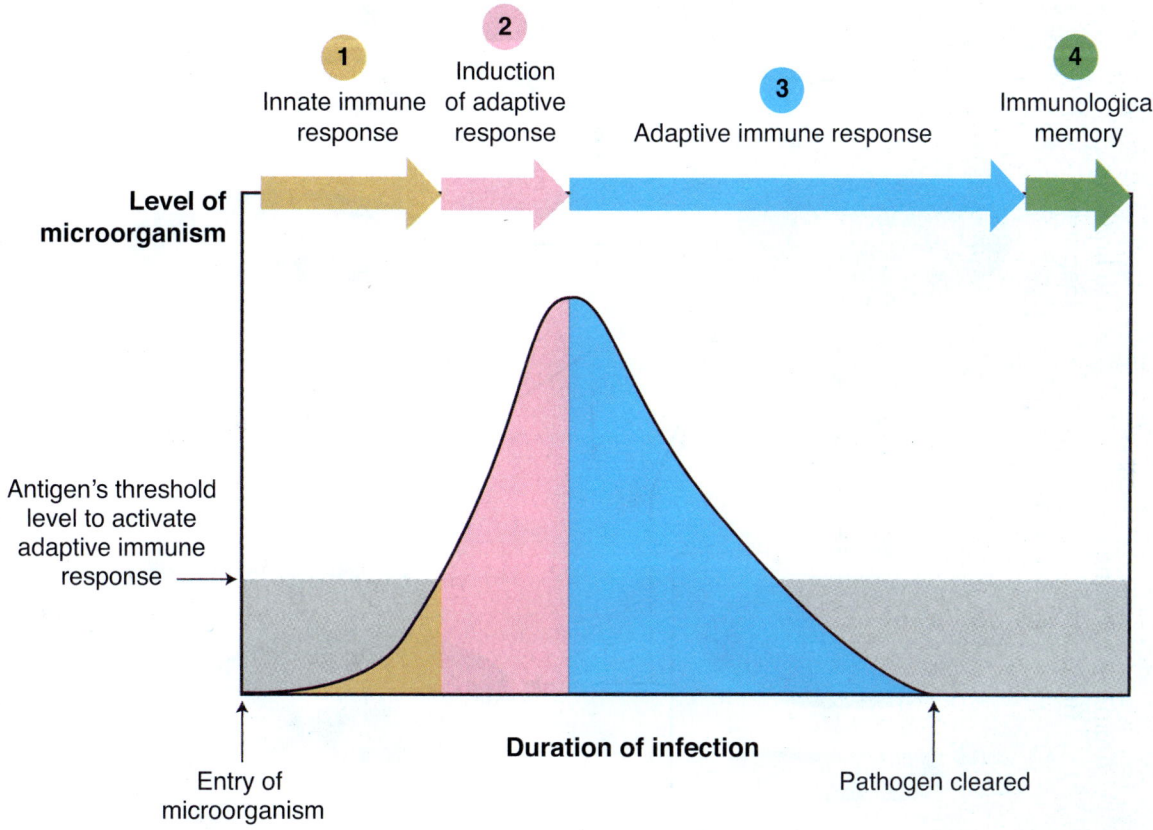

Figure 1-1. Timeline of the Immune Response to an Acute Infection

The innate and adaptive immune responses do not act independently of one another; rather, they work by a positive feedback mechanism.

- Phagocytic cells recognize pathogens by binding PAMPs through various pattern-recognition receptors leading to phagocytosis.
- Phagocytic cells process and present antigen to facilitate stimulation of specific T lymphocytes with subsequent release of cytokines that trigger initiation of specific immune responses.
- T lymphocytes produce cytokines that enhance microbicidal activities of phagocytes.
- Cytokines released by phagocytes and T lymphocytes will drive differentiation of B lymphocytes into plasma cells and isotype switching.
- Antibodies will aid in the destruction of pathogen through opsonization, complement activation and antibody-dependent cellular cytotoxicity.

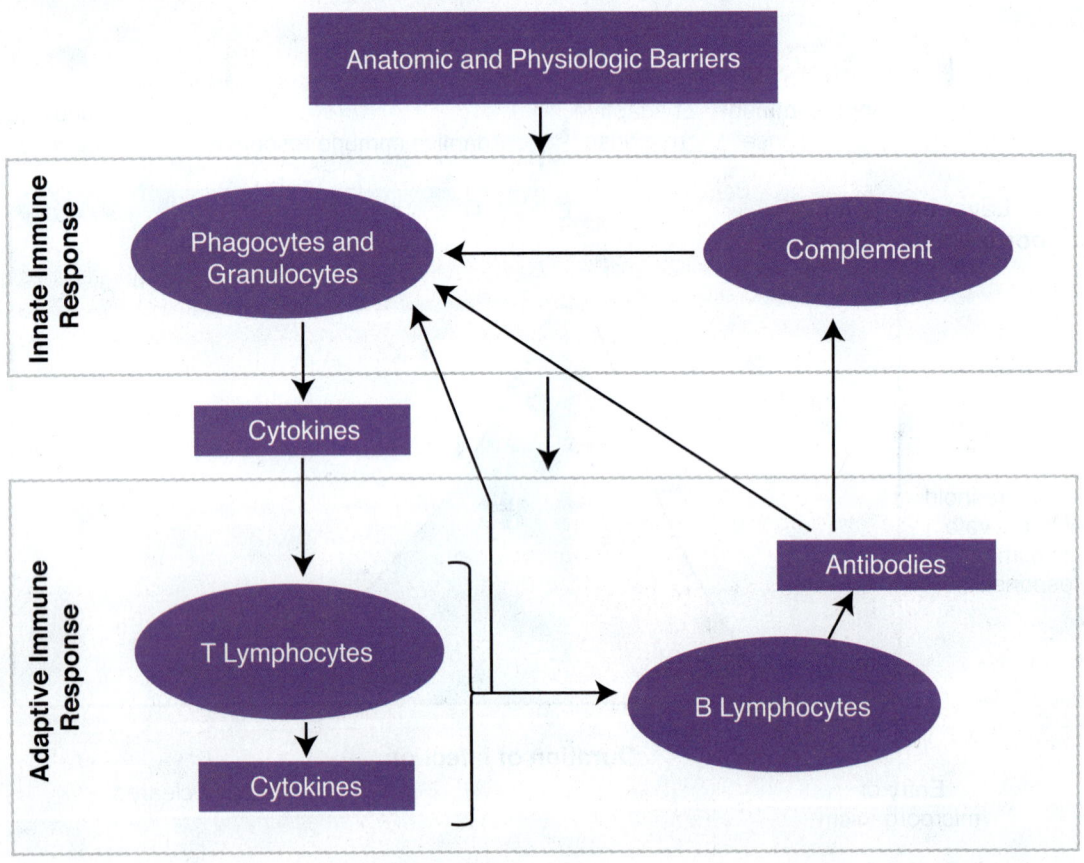

Figure 1-2. Interaction between Innate and Adaptive Immune Responses

Ontogeny of the Immune Cells 2

Learning Objectives

❏ Explain information related to origin and function of cells of the immune system

❏ Explain information related to antigen recognition molecules of lymphocytes

❏ Answer questions about the generation of receptor diversity

ORIGIN

Hematopoiesis involves the production, development, differentiation, and maturation of the blood cells (erythrocytes, megakaryocytes and leukocytes) from **multipotent stem cells**. The site of hematopoiesis changes during development.

During embryogenesis and early fetal development, the yolk sac is the site of hematopoiesis. Once organogenesis begins, hematopoiesis shifts to the liver and spleen, and finally, to the bone marrow where it will remain throughout adulthood.

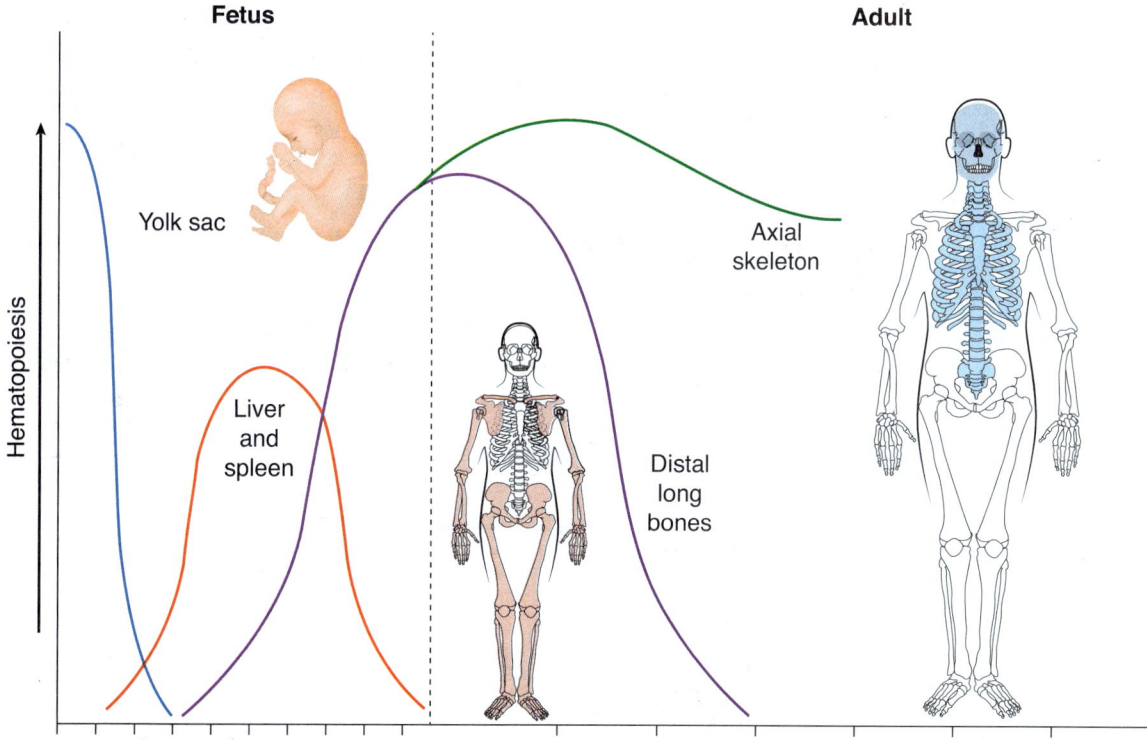

Figure 2-1. Sites of Hematopoiesis during Development

These **multipotent stem cells** found in the bone marrow have the ability to undergo asymmetric division. One of the two daughter cells will serve to renew the population of stem cells (**self-renewal**), while the other can give rise to either a common lymphoid progenitor cell or a common myeloid progenitor cell (**potency**). The multipotent stem cells will differentiate into the various lymphoid and myeloid cells in response to various cytokines and growth factors.

- The **common lymphoid progenitor** cell gives rise to B lymphocytes, T lymphocytes and natural killer (NK) cells.
- The **common myeloid progenitor cell** gives rise to erythrocytes, megakaryocytes/thrombocytes, mast cells, eosinophils, basophils, neutrophils, monocytes/macrophages and dendritic cells.

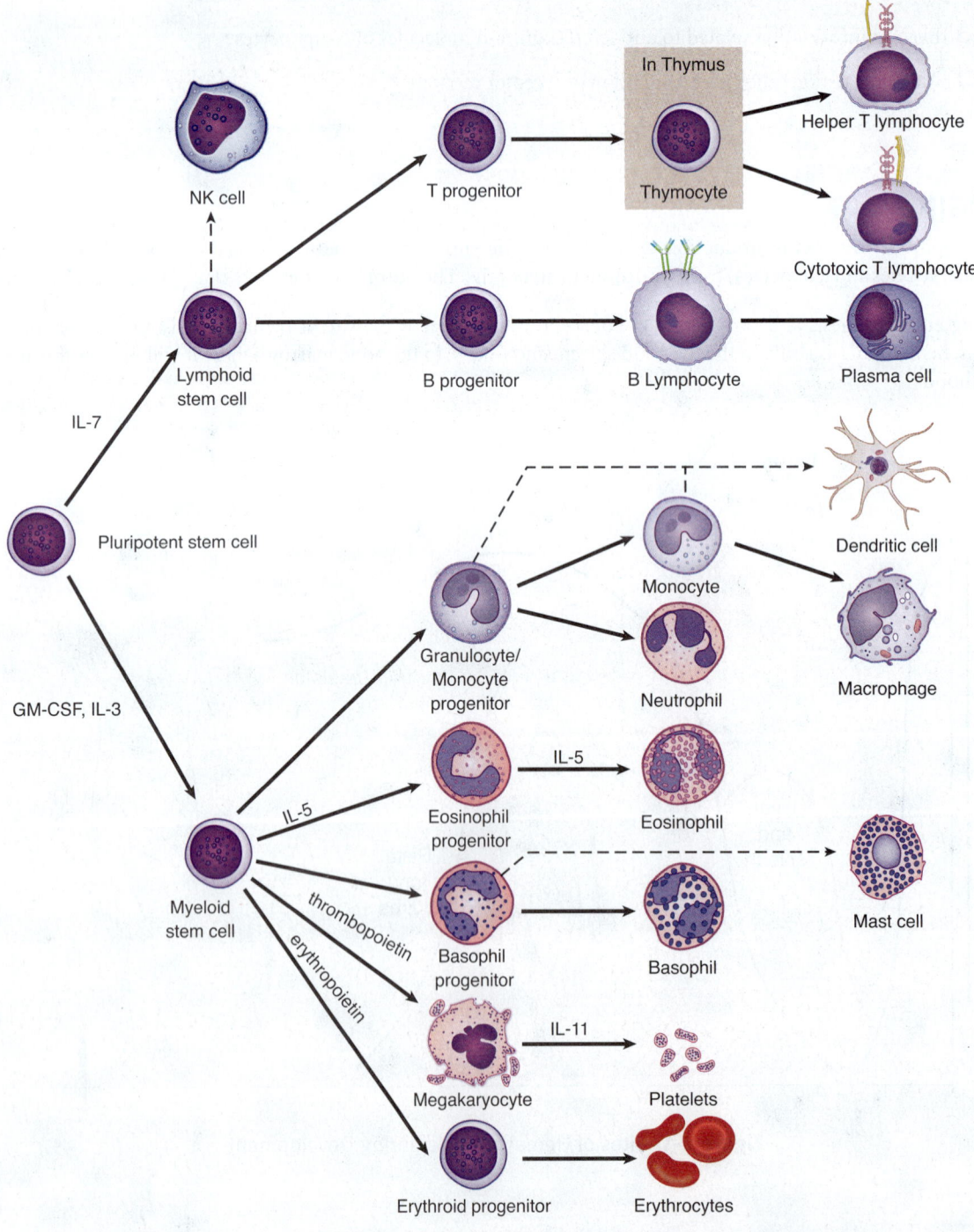

Figure 2-2. Ontogeny of Immune Cells

FUNCTION

The white blood cells of both the myeloid and lymphoid stem cells have specialized functions in the body once their differentiation in the bone marrow is complete. Cells of the myeloid lineage, except erythrocytes and megakaryocytes, perform non-specific, stereotypic responses and are members of the innate branch of the immune response. B lymphocytes and T lymphocytes of the lymphoid lineage perform focused, antigen-specific roles in immunity. Natural killer cells are also from the lymphoid lineage but participate in innate immunity.

Although B lymphocytes and T lymphocytes in the bloodstream are almost morphologically indistinguishable at the light microscopic level, they represent two interdependent cell lineages.

- **B lymphocytes** remain within the **bone marrow** to complete their development.
- **T lymphocytes** leave the bone marrow and undergo development within the **thymus.**

Both B and T lymphocytes have surface membrane receptors designed to bind to specific antigens; the generation of these receptors will be discussed in chapter 4.

- The **natural killer (NK) cell** (the third type of lymphocyte) is a large granular lymphocyte that recognizes tumor and virally infected cells through non-specific binding.

Table 2-1. White Blood Cells

Myeloid Cell	Tissue Location	Physical Description	Function
Neutrophil or polymorpho- nuclear (PMN) cell	Most abundant circulating blood cell	Granulocyte with a segmented, lobular nuclei (3–5 lobes) and small pink cytoplasmic granules	Phagocytic activity aimed at killing extracellular pathogens

Lymphoid Cell	Tissue Location	Physical Description	Function

Lymphocyte	Bloodstream, secondary lymphoid tissues	Large, dark-staining nucleus with a thin rim of cytoplasm
		
		Surface markers:
		
		B lymphocytes
		
		  — CD19, 20, 21
		
		T lymphocytes
		
		  — CD3
		
		Helper T cells
		
		  — CD4
		
		CTLs
		
		  — CD8
			No function until activated in the secondary lymphoid tissues

(Continue)

Lymphoid Cell	Tissue Location	Physical Description	Function
Plasma cell	Bloodstream, secondary lymphoid tissue and bone marrow	Small eccentric nucleus, intensely staining Golgi apparatus	Terminally differentiated B lymphocyte that secretes antibodies
Natural killer cell	Bloodstream	Lymphocyte with large cytoplasmic granules Surface markers: CD16, 56	Kills virally infected cells and tumor cells

Myeloid Cell	Tissue Location	Physical Description	Function
Monocyte	Circulating blood cell	Agranulocyte with a bean or kidney-shaped nucleus	Precursor of tissue macrophage
Macrophage	Resident in all tissues	Agranulocyte with a ruffled cytoplasmic membrane and cytoplasmic vacuoles and vesicles	• Phagocyte • Professional antigen presenting cell • T-cell activator
Dendritic cell	Resident in epithelial and lymphoid tissue	Agranulocyte with thin, stellate cytoplasmic projections	• Phagocyte • Professional antigen presenting cell • T-cell activator
Eosinophil	Circulating blood cell recruited into loose connective tissue of the respiratory and GI tracts	Granulocyte with bilobed nucleus and large pink cytoplasmic granules	• Elimination of large extracellular parasites • Type I hypersensitivity

(*Continue*)

Myeloid Cell	Tissue Location	Physical Description	Function
Mast cell	Reside in most tissues adjacent to blood vessels	Granulocyte with small nucleus and large blue cytoplasmic granule	• Elimination of large extracellular parasites • Type I hypersensitivity
Basophil	Low frequency circulating blood cell	Granulocyte with bilobed nucleus and large blue cytoplasmic granules	• Elimination of large extracellular parasites • Type I hypersensitivity

Laboratory evaluation of patients commonly involves assessment of white blood cell morphology and relative counts by examination of a blood sample. Changes in the morphology and proportions of white blood cells indicate the presence of some pathologic state. A standard white blood cell differential includes neutrophils, band cells (immature neutrophils), lymphocytes (B lymphocytes, T lymphocytes, and NK cells), monocytes, eosinophils and basophils.

Table 2-2. Leukocytes Evaluated in a WBC Differential

Cell Type	Adult Reference Range (%)
Neutrophils (PMNs)	50–70
Band cells (immature neutrophils)	0–5
Lymphocytes	20–40
Monocytes	5–10
Eosinophils	0–5
Basophils	<1

Lymphocyte Development and Selection

3

Learning Objectives

❑ Answer questions about selection of T and B lymphocytes

❑ Solve problems concerning innate immunity and components/barriers

ANTIGEN RECOGNITION MOLECULES OF LYMPHOCYTES

Each cell of the lymphoid lineage is clinically identified by the characteristic surface molecules that it possesses.

- The mature, naïve **B lymphocyte**, in its mature ready-to-respond form, expresses two isotypes of antibody or immunoglobulin called IgM and IgD within its surface membrane.
- The mature, naive **T cell** expresses a single genetically related molecule, called the **T-cell receptor** (**TCR**), on its surface.

Both of these types of antigen receptors are encoded within the immunoglobulin superfamily of genes and are expressed in literally millions of variations in different lymphocytes as a result of complex and random rearrangements of the cells' DNA.

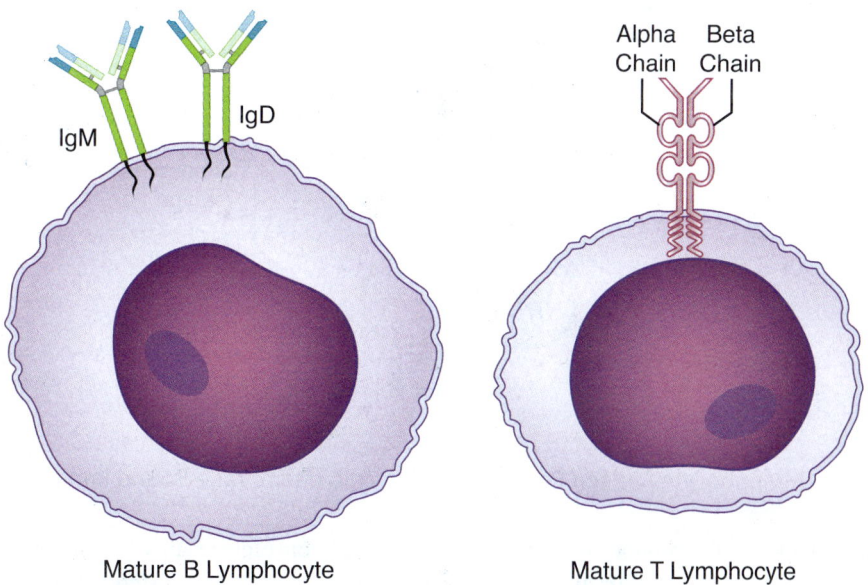

Mature B Lymphocyte   Mature T Lymphocyte

Figure 3-1. Antigen Receptors of Mature Lymphocytes

The antigen receptor of the B lymphocyte, or **membrane-bound immunoglobulin**, is a 4-chain glycoprotein molecule that serves as the basic monomeric unit for each of the distinct antibody molecules destined to circulate freely in the serum. This monomer has 2 identical halves, each composed of a **heavy chain** and a **light chain**. A cytoplasmic tail on the carboxy-terminus of each heavy chain extends through the plasma membrane and anchors the molecule to the cell surface. The two halves are held together by disulfide bonds into a shape resembling a "Y." Some flexibility of movement is permitted between the halves by disulfide bonds forming a **hinge region**.

On the N-terminal end of the molecule where the heavy and light chains lie side by side, an antigen binding site is formed whose 3-dimensional shape will accommodate the noncovalent binding of one, or a very small number, of related antigens. The unique structure of the antigen binding site is called the **idiotype** of the molecule. Although two classes (**isotypes**) of membrane immunoglobulin (IgM and IgD) are coexpressed on the surface of a mature, naïve B lymphocyte, only one idiotype or **antigenic specificity** is expressed per cell (although in multiple copies). Each individual is capable of producing hundreds of millions of unique idiotypes.

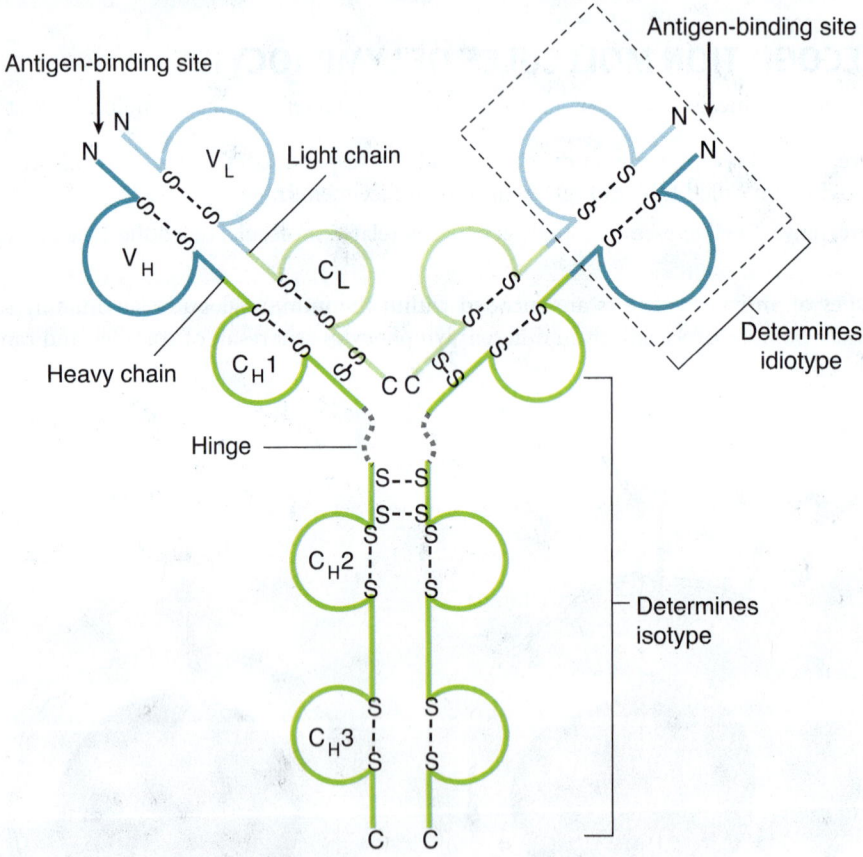

Figure 3-2. B-Lymphocyte Antigen Recognition Molecule (Membrane-Bound Immunoglobulin)

The antigen receptor of the T lymphocyte is composed of two glycoprotein chains, a beta and alpha chain that are similar in length. On the carboxy-terminus of the chains, a cytoplasmic tail extends through the membrane for anchorage. On the N-terminal end of the molecule, an antigen-binding site is formed between the two chains, whose three-dimensional shape will accommodate the binding of a small antigenic **peptide complexed to an MHC molecule** presented on the surface of an antigen-presenting cell. This groove forms the idiotype of the TCR. There is no hinge region present in this molecule, and thus its conformation is quite rigid.

The membrane receptors of B lymphocytes are designed to bind **unprocessed antigens** of almost any chemical composition, i.e., polysaccharides, proteins, lipids, whereas the TCR is designed to bind only **peptides complexed to MHC**. Also, although the B-cell receptor is ultimately modified to be secreted **antibody**, the TCR is never released from its membrane-bound location.

In association with these unique antigen-recognition molecules on the surface of B and T cells, accessory molecules are intimately associated with the receptors that function in signal transduction. Thus, when a lymphocyte binds to an antigen complementary to its idiotype, a cascade of messages transferred through its **signal transduction complex** will culminate in intracytoplasmic phosphorylation events leading to activation of the cell.

- In the B cell, this signal transduction complex is composed of two invariant chains, Ig-alpha and Ig-beta, and a B-cell co-receptor consisting of CD19, CD21 and CD81.

- The B-cell co-receptor is implicated in the attachment of several infectious agents. CD21 is the receptor for EBV and CD81 is the receptor for hepatitis C and *Plasmodium vivax*.

- In the T cell, the signal transduction complex is a multichain structure called CD3.

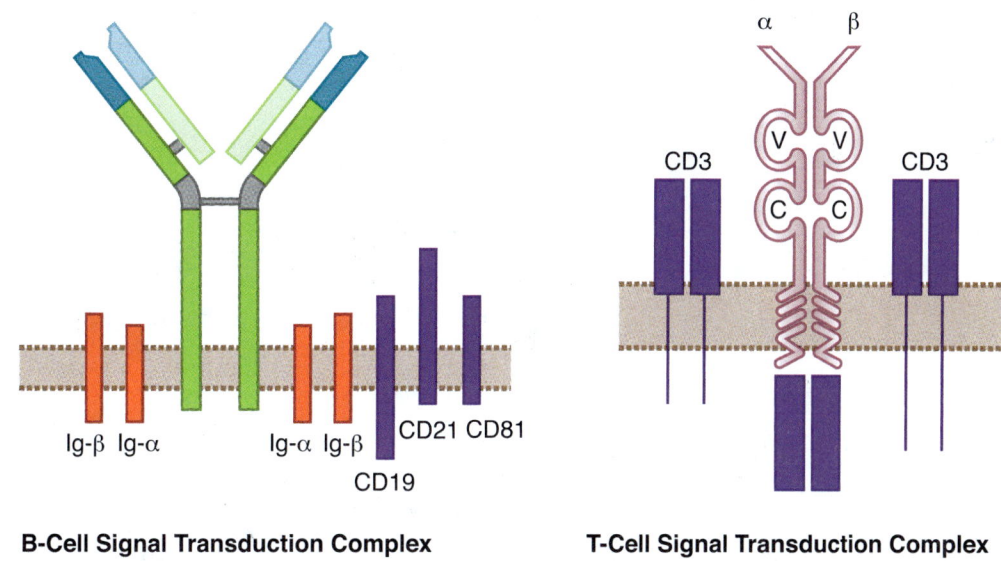

B-Cell Signal Transduction Complex **T-Cell Signal Transduction Complex**

Figure 3-3. Lymphocyte Signal Transduction

Table 3-1. B- versus T-Lymphocyte Antigen Receptors

Property	B-Cell Antigen Receptor	T-Cell Antigen Receptor
Molecules/Lymphocyte	100,000	100,000
Idiotypes/Lymphocyte	1	1
Isotypes/Lymphocyte	2 (IgM and IgD)	1 (α/β)
Is secretion possible?	Yes	No
Number of combining sites/ molecule	2	1
Mobility	Flexible (hinge region)	Rigid
Signal-transduction molecules	Ig-α, Ig-β, CD19, CD21	CD3

THE GENERATION OF RECEPTOR DIVERSITY

Because the body requires the ability to respond specifically to millions of potentially harmful agents it may encounter in a lifetime, a mechanism must exist to generate as many idiotypes of antigen receptors as necessary to meet this challenge. If each of these idiotypes were encoded separately in the germline DNA of lymphoid cells, it would require more DNA than is present in the entire cell. The generation of this necessary diversity is accomplished by a complex and unique set of rearrangements of DNA segments that takes place during the maturation of lymphoid cells.

It has been discovered that individuals inherit a large number of different segments of DNA which may be recombined and alternatively spliced to create unique amino acid sequences in the N-terminal ends (**variable domains**) of the chains that compose their antigen recognition sites. For example, to produce the **heavy chain variable domains** of their antigen receptor, B-lymphocyte progenitors select randomly and in the absence of stimulating antigen to recombine 3 gene segments designated variable (V), diversity (D), and joining (J) out of hundreds of germline-encoded possibilities to produce unique sequences of amino acids in the variable domains (VDJ recombination).

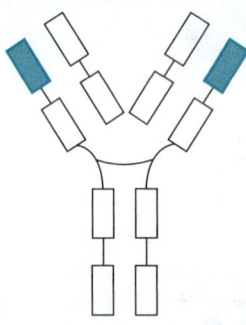

Note

VDJ rearrangements in DNA produce the diversity of heavy chain variable domains.

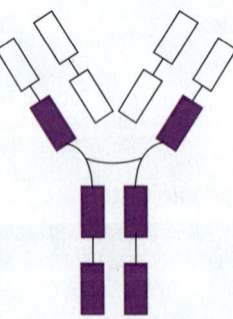

Note

mRNA molecules are created which join this variable domain sequence to μ or δ constant domains.

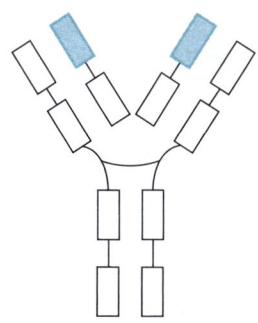

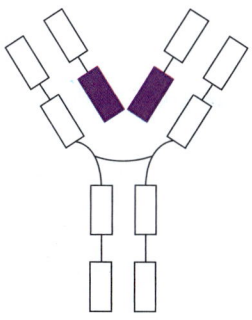

Next, the B-lymphocyte progenitor performs random rearrangements of two types of gene segments (V and J) to encode the **variable domain amino acids of the light chain.** An analogous random selection is made during the formation of the alpha-chain of the TCR. The enzymes responsible for these gene rearrangements are encoded by the genes *RAG1* and *RAG2*. The *RAG1* and *RAG2* gene products are two proteins found within the recombinase, a protein complex that includes a repair mechanism as well as DNA-modifying enzymes.

While heavy chain gene segments are undergoing recombination, the enzyme **terminal deoxyribonucleotidyl transferase** (Tdt) randomly inserts bases (without a template on the complementary strand) at the junctions of V, D, and J segments (**N-nucleotide addition**). The random addition of the nucleotide generates junctional diversity.

Bridge to Pathology

Tdt is used as a marker for early stage T- and B-cell development in acute lymphoblastic leukemia.

When the light chains are rearranged later, Tdt is not active, though it is active during the rearrangement of all gene segments in the formation of the TCR. This generates even more diversity than the random combination of V, D, and J segments alone.

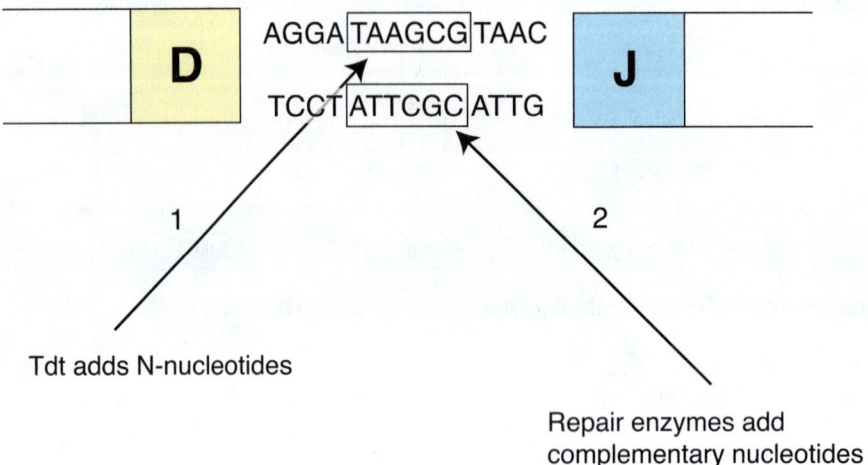

Figure 3-4. Function of Tdt

Needless to say, many of these gene segment rearrangements result in the production of truncated or nonfunctional proteins. When this occurs, the cell has a second chance to produce a functional strand by rearranging the gene segments of the homologous chromosome. If it fails to make a functional protein from rearrangement of segments on either chromosome, the cell is induced to undergo **apoptosis** or programmed cell death.

In this way, the cell has two chances to produce a functional heavy (or β) chain. A similar process occurs with the light (or α) chain. Once a functional product has been achieved by one of these rearrangements, the cell shuts off the rearrangement and expression of the other allele on the homologous chromosome—a process known as **allelic exclusion**. This process ensures that B and T lymphocytes synthesize only **one specific antigen-receptor per cell**.

Because any heavy (or β) chain can associate with any randomly generated light (or α) chain, one can multiply the number of different possible heavy chains by the number of different possible light chains to yield the total number of possible idiotypes that can be formed. This generates yet another level of diversity.

Table 3-2. Mechanisms for Generating Receptor Diversity

Mechanism	Cell in Which It Is Expressed
Existence in genome of multiple V, D, J segments	B and T cells
VDJ recombination	B and T cells
N-nucleotide addition	B cells (only heavy chain) T cells (all chains)
Combinatorial association of heavy and light chains	B and T cells
Somatic hypermutation	B cells only, after antigen stimulation (see chapter 7)

Downstream on the germline DNA from the rearranged segments, are encoded the amino acid sequences of all the constant domains of the chain. These domains tend to be similar within the classes or isotypes of immunoglobulin or TCR chains and are thus called **constant domains**.

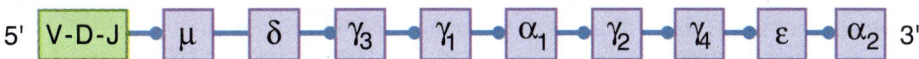

5' | V-D-J | — | μ | — | δ | — | γ_3 | — | γ_1 | — | α_1 | — | γ_2 | — | γ_4 | — | ε | — | α_2 | 3'

Figure 3-5. Immunoglobulin Heavy Chain DNA

The first set of constant domains for the heavy chain of immunoglobulin that is transcribed is that of IgM and next, IgD. These two sets of domains are alternatively spliced to the variable domain product at the RNA level. There are only two isotypes of light chain constant domains, named κ and λ, and one will be combined with the product of light chain variable domain rearrangement to produce the other half of the final molecule. Thus, the B lymphocyte produces IgM and IgD molecules with identical idiotypes and inserts these into the membrane for antigen recognition.

SELECTION OF T AND B LYMPHOCYTES

As lymphoid progenitors develop in the bone marrow, they make random rearrangements of their germline DNA to produce the unique idiotypes of antigen-recognition molecules that they will use throughout their lives. The bone marrow, therefore, is considered a **primary lymphoid organ** in humans because it supports and encourages these early developmental changes. B lymphocytes complete their entire formative period in the bone marrow and can be identified in their progress by the immunoglobulin chains they produce.

B Lymphocyte Development

In essence, the rearrangement of the gene segments and the subsequent production of immunoglobulin chains drive B-cell development.

Because these gene segment rearrangements occur randomly and in the absence of stimulation with foreign antigen, it stands to reason that many of the idiotypes of receptors produced could have a binding attraction or **affinity** for normal body constituents. These cells, if allowed to develop further, could develop into self-reactive lymphocytes that could cause harm to the host. Therefore, one of the key roles of the bone marrow stroma and interdigitating cells is to remove such potentially harmful products. Cells whose idiotype has too great an affinity for normal cellular molecules are either deleted in the bone marrow (**clonal deletion**) or inactivated in the periphery (**clonal anergy**). Anergic B cells express high levels of IgD on their surface rendering them inactive. The elimination of self-reactive cells in the bone marrow is intended to minimize the number of self-reactive B-lymphocytes released to the periphery, only those cells that are **selectively unresponsive** (**tolerant**) to self-antigens are allowed to leave the bone marrow.

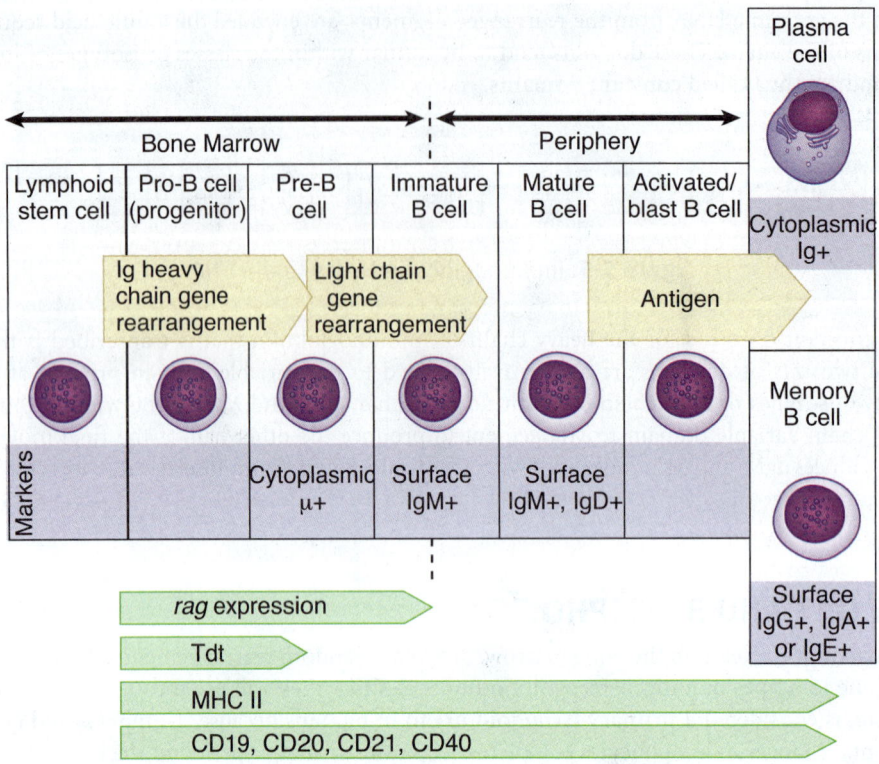

Figure 3-6. B-Cell Differentiation

T Lymphocyte Development

Immature lymphocytes destined to the T-cell lineage leave the bone marrow and proceed to the **thymus**, the second **primary lymphoid organ** dedicated to the maturation of T cells. These pre-thymic cells are referred to as **double negative** T lymphocytes since they do not express CD4 or CD8 on their surface. The thymus is a bilobed structure located above the heart; it consists of an outer **cortex** packed with immature T cells and an inner **medulla** into which cells pass as they mature. Both the cortex and medulla are laced with a network of epithelial cells, dendritic cells, and macrophages, which interact physically with the developing thymocytes.

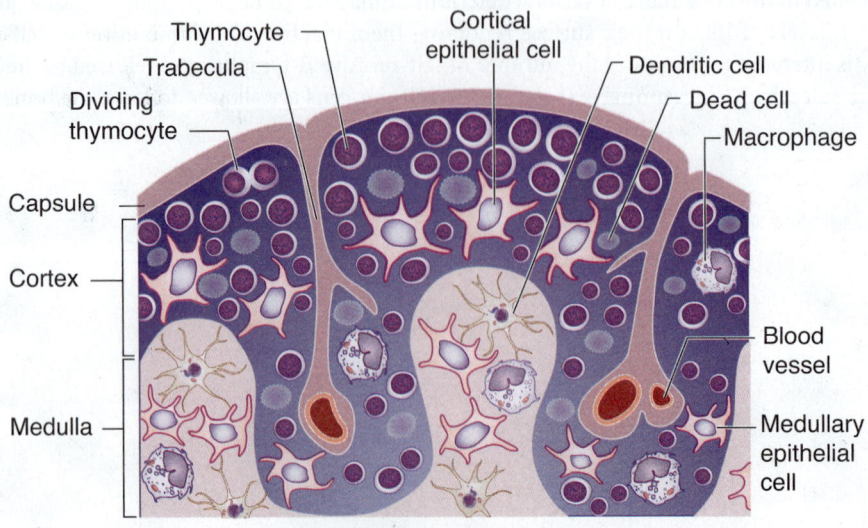

Figure 3-7. Structure of the Thymus

Within the cortex, the thymocytes will begin to rearrange the beta and alpha chains of the T-cell receptor (TCR) while coexpressing the CD3 complex as well as the CD4 and CD8 co-receptors; these thymocytes are collectively referred to as being **double positive**. As the developing thymocytes begin to express their TCRs, they are subjected to a rigorous two-step selection process. Because the TCR is designed to bind antigenic peptides presented on the surface of **antigen-presenting cells** (APCs) in the body, a selection process is necessary to remove those cells that would bind to normal self-antigens and cause **autoimmunity,** as well as those that have no attraction whatsoever for the surfaces of APCs. This is accomplished by exposure of developing thymocytes to high levels of a unique group of membrane-bound molecules known as **major histocompatibility complex** (MHC) antigens.

The MHC is a collection of highly polymorphic genes on the short arm of chromosome 6 in the human. There are two major classes of cell-bound MHC gene products: I and II. Both class I and class II molecules are expressed at high density on the surface of cells of the thymic stroma. MHC gene products are also called human leukocyte antigens (HLA).

- **Class I** MHC gene products: HLA-A, HLA-B, HLA-C
- **Class II** MHC gene products: HLA-DM, HLA-DP, HLA-DQ, HLA-DR

Table 3-3. Class I and II Gene Products

Class I Gene Products			Class II Gene Products			
HLA-A	HLA-B	HLA-C	HLA-DM*	HLA-DP	HLA-DQ	HLA-DR

*HLA-DM is not a cell surface molecule but functions as a molecular chaperone to promote proper peptide loading.

Class I molecules are expressed on all nucleated cells in the body, as well as platelets. They are expressed in **codominant** fashion, meaning that each cell expresses 2 A, 2 B, and 2 C products (one from each parent).

- The molecules (A, B, and C) consist of an a heavy chain with three extracellular domains and an intracyto-plasmic carboxy-terminus.
- A second light chain, β_2-microglobulin, is not encoded within the MHC and functions in peptide-loading and transport of the class I antigen to the cell surface.
- A groove between the first two extracellular domains of the α chain is designed to accommodate small peptides to be presented to the TCR.

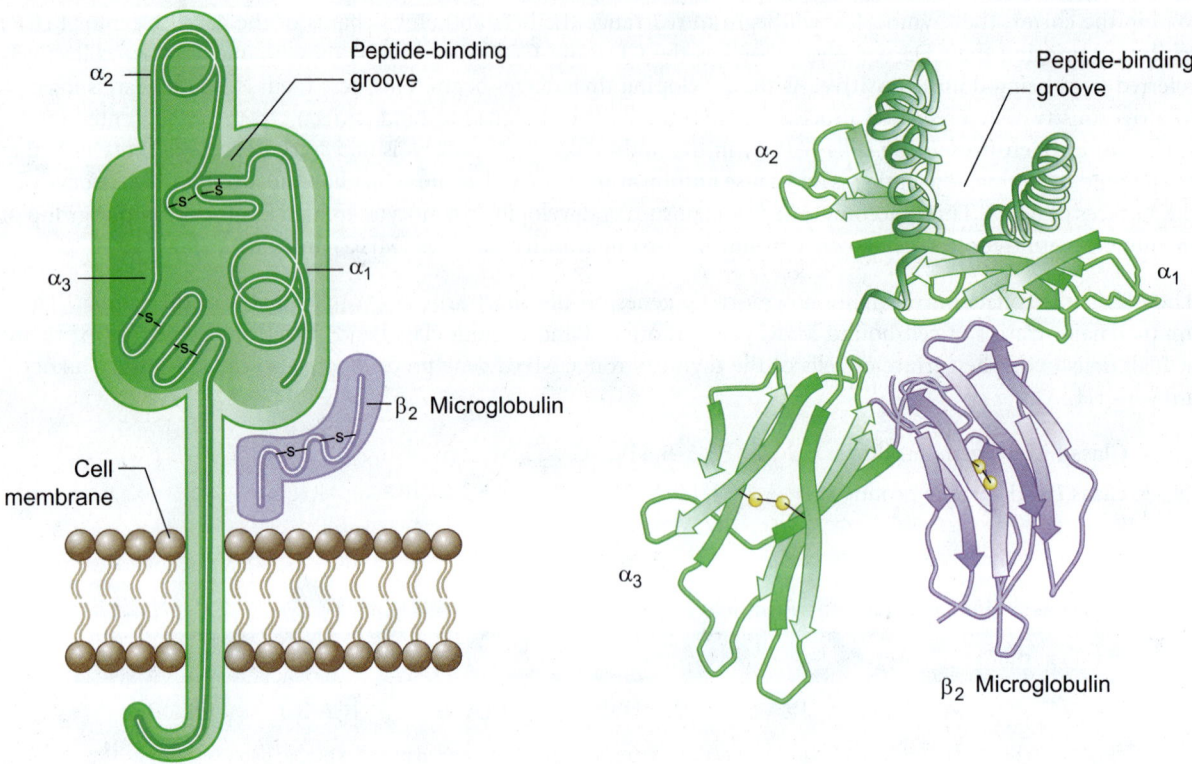

Figure 3-8. Class I MHC Molecule (left) and X-Ray Crystallographic Image (right) of Class I MHC Peptide-Binding Groove

Class II MHC molecules are expressed (also **codominantly**) on the professional antigen-presenting cells of the body (primarily the macrophages, B lymphocytes, and dendritic cells).

- The molecules are two chain structures of similar length, called α and β, each possessing two extracellular domains and one intracytoplasmic domain.
- A groove that will accommodate peptides to be presented to the TCR is formed at the N-terminal end of both chains.

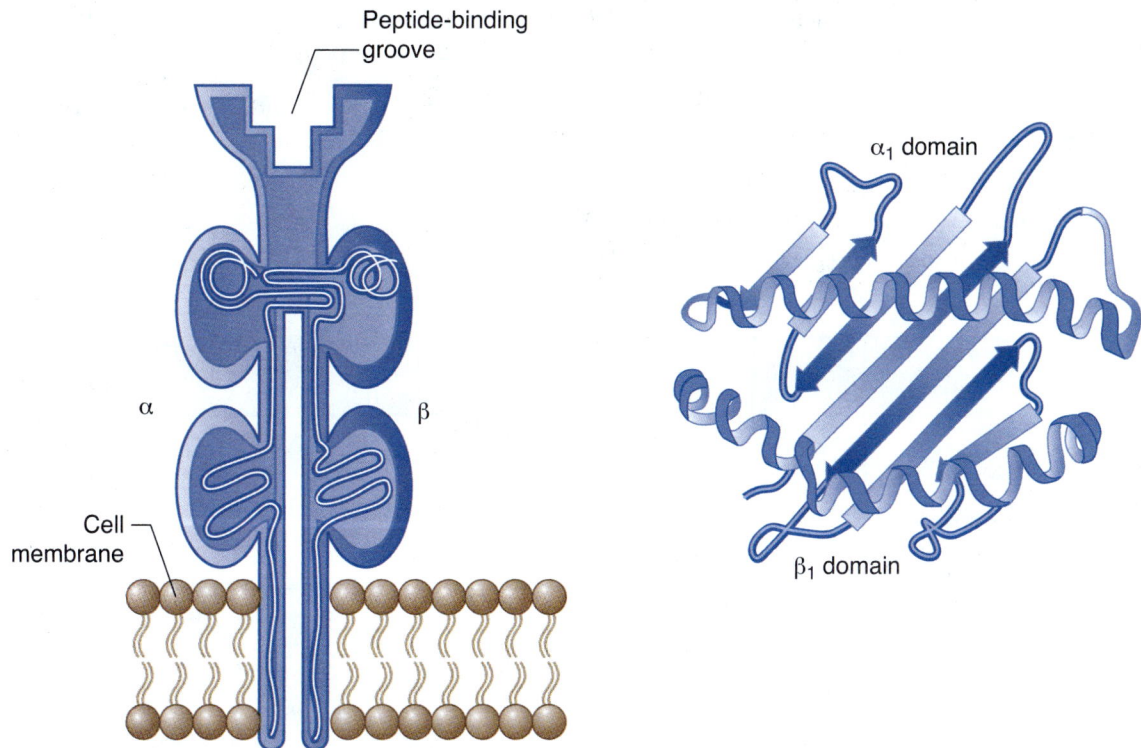

Figure 3-9. Class II MHC Molecule (left), and X-ray Crystallographic Image (right) of Class II MHC Peptide-Binding Groove

Within the thymus, each of these MHC products, loaded with normal self-peptides, is presented to the developing double positive thymocytes.

- Those that have TCRs capable of binding with low affinity will receive a **positive selection** signal to divide and establish clones that will eventually mature in the medulla.
- Those that fail to recognize self-MHC at all will not be encouraged to mature (**failure of positive selection**).
- Those that bind too strongly to self MHC molecules and self-peptide will be induced to undergo apoptosis (**negative selection**) because these cells would have the potential to cause autoimmune disease.

Although double positive thymocytes co-express **CD4** and **CD8**, the cells are directed to express only CD8 if their TCR binds class I molecules, and only CD4 if their TCR binds class II molecules. At this point in T-cell development, the thymocytes are referred to as being **single positive**.

This selection process is an extraordinarily rigorous one. A total of 95–99% of all T-cell precursors entering the thymus are destined to die there. Only those with TCRs appropriate to protect the host from foreign invaders will be permitted to exit to the periphery: CD4+ cells that recognize class II MHC are destined to become **"helper" T cells** (Th), and CD8+ cells that recognize class I MHC are destined to become **cytotoxic T lymphocytes** (CTLs).

While most self-reactive T cells will be deleted in the thymus, a small population of these T cells will instead differentiate into regulatory T cells (Tregs). Tregs inhibit self-reactive Th1 cells in the periphery.

- Identified by their constitutive expression of CD25 on the surface and by the expression of the transcription factor FoxP3
- Secrete IL-10 and TGF-β which inhibit inflammation
- Shown to be critical in the prevention of autoimmunity

Tregs will leave the thymus and serve in a peripheral tolerance.

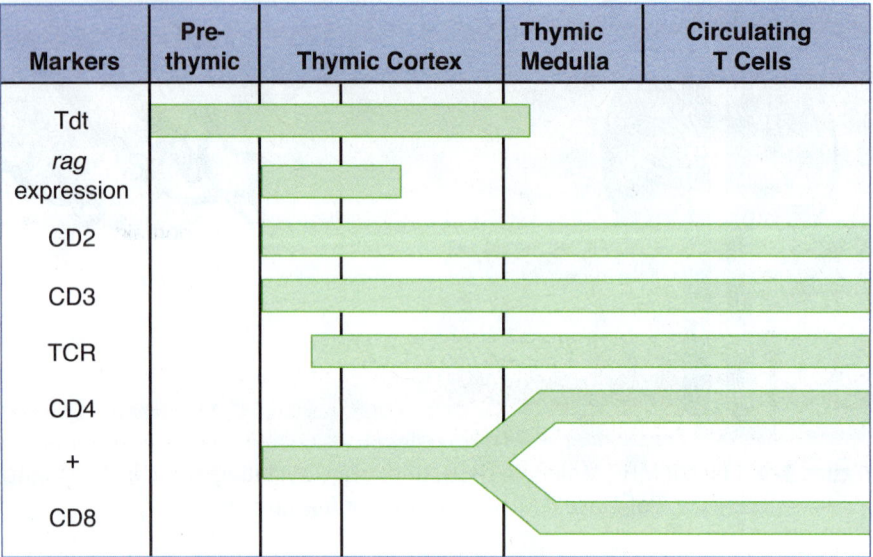

Figure 3-10. Human T-Cell Differentiation

Learning Objectives

- ❏ Describe the basic concepts of innate immunity
- ❏ Understand the role of physical and physiological barriers in the function of the innate immune response
- ❏ Decsribe the cells involved in innate immunity
- ❏ Answer questions about inflammatory response

INNATE IMMUNITY

The innate immune system is an important part of any immune response. It is responsible for reacting quickly to invading microbes and for keeping the host alive while the adaptive immune system is developing a very specific response. The innate immune defenses are all present at birth; they have a very limited diversity for antigen, and they attack the microbes with the same basic vigor no matter how many times they have seen the same pathogen.

The innate immune system handles pathogens in two general ways:

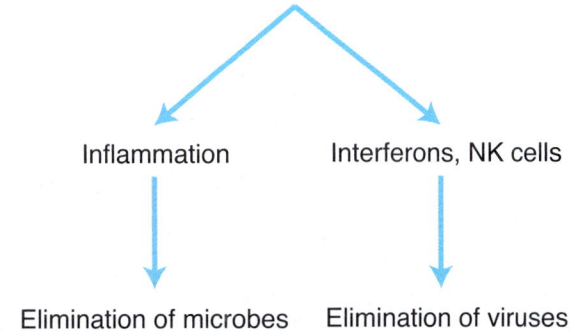

Figure 4-1. Pathogen Clearance by the Innate Immune System

Microbes may gain access to the tissues if the physical barriers are breached. In the tissues, they come in contact with phagocytic cells such as neutrophils, macrophages and dendritic cells, which will produce chemical messengers called **cytokines** that can initiate an inflammatory response.

Many times the innate immune components are enough to eliminate the pathogen, but not always. The pathogens may gain access to the blood, in which the alternate pathway for complement activation may provide some additional help. But this is where the adaptive immune system may have to take over to resolve the infection and eliminate the pathogen.

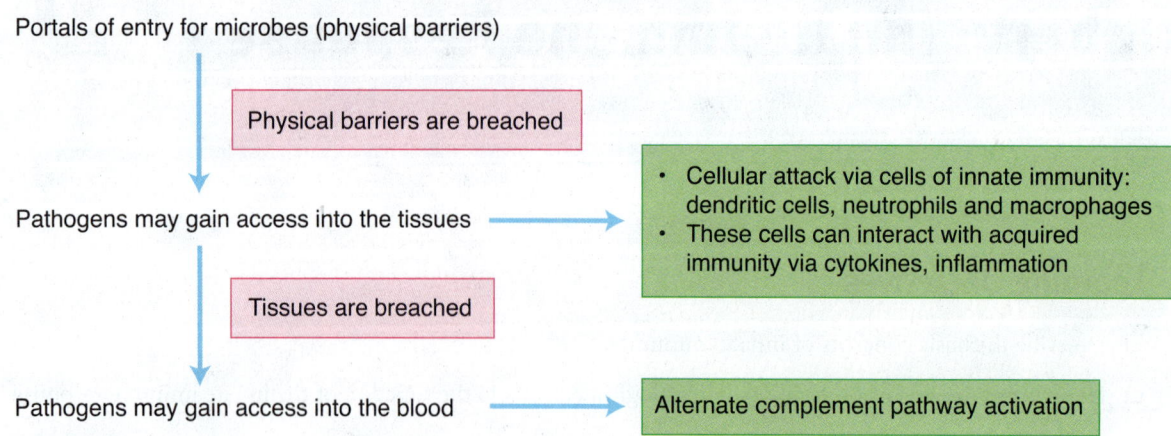

Portals of entry for microbes (physical barriers)

Physical barriers are breached

Pathogens may gain access into the tissues →
- Cellular attack via cells of innate immunity: dendritic cells, neutrophils and macrophages
- These cells can interact with acquired immunity via cytokines, inflammation

Tissues are breached

Pathogens may gain access into the blood → Alternate complement pathway activation

Figure 4-2. Entry Sites for Pathogens

INNATE IMMUNE COMPONENTS/BARRIERS

There are several components to the innate immune response that are essential for this early defense against pathogens. They will be introduced here and discussed in more depth later in this chapter. They include **physical (anatomic) barriers, physiologic barriers, innate cellular response**, and **inflammation**.

Anatomic Barriers

The main portals of entry for most pathogens are the skin, the respiratory tract, and the GI tract. All of these surfaces are lined with epithelial cells that can produce a few antimicrobial products such as defensins and interferons. They may also contain a number of specialized intra-epithelial lymphocytes (IEL) called $\gamma\delta$ T cells. These specialized T cells are considered part of innate immunity as they can only recognize shared microbial structures.

- The skin is a great physical barrier as most pathogens can't invade intact skin. The pH of the skin is also slightly acidic and can retard the growth of pathogenic organisms.
- The respiratory tract is lined with cilia that physically attempt to remove microbes as they enter. Saliva and mucous are also difficult environments for microbes to live in, as there are many antimicrobial enzymes and chemicals within those entities.
- The GI tract is also a mucous membrane with similar properties to the respiratory tract; however, pathogens that enter here must first survive a trip through the stomach with a highly acidic pH that kills many micro-organisms. See also the discussion of IgA later in its role of preventing bacterial attachments.

Physiologic Barriers

Physiologic barriers include the following components:

- **Temperature**
  - Many microbial pathogens can't survive much past human body temperature. When the inflammatory response is initiated in the local tissues, cytokines may act systemically to alter the temperature set point in the hypothalamus resulting in fever.
- **pH**
  - The acidic pH of the stomach impedes the growth and transmission to the gut of many pathogens.
  - The skin is also acidic and retards the growth of many microorganisms.

- **Chemical**
  - Lysozyme present in secretions such as tears, saliva, breast milk and mucous can break down the cell wall peptidoglycan of bacteria.
  - Defensins found within phagocytes can form pores in bacteria and fungi.
- **Interferons**
  - IFN-α and IFN-β are anti-viral interferons. They have a direct anti-viral effect by transiently inhibiting nascent protein synthesis in cells.

Innate Cellular Response

Phagocytic cells (monocytes/macrophages, neutrophils and dendritic cells) are part of the first line of defense against invading pathogens. They recognize pathogens via shared molecules that are not expressed on host cells. They are responsible for controlling the infections and sometimes are even capable of eradicating them.

Receptors of the innate immune system are referred to as **pattern recognition receptors (PRRs)**. PRRs recognize **pathogen-associated molecular patterns (PAMPs)**, molecules that are shared by pathogens of the same type (bacterial LPS, n-formyl peptides etc.) or **damage-associated molecular patterns (DAMPs)** released from dying or damaged cells. These receptors are present intrinsically, encoded in the germline genes, and are not generated through somatic recombination as the lymphocyte receptors are generated.

The innate immune system can recognize <1,000 patterns on various pathogens, compared to the adaptive immune system (B and T cells) which can recognize over 1 billion specific sequences on pathogens.

Inflammasome

The inflammasome is an important part of the innate immune system. It is expressed in myeloid cells as a signalling system for detection of pathogens and stressors. Activation of the inflammasome results in the production of IL-1b and IL-18, which are potent inflammatory cytokines.

Table 4-1. Receptors of the Innate Immune System

Receptor Type	Location in Cell	Receptor Name	Pathogen Target	Downstream Effects
Toll-like receptors (TLR)	Extracellular	TLR-1, 2, 6	Bacterial lipopeptides	Activation of transcription factors (including NF-κB) which results in the transcription of cytokines, adhesion molecules, and enzymes that are antimicrobial
		TLR-2	Bacterial peptidoglycan	
		TLR-4	Lipopolysaccharide (LPS)	
		TLR-5	Flagellin	
	Intracellular (endosomal)	TLR-3	DS RNA	
		TLR-7,8	SS RNA	
		TLR-9	Unmethylated CpG oligonucleotides	

(Continue)

Receptor Type	Location in Cell	Receptor Name	Pathogen Target	Downstream Effects
NOD-like receptors (NLR)	Intracellular (cytosolic)	NOD1, NOD2	Components of bacterial PG	Signals via NF-κB result in macrophage activation
		NLRP-3	Microbial products and molecules from damaged or dying cells (ATP, uric acid crystals, reactive oxygen species)	Inflammasome NLRP-3 (sensor) + adaptor protein links procaspase 1 and activates it to caspase 1; it is the caspase that cleaves the pro-IL-1β to generate IL-1β
RIG-like receptors (RLR)	Cytoplasmic	RIG-1, MDA-5	Viral RNA	Interferon production

Table 4-2. Myeloid Cells

Myeloid Cell	Tissue Location	Identification	Function
Monocyte	Bloodstream, 0–900/µL	Kidney bean-shaped nucleus, CD14 positive	Phagocytic, differentiate into tissue macrophages
Macrophage	Tissues	Ruffled membrane, cytoplasm with vacuoles and vesicles, CD14 positive	Phagocytosis, secretion of cytokines
Neutrophil	Bloodstream, 1,800–7,800/µL	Multilobed nucleus; small light pink to purple granules CD14 positive	Phagocytosis and activation of bactericidal mechanisms

Cells of Innate Immunity

Neutrophils

- Circulating phagocytes
- Short lived
- Rapid response, not prolonged defense

Monocytes/Macrophages

- Monocytes circulate in the blood, become macrophages in the tissues
- Provide a prolonged defense
- Produce cytokines that initiate and regulate inflammation
- Phagocytose pathogens
- Clear dead tissue and initiate tissue repair
- Macophages will develop along one of two different pathways

Table 4-3. Pathways for Macrophage Activation

Classical M1	Alternative M2
Induced by innate immunity (TLRs, IFN-γ)	Induced by IL-4, IL-13
Phagocytosis, initiate inflammatory response	Tissue repair and control of inflammation

Table 4-4. Additional Myeloid Cells

Myeloid Cell	Tissue Location	Identification	Function
Dendritic Cells	Epithelia, tissues	Long cytoplasmic arms CD14 positive	Antigen capture, transport, and presentation, initiate inflammation
Mast Cells	Tissues, mucosa, epithelia	Small nucleus, cytoplasm packed with large blue granules	Release of granules containing histamine, etc., during allergic responses
Natural killer Lymphocyte	Lymph nodes, spleen, mucosal-associated lymphoid tissues, bone marrow	Lymphocytes with large cytoplasmic granules CD16 + CD56 positive	Kill tumor/virus cell targets or antibody-coated target cells, secretion of IFN-γ

Dendritic cells (DCs)

- Found in all tissues
- Antigen processing and presentation
- Two major functions: initiate inflammatory response and stimulate adaptive immune response

Mast cells

- Skin, mucosa
- Two pathways for activation: innate TLRs and antibody-dependent (IgE)

Natural killer cells (NK cells)

- Blood, periphery
- Direct lysis of cells, secretion of IFN-γ

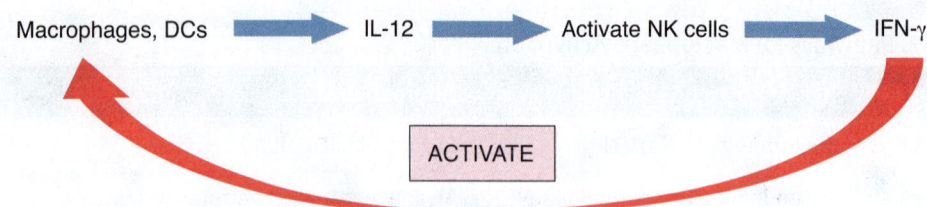

Figure 4-3. Collaboration of Macrophages and NK Cells

INFLAMMATORY RESPONSE

Complement

The complement system is a set of interacting proteins released into the blood after production in the liver. The components act together as zymogens, activating one another in cascade fashion after initiation from a variety of stimuli. Three pathways of activation occur in the body and culminate similarly in the production of important split products that mediate inflammation, enhance phagocytosis by opsonization, and cause lysis of particles by membrane pore formation.

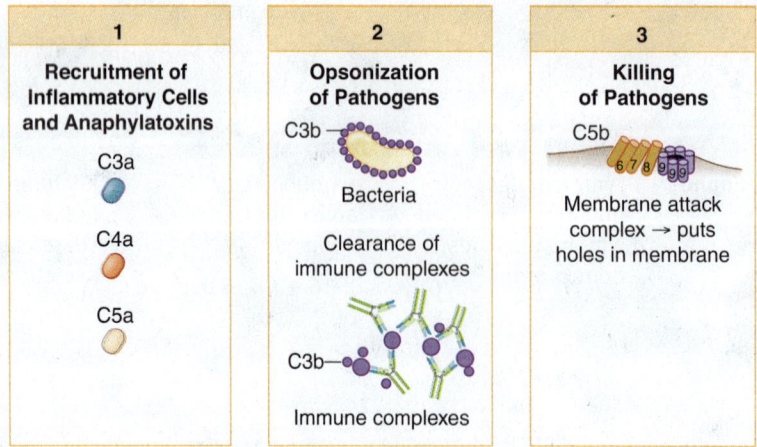

Figure 4-4. Three Functions of the Complement System

Two of the pathways are considered part of the innate immune system: the alternate pathway and the lectin-binding or mannose-binding pathway (MBP). The alternate pathway for complement activation is shown below; the MBP activates the classical complement pathway but without the use of antibody, and is therefore considered part of innate immunity. The MBP is activated when mannose-binding lectin binds to carbohydrates on the pathogen.

The alternative pathway of complement activation is probably the more primitive of the pathways because it is initiated by simple attraction of the early factors to the surfaces of microbes. Bacterial polysaccharides and the lipopolysaccharide of the cell envelope of gram-negative bacteria both serve as potent, initiating stimuli.

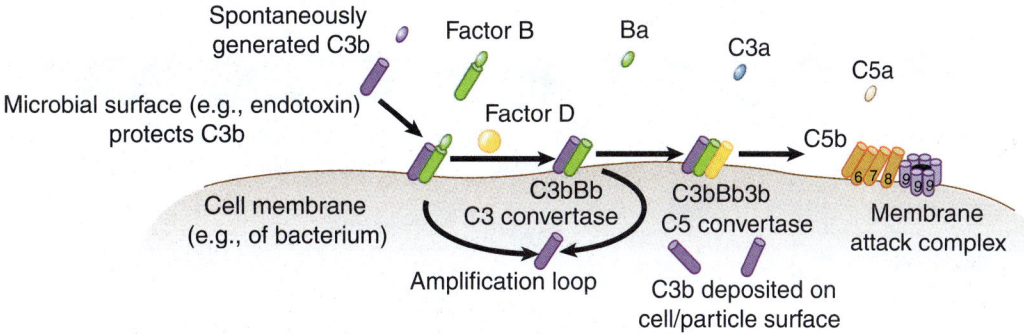

Figure 4-5. The Alternative Complement Pathway

Acute Inflammatory Response

Antigens are normally introduced into the body across the mucosa or the epithelia. The **acute inflammatory response** is often the first response to this invasion and represents a response of the innate immune system to block the challenge.

The first step in the acute inflammatory response is activation of the vascular endothelium in the breached epithelial barrier. Cytokines and other inflammatory mediators released in the area as a result of tissue damage induce expression of selectin-type adhesion molecules on the endothelial cells. Neutrophils are the first cells to bind to the inflamed endothelium and extravasate into the tissues, peaking within 6 hours. Monocytes, macrophages, and even eosinophils may arrive 5-6 hours later in response to neutrophil-released mediators.

The extravasation of phagocytes into the area requires **four sequential, overlapping steps**:

Step 1: Rolling

Phagocytes attach loosely to the endothelium by low-affinity, selectin-carbohydrate interactions. E-selectin molecules on the endothelium bind to mucin-like adhesion molecules on the phagocyte membrane and bind the cell briefly, but the force of blood flow into the area causes the cell to detach and reattach repeatedly, rolling along the endothelial surface until stronger binding forces can be elicited.

Step 2: Activation by chemo-attractants

Chemokines released in the area during inflammation, such as interleukin 8 (IL-8), complement split product C5a, and N-formyl peptides produced by bacteria bind to receptors on the phagocyte surface and trigger a G-protein–mediated activating signal. This signal induces a conformational change in integrin molecules in the phagocyte membrane that increases their affinity for immunoglobulin-superfamily adhesion molecules on the endothelium.

Step 3: Arrest and adhesion

Interaction between integrins and Ig-superfamily cellular adhesion molecules (Ig-CAMs) mediates the tight binding of the phagocyte to the endothelial cell. These integrin-IgCAM interactions also mediate the tight binding of phagocytes and their movement through the extracellular matrix.

Step 4: Transendothelial migration

The phagocyte extends pseudopodia through the vessel wall and extravasates into the tissues.

Once in the tissues, neutrophils express increased levels of receptors for chemoattractants and exhibit chemotaxis migrating up a concentration gradient toward the attractant. Neutrophils release chemoattractive factors that call in other phagocytes.

Table 4-5. Chemoattractive Molecules

Chemoattractive Molecule	Origin
Chemokines (IL-8)	Tissue mast cells, platelets, neutrophils, **monocytes**, **macrophages**, eosinophils, basophils, lymphocytes
Complement split product C5a	Classical or alternative pathways
Leukotriene B$_4$	Membrane phospholipids of macrophages, monocytes, neutrophils, mast cells → arachidonic acid cascade → lipoxygenase pathway
Formyl methionyl peptides	Released from microorganisms

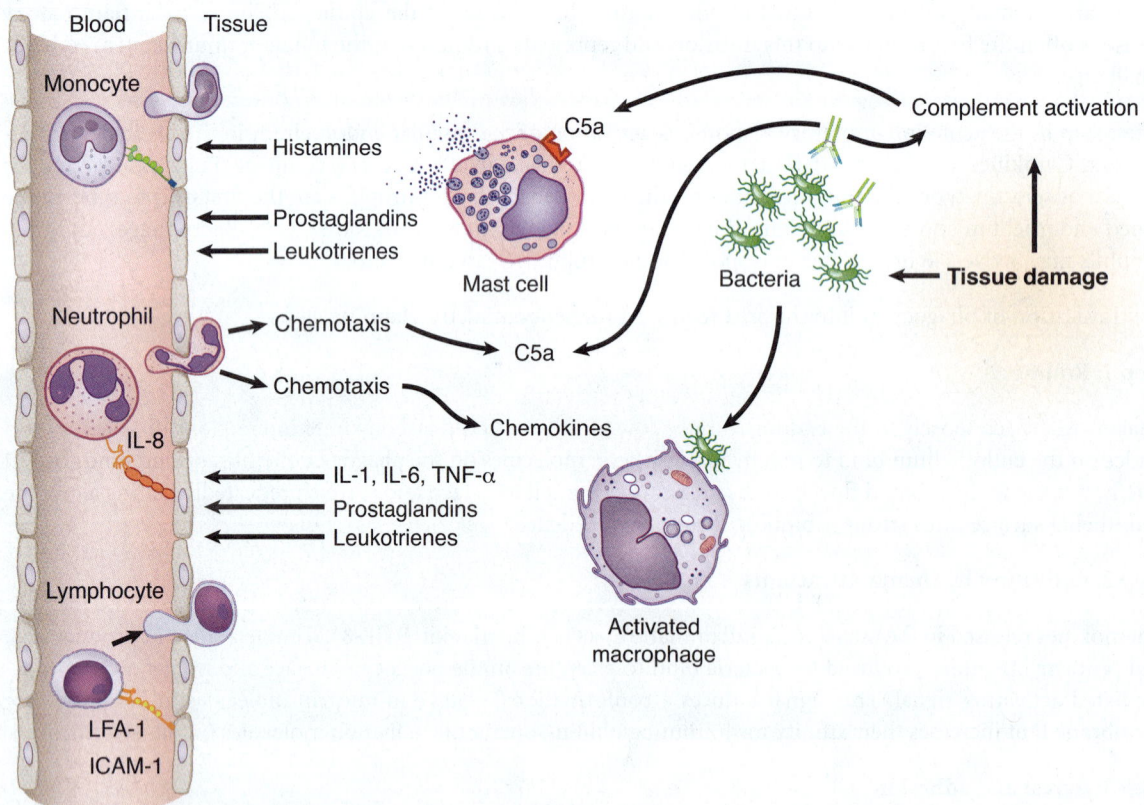

Figure 4-6. Acute Inflammatory Response

Phagocytosis

Once chemotaxis of phagocytic cells into the area of antigen entry is accomplished, these cells ingest and digest particulate debris, such as microorganisms, host cellular debris, and activated clotting factors. This process, called phagocytosis, involves the following:

- Extension of pseudopodia to engulf attached material
- Fusion of the pseudopodia to trap the material in a phagosome
- Fusion of the phagosome with a lysosome to create a phagolysosome
- Digestion
- Exocytosis of digested contents

Neutrophils release granule contents into extracellular milieu during phagocytosis and inflammation in which the neutrophils die, forming what is known as pus. They extrude nuclear contents, histones, neutrophil extracellular traps (NETs) which function to:

- Trap and kill pathogens
- May damage tissues when enzymes, ROS get released into tissues

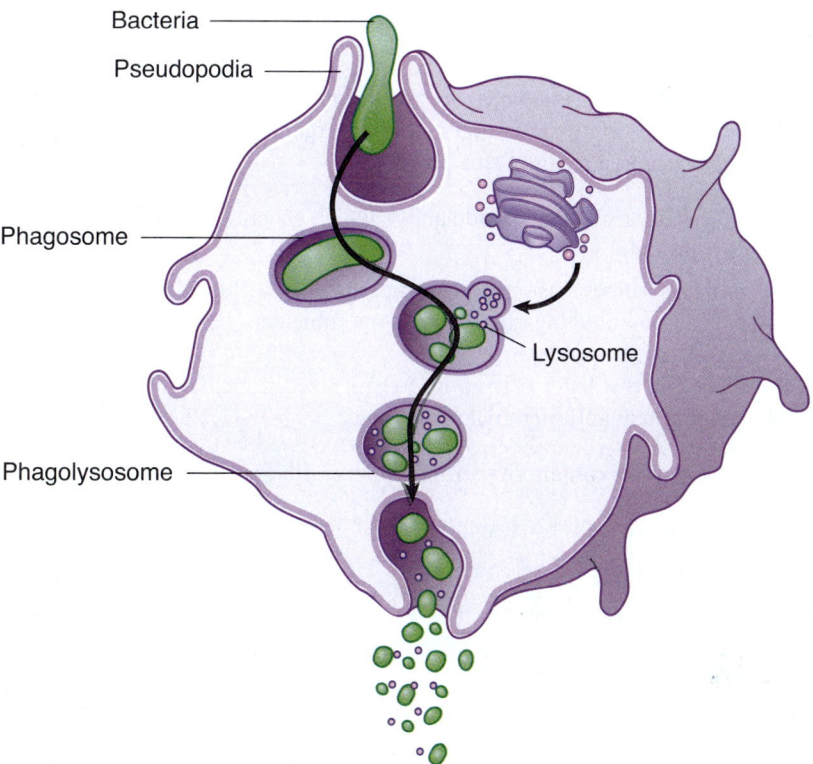

Figure 4-7. Phagocytosis

Opsonization

Both macrophages and neutrophils have membrane receptors for certain types of antibody (IgG) and certain complement components (C3b). If an antigen is coated with either of these materials, adherence and phagocytosis may be enhanced by up to 4,000-fold. Thus, antibody and complement are called **opsonins**, and the means by which they enhance phagocytosis is called opsonization.

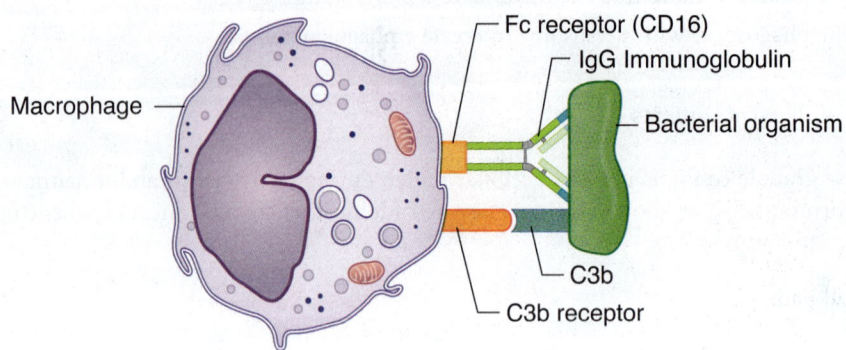

Figure 4-8. Opsonization of Bacteria with Antibody and Complement C3b

Intracellular Killing

During phagocytosis, a metabolic process known as the respiratory burst activates a membrane-bound oxidase that generates oxygen metabolites, which are toxic to ingested microorganisms. Two oxygen-dependent mechanisms of intracellular digestion are activated as a result of this process.

- NADPH oxidase reduces oxygen to superoxide anion, which generates hydroxyl radicals and hydrogen peroxide, which are microbicidal.
- Myeloperoxidase in the lysosomes acts on hydrogen peroxide and chloride ions to produce hypochlorite (the active ingredient in household bleach), which is microbicidal.

Additionally, reactive nitrogen intermediates play an important role. Inducible nitric oxide synthase converts arginine to nitric oxide, which has potent antimicrobial properties.

The lysosomal contents of phagocytes contain oxygen-independent degradative materials:

- Lysozyme digests bacterial cell walls by cleaving peptidoglycan
- Defensins form channels in bacterial cell membranes
- Lactoferrin chelates iron
- Hydrolytic enzymes

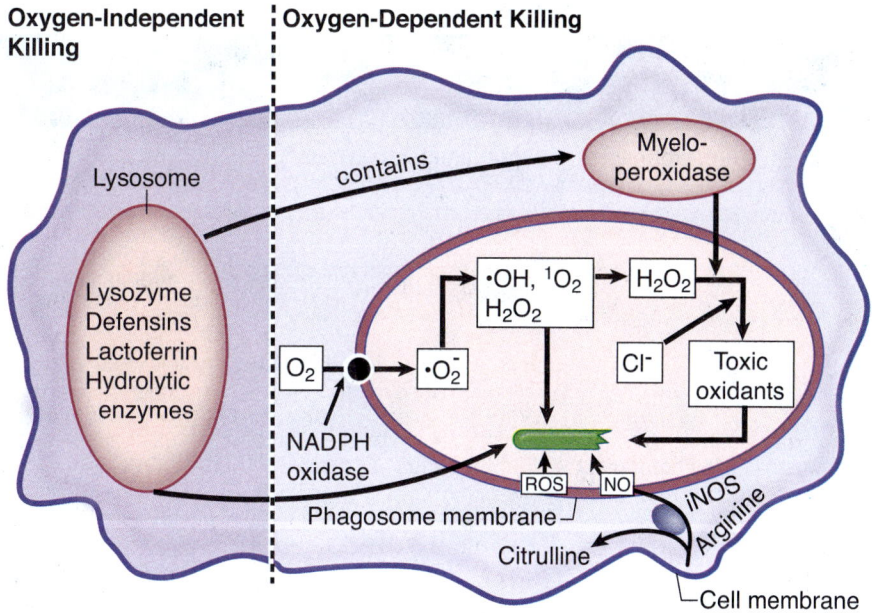

Figure 4-9. Metabolic Stimulation and Killing Within the Phagocyte

Systemic Inflammation

During the acute inflammatory response, pro-inflammatory cytokines such as IL-1, IL-6 and TNF-α are produced. These cytokines have systemic effects on the tissues, including fever, production of acute phase proteins, and leukocytosis.

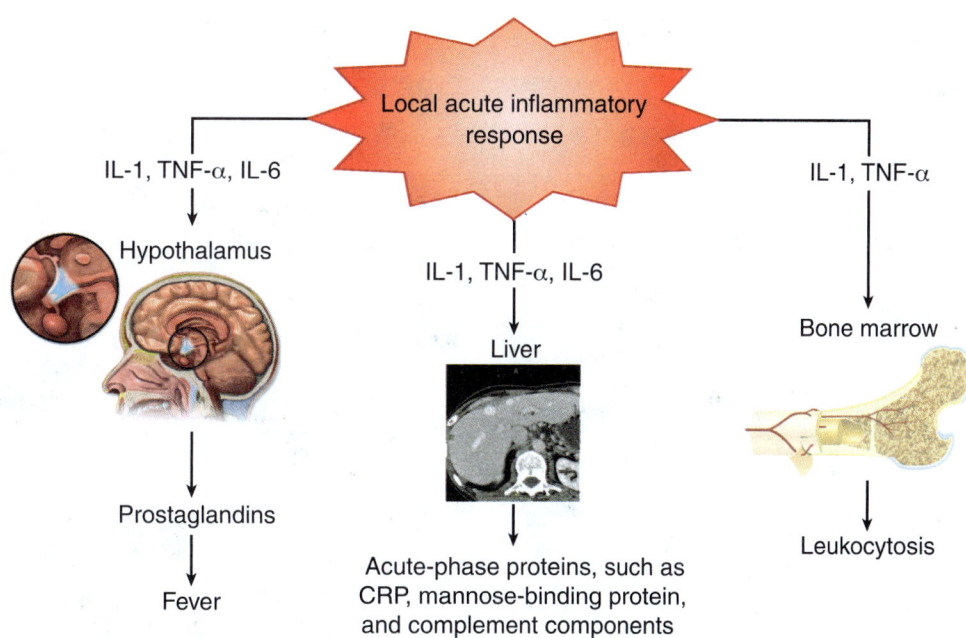

Figure 4-10. Systemic Inflammatory Response

Table 4-6. Cytokines Involved in Innate Immunity*

Cytokine(s)		Cell Secreted by	Target Cells/ Tissues	Activity
Pro-inflam- matory cytokines	IL-1	Macrophages	Hypothalmus	Fever
			Endothelial cells	Increases expression of ICAMs
			Liver	Stimulates production of acute phase proteins
	IL-6	Macrophages	Liver	Synthesis of acute phase proteins
	TNF-α	Macrophages	Hypothalamus	Fever
			Endothelial cells	Increases expression of ICAMs
			Liver	Stimulates production of acute phase proteins
			Neutrophils	Activation
			Tumor cells	Apoptosis
			Fat, muscle	Cachexia
Chemokine	IL-8	Macrophages	Leukocytes	Induces adherence to endothelium, chemotaxis, extravasation
IL-12		Macropages, dendritic cells	NK cells	IFN-γ production
IL-15		Macrophages	NK cells	Proliferation
IL-18		Macrophages		IFN-γ synthesis
Regulatory	IL-10	Macro- phages, den- dritic cells	Macrophages, dendritic cells	Inhibition of IL-12 production, decreased expression of co-stimulatory molecules, de- creased class II MHC expression
Type I IFNs	IFN-α	Dendritic cells, macro- phages	All cells	Transient inhibition of protein synthesis, increased class I MHC expression
			NK cells	Activation
	IFN-β	Fibroblasts	All cells	Transient inhibition of protein synthesis, increased class I MHC expression
			NK cells	Activation
TGF-β		Macro- phages, lymphocytes, etc.		Anti-inflammatory

*Only the innate functions of these cytokines are described here. Many of these cytokines have important functions in the regulation of the adaptive immune response; those will be discussed in subsequent chapters.

Innate Response to Viruses

The innate response to viruses is unique in that it is geared toward eliminating these intracellular pathogens. The two major mechanisms for dealing with viral infections are IFN-α/β and NK cells.

Interferons

Interferons (IFNs) are a family of eukaryotic cell proteins classified according to the cell of origin. IFN-α and IFN-β are produced by a variety of virus-infected cells. They do the following:

- Act on target cells to inhibit viral replication, not the virus
- Are not virus-specific

Interferon inhibits viral protein synthesis:

- Activation of an RNA endonuclease, which digests viral RNA
- Phosphorylation of protein kinase, which inactivates eIF2, inhibiting viral protein synthesis

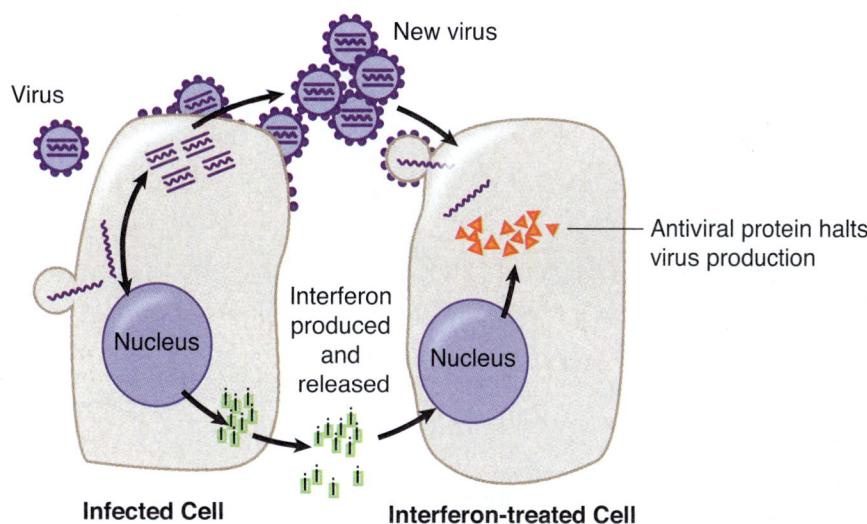

Figure 4-11. Interferon Production

NK Cells

NK cells are members of the innate branch of the immune response. They exhibit the capacity to kill virally infected cells and tumor cells. They kill via the same mechanisms of inducing apoptosis observed with CTLs (granzymes, perforin). NK activity is increased in the presence of interferons (IFNs) α and β, and IL-12.

NK cells share a common early progenitor with T cells, but they do not develop in the thymus. They do not express antigen-specific receptors or CD3. The markers used clinically to enumerate NK cells include CD16 (FcRγ) and CD56 (CAM). Their recognition of targets is not MHC-restricted, and their activity does not generate immunologic memory.

NK cells employ two categories of receptor: **killer activating receptor (KAR)** and **killer inhibitory receptor (KIR)**. If only KARs are engaged, the target cells will be killed. If both the KIRs and the KARs are ligated, the target cell lives. Therefore the inhibitory signals trump the activation signals.

NKG2D is the major KAR expressed by NK cells. There are many ligands for KARs; the MIC glycoproteins are one type. MIC proteins are stress proteins that are expressed only when cells are infected or undergoing transformation. Upon the binding of KAR to a MIC protein, NK cells become cytotoxic, resulting in death of the target cell.

The KIRs activate protein tyrosine phosphatases which inhibit intracellular signaling and activation by removing tyrosine residues from various signaling molecules. The KIRs on the NK cell bind to a specialized type of MHC class I antigens called HLA-E. HLA-E has a ubiquitous tissue distribution, as do the other class I HLA molecules. The HLA-E molecules bind to peptides derived from the leader sequence of HLA-A, -B and –C. HLA-E requires a bound peptide for proper expression within a cell. Therefore, the amount of HLA-E expression on a cell is indicative of the overall well-being of the cell. During viral infections or in transformed cells, the amount of class I HLA expression may be decreased, which would prevent the leader sequences from binding to HLA-E. This would decrease the expression of HLA-E, and make cells susceptible to NK mediated killing.

Interestingly, when NK cells are activated through the FcR (CD16), only one signal is required because the antibody signals that there is an active infection. This occurs through a mechanism called antibody-dependent cell-mediated cytotoxicity (ADCC) (see chapter 8).

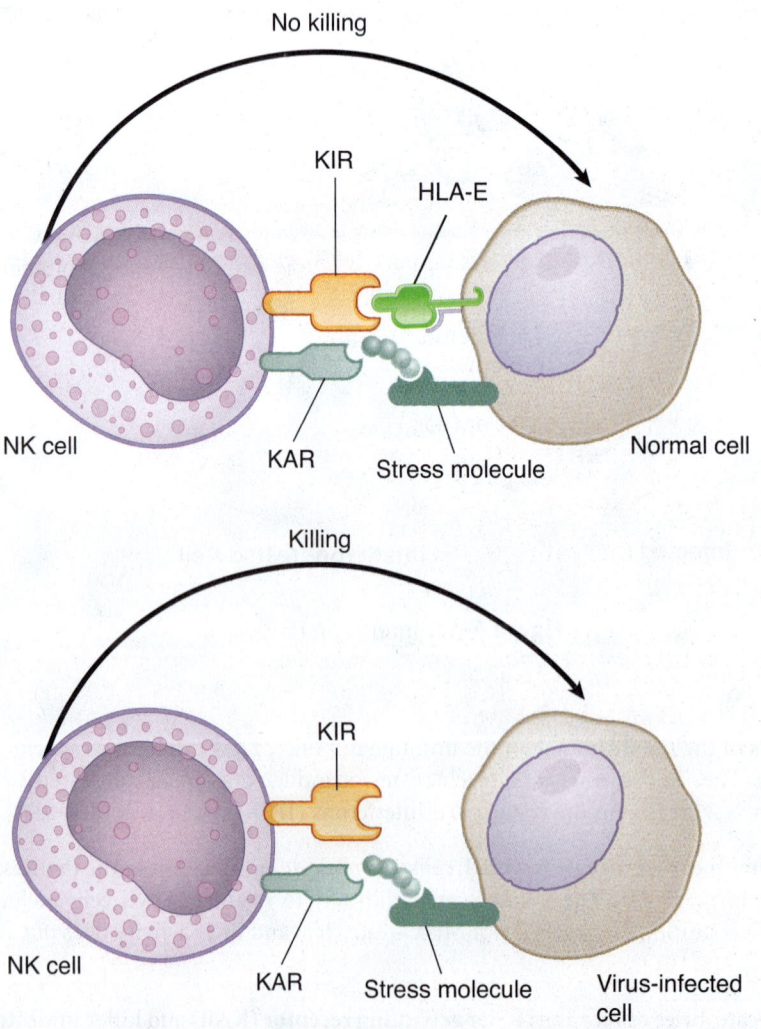

Figure 4-12. Activation of NK Cells

Learning Objectives

❏ Solve problems concerning structure of and migration to secondary lymphoid tissue

❏ Demonstrate understanding of the structure of secondary lymphoid tissue

❏ Understand antigen processing and presentation

MIGRATION TO THE SECONDARY LYMPHOID TISSUE

Within a few hours of the initiation of the acute inflammatory response, the professional APCs that have phagocytosed and processed the invading antigen begin to leave the area via lymphatic vessels. Dendritic cells are probably the most efficient of these cells and retract their membranous processes to round up and begin the journey to the closest lymph node (Figure 5-1).

As discussed earlier, dendritic cells and other phagocytes such as macrophages bind to antigens via PRRs, with a limited diversity, such as the TLRs. The activation of the TLRs induces an acute inflammatory response in the tissue, leading to the production of pro-inflammatory cytokines. These cytokines cause a change in the phenotype of the phagocyte which eventually alters their migration pattern and enhances their function.

Activated dendritic cells will begin to express a chemokine receptor called CCR7. CCR7 is activated by chemokines that are produced by the endothelium.

- Chemokines bind to CCR7 on DCs, allowing them to exit the tissue.
- Upon activation, DCs switch focus from antigen-capture to antigen-presentation.
- Activated DCs concentrate in draining lymph nodes and become trapped in the paracortex.
- Naive T cells expressing CCR7 bind to chemokines on HEVs and migrate to the paracortex.

Considering the vast number of pathogens that enter the body, it would be a nearly impossible task for the lymphoid cells to travel to all body sites to protect the host. Thus, the antigens are taken to the secondary lymphoid tissues where the lymphocytes constantly recirculate in order to come into contact with their specific antigen.

If the initial tissue damage is sufficient, these cells can also be flushed into blood vessels, ultimately becoming trapped in the vascular sinusoids of the spleen. Regardless, the secondary lymphoid organs (lymph nodes and spleen) are the sites where naive, mature lymphocytes will first be exposed to their specific antigens.

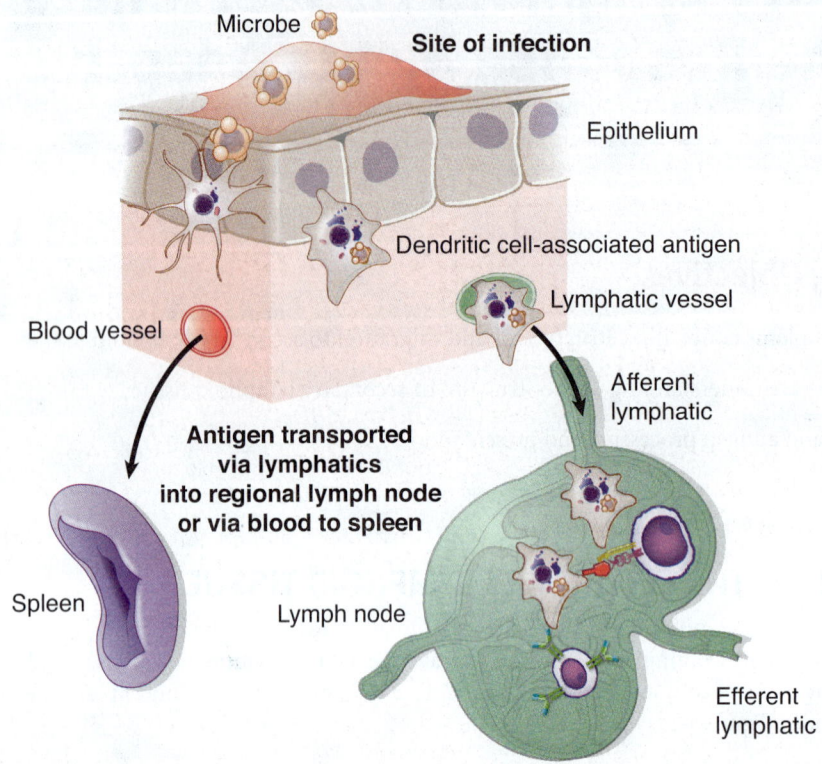

Figure 5-1. Transportation of Antigen to the Secondary Lymphoid Organs

STRUCTURE OF THE SECONDARY LYMPHOID TISSUE

Lymph nodes are small nodular aggregates of secondary lymphoid tissue found along the lymphatic channels of the body. They are designed to initiate immune responses to tissue-borne antigens.

- Each lymph node is surrounded by a fibrous capsule that is punctured by afferent lymphatics, which bring lymph into the subcapsular sinus.

- The fluid percolates through an outer cortex area that contains aggregates of cells called follicles.

- The lymph then passes into the inner medulla and the medullary sinus before leaving the node through the hilum in an efferent lymphatic vessel.

- Ultimately, lymph from throughout the body is collected into the thoracic duct, which empties into the vena cava and returns it to the blood.

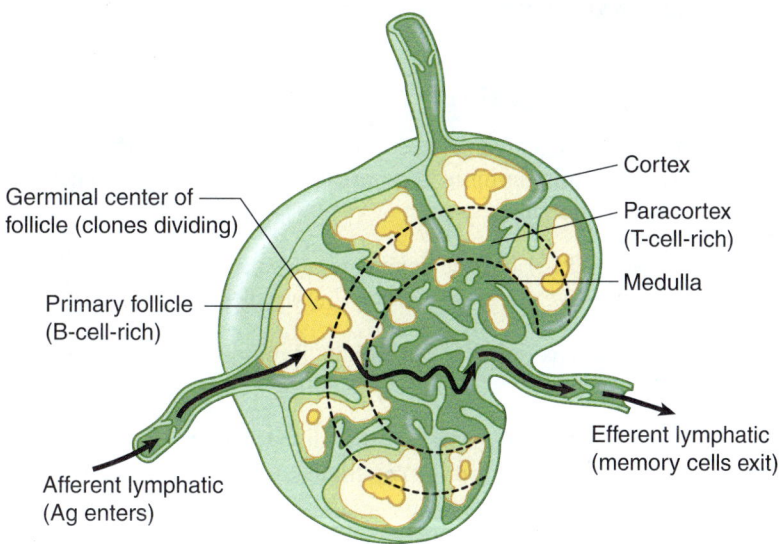

Figure 5-2. Compartmentalization of a Lymph Node

The spleen is the secondary lymphoid organ that initiates immune responses to bloodborne antigens. A single splenic artery enters the capsule at the hilum and branches into arterioles, which become surrounded by cuffs of lymphocytes known as the **periarteriolar lymphoid sheaths (PALS)**. Lymphoid follicles surrounded by a rim of lymphocytes and macrophages are attached nearby. This constitutes the white pulp. The arterioles ultimately end in vascular sinusoids, which make up the red pulp. From here, venules collect blood into the splenic vein, which empties into the portal circulation.

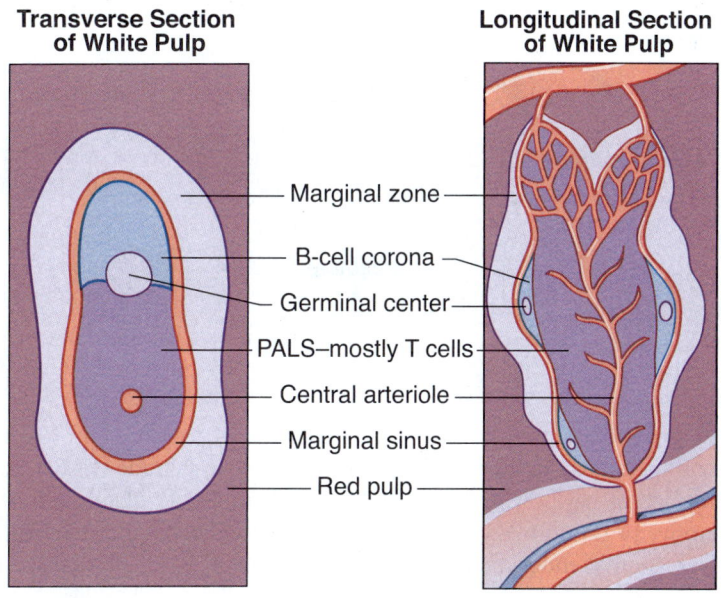

Figure 5-3. Structure of the Spleen

ANTIGEN PROCESSING AND PRESENTATION

Exogenous Pathway of MHC Loading

Although some small, easily digestible antigens are almost totally degraded and exocytosed by phagocytes, the critical first step in the elicitation of the adaptive immune response to a primary antigenic challenge is the processing of antigen for the presentation to naive T lymphocytes.

Professional antigen-presenting cells (APCs) include dendritic cells, macrophages, and B cells; their job is to load partially degraded peptides into the groove of the MHC class II molecules.

The APCs have slightly different functions to help elicit unique immune responses required to eliminate various types of pathogens.

- **Dendritic cells** are the most prolific of the APCs, as they do not have to be activated in order to present antigen to T cells. They constitutively express the co-stimulatory molecules needed to activate the T cells.
- **Macrophages** help activate the Th1 response by digesting microbes and presenting them to the T cells to elicit a cell-mediated immune response (see chapter 8).
- **B cells** present specific protein antigens to T cells to help elicit a humoral immune response or a Th2 response (see chapter 7). B cells are unique, as they are the only APCs that specifically recognize antigen via the B cell receptors (of surface bound antibody).

Table 5-1. APC Expression of Co-stimulatory Molecules, Class II MHC, and Function

APC	Expression of Co-stimulatory Molecules	Expression of HLA Class II	Major Function
Dendritic cells	Constitutive: B7 (B7.2)*, CD40 Inducible: IFN-γ, TLR's	Constitutive but upregulated by IFN-γ	Activation of naïve Th cells
Macrophages	Constitutive: B7 (B7.2), CD40 Inducible: IFN-γ, TLR's	Negative or low level expression but induced by IFN-γ	Initiation and effector phase of the T_h1 response for cell mediated immunity
B cells	Constitutive: CD40 Inducible: T cells, B7	Constitutive but upregulated by IL-4	Initiation of the T_h2 response for humoral immunity

*B7.2 is also called CD86.

When MHC class II molecules are produced in the endoplasmic reticulum of an APC, a protein called the invariant chain (Ii) is synthesized at the same time. The Ii has a class II invariant chain peptide (CLIP) that binds with high affinity to the peptide binding cleft of newly synthesized MHC class II molecule. The Ii with its associated CLIP blocks the peptide-binding groove so no normal cellular peptides can accidentally be attached. The CLIP + Ii is transported in a vesicle to the location of endocytic vesicles containing the ingested, internalized peptides.

A molecule called HLA-DM is found within the late endosome (lysosomal compartment). It is the job of HLA-DM to exchange the CLIP for a phagocytosed peptide that will bind to the MHC class II molecule with even higher affinity than the CLIP. Once exchanged for the CLIP, the peptide is loaded on the MHC class II molecule and the complex is transported to the cell surface, where it will be accessible for interaction with any T lymphocyte with a complementary TCR. If, however, the class II molecule does not find a peptide that it can bind with even higher affinity than the CLIP, the empty class II molecule is unstable and degraded, and will thus never make it to the cell surface.

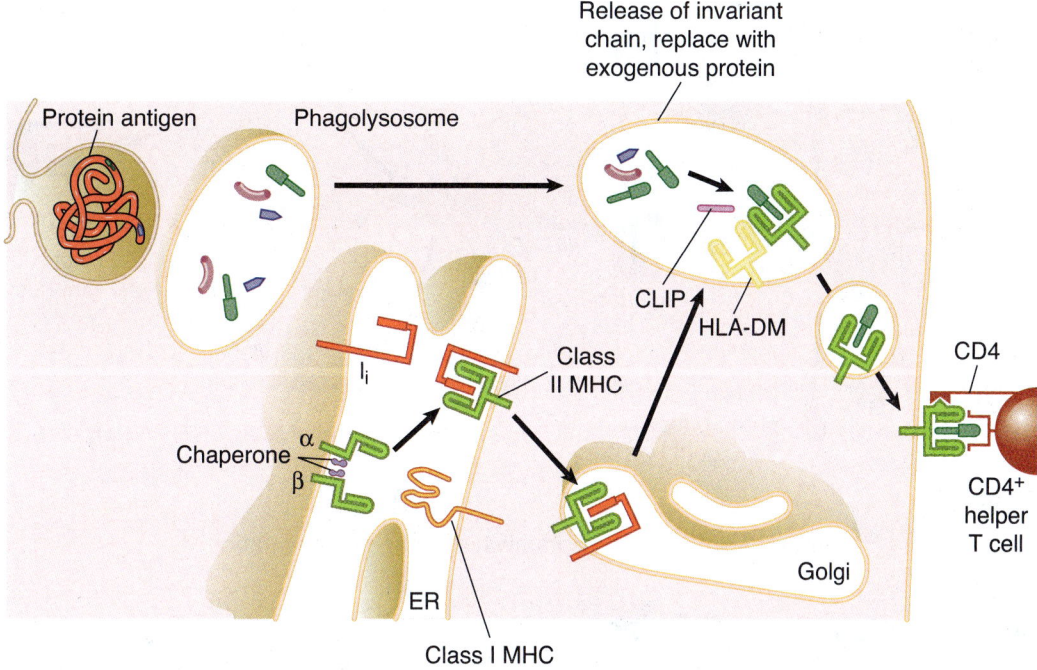

Figure 5-4. Exogenous Pathway of Antigen Presentation

Endogenous Pathway of MHC Loading

The endogenous pathway of antigen-processing handles threats to the host which are intracellular. These might include viruses, altered/mutated genes (from tumors), or even peptides from phagocytosed pathogens that may escape or be transported out of phagosomes into the host cell cytoplasm. Intracellular proteins are routinely targeted by ubiquitin and degraded in proteasomes.

The peptides from these proteins are transported through a peptide transporter known as the **TAP complex (transporter of antigen processing)**, and into the endoplasmic reticulum, where they have the opportunity to bind to freshly synthesized MHC class I molecules.

- The TAP complex includes the TAP proteins that form the tunnel through which the proteins travel and a bridging protein called tapasin.
- Tapasin bridges the TAP transporter to the MHC class I molecule so that as these peptides enter the endoplasmic reticulum, they are easily bound by the newly synthesized and empty class I molecules.
- The peptide-MHC class I complexes are then transported to the cell membrane where they may be presented to CD8+ T lymphocytes (see chapter 8).

Just as with the MHC class II molecules, MHC class I is unstable without the addition of peptide and will not be expressed at the cell surface without the addition of peptide.

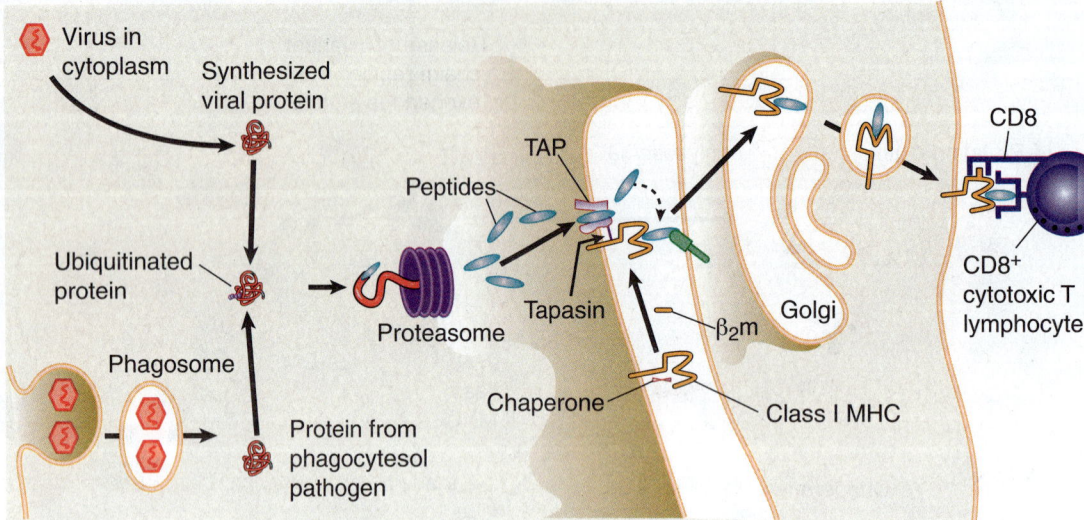

Figure 5-5. Endogenous Pathway of Antigen Presentation

Cross Presentation (Cross Priming)

In addition to presenting antigens on MHC class II molecules to CD4+ T cells, dendritic cells also have a role in presenting antigens to CD8+ T cells in a process called **cross presentation**. As professional phagocytes, dendritic cells are able to ingest a virally MHC class I infected cell in toto and present viral antigens within a molecule to CD8+ T cells. Therefore, DCs may activate or prime both CD4+ T cells and CD8+ T cells specific for the same pathogen. This activation may occur in close proximity, which is important for the activation of naïve CD8+ T cells into activated CTLs and memory cells. This occurs via the activation of CD4+ T cells and the production of cytokines such as IL-2 (see chapter 8).

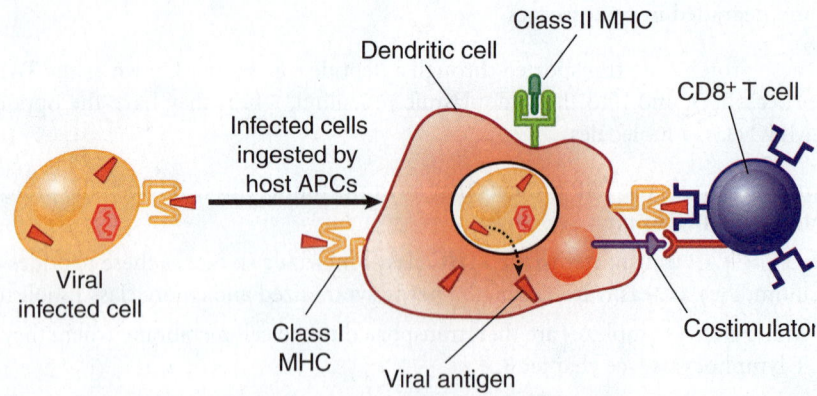

Figure 5-6. Cross-Priming

Secondary Lymphoid Tissue: B and T Lymphocyte Activation

6

Learning Objectives

❏ Answer questions about antigen processing and presentation

❏ Explain activation of T and B lymphocytes

ACTIVATION OF T LYMPHOCYTES

Once antigen is processed and presented to a T cell, the adaptive immune response is initiated. These interactions occur within the secondary lymphoid tissue. The purpose of these interactions is to generate effector cells, which will ultimately result in the elimination of the infection.

In order to generate specific effector cells, the activation of T cells via the TCR must go through several checkpoints to ensure antigen specificity and eventual T-cell activation.

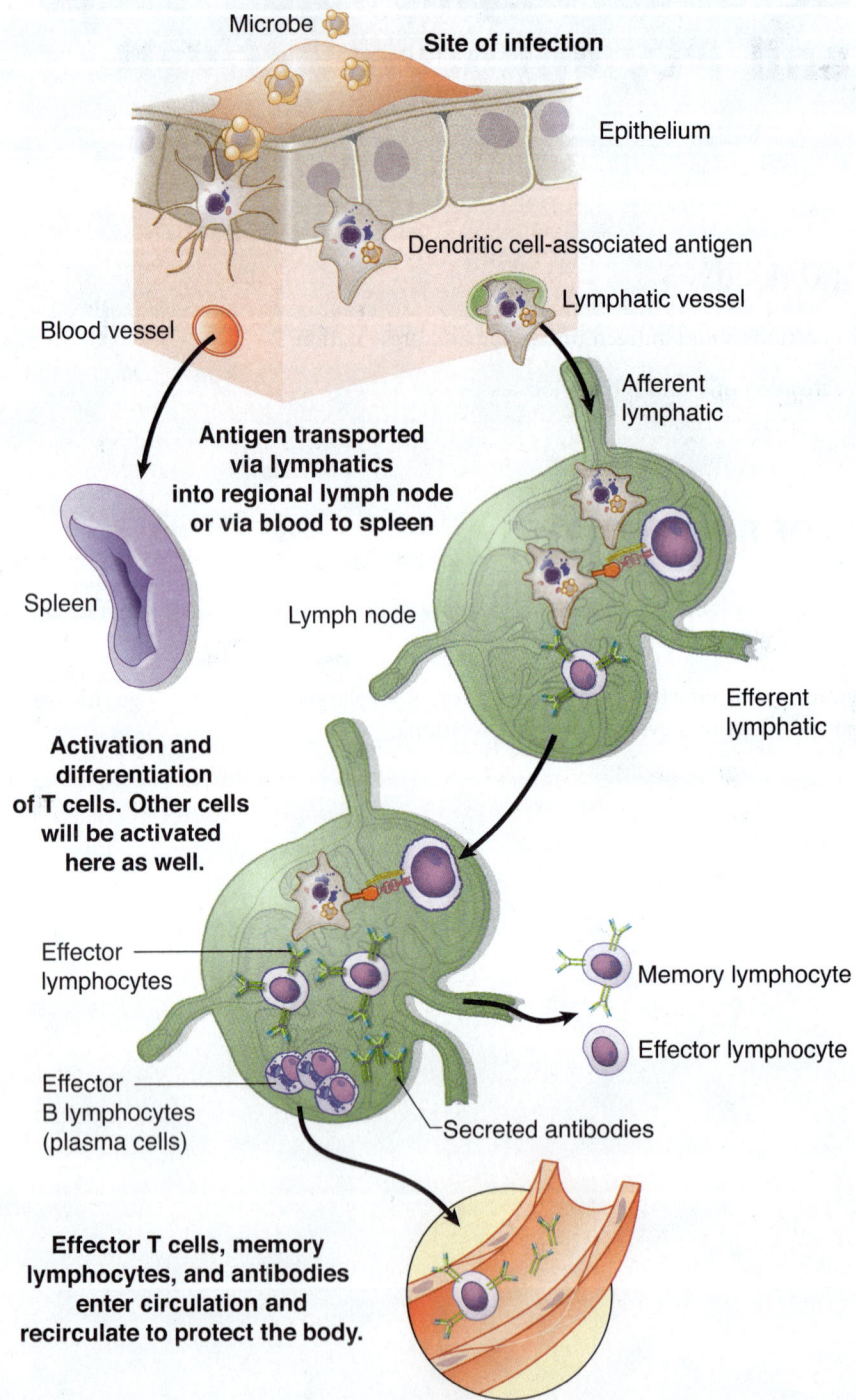

Microbe

Site of infection

Epithelium

Dendritic cell-associated antigen

Lymphatic vessel

Blood vessel

Afferent lymphatic

Antigen transported via lymphatics into regional lymph node or via blood to spleen

Spleen

Lymph node

Efferent lymphatic

Activation and differentiation of T cells. Other cells will be activated here as well.

Effector lymphocytes

Memory lymphocyte

Effector lymphocyte

Effector B lymphocytes (plasma cells)

Secreted antibodies

Effector T cells, memory lymphocytes, and antibodies enter circulation and recirculate to protect the body.

Figure 6-1. Production of Effector Cells in the Secondary Lymphoid Organs

The binding of the TCR of the mature, naive T cell to the MHC peptide complex of the APC provides the first signal to the T cell to begin its activation. This provides the antigenic specificity of the response. The interaction is stabilized by the coreceptors CD4 and CD8 which bind to MHC class II and MHC class I molecules, respectively.

Intimately associated with the T cell receptor is the CD3 signal transduction complex. Interaction of cell adhesion molecules on the surface of the APCs and T cells allows for the formation of the immune synapse.

The costimulatory molecules B7-1 (CD80) and B7-2 (CD86) on APCs bind to CD28 on the mature, naïve T cells, providing the second signal necessary for successful activation. Under normal conditions, B7 is expressed at low levels on APCs. In the presence of infection or inflammation, the expression will increase, enhancing activation of the mature, naïve T cells. Later in the immune response, B7 will preferentially bind to CTLA-4 or PD-1, effectively turning off the T-cell response.

Cytokines secreted by APCs and the activating T cells themselves induce the proliferation (**clonal expansion**) and differentiation of the T cells into **effector cells** and **memory cells**.

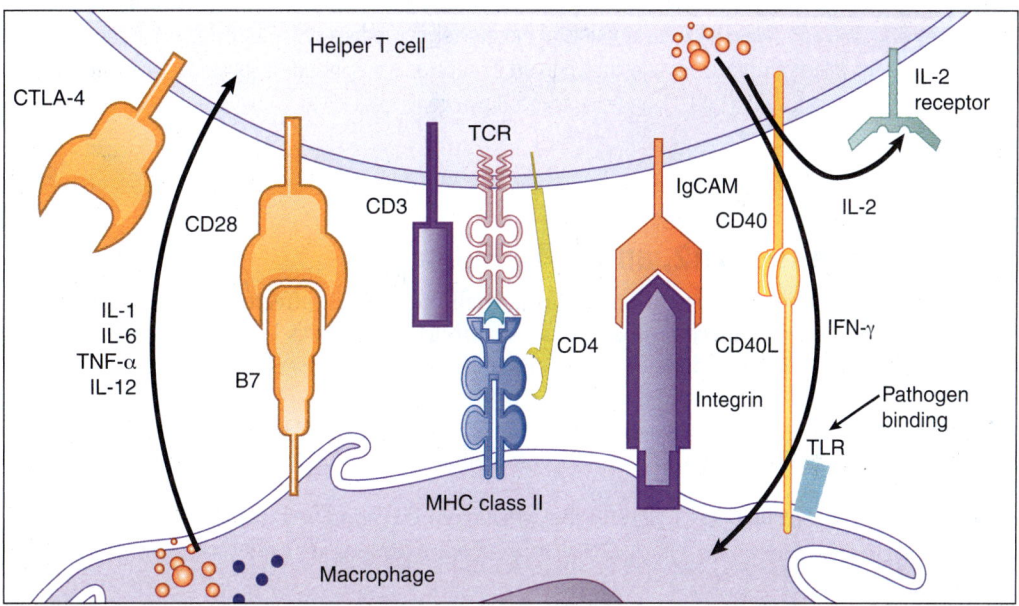

Figure 6-2. Helper T Cell and Macrophage Adhesion

Several surface molecules are involved in the activation of mature, naive T lymphocytes:

- **First (primary) signal**: recognition of the MHC:peptide complex by the T cell receptor and coreceptors (CD4 and CD8)
- **Second (costimulatory) signal**: recognition of B7 by CD28

The activated CD4+ (helper) T lymphocytes will begin to produce and secrete cytokines and increase surface expression of cytokine receptors. The first cytokine produced is IL-2, an autocrine signal, which induces T-cell proliferation by binding to a high affinity IL-2 receptor found on the same cells. Unlike helper T lymphocytes, activated CD8+ T lymphocytes secrete low levels of IL-2 and are dependent on the helper T lymphocytes for their proliferation and differentiation.

Clinical Correlate

Superantigens are viral and bacterial proteins that cross-link the variable β domain of a T-cell receptor to an α chain of a class II MHC molecule outside the normal peptide-binding groove. This cross-linkage provides an activating signal that induces T-cell activation and proliferation, in the absence of antigen-specific recognition of peptides in the MHC class II groove.

Because superantigens bind outside of the antigen-binding cleft, they activate any clones of T cells expressing a particular variable β sequence and thus cause polyclonal activation of T cells, resulting in the overproduction of IFN-γ. This, in turn, activates macrophages, resulting in overexpression of proinflammatory cytokines (IL-1, IL-6 and TNF-α). Excess amounts of these cytokines induce systemic toxicity. Molecules produced during infectious processes and known to act as superantigens include staphylococcal enterotoxins, toxic-shock syndrome toxin-1 (TSST-1), and streptococcal pyrogenic exotoxins.

Development of the Th1, Th2, and Th17 Subsets

Helper T lymphocytes serve as the orchestrators of virtually all the possible **effector mechanisms** that will arise to destroy the pathogen. The effector mechanisms that are controlled by Th cells include antibody synthesis, macrophage activation and CTL killing. The "decision" as to which of these mechanisms should be engaged is based on the characteristics of the invading pathogen and is controlled by the differentiation of specialized classes of helper T cells. All CD4+ T cells require recognition of their specific antigen complexed to MHC class II by their TCR (first signal) and costimulation through the binding of B7 on the professional APC by CD28 (costimulatory signal).

There are three major classes of helper T (Th) cell that arise from the same precursor, the naive Th lymphocyte (or Th0 cell):

- Th1
- Th2
- Th17

The pattern of differentiation is determined by the antigen or type of pathogen causing the infection, the cytokines produced in response to the antigen, and the transcription factors stimulated by the cytokines.

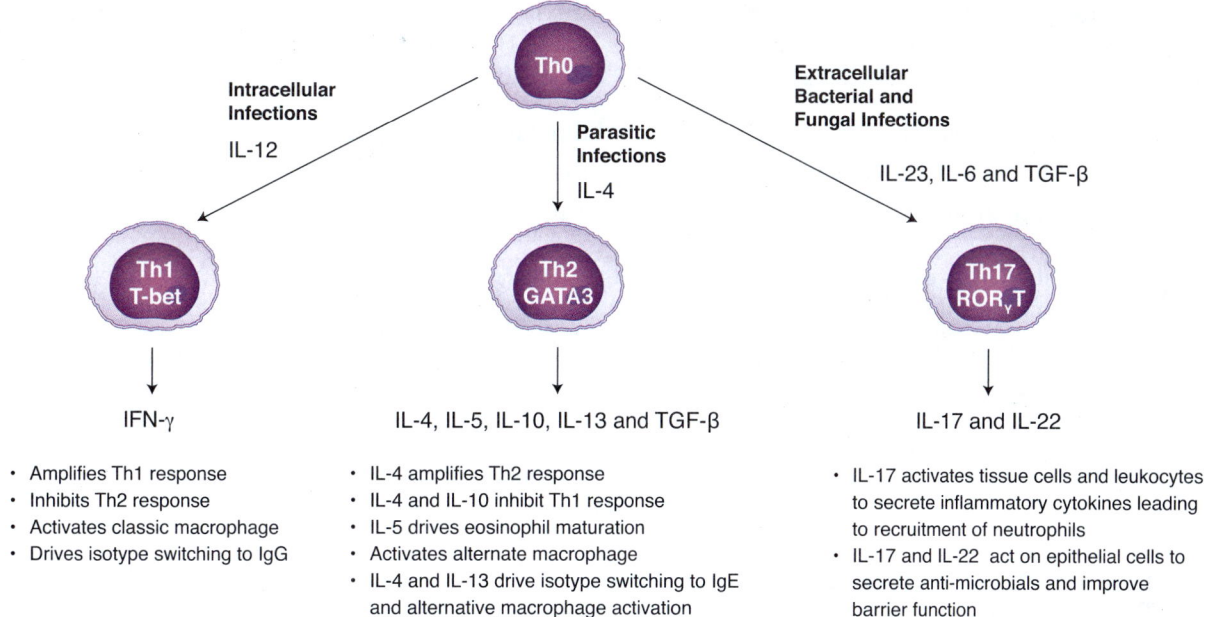

Figure 6-3. Subsets of Helper T Cells

Differentiation of a Th0 cell into a Th1 cell is stimulated by intracellular pathogens (e.g., viruses and intracellular bacteria). These pathogens induce a strong innate immune response with the resultant production of **IL-12** by macrophages and **IFN-γ** by NK cells increasing the expression of the transcription factor T-bet.

In turn, Th1 cells secrete high levels of the inflammatory cytokine IFN-γ which does the following:

- Amplifies the Th1 response
- Inhibits the Th2 response
- Activates classical macrophage
- Enhances isotype switching to IgG

Differentiation of a Th0 cell into a Th2 cell seems to be encouraged in response to large extracellar parasites such as helminths or allergens. Due to the inability to phagocytose these pathogens, there is not significant macrophage or NK-cell stimulation. In this way, naive Th0 cells seem to produce IL-4 constitutively, and in the absence of IL-12 stimulation, these cells will upregulate their production of IL-4 to encourage differentiation into Th2 cells by induction of the transcription factor GATA-3. Additional IL-4 is produced by the activation of mast cells and eosinophils by the helminths or allergens further driving differentiation into Th2 cells.

Several cytokines are produced by Th2 cells, including IL-4, IL-5, IL-10, IL-13 and TGF-β.

- IL-4 causes B lymphocytes to isotype switch predominantly to IgE, which will bind to mast cells, eosinophils and basophils.
- In collaboration with IL-13, IL-4 enhances alternative macrophage activation for tissue repair and increased intestinal mucus secretion and peristalsis.
- The combination of IL-4, IL-10, and IL-13 together promotes a Th2 response while inhibiting the Th1 response.
- IL-5 drives maturation and activation of eosinophils.

Differentiation of a Th0 cell into a Th17 cell occurs in the presence of extracellular bacterial and fungal infections. Local cells react to the infection by secreting IL-1, IL-6, IL-23, and TGF-β, inducing the expression of the transcription factor RORγ-T in the Th17 cells. The activated Th17 cells will in turn secrete the cytokines IL-17 and IL-22.

- IL-17 induces local cells to increase chemokine production recruiting neutrophils.
- IL-22 stabilizes interactions between cells in the endothelium decreasing permeability.
- IL-17 and IL-22 induce secretion of anti-microbials by the endothelium.

Another population of T cells that arises from the Th0 is the T regulatory cell (T_{Reg} cell). T_{Reg} cells regulate (inhibit) Th1 cell function.

- Identified by their constitutive expression of CD25 on the surface and by the expression of the transcription factor FoxP3
- Secrete inflammation inhibiting cytokines such as IL-10 and TGF-β
- Have been shown to be critical for the prevention of autoimmunity

Development of Cytotoxic T Lymphocytes

Like CD4+ T cells, CD8+ T cells require both a primary and a costimulatory signal to become activated. The main difference between them is that CD8+ T cells recognize their specific antigen presented by MHC class I molecules and rely upon the cytokines produced by T helper cells to proliferate and ultimately differentiate into cytotoxic T lymphocytes (CTLs).

Clinical Correlate

Tuberculoid vs. Lepromatous Leprosy

The progression of disease with *Mycobacterium leprae* in humans is a well-documented example of the crucial balance between Th1 and Th2 subsets. Leprosy is not a single clinical entity, but rather a spectrum of diseases, with tuberculoid and lepromatous forms at the far poles.

- In **tuberculoid leprosy**, the patient has a strong Th1 response, which eradicates the intracellular pathogens by granuloma formation. There is some damage to skin and peripheral nerves, but the disease progresses slowly, if at all, and the patient survives.
- In **lepromatous leprosy**, the Th2 response is turned on, and because of reciprocal inhibition, the cell-mediated response is depressed. Patients develop antibodies to the pathogen that are not protective, and the mycobacteria multiply inside macrophages, sometimes reaching levels of 1010 per gram of tissue. Hypergammaglobulinemia may occur, and these cases frequently progress to disseminated and disfiguring infections.

ACTIVATION OF B LYMPHOCYTES

As mature naive B lymphocytes leave the bone marrow following successful rearrangement of their membrane immunoglobulin receptor genes, they recirculate throughout the body, attracted to **follicular areas** of the lymph nodes and spleen. If antigen entering these secondary lymphoid organs binds to and cross-links the idiotypes of the immunoglobulin, this provides the first signal for the activation of the B lymphocyte.

The antigens that B lymphocytes encounter are divided into two categories: **thymus-independent** (TI) antigens and **thymus-dependent** (TD) antigens.

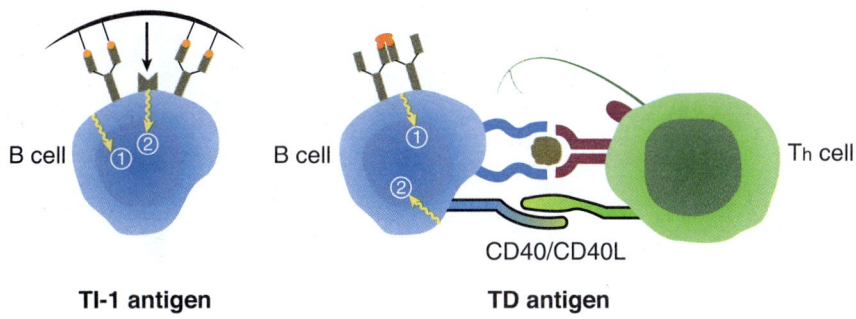

TI-1 antigen   **TD antigen**

Figure 6-4. TI versus TD Antigens

TI-Antigen Activated B Lymphocytes

Certain mature, naïve B lymphocytes are capable of being activated by macromolecules such as lipids, polysaccharides, and lipopolysaccharides without having to interact with helper T cells. These antigens are called **thymus-independent (TI) antigens**, and they directly stimulate B cells to proliferate and differentiate into plasma cells.

- The response to TI antigens is generally **weaker** than the response to TD antigens, resulting primarily in the **secretion of IgM antibodies** and the **absence of immunologic memory**.
- TI antigens may also act as B-cell **mitogens**, directly causing mitosis regardless of the cell's antigenic specificity.
- B lymphocytes activated by TI antigens are found in the spleen and mucosa.
- The marginal zone B cells are found in the periphery of the splenic white pulp and the B-1 cells in association with the mucosa and peritoneum.

TD-Antigen Activated B Lymphocytes

Most antigens introduced in the body fall into the category of **thymus-dependent (TD) antigens**. Response to such molecules requires the direct contact of B cells with helper T cells and are influenced by **cytokines** secreted by these cells. After the cross-linking of receptors on the B-cell surface with antigen, the material is endocytosed and processed via the exogenous pathway to generate an MHC class II:peptide complex, which is then inserted into the membrane of the professional APCs.

Simultaneously, expression of B7 is upregulated on the B lymphocytes, making the cells effective presenters of antigen to CD4+ T cells in the area. Once a CD4+ T cell recognizes its specific peptide displayed on MHC class II molecules, the two cells form a **conjugate**.

- The CD4+ T cell is activated and differentiates into a helper T cell.
- The helper T cells rearrange their Golgi apparatus toward the junction with the B cell leading to the directional release of cytokines.
- Expression of CD40L on the surface of the helper T cell is upregulated and interacts with CD40 on the B cell to provide the second signal for B-cell activation.
- The B cells respond by proliferating and differentiating into plasma cells and memory B cells.

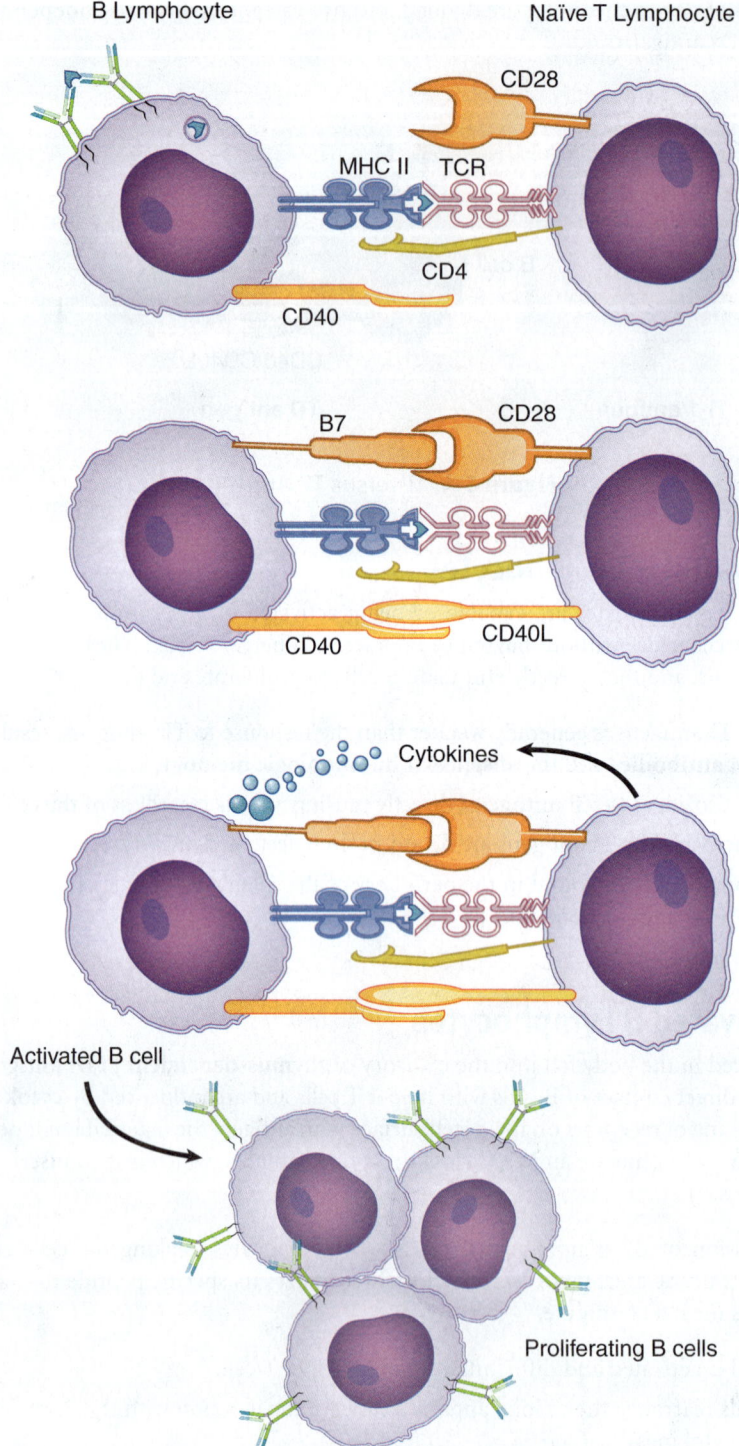

Figure 6-5. Steps in T-Cell-Dependent B-Cell Activation

B lymphocytes activated by TD antigens are released in two subsequent waves.

- The primary wave of activated B lymphocytes is comprised of strictly IgM-secreting plasma cells which leave the secondary lymphoid tissue shortly after being activated.

- The second wave of activated B lymphocytes remains within the follicles of the secondary lymphoid tissue undergoing clonal expansion producing the germinal center. During the expansion, the clones will undergo affinity maturation and isotype switching.

Affinity Maturation

During the activation of B lymphocytes by helper T cells, intense proliferation of the B cells results in the formation of **germinal centers** in the follicles of the secondary lymphoid tissues. These are clones of proliferating, antigen-specific cells. During the intense proliferative response of the B cell, random mutations in the coding of the variable domain region may occur. This is called **somatic hypermutation** and creates single point mutations in the antibody idiotype. If these slightly altered idiotypes have increased affinity for the antigen, then the cell expressing them will be at a selective advantage in competing to bind antigen.

Because binding antigen serves as the first signal for proliferation, over time clones of cells with higher receptor affinity will begin to predominate in the germinal center. This **clonal selection** results in the predominance of clones capable of producing antibodies with increasing affinity for the antigen, a process known as **affinity maturation**.

This means that although isotype switching will necessarily **decrease the avidity** of the preponderance of antibody molecules as the immune response evolves, this will be substituted by an **increase in antibody affinity** over time.

Isotype Switching

Although all of the antibody molecules secreted by a clone of B lymphocytes will have an identical idiotype (*see* chapter 3), the B cell is induced to make new classes (**isotypes**) of immunoglobulin in response to cytokine-directed instruction from the helper T cells.

As the B lymphocyte receives cytokine signals from the helper T cells in the secondary lymphoid organs, it is induced to undergo **isotype switching**, changing the heavy-chain constant domains to classes of antibodies with new and different effector functions. It does this by rearranging the DNA encoding the constant regions of the heavy chain by activating switch regions that cause the intervening DNA to be looped out, excised, and degraded. The idiotype is then joined to a new constant region domain, resulting in an antibody molecule with identical antigenic specificity but a new effector function. This isotype switch is **one-way**; the excised DNA is degraded so a cell that has begun to produce an isotype downstream from IgM coding can never produce IgM again.

This is why IgM is the principal immunoglobulin of the **primary immune response** when antigen is first encountered, and it is replaced in later responses by antibodies of different isotypes. Although IgM antibodies are occasionally produced at low levels during secondary and later immunologic responses, they are always produced by cells encountering that antigen for the first time; namely, mature, naive B cells newly emerging from the bone marrow.

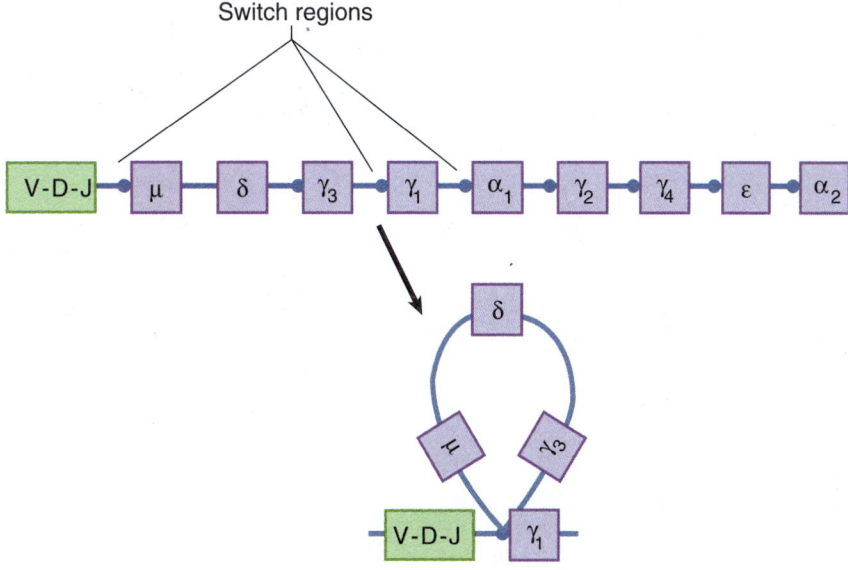

Figure 6-6. Immunoglobulin Heavy Chain Switching

Learning Objectives

❏ Explain information related to the primary humoral response

❏ Answer questions about antibodies of secondary immune responses

PRIMARY HUMORAL RESPONSE

The first isotype of immunoglobulin that can be produced by a B cell with or without T-cell help is IgM. This is because coding for the constant domains of the heavy chain of IgM (μ chains) are the first sequences downstream from the coding for the idiotype of the molecule.

The IgM molecule on the surface of the B cell is a monomer, but the secreted form of this molecule is a **pentamer**, held together in an extremely compact form by a **J chain** synthesized by the cell.

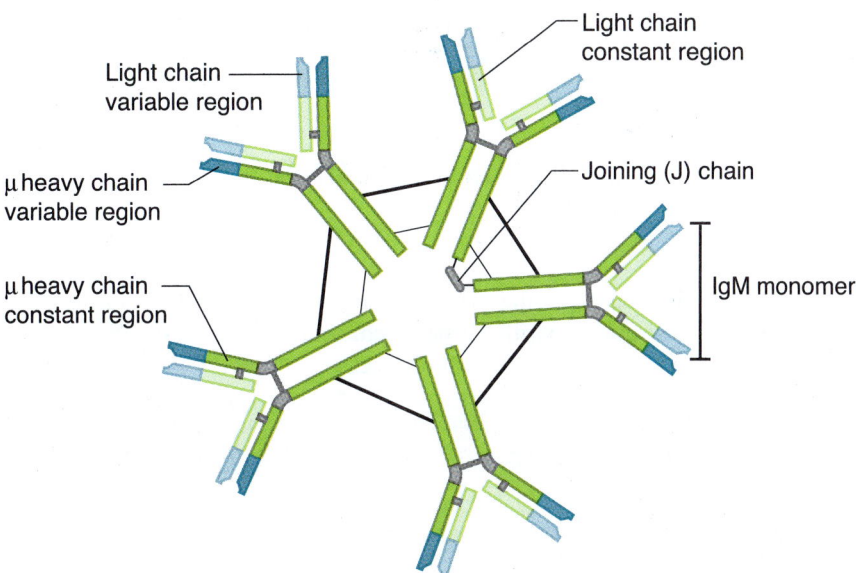

Light chain variable region

Light chain constant region

μ heavy chain variable region

Joining (J) chain

μ heavy chain constant region

IgM monomer

Figure 7-1. IgM Pentamer

The design of the IgM pentamer maximizes its effect critical to the body early during antigenic challenge. Because of its multimeric structure (5 of the Y-shaped monomers joined into one unit), plasma IgM has 5 times the capacity for binding antigenic epitopes. The valence of the molecule is therefore 10. In other words, 10 identical epitopes can be simultaneously bound, as compared with 2 for the monomeric structure.

This design makes IgM the most effective immunoglobulin isotype at "sponging" the free antigen out of the tissues, and proves critical—as the humoral response evolves—in trapping antigen so it can be presented to the lymphocytes that will ultimately refine the choice of effector mechanism. Although the affinity (binding strength) of the idiotype for the epitope may not be strong early in the immune response, the IgM molecule possesses the highest avidity (number of antigen-binding sites available to bind epitopes) of any immunoglobulin molecule produced in the body.

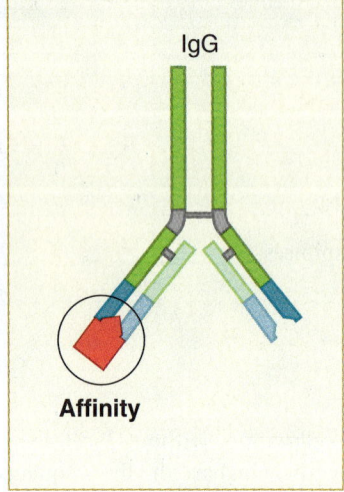
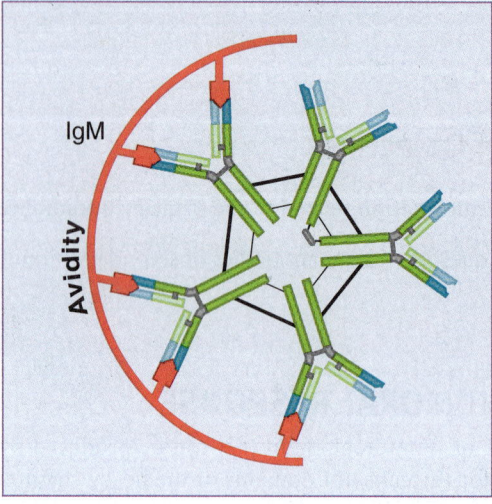

Figure 7-2. Affinity and Avidity

The multimeric structure of IgM also makes it the most effective antibody at activating complement, a set of serum proteases important in mediating inflammation and antigen removal. Serum IgM is incapable of binding to cellular Fc receptors and thus cannot act as an opsonin chapter 4) or a mediator of antibody-dependent cell-mediated cyto-toxicity (ADCC) (see chapter 8).

ANTIBODIES OF SECONDARY IMMUNE RESPONSES

Class Switching to IgG

The preponderant isotype of immunoglobulin that begins to be produced after IgM during the primary immune response is IgG. IgG is a monomeric molecule with a γ **heavy chain** and a new set of effector functions. A majority of IgG is produced in response to IFN-γ produced by the Th1 cells.

IgG exists in 4 different **subisotypes** (subclasses) in humans, IgG1, IgG2, IgG3, and IgG4, each of which exhibits a slightly different capacity in effector function. In general, however, IgG has the following characteristics:

- Activates complement
- Acts as an opsonin, enhancing phagocytosis
- Neutralizes pathogen and toxins
- Mediates ADCC

IgG is also actively transported across the placenta by receptor-mediated transport and thus plays a crucial role in protection of the fetus during gestation.

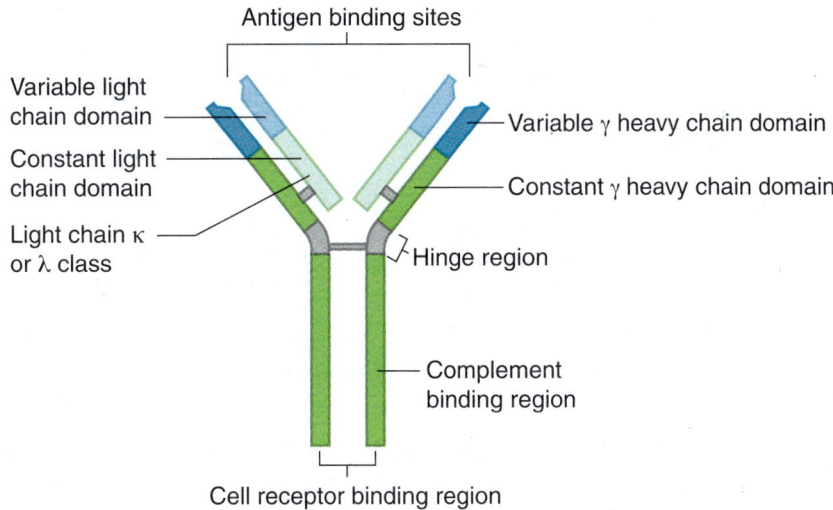

Antigen binding sites

Variable light chain domain

Constant light chain domain

Light chain κ or λ class

Variable γ heavy chain domain

Constant γ heavy chain domain

Hinge region

Complement binding region

Cell receptor binding region

Figure 7-3. Basic Structure of IgG

Class Switching to IgA

Another isotype of antibody that can be produced following class switching is IgA, though it is more commonly produced in the submucosa than in the lymph nodes and spleen. IgA generally exists as a **dimer**, held together by a J chain similar to that produced with IgM. IgA has the following characteristics:

- Serves as a major protective **defense of the mucosal surfaces of the body**
- Any pathogen that infects the mucosa will induce IgA production by the secretion of TGF-β by infected cells and to a lesser extent, IL-5.
- Functions as a neutralizing antibody by inhibiting the binding of toxins or pathogens to the mucosa of the digestive, respiratory, and urogenital systems (sole function)
- Does not activate complement, act as an opsonin, or mediate ADCC
- Exists in two isotypes, IgA1 and IgA2

The **classical pathway** is activated by antigen-antibody complexes and is probably the more phylogenetically advanced system of activation. Both IgG and IgM can activate the system by this pathway, although IgM is the more efficient.

Although the complement cascade is considered a component of the innate immune response, its overlapping stimulation of effector functions of cells of the adaptive immune response, as well as its role in enhancement of inflammation, make it a critical effector system for removal of extracellular invaders and concentration of antigens into the secondary lymphoid organs, where the adaptive immune responses are elicited.

The homing of specific memory cells to epithelial and mucosal surfaces leads to the production of specialized lymphoid aggregations along these barriers. Collectively referred to as **mucosal-associated lymphoid tissues** (MALT), they include the tonsils and Peyer patches, as well as numerous, less well-organized lymphoid accumulations in the lamina propria. Th2 cells in these sites are dedicated to providing help for class switching to IgA. Most IgA-secreting B lymphocytes and plasma cells in the body will be found in these locations.

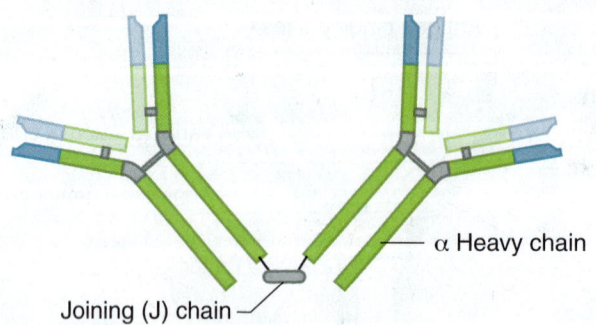

Figure 7-4. The IgA Dimer

Secretory IgA (that which is released across the mucosa of the respiratory, digestive, and urogenital tracts) differs from serum IgA in an important fashion. As the IgA dimer is produced by plasma cells and B lymphocytes, it becomes bound to poly-Ig receptors on the basolateral side of the epithelia, is endocytosed, and is released into the lumen bound to a secretory piece that is the residue of the receptor. The **secretory component** thus serves an important function in transepithelial transport, and once in the lumen of the tract, has a function in protecting the molecule from proteolytic cleavage.

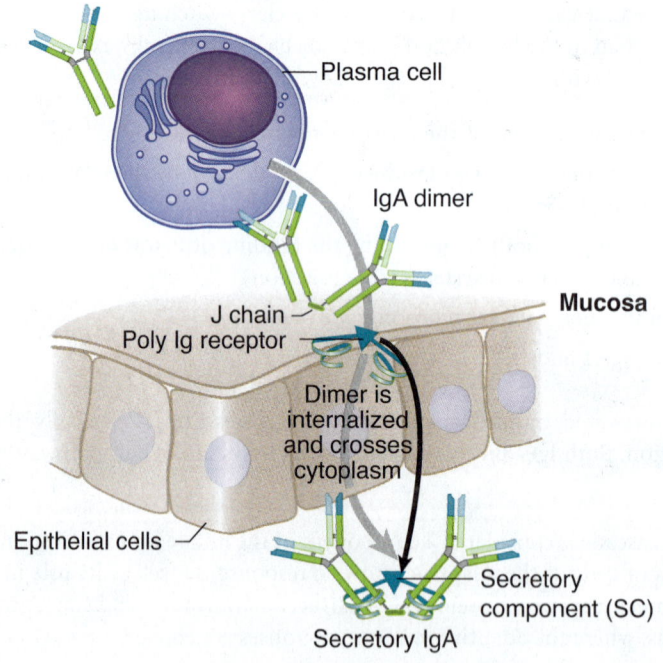

Figure 7-5. Secretory IgA

Class Switching to IgE

IgE binds directly to Fcε receptors present on mast cells, eosinophils and basophils, and is involved in elicitation of protective immune responses against parasites and allergens (see chapter 12). It does not activate complement or act as an opsonin. Its heavy chain is called the ε chain.

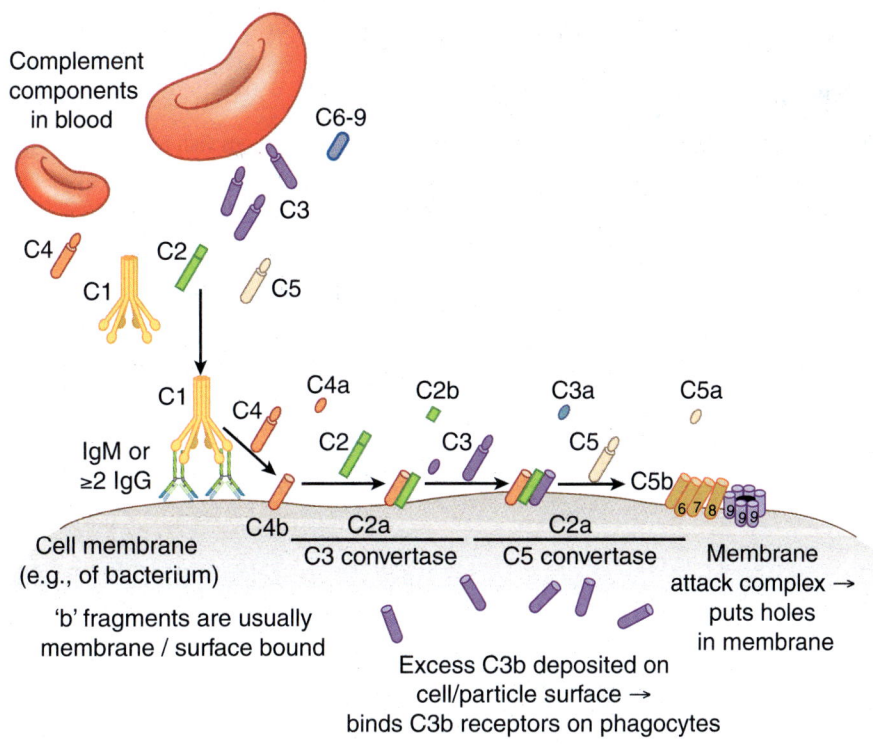

Figure 7-6. The Classical Complement Pathway

Table 7-1. Biologic Functions of the Antibody Isotypes

	IgM	IgG	IgA	IgD	IgE
Heavy chain	μ	γ	α	δ	ε
Adult serum levels (in mg/dL)	45–250	620–1,400	80–350	Trace	Trace
Functions					
Complement activation, classic pathway	+	+	–	–	–
Neutralization	+/–	+	+	–	–
Opsonization	–	+	–	–	–
Antibody-dependent cell-mediated cytotoxicity (ADCC)	–	+	–	–	+/–
Placental transport	–	+	–	–	–
Naive B-cell antigen receptor	+	–	–	+	–
Memory B-cell antigen receptor (one only)	–	+	+	–	+
Trigger mast cell granule release	–	–	–	–	+

Clinical Correlate

Immunodeficiencies Involving B Lymphocytes

Patients with B-cell deficiencies usually present with recurrent pyogenic infections with extracellular pathogens. The absence of immunoglobulins for opsonization and complement activation is a major problem (see chapter 11).

- T-cell immune system is intact.

- T-cell activities against intracellular pathogens, delayed-type hypersensitivity, and tumor rejection are normal (see chapter 8).

Cell-Mediated Immunity 8

Learning Objectives

❑ Describe the role of macrophages, B cells, cytotoxic T lymphocytes, and NK cells

❑ Demonstrate understanding of antibody dependent cell-mediated cytotoxicity

CELL-MEDIATED IMMUNITY

Cell-mediated immunity has evolved to battle two different types of pathogens:

- **Facultative intracellular pathogens**, which have adapted to living inside of phagocytic cells that are designed to kill them
- **Obligate intracellular pathogens**, which can't replicate outside of host cells

Cell-mediated immunity is dictated by the Th1 response and is mediated primarily via macrophages and CD8+ T cells. While the Th1 response is geared toward eliminating intracellular pathogens, Th cells—in general—direct all aspects of the immune system.

The primary mechanism by which Th cells direct all aspects of immunity is the secretion of cytokines. NK cells also have a role in this type of immunity; they were covered in chapter 4 and will be reviewed here.

MACROPHAGES/B CELLS

The Th1 response activates both macrophages and B cells via the cytokine IFN-γ. IFN-γ activates classical M1 macrophages to eradicate intracellular pathogens and induces B cells to class switch to produce opsonizing IgG antibodies that can assist the macrophages with phagocytosis.

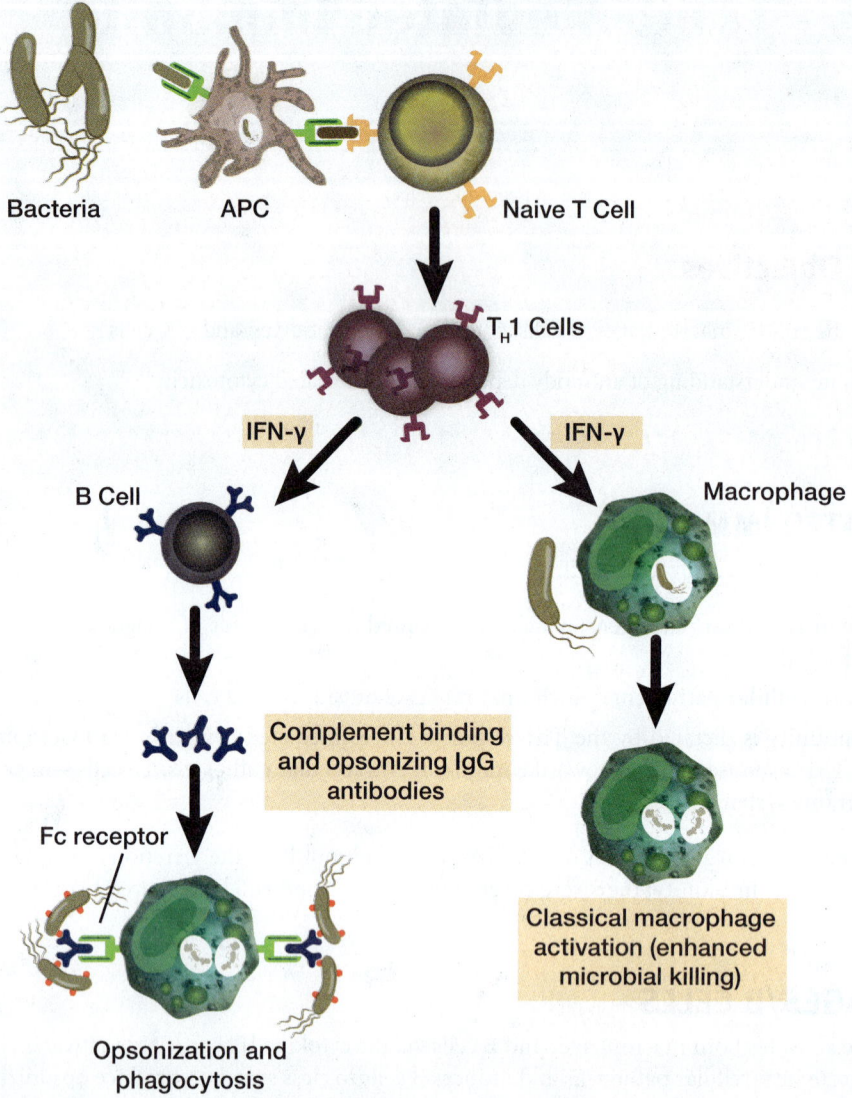

Figure 8-1. Cell-Mediated Immunity

Macrophage-Th Cell Interaction

The binding of the TCR of the naive Th cell to the MHC class II–peptide complex of the macrophage provides the first signal to the T cell to begin its activation. This provides the antigenic specificity of the response. Co-stimulatory molecules on macrophage provide the second signal, and cytokines secreted by the macrophage and the activating T cells themselves induce the proliferation (clonal expansion) and differentiation of the T cells into effector cells and memory cells. Effector cells leave the secondary lymphoid tissue, enter into circulation, and travel to the site of the infection.

Table 8-1. Summary of Macrophage Molecules and Function

Cell	CD Markers	MHC class I	Effector Mechanisms
Macrophage	CD14 (LPS receptor)	no	Nitric oxide, oxygen radicals, TNF-α

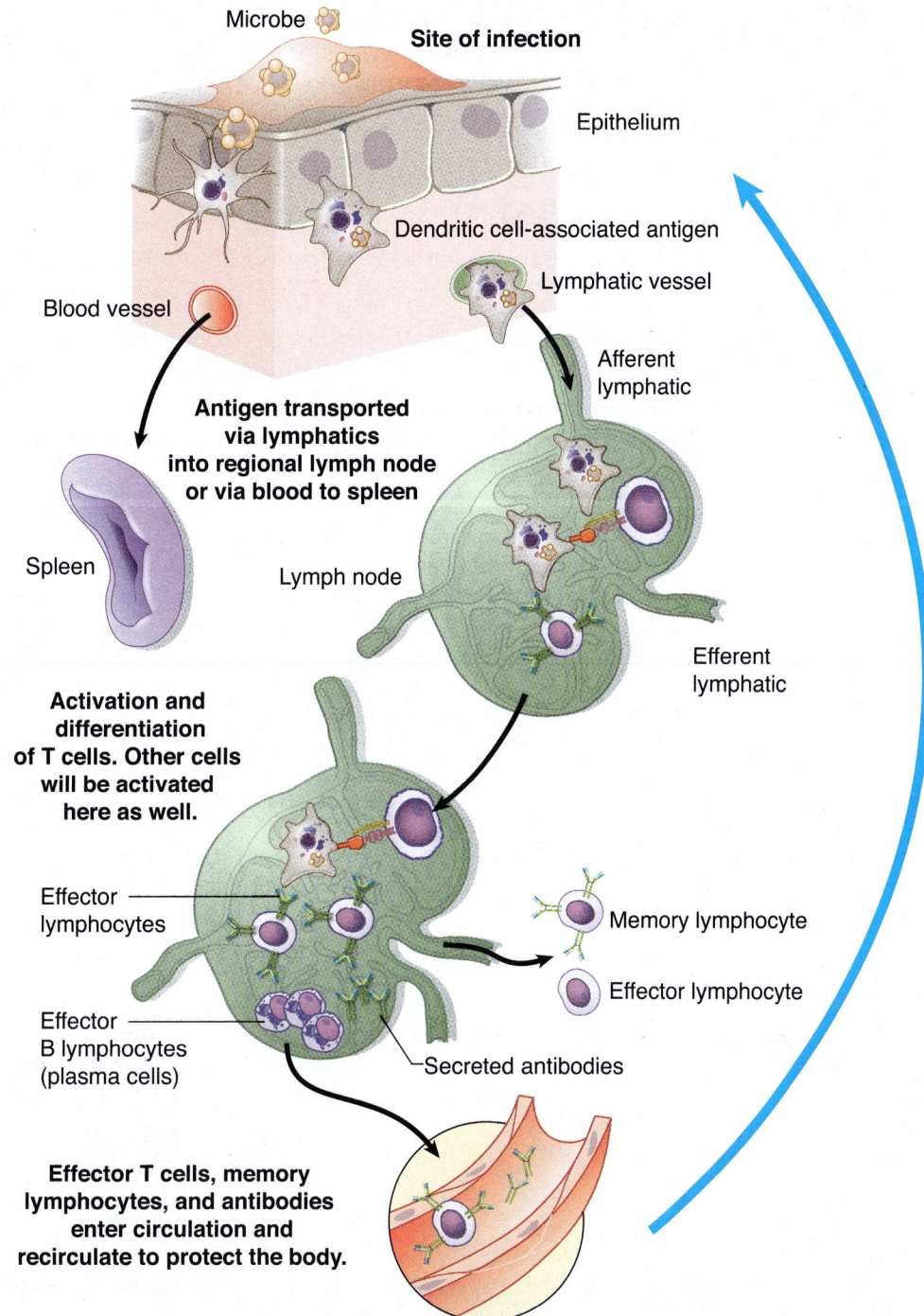

Figure 8-2. Migration of Effector Cells to the Site of Infection

The proliferation of naïve T cells in response to antigen recognition is mediated principally by an autocrine growth pathway, in which the responding T cell secretes its own growth-promoting cytokines and also expresses receptor molecules for these factors. IL-2 is the most important growth factor for T cells and stimulates the proliferation of clones of T cells specific to that antigen. Additionally, the T cells provide IFN-γ, which promotes macrophage activation that also helps to activate Th cells. The production of IL-12 by the macrophage also helps to activate the Th cells. Together, IL-12 and IFN-γ also help to promote the differentiation of the naïve Th cell into a Th1 cell.

The reaction mediated by the Th1 cell via macrophage and CD8+ T cell activation is often referred to as the delayed-type hypersensitivity (DTH) reaction. Although this is the normal response of the body to intracellular pathogens, it is the exact same mechanism of cellular interactions and cytokine production as a hypersensitivity to poison ivy or nickel (see chapter 12).

CYTOTOXIC T LYMPHOCYTES (CTLS)

CTLs recognize the cell they will ultimately kill by interaction between their TCR and the MHC class I peptide complex on the surface of the target cell.

- If the cell in question is performing **normal functions** and therefore producing normal "self" peptides, there should be no CD8+ T cells that have a complementary TCR structure.

- If the cell is **infected with an intracellular pathogen or is expressing neoantigens reflective of tumor transformation**, some small proportion of those CD8+ T cells generated from the thymus should be capable of binding their TCRs to this MHC class I/non-self-peptide complex.

Unfortunately, because of the extreme polymorphism of the HLA (MHC) system in humans, when tissues are transplanted between nonidentical individuals, cells of the transplant are often targeted by CTLs as abnormal. In spite of the fact that they may only be presenting normal cellular peptides, in these cases the HLA molecules themselves are different enough to elicit an immune response (*see* chapter 13). CTLs are capable of differentiation and cloning by themselves in the presence of the appropriate MHC class I non-self peptide complex stimulus, but are much more effective in so doing if they are assisted by signals from Th1 cells. The Th1 cell secretes IL-2, which acts on CD8+ cells to enhance their differentiation and cloning. This occurs via cross priming as discussed in chapter 5. Additionally, interferons produced in the area will increase the expression of MHC molecules to make target cells more susceptible to killing.

CTLs kill their target cells by the delivery of toxic granule contents that induce the apoptosis of the cell to which they attach. This process occurs in four phases:

- Attachment to the target cell (mediated by TCR, CD8, and LFA-1 integrin)
- Activation (cytoskeletal rearrangement to concentrate granules against attached target cell)
- Exocytosis of granule contents (perforin and granzymes)
- Detachment from the target cell

The death of the target cell may be mediated in distinct fashions. First, perforin present in the CTL granules creates pores in the membrane of the target cell through which granzymes (serine proteases) enter the cell, inducing the activation of caspases, which activate the "death domain." Second, cytokines such as IFN-γ with TNF-α or TNF-β can induce apoptosis. Furthermore, activated CTLs express a membrane protein called Fas ligand (FasL), which may bind to its complementary structure, Fas, on the target cell. When this occurs, caspases are induced and death results.

Table 8-2. Summary of Cytotoxic T-Cell Markers and Function

Cell	CD Markers	MHC class I	Effector Mechanisms
CTL	CD8, CD3, TCR, CD2	Yes	Perforin, granzymes, cytokines

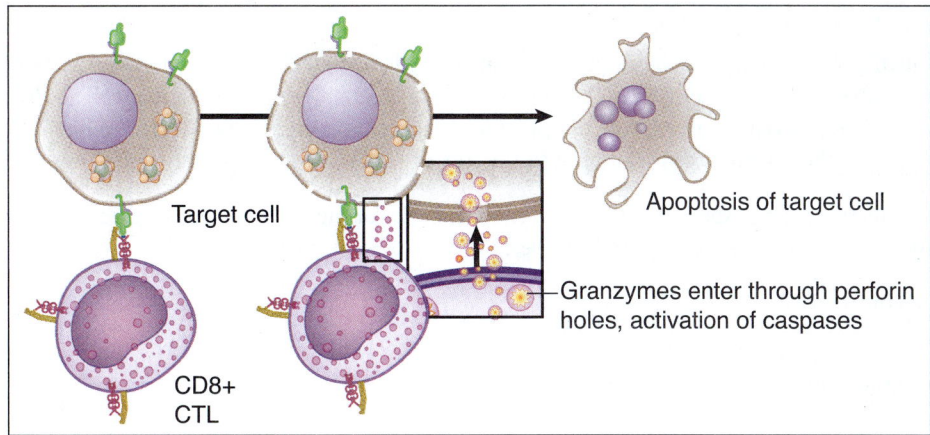

A: Perforin and Granzymes

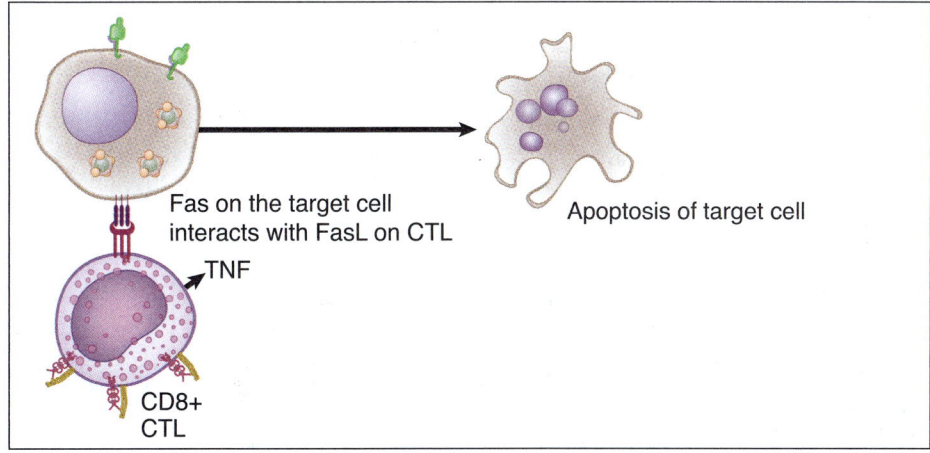

B: Fas/FasL Interaction

Figure 8-3. Mechanisms of Cytotoxic T-Cell Killing

NK CELLS

Another cell-mediated effector mechanism enhanced by the action of Th1 cells is NK cell-killing. Since the innate function of NK cells was discussed in chapter 4, the table below summarizes that information.

Table 8-3. Summary of NK Cell Markers and Function

Cell	CD Markers	MHC class I	Effector Mechanisms
NK	CD16 (FcR)* CD56 (CAM)	Inhibited by the normal expression of class I MHC via HLA-E.	Perforin, granzymes, cytokines (identical to CTL)**

*Keep in mind that CD16 is an FcR and is present on cells other than NK cells.

**The effector mechanisms of NK cell killing are identical to CTLs; the only difference between them is how they recognize the antigen.

ADCC

A final mechanism of cytotoxicity which bridges humoral and cell-mediated effector systems in the body is antibody-dependent cell-mediated cytotoxicity (ADCC). A number of cells with cytotoxic potential (NK cells, macrophages, neutrophils, and eosinophils) have membrane receptors for the Fc region of IgG (aka CD16). When IgG is specifically bound to a target cell, the cytotoxic cells can bind to the free Fc "tail" and subsequently cause lysis of the target cell.

Although these effectors are not specific for antigen, the specificity of the idiotype of the antibody directs their cytotoxicity. The mechanism of target cell killing in these cases may involve the following:

- Lytic enzymes
- Tumor necrosis factor
- Perforin/granzymes

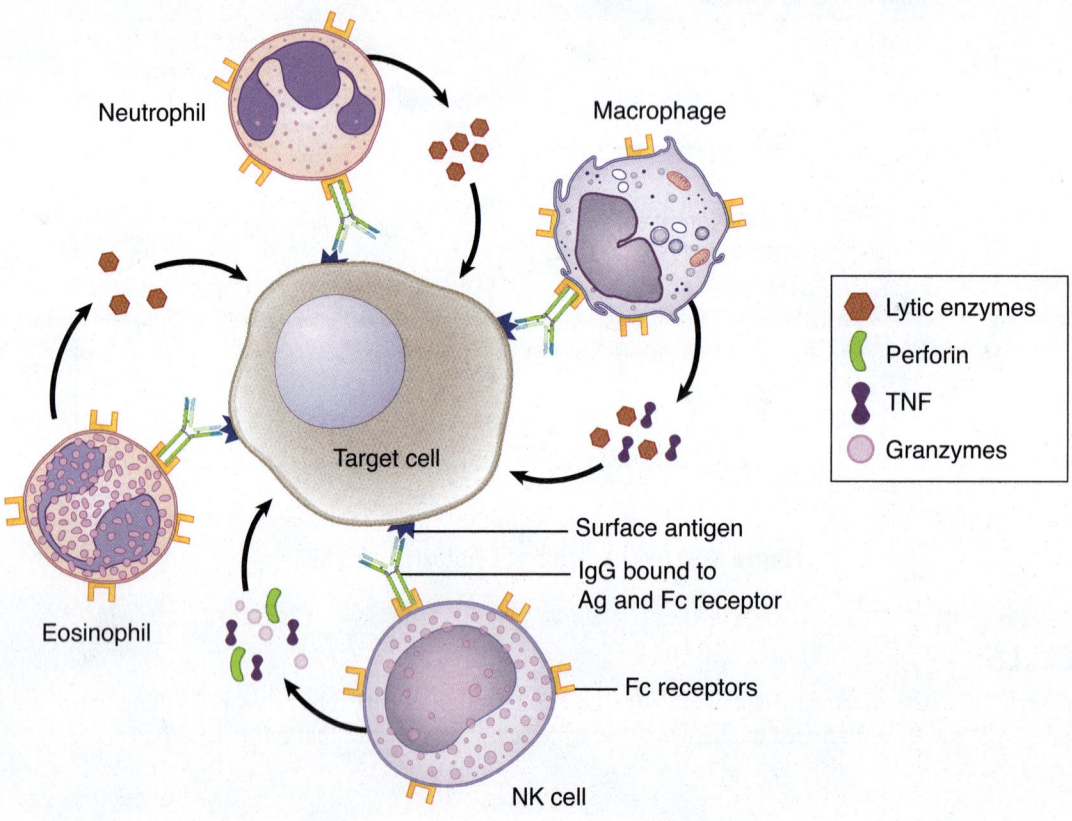

Figure 8-4. Antibody-Dependent Cell-Mediated Cytotoxicity

Immunodiagnostics 9

Learning Objectives

❏ Describe the role of serology in the diagnosis of disease

❏ Understand the process of agglutination

❏ Answer questions concerning ABO blood testing

❏ Explain the use of labelled antibodies in diagnosis

SEROLOGY

Serology is an important diagnostic tool for many diseases including infections and autoimmune disorders. The interaction of antigen and antibody that occurs in vivo and in clinical laboratory settings provides the basis for all serologically based tests.

IgM and IgG

IgM is the principal immunoglobulin of the primary immune response when antigen is first encountered. It is replaced in later responses by antibodies of different isotypes, mostly IgG in the serum. Although IgM antibodies are occasionally produced at low levels during secondary and later immunologic responses, they are always produced by cells encountering that antigen for the first time.

IgM is extremely important in diagnosis of recent infections and infections in neonates or fetuses. For example, a patient with IgM antibodies to the core antigen of HBV (HBcAb) is an important diagnostic tool because it suggests a recent or acute infection and may also be found in the window period when other antibodies may not be detectable.

Also, we can make certain assumptions based on serology using IgM in the diagnoses of neonatal or fetal infections. For example, a neonate that is making IgM specific for a virus such as rubella is infected with the virus rather than immune or protected by maternal antibodies. This is because IgM does not cross the placenta. Therefore, the only way a neonate or fetus can be producing IgM specific for a certain pathogen is if the neonate or fetus were infected with that agent.

The predominant isotype of immunoglobulin that begins to be produced after IgM during the primary immune response is IgG.

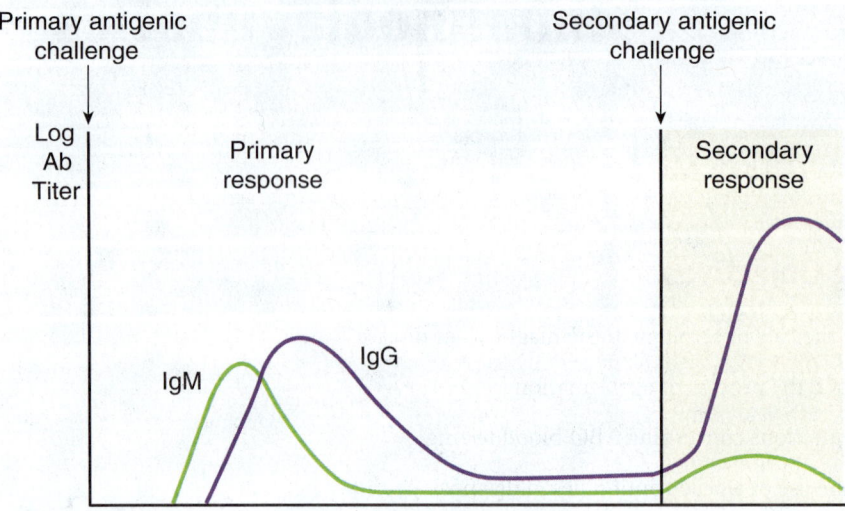

Figure 9-1. Primary and Secondary Antibody Responses

Ideotype, Isotype, and Allotype

The unique pocket created by the variable regions of the light chain and the heavy chain is called the **idiotype** of the antibody. It is the region that is specific for antigen. It is both extremely diverse and specific. Each individual is capable of producing hundreds of millions of unique idiotypes.

The **isotype** of the antibody is determined by the constant region and is encoded by the heavy chain genes. The isotype of the antibody determines its function.

The **allotype** of an antibody is an allelic difference in the same antibody isotypes that differ between people. For example, 2 individuals with the same IgG have subtle differences in their immunoglobulins due to heterogeneity which tends to be specific for individuals. A patient receiving pooled gamma globulins might react to these allotypic differences in the constant regions which may result in type III hypersensitivity reactions.

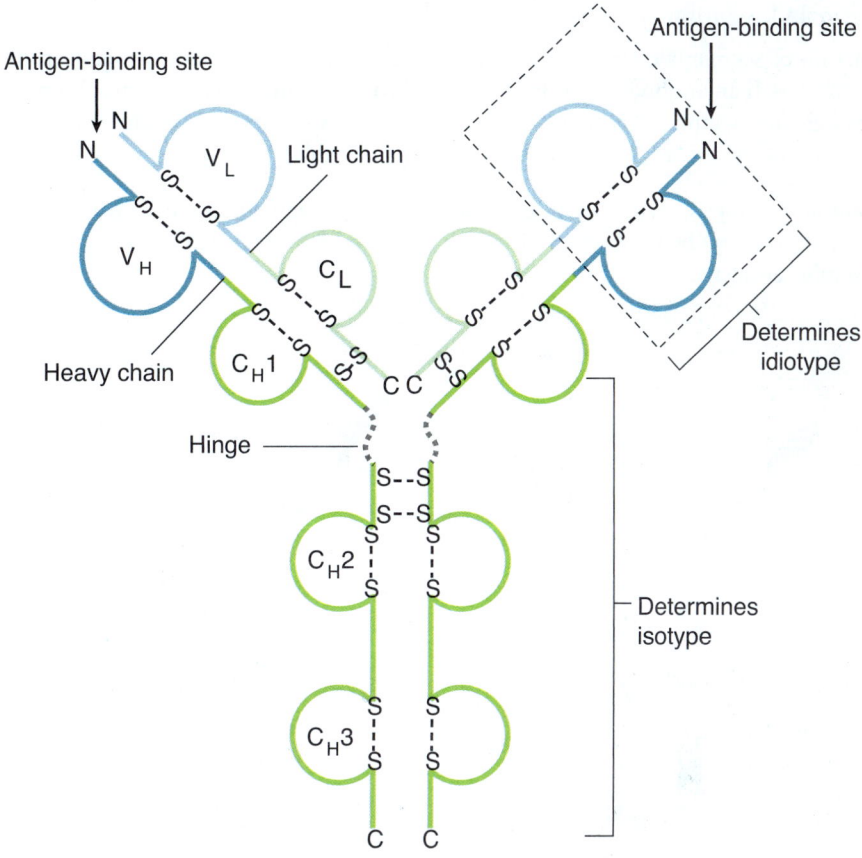

Figure 9-2. B-Lymphocyte Antigen Recognition Molecule (Membrane-Bound Immunoglobulin)

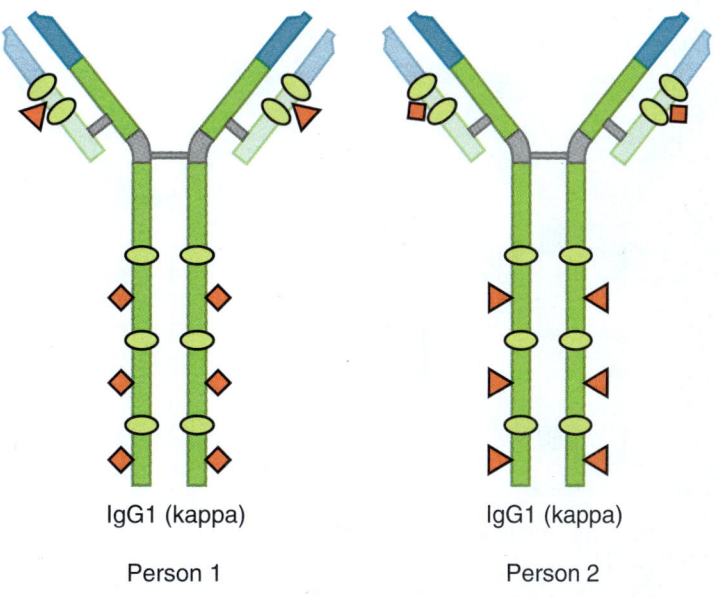

IgG1 (kappa)　　　　IgG1 (kappa)

Person 1　　　　　　Person 2

Figure 9-3. Allotypes

Papain versus Pepsin Digestion

The biologic function of segments of the antibody molecule was first elucidated by digestion of these molecules with proteolytic enzymes. If an antibody molecule is digested with papain, cleavage occurs above the disulfide bonds that hold the heavy chains together. This generates three separate fragments, two of which are called Fab (fragment antigen binding), and one of which is called Fc (fragment crystallizable).

Cleavage of the antibody molecule with pepsin generates one large fragment called F(ab′)2 and a digested Fc fragment. The bridging of antigens by antibody molecules is required for agglutination of particulate antigens or the precipitation of soluble antigens.

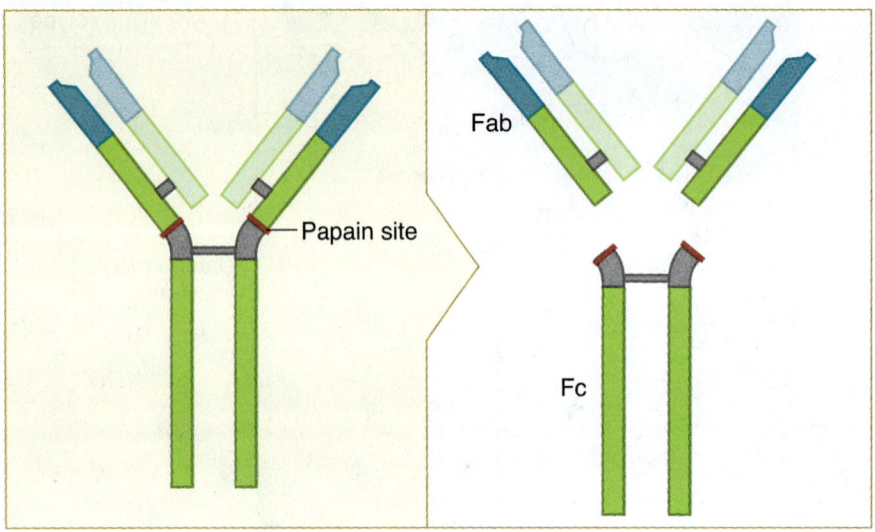

Proteolytic Cleavage with Papain

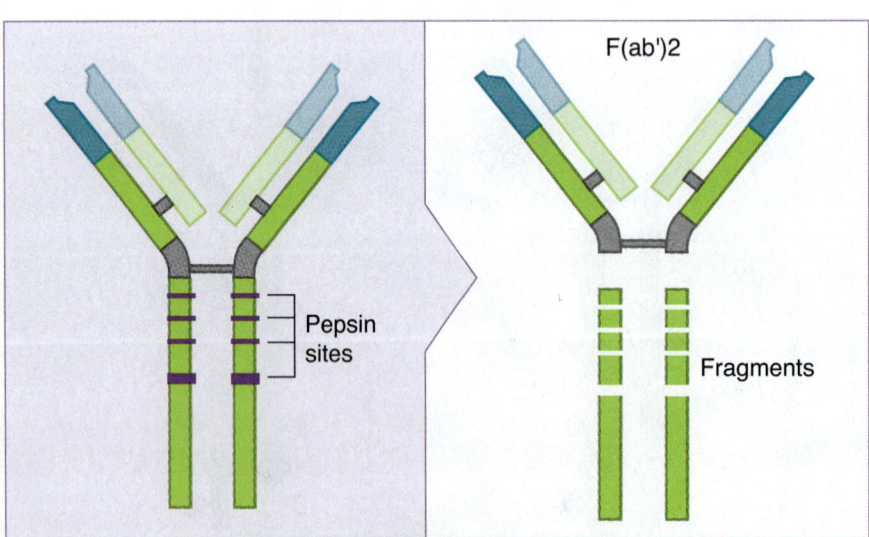

Proteolytic Cleavage with Pepsin

Figure 9-4. Proteolytic Cleavage of Immunoglobulin by Papain/Pepsin

Zone of Equivalence

Interaction of antigen and antibody occurs in vivo, and in clinical settings it provides the basis for all serologically based assays. The formation of immune complexes produces a visible reaction that is the basis of precipitation and agglutination assays. Agglutination and precipitation are maximized when multiple antibody molecules share the binding of multiple antigenic determinants, a condition known as **equivalence**.

In vivo, the precipitation of such complexes from the blood is critical to the trapping of pathogens and the initiation of the immune response in the secondary lymphoid organs, as well as the initiation of the pathologic phase of many immune complex-mediated diseases. In vitro, the kinetics of such reactions can be observed by titration of antigen against its specific antibody.

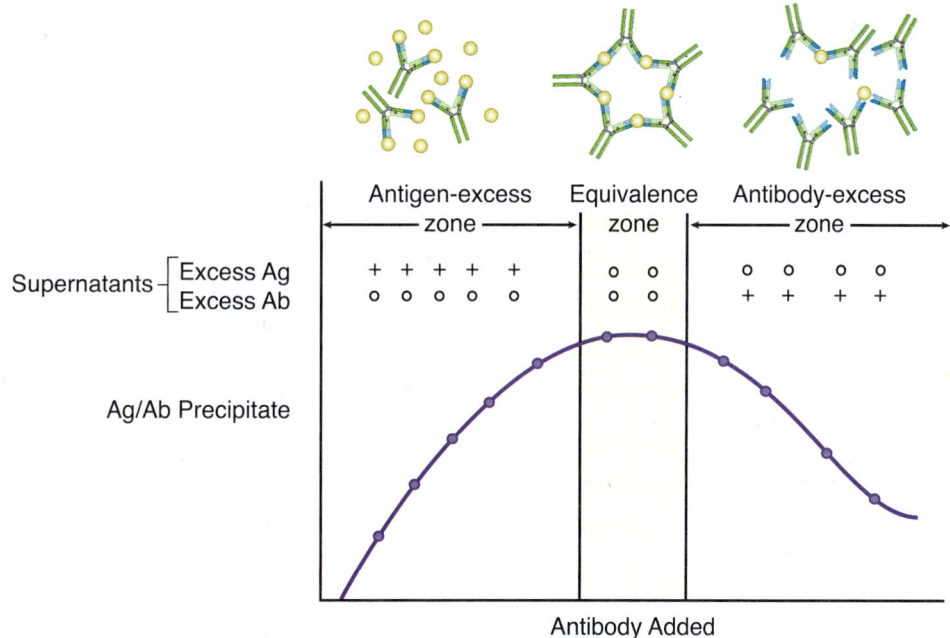

Figure 9-5. Precipitation of Ag–Ab Complexes during Titration of Ag with Ab

This figure demonstrates the normal progression of the antibody response during many infectious diseases.

- At the **start of the infection**, the patient is in a state of antigen excess; the pathogen is proliferating in the host and the development of specific antibodies has not yet begun.
- As the patient begins to make an **adequate antibody response**, he enters the equivalence zone; all available antigen is complexed with antibody, and neither free antigen nor free antibody can be detected in the serum.
- Finally, as the **infection is resolved**, the patient enters the antibody excess zone, when more antibody is being produced than is necessary to precipitate all available antigen.

The clinical demonstration of this phenomenon is most easily seen in our use of the serologic diagnosis of hepatitis B infection.

- Early in the course of this infection, HBsAg is easily detectable in the blood. The patient is in the antigen excess zone for this antigen.
- As the patient enters the window period (the equivalence zone), the HBsAg disappears from the circulation because it is being removed by antibody precipitation.
- Finally, antibody titers (HBsAb) rise in the serum as the patient enters the antibody excess zone and resolves the infection.

Although the "window period" in the hepatitis B infection is used exclusively to note the absence of HBsAg and HBsAb from the serum (only antigen–antibody response that has a clinical significance in the prognosis of disease). An equivalence zone is a universal stage in the development of any antibody–antigen interaction.

Monoclonal versus Polyclonal Antiserum

Polyclonal antiserum is generally produced in an individual naturally during any type of infection. It represents many different clones of B cells that are making antibodies to many different epitopes on an antigen; therefore a heterogenous complex mixture of antibodies is produced. Alternatively, polyclonal antiserum can be produced by inoculating an animal such as a mouse, rabbit or goat. This is done to produce commercial antiserum that can be purchased and utilized in laboratories.

Monoclonal antibodies are produced by one clone of B cells with specificity for the exact same epitope on an antigen. Monoclonal antibodies are produced in the laboratory and are used in all aspects of medicine from diagnostics to treatments for various types of cancer and autoimmune diseases.

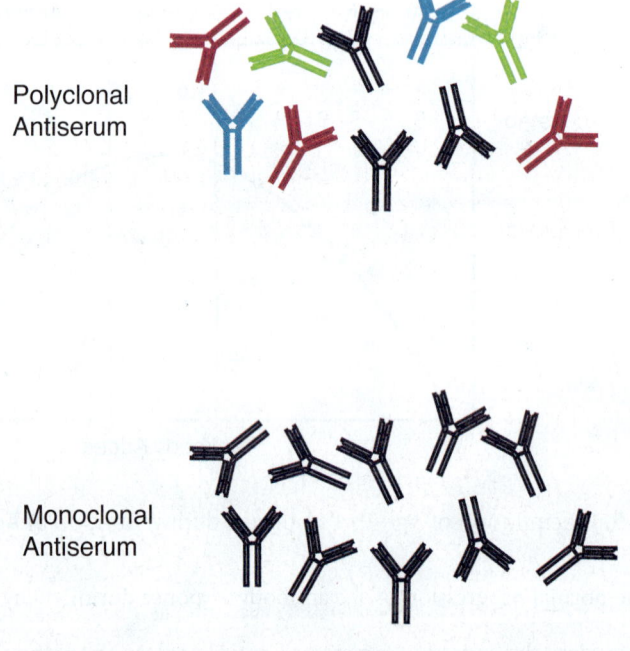

Polyclonal Antiserum

Monoclonal Antiserum

Figure 9-6. Polyclonal versus Monoclonal Antibodies

Direct versus Indirect Serologic Tests

Direct serologic testing utilizes a known antiserum in order to detect an unknown antigen, either foreign or self. Direct tests are qualitative and provide results relatively quickly. They are used mostly for screening purposes.

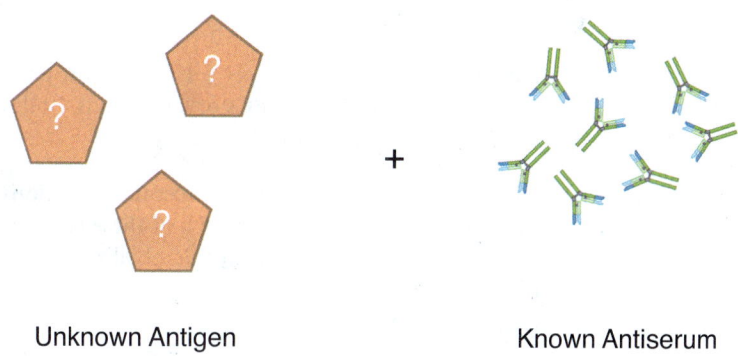

Figure 9-7. Direct Serologic Test

Indirect serologic testing utilizes antibodies from the patient that may be specific for either self or foreign antigen. This test is based on the concept that antibodies are produced in response to a specific disease state. Indirect tests may be qualitative and used for screening purposes or quantitative, which provides the amount of antibody in the patient's serum. Quantitative tests are also called antibody titers. A titer is often done to follow the progression of disease in a patient by looking for an increase or decrease in the level of antibodies. A titer involves diluting the patient's serum out to see how dilute the serum can be and still detect antigens in a solution.

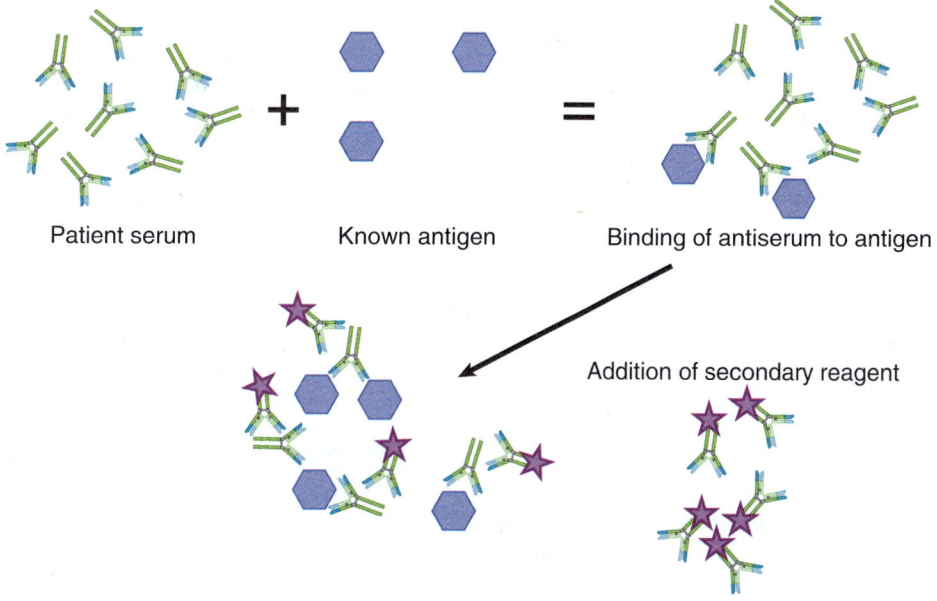

Figure 9-8. Indirect Serologic Test

Most immunologic tests can be performed using direct or indirect measures. Indirect tests are generally more specific, resulting in fewer false-positives. The Coombs, ELISA, and fluorescent antibody tests are all examples of tests that can be utilized in either a direct or indirect manner.

AGGLUTINATION

Agglutination tests are widespread in clinical medicine and are simply a variation on precipitation reactions. In agglutination reactions, the antigen is a particulate antigen such as RBCs or latex beads. Both will clump up to form of a lattice of antibody-bound particles in the presence of appropriate antibodies.

- Latex bead agglutination tests are available for the diagnosis of cerebrospinal infections such as *Haemophilus, pneumococcus, meningococcus, and Cryptococcus*. In each of these cases, antibodies against these organisms are conjugated to latex beads, and the presence of microbial antigens in the CSF is detected by the subsequent agglutination of those beads.
- RBC agglutination reactions are important in defining ABO blood groups, diagnosing Epstein-Barr virus infection (the monospot test), and identifying Coombs test for Rh incompatibility.

Coombs Test

Two variations of the Coombs test exist. The **direct Coombs** is designed to identify maternal anti-Rh antibodies that are already bound to infant RBCs or antibodies bound to RBCs in patients with autoimmune hemolytic anemia.

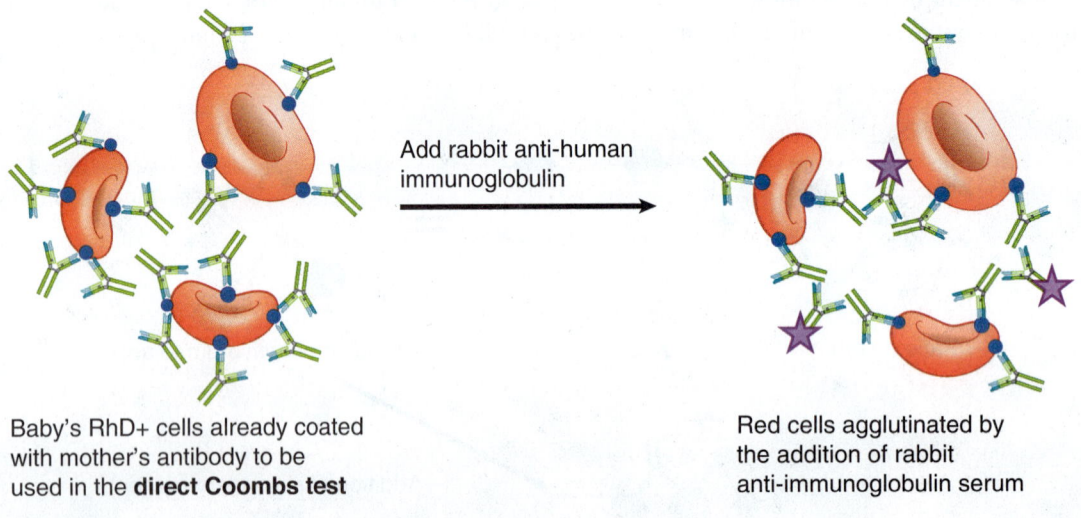

Add rabbit anti-human immunoglobulin

Baby's RhD+ cells already coated with mother's antibody to be used in the **direct Coombs test**

Red cells agglutinated by the addition of rabbit anti-immunoglobulin serum

Figure 9-9. Direct Coombs Test

The **indirect Coombs test** is designed to identify Rh-negative mothers who are producing anti-Rh antibodies of the IgG isotype, which may be transferred across the placenta harming Rh-positive fetuses. The indirect Coombs is also used in the diagnosis of transfusion reactions.

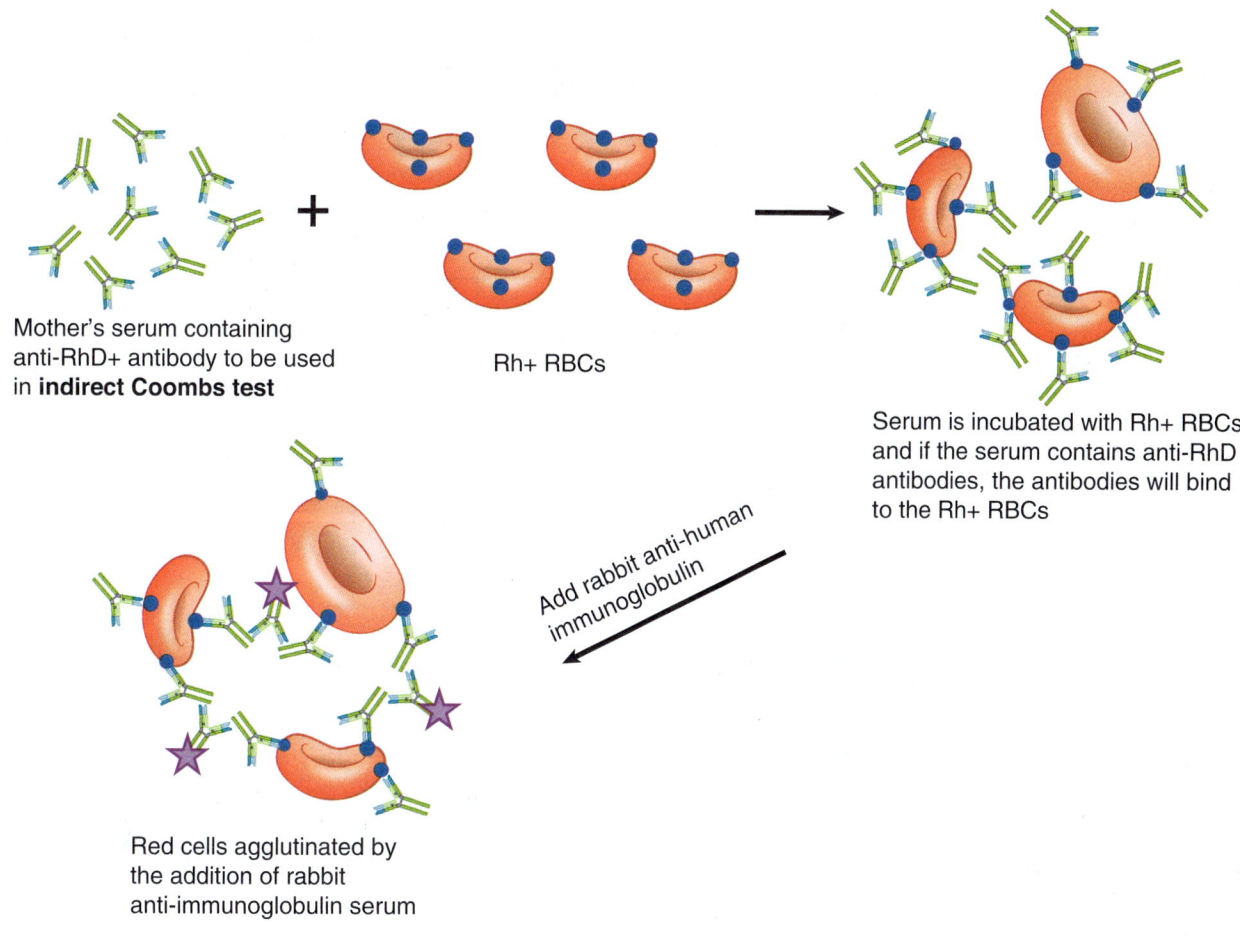

Mother's serum containing
anti-RhD+ antibody to be used
in **indirect Coombs test**

Rh+ RBCs

Serum is incubated with Rh+ RBCs
and if the serum contains anti-RhD
antibodies, the antibodies will bind
to the Rh+ RBCs

Add rabbit anti-human
immunoglobulin

Red cells agglutinated by
the addition of rabbit
anti-immunoglobulin serum

Figure 9-10. Indirect Coombs Test

ABO TESTING

ABO blood typing is a uniform first step in all tissue transplantation because ABO incompatibilities will cause hyper-acute graft rejection in the host. The ABO blood group antigens are a group of glycoprotein molecules expressed on the surface of erythrocytes and endothelial cells. Natural isohemagglutinins (IgM antibodies that will agglutinate the glycoprotein molecules on the red blood cells of nonidentical individuals) are produced in response to similar molecules expressed on the intestinal normal flora. A person is protected by self-tolerance from producing antibodies that would agglutinate his own red blood cells, but will produce those agglutinins that will react with the red blood cells from other individuals.

A: agglutination
N: no agglutination

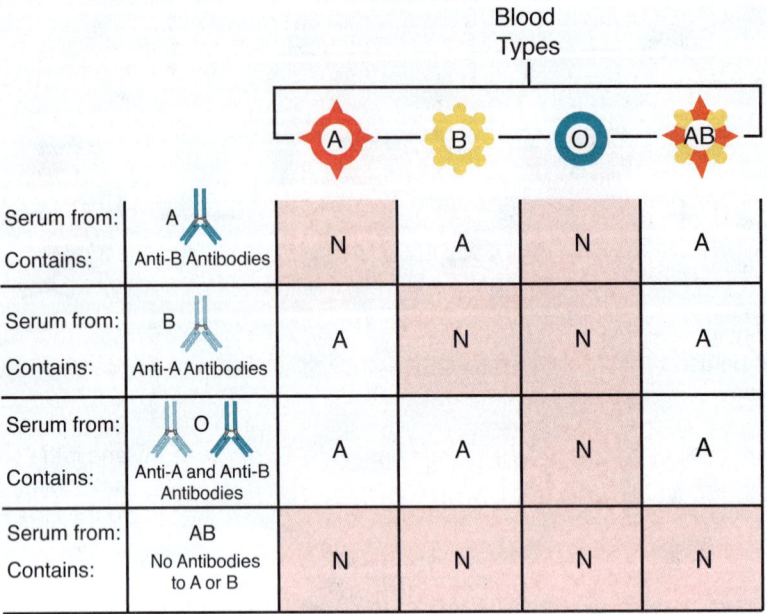

Figure 9-11. Agglutination Test for Blood Typing

LABELED ANTIBODY SYSTEMS

Labeled antibody systems are utilized for the detection of antigens, which may be either self or foreign. These antigens can be visualized using a combination of specific antibody that is labeled or tagged with a compound used for its detection. Common tags include fluorescent compounds and enzymes.

Each of the following discussed is an example of a labeled antibody system. Additionally, fluorescent antibody tests and ELISAs can be done using either direct or indirect tests as described previously.

Fluorescent Antibody Tests

The **direct fluorescent antibody test (DFA)** is used to detect and localize antigen in the patient. The tissue sample to be tested is treated with antibodies against that particular antigen that have been labeled with a fluorescent dye. If the antigen is present in the tissues, the fluorescent-labeled antibodies will bind, and their binding can be detected with a microscope. Variations of this test are used to diagnose respiratory syncytial virus, herpes simplex 1 and 2, rabies in animal tissues, and *Pneumocystis* infections.

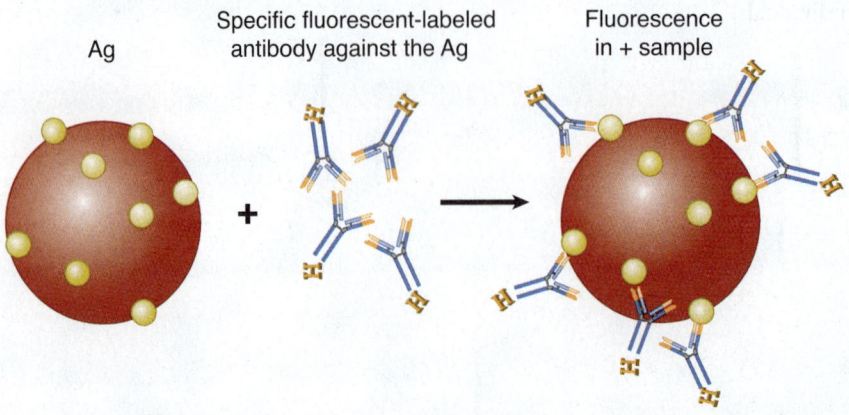

Figure 9-12. Direct Fluorescent Antibody (DFA) Test

The **indirect fluorescent antibody test (IFA)** is used to detect pathogen-specific antibodies in the patient. In this case, a laboratory-generated sample of infected tissue is mixed with serum from the patient. A fluorescent labeled anti-immunoglobulin is then added. If binding of antibodies from the patient to the tissue sample occurs, then the fluorescent antibodies can be bound and detected by microscopy. This technique can be used to detect autoantibodies in various autoimmune diseases.

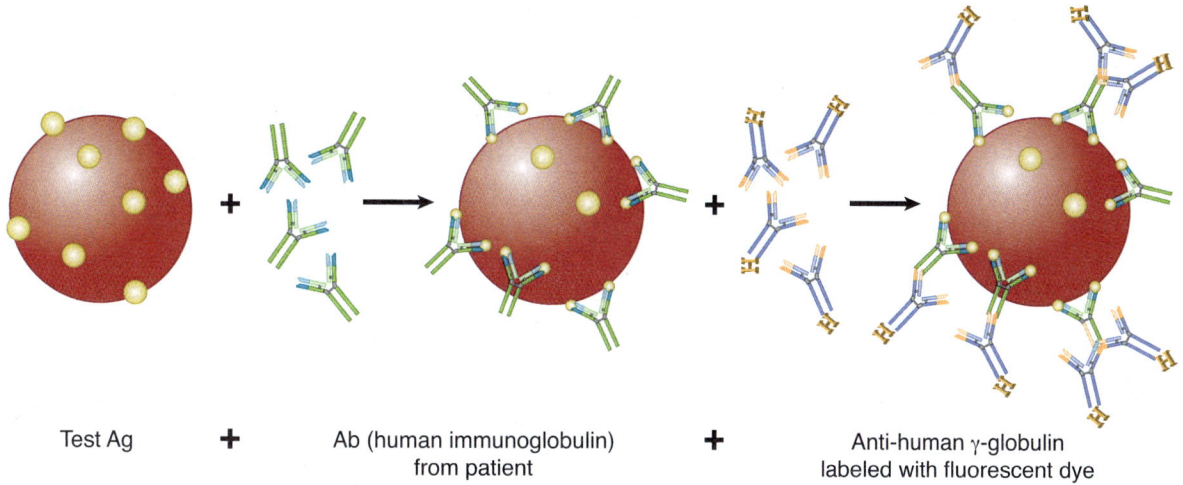

Test Ag   **+**   Ab (human immunoglobulin)   **+**   Anti-human γ-globulin
                      from patient   labeled with fluorescent dye

Figure 9-13. Indirect Fluorescent Antibody (IFA) Test

If the test Ag is fluorescent following these steps,
then the patient's serum had antibody against this antigen.

Enzyme-linked Immunosorbent Assay (ELISA)

The ELISA is an extremely sensitive test (as little as 10^{-9} g of material can be detected). It can be used to detect the presence of hormones, drugs, antibiotics, serum proteins, infectious disease antigens, and tumor markers. It does so by utilizing a chromogenic substrate that undergoes an enzyme-mediated color change.

In the screening test for HIV infection, the ELISA is used with the p24 capsid antigen coated onto microtiter plates. The serum from the patient is then added, followed by addition of an enzyme-labeled antihuman immunoglobulin. Finally, the chromogenic substrate is added, and the production of a color change in the well can be observed.

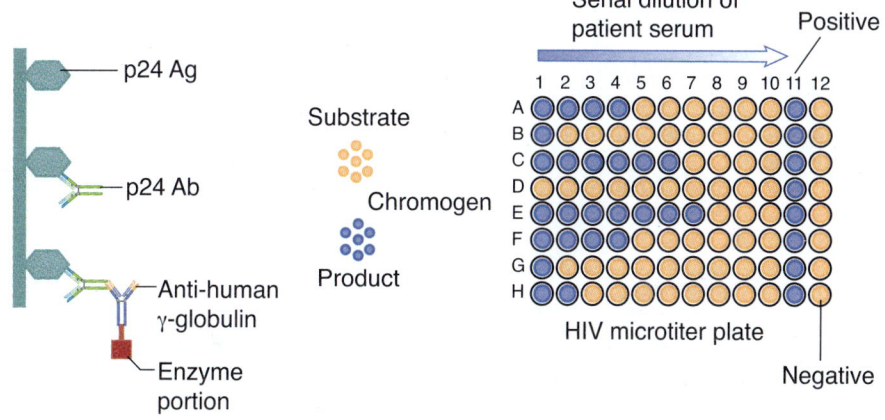

Figure 9-14. ELISA Test

Learning Objectives

❏ Explain information related to vaccinations and secondary/subsequent responses

❏ Differentiate between killed, live, and component of vaccines

❏ Differentiate between bacterial and viral vaccines

❏ Answer questions about acquisition of immunoglobulins in the fetus and neonate

VACCINATION

Vaccination is a true milestone of medicine and has saved countless lives from preventable diseases. The concept dates back into the 1100s when the Chinese practiced the art of variolation. However, the practice is credited to Edward Jenner in 1798, when he used a strain of cowpox virus to protect a child from smallpox.

This chapter will discuss the science behind vaccination as well as a summary of the types of vaccine currently used in medicine.

SECONDARY AND SUBSEQUENT RESPONSES

When an antigen is introduced into the system a second time, the response of lymphocytes is accelerated and the result amplified over that of the primary immune response. The increased speed of this response is due to the presence of the memory-cell progeny of the primary response throughout the body. The increased amplitude of effector production is due to the fact that activation and cloning begin from a much larger pool of respondents.

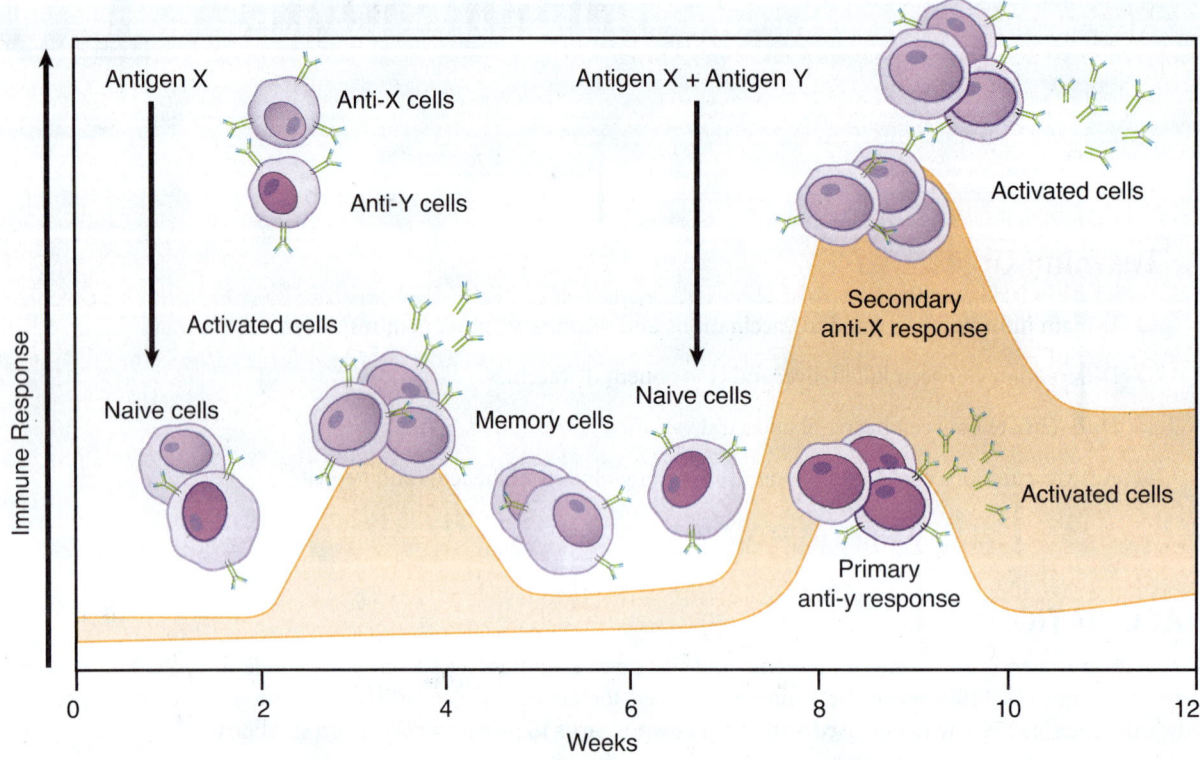

Figure 10-1. Primary and Secondary Immune Responses

Table 10-1. Primary versus Secondary Immune Response

Feature	Primary Response	Secondary Response
Time lag after immunization	5–10 days	1–3 days
Peak response	Small	Large
Antibody isotype	IgM, then IgG	Increasing IgG, IgA, or IgE
Antibody affinity	Variable to low	High (affinity maturation)
Inducing agent	All immunogens	**Protein** antigens
Immunization protocol	High dose of antigen (often with adjuvant)	Low dose of antigen (often without adjuvant)

TYPES OF IMMUNITY

Immunity to infectious organisms can be achieved by active or passive immunization. The goal of passive immunization is transient protection or alleviation of an existing condition, whereas the goal of active immunization is the elicitation of protective immunity and immunologic memory. Active and passive immunization can be achieved by both natural and artificial means.

Table 10-2. Types of Immunity

Type of Immunity	Acquired Through	Examples
Natural	Passive means	Placental IgG transport, colostrum
Natural	Active means	Recovery from infection
Artificial	Passive means	Horse antivenin against black widow spider bite, snake bite
		Horse antitoxin against botulism, diphtheria
		Pooled human immune globulin versus hepatitis A and B, measles, rabies, varicella zoster or tetanus
		"Humanized" monoclonal antibodies versus RSV*
Artificial	Active means	Hepatitis B component vaccine
		Diphtheria, tetanus, pertussis toxoid vaccine
		Haemophilus capsular vaccine
		Polio live or inactivated vaccine
		Measles, mumps, rubella attenuated vaccine
		Varicella attenuated vaccine

*Monoclonal antibodies prepared in mice but spliced to the constant regions of human IgG

Passive Immunotherapy

Passive immunotherapy may be associated with several risks:

- Introduction of antibodies from other species can generate IgE antibodies, which may cause systemic anaphylaxis. The generation of IgE after infusion with even human gamma globulins is particularly an issue in persons with selective IgA deficiency (1:700 in population) as IgA is a molecule they have not encountered before. These patients can, however, be given IgA depleted globulins.

- Introduction of antibodies from other species can generate IgG or IgM anti-isotype antibodies, which form complement-activating immune complexes, leading to possible type III hypersensitivity reactions.

- Introduction of antibodies from humans can elicit responses against minor immunoglobulin polymorphisms or allotypes.

TYPES OF VACCINE

Live Vaccines

- **Attenuated** (attenuated = weak)
  - Comprised of **live** organisms which lose capacity to cause disease but still replicate in the host
  - Best at stimulating both a humoral and cell mediated immune response, as they mimic the natural infection and typically elicit lifelong immunity
  - Typically, one dose provides immunity but two doses are used to ensure seroconversion in most individuals
  - Dangerous for immunocompromised patients because even attenuated viruses can cause them significant disease; since attenuated vaccines are comprised of live organisms, there is slight potential to revert back to a virulent form
  - Live viral vaccines:
    - Recommended in the United States:
      - Measles, mumps and rubella (MMR)
      - Varicella zoster (VZV) (for both chicken pox and zoster [shingles])
      - Rotavirus
      - Influenza (flu-mist)
    - Available in the United States but recommended only under special circumstances:
      - Polio (sabin)
      - Smallpox
      - Yellow fever
- **Non-attenuated**
  - Used by U.S. military against adenovirus types 4 and 7
  - Enteric coated, live, non-attenuated virus preparation
  - Produces an asymptomatic intestinal infection, thereby inducing mucosal IgA memory cells; these cells then populate the mucosal immune system throughout the body
  - Vaccine recipients are thus protected against adenovirus acquired by aerosol, which could otherwise produce pneumonia (this is the **only example** of a live non-attenuated vaccine that is used)

Killed Vaccines

- Utilize organisms that are killed so they can **no longer** replicate in the host
- Inactivated by chemicals rather than heat, as heat will often denature the immunogenic epitopes
- Typically require several doses to achieve desired response
- Predominantly produce humoral immunity
- Killed (inactivated) vaccines:
  - Rabies
  - Influenza
  - Polio (Salk)
  - Hepatitis A

Toxoid Vaccines

- Made from inactivated exotoxins from toxigenic bacteria
- Prevent disease but not infection
- Toxoid vaccines:
  - Diphtheria, tetanus, and acellular pertussis (DTaP)*

*The DTaP vaccine prep is composed of toxoids from both diphtheria and tetanus, while the pertussis is comprised of whole inactivated pertussis. The DTaP vaccine is considered safe with few side effects, and is the vaccine currently used in the United States.

Polysaccharide Vaccines

- Comprised of the capsular polysaccharide found in many bacteria
- Are only capable of producing IgM because of the inability of polysaccharide to activate Th cells (which require protein to become activated)
- Have largely been replaced with conjugate vaccines (see below)
- Polysaccharide vaccine(s):
  - *Streptococcus pneumoniae*, pneumococcal polysaccharide (PPSV23)
    - Comprised of 23 capsular serotypes of the most invasive and common strains of *S. pneumoniae*
    - Indicated for use in adults age >65 or special circumstances, i.e., splenectomy, COPD

Conjugate Vaccines

- Comprised of capsular polysaccharide conjugated to protein (usually a toxoid; this creates a T cell-dependent immune response with class switching
- Creates a booster response to multiple doses
- Conjugate vaccines:
  - *Haemophilus influenzae type b* (Hib)
  - *Streptococcus pneumoniae*, Pneumococcal conjugate (PCV13)
    - Comprised of 13 capsular serotypes
    - Indicated for use in infants
  - *Neisseria meningitidis*

Component Vaccines

- Comprised of an immunodominant protein from the virus that is grown in yeast cells
  - For example, in the hepatitis B vaccine, the gene coding for the HBsAg is inserted into yeast cells, which then releases this molecule into the culture medium; the molecule is then purified and used as the immunogen in the vaccine
- Component vaccines:
  - HBV
    - Hepatitis B surface antigen
- HPV
  - Quadrivalent vaccine with serotypes 6, 11, 16 and 18
  - 9-valent vaccine (Gardasil 9) to prevent >90% of cancers, as opposed to the quadrivalent vaccine which can protect up to 70% of cancers; contains serotypes 6, 11, 16, 18, 31, 33, 45, 52 and 58
    - Released in February 2015

ACQUISITION OF IMMUNOGLOBULINS IN THE FETUS AND NEONATE

Persistence of maternal Ab affects vaccinations.

- Live attenuated virus vaccines are given only age >12 months because residual maternal antibodies would inhibit replication and the vaccine would fail.

- When children are at exceptionally high risk for exposure to a pathogen, this rule is sometimes broken, but administration of vaccine at age <6–9 months is almost always associated with the need for repeated booster inoculations.

- IgM is the only isotype useful in diagnosing infections in neonates.

- Normal infants have few infections during first few months because of maternal IgG.

- Children with immune deficiencies don't become ill until maternal IgG is low.

- Infants have 20% of adult IgA at age 12 months, so colostrum is important.

Hypersensitivity and Autoimmune Disease

11

Learning Objectives

❏ Differentiate type I (immediate), type II (antibody-mediated), type III (immune complex), and type IV (T-cell-mediated) hypersensitivity

❏ Answer questions about the pathogenesis of autoimmunity

Hypersensitivity diseases are conditions in which tissue damage is caused by immune responses. They may result from uncontrolled or excessive responses against **foreign** antigens or from a **failure of self-tolerance**, in which case they are called **autoimmune diseases**.

The 2 principal factors which determine the clinical and pathologic consequences of such conditions are the **type of immune response** elicited and the **nature and location of the inciting antigen**.

What the hypersensitivity reactions have in common:

- The first exposure to the antigen "sensitizes" lymphocytes.
- Subsequent exposures elicit a damaging reaction.
- The response is specific to a particular antigen or a cross-reacting substance.

Hypersensitivity diseases are classified on the basis of the effector mechanism responsible for tissue injury, and four types are commonly recognized.

Table 11-1. Classification of Immunologic Diseases

Type of Hypersensitivity	Immune Mechanisms	Mechanisms of Tissue Injury
Immediate (type I)	Activation of Th2 cells resulting in the production of IgE which in turn binds to Fc R on mast cells, basophils and eosinophils	**Immediate reaction** • Degranulation and release of vasoactive amines (ie. histamine) and proteases **Late-phase reaction** • Synthesis and secretion of prostaglandins and leukotrienes • Cytokine-induced inflammation and leukocyte recruitment
Antibody-mediated (type II)	IgM and IgG against surface (cell surface or extracellular matrix)	**Complement-mediated (cytotoxic)** • Opsonization and enhances phagocytosis • Recruitment and activation of inflammatory cells **Non-cytotoxic** • Change in physiologic behavior of a cell
Immune complex–mediated (type III)	Deposition of immune complexes comprised of IgM or IgG and soluble antigen	Complement-mediated recruitment and activation of inflammatory cells resulting in some combination of arthritis, vasculitis and/or nephritis.
Delayed-type hypersensitivity (type IV)	Inflammatory cytokines, IFN-γ and IL-17, produced by CD4+ Th1 and Th17 cells, respectively.	**Cytokine-mediated tissue damage** • IFN-γ activation of macrophage • IL-17 recruitment and activation of neutrophil **Direct killing** • CTL-mediated cellular death
		CD8+ CTLs (T-cell-mediated cytolysis) Direct target cell killing, cytokine-mediated inflammation

TYPE I (IMMEDIATE) HYPERSENSITIVITY

Type I is the only type of hypersensitivity mediated by IgE antibodies and mast cells. It is manifested within minutes of the reexposure to an antigen. The IgE response is the normal protective response against many metazoan parasites, which are too large to be phagocytized or killed by other cytopathic mechanisms. Approximately 20% of all individuals in the United States, however, display this immune response against harmless environmental antigens, such as pet dander or pollen; these responses are called **atopic** or **allergic** responses.

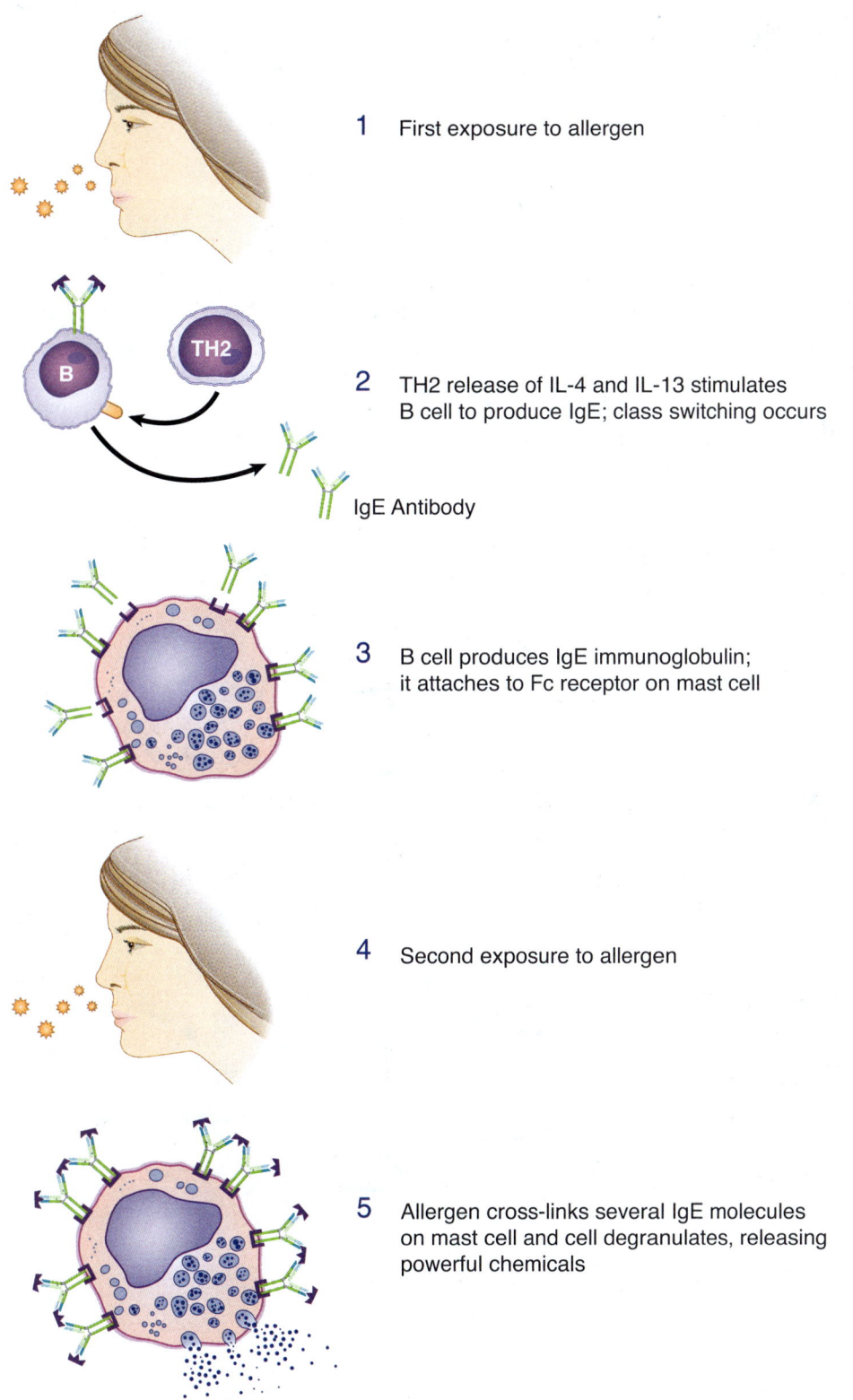

1   First exposure to allergen

2   TH2 release of IL-4 and IL-13 stimulates
     B cell to produce IgE; class switching occurs

IgE Antibody

3   B cell produces IgE immunoglobulin;
     it attaches to Fc receptor on mast cell

4   Second exposure to allergen

5   Allergen cross-links several IgE molecules
     on mast cell and cell degranulates, releasing
     powerful chemicals

Figure 11-1. Development of the Immediate Hypersensitivity Reaction

The effector cells of the immediate hypersensitivity reaction are mast cells, basophils, and eosinophils. The soluble substances they release into the site cause the symptoms of the reaction. Approximately 2-4 hours after the immediate response to release of these mediators, a **late-phase reaction** is mediated by products of the arachidonic acid cascade.

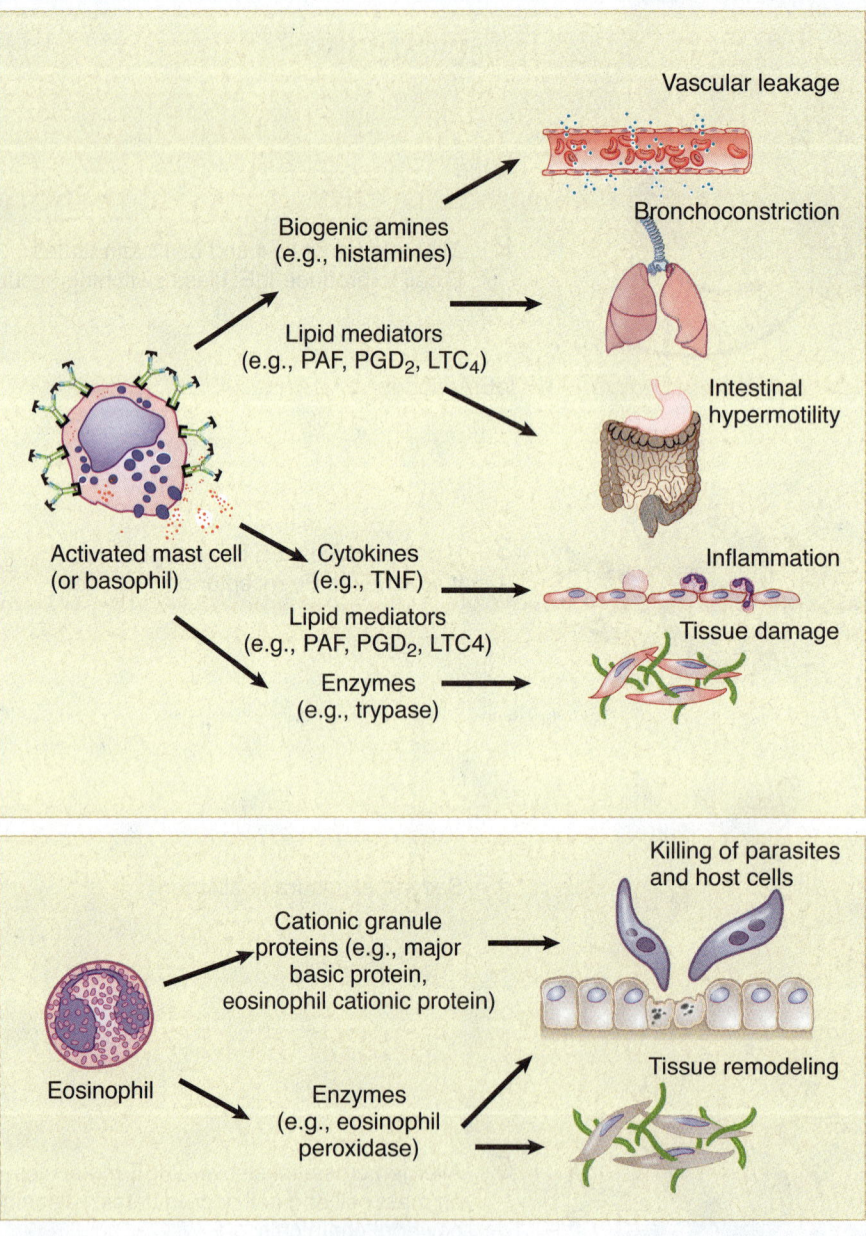

Figure 11-2. Mediators of Type I Hypersensitivity

Table 11-2. Mast Cell Mediators

Mediators Stored and Released	Effect
Histamine	Smooth muscle contraction; increased vascular permeability
Heparin	Anticoagulant
Eosinophil chemotactic factor A (multiple chemokines)	Chemotactic
Mediators Newly Synthesized from Arachidonic Acid	**Effect**
Prostaglandin D_2, E_2, $F_{2\alpha}$	Increased smooth muscle contraction and vascular permeability
Leukotrienes C_4, D_4, E_4 (lipoxygenase pathway)	Increased smooth muscle contraction and vascular permeability
Leukotriene B_4	Chemotactic for neutrophils

Table 11-3. Allergic Diseases Due to Specific Allergens and Their Clinical Manifestations

Allergic Disease	Allergens	Clinical Findings
Allergic rhinitis (hay fever)	Trees, grasses, dust, cats, dogs, mites	Edema, irritation, mucus in nasal mucosa
Systemic anaphylaxis	**Insect stings, drug reactions** Latex allergy (systemic)	Bronchial and tracheal constriction, complete vasodilation and death
Food allergies	Milk, eggs, fish, cereals, grains	Hives and gastrointestinal problems
Wheal and flare	In vivo skin testing for allergies	Local skin edema, reddening, vasodilation of vessels
Asthma	Inhaled materials	Bronchial and tracheal constriction, edema, mucus production, massive inflammation

TYPE II (ANTIBODY-MEDIATED) HYPERSENSITIVITY

Antibodies against cell surface or extracellular matrix antigens cause diseases that are **specific to the tissues** where those antigens are present; they are not usually systemic. In most cases, these antibodies are **autoantibodies**, but they may be produced against a foreign antigen that is cross-reactive with self-components of tissues.

These antibodies can cause tissue damage by three main mechanisms:

- Opsonization of cells
- Activation of the complement system which recruit neutrophils and macrophages that cause tissue damage
- Possible binding to normal cellular receptors and interference with their function

In some types of type II hypersensitivity, complement is activated and/or ADCC is active (e.g., hemolytic disease of the newborn [HDNB]). In other types, cell function is altered in the absence of complement activation and ADCC (e.g., myasthenia gravis and Graves disease). Eventually, as these diseases progress, complexes of antigen and antibody may cause localized damage, but they **do not circulate** so the damage is localized to the specific tissue.

Table 11-4. Type II Hypersensitivities

Disease	Target Antigen	Mechanism of Pathogenesis	Clinical Manifestations
Cytotoxic			
Autoimmune hemolytic anemia (HDNB)	RBC membrane proteins (Rh, I Ags)	Opsonization, phagocytosis, and complement-mediated destruction of RBCs	Hemolysis, anemia
Acute rheumatic fever	**Streptococcal cell-wall Ag;** Ab cross-reacts with myocardial Ag	Inflammation, macrophage activation	**Myocarditis, arthritis**
Goodpasture syndrome	**Type IV collagen** in basement membranes of kidney glomeruli and lung alveoli	Complement- and Fc-receptor–mediated inflammation	**Nephritis,** lung hemorrhage, **linear Ab deposits**
Transfusion reaction	ABO blood glycoproteins	IgM isohemagglutinins formed naturally in response to normal bacterial flora cause opsonization + complement activation	Hemolysis
Autoimmune thrombocytopenic purpura	Platelet membrane proteins	Ab-mediated platelet destruction through opsonization and complement activation	Bleeding
Non-cytotoxic			
Myasthenia gravis	**Acetylcholine receptor**	Ab inhibits acetylcholine binding, downmodulates receptors	**Muscle weakness, paralysis**
Graves disease	**TSH receptor**	Ab-mediated stimulation of TSH receptors	**Hyperthyroidism followed by hypothyroidism**
Type II (insulin-resistant) diabetes	Insulin receptor	Ab inhibits binding of insulin	Hyperglycemia
Pernicious anemia	Intrinsic factor of gastric parietal cells	Neutralization of intrinsic factor, decreased absorption of vitamin B12	Abnormal erythropoiesis, anemia

An important example of type II hypersensitivity is **HDNB**, also known as erythro-blastosis fetalis. In the fetus, this disease is due to transport of IgG specific for one of the Rhesus (Rh) protein antigens (RhD) across the placenta.

About 85% of people are Rh+. If a pregnant woman is Rh– and the father is Rh+, there is a chance that the fetus will also be Rh+. This situation will pose no problem in the first pregnancy, as the mother's immune system will not usually encounter fetal blood cell antigens until placental separation at the time of birth. At that time, however, Rh+ fetal red blood cells will enter the maternal circulation and stimulate a T-dependent immune response, eventually resulting in the generation of memory B cells capable of producing IgG antibody against RhD.

In a subsequent pregnancy with another Rh+ fetus, this maternal IgG can be transported across the placenta, react with fetal Rh+ red cells, and activate complement, producing hemolytic disease. Hemolytic disease of the newborn can be prevented by treating the Rh– mother with RhoGAM^{TM}, a preparation of human anti-RhD antibody, at 28 weeks of gestation and again within 72 hours after birth. This antibody effectively eliminates the fetal Rh+ cells before they can generate RhD-specific memory B cells in the mother. Anti-RhD antibody should be given to any Rh– individual following any termination of pregnancy.

TYPE III (IMMUNE COMPLEX) HYPERSENSITIVITY

The immune complexes that cause disease may involve either self or foreign antigens bound to antibodies. These immune complexes are filtered out of the circulation in the small vasculature, so their sites of ultimate damage do not reflect their sites of origin. These diseases tend to be systemic, with little tissue or organ specificity.

Table 11-5. Examples of Type III Hypersensitivities

Disease	Antigen Involved	Clinical Manifestations
Systemic lupus erythematosus[+]	**dsDNA**, Sm, other nucleoproteins	Nephritis, arthritis, vasculitis, **butterfly facial rash**
Poststreptococcal glomerulonephritis	Streptococcal cell wall Ags (may be "planted" in glomerular basement membrane)	Nephritis, **"lumpy-bumpy" deposits**
Arthus reaction	Any injected protein	Local pain and edema
Serum sickness	Various proteins	Arthritis, vasculitis, nephritis
Polyarteritis nodosa	Hepatitis B virus Ag	Systemic vasculitis

[+]Other autoimmune diseases correlated with production of antinuclear antibodies include diffuse systemic sclerosis (antibodies to DNA topoisomerase 1), limited scleroderma (CREST; antibodies to centromeric proteins) and Sjögren syndrome (antibodies to ribonucleoproteins).

TYPE IV (T-CELL–MEDIATED) HYPERSENSITIVITY

T lymphocytes may cause tissue injury by triggering delayed-type hypersensitivity (DTH) reactions or by directly killing target cells. These reactions are elicited by CD4+ Th1, Th17 cells, or CD8+ CTLs, which activate macrophages, recruit neutrophils, and induce inflammation. These T cells may be autoreactive or specific against foreign protein antigens bound to tissues. T-cell-mediated tissue injury is common during the protective immune response against persistent intracellular microbes.

Table 11-6. Examples of Type IV Hypersensitivities

Disease	Specificity of Pathogenic T Cells	Clinical Manifestations
Tuberculin test	PPD (tuberculin & mycolic acid)	Indurated skin lesion (granuloma)
Contact dermatitis	Nickel, poison ivy/oak catechols, hapten/carrier	Vesicular skin lesions, pruritus, rash
	Latex allergy (on skin)	
Hashimoto thyroiditis*	Unknown Ag in thyroid	**Hypothyroidism**
Multiple sclerosis	Myelin Basic Protein	Progressive demyelination, blurred vision, paralysis
Rheumatoid arthritis*	Unknown Ag in joint synovium (type II collagen?)	Rheumatoid factor (IgM against Fc region of IgG), alpha-cyclic citrullinated peptide (α-CCP) antibodies, chronic arthritis, inflammation, destruction of articular cartilage and bone
Insulin-dependent diabetes mellitus (type I)*	Islet-cell antigens, insulin, glutamic acid decarboxylase, others	Chronic inflammation and destruction of β cells, polydipsia, polyuria, polyphagia, ketoacidosis
Guillain-Barré syndrome*	Peripheral nerve myelin or gangliosides	Ascending paralysis, peripheral nerve demyelination
Celiac disease	CD4+ cells—gliadin, CD8+ cells—HLA class I-like molecule expressed during stress	Gluten-sensitive enteropathy
Crohn disease	Unknown Ag, commensal bacteria?	Chronic intestinal inflammation due to Th1 and Th17 cells, obstruction

*Diseases classified at type IV pathologies in which autoantibodies are present and used as clinical markers

THE PATHOGENESIS OF AUTOIMMUNITY

The key factor in the development of autoimmunity is the recognition of self-antigens by autoreactive lymphocytes, which then become activated, proliferate, and differentiate to produce effector cells and cytokines that cause tissue injury. Autoimmunity must initially result from a failure of mechanisms of **central tolerance,** as cells are "educated" in the bone marrow and thymus (see chapter 3).

Self-reactive lymphocytes that escaped central tolerance are subject to the different mechanisms of peripheral tolerance. The three primary mechanisms that induce peripheral tolerance are anergy, deletion and supression.

B lymphocytes that recognize self-antigen in the absence of the T-cell signaling become anergic and express high levels of IgD on their surface, excluding them from secondary lymphoid tissues. Anergic B lymphocytes are then unable to receive the signals necessary for survival and undergo apoptosis. Additionally, B lymphocytes have inhibitory receptors that can be engaged when self-antigen is recognized suppressing their activity.

Similar to self-reactive B lymphocytes, T lymphocytes that recognize self-antigen in the absence of the appropriate costimulatory signals are subject to anergy or deletion. Anergy is the result of a breakdown in either TCR signaling or the binding of an inhibitory receptor, CTLA-4 or PD-1. Deletion of self-reactive T lymphocytes is due to apoptosis by activation of the caspase signaling pathway or the Fas signaling pathway.

Self-reactive T lymphocytes are also subject to suppression by Tregs. Although a majority of Tregs are generated during central tolerance, some arise in the periphery. Tregs secrete IL-10 and TGF-beta that inhibit the activation of lymphocytes, macrophage and dendritic cells. CTLA-4 is expressed at high levels on Tregs and is thought to bind to and sequester the costimulatory molecule B7 which would otherwise be used to activate T lymphocytes.

Development of autoimmune disease is due to a combination of genetic and environmental factors as well as hormonal triggers. Among the strongest genetic associations with the development of autoimmune disease are the **HLA genes**. Also known to contribute to autoimmunity are polymorphisms in non-HLAgenes.

Table 11-7. Examples of HLA-Linked Immunologic Diseases

Disease	HLA Allele
Rheumatoid arthritis	DR4
Insulin-dependent diabetes mellitus	DR3/DR4
Multiple sclerosis, Goodpasture's	DR2
Systemic lupus erythematosus	DR2/DR3
Ankylosing spondylitis, psoriasis, inflammatory bowel disease, reactive arthritis	B27
Celiac disease	DQ2 or DQ8
Graves disease	B8

Infections and tissue injury may alter the way that self-antigens are presented to lymphocytes and serve as an inciting factor in the development of disease. Because autoimmune reactions against one self-antigen may injure other tissues and expose other potential self-antigens for recognition, autoimmune diseases tend to be chronic and progressive.

Transplantation 12

Learning Objectives

❏ Use knowledge of mechanisms of graft rejection

❏ Answer questions about graft versus host disease

OVERVIEW

Transplantation is the process of taking cells, tissues, or organs (a **graft**) from one individual (the **donor**) and implanting them into another individual or another site in the same individual (the **host** or **recipient**). **Transfusion** is a special case of transplantation and the most frequently practiced today, in which circulating blood cells or plasma are infused from one individual into another. As we have seen in previous chapters, the immune system is elaborately evolved to recognize minor differences in self antigens that reflect the invasion of harmful microbes or pathologic processes, such as cancer. Unfortunately, it is this same powerful mechanism of self-protection which thwarts tissue transplantation because tissues derived from other individuals are recognized as **"altered-self"** by the educated cells of the host's immune system.

Types of Graft Tissue

Several different types of grafts are used in medicine:

- Autologous grafts (or **autografts**) are those where tissue is moved from one location to another in the same individual (skin grafting in burns or coronary artery replacement with saphenous veins).
- **Isografts (or syngeneic grafts)** are those transplanted between genetically identical individuals (monozygotic twins).
- **Allogeneic** grafts are those transplanted between genetically different members of the same species (kidney transplant).
- **Xenogeneic** grafts are those transplanted between members of different species (pig heart valves into human).

MECHANISMS OF GRAFT REJECTION

The recognition of transplanted cells as self or foreign is determined by the extremely polymorphic genes of the major histocompatibility complex, which are expressed in a **codominant** fashion. This means that each individual inherits a complete set or **haplotype** from each parent and virtually assures that two genetically unrelated individuals will have distinctive differences in the antigens expressed on their cells. The net result is that all grafts except autografts are ultimately identified as foreign invading proteins and destroyed by the process of **graft rejection**. Even syngeneic grafts between identical twins can express recognizable antigenic differences due to somatic mutations that occur during the development of the individual. For this reason, all grafts except autografts must be followed by some degree of lifelong immunosuppression of the host to attempt to avoid rejection reactions.

The time sequence of allograft rejection differs depending on the tissue involved but always displays specificity and memory. As the graft becomes vascularized, CD4+ and CD8+ cells that migrate into the graft from the host become sensitized and proliferate in response to both major and minor histocompatibility differences. In the **effector phase** of the rejection, Th cytokines play a critical role in stimulating macrophage, cytotoxic T cell, and even antibody-mediated killing. Interferons and TNF-α and -β all increase the expression of class I MHC molecules in the graft, and IFN- increases the expression of class II MHC as well, increasing the susceptibility of cells in the graft to MHC-restricted killing.

Note

MHC alleles are expressed codominantly.

Four different classes of allograft rejection phenomena are classified according to their time of activation and the type of effector mechanism that predominates.

Hyperacute Graft Rejection

- Occurs within minutes to hours
- Due to pre-formed antibodies due to transfusions, multi-parity, or previous organ transplants (type II cytotoxic hypersensitivity)
- Antibodies bind to the grafted tissue and activate complement and the clotting cascade resulting in thrombosis and ischemic necrosis
- Rare because of cross-matching blood, **but common vignette**

Acute Graft Rejection

- Occurs within days to weeks; the timing and mechanism are similar to a primary immune response
- Induced by alloantigens (predominantly MHC) in the graft
- Both CD4 and CD8 T cells play a role as well as antibodies (think normal immune response)
- Immunosuppressive therapy works to prevent this type of graft rejection mainly

Accelerated Acute Graft Rejection

- Occurs within days; the timing and mechanism are similar to a memory response.

Chronic Graft Rejection

- Occurs within months to years
- Predominantly T cell mediated
- Difficult to treat and usually results in graft rejection
- Etiology not well understood, possibly triggered by viral infections

GRAFT VERSUS HOST DISEASE

A special case of tissue transplantation occurs when the grafted tissue is bone marrow. Because the bone marrow is the source of pluripotent hematopoietic stem cells, it can be used to reconstitute myeloid, erythroid, and lymphoid cells in a recipient who has lost these cells as a result of malignancy or chemotherapeutic regimens. Because the bone marrow is a source of some mature T lymphocytes, it is necessary to remove these cells before transplantation to avoid the appearance of **graft-versus-host disease** in the recipient. In this special case of rejection, any mature T cells remaining in the bone marrow inoculum can attack allogeneic MHC-bearing cells of the recipient and cause widespread epithelial cell death accompanied by rash, jaundice, diarrhea, and gastrointestinal hemorrhage.

Appendix I: CD Markers

CD Designation	Cellular Expression	Known Functions
CD2 (LFA-2)	T cells, thymocytes, NK cells	Adhesion molecule
CD3	T cells, thymocytes	Signal transduction by the TCR
CD4	Th cells, thymocytes, monocytes, and macrophages	Coreceptor for TCR-MHC II interaction, receptor for HIV
CD8	CTLs, some thymocytes	Coreceptor for MHC class I–restricted T cells
CD14 (LPS receptor)	Monocytes, macrophages, granulocytes	Binds LPS
CD16 (Fc receptor)	NK cells, macrophages, neutrophils	Opsonization ADCC
CD18	Leukocytes	Cell adhesion molecule (missing in leukocyte adhesion deficiency)
CD19	B cells	Coreceptor with CD21 for B-cell activation (signal transduction)
CD20	Most or all B cells	Unknown role in B-cell activation
CD21 (CR2, C3d receptor)	Mature B cells	Receptor for complement fragment C3d, forms coreceptor complex with CD19, Epstein-Barr virus receptor
CD25	Activated Th cells and T_{Reg}	Alpha chain of IL-2 receptor
CD28	T cells	T-cell receptor for costimulatory molecule B7
CD34	Precursors of hematopoietic cells, endothelial cells in HEV	Cell–cell adhesion, binds L-selectin
CD40	B cells, macrophages, dendritic cells, endothelial cells	Binds CD40L, role in T-cell–dependent B cell, macrophage, dendritic cell and endothelial cell activation
CD56	NK cells	Cell adhesion
CD152 (CTLA-4)	Activated T cells	Negative regulation: competes with CD28 for B7 binding

APPENDIX II: Cytokines

Cytokine	Secreted by	Target Cell/Tissue	Activity
Interleukin (IL)-1	Monocytes, macrophages, B cells, dendritic cells, endothelial cells, others	Th cells	Costimulates activation
		B cells	Promotes maturation and clonal expansion
		NK cells	Enhances activity
		Endothelial cells	Increases expression of ICAMs
		Macrophages and neutrophils	Chemotactically attracts
		Hepatocytes	Induces synthesis of acute-phase proteins
		Hypothalamus	Induces fever
IL-2	Th cells	Antigen-primed Th and CTLs	Induces proliferation, enhances activity
IL-3	Th cells, NK cells	Hematopoietic cells (myeloid)	Supports growth and differentiation
IL-4	Th2 cells	Antigen-primed B cells	Costimulates activation
		Activated B cells	Stimulates proliferation and differentiation, induces class switch to IgE
IL-5	Th2 cells and mast cells	Bone marrow cells	Induces eosinophil differentiation
IL-6	Monocytes, macrophages, Th2 cells, bone marrow stromal cells	Proliferating B cells	Promotes terminal differentiation into plasma cells
		Plasma cells	Stimulates Ab secretion
		Myeloid stem cells	Helps promote differentiation
		Hepatocytes	Induces synthesis of acute-phase proteins

(*Continue*)

Cytokine	Secreted by	Target Cell/Tissue	Activity
IL-7	Bone marrow, thymic stromal cells	Lymphoid stem cells	Induces differentiation into progenitor B and T cells
IL-8	Macrophages, endothelial cells	Neutrophils	Chemokine, induces adherence to endothelium and extravasation into tissues
IL-10	Th2 cells T$_{Reg}$ cells	Macrophages	Suppresses cytokine production by Th1 cells
IL-11	Bone marrow stroma	Bone marrow	↑ platelet count
IL-12	Macrophages, B cells	Activated CD8+ cells	Acts synergistically with IL-2 to induce differentiation into CTLs
		NK and LAK cells and activated Th1 cells	Stimulates proliferation
IL-13	Th2 cell	B cells	Induces isotype switch to IgE
IL-17	Th17 cells	Fibroblasts, endothelial cells, macrophages	Increases inflammation.Attracts PMNs, induces IL-6, IL-1, TGFβ, TNFα, IL-8
IL-18	Macrophages	IFN-γ synthesis	NK cells, Th cells, IFN-γ synthesis
Interferon-α (type I)	Leukocytes	Uninfected cells	Inhibits viral replication
IL-22	Th17	Endothelium	Stabilizes endothelial barrier, induces secretion of microbials
Interferon-β (type I)	Fibroblasts	Uninfected cells	Inhibits viral replication
Interferon-γ (type II)	Th1, CTLs, NK cells	Macrophages	Enhances activity
		Many cell types	Increases expression of classes I and II MHC
		Proliferating B cells	Induces class switch to IgG2a, blocks IL-4−induced class switch to IgE and IgG1
		Th2 cells	Inhibits proliferation
		Phagocytic cells	Mediates effects important in DTH, treatment for CGD
Transforming growth factor-β	Platelets, macrophages, lymphocytes, mast cells	Proliferating B cells	Induces class switch to IgA

(Continue)

Cytokine	Secreted by	Target Cell/Tissue	Activity
Tumor necrosis factor-α	Macrophages, NK cells	Tumor cells	Has cytotoxic effect
		Inflammatory cells	Induces cytokine secretion, causes cachexia of chronic inflammation
Tumor necrosis factor-β	Th1 and CTL	Tumor cells	Has cytotoxic and other effects, like TNF-α
		Macrophages and neutrophils	Enhances phagocytic activity
Granulocyte colony-stimulating factor (G-CSF)	Macrophages and Th cells	Bone marrow granulocyte precursors	Induce proliferation, used clinically to counteract neutropenia following ablative chemotherapy
Granulocyte–macrophage colony-stimulating factor (GM-CSF)	Macrophages and Th cells	Bone marrow granulocyte and macrophage precursors	Induces proliferation; used clinically to counteract neutropenia following ablative chemotherapy

Pathology

Fundamentals of Pathology

Learning Objectives

❑ Define etiology, pathogenesis, morphology, and clinical significance of disease

❑ List techniques for staining pathologic specimens

OVERVIEW OF PATHOLOGY

Definitions

- The study of the essential nature of disease, including symptoms/signs, pathogenesis, complications, and morphologic consequences including structural and functional alterations in cells, tissues, and organs
- The study of all aspects of the disease process focusing on the pathogenesis leading to classical structural changes (gross and histopathology) and molecular alterations

The **etiology** (cause) of a disease may be genetic or environmental. The **pathogenesis** of a disease defines the temporal sequence and the patterns of cellular injury that lead to disease. **Morphologic** changes of the disease process include both gross changes and microscopic changes. The **clinical significance** of a disease relates to its signs and symptoms, disease course including complications, and prognosis.

Methods Used

Gross examination of organs on exam questions has two major components: identifying the organ and identifying the pathology. Useful gross features include consideration of size, shape, consistency, and color.

Microscopic examination of tissue

- In light microscopic examination of tissue, **hematoxylin and eosin (H&E)** is considered the gold standard stain and is used routinely in the initial microscopic examination of pathologic specimens.

Table 1-1. Structures Stained by Hematoxylin and Eosin

Hematoxylin	Eosin
Stains blue to purple	Stains pink to red
• Nuclei	• Cytoplasm
• Nucleoli	• Collagen
• Bacteria	• Fibrin
• Calcium	• RBCs
	• Thyroid colloid

The common denominator of the features shown in Table 1-1 is that hematoxylin binds nucleic acids and calcium salts, while eosin stains the majority of proteins (both extracellular and intracellular).

- **Other histochemical stains** (chemical reactions): Prussian blue (stains iron), Congo red (stains amyloid), acid fast (Ziehl-Neelsen, Fite) (stains acid-fast bacilli), periodic acid-Schiff (PAS, stains high carbohydrate content molecules), Gram stain (stains bacteria), trichrome (stains cells and connective tissue), and reticulin (stains collagen type III molecules).

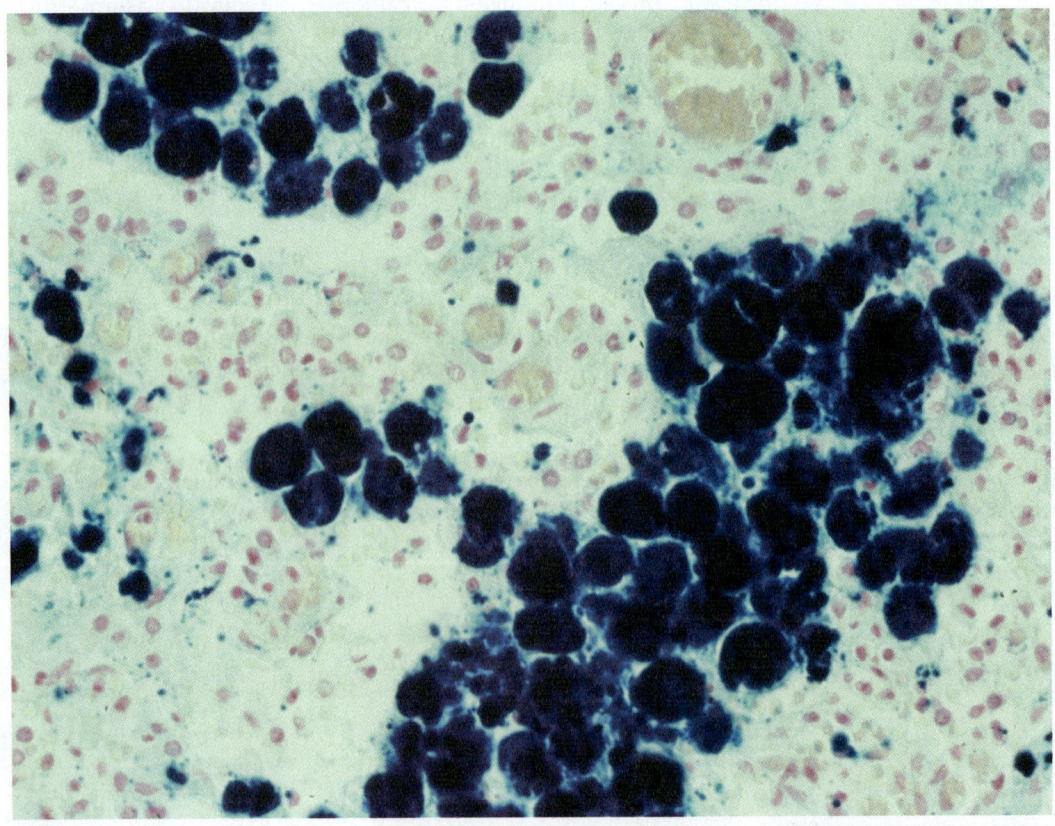

Figure 1-1. Prussian Blue Stain Showing Hemosiderin, Which Results from RBC Breakdown Within Macrophages

© Katsumi M. Miyai, M.D., Ph.D.; Regents of the University of California. Used with permission.

- **Immunohistochemical (antibody) stains** include cytokeratin (stains epithelial cells), vimentin (stains cells of mesenchymal origin except the three muscle types; stains many sarcomas), desmin (stains smooth, cardiac, and skeletal myosin), prostate specific antigen, and many others.

Ancillary techniques include **immunofluorescence microscopy (IFM)**, typically used for renal and autoimmune disease, and **transmission electron microscopy (EM)**, used for renal disease, neoplasms, infections, and genetic disorders.

Molecular techniques include protein electrophoresis, Southern and Western blots, polymerase chain reaction (PCR), and cytogenetic analysis (karyotyping, in situ hybridization studies).

Cellular Injury and Adaptation 2

Learning Objectives

❏ Explain causes of cellular injury

❏ Demonstrate understanding of cellular changes during injury and cell death

❏ Answer questions about cellular adaptive responses to injury

❏ Describe cellular alterations during injury

CAUSES OF CELLULAR INJURY

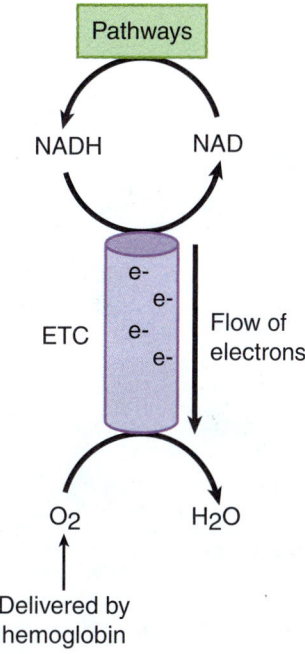

Figure 2-1. Overview of the Electron Transport Chain

Hypoxia is the most common cause of injury; it occurs when lack of oxygen prevents the cell from synthesizing sufficient ATP by aerobic oxidation. Major mechanisms leading to hypoxia are ischemia, cardiopulmonary failure, and decreased oxygen-carrying capacity of the blood (e.g., anemia). **Ischemia**, due to a loss of blood supply, is the most common cause of hypoxia, and is typically related to decreased arterial flow or decreased venous outflow (e.g., atherosclerosis, thrombus, thromboembolus).

Pathogens (viruses, bacteria, parasites, fungi, and prions) can injure the body by direct infection of cells, production of toxins, or host inflammatory response.

Immunologic dysfunction includes hypersensitivity reactions and autoimmune diseases.

Congenital disorders are inherited genetic mutations (e.g., inborn errors of metabolism).

Chemical injury can occur with drugs, poisons (cyanide, arsenic, mercury, etc.), pollution, occupational exposure (CCl_4, asbestos, carbon monoxide, etc.), and social/lifestyle choices (alcohol, smoking, IV drug abuse, etc.)

Physical forms of injury include trauma (blunt/penetrating/crush injuries, gunshot wounds, etc.), burns, frostbite, radiation, and pressure changes.

Nutritional or vitamin imbalance

- **Inadequate calorie/protein intake** can cause marasmus (decrease in total caloric intake), and kwashiorkor (decrease in total protein intake).
- **Excess caloric intake** can cause obesity (second leading cause of premature preventable death in the United States) and atherosclerosis.
- **Vitamin deficiencies** can be seen with vitamin A (night blindness, squamous metaplasia, immune deficiency), vitamin C (scurvy), vitamin D (rickets and osteomalacia), vitamin K (bleeding diathesis), vitamin B12 (megaloblastic anemia, neuropathy, and spinal cord degeneration), folate (megaloblastic anemia and neural tube defects), and niacin (pellagra [diarrhea, dermatitis, and dementia]).
- **Hypervitaminosis** is less commonly a problem but can result in tissue specific abnormalities.

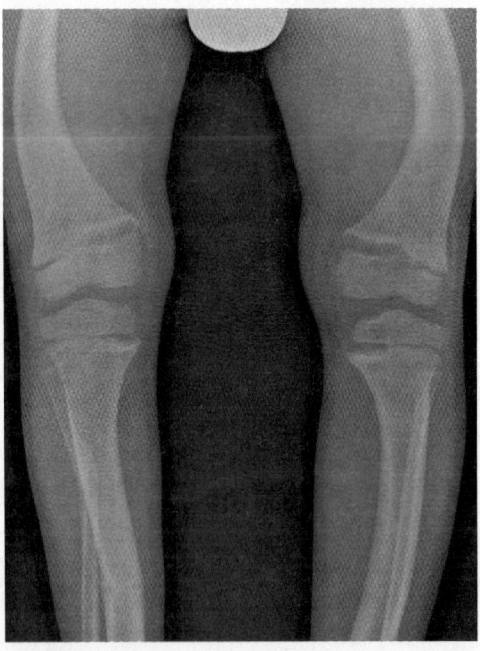

Figure 2-2. Radiograph of a Child with Rickets Shows Bowed Legs

© Dr. Angela Byrne, Radiopaedia.org. Used with permission.

CELLULAR CHANGES DURING INJURY

Cellular responses to injury include adaptation (hypertrophy or atrophy, hyperplasia or metaplasia), reversible injury, and irreversible injury and cell death (necrosis, apoptosis, or necroptosis).

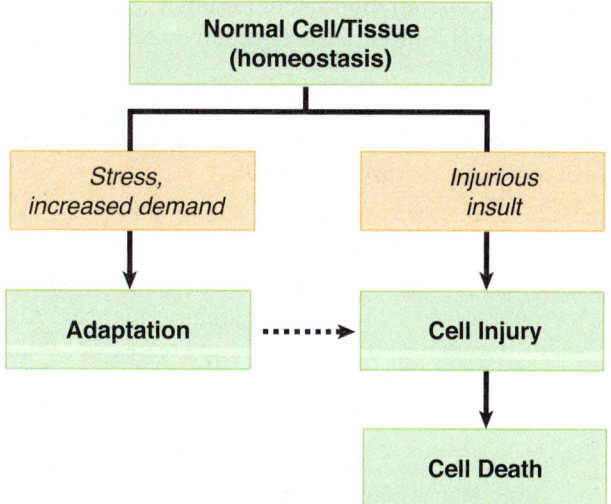

Figure 2-3. Cellular Response to Stress and Injurious Stimuli

The **cellular response to injury depends on several important factors**, including the type of injury, duration (including pattern) of injury, severity and intensity of injury, type of cell injured, the cell's metabolic state, and the cell's ability to adapt.

The **critical intracellular targets that are susceptible to injury** are DNA, production of ATP via aerobic respiration, cell membranes, and protein synthesis.

Note

Protective Factors against free radicals include:

- Antioxidants
- Vitamins A, E, and C
- Superoxide dismutase
- Superoxide → hydrogen peroxide
- Glutathione peroxidase
- Hydroxyl ions or hydrogen peroxide → water
- Catalase
- Hydrogen peroxide → oxygen and water

Important mechanisms of cell injury are as follows:

- Damage to DNA, proteins, lipid membranes, and circulating lipids (LDL) can be caused by oxygen-derived free radicals, including superoxide anion ($O_2^{\cdot-}$), hydroxyl radical ($OH^\cdot$), and hydrogen peroxide (H_2O_2).

- ATP depletion: Several key biochemical pathways are dependent on ATP. Disruption of Na^+/K^+ or Ca^{++} pumps cause imbalances in solute concentrations. Additionally, ATP depletion increases anaerobic glycolysis that leads to a decrease in cellular pH. Chronic ATP depletion causes morphological and functional changes to the ER and ribosomes.

- Increased cell membrane permeability: Several defects can lead to movement of fluids into the cell, including formation of the membrane attack complex via complement, breakdown of Na+/K+ gradients (i.e., causing sodium to enter or potassium to leave the cell), etc.

- Influx of calcium can cause problems because calcium is a second messenger, which can activate a wide spectrum of enzymes. These enzymes include proteases (protein breakdown), ATPases (contributes to ATP depletion), phospholipases (cell membrane injury), and endonucleases (DNA damage).

- Mitochondrial dysfunction causes decreased oxidative phosphorylation and ATP production, formation of mitochondrial permeability transition (MPT) channels, and release of cytochrome c (a trigger for apoptosis).

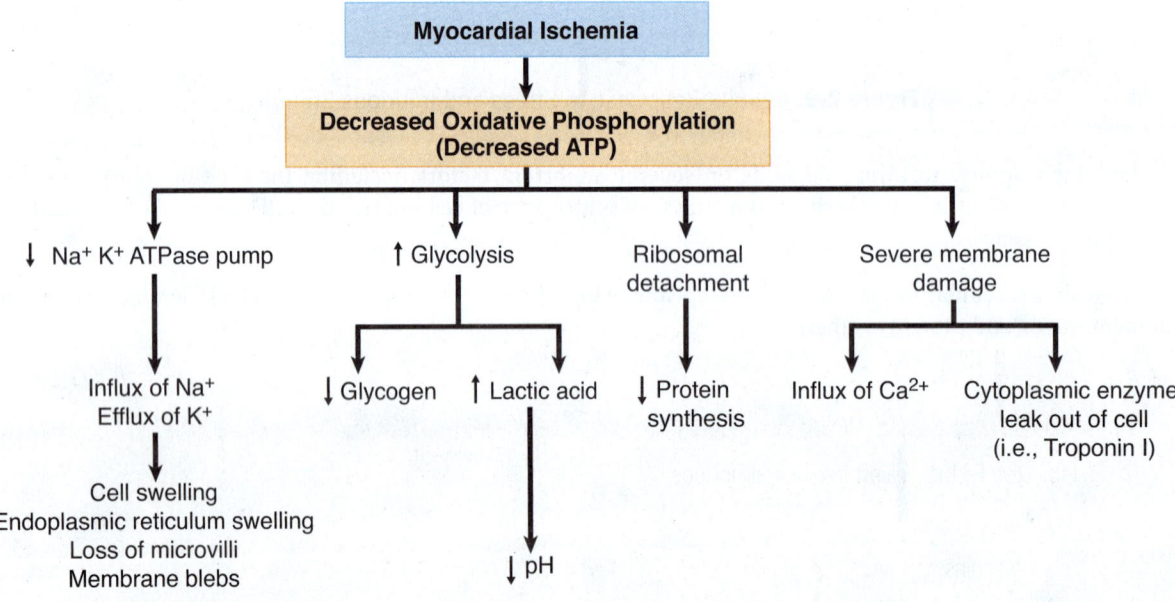

Figure 2-4. Classic Example of Cellular Injury Caused by Hypoxia

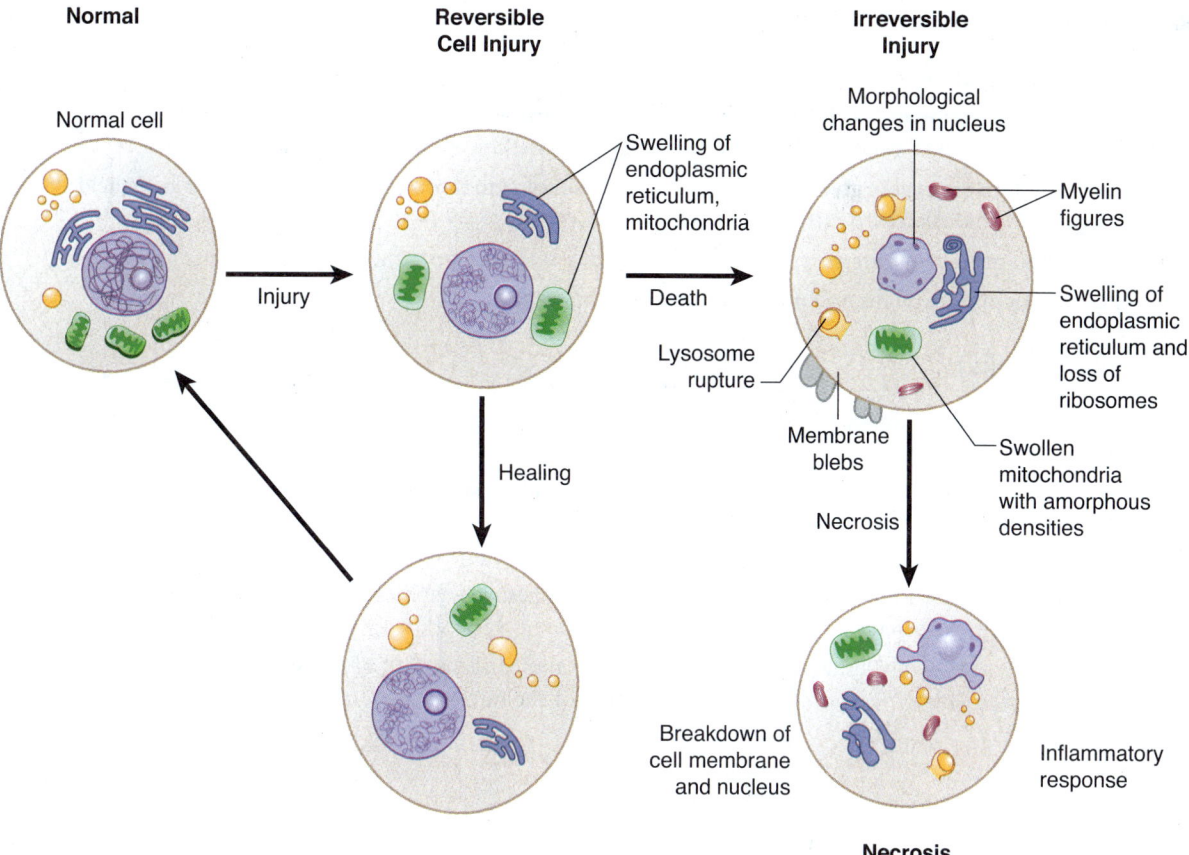

Figure 2-5. Cell Injury

Clinical Correlate

The loss of membrane integrity (cell death) allows intracellular enzymes to leak out, which can then be measured in the blood. Detection of these proteins in the circulation serves as a clinical marker of cell death and organ injury. Clinically important examples:

- Myocardial injury: troponin (most specific), CPK-MB, lactate dehydrogenase (LDH)
- Hepatitis: transaminases
- Pancreatitis: amylase and lipase
- Biliary tract obstruction: alkaline phosphatase

Reversible cell injury:

- **Decreased synthesis of ATP** by oxidative phosphorylation.

- **Decreased function of Na$^+$K$^+$ ATPase membrane pumps**, which in turn causes influx of Na+ and water, efflux of K$^+$, cellular swelling (hydropic swelling), and swelling of the endoplasmic reticulum.

- The **switch to anaerobic glycolysis** results in depletion of cytoplasmic glycogen, increased lactic acid production, and decreased intracellular pH.

- **Decreased protein synthesis** leads to detachment of ribosomes from the rough endoplasmic reticulum.

- **Plasma-membrane blebs and myelin figures** may be seen.

Irreversible cell injury:

- **Severe membrane damage** plays a critical role in irreversible injury, allows a massive influx of calcium into the cell, and allows efflux of intracellular enzymes and proteins into the circulation.

- **Marked mitochondrial dysfunction** produces mitochondrial swelling, large densities seen within the mitochondrial matrix, irreparable damage of the oxidative phosphorylation pathway, and an inability to produce ATP.

- **Rupture of the lysosomes** causes release of lysosomal digestive enzymes into the cytosol and activation of acid hydrolases followed by autolysis.

- **Nuclear changes** can include pyknosis (degeneration and condensation of nuclear chromatin), karyorrhexis (nuclear fragmentation), and karyolysis (dissolution of the nucleus).

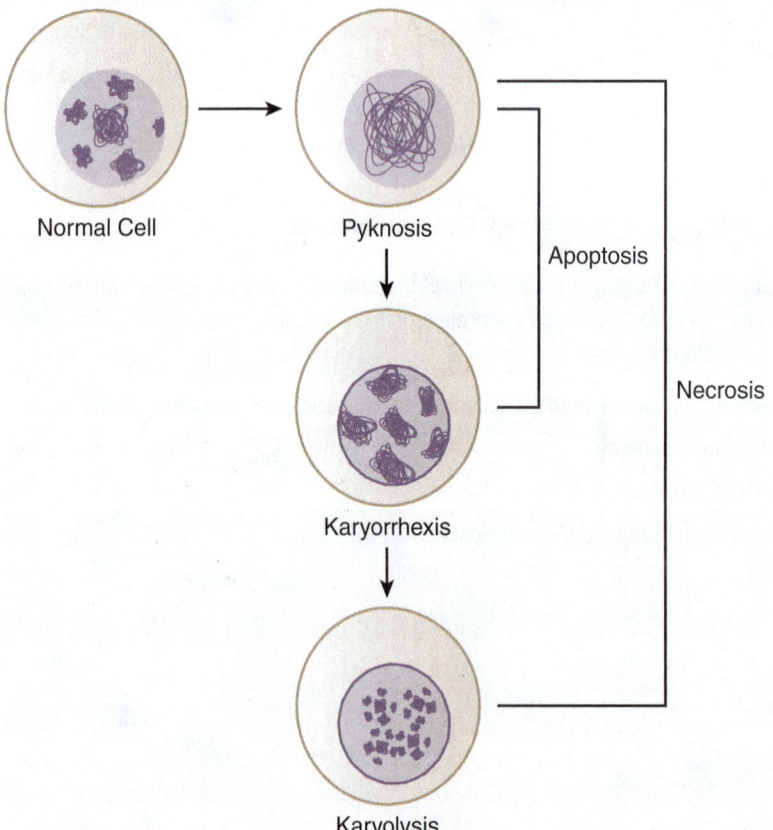

Normal Cell   Pyknosis

Apoptosis

Necrosis

Karyorrhexis

Karyolysis

Figure 2-6. Nuclear Changes in Irreversible Cell Injury

CELL DEATH

Morphologic types of necrosis (cell death in living tissue, often with an inflammatory response) are as follows:

> **Note**
>
> Liquefaction by leukocyte enzymes is called suppuration, and the resultant fluid is called pus.

- **Coagulative necrosis**, the most common form of necrosis, is most often due to ischemic injury (infarct). It is caused by the denaturing of proteins within the cytoplasm. Microscopic examination shows loss of the nucleus but preservation of cellular shape. Coagulative necrosis is common in most organs, including the heart, liver, and kidney, but not the brain.

- **Liquefaction necrosis** results from cellular destruction by hydrolytic enzymes, leading to autolysis (release of proteolytic enzymes from injured cells) and heterolysis (release of proteolytic enzymes from inflammatory cells). Liquefaction necrosis occurs in abscesses, brain infarcts, and pancreatic necrosis.

- **Caseous necrosis** is a combination of coagulation and liquefaction necrosis. The gross appearance is soft, friable, and "cheese-like." Caseous necrosis is characteristic of granulomatous diseases, including tuberculosis.

- **Fat necrosis** is caused by the action of lipases on adipocytes and is characteristic of acute pancreatitis. On gross examination fat necrosis has a chalky white appearance.

- **Fibrinoid necrosis** is a form of necrotic connective tissue that histologically resembles fibrin. On microscopic examination fibrinoid necrosis has an eosinophilic (pink) homogeneous appearance. It is often due to acute immunologic injury (e.g., hypersensitivity type reactions II and III) and vascular hypertensive damage.

- **Gangrenous necrosis** is a gross term used to describe dead tissue. Common sites of involvement include lower limbs, gallbladder, GI tract, and testes. Dry gangrene has coagulative necrosis for the microscopic pattern, while wet gangrene has liquefactive necrosis.

> **Note**
>
> Necrotic tissue within the body evokes an inflammatory response that removes the dead tissue and is followed by healing and tissue repair. Necrotic debris may also undergo dystrophic calcification.

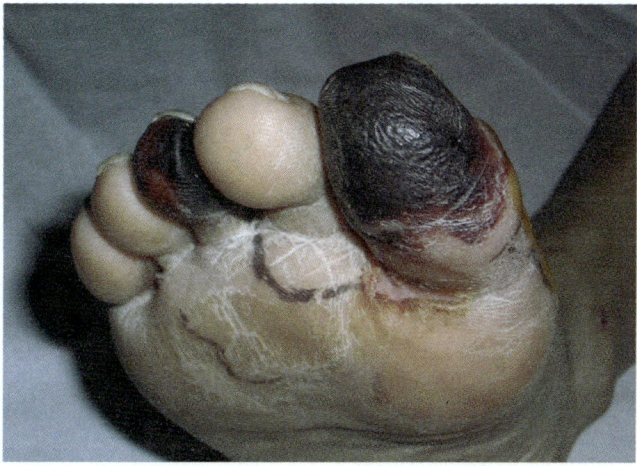

Figure 2-7. Gangrenous Necrosis Affects the First and Third Toes of a Diabetic Foot

© Richard P. Usatine, M.D. Used with permission.

Apoptosis is a specialized form of programmed cell death without an inflammatory response. It is an active process regulated by proteins that often affects only single cells or small groups of cells.

- In **morphologic appearance,** the cell shrinks in size and has dense eosinophilic cytoplasm. Next, nuclear chromatin condensation (pyknosis) is seen that is followed by fragmentation of the nucleus (karyorrhexis). Cytoplasmic membrane blebs form next, leading eventually to a breakdown of the cell into fragments (apoptotic bodies). Phagocytosis of apoptotic bodies is by adjacent cells or macrophages.

- **Stimuli for apoptosis** include cell injury and DNA damage, lack of hormones, cytokines, or growth factors, and receptor-ligand signals such as Fas binding to the Fas ligand and tumor necrosis factor (TNF) binding to TNF receptor 1 (TNFR1).

- **Apoptosis is regulated by proteins.** The protein bcl-2 (which inhibits apoptosis) prevents release of cytochrome c from mitochondria and binds pro-apoptotic protease activating factor (Apaf-1). The protein p53 (which stimulates apoptosis) is elevated by DNA injury and arrests the cell cycle. If DNA repair is impossible, p53 stimulates apoptosis.

- **Execution of apoptosis** is mediated by a cascade of caspases (cysteine aspartic acid proteases). The caspases digest nuclear and cytoskeletal proteins and also activate endonucleases.

- **Physiologic examples of apoptosis** include embryogenesis (organogenesis and development), hormone-dependent apoptosis (menstrual cycle), thymus (selective death of lymphocytes).

- **Pathologic examples of apoptosis** include viral diseases (viral hepatitis [Councilman body]), graft-versus-host disease, and cystic fibrosis (duct obstruction and pancreatic atrophy).

Clinical Correlate

If the cells in the interdigital space fail to undergo apoptosis, the fetus will be born with webbed hands and/or webbed feet, a condition known as *syndactyly*.

Another example is the hormone-dependent apoptosis prior to menstruation; programmed cell death plays a role in endometrial gland morphological changes.

Serum enzyme markers of cell damage include aspartate aminotransferase (AST) (liver injury), alanine aminotransferase (ALT) (liver injury), creatine kinase (CK-MB) (heart injury), and amylase and lipase (pancreatic injury; amylase also rises with salivary gland injury).

CELLULAR ADAPTIVE RESPONSES TO INJURY

In general, cellular adaptation is a potentially reversible change in response to the environment.

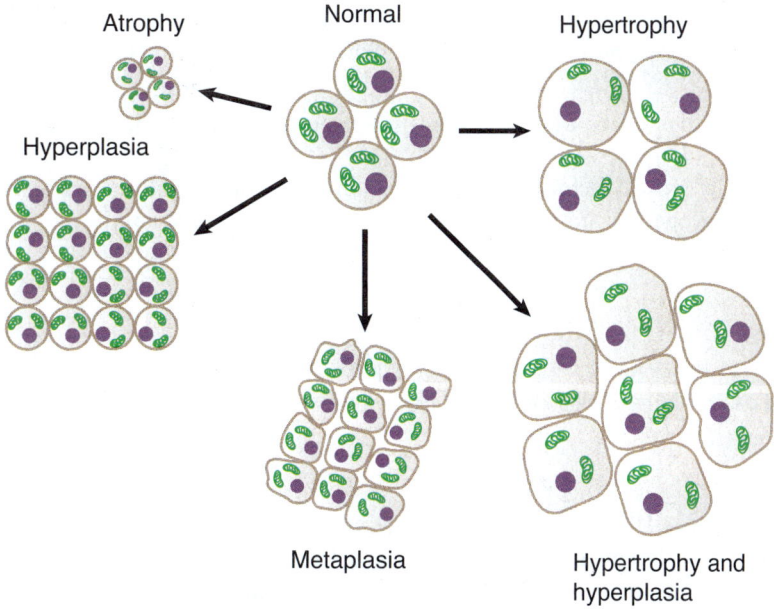

Figure 2-8. Cellular Adaptive Responses to Cell Injury

Atrophy is a decrease in cell/organ size and functional ability. Causes of atrophy include decreased workload/disuse (immobilization); ischemia (atherosclerosis); lack of hormonal or neural stimulation, malnutrition, and aging.

Light microscopic examination shows small shrunken cells with lipofuscin granules. Electron microscopy shows decreased intracellular components and autophagosomes.

Hypertrophy is an increase in cell size and functional ability due to increased synthesis of intracellular components.

Causes of hypertrophy include:

- Increased mechanical demand can be physiologic (striated muscle of weight lifters) or pathologic (cardiac muscle in hypertension).
- Increased endocrine stimulation plays a role in puberty (growth hormone, androgens/estrogens, etc.), gravid uterus (estrogen), and lactating breast (prolactin and estrogen).

Hypertrophy is mediated by growth factors, cytokines, and other trophic stimuli and leads to increased expression of genes and increased protein synthesis.

Hypertrophy and hyperplasia often occur together.

Hyperplasia is an increase in the number of cells in a tissue or organ. Some cell types are unable to exhibit hyperplasia (e.g., nerve, cardiac, skeletal muscle cells).

- Physiologic causes of hyperplasia include compensatory mechanisms (e.g., after partial hepatectomy), hormonal stimulation (e.g., breast development at puberty), and antigenic stimulation (e.g., lymphoid hyperplasia).
- Pathologic causes of hyperplasia include endometrial hyperplasia and prostatic hyperplasia of aging.

Hyperplasia is mediated by growth factors, cytokines, and other trophic stimuli; increased expression of growth-promoting genes (proto-oncogenes); and increased DNA synthesis and cell division.

Clinical Correlate

Residence at high altitude, where oxygen content of air is relatively low, leads to compensatory hyperplasia of red blood cell precursors in the bone marrow and an increase in the number of circulating red blood cells (secondary polycythemia).

Metaplasia is a reversible change of one fully differentiated cell type to another, usually in response to irritation. It has been suggested that the replacement cell is better able to tolerate the environmental stresses. For example, bronchial epithelium undergoes squamous metaplasia in response to the chronic irritation of tobacco smoke.

The proposed mechanism is that the reserve cells (or stem cells) of the irritated tissue differentiate into a more protective cell type due to the influence of growth factors, cytokines, and matrix components.

Clinical Correlate

Barrett's esophagus is a classic example of metaplasia. The esophageal epithelium is normally squamous, but it undergoes a change to intestinal epithelium (columnar) when it is under constant contact with gastric acid.

OTHER CELLULAR ALTERATIONS DURING INJURY

Pathologic Accumulations

- **Lipids** that can accumulate intracellularly include triglycerides (e.g., fatty change in liver cells), cholesterol (e.g., atherosclerosis, xanthomas), and complex lipids (e.g., sphingolipid accumulation).
- **Proteins** can accumulate in proximal renal tubules in proteinuria and can form Russell bodies (intracytoplasmic accumulation of immunoglobulins) in plasma cells.
- **Glycogen storage diseases** (*See* Genetic Disorders chapter.)
- **Exogenous pigments** include anthracotic pigmentation of the lung (secondary to the inhalation of carbon dust), tattoos, and lead that has been ingested (e.g., gingival lead line, renal tubular lead deposits).

Endogenous pigments

- **Lipofuscin** is a wear-and-tear pigment that is seen as perinuclear yellow-brown pigment. It is due to indigestible material within lysosomes and is common in the liver and heart.

- **Melanin** is a black-brown pigment derived from tyrosine found in melanocytes and substantia nigra.

- **Hemosiderin** is a golden yellow-brown granular pigment found in areas of hemorrhage or bruises. Systemic iron overload can lead to hemosiderosis (increase in total body iron stores without tissue injury) or hemochromatosis (increase in total body iron stores with tissue injury). Prussian blue stain can identify the iron in the hemosiderin.

- **Bilirubin** accumulates in newborns in the basal ganglia, causing permanent damage (kernicterus).

  Hyaline change is a nonspecific term used to describe any intracellular or extracellular alteration that has a pink homogenous appearance (proteins) on H&E stains.

- Examples of **intracellular hyaline** include renal proximal tubule protein reabsorption droplets, Russell bodies, and alcoholic hyaline.

- Examples of **extracellular hyaline** include hyaline arteriolosclerosis, amyloid, and hyaline membrane disease of the newborn.

Pathologic forms of calcification

- **Dystrophic calcification** is the precipitation of calcium phosphate in dying or necrotic tissues. Examples include fat necrosis (saponification), psammoma bodies (laminated calcifications that occur in meningiomas and papillary carcinomas of the thyroid and ovary), Mönckeberg medial calcific sclerosis in arterial walls, and atherosclerotic plaques.

- **Metastatic calcification** is the precipitation of calcium phosphate in normal tissue due to hypercalcemia (supersaturated solution). The many causes include hyperparathyroidism, parathyroid adenomas, renal failure, paraneoplastic syndrome, vitamin D intoxication, milk-alkali syndrome, sarcoidosis, Paget disease, multiple myeloma, metastatic cancer to the bone. The calcifications are located in the interstitial tissues of the stomach, kidneys, lungs, and blood vessels.

Inflammation 3

Learning Objectives

❏ Solve problems concerning acute and chronic inflammation

❏ Describe tissue responses to infectious agents

ACUTE INFLAMMATION

Acute inflammation is an immediate response to injury or infection, which is part of innate immunity.

- Short duration in normal host
- Cardinal signs of inflammation include rubor (redness); calor (heat); tumor (swelling); dolor (pain); functio laesa (loss of function).

The important components of acute inflammation are hemodynamic changes, **neutrophils**, and chemical mediators.

Hemodynamic Changes

- Initial transient vasoconstriction
- Massive vasodilatation mediated by histamine, bradykinin, and prostaglandins
- Increased vascular permeability
  - Chemical mediators of increased permeability include vasoactive amines (histamine and serotonin), bradykinin (an end-product of the kinin cascade), leukotrienes (e.g., LTC4, LTD4, LTE4).
  - The mechanism of increased vascular permeability involves endothelial cell and pericyte contraction; direct endothelial cell injury; and leukocyte injury of endothelium.
- Blood flow slows (stasis) due to increased viscosity, allows neutrophils to marginate

Neutrophils

- Life span in tissue 1–2 days
- Synonyms: segmented neutrophils, polymorphonuclear leukocytes (PMN)
- Primary (azurophilic) granules contain myeloperoxidase, phospholipase A2, lysozyme (damages bacterial cell walls by catalyzing hydrolysis of 1,4-beta-linkages), and acid hydrolases. Also present are elastase, defensins (microbicidal peptides active against many gram-negative and gram-positive bacteria, fungi, and enveloped viruses), and bactericidal permeability increasing protein (BPI).
- Secondary (specific) granules contain phospholipase A2, lysozyme, leukocyte alkaline phosphatase (LAP), collagenase, lactoferrin (chelates iron), and vitamin B12-binding proteins.
- **Macrophages** (life span in tissue compartment is 60–120 days) have acid hydrolases, elastase, and collagenase.

Neutrophil margination and adhesion. Adhesion is mediated by complementary molecules on the surface of neutrophils and endothelium.

- In **step 1**, the endothelial cells at sites of inflammation have increased expression of *E-selectin* and *P-selectin*.
- In **step 2**, neutrophils weakly bind to the endothelial selectins and roll along the surface.
- In **step 3**, neutrophils are stimulated by chemokines to express their integrins.
- In **step 4**, binding of the integrins to cellular adhesion molecules (ICAM-1 and VCAM-1) allows the neutrophils to firmly adhere to the endothelial cell.

Modulation of adhesion molecules in inflammation occurs as follows. The fastest step involves redistribution of adhesion molecules to the surface; for example, P-selectin is normally present in the Weibel-Palade bodies of endothelial cells and can be mobilized to the cell surface by exposure to inflammatory mediators such as histamine and thrombin.

- Additionally, synthesis of adhesion molecules occurs. For example, proinflammatory cytokines IL-1 and TNF induce production of E-selectin, ICAM-1, and VCAM-1 in endothelial cells.
- There can also be increased binding affinity, as when chemotactic agents cause a conformational change in the leukocyte integrin LFA-1, which is converted to a high-affinity binding state.

Defects in adhesion can be seen in diabetes mellitus, corticosteroid use, acute alcohol intoxication, and leukocyte adhesion deficiency (autosomal recessive condition with recurrent bacterial infections).

In **emigration (diapedesis),** leukocytes emigrate from the vasculature (postcapillary venule) by extending pseudopods between the endothelial cells. They then move between the endothelial cells, migrating through the basement membrane toward the inflammatory stimulus.

Chemotaxis is the attraction of cells toward a chemical mediator that is released in the area of inflammation. Important chemotactic factors for neutrophils include bacterial products such as *N*-formyl-methionine and host derived molecules such as leukotriene B4 (LTB4), complement system product C5a, and α-chemokines (IL-8).

Phagocytosis and degranulation. Opsonins coat microbes to enhance their detection and phagocytosis. Important opsonins include the Fc portion of IgG isotypes, complement system product C3b, and plasma proteins such as collectins (which bind to bacterial cell walls).

Engulfment occurs when the neutrophil sends out cytoplasmic processes that surround the bacteria. The bacteria are then internalized within a phagosome. The phagosome fuses with lysosomes (degranulation).

Defects in phagocytosis and degranulation include Chédiak-Higashi syndrome, an autosomal recessive condition characterized by neutropenia. The neutrophils have giant granules (lysosomes) and there is a defect in chemotaxis and degranulation.

Intracellular killing.

In oxygen-dependent killing, respiratory burst requires oxygen and NADPH oxidase and produces superoxide, hydroxyl radicals, and hydrogen peroxide. Myeloperoxidase requires hydrogen peroxide and halide (Cl–) and produces HOCl (hypochlorous acid).

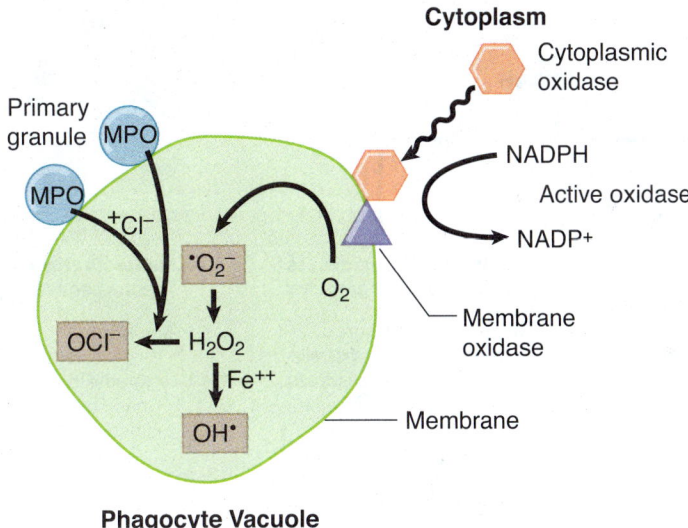

Figure 3-1. Oxygen-Dependent Killing

Oxygen-independent killing involves lysozyme, lactoferrin, acid hydrolases, bactericidal permeability increasing protein (BPI), and defensins.

Deficiencies of oxygen-dependent killing include:

- Chronic granulomatous disease of childhood can be X-linked or autosomal recessive. It is characterized by a deficiency of NADPH oxidase, lack of superoxide and hydrogen peroxide, and recurrent bacterial infections with catalase-positive organisms (*S. aureus*). The nitroblue tetrazolium test will be negative.
- Myeloperoxidase deficiency is an autosomal recessive condition characterized by infections with *Candida*. In contrast to chronic granulomatous disease, the nitroblue tetrazolium test will be positive.

Chemical Mediators of Inflammation

Vasoactive amines

- **Histamine** is produced by basophils, platelets, and mast cells. It causes vasodilation and increased vascular permeability. Triggers for release include IgE-mediated mast cell reactions, physical injury, anaphylatoxins (C3a and C5a), and cytokines (IL-1).
- **Serotonin** is produced by platelets and causes vasodilation and increased vascular permeability.

Kinin system

- Activated Hageman factor (factor XII) converts prekallikrein → kallikrein
- Kallikrein cleaves high molecular weight kininogen (HMWK) →bradykinin
- Effects of bradykinin include increased vascular permeability, pain, vasodilation, bronchoconstriction, and pain

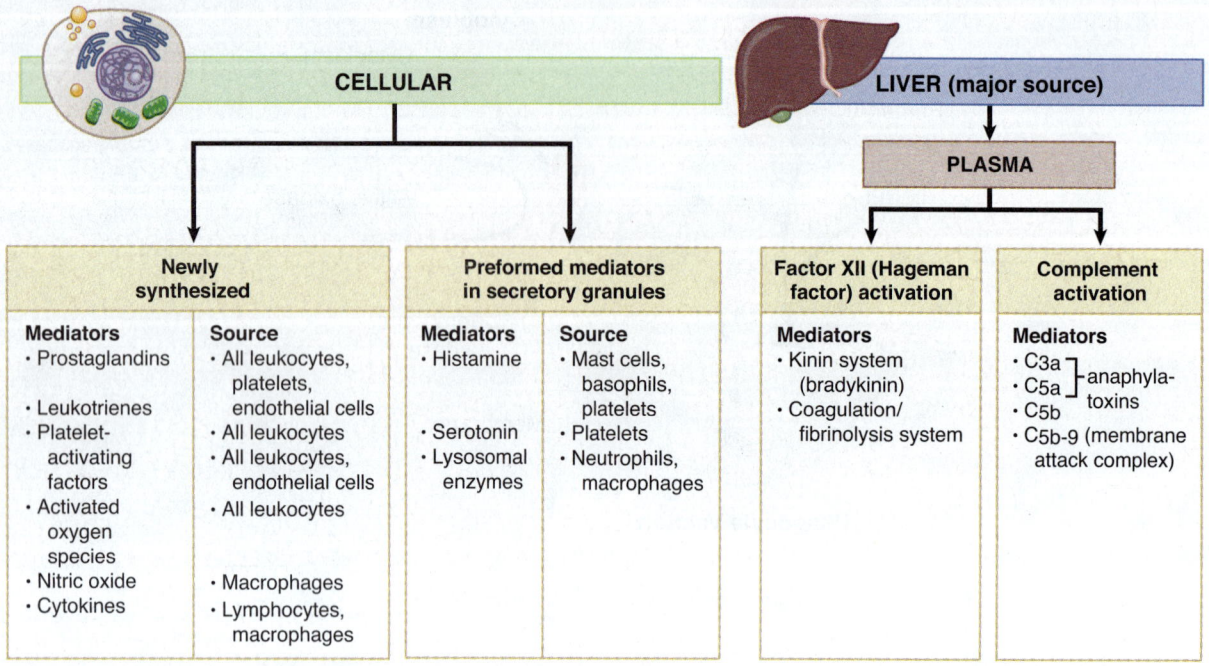

Figure 3-2. Sources of Chemical Mediators of Inflammation

Arachidonic acid products

- **Cyclooxygenase pathway**
  - Thromboxane A2 is produced by platelets and causes vasoconstriction and platelet aggregation.
  - Prostacyclin (PGI2) is produced by vascular endothelium and causes vasodilation and inhibition of platelet aggregation.
  - Prostaglandin E_2 causes pain.
  - Prostaglandins PGE2, PGD2, and PGF2 cause vasodilatation.

- **Lipoxygenase pathway**

  Leukotriene B4 (LTB4) causes neutrophil chemotaxis, while leukotriene C4, D4, E4 cause vasoconstriction. Lipoxins are antiinflammatory products which inhibit neutrophil chemotaxis.

In a Nutshell

Mediators of Pain

- Bradykinin
- Prostaglandins (E_2)

Important products in the complement cascade include C5b-C9 (membrane attack complex), C3a,C5a (anaphylatoxins stimulate the release of histamine), C5a (leukocyte chemotactic factor), and C3b (opsonin for phagocytosis).

Cytokines

- IL-1 and TNF cause fever and induce acute phase reactants; enhance adhesion molecules; and stimulate and activate fibroblasts, endothelial cells, and neutrophils.
- IL-8 is a neutrophil chemoattractant produced by macrophages.

In a Nutshell

Mediators of Fever

- Cytokines IL-1, IL-6, and TNF-α
- Prostaglandins

Four Outcomes of Acute Inflammation

- Complete resolution with regeneration
- Complete resolution with scarring
- Abscess formation
- Transition to chronic inflammation

CHRONIC INFLAMMATION

Causes of chronic inflammation include the following:

- Following a bout of acute inflammation
- Persistent infections
- Infections with certain organisms, including viral infections, mycobacteria, parasitic infections, and fungal infections
- Autoimmune diseases
- Response to foreign material
- Response to malignant tumors

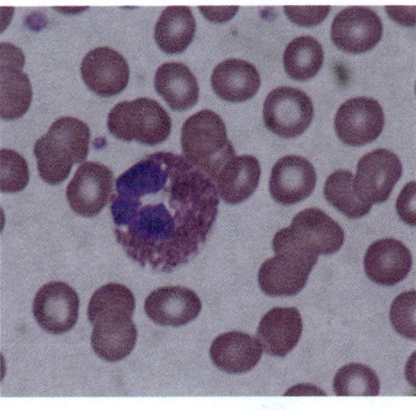

Bilobed nucleus, large granules (pink)
Eosinophil
Source: commons.wikimedia.org (Bobjgalindo)

There are several **important cells** in chronic inflammation.

- **Macrophages** are derived from blood monocytes. Tissue-based macrophages (life span in connective tissue compartment is 60–120 days) are found in connective tissue (histiocyte), lung (pulmonary alveolar macrophages), liver (Kupffer cells), bone (osteoclasts), and brain (microglia). During inflammation circulating monocytes emigrate from the blood to the periphery and differentiate into macrophages.
    - Respond to chemotactic factors: C5a, MCP-1, MIP-1α, PDGF, TGF-β
    - Secrete a wide variety of active products (monokines)
    - May be modified into epithelioid cells in granulomatous processes
- **Lymphocytes** include B cells and plasma cells, as well as T cells. Lymphotaxin is the lymphocyte chemokine.
- **Eosinophils** play an important role in parasitic infections and IgE-mediated allergic reactions. The eosinophilic chemokine is eotaxin. Eosinophil granules contain major basic protein, which is toxic to parasites.
- **Basophils** contain similar chemical mediators as mast cells in their granules. Mast cells are present in high numbers in the lung and skin. Both basophils and mast cells play an important role in IgE-mediated reactions (allergies and anaphylaxis) and can release histamine.

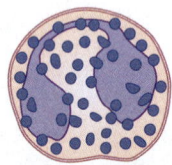

Bilobed nucleus, large granules (blue)
Basophil

Chronic granulomatous inflammation is a specialized form of chronic inflammation characterized by small aggregates of modified macrophages (epithelioid cells and multinucleated giant cells) usually populated by CD4+ Th1 lymphocytes.

Composition of a granuloma is as follows:

- Epithelioid cells, located centrally, form when IFN-γ transforms macrophages to epithelioid cells. They are enlarged cells with abundant pink cytoplasm.
- Multinucleated giant cells, located centrally, are formed by the fusion of epithelioid cells. Types include Langhans-type giant cell (peripheral arrangement of nuclei) and foreign body type giant cell (haphazard arrangement of nuclei).
- Lymphocytes and plasma cells are present at the periphery.
- Central necrosis occurs in granulomata due to excessive enzymatic breakdown and is commonly seen in *Mycobacterium tuberculosis* infection as well as fungal infections and a few bacterial infections. Because of the public health risk of tuberculosis, necrotizing granulomas should be considered tuberculosis until proven otherwise.

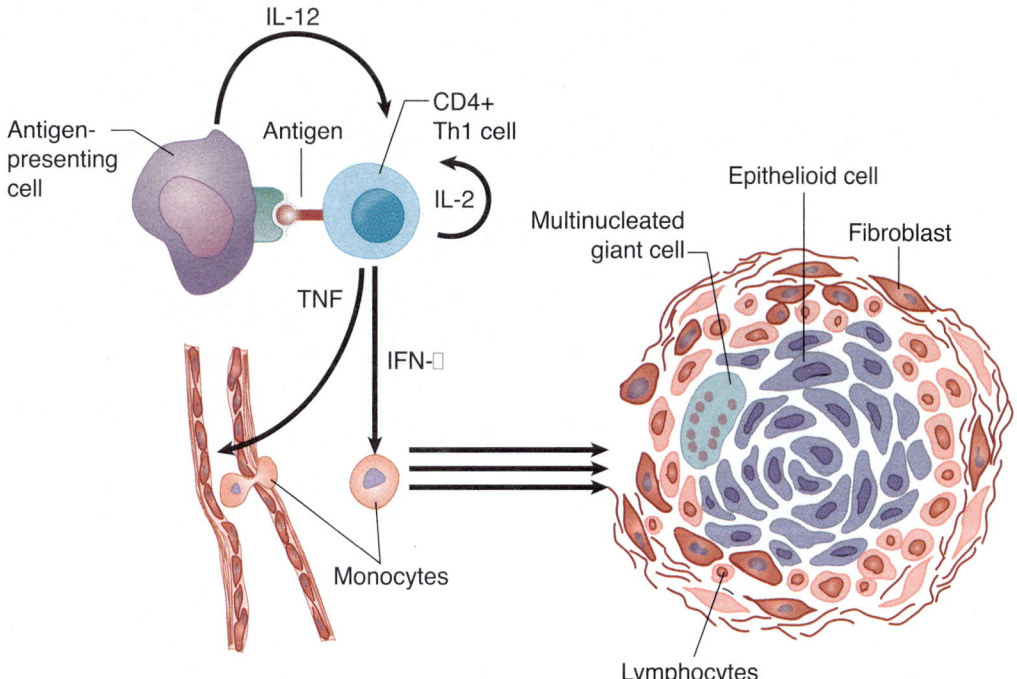

Figure 3-3. Granuloma Formation

Granulomatous diseases include tuberculosis (caseating granulomas), cat-scratch fever, syphilis, leprosy, fungal infections (e.g., coccidioidomycosis), parasitic infections (e.g., schistosomiasis), foreign bodies, beryllium, and sarcoidosis.

TISSUE RESPONSES TO INFECTIOUS AGENTS

Infectious diseases are very prevalent worldwide and are a major cause of morbidity and mortality. Infectious agents tend to have **tropism** for specific tissues and organs.

There are **six major histologic patterns:**

- **Exudative inflammation** is acute inflammatory response with neutrophils. Examples include bacterial meningitis, bronchopneumonia, and abscess.
- **Necrotizing inflammation** occurs when a virulent organism produces severe tissue damage and extensive cell death. Examples include necrotizing fasciitis and necrotizing pharyngitis.
- **Granulomatous inflammation.** Granulomatous response predominates with slow-growing organisms such as mycobacteria, fungi, and parasites.
- **Interstitial inflammation** is a diffuse mononuclear interstitial infiltrate that is a common response to viral infectious agents. Examples include myocarditis (Coxsackie virus) and viral hepatitis.
- **Cytopathic/cytoproliferative** inflammation refers to inflammation in which the infected/injured cell is altered. The changes may include intranuclear/cytoplasmic inclusions (cytomegalic inclusion disease, rabies [Negri body]); syncytia formation (respiratory syncytial virus and herpes virus); and apoptosis (Councilman body in viral hepatitis).
- **No inflammation.** An inflammatory response to microbes cannot occur in severely immunosuppressed individuals due to primary immunodeficiencies or acquired immunodeficient states (e.g., AIDS).

Learning Objectives

❏ Demonstrate understanding of regeneration and healing

❏ Answer questions about aberrations in wound healing

REGENERATION AND HEALING

Regeneration and healing of damaged cells and tissues starts almost as soon as the inflammatory process begins. Tissue repair involves five overlapping processes:

- Hemostasis (coagulation, platelets)
- Inflammation (neutrophils, macrophages, lymphocytes, mast cells)
- Regeneration (stem cells and differentiated cells)
- Fibrosis (macrophages, granulation tissue [fibroblasts, angiogenesis], type III collagen)
- Remodeling (macrophages, fibroblasts, converting collagen III to I)

The extracellular matrix (ECM) is an important tissue scaffold with two forms, the interstitial matrix and the basement membrane (type IV collagen and laminin). There are three ECM components:

- Collagens and elastins
- Gels (proteoglycans and hyaluronan)
- Glycoproteins and cell adhesion molecules

Different tissues have different **regenerative** capacities.

- **Labile cells** (primarily stem cells) regenerate throughout life. Examples include surface epithelial cells (skin and mucosal lining cells), hematopoietic cells, stem cells, etc.
- **Stable cells** (stem cells and differentiated cells) replicate at a low level throughout life and have the capacity to divide if stimulated by some initiating event. Examples include hepatocytes, proximal tubule cells, endothelium, etc.
- **Permanent cells** (few stem cells and/or differentiated cells with the capacity to replicate) have a very low level of replicative capacity. Examples include neurons and cardiac muscle.

Scar formation occurs in a series of steps when repair cannot be effected by regeneration.

- Angiogenesis is promoted by vascular endothelial growth factor (VEGF) and the fibroblast growth factor (FGF) family of growth factors
- Platelet-derived growth factor (PDGF), fibroblast growth factor 2 (FGF-2), and transforming growth factor β (TGF-β) drive fibroblast activation
- TGF-β, PDGF, and FGF drive ECM deposition. Cytokines IL-1 and IL-13 stimulate collagen production.

Types of Wound Healing

Primary union (**healing by first intention**) occurs when wounds are closed physically with sutures, metal staples, dermal adhesive, etc.

Secondary union (**healing by secondary intention**) occurs when wounds are allowed to heal by wound contraction and is mediated by myofibroblasts at the edge of the wound.

Note

Clinicians make decisions about wound healing techniques based on clinical information and the size of the tissue defect.

Repair in specific organs occurs as follows:

- **Liver:** Mild injury is repaired by regeneration of hepatocytes, sometimes with restoration to normal pathology. Severe or persistent injury causes formation of regenerative nodules that may be surrounded by fibrosis, leading to hepatic cirrhosis.
- In the **brain**, neurons do not regenerate, but microglia remove debris and astrocytes proliferate, causing gliosis.
- Damaged **heart muscle** cannot regenerate, so the heart heals by fibrosis.
- In the **lung**, type II pneumocytes replace type I pneumocytes after injury.
- In **peripheral nerves**, the distal part of the axon degenerates while the proximal part regrows slowly, using axonal sprouts to follow Schwann cells to the muscle.

ABERRATIONS IN WOUND HEALING

- **Delayed wound healing** may be seen in wounds complicated by foreign bodies, infection, ischemia, diabetes, malnutrition, scurvy, etc.
- **Hypertrophic scar** results in a prominent scar that is localized to the wound, due to excess production of granulation tissue and collagen. It is common in burn patients.
- **Keloid formation** is a genetic predisposition that is common in African Americans. It tends to affect the earlobes, face, neck, sternum, and forearms, and it may produce large tumor-like scars extending beyond the injury site. There is excess production of collagen that is predominantly type III.

Circulatory Pathology 5

Learning Objectives

❑ Use knowledge of edema, hemostasis, and bleeding disorders to solve problems

❑ Answer questions about thrombosis, embolism, and infarction

❑ Solve problems concerning shock

EDEMA

Edema is the presence of excess fluid in the intercellular space. It has many causes.

- **Increased hydrostatic pressure** causes edema in congestive heart failure (generalized edema), portal hypertension, renal retention of salt and water, and venous thrombosis (local edema).
- **Hypoalbuminemia and decreased colloid osmotic pressure** cause edema in liver disease, nephrotic syndrome, and protein deficiency (e.g., kwashiorkor).
- **Lymphatic obstruction** (lymphedema) causes edema in tumor, following surgical removal of lymph node drainage, and in parasitic infestation (filariasis → elephantiasis).
- **Increased endothelial permeability** causes edema in inflammation, type I hypersensitivity reactions, and with some drugs (e.g., bleomycin, heroin, etc.).
- **Increased interstitial sodium** causes edema when there is increased sodium intake, primary hyperaldosteronism, and renal failure.
- Specialized forms of tissue swelling due to **increased extracellular glycosaminoglycans** also occur, notably in pretibial myxedema and exophthalmos (Graves disease).

  Anasarca is severe generalized edema. **Effusion** is fluid within the body cavities.

Types of Edema Fluid

- **Transudate** is edema fluid with low protein content.
- **Exudate** is edema fluid with high protein content and cells. Types of exudates include purulent (pus), fibrinous, eosinophilic, and hemorrhagic.
- **Lymphedema** related to lymphatic obstruction leads to accumulation of protein-rich fluid which produces a non-pitting edema.
- **Glycosaminoglycan-rich** edema fluid shows increased hyaluronic acid and chondroitin sulfate, and causes myxedema.

  Active hyperemia versus congestion (passive hyperemia): an excessive amount of blood in a tissue or organ can accumulate secondary to vasodilatation (active, e.g., inflammation) or diminished venous outflow (passive, e.g., hepatic congestion).

HEMOSTASIS AND BLEEDING DISORDERS

Hemostasis is a sequence of events leading to the cessation of bleeding by the formation of a stable fibrin-platelet hemostatic plug. It involves interactions between the vascular wall, platelets, and the coagulation system.

Note

Clotting is a balance between two opposing forces: those favoring the formation of a stable thrombus versus those factors causing fibrinolysis of the clot.

Vascular Wall Injury

Transient vasoconstriction is mediated by endothelin-1. Thrombogenic factors include a variety of processes:

- Changes in blood flow cause turbulence and stasis favor clot formation.
- Release of tissue factor from injured cells activates factor VII (extrinsic pathway).
- Exposure of thrombogenic subendothelial collagen activates factor XII (intrinsic pathway).
- Release of von Willebrand factor (vWF) binds to exposed collagen and facilitates platelet adhesion.
- Decreased endothelial synthesis of antithrombogenic substances (prostacyclin, nitric oxide [NO2], tissue plasminogin activator, and thrombomodulin)

Bridge to Pharmacology

Aspirin irreversibly acetylates cyclooxygenase, preventing platelet production of thromboxane A2.

Platelets

Platelets are derived from megakaryocytes in the bone marrow. They form a thrombus through a series of steps.

- **Step 1: Platelet adhesion** occurs when vWF adheres to subendothelial collagen and then platelets adhere to vWF by glycoprotein Ib.
- **Step 2: Platelet activation** occurs when platelets undergo a shape change and degranulation occurs. Platelets synthesize thromboxane A2. Platelets also show membrane expression of the phospholipid complex, which is an important substrate for the coagulation cascade.
- **Step 3: Platelet aggregation** occurs when additional platelets are recruited from the bloodstream. ADP and thromboxane A2 are potent mediators of aggregation. Platelets bind to each other by binding to fibrinogen using GPIIb-IIIa.

  Laboratory tests for platelets include platelet count (normal 150,000–400,000 mm3) and platelet aggregometry.

  Bernard-Soulier syndrome and Glanzmann thrombasthenia present as mucocutaneous bleeding in childhood.

Table 5-1. Contents of Platelet Alpha Granules and Dense Bodies

Alpha Granules	Dense Bodies
• Fibrinogen	• ADP (potent platelet aggregator)
• Fibronectin	• Calcium
• Factor V and vWF	• Histamine and serotonin
• Platelet factor 4	• Epinephrine
• Platelet-derived growth factor (PDGF)	

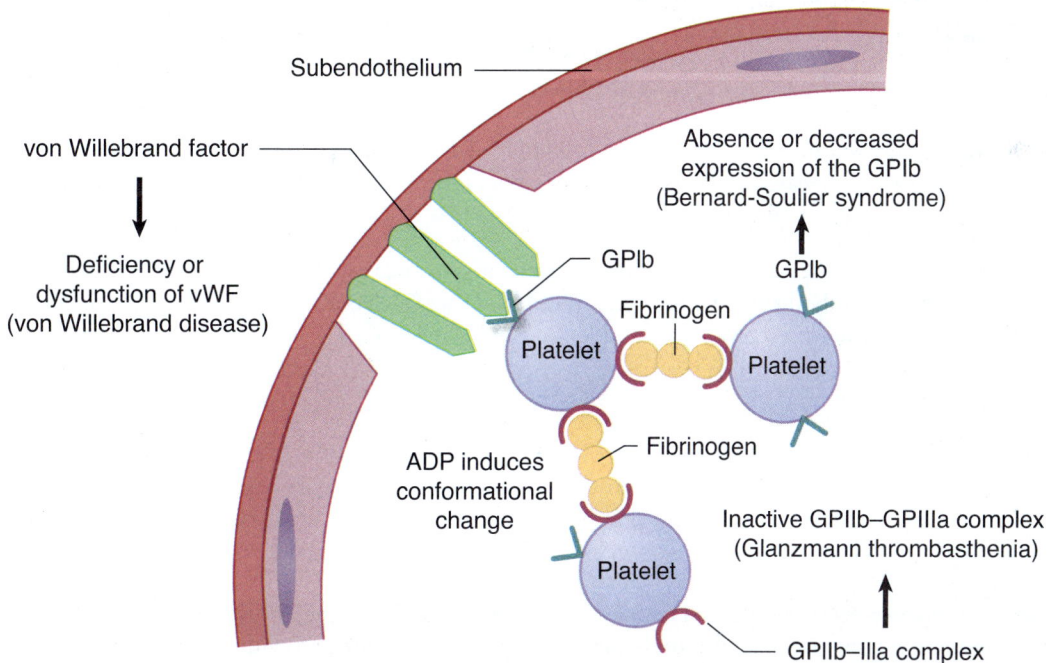

Figure 5-1. Platelet Aggregation

Table 5-2. Common Platelet disordersPlatelet Disorders

Thrombocytopenia	Qualitative Defects
Decreased production • Aplastic anemia (drugs, virus, etc.) • Tumor	• von Willebrand disease • Bernard-Soulier syndrome • Glanzmann thrombasthenia • Drugs (aspirin) • Uremia
Increased destruction • Immune thrombocytopenia (ITP) • Thrombotic thrombocytopenic purpura (TTP) • Disseminated intravascular coagulation (DIC) • Hypersplenism	

Immune thrombocytopenia purpura (ITP) is an immune-mediated attack (usually IgG antiplatelet antibodies) against platelets leading to decreased platelets (thrombocytopenia) which result in petechiae, purpura (bruises), and a bleeding diathesis (e.g., hematomas).

The etiology involves antiplatelet antibodies against platelet antigens such as GPIIb-IIIa and GPIb-IX (type II hypersensitivity reaction). The antibodies are made in the spleen, and the platelets are destroyed peripherally in the spleen by macrophages, which have Fc receptors that bind IgG-coated platelets.

Forms of ITP include:

- Acute ITP, seen in children following a viral infection and is a self-limited disorder.
- Chronic ITP, usually seen in women in their childbearing years and may be the first manifestation of systemic lupus erythematosus (SLE). Clinically, it is characterized by petechiae, ecchymoses, menorrhagia, and nosebleeds.

Lab studies usually show decreased platelet count and prolonged bleeding time but normal prothrombin time and partial thromboplastin time. Peripheral blood smear shows thrombocytopenia with enlarged immature platelets (megathrombocytes). Bone marrow biopsy shows increased numbers of megakaryocytes with immature forms.

Treatment is corticosteroids, which decrease antibody production; immunoglobulin therapy, which floods Fc receptors on splenic macrophages; and/or splenectomy, which removes the site of platelet destruction and antibody production.

Thrombotic thrombocytopenic purpura (TTP) is a rare disorder of hemostasis in which there is widespread intravascular formation of fibrin-platelet thrombi. It is sometimes associated with an acquired or inherited deficiency of the enzyme ADAMTS13, responsible for cleaving large multimers of von Willebrand factor.

Clinically, TTP most often affects adult women. The inclusion criteria are microangiopathic hemolytic anemia and thrombocytopenia, with or without renal failure or neurologic abnormalities. Pathology includes widespread formation of platelet thrombi with fibrin (hyaline thrombi) leading to intravascular hemolysis (thrombotic microangiopathy).

Lab studies typically show decreased platelet count and prolonged bleeding time but normal prothrombin time and partial thromboplastin time. Peripheral blood smear shows thrombocytopenia, schistocytes, and reticulocytosis. Treatment is plasma exchange.

Hemolytic uremic syndrome (HUS) is a form of thrombotic microangiopathy due to endothelial cell damage. It occurs mostly in children, typically after a gastroenteritis (typically due to Shiga toxin-producing *E. coli 0157:H7*).

Typical HUS presents with abdominal pain, diarrhea (an atypical variant is diarrhea-negative), microangiopathic hemolytic anemia, thrombocytopenia, and renal failure. Renal involvement is seen more commonly than in TTP. The kidney shows fibrin thrombi in the glomeruli. Renal glomerular endothelial cells are targeted by the bacterial toxin. Glomerular scarring may ensue.

Treatment is supportive (fluid management, dialysis, erythrocyte transfusions); plasma exchange is only used for atypical cases.

Coagulation factors. The majority of the clotting factors are produced by the liver. The factors are proenzymes that must be converted to the active form. Some conversions occur on a phospholipid surface, and some conversions require calcium.

- The **intrinsic coagulation pathway** is activated by the contact factors, which include contact with subendothelial collagen, high molecular weight kininogen (HMWK), and kallikrein.
- The **extrinsic coagulation pathway** is activated by the release of tissue factor.

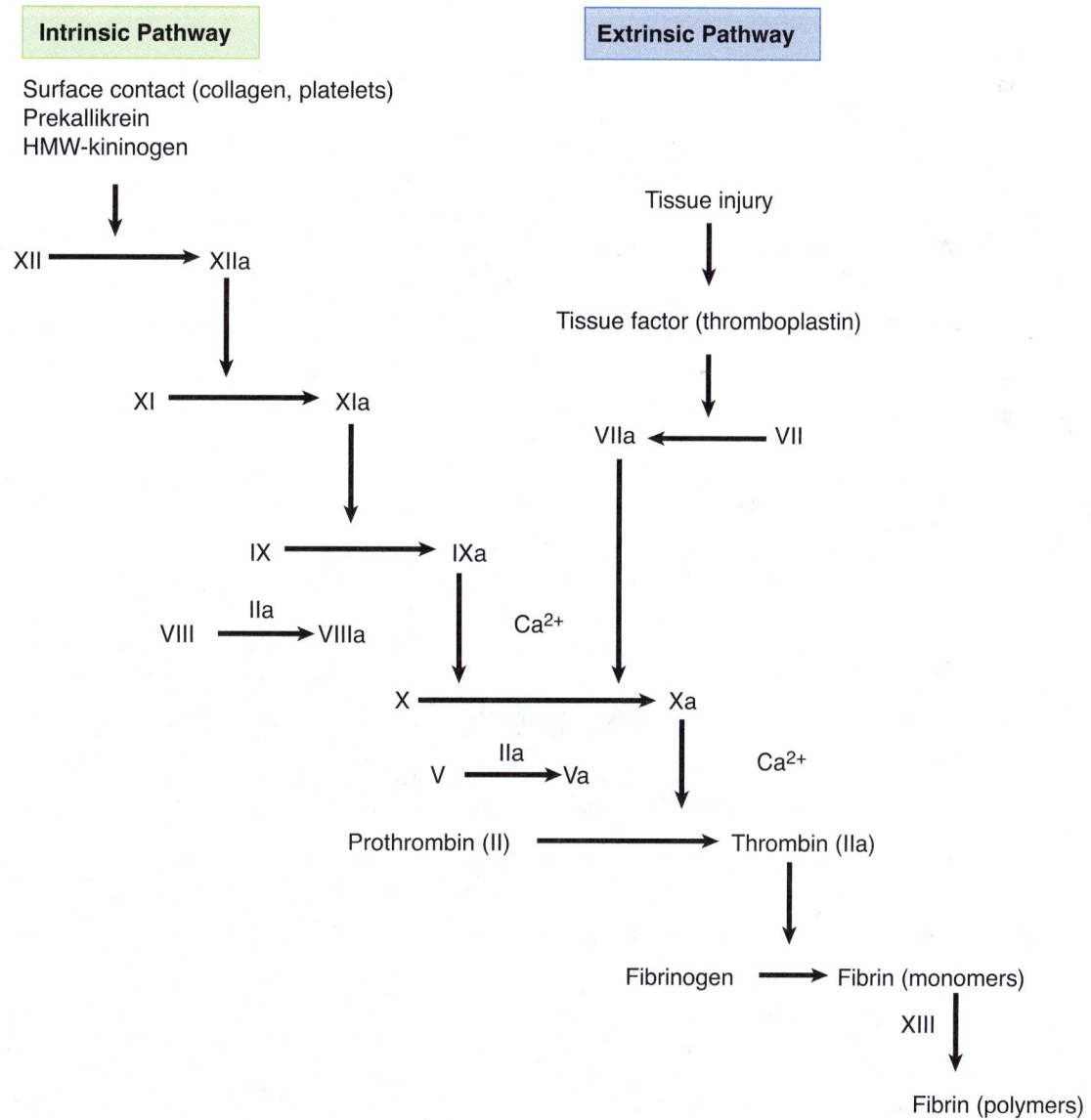

Figure 5-2. Coagulation Cascade

Lab tests for coagulation include the following:

- Prothrombin time (PT), which tests the extrinsic and common coagulation pathways (more specifically, it tests factors VII, X, V, prothrombin, and fibrinogen). The international normalized ratio (INR) standardizes the PT test so that results throughout the world can be compared. A longer time means blood takes longer to clot.
- Partial thromboplastin time (PTT), which tests the intrinsic and common coagulation pathways (more specifically, it tests factors XII, XI, IX, VIII, X, V, prothrombin, and fibrinogen).
- Thrombin time (TT), which tests for adequate fibrinogen levels.
- Fibrin degradation products (FDP), which tests the fibrinolytic system (increased with DIC).

  Hemophilia A (classic hemophilia) is an X-linked recessive condition resulting from a deficiency of factor VIII. Clinically, hemophilia A predominately affects males. Symptoms vary depending on the degree of deficiency.
- Newborns may develop bleeding at the time of circumcision.
- Other problems include spontaneous hemorrhage into joints (hemarthrosis), easy bruising and hematoma formation after minor trauma, and severe prolonged bleeding after surgery or lacerations.

Laboratory studies typically show normal platelet count and normal bleeding time, normal PT and prolonged PTT. Treatment is factor VIII concentrate.

Hemophilia B (Christmas disease) is an X-linked recessive condition resulting from a deficiency of factor IX that is clinically identical to hemophilia A. Treatment is recombinant factor IX.

Acquired coagulopathies include vitamin K deficiency (decreased synthesis of factors II, VII, IX, X, and protein C & S) and liver disease (decreased synthesis of virtually all clotting factors).

Von Willebrand disease is an autosomal dominant bleeding disorder characterized by a deficiency or qualitative defect in von Willebrand factor. vWF is normally produced by endothelial cells and megakaryocytes. Clinical features include spontaneous bleeding from mucous membranes, prolonged bleeding from wounds, and menorrhagia in young females. Hemarthrosis is uncommon.

Lab studies show normal platelet count, a prolonged bleeding time, normal PT, and often prolonged PTT. Abnormal platelet response to ristocetin (adhesion defect) is an important diagnostic test. Treatment for mild classic cases (type I) is desmopressin (an antidiuretic hormone analog), which releases vWF from Weibel-Palade bodies of endothelial cells.

Note

Von Willebrand disease is the most common inherited bleeding disorder.

Disseminated intravascular coagulation (DIC) is always secondary to another disorder. Causes are diverse.

- Obstetric complications can cause DIC because placental tissue factor activates clotting.
- Gram-negative sepsis can cause DIC because tumor necrosis factor activates clotting.
- Microorganisms (especially meningococcus and rickettsiae)
- AML M3 (cytoplasmic granules in neoplastic promyelocytes activate clotting)
- Adenocarcinomas (mucin activates clotting)

DIC causes widespread microthrombi with consumption of platelets and clotting factors, causing hemorrhage. Laboratory studies show decreased platelet count, prolonged PT/PTT, decreased fibrinogen, and elevated fibrin split products (D dimers). Treat the underlying disorder.

THROMBOSIS

Thrombosis is the pathologic formation of an intravascular fibrin-platelet thrombus during life. Factors involved in thrombus formation (**Virchow's triad**) include:

- Endothelial injury due to atherosclerosis, vasculitis, or many other causes
- Alterations in laminar blood flow predisposing for DIC occur with stasis of blood (e.g., immobilization); turbulence (e.g., aneurysms); and hyperviscosity of blood (e.g., polycythemia vera)
- Hypercoagulability of blood can be seen with clotting disorders (factor V Leiden; deficiency of antithrombin III, protein C, or protein S); tissue injury (postoperative and trauma); neoplasia; nephrotic syndrome; advanced age; pregnancy; and oral contraceptives (estrogen increases synthetic activity of the liver, including clotting factors)

Table 5-3. Comparison of a Thrombus with a Blood Clot

	Thrombus	Blood Clot
Location	Intravascular	Extravascular or intravascular (postmortem)
Composition	Platelets	Lacks platelets
	Fibrin	Fibrin
	RBCs and WBCs	RBCs and WBCs
Lines of Zahn	Present	Absent
Shape	Has shape	Lacks shape

Common locations of thrombus formation include coronary and cerebral arteries; heart chambers in atrial fibrillation or post-MI (mural thrombus); aortic aneurysms; heart valves (vegetations); and deep leg veins (DVTs).

Outcomes of thrombosis include vascular occlusion and infarctions; embolism; thrombolysis; and organization and recanalization.

EMBOLISM

An embolism is any intravascular mass that has been carried down the bloodstream from its site of origin, resulting in the occlusion of a vessel. There are many types of emboli:

- **Thromboemboli:** most common (98%)
- Atheromatous emboli (severe atherosclerosis)
- Fat emboli (bone fractures and soft tissue trauma)
- Bone marrow emboli (bone fractures and cardiopulmonary resuscitation [CPR])
- Gas emboli cause decompression sickness ("the bends" and caisson disease) when rapid ascent results in nitrogen gas bubbles in the blood vessels
- Amniotic fluid emboli are a complication of labor that may result in DIC; fetal squamous cells are seen in the maternal pulmonary vessels
- Tumor emboli (metastasis)
- Talc emboli (IV drug abuse)
- Bacterial/septic emboli (infectious endocarditis)

Pulmonary emboli (PE) are often clinically silent and are the most commonly missed diagnosis in hospitalized patients. They are found in almost 50% of all hospital autopsies. Most PE (95%) arise from deep leg vein thrombosis (DVT) in the leg; other sources include the right side of the heart and the pelvic venous plexuses of the prostate and uterus.

Diagnosis of a PE can be established when V/Q lung shows a scan V/Q mismatch. Doppler ultrasound of the leg veins can be used to detect a DVT. Additionally, plasma D-dimer ELISA test is elevated.

Most cases are clinically silent and resolve.

Clinical Correlate

The classic presentation of pulmonary embolism, which occurs in <20% of patients, includes hemoptysis, dyspnea, and chest pain.

Infarction is more common in patients with cardiopulmonary compromise. Symptoms include shortness of breath, hemoptysis, pleuritic chest pain, and pleural effusion. On gross examination there is typically a hemorrhagic wedge-shaped infarct. The infarction heals by regeneration or scar formation.

- Sudden death can occur when large emboli lodge in the bifurcation (saddle embolus) or large pulmonary artery branches.
- Chronic secondary pulmonary hypertension is caused by recurrent PEs, which increase pulmonary resistance and lead to secondary pulmonary hypertension.

INFARCTION

Infarction is a localized area of necrosis secondary to ischemia. Common sites of infarction include heart, brain, lungs, intestines, kidneys. Infarcts have multiple causes.

- Most infarcts (99%) result from thrombotic or embolic occlusion of an artery or vein.
- Less common causes include vasospasm and torsion of arteries and veins (e.g., volvulus, ovarian, and testicular torsion).

On gross examination infarctions typically have a wedge shape, with the apex of the wedge tending to point to the occlusion.

- **Anemic infarcts (pale or white color)** occur in solid organs with a single blood supply such as the spleen, kidney, and heart.
- **Hemorrhagic infarcts (red color)** occur in organs with a dual blood supply or collateral circulation, such as the lung and intestines, and can also occur with venous occlusion (e.g., testicular torsion).

Microscopic pathology of infarction can show either coagulative necrosis (most organs) or liquifactive necrosis (brain). The general sequence of tissue changes after infarction is as follows:

ischemia → coagulative necrosis → inflammation → granulation tissue → fibrous scar

SHOCK

Shock is characterized by vascular collapse and widespread hypoperfusion of cells and tissue due to reduced blood volume, cardiac output, or vascular tone. The cellular injury is initially reversible; if the hypoxia persists, the cellular injury becomes irreversible, leading to the death of cells and the patient.

Major Causes of Shock

- **Cardiogenic shock** (pump failure) can be due to myocardial infarction, cardiac arrhythmias, pulmonary embolism, and cardiac tamponade.
- **Hypovolemic shock** (reduced blood volume) can be due to hemorrhage, fluid loss secondary to severe burns, and severe dehydration.
- **Septic shock** (viral or bacterial infection) causes cytokines to trigger vasodilatation and hypotension, acute respiratory distress syndrome (ARDS), DIC, and multiple organ dysfunction syndrome. Mortality rate is 20%.
- **Neurogenic shock** (generalized vasodilatation) can be seen with anesthesia and brain or spinal cord injury.
- **Anaphylactic shock** (generalized vasodilatation) is a type I hypersensitivity reaction.

Stages of Shock

The stages of shock are arbitrarily defined as follows.

- **Stage I: compensation**

  Perfusion to vital organs is maintained by reflex mechanisms. Compensation is characterized by increased sympathetic tone, release of catecholamines, and activation of the renin-angiotensin system.
- **Stage II: decompensation**

  There is a progressive decrease in tissue perfusion, leading to potentially reversible tissue injury with development of a metabolic (lactic) acidosis, electrolyte imbalances, and renal insufficiency.
- **Stage III: irreversible tissue injury and organ failure**

  This ultimately results in death.

The organs show various manifestations of shock:

- Kidneys show fibrin thrombi in glomeruli and ultimately, acute tubular failure ensues, which causes oliguria and electrolyte imbalances.
- Lungs undergo diffuse alveolar damage ("shock lung").
- Intestines show superficial mucosal ischemic necrosis and hemorrhages, and with prolonged injury, bacteremia may ensue.

Learning Objectives

❏ Answer questions about disorders involving an extra autosome and chromosomal deletions

❏ Demonstrate understanding of Mendelian disorders, autosomal recessive/dominant, and x-linked recessive/dominant conditions

❏ Solve problems concerning triplet repeat mutations

❏ Explain information related to mitochondrial DNA disorders and multifactorial inheritance

DISORDERS INVOLVING AN EXTRA AUTOSOME

Down syndrome (trisomy 21).

The most common **karyotype** is 47, XX, +21. Down syndrome is the **most common of the chromosomal disorders**. The risk increases with maternal age to an incidence of 1 in 25 live births in women age ≥45. The pathogenesis involves meiotic nondisjunction (95%), Robertsonian translocation (4%), or mosaicism due to mitotic nondisjunction during embryogenesis (1%).

Clinical findings can include intellectual disability; mongoloid facial features (flat face, low-bridged nose, and epicanthal folds); Brushfield spots (speckled appearance of the iris); muscular hypotonia; broad short neck; palmar (simian) crease; and congenital heart defects. Endocardial cushion defect, if present, leads to the formation of an atrioventricular canal (a common connection between all four chambers of the heart). Additional clinical problems that can develop include duodenal atresia ("double-bubble" sign); Hirschsprung disease; increased risk (15–20 fold) of acute lymphoblastic leukemia (ALL); and Alzheimer disease (by age 40 virtually all will develop Alzheimer disease).

Prenatal tests include maternal serum tests, ultrasonography, amniocentesis, and chorionic villus sampling.

Median life expectancy is 47 years.

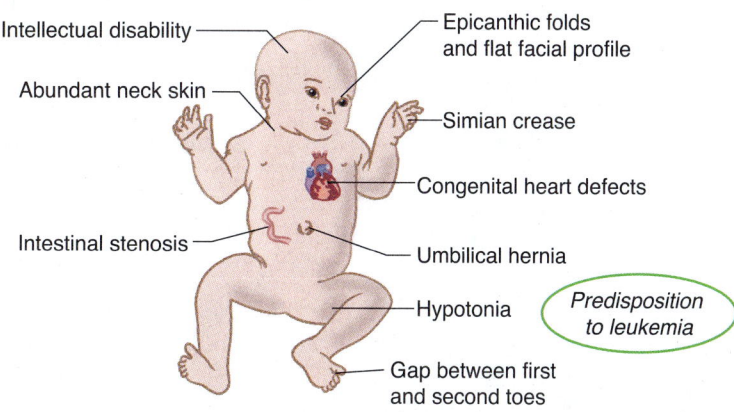

Figure 6-1. Down Syndrome

Edwards syndrome (trisomy 18) is caused by nondisjunction. The risk increases with maternal age.

Clinical findings can include intellectual disability; low-set ears and micrognathia; congenital heart defects; overlapping flexed fingers; and rocker-bottom feet. There is a very poor prognosis due to severe congenital malformations.

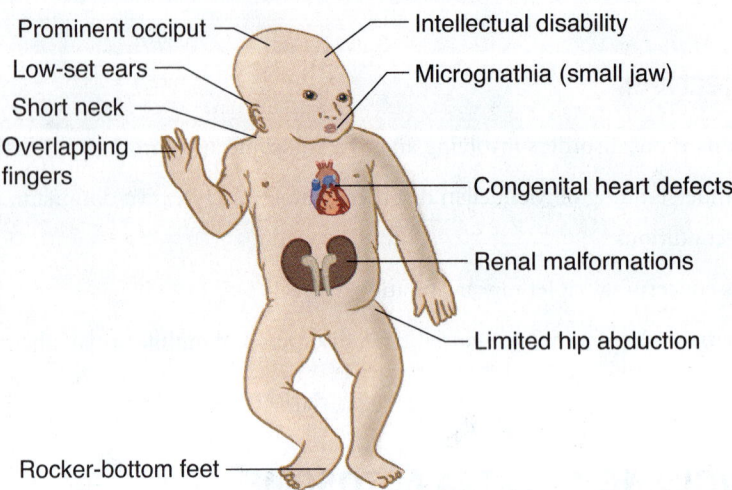

Prominent occiput
Low-set ears
Short neck
Overlapping fingers

Intellectual disability
Micrognathia (small jaw)
Congenital heart defects
Renal malformations
Limited hip abduction

Rocker-bottom feet

Figure 6-2. Edwards Syndrome

Patau syndrome (trisomy 13) is caused by nondisjunction. The risk increases with maternal age.

Clinical findings can include intellectual disability; cleft lip and/or palate; cardiac defects; renal abnormalities; microcephaly; holoprosencephaly; and polydactyly. The very poor prognosis is due to severe congenital malformations.

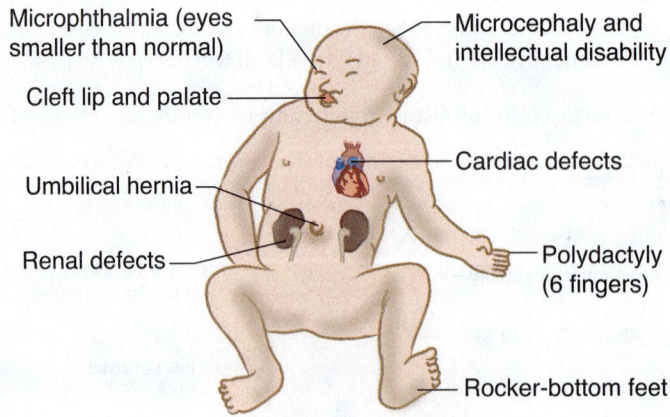

Microphthalmia (eyes smaller than normal)
Cleft lip and palate
Umbilical hernia
Renal defects

Microcephaly and intellectual disability
Cardiac defects
Polydactyly (6 fingers)
Rocker-bottom feet

Figure 6-3. Patau Syndrome

DISORDERS INVOLVING CHROMOSOMAL DELETIONS

Cri du chat syndrome is due to deletion of the short arm of chromosome 5. Clinical findings include a characteristic high-pitched catlike cry; intellectual disability; congenital heart disease; and microcephaly. **Microdeletions** include 13q14 (retinoblastoma gene) and 11p13 (WAGR complex [Wilms tumor, aniridia, genitourinary anomalies, and intellectual disability [previously known as mental retardation]]). Microdeletions are too small to be detected by karyotyping and require molecular techniques for detection.

DISORDERS INVOLVING SEX CHROMOSOMES

Klinefelter syndrome is caused by meiotic nondisjunction and is a common cause of male hypogonadism. The most common karyotype is 47,XXY. Lab studies show elevated FSH and LH with low levels of testosterone. Clinical findings include testicular atrophy, infertility due to azoospermia, eunuchoid body habitus, high-pitched voice; female distribution of hair; and gynecomastia.

> **Note**
>
> The presence of a Y chromosome determines male phenotype due to the presence of the testes-determining factor gene (also called the sex-determining region Y [SRY]) on the Y chromosome.

Turner syndrome is a common cause of female hypogonadism. The most common karyotype is 45,X. The second X chromosome is necessary for oogenesis and normal development of the ovary. Clinically, patients fail to develop secondary sex characteristics and have short stature with widely spaced nipples. Other features include gonadal dysgenesis with atrophic streak ovaries; primary amenorrhea; and infertility.

Clinical features involving other organ systems include cystic hygroma and webbing of the neck; hypothyroidism; congenital heart disease (preductal coarctation of the aorta and bicuspid aortic valve); and hydrops fetalis. Females with 45,X/46,XY mosaicism are at risk for gonadoblastoma.

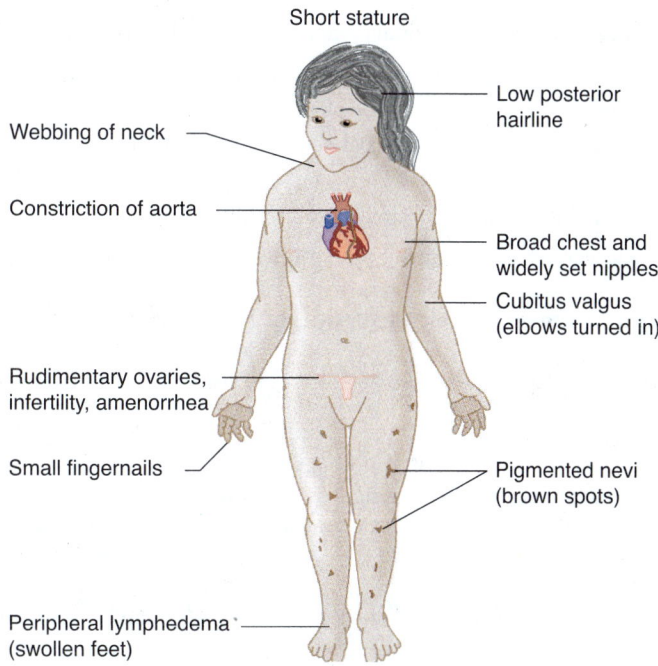

Figure 6-4. Turner Syndrome

MENDELIAN DISORDERS

Mendelian disorders are characterized by single gene mutations. Common types of mutations include point mutations and frameshift mutations.

- **Point mutations** occur with a single nucleotide base substitution, which may produce a variety of effects. The form of point mutation called synonymous mutation (silent mutation) occurs when a base substitution results in a codon that codes for the same amino acid. The form of point mutation called missense mutation occurs when a base substitution results in a new codon and a change in amino acids. The form of point mutation called a nonsense mutation occurs when a base substitution produces a stop codon and therefore produces a truncated protein.

- **Frameshift mutations** occur when insertion or deletion of bases leads to a shift in the reading frame of the gene.

The location of a mutation will alter its potential effects. Mutations involving coding regions of DNA may result in abnormal amino acid sequences; decreased production of the protein; truncated or abnormally folded protein; or altered or lost function of the protein. Mutations of promoter or enhancer regions may interfere with transcription factors, resulting in decreased transcription of the gene.

Patterns of inheritance for genetic diseases show wide variation, and the genetic pattern of a disease may be classified as autosomal dominant; autosomal recessive; X-linked recessive; X-linked dominant; triplet repeat mutations; genomic imprinting; mitochondrial; or multifactorial.

AUTOSOMAL RECESSIVE DISORDERS

Cystic fibrosis (CF) is the most common lethal genetic disorder in Caucasians. It is due to mutation of the chloride channel protein, cystic fibrosis transmembrane conductance regulator (CFTR), whose *CFTR* gene is located on chromosome 7 and most commonly has been damaged by a deletion of the amino acid phenylalanine at position 508 (ΔF508). The defective chloride channel protein leads to abnormally thick viscous mucus, which obstructs the ducts of exocrine organs.

The **distribution of disease** reflects the distribution of eccrine sweat glands and exocrine glands.

- In the lungs, CF may cause recurrent pulmonary infections; chronic bronchitis; and bronchiectasis.
- In the pancreas, CF may cause plugging of pancreatic ducts resulting in atrophy and fibrosis; and pancreatic insufficiency leading to fat malabsorption, malodorous steatorrhea, and deficiency of fat-soluble vitamins.
- In the male reproductive system, CF may be associated with absence or obstruction of the vas deferens and epididymis, which often leads to male infertility.
- In the liver, plugging of the biliary canaliculi may result in biliary cirrhosis.
- In the GI tract, the thick secretions may cause small intestinal obstruction (meconium ileus).

Diagnosis can be established with a sweat test (elevated NaCl) or DNA probes.

Phenylketonuria (PKU) is due to deficiency of phenylalanine hydroxylase, resulting in toxic levels of phenylalanine and a lack of tyrosine.

Clinically, affected children are normal at birth but, if undiagnosed and untreated, develop intellectual development disorder by age 6 months. The lack of tyrosine causes light-colored skin and hair, since melanin is a tyrosine derivative. Affected children may have a mousy or musty odor to the sweat and urine (secondary to metabolite [phenylacetate] accumulation).

Screening for PKU is done at birth. Treatment is dietary restriction of phenylalanine, including avoidance of the artificial sweetener aspartame.

Bridge to Biochemistry

Phenylalanine hydroxylase converts phenylalanine into tyrosine.

Alkaptonuria (ochronosis) occurs when deficiency of homogentisic acid oxidase results in the accumulation of homogentisic acid. The homogentisic acid has an affinity for connective tissues (especially cartilage), resulting in a black discoloration (as a consequence of oxidation of homogentisic acid).

Clinical features include urine that is initially pale yellow but turns black upon standing, and black-stained cartilage, which causes discoloration of the nose and ears. Alkaptonuria also predisposes for early onset of degenerative arthritis.

Albinism is caused by a lack of the enzyme tyrosinase needed for melanin production. Affected individuals show deficiency of melanin pigmentation in the skin, hair follicles, and eyes (oculocutaneous albinism), with resulting increased risk of basal cell and squamous cell carcinomas.

The **glycogen storage diseases** are a group of rare diseases that have in common a deficiency of one of the enzymes necessary for the metabolism of glycogen, which results in the accumulation of glycogen in the liver, heart, and skeletal muscle.

- **Type I (von Gierke disease)** is due to a deficiency of *glucose-6-phosphatase*, and is characterized clinically by hepatomegaly and hypoglycemia.
- **Type II (Pompe disease)** is due to a deficiency of *lysosomal α-1, 4-glucosidase (acid maltase)*, and is characterized clinically by hepatomegaly, skeletal muscle hypotonia, cardiomegaly, and death from cardiac failure by age 2 years.
- **Type V (McArdle syndrome)** is due to a deficiency of *muscle glycogen phosphorylase*, and is characterized clinically by exercise-induced muscle cramps.

  Tay-Sachs disease is due to a deficiency of hexosaminidase A (due to mutation of *HEXA* gene on chromosome 15), which leads to the accumulation of GM_2 ganglioside in the lysosomes of the CNS and retina. Tay-Sachs is common in Ashkenazi Jews (1 in 30 carrier rate).

  The distribution of disease involves the retina (cherry-red spot due to accentuation of the macula) and central nervous system (dilated neurons with cytoplasmic vacuoles). Affected children are normal at birth, but by six months show onset of symptoms (progressive mental deterioration and motor incoordination) that progress to death by age 2-3 years. **Electron microscopy** shows distended lysosomes with whorled membranes; the diagnosis can also be established with enzyme assays and DNA probes.

Niemann-Pick disease is caused by a deficiency of sphingomyelinase, which leads to the accumulation of sphingomyelin within the lysosomes of the CNS and reticuloendothelial system (monocytes and macrophages located in reticular connective tissue). Niemann-Pick is common in Ashkenazi Jews (note similarity to Tay-Sachs disease).

The distribution of disease depends on the form of disease, but can involve the retina (cherry-red spot, note similarity to Tay-Sachs disease); central nervous system (distended neurons with a foamy cytoplasmic vacuolization, note similarity to Tay-Sachs disease); and reticuloendothelial system (hepatosplenomegaly, lymphadenopathy, and bone marrow involvement; note difference from Tay-Sachs disease).

In Neimann-Pick **types A and B**, there is a mutation affecting an enzyme that metabolizes lipids; organomegaly occurs, and with type A, there is severe neurologic damage. In **type C**—the most common form—a defect in cholesterol transport causes ataxia, dysarthria, and learning difficulties. All forms are lethal, usually before adulthood.

Gaucher disease is the most common lysosomal storage disorder. Deficiency of glucocerebrosidase leads to the accumulation of glucocerebroside, predominately in the lysosomes of the reticuloendothelial system (monocytes and macrophages located in reticular connective tissue).

Type I represents 99% of cases and presents in adulthood with hepatosplenomegaly; thrombocytopenia/pancytopenia secondary to hypersplenism; lymphadenopathy; and bone marrow involvement that may lead to bone pain, deformities, and fractures. Central nervous system manifestations occur in **types II and III**.

The characteristic **Gaucher cells** are enlarged macrophages with a fibrillary (tissue paper–like) cytoplasm. Diagnosis can be established with biochemical enzyme assay of glucocerebrosidase activity.

Mucopolysaccharidosis (MPS) is a group of lysosomal storage disorders characterized by deficiencies in the lysosomal enzymes required for the degradation of mucopolysaccharides (glycosaminoglycans).

Clinical features include intellectual disability; cloudy cornea; hepatosplenomegaly; skeletal deformities and coarse facial features; joint abnormalities; and cardiac lesions. MPS I (Hurler syndrome) is the severe form and is due to deficiency of α-L-iduronidase. MPS II (Hunter syndrome) is a milder form; it shows X-linked recessive inheritance and is due to a deficiency of L-iduronate sulfatase.

AUTOSOMAL DOMINANT DISORDERS

Familial hypercholesterolemia is the most common inherited disorder (incidence 1 in 500) and is due to a mutation in the low density lipoprotein (LDL) receptor gene (LDLR) on chromosome 19. The mutations in the LDL receptor cause increased levels of circulating cholesterol, loss of feedback inhibition of HMG-coenzyme A (HMG-CoA) reductase, and increased phagocytosis of LDL by macrophages.

Clinical features include elevated serum cholesterol (heterozygotes have elevations of 2–3 times the normal level and homozygotes have elevations of 5–6 times the normal level), skin xanthomas (collections of lipid-laden macrophages), xanthelasma around the eyes, and premature atherosclerosis (homozygotes often develop myocardial infarctions in late teens and twenties).

Marfan syndrome is due to a mutation of the **fibrillin** gene (*FBN1*) on chromosome 15q21. Fibrillin is a glycoprotein that functions as a scaffold for the alignment of elastic fibers.

Clinical features include skeletal changes (tall, thin build with long extremities, hyperextensible joints, pectus excavatum [inwardly depressed sternum], and pectus carinatum [pigeon breast]) and abnormal eyes (ectopia lentis, characterized by bilateral subluxation of the lens). The cardiovascular system is also particularly vulnerable; it may show cystic medial degeneration of the media of elastic arteries with a loss of elastic fibers and smooth muscle cells with increased risk of dissecting aortic aneurysm (a major cause of death), dilatation of the aortic ring potentially leading to aortic valve insufficiency, and/or mitral valve prolapse.

Ehlers-Danlos syndrome (EDS) is a group of inherited connective tissue diseases that have in common a defect in collagen structure or synthesis. Clinically, the disease causes hyperextensible skin that is easily traumatized and hyperextensible joints secondary to effects on the joints and adjacent ligaments.

Note

Disorders of collagen biosynthesis include scurvy, osteogenesis imperfecta, Ehlers-Danlos syndrome, Alport syndrome, and Menkes disease.

Neurofibromatosis

Type 1 (**von Recklinghausen disease**) neurofibromatosis (90% of cases) has an incidence of 1 in 3,000. The condition is due to a mutation of the tumor suppressor gene *NF1* located on chromosome 17 (17q11.2). The normal gene product (neurofibromin) inhibits p21 ras oncoprotein.

- Affected individuals characteristically have multiple neurofibromas and benign tumors of peripheral nerves that are often numerous and may be disfiguring. The plexiform variant of the neurofibromas are diagnostic.
- Rarely (3%), malignant transformation of a neurofibroma may occur.
- Other clinical features include pigmented skin lesions (6 or more "cafe-au-lait spots" that are light brown macules usually located over nerves); pigmented iris hamartomas (Lisch nodules); and increased risk of meningiomas and pheochromocytoma, an adrenal tumor that also occurs with von Hippel-Lindau disease and MEN 2.

Type 2 (**bilateral acoustic**) neurofibromatosis (10% of cases) has an incidence of 1 in 45,000.

- There is a mutated tumor suppressor gene *NF-2* (22q12.2) on chromosome 22.
- The normal gene product (merlin) is a critical regulator of contact-dependent inhibition of proliferation.
- Clinical features include vestibular schwannomas (acoustic neuromas), and increased risk of meningioma and ependymomas.

TRIPLET REPEAT MUTATIONS

Fragile X syndrome is due to triplet nucleotide repeat mutations, so that the nucleotide sequence CGG repeats typically hundreds to thousands of times. The mutation occurs in the *FMR-1* gene (fragile X mental retardation-1) on the X chromosome (Xq27.3), and the disease behaves as an X-linked dominant disease that causes intellectual disability in all affected males and 50% of female carriers. The characteristic phenotype includes elongated face with a large jaw, large everted ears, and macroorchidism. The condition can be diagnosed with DNA probe analysis.

Huntington disease is due to a triplet repeat mutation (CAG) of the *HTT* gene that produces an abnormal protein (huntingtin), which is neurotoxic and causes atrophy of the caudate nucleus. Huntington disease has an early onset (age range: 20–50 years) of progressive dementia with choreiform movements.

MITOCHONDRIAL DNA DISORDERS

Mitochondrial DNA codes for mitochondrial oxidative phosphorylation enzymes; inheritance is only from mother to child, because only the ovum contributes mitochondria to the zygote. Examples include:

- **Leber hereditary optic neuropathy** causes loss of retinal cells, which leads to central vision loss.
- **Myoclonic epilepsy with ragged red fibers (MERRF)** is a mitochondrial disorder characterized by epilepsy, ataxia, peripheral neuropathy and deterioration in cognitive ability. Sensorineural hearing loss and ocular dysfunction can also develop. Patients have short stature and cardiomyopathy. On muscle biopsy, ragged red fibers are seen on Gomori trichrome staining due to the accumulation of mitochondria.

MULTIFACTORIAL INHERITANCE

Multifactorial inheritance refers to disease caused by a combination of multiple minor gene mutations and environmental factors. Examples include open neural tube defects and type 2 diabetes mellitus.

Immunopathology

Learning Objectives

❑ Explain information related to hypersensitivity reactions and autoimmune diseases

❑ Answer questions about primary/secondary immune deficiency syndromes

❑ Demonstrate understanding of AIDS

❑ Answer questions about immunology of transplant rejection

HYPERSENSITIVITY REACTIONS

(This material is included here for reinforcement. It is also covered in the Immunology Lecture Notes.)

Type I (immediate) hypersensitivity reactions (**anaphylactic type**) are characterized by IgE-dependent release of chemical mediators from mast cells and basophils. Cross-linking of IgE bound to antigen to IgE Fc receptors on the surface of mast cells and basophils causes degranulation. This binding triggers release of chemical mediators that include histamine and heparin; eosinophil chemotactic factor; leukotriene B4 and neutrophil chemotactic factor; and prostaglandin D4, platelet-activating factor (PAF), and leukotrienes C4 and D4. Influx of eosinophils amplifies and perpetuates the reaction. Effects may be systemic (anaphylaxis, as for example due to bee stings or drugs) or localized (food allergies, atopy, and asthma).

Type II hypersensitivity reactions (antibody-mediated) are mediated by IgG or IgM antibodies directed against a specific target cell or tissue. Reactions can take several forms.

- In complement-dependent cytotoxicity, fixation of complement results in osmotic lysis or opsonization of antibody-coated cells; examples include autoimmune hemolytic anemia, transfusion reactions, and erythroblastosis fetalis.
- In antibody-dependent cell-mediated cytoxicity (ADCC), cytotoxic killing of an antibody-coated cell occurs; an example is pernicious anemia. Antireceptor antibodies can activate or interfere with receptors; examples include Graves disease and myasthenia gravis.

Type III hypersensitivity reactions (**immune complex disease**) are characterized by the formation of in situ or circulating antibody-antigen immune complexes, which deposit in tissue resulting in inflammation and tissue injury. Examples include serum sickness, systemic lupus erythematosus (SLE), and glomerulonephritis.

Type IV hypersensitivity reactions (**cell-mediated type**) are mediated by sensitized T lymphocytes. In delayed type hypersensitivity, CD4+ TH1 lymphocytes mediate granuloma formation; examples include the PPD skin test and tuberculosis.

In cytotoxic T-cell–mediated hypersensitivity, CD8+ T-cell lymphocytes destroy antigen-containing cells; examples include type 1 diabetes, virus-infected cells, immune reaction to tumor-associated antigens, and graft rejection.

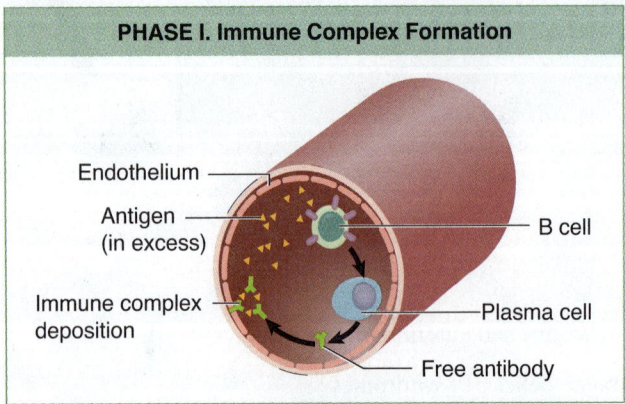

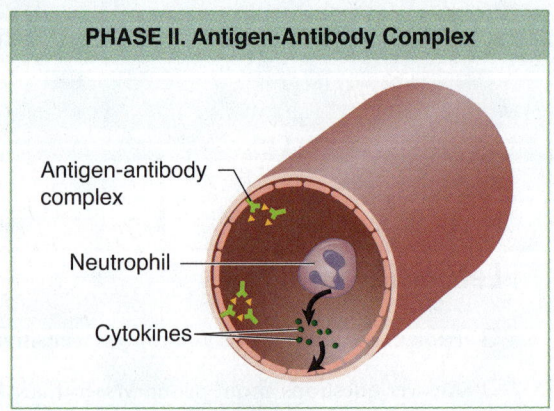

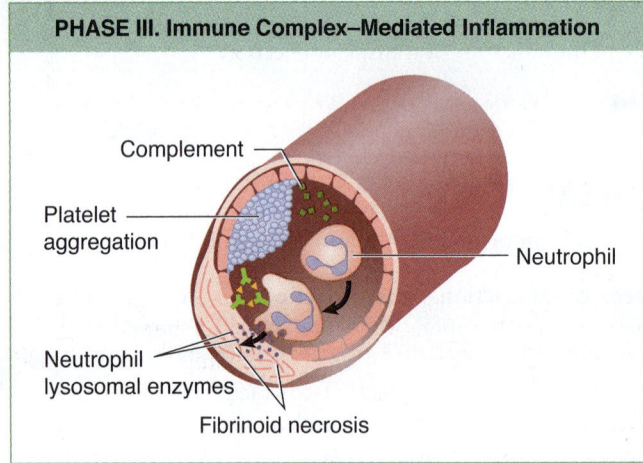

Figure 7-1. Type III Hypersensitivity

AUTOIMMUNE DISEASES

Systemic lupus erythematosus (SLE) is a chronic systemic autoimmune disease characterized by loss of self-tolerance and production of autoantibodies. Females are affected much more often than males (M:F = 1:9); peak incidence is age 20–45; and African Americans are affected more often than Caucasians. The mechanism of injury in lupus is a mix of type II and III hypersensitivity reactions.

- Important **autoantibodies** that may be detected in the sera from lupus patients include antinuclear antibody (ANA) (>95%); anti-dsDNA (40–60%); anti-Sm (20–30%); antihistone antibodies; nonhistone nuclear RNA proteins; and blood cells.

- SLE affects **many organ systems**.

  - Hematologic (type II hypersensitivity reaction) manifestations can include hemolytic anemia, thrombocytopenia, neutropenia, and lymphopenia.

  - Skeletal manifestations include an arthritis characterized by polyarthralgia and synovitis without joint deformity (type III hypersensitivity reaction).

  - Skin (type III hypersensitivity reaction) manifestations can include a malar "butterfly" rash; maculopapular rash; and ulcerations and bullae formation.

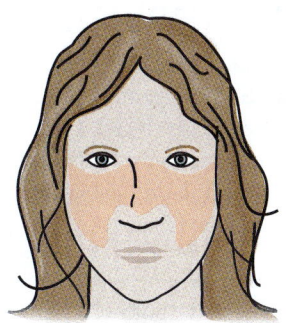

Butterfly Rash

- o Serosal surfaces may also be affected, with resulting pericarditis, pleuritis, or pleural effusions (type III hypersensitivity reaction).
- o Central nervous system manifestations include focal neurologic symptoms, seizures, and psychosis (type III hypersensitivity reaction).
- o Cardiac manifestations include Libman-Sacks endocarditis (nonbacterial verrucous endocarditis) (type III hypersensitivity reaction).
- Of particular importance are the renal manifestations (type III hypersensitivity) which involve various types of nephritis.
- Lupus is treated with **steroids** and **immunosuppressive agents**. It tends to have a chronic, unpredictable course with remissions and relapses. The 10-year survival is 85%, with death frequently being due to renal failure or infections.

Sjögren syndrome (sicca syndrome) is an autoimmune disease characterized by destruction of the lacrimal and salivary glands, resulting in the inability to produce saliva and tears. Females are affected more often than males, with typical age 30–50.

Clinical manifestations include keratoconjunctivitis sicca (dry eyes) and corneal ulcers; xerostomia (dry mouth); and Mikulicz syndrome (enlargement of the salivary and lacrimal glands). Sjögren syndrome is often associated with rheumatoid arthritis and other autoimmune diseases. The characteristic autoantibodies are the anti-ribonucleoprotein antibodies SS-A (Ro) and SS-B (La). There is an increased risk of developing non-Hodgkin lymphoma.

Scleroderma (progressive systemic sclerosis) is an autoimmune disease characterized by fibroblast stimulation and deposition of collagen in the skin and internal organs. It affects females more than males, with typical age range of 20 to 55 years. The pathogenesis involves activation of fibroblasts by cytokines interleukin 1 (IL-1), platelet-derived growth factor (PDGF), and/or fibroblast growth factor (FGF) with the resulting activated fibroblasts causing fibrosis.

- **Diffuse scleroderma** has anti-DNA topoisomerase I antibodies (Scl-70) (70%), widespread skin involvement, and early involvement of the visceral organs. Organs that can be affected include the esophagus (dysphagia), GI tract (malabsorption), lungs (pulmonary fibrosis which causes dyspnea on exertion), heart (cardiac fibrosis which may manifest as arrhythmias), and kidney (fibrosis that may manifest as renal insufficiency).
- **Localized scleroderma** (CREST syndrome) has anti-centromere antibodies, skin involvement of the face and hands, late involvement of visceral organs, and a relatively benign clinical course.

Dermatomyositis and polymyositis. See Skeletal Muscle chapter.

Mixed connective tissue disease is an overlap condition with features of systemic lupus erythematosus, systemic sclerosis, and polymyositis. Antiribonucleoprotein antibodies are nearly always positive.

PRIMARY IMMUNE DEFICIENCY SYNDROMES

X-linked agammaglobulinemia of Bruton is an immunodeficiency characterized by a developmental failure to produce mature B cells and plasma cells, resulting in agammablobulinemia. The condition occurs because of loss of function mutations of B-cell Bruton tyrosine kinase (BTK). Clinically, the disease affects male infants who have recurrent infections beginning at 6 months of life due to the loss of passive maternal immunity. Common infections include pharyngitis, otitis media, bronchitis, and pneumonia; common infecting organisms include *H. influenza*, *S. pneumococcus*, and *S. aureus*.

Common variable immunodeficiency is a group of disorders characterized by defects in B-cell maturation that can lead to defective IgA or IgG production. Clinically, both sexes are affected with onset in childhood of recurrent bacterial infections and with increased susceptibility to *Giardia lamblia*. Complications include increased frequency of developing autoimmune disease, non-Hodgkin lymphoma, and gastric cancer.

DiGeorge syndrome is an embryologic failure to develop the 3rd and 4th pharyngeal pouches, resulting in the absence of the parathyroid glands and thymus. Clinical findings can include neonatal hypocalcemia and tetany, T-cell deficiency, and recurrent infections with viral and fungal organisms.

Severe combined immunodeficiency (SCID) is a combined deficiency of cell-mediated and humoral immunity that is often caused by a progenitor-cell defect. The modes of inheritance are variable and can include X-linked (mutation of the common [gamma] chain of the interleukin receptors IL-2, IL-4, IL-7, IL-9, IL-15, and IL-21) and autosomal recessive (deficiency of adenosine deaminase). Clinical features include recurrent infections with bacteria, fungi, viruses, and protozoa; susceptibility to *Candida*, cytomegalovirus (CMV), and *Pneumocystis jirovecii* infections, and adverse reactions to live virus immunizations. SCID is treated with hematopoietic stem cell transplantation since the prognosis without treatment is death of most infants within a year.

Complement system disorders can involve a variety of factors, with deficiencies of different factors producing different clinical patterns.

In both the classical and alternate pathways, C3 deficiency causes both recurrent bacterial infections and immune complex disease, while C5, C6, C7, and C8 deficiencies cause recurrent meningococcal and gonococcal infections.

- In the classical pathway only, C1q, C1r, C1s, C2, and C4 deficiencies cause marked increases in immune complex diseases, including infections with pyogenic bacteria.
- In the alternate pathway, Factor B and properdin deficiencies cause increased neisserial infections. Deficiencies in complement regulatory proteins can cause C1-INH deficiency (hereditary angioedema), which is characterized clinically by edema at mucosal surfaces with low C2 and C4 levels.

MHC class II deficiency can be caused by defects in positive selection of thymocytes. Few CD4+ lymphocytes develop and as a result, patients suffer from severe immunodeficiency. Mutations in genes (i.e., *CIITA*) that encode proteins that regulate MHC class II gene expression are the cause. CD8+ T cells are unaffected.

Hyper IgM syndrome is characterized by normal B and T lymphocyte numbers and normal to elevated IgM levels but significantly decreased IgA, IgG and IgE levels. Mutations in the gene for CD40 ligand result in the most common form of X-linked hyper IgM syndrome.

Selective IgA deficiency has unknown genetic etiology. Many affected individuals appear healthy while others have significant illness. Sinopulmonary infections, diarrhea and adverse reactions to transfusions can occur. Levels of IgA are undetectable whereas levels of other isotypes are normal. There is an association with autoimmune disease.

Phagocyte deficiencies (See chapter 3.)

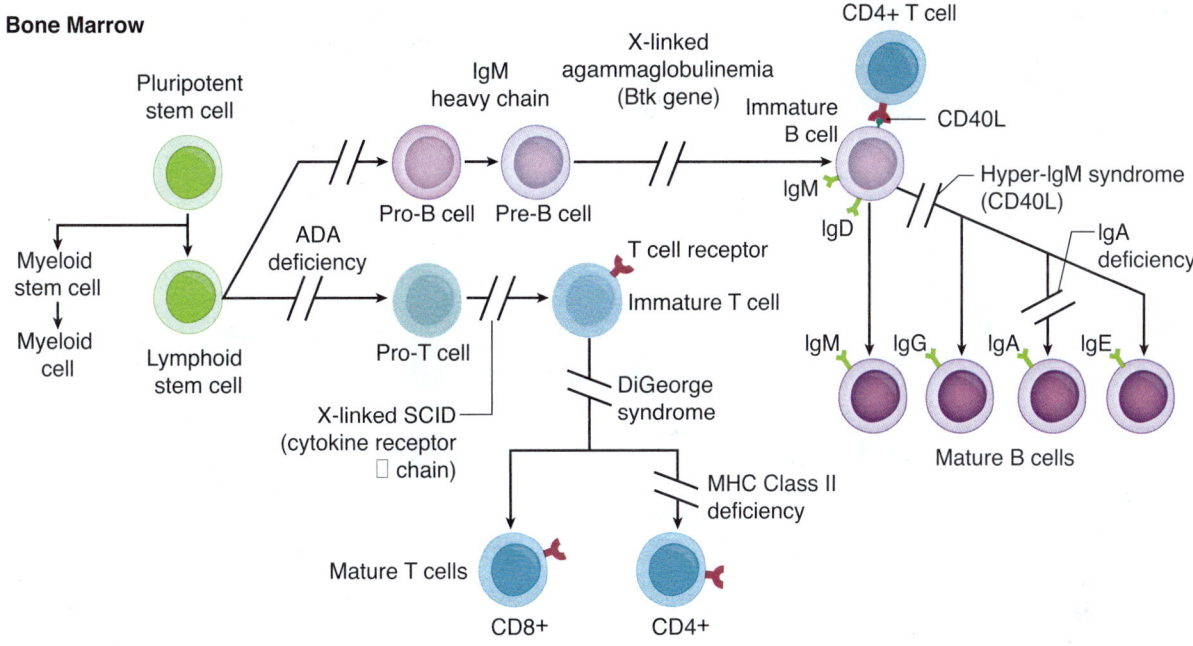

Figure 7-2. Primary Immune Deficiency Syndromes

SECONDARY IMMUNE DEFICIENCY SYNDROMES

Systemic diseases that can cause secondary immunodeficiency include diabetes mellitus, collagen vascular disease (e.g., systemic lupus erythematosus), and chronic alcoholism. Secondary immunodeficiency is more common.

ACQUIRED IMMUNODEFICIENCY SYNDROME (AIDS)

AIDS can be diagnosed when a person is HIV-positive and has CD4 count <200 cells/mL, **or** when a person is HIV-positive and has an AIDS-defining disease. Males are affected more frequently than females.

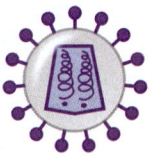

Retrovirus

The *human immunodeficiency virus* (HIV) is an enveloped RNA retrovirus that contains reverse transcriptase. HIV infects CD4-positive cells, including CD4+ T lymphocytes, all macrophages, lymph node follicular dendritic cells, and Langerhans cells. The mechanism of infection is by binding of CD4 by the viral gp120, followed by entry into cell by fusion, which requires gp41 and coreceptors CCR5 (β-chemokine receptor 5) and CXCR4 (α-chemokine receptor).

Transmission of HIV can occur by many mechanisms, including sexual contact (most common mode, including both homosexual transmission and an increasing rate of heterosexual transmission, with important cofactors including herpes and syphilis infection); parenteral transmission; IV drug use; blood transfusions (including those done in hemophiliacs); accidental needle sticks in hospital workers; and vertical transmission.

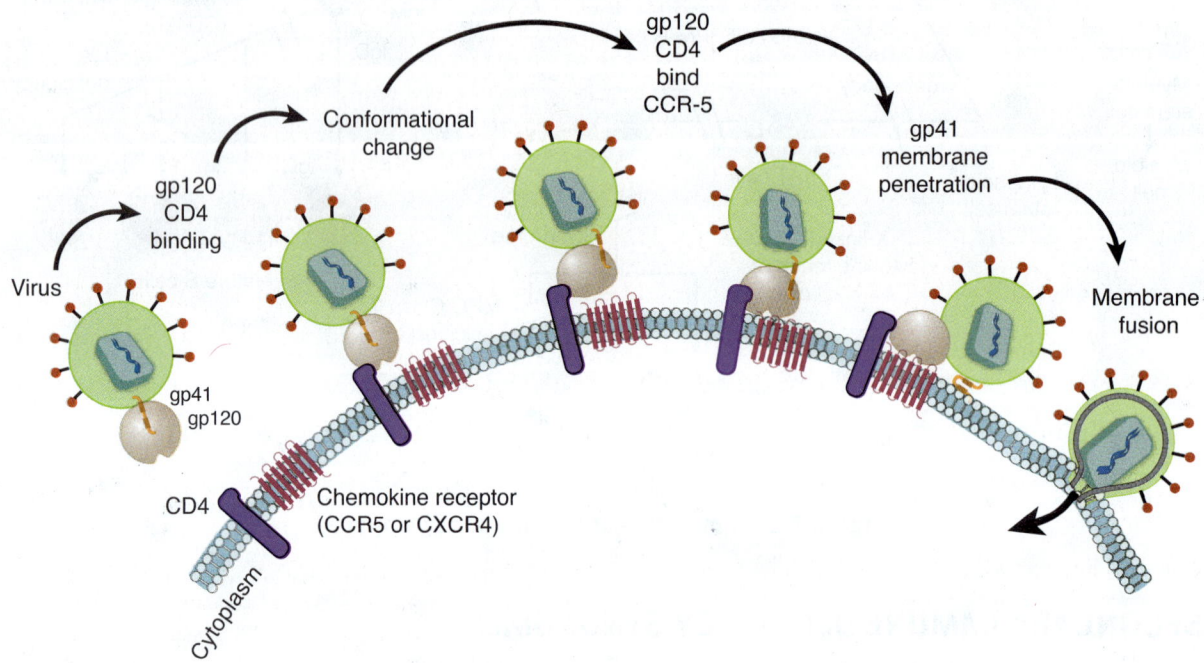

Figure 7-3. Mechanisms of HIV Infection

Note
Macrophages and follicular dendritic cells are reservoirs for the virus.

Diagnosis. The CDC recommends initial testing with an antigen/antibody combination immunoassay, followed by a confirmatory HIV-1/HIV-2 antibody differentiation immunoassay. If the confirmatory test is negative, testing with an HIV-1 nucleic acid test is done. Treatment varies, and can include combination antiretroviral treatment, reverse transcriptase inhibitors, protease inhibitors, and prophylaxis for opportunistic infections based on CD4 count.

Note
The CD4+ cell count is used to determine the health of the immune system and for recommendations on instituting prophylaxis for opportunistic diseases. Viral load is followed to assess treatment efficacy.

The clinical manifestations of HIV infection vary over time.

- The **acute phase** is characterized by viremia with a reduction in CD4 count, mononucleosis-like viral symptoms and lymphadenopathy, and seroconversion.

- The **latent phase** is characterized by asymptomatic or persistent generalized lymphadenopathy with continued viral replication in the lymph nodes and spleen, low level of virus in the blood, and minor opportunistic infections including oral thrush (candidiasis) and herpes zoster. The average duration of latent phase is 10 years.
- **Progression to AIDS** (third phase) occurs with reduction of CD4 count to <200 cells/mL, which is accompanied by reemergence of viremia and development of AIDS-defining diseases, possibly to eventual death.

Table 7-1. Opportunistic Infection and Common Sites of Infection in AIDS Patients

Opportunistic Infection	Common Sites of Infection
Pneumocystis jiroveci	Lung (pneumonia), bone marrow
Mycobacterium tuberculosis	Lung, disseminated
Mycobacterium avium-intracellulare	Lung, GI tract, disseminated
Coccidioidomycosis	Lung, disseminated
Histoplasmosis	Lung, disseminated
Cytomegalovirus	Lung, retina, adrenals, and GI tract
Giardia lamblia	GI tract
Cryptosporidium	GI tract
Herpes simplex virus	Esophagus and CNS (encephalitis)
Candida	Oral pharynx and esophagus
Aspergillus	CNS, lungs, blood vessels
Toxoplasmosis	CNS
Cryptococcus	CNS (meningitis)
JC virus	CNS (progressive multifocal leukoencephalopathy)
Bartonella spp.	Skin, mucosa, bone (bacillary angiomatosis)

AIDS-Defining Diseases

Hairyleukoplakia is an Epstein-Barr virus (EBV)–associated condition due to infection of squamous cells. White plaques are present on the tongue.

Kaposi sarcoma is the most common neoplasm in AIDS patients. (*See* Vascular Pathology chapter.)

Oral manifestations include purplish lesions of gingiva and hard palate.

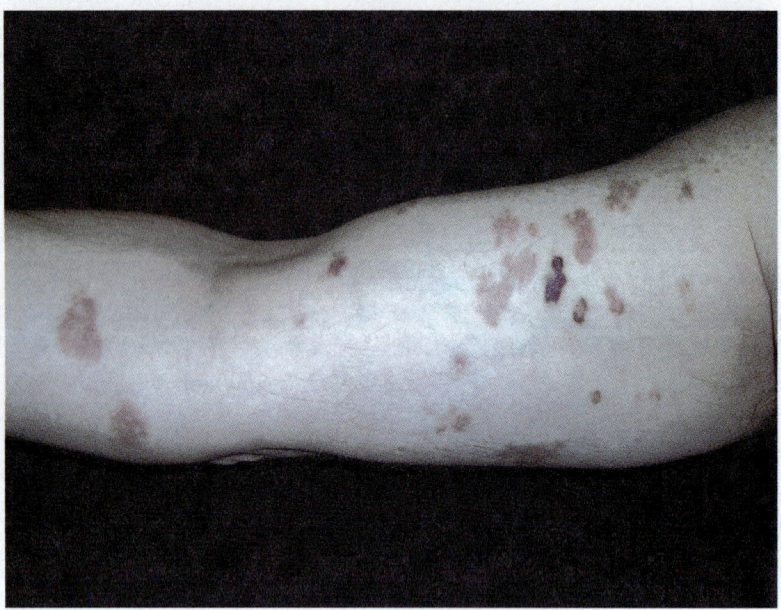

Figure 7-4. Kaposi Sarcoma in an AIDS Patient
© Richard P. Usatine, M.D. Used with permission.

Non-Hodgkin lymphomas tend to be high-grade B-cell lymphomas; extranodal CNS lymphomas are common.

Other AIDS-defining diseases include cervical cancer, HIV-wasting syndrome, AIDS nephropathy, and AIDS dementia complex.

Amyloidosis 8

Learning Objectives

❏ Answer questions about composition of amyloid

❏ Explain information related to systemic types of amyloid

❏ Demonstrate understanding of localized types of amyloid

COMPOSITION OF AMYLOID

Amyloidosis is a group of diseases characterized by the deposition of an extracellular protein that has specific properties.

- Individual molecular subunits form β-pleated sheets. Amorphous eosinophilic extracellular deposits of amyloid are seen on the H&E stain. These deposits stain red with the Congo red stain, and apple green birefringence of the amyloid is seen on the Congo red stain under polarized light.
- The fibrillary protein of amyloid varies with each disease. Also present in amyloid are serum amyloid P (SAP) and glycosaminoglycans (heparan sulfate).

SYSTEMIC TYPES OF AMYLOID

Primary amyloidosis has amyloid light chain (AL) amyloid, whose fibrillary protein is made of kappa or lambda light chains. Primary amyloidosis may be seen in plasma cell disorders (multiple myeloma, B-cell lymphomas, etc.) but most cases occur independent of other diseases.

Reactive systemic amyloidosis (secondary amyloidosis) has amyloid-associated (AA) protein, whose precursor is serum amyloid A (SAA), an acute phase reactant produced by the liver which is elevated with ongoing chronic inflammation and neoplasia. Reactive systemic amyloidosis can be seen with a wide variety of chronic diseases, including rheumatoid arthritis, systemic lupus erythematosus, tuberculosis, bronchiectasis, osteomyelitis, inflammatory bowel disease, and cancer.

Clinical Correlate

Carpal tunnel syndrome is caused when fibrosis, edema, or another pathologic process compresses and damages the median nerve within the tunnel formed by the carpal bones and flexor retinaculum.

Familial Mediterranean fever has AA type amyloid with fibrillary protein composed of serum amyloid A (SAA). This autosomal recessive disease is characterized by recurrent inflammation, fever, and neutrophil dysfunction.

Hemodialysis-associated amyloidosis has Aβ2M type amyloid with precursor protein β2-microglobulin. This form of amyloidosis may cause carpal tunnel syndrome and joint disease.

LOCALIZED TYPES OF AMYLOID

Senile cerebral amyloidosis (Alzheimer disease) has Aβ type amyloid with fibrillary protein composed of β-amyloid precursor protein (βAPP). It is found in Alzheimer plaques and in cerebral vessels.

Senile cardiac/systemic amyloidosis has ATTR type amyloid with fibrillary protein composed of transthyretin. This type of amyloidosis is seen in men older than 70 years and may cause heart failure as a result of restrictive/infiltrative cardiomyopathy.

Endocrine type amyloidosis is seen in medullary carcinoma of the thyroid (procalcitonin), adult-onset diabetes (amylin), and pancreatic islet cell tumors (amylin).

CLINICAL FEATURES

In **systemic forms** of amyloidosis, the kidney is the most commonly involved organ, and patients may experience nephrotic syndrome and/or progressive renal failure. Cardiac involvement may cause restrictive cardiomyopathy and conduction disturbances. Other clinical features include hepatosplenomegaly and involvement of the gastrointestinal tract, which may produce tongue enlargement (macroglossia, primarily in AL type) and malabsorption.

Diagnosis in systemic forms of amyloidosis can be established with biopsy of the rectal mucosa, gingiva, or the abdominal fat pad; Congo red stain shows apple green birefringence under polarized light of amyloid deposits. AL amyloidosis is diagnosed by serum and urinary protein electrophoresis and immunoelectrophoresis. Proteomic analysis is another diagnostic tool.

Principles of Neoplasia

Learning Objectives

❑ Use knowledge of epidemiology of neoplasias

❑ Answer questions about carcinogenic agents

❑ Solve problems concerning carcinogenesis

❑ Answer questions about diagnosis of cancer

DEFINITION

In **neoplasia**, an abnormal cell or tissue grows more rapidly than normal cells or tissue; it does so by acquiring multiple genetic changes over time and by continuing to grow after the stimuli that initiated the new growth have been removed.

EPIDEMIOLOGY

Cancer is the **second leading cause of death** in the United States. In 2015, the estimated number of new cancers diagnosed was 1,658,370, and the estimated number of deaths from cancer was 589,430.

In men, the sites with the highest new cancer rates are (in order of decreasing frequency):

- Prostate
- Lung and bronchus
- Colon and rectum

These same sites have the highest mortality rate, although lung and bronchus cancers more commonly cause death than prostate cancer.

In women, the sites with the highest new cancer rates are (in order of decreasing frequency):

- Breast
- Lung and bronchus
- Colon and rectum

These same sites have the highest mortality rate, although lung and bronchus cancers more commonly cause death than breast cancer.

In children, the most common cancers are acute lymphocytic leukemia, CNS malignancy, neuroblastoma, and non-Hodgkin lymphoma.

Predisposition to cancer involves many factors. Geographic and racial factors can be important:

- Stomach cancer is **much more prevalent** in Japan than in the United States.
- Breast cancer is **much more prevalent** in the United States than in Japan.
- Liver hepatoma is **much more prevalent** in Asia than in the United States.
- Prostate cancer is **more prevalent** in African Americans than in Caucasians.

Heredity predisposition can be seen in many cancers, including familial retinoblastoma, multiple endocrine neoplasia, and familial polyposis coli.

Acquired preneoplastic disorders also affect cancer incidence, with examples including cervical dysplasia (characterized by changes in cell size and shape), endometrial hyperplasia, cirrhosis, inflammatory bowel disease, and chronic atrophic gastritis.

CARCINOGENIC AGENTS

Chemical carcinogens. Carcinogenesis is a multistep process involving a sequence of initiation (mutation) followed by promotion (proliferation). Initiators can be either direct-acting chemical carcinogens (mutagens which cause cancer directly by modifying DNA) or indirect-acting chemical carcinogens (procarcinogens which require metabolic conversion to form active carcinogens). Promotors cause cellular proliferation of mutated (initiated) cells, which may lead to accumulation of additional mutations.

- **Clinically important chemical carcinogens** are numerous, and include nitrosamines (gastric cancer), cigarette smoke (multiple malignancies), polycyclic aromatic hydrocarbons (bronchogenic carcinoma), asbestos (bronchogenic carcinoma, mesothelioma), chromium and nickel (bronchogenic carcinoma), arsenic (squamous cell carcinomas of skin and lung, angiosarcoma of liver), vinyl chloride (angiosarcoma of liver), aromatic amines and azo dyes (hepatocellular carcinoma), alkylating agents (leukemia, lymphoma, other cancers), benzene (leukemia), and naphthylamine (bladder cancer). Potential carcinogens are screened by the Ames test, which detects any mutagenic effects of potential carcinogens on bacterial cells in culture; mutagenicity *in vitro* correlates well with carcinogenicity in vivo.

Radiation. Ultraviolet B sunlight is the most carcinogenic because it produces pyrimidine dimers in DNA, leading to transcriptional errors and mutations of oncogenes and tumor suppressor genes, thereby increasing the risk of skin cancer. Xeroderma pigmentosum is an autosomal recessive inherited defect in DNA repair, in which the pyrimidine dimers formed with ultraviolet B sunlight cannot be repaired; this defect predisposes to skin cancer. Ionizing radiation includes x-rays and gamma rays, alpha and beta particles, protons, and neutrons. Cells in mitosis or the G2 phase of the cell cycle are most sensitive to radiation. Radiation causes cross-linking and chain breaks in nucleic acids. Atomic bomb survivors experienced an increased incidence of leukemias, thyroid cancer, and other cancers. Uranium miners historically had increased lung cancer, related to inhalation of radioactive radon, which is a decay product of uranium.

Oncogenic viruses.

RNA oncogenic viruses. Human T-cell leukemia virus (HTLV-1) causes adult T-cell leukemia/lymphoma.

DNA oncogenic viruses include the following:

- Hepatitis B virus (hepatocellular carcinoma)
- Epstein-Barr virus (EBV), which has been implicated in Burkitt lymphoma, B-cell lymphomas in immunosuppressed patients, nasopharyngeal carcinoma

- Human papilloma virus (HPV), which causes benign squamous papillomas (warts-condyloma acuminatum) and a variety of carcinomas (cervical, vulvar, vaginal, penile, and anal)
- Kaposi-sarcoma-associated herpesvirus (HHV8) which causes Kaposi sarcoma

Loss of immune regulation. Immunosurveillance normally destroys neoplastic cells via recognition of "non-self" antigens, and both humoral and cell-mediated immune responses play a role. Patients with immune system dysfunction have an increased number of neoplasms, especially malignant lymphomas.

CARCINOGENESIS

Carcinogenesis is a multistep process, and development of all human cancers appears to require the accumulation of multiple genetic changes. These changes can involve either inherited germline mutations or acquired mutations. Once a single severely mutated cell forms, monoclonal expansion of the cell's line can cause a tumor. Most important mutations in tumorogenesis involve growth promoting genes (proto-oncogenes), growth inhibiting tumor suppressor genes, or the genes regulating apoptosis and senescence.

Activation of growth promoting oncogenes. Proto-oncogenes are normal cellular genes involved with growth and cellular differentiation. Oncogenes are derived from proto-oncogenes by either a change in the gene sequence, resulting in a new gene product (oncoprotein), or a loss of gene regulation resulting in overexpression of the normal gene product. Mechanisms of oncogene activation include point mutations, chromosomal translocations, gene amplification, and insertional mutagenesis. Activated oncogenes lack regulatory control and are overexpressed, resulting in unregulated cellular proliferation.

Inactivation of tumor suppressor genes. Tumor suppressor genes encode proteins that regulate and suppress cell proliferation by inhibiting progression of the cell through the cell cycle. The mechanism of action of tumor suppressor genes may vary. As examples, p53 prevents a cell with damaged DNA from entering S-phase, while Rb prevents the cell from entering S-phase until the appropriate growth signals are present.

- **Knudson's "two hit hypothesis"** states that at least 2 tumor suppressor genes must be inactivated for oncogenesis. In cancers arising in individuals with inherited germline mutations, the "first hit" is the inherited germline mutation and the "second hit" is an acquired somatic mutation. Examples of inherited germline mutations include familial retinoblastoma (in which germline mutation of *RB1* on chromosome 13 is associated with a high rate of retinoblastoma and osteosarcoma) and Li-Fraumini syndrome (in which germline mutation of *TP53* on chromosome 17 is associated with a high rate of many types of tumors).

Regulation of apoptosis. Tumor genesis related to changes in regulation of apotosis occurs in the follicular lymphomas that have the translocation t(14;18). Normally, Bcl-2 prevents apoptosis (programmed cell death). In the follicular lymphomas with this translocation, the Bcl-2 regulator of apoptosis is overexpressed, because the translocation connects the immunoglobulin heavy chain gene on chromosome 14 (which turns on easily in B lymphocytes) to the *BCL2* gene on chromosome 18, thereby leading to a situation in which lymphocytes fail to die as expected and instead produce a tumor.

DIAGNOSIS OF CANCER

Table 9-1. General Features of Benign versus Malignant Neoplasms

	Benign	Malignant
Gross	• Small size • Slow growing • Encapsulated or well-demarcated borders	• Larger in size • Rapid growth • Necrosis and hemorrhage are commonly seen • Poorly demarcated
Micro	• Expansile growth with well-circumscribed borders • Tend to be well differentiated • Resemble the normal tissue counterpart from which they arise • Noninvasive and never metastasize	• Vary from well to poorly (anaplastic) differentiated • Tumor cells vary in size and shape (pleomorphism) • Increased nuclear to cytoplasmic ratios • Nuclear hyperchromasia and prominent nucleoli • High mitotic activity with abnormal mitotic figures • Invasive growth pattern • Has potential to metastasize

Histologic diagnosis of cancer. Microscopic examination of tissue or cells is required to make the diagnosis of cancer. Material suitable for diagnosis of a tumor may be obtained by complete excision, biopsy, fine needle aspiration, or cytologic smears (Pap test).

- **Immunohistochemistry** may be helpful in confirming the tissue of origin of metastatic or poorly differentiated tumors. The technique uses monoclonal antibodies that are specific for a cellular component. Among the many antibodies that are clinically useful are:
  - All of the serum tumor markers
  - Thyroglobulin (thyroid cancers)
  - S100 (melanoma and neural tumors)
  - Actin (smooth and skeletal muscle)
  - CD markers (lymphomas/leukemias)
  - Estrogen receptors (breast cancer)
  - Intermediate filaments
- **Ancillary tests** for the diagnosis of cancer include electron microscopy, flow cytometry, cytogenetics, and PCR/DNA probes.

Serum tumor markers. Tumor markers are usually normal cellular components that are increased in neoplasms but may also be elevated in nonneoplastic conditions. Serum tumor markers are used for screening (e.g., prostate specific antigen [PSA]) for cancer, monitoring treatment efficacy, and detecting recurrence of cancers.

- **Clinically useful tumor markers** include alpha-fetoprotein (AFP, used for hepatoma, nonseminomatous testicular germ cell tumors); beta human chorionic gonadotropin (hCG, used for trophoblastic tumors, choriocarcinoma); calcitonin (used for medullary carcinoma of the thyroid); carcinoembryonic antigen (CEA, used for carcinomas of the lung, pancreas, stomach, breast, and colon); CA-125 (used for malignant ovarian epithelial tumors); CA19-9 (used for malignant pancreatic adenocarcinoma); placental alkaline phosphatase (used for seminoma); and prostate specific antigen (PSA, used for prostate cancer).

> **Note**
>
> Most neoplasms (90%) arise from epithelium, with the remainder from mesenchymal cells.

Grading and staging. Tumor grade is a histologic estimate of the malignancy of a tumor, and typically uses criteria such as the degree of differentiation from low grade (well-differentiated) to high grade (poorly differentiated/anaplastic) and the number of mitoses.

Tumor stage is a clinical estimate of the extent of tumor spread. TNM staging system criteria is used for most tumor types:

- **T** indicates the size of the primary tumor.
- **N** indicates extent of regional lymph node spread.
- **M** indicates the presence or absence of metastatic disease.

In general, staging is a better predictor of prognosis than tumor grade.

Tumor progression refers to the tendency of a tumor to become more malignant over time. This progression can be related to both natural selection (evolution of a more malignant clone over time due to a selective growth advantage) and genetic instability (malignant cells are more prone to mutate and accumulate additional genetic defects).

Metastasis. Lymphatic spread is the most common initial route of spread for epithelial carcinomas. Early hematogenous spread is typically seen with most sarcomas (e.g., osteogenic sarcoma), renal cell carcinoma (because of the proximity of the large renal vein), hepatocellular carcinoma (because of the presence of the hepatic sinusoids), follicular carcinoma of the thyroid, and choriocarcinoma (because of its propensity to seek vessels). Seeding of body cavities and surfaces occurs in ovarian carcinoma. Transplantation via mechanical manipulation (e.g., surgical incision, needle tracts) may occur but is relatively rare.

Learning Objectives

❏ Solve problems concerning disorders of pigmentation

❏ Answer questions about melanocytic tumors

❏ Explain information related to epidermal and dermal lesions

❏ Explain information related to malignant tumors

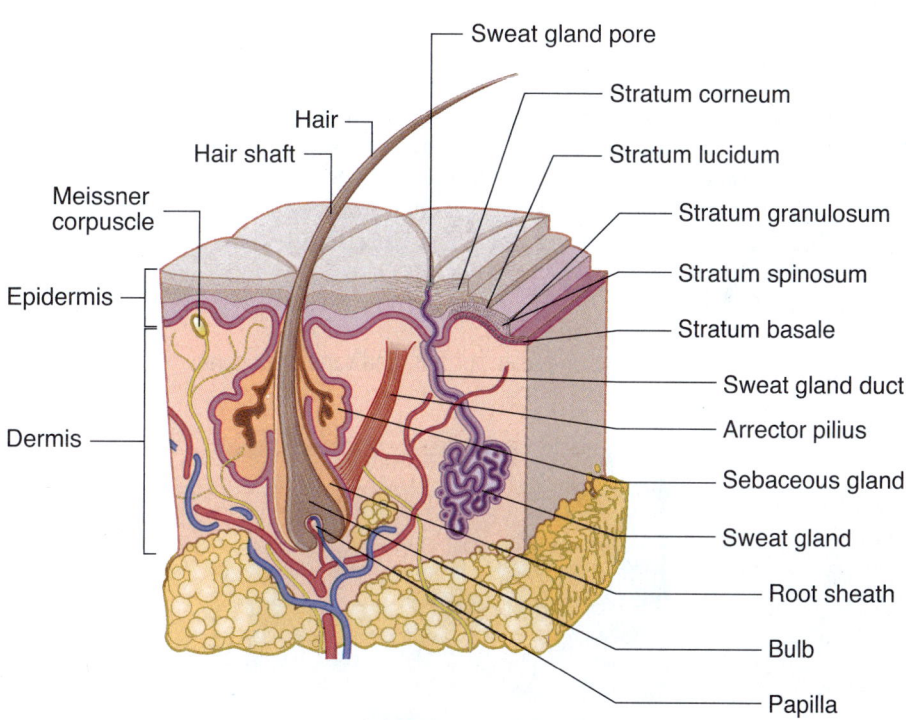

Figure 10-1. Skin

DISORDERS OF PIGMENTATION

Vitiligo causes irregular, completely depigmented skin patches. It is common and can affect any race; there may also be a familial predisposition. The disease has an unknown etiology that is possibly autoimmune. Microscopically, affected areas are devoid of epidermal melanocytes.

Melasma causes irregular blotchy patches of hyperpigmentation on the face; it is associated with sun exposure, oral contraceptive use, and pregnancy ("mask of pregnancy") and may regress after pregnancy.

Freckles (ephelides) are light brown macules on the face, shoulders, and chest. They are common in fair-skinned children and tend to darken and fade with the seasons due to sunlight exposure. Microscopically, freckles are characterized by increased melanin deposition in the basal cell layer of the epidermis with a normal number of melanocytes.

Benign **lentigo** is a localized proliferation of melanocytes which cause small, oval, light brown macules. Microscopically, benign lentigos show linear melanocytic hyperplasia.

MELANOCYTIC TUMORS

Congenital nevi (birthmarks) are present at birth; giant congenital nevi have increased risk of developing melanoma.

Nevocellular nevus (mole) is a benign tumor of melanocytes (melanocytic nevus cells) that is clearly related to sun exposure. Types of nevi include junctional, compound, and intradermal. Nevi have uniform tan to brown color with sharp, well-circumscribed borders and tend to be stable in shape and size. Malignant transformation is uncommon.

Dysplastic nevi (BK moles) are larger and more irregular than common nevi, and they may have pigment variation. Microscopically, the nevus exhibits cytological and architectural atypia. Dysplastic nevus syndrome is autosomal dominant (*CMM1* locus on chromosome 1); patients often have multiple dysplastic nevi; and there is increased risk of developing melanoma.

Malignant melanoma is a malignancy of melanocytes whose incidence is increasing at a rapid rate, with peak in ages 40–70. Risk factors include chronic sun exposure, sunburn, fair skin, dysplastic nevus syndrome, and familial melanoma (associated with loss of function mutation of the p16 tumor suppressor gene, *CDKN2A*, on chromosome 9; somatic mutations of *NRAS* and *BRAF* also occur). Melanomas characteristically form skin lesions of large diameter with asymmetric and irregular borders and variegated color; the lesions may be macules, papules, or nodules. Melanomas on males have increased frequency on the upper back; females have increased frequency on the back and legs.

Note the size, irregular borders, and variegated color.

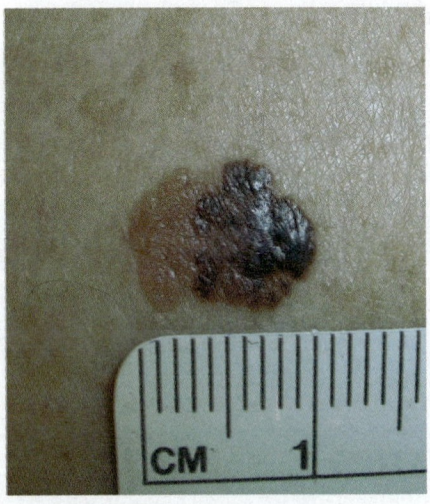

Figure 10-2. Melanoma
© Richard P. Usatine, M.D. Used with permission.

The **prognosis** of melanomas is determined by TNM staging; T status is based on the depth of invasion (Breslow thickness measured histologically in millimeters).

Local disease is treated with wide surgical excision and sometimes sentinel node biopsy. Systemic disease is treated with chemotherapy or immunotherapy. Metastases may occur after years of dormancy.

EPIDERMAL AND DERMAL LESIONS

Acanthosis nigricans causes thickened, hyperpigmented skin of the posterior neck, axillae, and groin; it is often associated with obesity and hyperinsulinism. On rare occasions it is associated with internal malignancy (stomach and other gastrointestinal malignancies).

Seborrheic keratoses are benign squamoproliferative neoplasms that are very common in middle-aged and elderly individuals; they may occur on the trunk, head, neck, and the extremities. The lesions are tan to brown coin-shaped plaques that have a granular surface with a "stuck on" appearance, characterized microscopically by basaloid epidermal hyperplasia and "horn cysts" (keratin-filled epidermal pseudocysts). They are usually left untreated, but may be removed if they become irritated or for cosmetic purposes. The sign of Leser-Trélat (paraneoplastic syndrome) is the sudden development of multiple lesions which may accompany an internal malignancy.

Psoriasis is an autoimmune disorder with a clear genetic component that causes increased proliferation and turnover of epidermal keratinocytes; it affects 1% of the U.S. population. The most common form is psoriasis vulgaris. Common sites of involvement include the knees, elbows, and scalp; the classic skin lesion is a well-demarcated erythematous plaque with a silvery scale. Removal of scale results in pinpoint bleeding (Auspitz sign). Nail beds show pitting and discoloration. Psoriasis may be associated with arthritis, enteropathy, and myopathy.

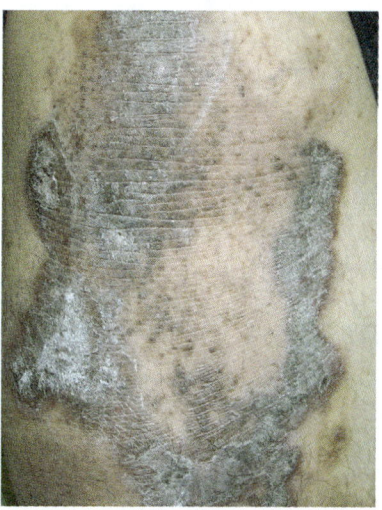

Figure 10-3. The Silvery Plaques of Psoriasis
© Richard P. Usatine, M.D. Used with permission.

- **Microscopically,** the lesions show epidermal hyperplasia (acanthosis), patchy hyperkeratinization with parakeratosis, uniform elongation and thickening of the rete ridges, thinning of the epidermis over the dermal papillae, and Munro microabscesses.
- Treatment is topical steroids and ultraviolet irradiation; severe systemic disease may be treated with methotrexate.

Pemphigus is a rare, potentially fatal autoimmune disorder that is characterized by intraepidermal blister formation. Pemphigus vulgaris is the most common form. The pathogenesis involves the production of autoantibodies directed against a part of the keratinocyte desmosome called desmoglein 3, with resulting loss of intercellular adhesion (acantholysis) and blister formation. Pemphigus causes mucosal lesions and easily ruptured, flaccid blisters. Oral involvement is common.

- Microscopic examination shows intraepidermal acantholysis; the acantholysis leaves behind a basal layer of keratinocytes, which has a tombstone-like arrangement. Immunofluorescence shows a net-like pattern of IgG staining between the epidermal keratinocytes that create bullae.
- Treatment is with immunosuppression.

Bullous pemphigoid is a relatively common autoimmune disorder of older individuals characterized by subepidermal blister formation with tense bullae that do not rupture easily. The condition results from production of autoantibodies directed against a part of the keratinocyte hemidesmosome called *bullous pemphigoid antigens 1 and 2*. Immunofluorescence shows linear deposits of IgG at the dermal-epidermal junction.

Dermatitis herpetiformis is a rare immune disorder that is often associated with celiac sprue; it is characterized by subepidermal blister formation with itchy, grouped vesicles and occasional bullae on the extensor surfaces. Production of IgA antibodies directed against gliadin and other antigens deposit in the tips of the dermal papillae and result in subepidermal blister formation. Routine microscopy shows microabscesses at the tips of the dermal papillae that can lead to eventual subepidermal separation results in blister formation; immunofluorescence shows granular IgA deposits at the tips of the dermal papillae. Dermatitis herpetiformis often responds to a gluten-free diet.

Xerosis is a common cause of pruritus and dry skin in the elderly that is due to decreased skin lipids. Cancer patients receiving epidermal growth factor receptor inhibitor are susceptible. Treatment is with emollients.

Eczema is a group of related inflammatory skin diseases characterized by pruritus and epidermal spongiosis (edema).

- Acute eczema causes a vesicular, erythematous rash.
- Chronic eczema develops following repetitive scratching, and is characterized by dry, thickened, hyperkeratotic skin.
- Atopic dermatitis is often inherited. Defects in the keratinocyte barrier are due to mutations in the filaggrin gene (*FLG*).
- Contact dermatitis can be either allergic type (poison ivy, nickel in jewelry) or photodermatitis type (such as photosensitivity reaction after tetracycline).

Polymorphous light eruption is the most common idiopathic form of photodermatosis and causes pruritic erythematous macules, papules, plaques, or vesicles on exposure to sunlight. There is dermal edema and inflammation.

Verrucae (warts) are caused by human papillomavirus. Verruca vulgaris is the most common type.

Cutaneous lupus erythematosus may be acute (facial butterfly rash), subacute (photosensitive rash on anterior chest, upper back and upper extremities), or chronic (discoid plaques, usually above the neck). Direct immunofluorescence shows deposition of immunoglobulin and complement at the dermal-epidermal junction. Serologies for autoantibodies and clinical correlation help establish the diagnosis.

Erythema multiforme is a hypersensitivity skin reaction to infections (*Mycoplasma pneumoniae*, herpes simplex) or drugs (sulfonamides, penicillin, barbiturates, phenytoin) characterized by vesicles, bullae, and "targetoid" erythematous lesions. The most severe form is Stevens-Johnson syndrome, which has extensive involvement of skin and mucous membranes.

Pityriasis rosea causes a pruritic rash that starts with an oval-shaped "herald patch" and progresses to a papular eruption of the trunk to produce a "Christmas tree" distribution. It is clinically diagnosed, self-limiting and possibly a viral exanthem.

Granuloma annulare is a chronic inflammatory disorder that causes papules and plaques. Palisaded granulomas are present microscopically. The pathogenesis is immunologic, but most cases occur in healthy patients.

Erythema nodosum causes raised, erythematous, painful nodules of subcutaneous adipose tissue, typically on the anterior shins, which can be associated with granulomatous diseases and streptococcal infection.

Epidermoid cyst is a common benign skin cyst lined with stratified squamous epithelium and filled with keratin debris.

MALIGNANT TUMORS

Squamous cell carcinoma (SCC) has peak incidence at age 60. Risk factors include chronic sun exposure (ultraviolet UVB); fair complexion; chronic skin ulcers or sinus tracts; long-term exposure to hydrocarbons, arsenic, burns, and radiation; immunosuppression; and xeroderma pigmentosum.

- Precursors include actinic keratosis (a sun-induced dysplasia of the keratinocytes that causes rough, red papules on the face, arms, and hands) and Bowen disease (squamous cell carcinoma *in situ*).
- **Squamous cell carcinoma** occurs on sun-exposed areas (face and hands) and causes a tan nodular mass which commonly ulcerates. Microscopic examination shows nests of atypical keratinocytes that invade the dermis, (oftentimes) formation of keratin pearls, and intercellular bridges (desmosomes) between tumor cells. Squamous cell carcinoma of the skin rarely metastasizes and complete excision is usually curative.
- A variant is **keratoacanthoma** (well differentiated Squamous cell carcinoma), which causes rapidly growing, dome-shaped nodules with a central keratin-filled crater; these are often self-limited and may regress spontaneously.

Basal cell carcinoma (BCC) is the most common tumor in adults in the Western world; it is most common in middle-aged or elderly individuals and arises from the basal cells of hair follicles. Risk factors include chronic sun exposure, fair complexion, immunosuppression, and xeroderma pigmentosum.

BCC occurs on sun-exposed, hair-bearing areas (face), and may form pearly papules; nodules with heaped-up, translucent borders, telangiectasia, or ulcers (rodent ulcer). Microscopically, BCCs show invasive nests of basaloid cells with a palisading growth pattern.

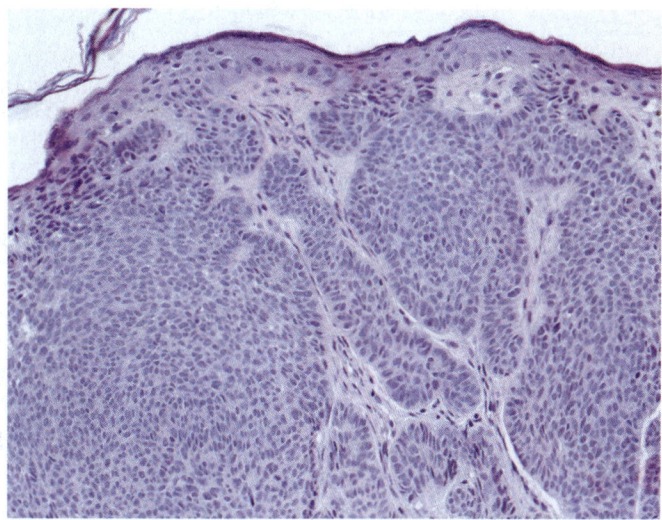

Figure 10-4. Basal Cell Carcinoma
© Gregg Barré, M.D. Used with permission.

BCC grows slowly and rarely metastasizes, but it may be locally aggressive. Shave biopsies have a 50% recurrence rate, but complete excision is usually curative. Mutations affecting the Hedgehog pathway are seen in sporadic and familial cases.

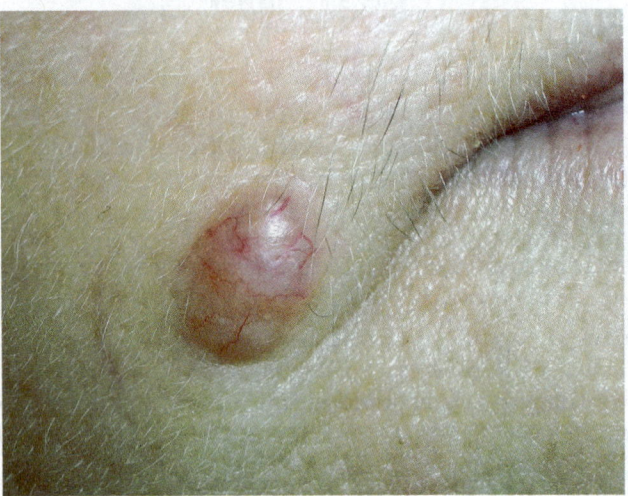

Figure 10-5. Pearly Papule Characteristic of a Basal Cell Carcinoma

© Richard P. Usatine, M.D. Used with permission.

Red Blood Cell Pathology: Anemias 11

Learning Objectives

❏ Explain information related to red blood cell morphology

❏ Solve problems using knowledge of microcytic, normocytic, and macrocytic anemias

❏ Demonstrate understanding of polycythemia vera

RED BLOOD CELL MORPHOLOGY

Red Cell Shapes

Abnormal size is called anisocytosis (*aniso* means unequal). Abnormal shape is called poikilocytosis (*poikilo* means various). **Elliptocytes** may be seen in hereditary elliptocytosis. **Spherocytes** result from decreased erythrocyte membrane, and they may be seen in hereditary spherocytosis and in autoimmune hemolytic anemia. **Target cells** result from increased erythrocyte membrane, and they may be seen in hemoglobinopathies, thalassemia, and liver disease. **Acanthocytes** have irregular spicules on their surfaces; numerous acanthocytes can be seen in abetalipoproteinemia. **Echinocytes** (burr cells) have smooth undulations on their surface; they may be seen in uremia or more commonly as an artifact.

Schistocytes are erythrocyte fragments (helmet cells are a type of schistocyte); they can be seen in microangiopathic hemolytic anemias or traumatic hemolysis. **Bite cells** are erythrocytes with "bites" of cytoplasm being removed by splenic macrophages; they may be seen in G6PD deficiency. **Teardrop cells** (dacrocytes) may be seen in thalassemia and myelofibrosis. **Sickle cells** (drepanocytes) are seen in sickle cell anemia. **Rouleaux** ("stack of coins") refers to erythrocytes lining up in a row. Rouleaux are characteristic of multiple myeloma.

Red Cell Inclusions

Basophilic stippling results from cytoplasmic remnants of RNA; it may indicate reticulocytosis or lead poisoning. **Howell-Jolly bodies** are remnants of nuclear chromatin that may occur in severe anemias or patients without spleens. **Pappenheimer bodies** are composed of iron, and they may be found in the peripheral blood following splenectomy. **Ring sideroblasts** have iron trapped abnormally in mitochondria, forming a ring around nucleus; they can be seen in sideroblastic anemia. **Heinz bodies** result from denatured hemoglobin; they can be seen with glucose-6-phosphate dehydrogenase deficiency.

ANEMIAS

Anemia is a reduction below normal limits of the total circulating red cell mass. Signs of anemia include palpitations, dizziness, angina, pallor of skin and nails, weakness, claudication, fatigue, and lethargy.

- **Reticulocytes** are immature, larger red cells (macrocytic cells) that are spherical and have a bluish color (polychromasia) due to free ribosomal RNA. Reticulocytes do not have a nucleus; note that any erythrocyte with a nucleus (nRBC) in peripheral blood is abnormal. Reticulocyte maturation to a mature erythrocyte takes about 1 day. The reticulocyte count is the percentage of red immature cells present in peripheral blood (normal 0.5–1.5%).

Classification of anemia can be based on color: normochromic anemias have normal red cell color (central pallor of about a third the diameter of the erythrocyte); hypochromic anemias have decreased color (seen as an increased central pallor of erythrocyte); and hyperchromic anemias, while theoretically possible, are usually instead called spherocytosis and have increased color (loss of central pallor of erythrocyte). Classification of anemia can also be based on size (MCV, or mean corpuscular volume).

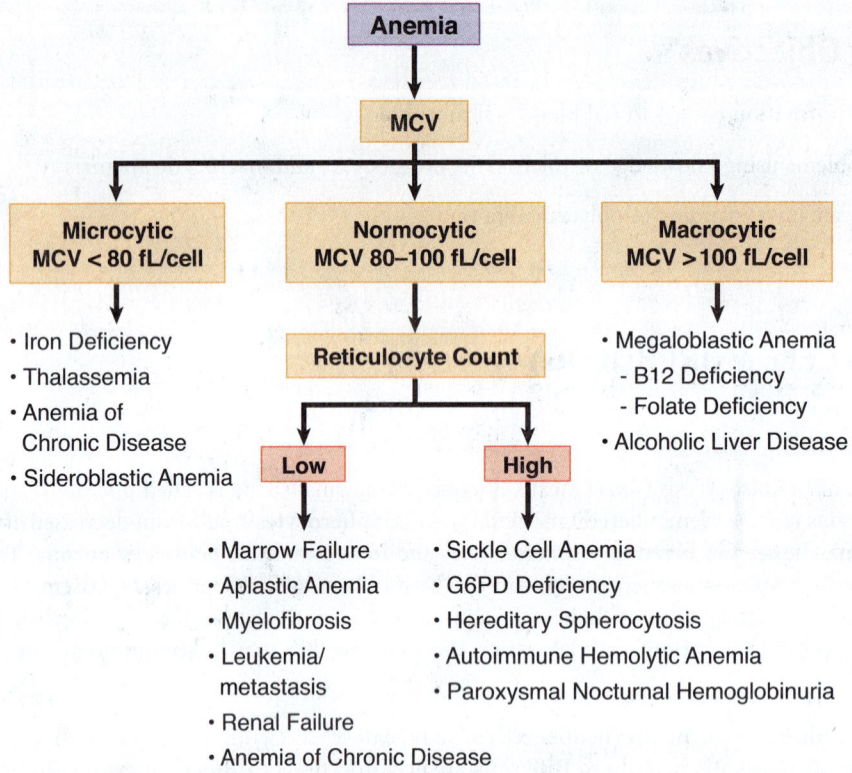

Figure 11-1. Classification of Anemias Based on MCV

The pathogenesis of anemia varies with the underlying disease. Blood loss can cause anemia. **Hemolytic anemias** are also important, and include hereditary spherocytosis, glucose-6-phosphate dehydrogenase deficiency, sickle cell disease, hemoglobin C disease, thalassemia, and paroxysmal nocturnal hemoglobinuria. **Immunohemolytic anemias**, which are hemolytic anemias with an immune component to the pathology, include autoimmune hemolytic anemia (AIHA), cold AIHA, incompatible blood transfusions, and hemolytic disease of the newborn. **Anemias of diminished erythropoiesis** include megaloblastic anemia (B12 and folate deficiencies), iron deficiency anemia, anemia of chronic disease, aplastic anemia, myelophthisic anemia, and sideroblastic anemia.

MICROCYTIC ANEMIAS

Iron Deficiency Anemia

Iron physiology. Functionally available iron is normally found in hemoglobin, myoglobin, and enzymes (catalase and cytochromes). Additionally, ferritin is the physiological storage form (plasma ferritin is normally close to the total body Fe), and hemosiderin (Prussian blue positive) is iron precipitated in tissues in the form of degraded ferritin mixed with lysosomal debris.

Iron is transported in the blood stream by transferrin. Transferrin saturation is reported as a percentage; it represents the ratio of the serum iron to the total iron-binding capacity, multiplied by 100.

Dietary deficiency of iron is seen in elderly populations, children, and the poor. Increased demand for iron is seen in children and pregnant women. Additionally, iron deficiency can develop because of decreased absorption, either due to generalized malabsorption or more specifically after gastrectomy (due to decreased acid, which is needed for ferrous absorption) or when there is decreased small intestinal transit time (causing "dumping syndrome"). Iron deficiency can also be due to chronic blood loss due to gynecologic (menstrual bleeding) or gastrointestinal causes (in the United States, think carcinoma; in the rest of the world, think hookworm).

Other clinical features of iron deficiency include increased free erythrocyte protoporphyrin (FEP), oral epithelial atrophy if Plummer-Vinson syndrome is present, koilonychia (concave or spoon nails with abnormal ridging and splitting), and pica (eating nonfood substances, e.g. dirt).

Anemia of chronic disease (AOCD)(or anemia of inflammation) is characterized by iron being trapped in bone marrow macrophages, leading to decreased utilization of endogenous iron stores. Laboratory studies show increased serum ferritin with decreased total iron binding capacity.

Thalassemia syndromes are quantitative, not qualitative, abnormalities of hemoglobin. α-thalassemia has decreased α-globin chains with relative excess β chains, while β-thalassemia has decreased β-globin chains with relative excess α chains. It is hypothesized that the thalassemia genes have been selectively preserved in the human genome because the thalassemias provide a protective advantage to carriers exposed to diseases such as malaria.

Note
Composition of hemoglobins: • HbA (2 alpha, 2 beta)   • HbA2 (2 alpha, 2 delta)   • HbF (2 alpha, 2 gamma)   • Hb Barts (4 gamma)   • Hb H (4 beta)

α-**thalassemia.** There are a total of 4 α-globin chain genes, 2 from each parent. α-thalassemia is due to gene deletions in the α-globin chain genes, and the clinical manifestations depend upon the number of genes that are affected. α chains are normally expressed prenatally and postnatally; therefore, there is prenatal and postnatal disease. In normal individuals, 4 α genes ($\alpha\alpha/\alpha\alpha$) are present and 100% of the α chains are normal.

- In the **silent carrier state**, one deletion is present.
- In α-**thalassemia trait**, 2 deletions are present.
- **Hemoglobin H disease** is characterized by 3 deletions.
- **Hydrops fetalis** has 4 deletions and is lethal in utero.

β-**thalassemia.** There are a total of 2 β-globin chain genes. In contrast to the α-globin chain genes, the 2 β-globin chain genes are expressed postnatally only, and therefore there is only postnatal disease and not prenatal disease. The damage to the genes is mainly by point mutations, which form either some β chains ($\beta+$) or none ($\beta0$).

- β-**thalassemia minor** is seen when one of the β-globin chain genes has been damaged. The condition is asymptomatic.
- β-**thalassemia intermedia** causes varying degrees of anemia, but no transfusions are needed.
- β-**thalassemia major** (Cooley anemia). Patients are normal at birth, and symptoms develop at about 6 months as hemoglobin F levels decline. Severe hemolytic anemia results from decreased erythrocyte life span. This severe anemia causes multiple problems:
  - Intramedullary destruction results in "ineffective erythropoiesis."
  - Hemolysis causes jaundice and an increased risk of pigment (bilirubin) gallstones.

- Lifelong transfusions are required, which result in secondary hemochromatosis.
- Congestive heart failure (CHF) is the most common cause of death.

Erythroid hyperplasia in the bone marrow causes "crewcut" skull x-ray and increased size of maxilla ("chipmunk face"). The peripheral blood shows microcytic/hypochromic anemia with numerous target cells and increased reticulocytes. Hemoglobin electrophoresis shows increased hemoglobin F (90%), normal or increased hemoglobin A2, and decreased hemoglobin A. Treatment is hematopoietic stem cell transplantation.

Sideroblastic anemia is a disorder in which the body has adequate iron stores, but is unable to incorporate the iron into hemoglobin. It is associated with ring sideroblasts (accumulated iron in mitochondria of erythroblasts) in bone marrow.

NORMOCYTIC ANEMIAS

Anemias of blood loss. Acute blood loss may cause shock or death. If the patient survives, the resulting hemodilution caused by shift of water from the interstitium will lower the hematocrit. There will be a marked reticulocytosis in 5-7 days. Chronic blood loss, such as from the gastrointestinal tract or from the gynecologic system, may result in iron deficiency anemia.

Hemolytic anemias.

- In **intravascular (IV) hemolysis**, release of hemoglobin into the blood causes hemoglobinemia and hemoglobinuria; increased bilirubin from erythrocytes causes jaundice and an increased risk of pigment (bilirubin) gallstones. The hemoglobin may be oxidized to methemoglobin, which causes methemoglobinemia and methemoglobinuria. Markedly decreased (because they have been used up) hemoglobin-binding proteins in the blood, such as haptoglobin and hemopexin, are characteristic. No splenomegaly is seen.
- In **extravascular (EV) hemolysis**, splenomegaly results if the EV hemolysis occurs in the spleen and hepatomegaly results if the EV hemolysis occurs in the liver. EV hemolyis causes increased bilirubin and decreased haptoglobin, but not to the degree seen with intravascular hemolysis. In EV hemolysis, there is an absence of hemoglobinemia, hemoglobinuria, and methemoglobin formation.

Sickle cell disease is an inherited blood disorder leading to the formation of hemoglobin S and increased propensity for the affected red blood cells to become sickle-shaped and occlude small vessels. The genetic abnormality is a single nucleotide change that causes valine (neutral) to replace normal glutamic acid (acidic) at the sixth position of the β-globin chain. This biochemical change then makes a critical point on the surface of the hemoglobin molecule become hydrophobic, making it feel "sticky" to an adjacent hemoglobin molecule, thereby favoring hemoglobin precipitation in crystalline form.

Heterozygous (AS) genome causes sickle cell trait. About 8% of African Americans are heterozygous for hemoglobin S. Patients with sickle trait have fewer symptoms than those with sickle disease, and also have resistance to *Plasmodium falciparum* infection (malaria), which may be why the disease has remained in the human genetic pool. Homozygous (SS) genome causes clinical disease (sickle cell anemia).

There are several factors affecting formation of irreversibly sickled red blood cells.

- **Increased concentration** (dehydration) makes symptoms worse; decreased concentration of sickled hemoglobin (as is seen if a sickle cell patient also has a thalassemia) makes symptoms better.
- **Decreased pH** decreases oxygen affinity and makes symptoms worse.
- **Increased hemoglobin F** makes symptoms better (rationale for therapy with hydroxyurea, which increases blood hemoglobin F levels).
- The **presence of hemoglobin C** (SC: double-heterozygote individual) makes symptoms better.

Clinical features include increased erythrocyte destruction which causes a severe hemolytic anemia, accompanied by erythroid hyperplasia in the bone marrow and increased bilirubin leading to jaundice and gallstone (pigment) formation. Capillary thrombi result from sickle cells blocking small vessels and may cause vaso-occlusive (painful) crises; hand-foot syndrome (swelling) in children; and autosplenectomy, which is seen in older children and adults. Howell-Jolly bodies will appear in peripheral blood after autosplenectomy, and the lack of a functional spleen predisposes to increased incidence of infections (encapsulated organisms), increased incidence of *Salmonella* osteomyelitis (leg pain), leg ulcers, and risk of aplastic crisis (especially with *parvovirus B19* infection). Emergencies that may occur include priapism and acute chest syndrome.

For testing, hemoglobin electrophoresis is used to diagnose the disease, though genetic testing can be performed on amniotic fluid for prenatal diagnosis. Newborn screening is now mandatory in the United States and is commonly performed via high performance liquid chromatography. Treatment is hydroxyurea (to increase hemoglobin F) and hematopoietic stem cell transplantation.

Glucose-6-phosphate dehydrogenase deficiency (G6PD) is a genetic disorder affecting the hexose monophosphate shunt pathway. It results in decreased levels of the antioxidant glutathione (GSH), leaving erythrocytes sensitive to injury by oxidant stresses leading to hemolysis. In some variants, G6PD is not due to decreased synthesis but rather to defective protein folding, resulting in a protein having a decreased half-life. The condition has X-linked inheritance.

- In **African Americans (A− type)** with G6PD, the hemolysis is secondary to acute oxidative stress, such as oxidative drugs (primaquine, sulfonamides, anti-tuberculosis drugs), and more typically by viral or bacterial infections. The hemolysis is intermittent (even if the offending drug is continued) because only older erythrocytes have decreased levels of glucose-6-phosphate dehydrogenase.

- In individuals with G6PD of **Mediterranean type**, the disease is associated with favism due to ingestion of fava beans; more severe hemolysis occurs because all erythrocytes have decreased glucose-6-phosphate dehydrogenase activity in that there is both decreased synthesis and decreased stability.

- In **both forms**, the oxidation of hemoglobin forms **Heinz bodies**; these cannot be seen with normal peripheral blood stains (Wright-Giemsa) but can be visualized with supravital stains (methylene blue and crystal violet). The Heinz bodies are "eaten" by splenic macrophages (extravascular hemolysis), which may form "bite cell" erythrocytes that are visible on routine peripheral blood smears.

Hereditary spherocytosis (HS) is an autosomal dominant disorder caused by a defect involving ankyrin and spectrin in the erythrocyte membrane; this causes a decrease in the erythrocyte surface membrane (spherocytosis). Spherocytes are not flexible and are removed in the spleen by macrophages (i.e., extravascular hemolysis). This causes multiple problems, including splenomegaly with a mild to moderate hemolytic anemia, increased bilirubin and increased risk for jaundice and pigment gallstones secondary to chronic hemolysis, and increased risk for acute red-cell aplasia due to parvovirus B19 infection.

Autoimmune hemolytic anemia (AIHA) is most commonly warm AIHA, in which the antibodies are IgG that are usually against Rh antigens and are active at 37°C. Erythrocytes to which the antibodies attach are removed by splenic macrophages, which tends to induce splenomegaly as the spleen responds to the perceived need for increased phagocytosis.

The etiology varies; most cases are idiopathic, but some cases are related to autoimmune diseases such as systemic lupus erythematosus, chronic lymphocytic leukemia (CLL), small lymphocytic lymphoma (WDLL), or medications (penicillin).

Pyruvate kinase deficiency is the most common enzyme deficiency in the glycolytic pathway and involves the enzyme that normally converts phosphoenolpyruvate to pyruvate. Deficiency leads to decreased ATP with resulting damage to the erythrocyte membrane. Clinically, there is a hemolytic anemia with jaundice from birth.

Hereditary elliptocytosis is a mild, hereditary, hemolytic anemia caused by a defect in spectrin. It is characterized by osmotically fragile ovoid erythrocytes ("elliptocytes").

Aplastic anemia is the term used when marrow failure causes a pancytopenia of the blood. Idiopathic causes for aplastic anemia are most commonly seen; when the etiology is known, the aplastic anemia may be due to medications (alkylating agents, chloramphenicol), chemical agents (benzene, insecticides), infection (EBV, CMV, parvovirus, hepatitis), or whole body radiation (therapeutic or nuclear exposure).

MACROCYTIC ANEMIAS

The basic cause of **megaloblastic anemias** is impaired DNA synthesis (delayed mitoses) without impairment of RNA synthesis; this produces a nuclear-cytoplasmic asynchrony that affects all rapidly proliferating cell lines, including cells of the bone marrow, gastrointestinal tract, and gynecologic system. The erythrocytes are the most obvious rapidly proliferating cells that exhibit these changes, and specifically show megaloblastic maturation, with megaloblasts in bone marrow forming macro-ovalocytes in peripheral blood. Autohemolysis of the affected megaloblasts in bone marrow (ineffective erythropoiesis) will cause increased bilirubin and increased lactate dehydrogenase (LDH). White blood cell changes include giant metamyelocytes in bone marrow and hypersegmented neutrophils (>5 lobes) in peripheral blood. Note that platelets are not increased in size.

Megaloblastic anemia due to vitamin B12 (cobalamin) deficiency

- Dietary deficiency is rare because B12 is stored in the liver and it takes years to develop dietary deficiency; it is usually seen only in strict vegetarians (diet with no animal protein, milk, or eggs).

- Decreased absorption of vitamin B12 is more common and may be caused by decreased intrinsic factor associated with gastrectomy or pernicious anemia (an autoimmune gastritis); pancreatic insufficiency (pancreatic proteases normally break down B12-R complexes in duodenum); or intestinal malabsorption due to parasites (fish tapeworm [*Diphyllobothrium latum*]), bacteria (blind-loop syndrome), or Crohn's disease of the ileum.

- Clinically, B12 deficiency causes weakness due to anemia (megaloblastic anemia) and sore ("beefy") tongue due to generalized epithelial atrophy. Unlike folate deficiency, vitamin B12 deficiency can also cause the central nervous system effects of subacute combined degeneration of the spinal cord, characterized by demyelination of the posterior and lateral columns of the spinal cord; the posterior (sensory) tract damage causes loss of vibratory and position sense, while the lateral cord damage involves dorsal spinocerebellar tracts (arm and leg dystaxia) and corticospinal tracts (spastic paralysis).

- Lab tests show low serum B12, increased serum homocysteine, and increased methylmalonic acid in urine. Treatment is intramuscular vitamin B12, which will cause increased reticulocytes in about 5 days.

Megaloblastic anemia due to folate deficiency can be caused by multiple processes:

- **Decreased intake** in chronic alcoholics and the elderly
- **Decreased absorption** in the upper small intestine
- **Increased requirement for folate** during pregnancy and infancy
- Folate antagonists, e.g., methotrexate

Clinically, folate deficiency produces megaloblastic anemia without neurologic disease symptoms. Lab tests show low serum folate levels and increased serum homocysteine. Treatment is folate replacement.

POLYCYTHEMIA VERA

Polycythemia vera is caused by a clonal expansion of a multipotent myeloid stem cell that primarily produces extra erythrocytes. See discussion of myeloproliferative disorders in chapter 21.

Secondary polycythemia refers to increased red cell mass due to compromised ability of blood to supply oxygen to tissues. Causes include chronic obstructive pulmonary disease and cyanotic congenital heart disease. Erythropoietin levels can be appropriately high. Secondary polycythemia may also be caused by inappropriately high erythropoietin levels, with renal cell carcinoma excreting erythropoietin being the typical cause.

Relative polycythemia refers to an increased red cell count secondary to decreased plasma volume (typically due to dehydration). Red cell mass, erythropoietin, and blood oxygen content are normal.

Vascular Pathology 12

Learning Objectives

❏ Demonstrate understanding of the vasculitides

❏ Answer questions about arteriosclerosis, hypertension, aneurysms, and arteriovenous fistulas

❏ Explain information related to venous disease

❏ Demonstrate understanding of vascular neoplasms

THE VASCULITIDES

The vasculitides are a group of systemic disorders with vessel inflammation and myriad clinical presentations. There are many systems used to categorize them. The system below is based largely on the size of the vessels involved.

Large Vessel Vasculitides

Takayasu arteritis occurs in older adults (age >50). Initial symptoms may be nonspecific (fatigue) with a variable course to more severe symptoms (blindness) and involvement of the aortic arch. Microscopically, there is vessel wall thickening and variable inflammation (from a mononuclear adventitial infiltrate to medial necrosis with granulomas).

Giant cell arteritis was formerly called temporal arteritis, but the temporal arteries are not always involved. The vertebral and ophthalmic arteries and aorta are often involved. The typical presentation evolves from nonspecific symptoms (headache) to more severe symptoms (blindness). Microscopically, there are inner media granulomas in classic cases. Treatment is steroids and anti-TNF therapy.

In a Nutshell

Thromboangiitis obliterans (Buerger's disease) is often categorized with the vasculitides, but the main lesion is thrombosis; inflammation may extend from vessels into adjacent soft tissue and nerves. The disease, which presents with severe distal extremity pain and ulceration, is seen most often in young male cigarette smokers. Pharmacologic therapies have not been successful.

Medium Vessel Vasculitides

Kawasaki disease presents with mucocutaneous symptoms and cervical lymph node enlargement in children. Involvement of the coronary arteries leads to cardiovascular sequelae, which can be circumvented with immunoglobulin therapy. Microscopically, there is transmural vascular inflammation.

Polyarteritis nodosa is a systemic necrotizing vasculitis occurring most often in young adults (M > F). It has an association with hepatitis B virus. The clinical course is one of episodic nonspecific symptoms (low-grade fever).

Pulmonary involvement is rare; renal artery involvement can be fatal. Immunosuppressive therapy can achieve remission in most cases.

Small Vessel Vasculitides

Small vessel vasculitides include those that are ANCA (antineutrophil cytoplasmic antibody)-associated (**granulomatosis with polyangiitis**, formerly known as Wegener's granulomatosis; and **eosinophilic granulomatosis with polyangiitis**, formerly known as Churg-Strauss syndrome) and those that are mediated by immune complexes (e.g., anti-glomerular basement membrane disease and IgA vasculitis, also known as Henoch-Schönlein purpura).

Granulomatosis with polyangiitis typically occurs in middle-aged men; it is characterized by granulomas of the lung and upper respiratory tract, glomerulonephritis, and a necrotizing granulomatous vasculitis. PR3-ANCAs are present in most cases.

Eosinophilic granulomatosis with polyangiitis is associated with asthma, extravascular granulomas (respiratory tract), and a systemic vasculitis that features eosinophils; eosinophil counts may be extremely high in peripheral blood.

RAYNAUD DISEASE AND PHENOMENON

Primary Raynaud phenomenon (Raynaud disease) typically occurs in young women as episodic small artery vasospasm in the extremities, nose, or ears; it results in blanching and cyanosis of the fingers or toes upon stress or (more commonly) exposure to cold. The pathogenesis may involve CNS and intravascular factors.

Secondary Raynaud phenomenon is caused by arterial insufficiency secondary to an underlying disease such as scleroderma (CREST).

ARTERIOSCLEROSIS

Mönckeberg medial calcific sclerosis is a medial calcification of medium-sized (muscular) arteries, such as femoral, tibial, radial, and ulnar arteries. It is asymptomatic, but may be detected by x-ray.

Arteriolosclerosis refers to sclerosis of arterioles; it affects small arteries and arterioles. Microscopically, either hyaline arteriolosclerosis (pink, glassy arterial wall thickening with luminal narrowing seen in benign hypertension, diabetes, and aging) or hyperplastic arteriolosclerosis (smooth-muscle proliferation resulting in concentric ["onion skin"] wall thickening and luminal narrowing seen in malignant hypertension) may occur.

Atherosclerosis is a common vascular disorder characterized by lipid deposition and intimal thickening of large and medium-sized (elastic and muscular) arteries, resulting in fatty streaks and atheromatous plaques over a period of decades (a type of chronic inflammatory condition). Particularly likely to be affected are the aorta and a number of important muscular arteries (coronary, carotid, cerebral, renal, iliac, and popliteal arteries).

Risk factors for atherosclerosis are as follows:

Hyperlipidemia	Sedentary lifestyle
Hypertension	Stress (type A personality)
Smoking	Elevated homocysteine
Diabetes	Oral contraceptive use
Obesity	Increasing age
Male gender	Familial/genetic factors

- The earliest (clinically reversible) stage in atherosclerosis is the **fatty streak**, which is seen grossly as a flat, yellow intimal streak and is characterized microscopically by lipid-laden macrophages (foam cells).
- **Stable atheromatous plaques** have a dense fibrous cap, a small lipid core and less inflammation than their vulnerable counterparts. They cause chronic ischemia.

Vulnerable atheromatous plaques are at risk for rupture, thrombosis or embolization due to their composition (thin fibrous cap, large lipid core, dense inflammation).

Clinical complications of atherosclerosis are protean; these complications include ischemic heart disease (myocardial infarctions); cerebrovascular accidents (CVA); atheroemboli (transient ischemic attacks [TIAs] and renal infarcts); aneurysm formation; peripheral vascular disease; and mesenteric artery occlusion.

HYPERTENSION (HTN)

Hypertension is an elevated blood pressure leading to end-organ damage, or a sustained diastolic pressure >90 mm Hg and/or systolic pressure >140 mm Hg.

Hypertension is very common, affecting 25% of the U.S. population. African Americans tend to be more seriously affected than Caucasians, and the risk increases with age. Approximately 95% of cases of hypertension are idiopathic (essential); the remainder are due to secondary hypertension related to renal disease, pheochromocytoma, or other disease processes.

Mild to moderate elevations in blood pressure cause end-organ damage by damaging arterioles with hyaline arteriolosclerosis. Late manifestations of hypertension include concentric left ventricular hypertrophy; congestive heart failure; accelerated atherosclerosis; myocardial infarction; aneurysm formation, rupture, and dissection; intracerebral hemorrhage; and chronic renal failure.

Malignant (accelerated) hypertension accounts for 5% of the cases and is characterized by markedly elevated pressures (e.g., systolic pressure >180 mm Hg and/or diastolic >120 mm Hg), which can rapidly cause end-organ damage. Funduscopic examination may demonstrate retinal hemorrhages, exudates, and papilledema. See chapter 15 for a discussion of renal pathology. Malignant hypertension is a medical emergency; if untreated, most patients will die within 2 years from renal failure, intracerebral hemorrhage, or chronic heart failure.

ANEURYSMS AND ARTERIOVENOUS FISTULAS

Aneurysms are congenital or acquired weakness of the vessel wall media, resulting in a localized dilatation or outpouching. Complications include thrombus formation, thromboembolism, and compression of nearby structures. Rupture or dissection may cause sudden death.

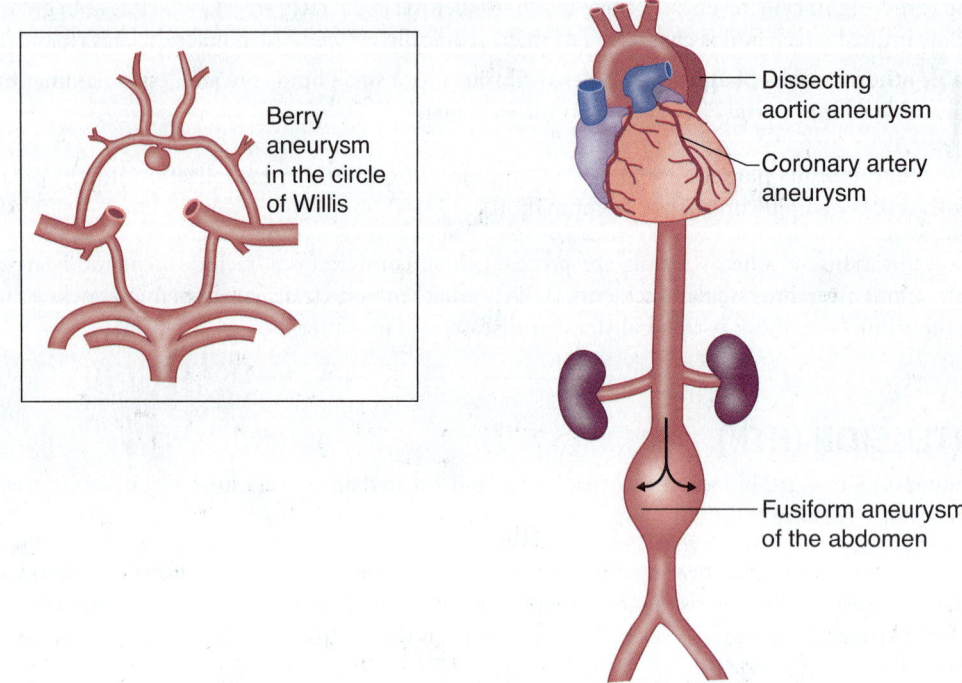

Figure 12-1. Location of Aneurysms

Atherosclerotic aneurysms are due to weakening of the media secondary to atheroma formation, and typically occur in the abdominal aorta below the renal arteries. They are associated with hypertension. Half of aortic aneurysms >6 cm in diameter will rupture within 10 years. Those >5 cm are treated surgically.

Syphilitic aneurysms involve the ascending aorta in tertiary syphilis (late stage). Syphilitic (luetic) aortitis causes an obliterative endarteritis of the vasa vasorum, leading to ischemia and smooth-muscle atrophy of the aortic media. Syphilitic aneurysms may dilate the aortic valve ring, causing aortic insufficiency.

Aortic dissecting aneurysm occurs when blood from the vessel lumen enters an intimal tear and dissects through the layers of the media. The etiology usually involves degeneration (cystic medial degeneration) of the tunica media. Aortic dissecting aneurysm presents with severe tearing pain. The dissecting aneurysm may compress and obstruct the aortic branches (e.g., renal or coronary arteries). Hypertension and Marfan syndrome are predisposing factors.

Berry aneurysm is a congenital aneurysm of the circle of Willis.

Microaneurysms are small aneurysms commonly seen in hypertension and diabetes.

Mycotic aneurysms are aneurysms usually due to bacterial or fungal infections.

Arteriovenous (AV) fistulas are a direct communication between a vein and an artery without an intervening capillary bed. They may be congenital or acquired (e.g., trauma). Potential complications include shunting of blood which may lead to high-output heart failure and risk of rupture and hemorrhage.

VENOUS DISEASE

Deep vein thrombosis (DVT) usually affects deep leg veins (90%), with iliac, femoral, and popliteal veins being particularly commonly affected. It is often asymptomatic and is consequently a commonly missed diagnosis. When symptomatic, it can produce unilateral leg swelling with warmth, erythema, and positive Homan sign (increased resistance to passive dorsiflexion of the ankle by the examiner). The diagnosis can be established with doppler "duplex" ultrasound. The major complication is pulmonary embolus.

Varicose veins are dilated, tortuous veins caused by increased intraluminal pressure. A variety of veins can be affected.

- **Superficial veins of the lower extremities** are particularly vulnerable due to a lack of structural support from superficial fat and/or incompetent valve(s). Varicosities of these superficial veins are very common (15% of the U.S. population); occur more frequently in females than males; and are common in pregnancy.

- **Esophageal varices** are due to portal hypertension (usually caused by cirrhosis) and may be a source of life-threatening hemorrhage.

- Varices of the anal region are commonly called **hemorrhoids**; are associated with constipation and pregnancy; and may be complicated by either bleeding (streaks of red blood on hard stools) or thrombosis (painful).

Venous insufficiency is more common in women than men, and the incidence increases with age. Lower extremities demonstrate edema, hyperpigmentation and ulceration due to venous hypertension and incompetent valves.

Vascular ectasias:

- **Nevus flammeus nuchae** is a neck "birthmark" or "stork bite" that regresses.
- **Port wine stain** is a vascular birthmark that does not regress.
- **Spider telangiectasias** occur on the face, blanch with pressure, and are associated with pregnancy.

VASCULAR NEOPLASMS

Hemangiomas are extremely common, benign vascular tumors. They are the most common tumor in infants appearing on the skin, mucous membranes, or internal organs. The major types are capillary and cavernous hemangiomas. Hemangiomas may spontaneously regress.

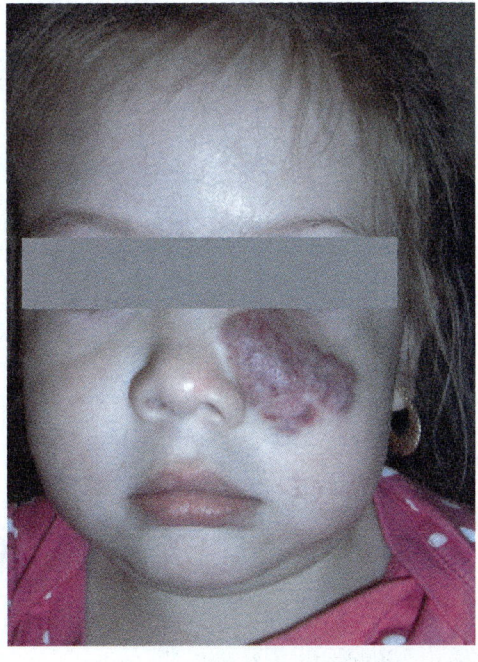

Figure 12-2. Hemangioma
© Richard P. Usatine, M.D. Used with permission.

Hemangioblastomas are associated with von Hippel-Lindau disease, which may cause multiple hemangioblastomas involving the cerebellum, brain stem, spinal cord, and retina, as well as renal cell carcinoma.

Glomus tumors (glomangioma) are benign, small, painful tumors of the glomus body that usually occur under fingernails.

Kaposi sarcoma is a malignant tumor of endothelial cells associated with Kaposi-sarcoma–associated virus (HHV8). The condition causes multiple red-purple patches, plaques, or nodules that may remain confined to the skin or may disseminate. Microscopically, there is a proliferation of spindle-shaped endothelial cells with slit-like vascular spaces and extravasated erythrocytes.

- The **classic European form** occurs in older men of Eastern European or Mediterranean origin, who develop red-purple skin plaques on the lower extremities.
- The **transplant-associated form** occurs in patients on immunosuppression for organ transplants; involves skin and viscera; may regress with reduction of immunosuppression.
- The **African form** occurs in African children and young men in whom generalized lymphatic spread is common.
- The **AIDS-associated form** is most common in homosexual male AIDS patients; it is an aggressive form with frequent widespread visceral dissemination. Common sites of involvement include skin, GI tract, lymph nodes, and lungs. This form of Kaposi sarcoma is responsive to chemotherapy and interferon-alpha, and only rarely causes death.

Angiosarcoma (hemangiosarcoma) is a malignant vascular tumor with a high mortality that most commonly occurs in skin, breast, liver, and soft tissues. Liver angiosarcomas are associated with vinyl chloride, arsenic, and thorotrast.

Cardiac Pathology 13

Learning Objectives

❑ Demonstrate understanding of ischemic heart disease

❑ Describe the characteristics of congestive heart failure

❑ Answer questions about valvular heart disease

❑ Explain the factors involved in myocarditis, congenital heart disease, and primary cardiomyopathies

❑ Demonstrate understanding of carcinoid heart disease, cardiac tumors and pericardial disease

ISCHEMIC HEART DISEASE

Cardiac ischemia is usually secondary to coronary artery disease (CAD); it is the most common cause of death in the United States. It is most often seen in middle-age men and postmenopausal women.

Angina pectoris is due to transient cardiac ischemia without cell death resulting in substernal chest pain.

- **Stable angina** (most common type) is caused by coronary artery atherosclerosis with luminal narrowing >75%. Chest pain is brought on by increased cardiac demand (exertional or emotional), and is relieved by rest or nitroglycerin (vasodilation).

- **Prinzmetal variant angina** is caused by coronary artery vasospasm and produces episodic chest pain often at rest; it is relieved by nitroglycerin (vasodilatation).

- **Unstable or crescendo angina** is caused by formation of a nonocclusive thrombus in an area of coronary atherosclerosis, and is characterized by increasing frequency, intensity, and duration of episodes; episodes typically occur at rest. This form of angina has a high risk for myocardial infarction.

  Myocardial infarction (MI) occurs when a localized area of cardiac muscle undergoes coagulative necrosis due to ischemia. It is the most common cause of death in the United States. The mechanism leading to infarction is coronary artery atherosclerosis (90% of cases). Other causes include decreased circulatory volume, decreased oxygenation, decreased oxygen-carrying capacity, or increased cardiac workload, due to systemic hypertension, for instance.

- **Distribution of coronary artery thrombosis.** The left anterior descending artery (LAD) is involved in 45% of cases; the right coronary artery (RCA) is involved in 35% of cases; and the left circumflex coronary artery (LCA) is involved in 15% of cases.

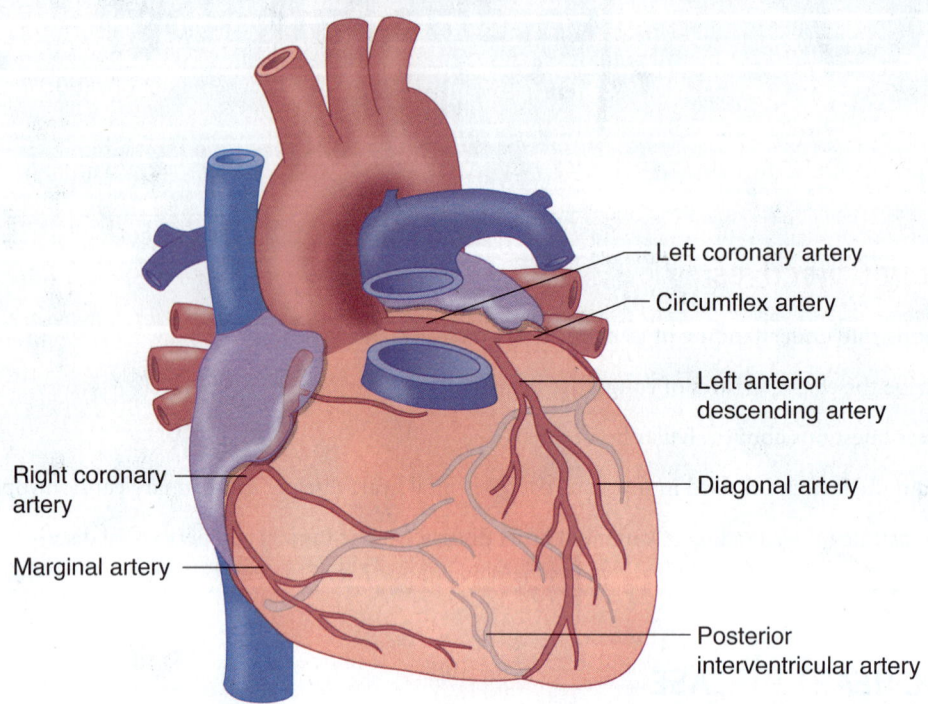

Figure 13-1. Arterial Supply to the Heart

Infarctions are classified as transmural, subendocardial, or microscopic.

- **Transmural** infarction (most common type) is considered to have occurred when ischemic necrosis involves >50% of myocardial wall. It is associated with regional vascular occlusion by thrombus.

- **Subendocardial** infarction is considered to have occurred when ischemic necrosis involves <50% of myocardial wall. It is associated with hypoperfusion due to shock. ECG changes are not noted. This type of infarction occurs in a setting of coronary artery disease with a decrease in oxygen delivery or an increase in demand.

- **Microscopic** infarction is caused by small vessel occlusion due to vasculitis, emboli, or spasm. ECG changes are not noted.

Clinical Correlate

Atypical presentation of MI with little or no chest pain is seen most frequently in elderly patients, diabetics, women, and post-surgical patients.

The clinical presentation of MI is classically a sudden onset of severe "crushing" substernal chest pain that radiates to the left arm, jaw, and neck. The pain may be accompanied by chest heaviness, tightness, and shortness of breath; diaphoresis, nausea, and vomiting; jugular venous distension (JVD); anxiety and often "feeling of impending doom."

- **Gross and microscopic** sequence of changes. The microscopic and gross changes represent a spectrum that is preceded by biochemical changes going from aerobic metabolism to anaerobic metabolism within minutes. The time intervals are variable and depend on the size of the infarct, as well as other factors.

Complications of MI include cardiac arrhythmias that may lead to sudden cardiac death; congestive heart failure; cardiogenic shock (>40–50% myocardium is necrotic); mural thrombus and thromboembolism; fibrinous pericarditis; ventricular aneurysm; and cardiac rupture. Cardiac rupture most commonly occurs 3–7 days after MI, and has effects that vary with the site of rupture: ventricular free wall rupture causes cardiac tamponade; interventricular septum rupture causes left to right shunt; and papillary muscle rupture causes mitral insufficiency.

Sudden cardiac death is defined to be death within 1 hour of the onset of symptoms. The mechanism is typically a fatal cardiac arrhythmia (usually ventricular fibrillation).

Coronary artery disease is the most common underlying cause (80%); other causes include hypertrophic cardiomyopathy, mitral valve prolapse, aortic valve stenosis, congenital heart abnormalities, and myocarditis.

Chronic ischemic heart disease is the insidious onset of progressive congestive heart failure. It is characterized by left ventricular dilation due to accumulated ischemic myocardial damage (replacement fibrosis) and functional loss of hypertrophied noninfarcted cardiac myocytes.

CONGESTIVE HEART FAILURE

Congestive heart failure (CHF) refers to the presence of insufficient cardiac output to meet the metabolic demand of the body's tissues and organs. It is the final common pathway for many cardiac diseases and has an increasing incidence in the United States. Complications include both **forward failure** (decreased organ perfusion) and **backward failure** (passive congestion of organs). Right- and left-sided heart failure often occur together.

- **Left heart failure** can be caused by ischemic heart disease, systemic hypertension, myocardial diseases, and aortic or mitral valve disease. The heart has increased heart weight and shows left ventricular hypertrophy and dilatation. The lungs are heavy and edematous. Left heart failure presents with dyspnea, orthopnea, paroxysmal nocturnal dyspnea, rales, and S3 gallop. Microscopically, the heart shows cardiac myocyte hypertrophy with "enlarged pleiotropic nuclei," while the lung shows pulmonary capillary congestion and alveolar edema with intra-alveolar hemosiderin-laden macrophages ("heart failure cells"). Complications include passive pulmonary congestion and edema, activation of the renin-angiotensin-aldosterone system leading to secondary hyperaldosteronism, and cardiogenic shock.

- **Right heart failure** is most commonly caused by left-sided heart failure, with other causes including pulmonary or tricuspid valve disease and *cor pulmonale*. Right heart failure presents with JVD, hepatosplenomegaly, dependent edema, ascites, weight gain, and pleural and pericardial effusions. Grossly, right ventricular hypertrophy and dilatation develop. Chronic passive congestion of the liver may develop and may progress to cardiac sclerosis/cirrhosis (only with long-standing congestion).

Clinical Correlate

Clinically, the degree of orthopnea is often quantified in terms of the number of pillows the patient needs in order to sleep comfortably (e.g., "three-pillow orthopnea").

VALVULAR HEART DISEASE

Degenerative calcific aortic valve stenosis is a common valvular abnormality characterized by age-related dystrophic calcification, degeneration, and stenosis of the aortic valve. It is common in congenital bicuspid aortic valves. It can lead to concentric left ventricular hypertrophy (LVH) and congestive heart failure with increased risk of sudden death. The calcifications are on the outflow side of the cusps. Treatment is aortic valve replacement.

Mitral valve prolapse has enlarged, floppy mitral valve leaflets that prolapse into the left atrium and microscopically show myxomatous degeneration. The condition affects individuals with Marfan syndrome. Patients are asymptomatic and a mid-systolic click can be heard on auscultation. Complications include infectious endocarditis and septic emboli, rupture of chordae tendineae with resulting mitral insufficiency, and rarely sudden death.

Rheumatic valvular heart disease/acute rheumatic fever

Rheumatic fever is a systemic recurrent inflammatory disease, triggered by a pharyngeal infection with Group A β-*hemolytic streptococci*. In genetically susceptible individuals, the infection results in production of antibodies that cross-react with cardiac antigens (type II hypersensitivity reaction). Rheumatic fever affects children (ages 5–15 years), and there is a decreasing incidence in the United States. Symptoms occur 2–3 weeks after a pharyngeal infection; laboratory studies show elevated antistreptolysin O (ASO) titers.

Diagnosis of rheumatic fever requires **two major** OR **one major and two minor criteria,** plus a preceding group A strep infection.

Clinical Correlate

Endocarditis involving the tricuspid valve is highly suggestive of IV drug use or central line bacteremia.

- **Acute rheumatic heart disease** affects myocardium, endocardium, and pericardium. The myocardium can develop myocarditis, whose most distinctive feature is the Aschoff body, in which fibrinoid necrosis is surrounded by macrophages (Anitschkow cells), lymphocytes, and plasma cells. Fibrinous pericarditis may be present. Endocarditis may be a prominent feature that typically involves mitral and aortic valves (forming fibrin vegetations along the lines of closure) and may also cause left atrial endocardial thickening (MacCallum plaques).

- **Chronic rheumatic heart disease** is characterized by mitral and aortic valvular fibrosis, characterized by valve thickening and calcification; fusion of the valve commissures; and damaged chordae tendineae (short, thickened, and fused). Complications can include mitral stenosis and/or regurgitation, aortic stenosis and/or regurgitation, congestive heart failure, and infective endocarditis.

Infectious bacterial endocarditis refers to bacterial infection of the cardiac valves, characterized by vegetations on the valve leaflets. Risk factors include rheumatic heart disease, mitral valve prolapse, bicuspid aortic valve, degenerative calcific aortic stenosis, congenital heart disease, artificial valves, indwelling catheters, dental procedures, immunosuppression, and intravenous drug use.

- **Acute endocarditis** is typically due to a *high virulence organism* that can colonize a normal valve, such as *Staphylococcus aureus*. Acute endocarditis produces large destructive vegetations (fibrin, platelets, bacteria, and neutrophils). The prognosis is poor, with mortality of 10–40%.

- **Subacute endocarditis** is typically due to a low virulence organism, such as *Streptococcus group viridians*, which usually colonizes a previously damaged valve. The disease course is typically indolent with <10% mortality.

- *Note: that there have been extensive revisions of dental prophylaxis for SBE over the past decades. Many cardiac conditions formerly requiring prophylaxis no longer do. Antibiotic regimens have also changed. See Details of SBE Dental Prophylaxis in chapter 2 of Microbiology (Part 4) for a complete discussion.*

Bridge to Microbiology

Viridans streptococci

- Alpha-hemolytic
- Bile-resistant
- Normal oral flora
- Optochin-resistant

Clinically, endocarditis presents with fever, chills, weight loss, and cardiac murmur. Embolic phenomena may occur, and may affect systemic organs; retina (Roth spots); and distal extremities (Osler nodes [painful, red subcutaneous nodules on the fingers and toes], Janeway lesions [painless, red lesions on the palms and soles], and splinter fingernail hemorrhages). Diagnosis is by serial blood cultures. Complications include septic emboli, valve damage resulting in insufficiency and congestive heart failure, myocardial abscess, and dehiscence of an artificial heart valve.

MYOCARDITIS

Myocarditis is caused by infectious (coxsackie A and B viruses, Chagas disease) and immune causes. Clinically, the patient may be asymptomatic or may suffer from acute heart failure or even dilated cardiomyopathy.

CONGENITAL HEART DISEASE

Congenital heart disease is the most common cause of childhood heart disease in the United States; 90% of cases are idiopathic and 5% are associated with genetic disease (trisomies, cri du chat, Turner syndrome, etc.), viral infection (especially congenital rubella), or drugs and alcohol.

Coarctation of the aorta is a segmental narrowing of the aorta.

- **Preductal coarctation** (infantile-type) is associated with Turner syndrome and causes severe narrowing of aorta proximal to the ductus arteriosus. It is usually associated with a patent ductus arteriosus (PDA), which supplies blood to aorta distal to the narrowing, and right ventricular hypertrophy (secondary to the need for the right ventricle to supply the aorta through the patent ductus arteriosus). It presents in infancy with congestive heart failure that is accompanied by weak pulses and cyanosis in the lower extremities; the prognosis is poor without surgical correction.

- **Postductal coarctation** (adult-type) causes stricture or narrowing of the aorta distal to the ductus arteriosus. It can present in a child or an adult with hypertension in the upper extremities, and hypotension and weak pulses in the lower extremities. Some collateral circulation may be supplied via the internal mammary and intercostal arteries; the effects of this collateral circulation may be visible on chest x-ray with notching of the ribs due to bone remodeling as a consequence of increased blood flow through the intercostal arteries.

Complications can include congestive heart failure (the heart is trying too hard), intracerebral hemorrhage (the blood pressure in the carotid arteries is too high), and dissecting aortic aneurysm (the blood pressure in the aortic route is too high).

Table 13-1. Left Versus Right Shunt Congenital Disease

Right → Left Shunt	Left → Right Shunt
Early cyanosis (blue babies)	Late cyanosis (blue kids)
Blood shunted past the lungs	Secondary pulmonary HTN → reversal of shunt (Eisenmenger syndrome)
• Tetralogy of Fallot • Transposition of the great vessels • Truncus arteriosus • Tricuspid atresia	• Ventricular septal defect • Atrial septal defect • Patent ductus arteriosus

Tetralogy of Fallot is the most common cause of congenital cyanotic heart disease. The classic tetrad includes **right ventricular outflow obstruction/stenosis; right ventricular hypertrophy; ventricular septal defect;** and **overriding aorta**. Clinical findings include cyanosis, shortness of breath, digital clubbing, and polycythemia. Progressive pulmonary outflow stenosis and cyanosis develop over time; treatment is surgical correction.

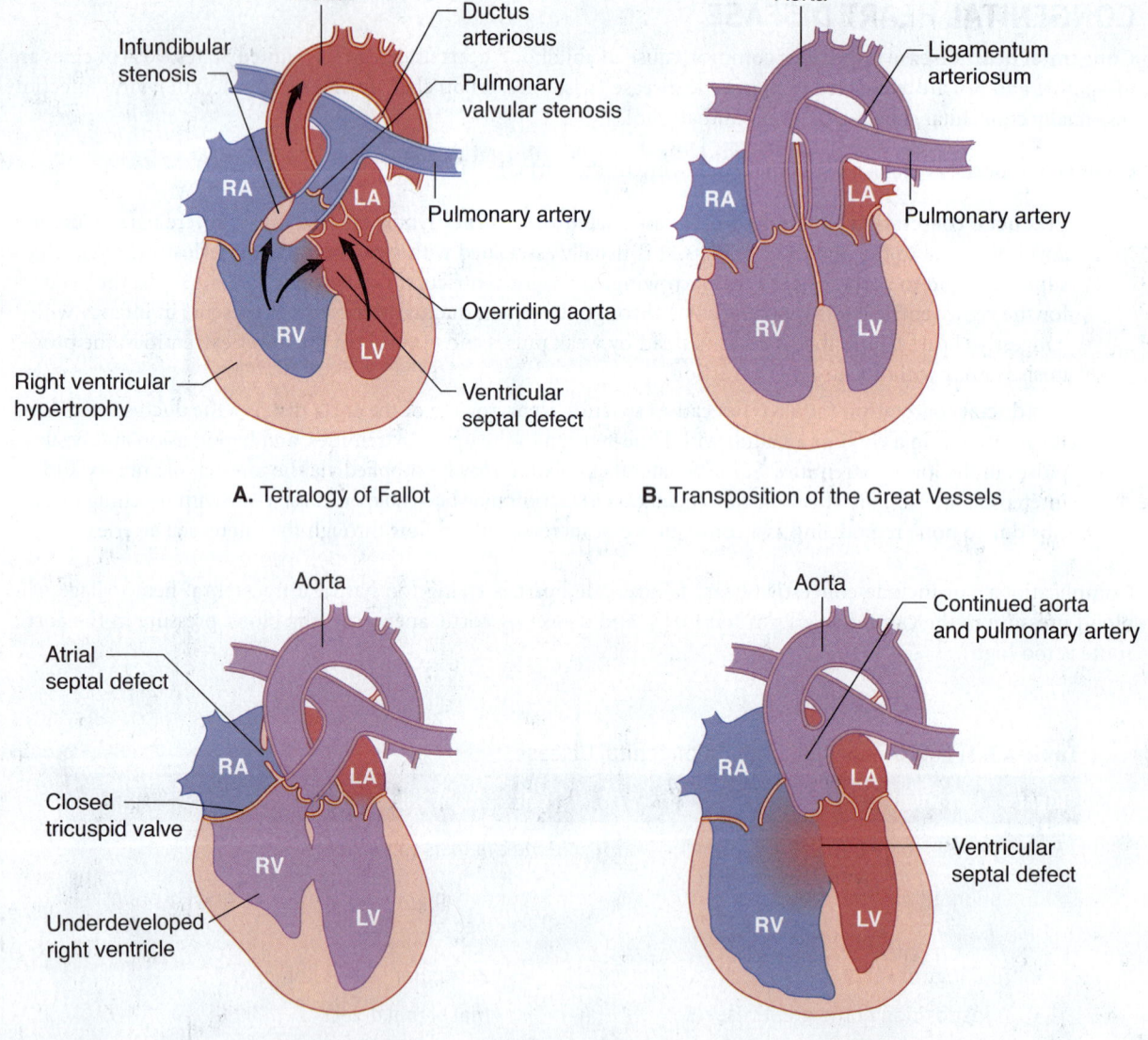

Figure 13-2. Common Forms of Cyanotic Congenital Heart Disease

Transposition of the great vessels is an abnormal development of the truncoconal septum whereby the aorta arises from the right ventricle, and the pulmonary artery arises from the left ventricle. The risk is increased in infants of diabetic mothers. Affected babies develop early cyanosis and right ventricular hypertrophy. To survive, infants must have mixing of blood by a VSD, ASD, or PDA. The prognosis is poor without surgery.

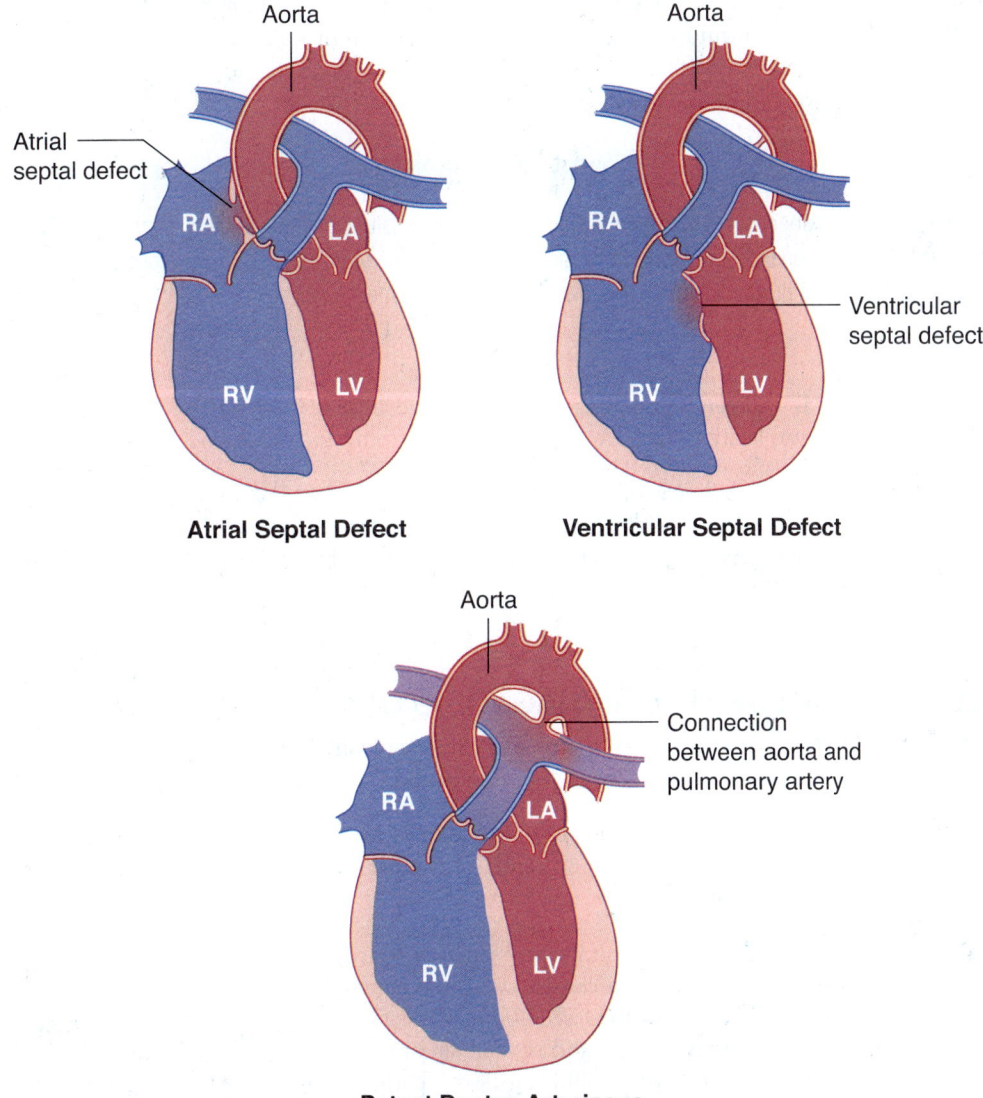

Atrial Septal Defect

Ventricular Septal Defect

Patent Ductus Arteriosus

Figure 13-3. Common Forms of Acyanotic Congenital Heart Disease

Truncus arteriosus is a failure to develop a dividing septum between the aorta and pulmonary artery, resulting in a common trunk. Blood flows from the pulmonary trunk to the aorta. Truncus arteriosus causes early cyanosis and congestive heart failure, with a poor prognosis without surgery.

Tricuspid atresia refers to the absence of a communication between the right atrium and ventricle due to developmental failure to form the tricuspid valve. Associated defects include right ventricular hypoplasia and an ASD. The prognosis is poor without surgery.

Ventricular septal defect (VSD), which consists of a direct communication between the ventricular chambers, is the second most common congenital heart defect (the most common is a bicuspid aortic valve).

- A **small ventricular septal defect** may be asymptomatic and close spontaneously, or it may produce a jet stream that damages the endocardium and increases the risk of infective endocarditis.
- A **large ventricular septal defect** may cause Eisenmenger complex, which is characterized by secondary pulmonary hypertension, right ventricular hypertrophy, reversal of the shunt, and late cyanosis.
- In **both types**, a systolic murmur can be heard on auscultation. Ventricular septal defects are commonly associated with other heart defects. Large ventricular septal defects can be surgically corrected.

Bridge to Embryology

In utero the ductus arteriosus is kept open by low arterial oxygen saturation and elevated prostaglandin E2 (PGE2) levels. Functional closure occurs in the first 2 days of life due to increased oxygen saturation and decreased PGE2. The ductus arteriosus becomes the ligamentum arteriosum.

Atrial septal defect (ASD) is a direct communication between the atrial chambers. The most common type is an ostium secundum defect. Complications include Eisenmenger syndrome and paradoxical emboli.

Patent ductus arteriosus (PDA) is a direct communication between the aorta and pulmonary artery due to the continued patency of the ductus arteriosus after birth. It is associated with prematurity and congenital rubella infections. Clinical findings include machinery murmur, late cyanosis, and congestive heart failure. Eisenmenger syndrome may develop as a complication.

PRIMARY CARDIOMYOPATHIES (DIAGNOSIS OF EXCLUSION)

Dilated cardiomyopathy (most common form) is cardiac enlargement with dilatation of all four chambers, resulting in progressive congestive heart failure (typical mode of presentation).

In cases of all types, the underlying etiology leads to destruction of myocardial contractility, which affects systolic function. Complications include mural thrombi and cardiac arrhythmias; prognosis is poor with 5-year survival of 25%. Treatment is heart transplantation.

Hypertrophic cardiomyopathy (also called asymmetrical septal hypertrophy, and idiopathic hypertrophic subaortic stenosis [IHSS]) is a common cause of sudden cardiac death in young athletes. The condition is an asymmetrical hypertrophy of cardiac muscle that causes decreased compliance affecting diastolic function. The muscle hypertrophy is due to the increased synthesis of actin and myosin, and on microscopic examination, the cardiac muscle fibers are hypertrophied and in disarray. Hypertrophic cardiomyopathy is most prominent in the ventricular septum, where it can obstruct the ventricular outflow tract. This can potentially lead to death during severe exercise when the cardiac outflow tract collapses, preventing blood from exiting the heart.

Restrictive cardiomyopathy (uncommon form) is caused by diseases which produce restriction of cardiac filling during diastole; etiologies include amyloidosis, sarcoidosis, endomyocardial fibroelastosis, and Loeffler endomyocarditis. In all of these diseases, increased deposition of material leads to decreased compliance, affecting diastolic function.

CARCINOID HEART DISEASE

Carcinoid heart disease is right-sided endocardial and valvular fibrosis secondary to serotonin exposure in patients with carcinoid tumors that have metastasized to the liver. It is a plaque-like thickening (endocardial fibrosis) of the endocardium and valves of the right side of the heart. Many patients experience carcinoid syndrome (also related to secretion of serotonin and other metabolically active products of the tumors), characterized by skin flushing, diarrhea, cramping, bronchospasm, wheezing, and telangiectasias.

CARDIAC TUMORS

Primary cardiac tumors are rare. The majority are benign; the malignant tumors are sarcomas. Treatment is excision.

- **Cardiac myxoma** is a benign tumor usually arising within the left atrium near the fossa ovalis in decades 3-6 of life; it can present like mitral valve disease.
- **Cardiac rhabdomyoma** is a benign tumor usually arising within the myocardium that is associated with tuberous sclerosis.

PERICARDIAL DISEASE

Pericarditis. There are two kinds of pericarditis, acute and chronic.

- **Acute pericarditis** is characterized by a fibrinous exudate (viral infection or uremia) or by a fibrinopurulent exudate (bacterial infection).
- **Chronic pericarditis** can occur when acute pericarditis does not resolve and adhesions form.

  Pericardial effusion may be serous (secondary to heart failure or hypoalbuminemia), serosanguineous (due to trauma, malignancy, or rupture of the heart or aorta) or chylous (due to thoracic duct obstruction or injury).

Tumors of the lung and breast may spread by **direct extension** to the pericardia.

Respiratory Pathology   14

Learning Objectives

❏ Demonstrate understanding of atelectasis and sarcoidosis

❏ Solve problems concerning pulmonary infections

❏ Answer questions about obstructive versus restrictive lung disease

❏ Demonstrate understanding of pulmonary and laryngeal neoplasias

❏ Explain information related to diseases of the pleural cavity

CONGENITAL CYSTIC LUNG LESIONS

The two most common malformations of the lung are **congenital cystic adenomatoid** *malformation* (CCAM) and **bronchopulmonary sequestration** (BPS). CCAM is a hamartomatous lesion, and BPS is a nonfunctioning bronchopulmonary segment separate from the tracheobronchial tree.

ATELECTASIS

Atelectasis refers to an area of collapsed or nonexpanded lung. It is reversible, but areas of atelectasis predispose for infection due to decreased mucociliary clearance.

The major types are as follows:

- **Obstruction/resorption atelectasis** is collapse of lung due to resorption of air distal to an obstruction; examples include aspiration of a foreign body, chronic obstructive pulmonary disease (COPD), and postoperative atelectasis.
- **Compression atelectasis** is atelectasis due to fluid, air, blood, or tumor in the pleural space.
- **Contraction (scar) atelectasis** is due to fibrosis and scarring of the lung.
- **Patchy atelectasis** is due to a lack of surfactant, as occurs in hyaline membrane disease of newborn or acute (adult) respiratory distress syndrome (ARDS).

PULMONARY INFECTIONS

In **bacterial pneumonia,** acute inflammation and consolidation (solidification) of the lung are due to a bacterial agent. Clinical signs and symptoms include fever and chills; productive cough with yellow-green (pus) or rusty (bloody) sputum; tachypnea; pleuritic chest pain; and decreased breath sounds, rales, and dullness to percussion.

Studies typically show elevated white blood cell count with a left shift (an increase in immature leukocytes). Chest x-ray for lobar pneumonia typically shows lobar or segmental consolidation (opacification), and for bronchopneumonia typically shows patchy opacification. Pleural effusion may also be picked up on chest x-ray.

In general, the keys to effective therapy are identification of the organism and early treatment with antibiotics.

Bridge to Anatomy

Pores of Kohn are collateral connections between alveoli through which infections and neoplastic cells can spread.

Lobar pneumonia is characterized by consolidation of an entire lobe. The infecting organism is typically *Streptococcus pneumoniae* (95%) or *Klebsiella*. The lancet-shaped diplococcus *Streptococcus pneumoniae* is alpha-hemolytic, bile soluble, and optochin sensitive.

The **four classic phases** of lobar pneumonia are **congestion** (active hyperemia and edema); **red hepatization** (neutrophils and hemorrhage); **grey hepatization** (degradation of red blood cells); and **resolution** (healing). In today's antibiotic era, these changes are not generally observed in practice.

Bronchopneumonia is characterized by scattered patchy consolidation centered on bronchioles; the inflammation tends to be bilateral, multilobar, and basilar, and particularly susceptible populations include the young, old, and terminally ill. Infecting organisms exhibit more variation than in lobar pneumonia, and include *Staphylococci*, *Streptococci*, *Haemophilus influenzae*, *Pseudomonas aeruginosa*, etc. Microscopic examination of tissue shows acute inflammation of bronchioles and surrounding alveoli. The diagnosis can often be established with sputum gram stain and sputum culture, but will sometimes require blood cultures.

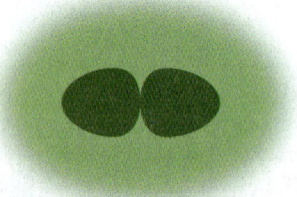

Figure 14-1. Streptococcus pneumoniae

Complications of pneumonia include fibrous scarring and pleural adhesions, lung abscess, empyema (pus in a body cavity), and sepsis.

Treatment of pneumonia is generally initial empiric antibiotic treatment, modified by the results of cultures and organism sensitivities.

Lung abscess is a localized collection of neutrophils (pus) and necrotic pulmonary parenchyma. The etiology varies with the clinical setting. **Aspiration** is the most common cause. It tends to involve right lower lobe and typically has mixed oral flora (often both anaerobic and aerobic) for infecting organisms.

Lung abscess may also occur following a pneumonia, especially one due to *S. aureus* or *Klebsiella*. Lung abscesses may also occur following airway obstruction (postobstructive) or deposition of septic emboli in the lung.

Complications of lung abscess include empyema, pulmonary hemorrhage, and secondary amyloidosis.

Atypical pneumonia is the term used for interstitial pneumonitis without consolidation. It is more common in children and young adults.

Infecting organisms that can cause atypical pneumonia include *Mycoplasma pneumoniae, influenza virus, parainfluenza virus, respiratory syncytial virus* (RSV) (which is especially important in young children), *adenovirus, cytomegalovirus* (CMV) (which is especially important in the immunocompromised), *varicella virus,* and many others.

Diagnosis. Chest x-ray typically shows diffuse interstitial infiltrates. An elevated cold agglutinin titer specifically suggests *Mycoplasma* as a cause, which is important to identify since antibiotic therapy for *Mycoplasma* exists. Lung biopsy, if performed, typically shows lymphoplasmacytic inflammation within the alveolar septa.

Complications include superimposed bacterial infections and Reye syndrome (potentially triggered by viral illness [influenza/varicella] treated with aspirin).

Tuberculosis (TB). The number of cases of TB is declining in the United States, but the proportion of cases in people born outside the country is rising. In this clinical setting, a positive PPD skin test may demonstrate that the person has been exposed to the mycobacterial antigens. Individuals who have received the BCG vaccine in some foreign countries may have a positive PPD test without being infected. In such cases chest x-ray and sputum smears and cultures are done.

Infection is usually acquired by inhalation of aerosolized bacilli.

Note

BCG (Bacillus Calmette-Guérin) is a tuberculosis vaccine prepared from a strain of attenuated live bovine tuberculosis bacillus, *Mycobacterium bovis.*

The **clinical presentation** of Mycobacterium tuberculosis includes fevers and night sweats, weight loss, cough, and hemoptysis.

Primary pulmonary TB develops on initial exposure to the disease. The Ghon focus of primary TB is characterized by subpleural caseous granuloma formation, either above or below the interlobar fissure. The term *Ghon complex* refers to the combination of the Ghon focus and secondarily-involved hilar lymph nodes with granulomas. Most primary pulmonary tuberculosis lesions (95%) will undergo fibrosis and calcification.

Progressive pulmonary TB can take several forms, including cavitary tuberculosis, miliary pulmonary tuberculosis, and tuberculous bronchopneumonia.

Secondary pulmonary TB (also known as postprimary or reactivation TB) occurs either with reactivation of an old, previously quiescent infection or with reinfection secondary to a second exposure to the mycobacteria. In secondary pulmonary TB, the infection often produces a friable nodule at the lung apex (Simon focus) secondary to the high oxygen concentration present at that site, since the upper parts of the lung typically ventilate more efficiently than the lower parts. Biopsy of affected tissues will typically show AFB-positive caseating granulomas.

Additionally, **dissemination to other organ systems** can occur in advanced TB via a hematogenous route that often results in a miliary pattern ("Miliary TB") within each affected organ. Sites that may become involved include meninges; cervical lymph nodes (scrofula) and larynx; liver/spleen, kidneys, adrenals, and ileum; lumbar vertebrae bone marrow (Pott disease); and fallopian tubes and epididymis. Note that aerobic tissues are favored due to aerobic requirements of Mycobacteria.

Nontuberculous mycobacteria. M. avium complex (MAC) typically occurs in AIDS patients with CD4 counts <50 cells/mm3 and presents as disseminated disease.

The diagnosis of TB requires identification of the bacilli. Positive sputum smear necessitates culture for species identification. Adequate treatment requires drug susceptibility testing.

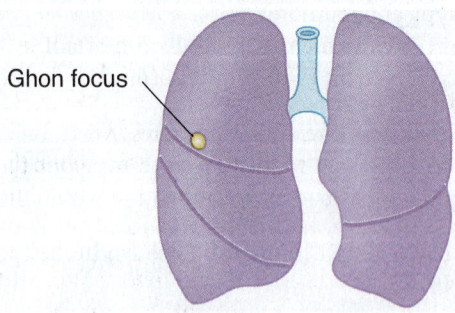

Ghon focus

Figure 14-2. Primary Tuberculosis

SARCOIDOSIS

Sarcoidosis is a systemic granulomatous disease of uncertain etiology. The disease affects females more than males, with typical age 20–60. It is most common in African American women. Clinical presentation varies. It may be asymptomatic, or presenting symptoms may include cough and shortness of breath; fatigue and malaise; skin lesions; eye irritation or pain; and fever or night sweats. Most often, the disease is first detected on chest x-ray as bilateral hilar lymphadenopathy or parenchymal infiltrates.

The noncaseating granulomas that are characteristic of sarcoidosis may occur in **any organ of the body**. In the lung, they typically form diffuse scattered granulomas; lymph node involvement may cause hilar and mediastinal adenopathy. Skin, liver and/or spleen, heart, central nervous system, bone marrow, and gastrointestinal tract are also frequent targets of the disease. Eye involvement can be seen in Mikulicz syndrome (involvement of the uvea and parotid).

The diagnosis of sarcoidosis can be suggested by clinical studies. In the laboratory, serum angiotensin converting enzyme (ACE), which is synthesized by endothelial cells and macrophages, may be elevated. X-ray studies frequently show bilateral hilar lymphadenopathy.

The prognosis is favorable with a variable clinical course. Most patients completely recover but some succumb to respiratory compromise.

OBSTRUCTIVE VERSUS RESTRICTIVE LUNG DISEASE

Table 14-1. Obstructive Versus Restrictive Lung Disease

Obstructive Airway Disease	Restrictive Lung Disease
Definition: Increased resistance to airflow secondary to obstruction of airways	Decreased lung volume and capacity
Pulmonary function tests (spirometry) FEV1/FVC ratio is decreased	Decreased TLC and VC
Examples: Chronic obstructive airway disease • Asthma • Chronic bronchitis • Emphysema • Bronchiectasis	Chest wall disorders • Obesity, kyphoscoliosis, polio, etc. Interstitial/infiltrative diseases • ARDS, pneumoconiosis • Pulmonary fibrosis

Table 14-2. Summary of Obstructive Versus Restrictive Pattern

Variable	Obstructive Pattern, e.g., Emphysema	Restrictive Pattern, e.g., Fibrosis
Total lung capacity	increased	decreased
FEV1	decreased	decreased
Forced vital capacity	normal or slightly decreased	decreased
FEV1/FVC	decreased	increased or normal
Peak flow	decreased	decreased
Functional residual capacity	increased	decreased
Residual volume	increased	decreased

OBSTRUCTIVE PULMONARY DISEASE

Chronic obstructive pulmonary disease (COPD) is a general term used to indicate chronic decreased respiratory function due to chronic bronchitis or emphysema. Both diseases are associated with smoking.

Chronic bronchitis is a clinical diagnosis made when a patient has a persistent cough and copious sputum production for at least 3 months in 2 consecutive years. It is highly associated with smoking (90%). Clinical findings include cough, sputum production, dyspnea, frequent infections, hypoxia, cyanosis, and weight gain.

Microscopic examination demonstrates hypertrophy and hyperplasia of bronchial mucous glands.

Complications include increased risk for recurrent infections; secondary pulmonary hypertension leading to right heart failure (cor pulmonale) and lung cancer.

Emphysema is the term used when destruction of alveolar septa results in enlarged air spaces and a loss of elastic recoil. The 4 types of emphysema are named for the anatomical distribution of the septal damage.

- In **centrilobular emphysema**, the damage is in the proximal portion of the acinus and the cause is cigarette smoking.
- In **panacinar emphysema**, the damage affects the entire acinus and the common cause is alpha-1 antitrypsin deficiency.
- In **distal acinar emphysema** (unknown cause), extension to the pleura causes pneumothorax.
- In **irregular emphysema**, post-inflammatory scarring involves the acinus in an irregular distribution.

   The etiology of emphysema involves a **protease/antiprotease imbalance**. On gross examination, the lungs are overinflated and enlarged, and have enlarged, grossly visible air spaces. Clinical findings include progressive dyspnea, pursing of lips and use of accessory respiratory muscles to breathe, barrel chest (increased anterior-posterior diameter), and weight loss.

Asthma is due to hyperreactive airways, which undergo episodic bronchospasm when triggered by certain stimuli.

- **Atopic (type I IgE-mediated hypersensitivity reaction) asthma** (most common form) usually affects children and young adults. There is often a positive family history.
- **Nonatopic asthma** is triggered by processes including respiratory infections (usually viral), stress, exercise, or cold temperatures.

- **Drug-induced asthma** affects about 10% of adults with a diagnosis of asthma. Aspirin is a key example of a precipitating drug.
- **Occupational asthma** is caused by workplace triggers including fumes and dusts.

An asthma attack is characterized by wheezing, severe dyspnea, and coughing. Problems with expiration cause lung overinflation. Status asthmaticus is a potentially fatal unrelenting attack of asthma.

Microscopic examination of sputum cytology may show Curschmann spirals (twisted mucus plugs admixed with sloughed epithelium), eosinophils, or Charcot-Leyden crystals (protein crystalloids from broken down eosinophils).

In patients dying from disease, autopsy findings include mucus plugs, increased mucous glands with goblet cell hyperplasia, inflammation (especially with eosinophils), edema; hypertrophy and hyperplasia of bronchial wall smooth muscle, and thickened basement membranes.

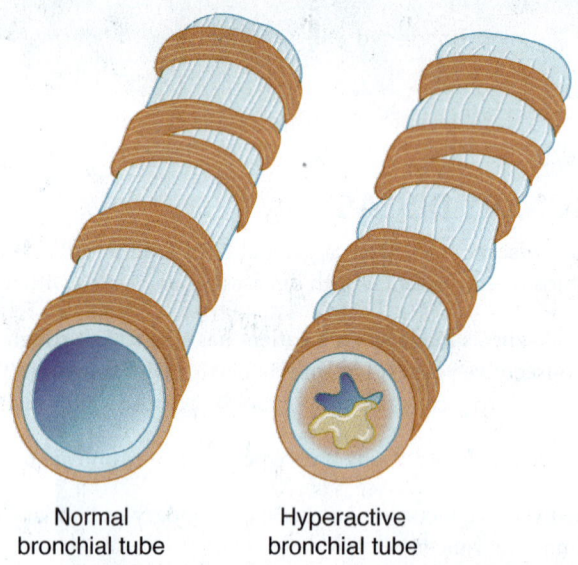

Normal
bronchial tube

Hyperactive
bronchial tube

Figure 14-3. Bronchial Changes in Asthma

Bronchiectasis is an abnormal permanent airway dilatation due to chronic necrotizing inflammation. Clinical findings include cough, fever, malodorous purulent sputum, and dyspnea. Causes are diverse, and include bronchial obstruction by foreign body, mucus, or tumor, necrotizing pneumonias, cystic fibrosis, and Kartagener syndrome.

- **Kartagener syndrome** is an autosomal recessive condition caused by immotile cilia due to a defect of dynein arms (primary ciliary dyskinesia). It is characterized clinically by bronchiectasis, chronic sinusitis, and situs inversus (a congenital condition where the major visceral organs are anatomically reversed compared with their normal anatomical positions).

On gross examination, bronchiectasis shows dilated bronchi and bronchioles extending out to the pleura. These changes may also be appreciated on chest x-ray. Complications include abscess, septic emboli, cor pulmonale, and secondary amyloidosis.

INFILTRATIVE RESTRICTIVE LUNG DISEASES (DIFFUSE INTERSTITIAL DISEASES)

Acute respiratory distress syndrome (ARDS) refers to diffuse damage of alveolar epithelium and capillaries, resulting in progressive respiratory failure that is unresponsive to oxygen treatment. Clinicians use the term *ARDS*, while pathologists use the term *diffuse alveolar damage (DAD)* to describe the pathologic changes.

ARDS may be caused by shock, sepsis, trauma, gastric aspiration, radiation, oxygen toxicity, drugs, or pulmonary infection. Activated neutrophils mediate cell damage. Clinically, patients show dyspnea, tachypnea, hypoxemia, cyanosis, and use of accessory respiratory muscles. X-rays show bilateral lung opacity ("white out").

On gross pathologic examination affected lungs are heavy, stiff, and noncompliant. Microscopically, there is intra-alveolar edema, and hyaline membranes line the alveolar spaces. In resolving cases there is proliferation of type II pneumocytes and interstitial inflammation and fibrosis.

Respiratory distress syndrome of the newborn (hyaline membrane disease of newborns) is caused by a deficiency of surfactant. It is associated with prematurity, maternal diabetes, multiple births, male gender, and cesarean section delivery. Clinically, infants are normal at birth but within a few hours develop increasing respiratory effort, tachypnea, nasal flaring, use of accessory muscles of respiration, an expiratory grunt, and cyanosis. Chest radiograph may demonstrate bilateral "ground-glass" reticulogranular densities. Autopsy findings include atelectasis and hyaline membranes.

- **Smoking-related pneumonitis.** Several entities have been identified.
  - Desquamative interstitial pneumonia features alveolar macrophages.
  - Respiratory bronchiolitis features bronchiolocentric macrophages.
  - Smoking-related interstitial fibrosis shows septal collagen deposition without significant associated inflammation.
- **Hypersensitivity pneumonitis.** After exposure to a sensitizing agent such as moldy hay, patients present with a febrile acute reaction or a chronic disease with weight loss. Biopsy shows peribronchiolar acute and chronic interstitial inflammation +/− noncaseating granulomas. The disease is immunologically mediated.
- **Eosinophilic pneumonia** describes a group of diseases with varying clinical features but a common histologic finding of a mixed septal inflammatory infiltrate and eosinophils within alveolar spaces. **Loeffler's syndrome** is a self-limiting type of eosinophilic pneumonia with peripheral blood eosinophilia.

  Occupation-associated pneumoconiosis is a common cause of chronic interstitial lung disease. It is considered separately here to show the full spectrum of disease since neoplasia may occur during its course.

- **Pneumoconioses** are fibrosing pulmonary diseases caused by inhalation of an aerosol (mineral dusts, particles, vapors, or fumes). Key factors affecting their development include the type of aerosol and its ability to stimulate fibrosis; the dose and duration of exposure; and the size of the particle, with only particles <10 microns entering the alveolar sac.
  - **Coal worker's pneumoconiosis** is an important pneumoconiosis that is due to anthracosis, in which carbon pigment (anthracotic pigment) from coal mining accumulates in macrophages along the pleural lymphatics and interstitium.
- **Asbestosis** is caused by members of a family of crystalline silicates. Occupations in which asbestos exposure may occur include shipyard work, insulation and construction industries, brake-lining manufacture.
  - **The pulmonary pathology of asbestosis** is a diffuse interstitial fibrosis that begins in the lower lobes; it causes slowly progressive dyspnea which may eventually be complicated by secondary pulmonary hypertension and cor pulmonale. Pulmonary biopsy may demonstrate asbestos bodies that have become coated with iron (ferruginous bodies). Otherwise, the findings are the same as usual interstitial pneumonia.
  - **Pleural involvement** may take the form of parietal pleural plaques (acellular type I collagen deposition) in a symmetrical distribution involving the domes of the diaphragm and posterolateral chest walls on chest x-ray. The apices and costophrenic angles are spared. Plaques on the anterior chest wall may be seen on CT. Fibrous pleural adhesions may occur on the visceral pleura.

- o **Lung cancer** is the most common tumor in asbestos-exposed individuals; there is a strong synergistic effect between smoking and asbestos exposure.

- o **Malignant mesothelioma** is a rare, highly malignant neoplasm associated with occupational exposure to asbestos in 90% of cases. It presents with recurrent pleural effusions, dyspnea, and chest pain. The tumor grossly encases and compresses the lung; microscopic exam exhibits carcinomatous and sarcomatous elements (biphasic pattern), while electron microscopy shows long, thin microvilli on some tumor cells. The prognosis of mesothelioma is poor. Other problems include increased risk of laryngeal, stomach, and colon cancers. Family members also have increased risk of cancer due to the worker bringing home clothing covered with asbestos fibers.

- **Silicosis** is due to exposure to silicon dioxide (silica). It is seen most frequently with occupational exposure (sandblasters, metal grinders, miners). The **pulmonary pathology** shows dense nodular fibrosis of the upper lobes which may progress to massive fibrosis; birefringent silica particles can be seen with polarized light. Patients present with insidious onset of dyspnea that is slowly progressive despite cessation of exposure. X-ray shows fibrotic nodules in the upper zones of the lungs. There is an increased risk of TB.

- **Berylliosis** is an allergic granulomatous reaction due to workplace exposure to beryllium in the nuclear, electronics, and aerospace industries. Genetic susceptibility appears to play a role, as does a type IV hypersensitivity reaction, resulting in granuloma formation. Clinically, acute exposure causes acute pneumonitis, while chronic exposure causes pulmonary noncaseating granulomas and fibrosis, hilar lymph node granulomas, and systemic granulomas

VASCULAR DISORDERS

Pulmonary edema is fluid accumulation within the lungs, usually due to imbalance of Starling forces or endothelial injury.

- Pulmonary edema due to **increased hydrostatic pressure** can be seen in left-sided heart failure, mitral valve stenosis, high altitude pulmonary edema, and fluid overload.

- Pulmonary edema due to **decreased oncotic pressure** can be seen in nephrotic syndrome and liver disease.

- Pulmonary edema due to **increased capillary permeability** can be due to infections, drugs (bleomycin, heroin), shock, and radiation.

The pathology grossly shows wet, heavy lungs (usually worse in lower lobes), while microscopic examination shows intra-alveolar fluid, engorged capillaries, and hemosiderin-laden macrophages (heart-failure cells).

Note

High altitude pulmonary edema is a hydrostatic-type pulmonary edema. Symptoms (i.e., cough and shortness of breath) resolve with descent and administration of oxygen.

Pulmonary emboli (PE) and pulmonary infarction (See chapter 5.)

Pulmonary hypertension is increased pulmonary artery pressure, usually due to increased vascular resistance or blood flow.

The etiology varies and can include chronic obstructive pulmonary disease and interstitial disease (hypoxic vasoconstriction); multiple ongoing pulmonary emboli; mitral stenosis and left heart failure; congenital heart disease with left to right shunts (atrial septal defect, ventricular septal defect, patent ductus arteriosus); and primary (idiopathic) pulmonary hypertension, typically in young women.

The pathology includes pulmonary artery atherosclerosis, small artery medial hypertrophy and intimal fibrosis, and plexogenic pulmonary arteriopathy. Pulmonary hypertension may also damage the heart, leading to right ventricular hypertrophy and then failure (cor pulmonale).

PULMONARY NEOPLASIA

Lung cancer is the leading cause of cancer death among both men and women; it has been increasing in women (increased smoking) in the past few decades. It occurs most commonly age 50–80. Major risk factors include cigarette smoking, occupational exposure (asbestosis, uranium mining, radiation, etc.), passive smoking, and air pollution. Clinical features include cough, sputum production, weight loss, anorexia, fatigue, dyspnea, hemoptysis, and chest pain. Obstruction may produce focal emphysema, atelectasis, bronchiectasis, or pneumonia.

Adenocarcinoma is more commonly seen in women and nonsmokers. Grossly, it causes a peripheral gray-white mass, and the tumor may develop in areas of parenchymal scarring (scar carcinoma). Microscopically, common patterns include acinar, papillary, mucinous, and solid. The precursor lesion—atypical adenomatous hyperplasia—progresses to adenocarcinoma in situ (noninvasive well-differentiated tumor <3 cm) and to minimally invasive tumor (invasion no more than 5 mm) before progressing to invasive adenocarcinoma.

Squamous cell carcinoma (SCC) is strongly related to smoking and affects males more than females. Squamous cell carcinoma arises from bronchial epithelium after a progression:

$$\text{metaplasia} \rightarrow \text{dysplasia} \rightarrow \text{carcinoma } \textit{in situ} \rightarrow \text{invasive carcinoma}$$

Pathologically, the tumor grossly causes a gray-white bronchial mass, usually centrally located. Microscopically, well-differentiated tumors show invasive nests of squamous cells with intercellular bridges (desmosomes) and keratin production ("squamous pearls").

Small cell carcinoma has a strong association with smoking, and affects males more than females. This neuroendocrine tumor is very aggressive, with rapid growth and early dissemination. Small cell carcinoma is commonly associated with paraneoplastic syndromes.

Pathologically, gross examination demonstrates central, gray-white masses. Microscopic examination shows small round or polygonal cells in clusters, and electron microscopy shows cytoplasmic dense-core neurosecretory granules.

Large cell carcinoma has large anaplastic cells without evidence of differentiation.

Intrathoracic spread of lung cancer is to lymph nodes, particularly hilar, bronchial, **tracheal, and mediastinal;** pleura **(adenocarcinoma);** and lung apex causing **Horner syndrome (Pancoast tumor).**

- Obstruction of the superior vena cava by tumor causes **superior vena cava syndrome,** characterized by distended head and neck veins, plethora, and facial and upper arm edema.
- **Esophageal obstruction** can cause dysphagia.
- Recurrent laryngeal **nerve involvement** causes hoarseness, while phrenic nerve damage causes diaphragmatic paralysis.

Extrathoracic sites of metastasis include adrenal (>50%), liver, brain, and bone.

Paraneoplastic syndromes

- Endocrine/metabolic syndromes include Cushing syndrome secondary to ACTH production, SIADH secondary to ADH production, and hypercalcemia secondary to PTH production (squamous cell carcinoma).
- Eaton-Lambert syndrome (*See* Skeletal Muscle and Peripheral Nerve Pathology chapter.)
- Acanthosis nigricans (*See* Skin Pathology chapter.)
- Hypertrophic pulmonary osteoarthropathy is characterized by periosteal new bone formation with clubbing and arthritis.

Treatment of non–small cell lung cancer is with surgery, and treatment of small cell lung cancer is with chemotherapy and radiation. Despite treatment, the prognosis is poor, with overall 5-year survival 16%.

Bronchial carcinoids occur in a younger age group (mean age 40 years) and typically produce a polypoid intrabronchial mass or plaque; it is characterized on light microscopy by small, round, uniform cells growing in nests (organoid pattern), and on electron microscopy by cytoplasmic dense-core neurosecretory granules. Atypical carcinoid is more aggressive than typical carcinoid.

Metastatic carcinoma is the most common malignant neoplasm in the lung. It typically causes multiple, bilateral, scattered nodules; common primary sites include breast, stomach, pancreas, and colon.

Hamartomas are benign tumors; they occur more commonly in middle-aged adults but also occur in children. They can appear as coin lesions on chest x-ray. Microscopically, they are comprised of nonencapsulated fibromyxoid tissue.

LARYNGEAL CANCER

Laryngeal squamous cell carcinoma causes hoarseness, difficulty swallowing, pain, hemoptysis, and eventual respiratory compromise. Risk factors include smoking, alcohol, and frequent cord irritation (professional singing or lecturing). Complications include direct extension, metastases, and infection.

DISEASES OF THE PLEURAL CAVITY

Pleural effusion is the accumulation of fluid in the pleural cavity.

- *Empyema* refers to pus in pleural space.
- *Chylothorax* refers to chylous fluid in the pleural space secondary to obstruction of the thoracic duct, usually by tumor.

Pneumothorax is the term used for air in the pleural cavity. It can be due to traumatic penetrating chest wall injuries or spontaneous rupture of apical blebs in typically tall young adults (spontaneous pneumothorax). The term **tension pneumothorax** is used if a life-threatening shift of thoracic organs across midline occurs.

Hemothorax is the presence of blood in the pleural cavity. Trauma is a common cause. There may be hypotension and shift of the trachea to the unaffected side.

Chylothorax is lymphatic fluid in the pleural cavity. Malignancy is a common cause.

Mesothelioma (See section on asbestosis earlier in this chapter.)

Renal Pathology 15

Learning Objectives

- ❏ Demonstrate understanding of congenital anomalies of the kidney
- ❏ Use knowledge of cystic disease to solve problems
- ❏ Describe epidemiology and course of urolithiasis
- ❏ Solve problems concerning chronic renal failure and tumors of the kidney
- ❏ Explain information related to ureteral disorders and urinary bladder pathology

CONGENITAL ANOMALIES OF THE KIDNEY

Renal agenesis

- **Bilateral agenesis** is incompatible with life. Ultrasound shows oligohydramnios.

Hypoplasia is failure of a kidney (usually unilateral) to develop to normal weight; the hypoplastic kidney has a decreased number of calyces and lobes.

Horseshoe kidney is a common congenital anomaly that is found in 1 in 600 abdominal x-rays. The kidneys show fusion, usually at the lower pole; affected individuals have normal renal function but may be predisposed to renal calculi.

Abnormal locations. The most common abnormal location is a pelvic kidney. The ectopic kidney usually has normal function. Tortuosity of ureters may predispose to pyelonephritis.

CYSTIC DISEASE

Autosomal recessive polycystic kidney disease (also called infantile polycystic kidney disease or renal dysgenesis Potter type I) is a rare autosomal recessive disease that presents in infancy with progressive and often fatal renal failure.

The kidneys are bilaterally enlarged and have a spongelike cut surface. The liver may have multiple hepatic cysts and cirrhosis may develop in childhood. Pulmonary hypoplasia is present to varying degrees.

Autosomal dominant polycystic kidney disease (also called adult polycystic kidney disease or renal dysgenesis Potter type III) is an autosomal dominant disease that affects 1 in 1,000.

Clinically, patients are asymptomatic with normal renal function until middle age, and then present with renal insufficiency, renal stones, hematuria, and hypertension or with abdominal masses and flank pain.

On gross pathologic examination, the kidneys have massive bilateral enlargement with large bulging cysts filled with serous, turbid, or hemorrhagic fluid. Microscopic examination shows functioning nephrons present between the cysts; the cysts arise from the tubular epithelial cells of the kidney.

Extrarenal manifestations include cysts of the liver, pancreas, and lungs; berry aneurysms of the circle of Willis; mitral valve prolapse; and colonic diverticula.

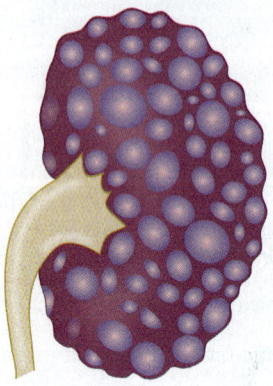

Figure 15-1. Adult Polycystic Disease

Renal dysplasia is the most common renal cystic disease in children, in whom it causes an enlarged renal mass with cartilage and immature collecting ducts. It may progress clinically to renal failure.

Acquired polycystic disease is seen in renal dialysis patients and is associated with a small risk of developing renal adenomas and renal cell carcinoma.

Simple retention cysts of the kidney are common in adults and occasionally cause hematuria.

Medullary diseases with cysts

- Medullary sponge kidney can cause nephrolithiasis but is otherwise innocuous.
- Nephronophthisis-medullary cystic disease complex presents as polyuria and polydipsia; it can progress to chronic renal failure in young adults. There are autosomal recessive forms. The cysts are in the cortex and the medulla.

GLOMERULAR DISEASES

Immune mechanisms play a role in the pathogenesis of most glomerular diseases, either via deposition of immune complexes or injury from antibodies. Glomerular diseases may be divided into those originating in the kidney and those caused by systemic disease (secondary).

Glomerular disease may present clinically as **nephrotic** or **nephritic syndrome**. Their clinical features are different.

Table 15-1. Clinical Syndromes in Glomerular Disease

Nephritic Syndrome	Nephrotic Syndrome
Hematuria (RBC casts)	Severe proteinuria (>3.5 g/day)
Hypertension	Hypoalbuminemia (<3 g/dL)
Azotemia	Generalized edema
Oliguria	Hyperlipidemia
Proteinuria (<3.5 g/day)	Lipiduria

Renal biopsy can yield a definitive diagnosis when light microscopy features are considered in concert with immunofluoresence (IF) and electron microscopy (EM).

PRIMARY GLOMERULOPATHIES (NEPHRITIC SYNDROME)

Acute poststreptococcal glomerulonephritis (APSGN) (or acute proliferative glomerulonephritis or postinfectious glomerulonephritis) is an immune complex disease that typically occurs 2-4 weeks after a streptococcal infection of the throat or skin. There is a decreasing incidence in the United States; children are affected more often than adults.

The infecting organism is most commonly β-hemolytic group A *streptococci*, but APSGN can also be caused by other bacteria, viruses, parasites, and even systemic diseases (SLE and polyarteritis nodosa). Clinically, it presents with nephritic syndrome with elevated antistreptolysin O (ASO) titers (when related to streptococcal infection) and low C3.

Renal biopsy. Light microscopy shows an infiltrate of neutrophils in the glomeruli; the process is diffuse, that is, it involves all the glomeruli. Immunofluorescence shows granular deposits of IgG and C3 throughout the glomerulus within the capillary walls and some mesangial areas. Electron microscopy shows subepithelial immune complex deposits (humps).

Treatment is conservative fluid management.

Rapidly progressive glomerulonephritis (RPGN) (crescentic glomerulonephritis) is group of diseases characterized by glomerular crescents and a rapid deterioration of renal function.

- **Anti-glomerular basement membrane antibody-mediated crescentic glomerulonephritis** has a peak incidence at age 20-40, and males are affected more frequently than females.

Pulmonary involvement is called **Goodpasture syndrome**. These patients have pulmonary hemorrhage and hemoptysis.

Renal biopsy findings include hypercellularity, crescents, and fibrin deposition in glomeruli. Immunofluorescence shows a smooth and linear pattern of IgG and C3 in the glomerular basement membrane (GBM). By electron microscopy, there are no deposits, but there is glomerular basement membrane disruption.

IgA nephropathy (Berger disease) is the most common cause of glomerulonephritis in the world. It affects children and young adults (mostly males).

IgA nephropathy is characterized by recurrent gross hematuria (a predominately nephritic presentation), whose onset may follow a respiratory infection. IgA nephropathy can be associated with celiac sprue and Henoch-Schönlein purpura or can be secondary to celiac sprue or liver disease.

The pathogenesis is unknown, but may be related to a possible entrapment of circulating immune complexes with activation of the alternate complement pathway; it may also be related to a genetic predisposition.

Membranoproliferative glomerulonephritis (MPGN) is a form of glomerular disease that affects both the glomerular mesangium and the basement membranes.

PRIMARY GLOMERULOPATHIES (NEPHROTIC)

Membranous glomerulonephritis is a common cause of nephrotic syndrome in adults that is mediated by immune complexes.

Most cases (85%) are idiopathic; in most of these cases, autoantibodies cross-react with podocyte antigens. Membranous glomerulonephritis may also be caused by drugs (penicillamine), infections (hepatitis virus B and C, syphilis, etc.), and systemic diseases (SLE, diabetes mellitus, etc.). It has also been associated with malignant carcinomas of the lung and colon, and there may be a genetic predisposition.

Renal biopsy shows diffuse thickening of the capillary walls. Basement membrane projections ("spikes") are seen on silver stains. Immunofluorescence shows a granular and linear pattern of IgG and C3. Electron microscopy shows subepithelial deposits along the basement membranes with effacement of podocyte foot processes.

The clinical course is variable and may lead to spontaneous remission, persistent proteinuria, or end-stage renal disease.

Minimal change disease (also called lipoid nephrosis and nil disease) is the most common cause of nephrotic syndrome in children. Peak incidence is age 2-6.

The diagnosis is one of exclusion. Light microscopy shows normal glomeruli with lipid accumulation in proximal tubule cells (lipoid nephrosis). Immunofluorescence is negative, with no immune deposits. Electron microscopy shows effacement of epithelial (podocyte) foot processes, microvillous transformation, and no immune complex deposits.

The prognosis is excellent because treatment with corticosteroids produces a dramatic response in children. The majority have a complete recovery.

Focal segmental glomerulosclerosis is a very common cause of nephrotic syndrome that occurs in all ages. African Americans are affected more frequently than Caucasians.

The condition may be idiopathic (primary), or it may be related to a wide variety of predisposing conditions including loss of renal tissue; preexisting glomerular diseases (such as IgA nephropathy); sickle cell anemia; heroin use; AIDS; or morbid obesity. Inherited and congenital forms occur.

SECONDARY GLOMERULONEPHRITIS

Secondary glomerulonephritis is glomerular disease that is secondary to other disease processes.

Diabetes causes nodular glomerulosclerosis, hyaline arteriolosclerosis, and diabetic microangiopathy. Clinically, diabetic patients may develop microalbuminuria that can progress to nephrotic syndrome.

Systemic lupus erythematosus can cause various patterns of damage to the kidney with clinical features that can include hematuria, nephritic syndrome, nephrotic syndrome, hypertension, and renal failure.

CHRONIC GLOMERULONEPHRITIS

End-stage renal disease is the final stage of many forms of glomerular disease. It is characterized by progressive renal failure, uremia, and ultimately death.

Clinical features include anemia, anorexia, malaise, proteinuria, hypertension, and azotemia. Urinalysis shows broad, waxy casts. On pathologic examination, the kidneys are grossly small and shrunken; microscopic exam shows hyalinization of glomeruli, interstitial fibrosis, atrophy of tubules, and a lymphocytic infiltrate.

Treatment is dialysis and renal transplantation.

TUBULOINTERSTITIAL NEPHRITIS

Tubulointerstitial nephritis is an acute or chronic inflammation of tubules and interstitium. It can be due to many causes, including medications, infections, acute pyelonephritis, systemic lupus erythematosus, lead poisoning, urate nephropathy, or multiple myeloma.

- **Acute pyelonephritis** refers to bacterial infections involving the renal pelvis, tubules, and interstitium. Pyelonephritis affects females much more than males, but the incidence increases in older males with prostatic hyperplasia. Ascending infection is the most common route of infection. Causative organisms include gram-negative enteric bacilli, *Escherichia coli*, *Proteus*, *Klebsiella*, and *Enterobacter*. Predisposing factors include urinary obstruction, vesicoureteral reflux, pregnancy, urethral instrumentation, diabetes mellitus, benign prostatic hyperplasia, and other renal pathology. Symptoms can include fever, chills, and malaise; dysuria, frequency, and urgency; and costovertebral angle tenderness. Urinalysis shows pyuria and white blood cell casts.

The kidney may be enlarged, and the cortical surface may show abscesses. Microscopically there is a neutrophilic insterstitial infiltrate. **Parenchymal abscesses** may be present. The tubules contain neutrophil casts.

- **Chronic pyelonephritis** can occur from chronic obstruction or in the setting of vesicoureteral reflux. Scarring can be seen at the upper and lower poles of the kidney, with associated calyceal blunting. Microscopically there is interstitial fibrosis and inflammation with thyroidization of the tubule. Some patients develop glomerulosclerosis. Renal insufficiency develops gradually.

- **Drug-induced tubular interstitial nephritis** is commonly caused by penicillins, other antibiotics, diuretics, and NSAIDs. Interstitial inflammation is characteristic and granulomas may be seen. This hypersensitivity reaction presents a couple of weeks after drug exposure with fever, eosinophilia, rash, and hematuria. Minimal proteinuria may be present. Recovery is expected after withdrawal of the drug.

- **Urate nephropathy** is caused by a deposition of urate crystals (secondary to leukemia treatment, lead poisoning, and gout) in renal tubules and interstitium. It may produce acute renal failure.

ACUTE TUBULAR INJURY

Acute tubular injury (ATI) is acute renal failure associated with potentially reversible injury to the tubular epithelium. It is the most common cause of acute renal failure in the United States. It is characterized by oliguria with elevation of blood urea nitrogen (BUN) and creatinine; metabolic acidosis and hyperkalemia; and dirty brown granular casts and epithelial casts on urinalysis.

- **Ischemic acute tubular necrosis** is the most common cause of ATI. The condition is due to decreased blood flow caused by severe hemorrhage, severe renal vasoconstriction, hypotension, dehydration, or shock.

- **Nephrotoxic ATN** has a large number of causes, including drugs (e.g., polymyxin, methicillin, gentamicin, sulfonamides); radiographic contrast agents; heavy metals (e.g., mercury, lead, gold); organic solvents (e.g., carbon tetrachloride, chloroform, methyl alcohol); ethylene glycol (antifreeze); mushroom poisoning; phenol; pesticides; and myoglobin.

The **prognosis** is excellent if the patient survives the underlying disease, and if the patient had no preexisting kidney disease.

UROLITHIASIS

Renal calculi occur in up to 6% of the population; men are affected more often than women.

Note
Calcium oxalate stones form in people with alkaline urine.
Uric acid and **cystine stones** form in people with acidic urine.

- **Stone composition.** Most (75%) stones are calcium oxalate stones. Magnesium ammonium phosphate ("struvite") stones are associated with infection by urea-splitting bacteria (proteus), and these stones often form large staghorn calculi. Uric acid stones are seen in gout, leukemia, and in patients with acidic urine. Cystine stones are uncommon.

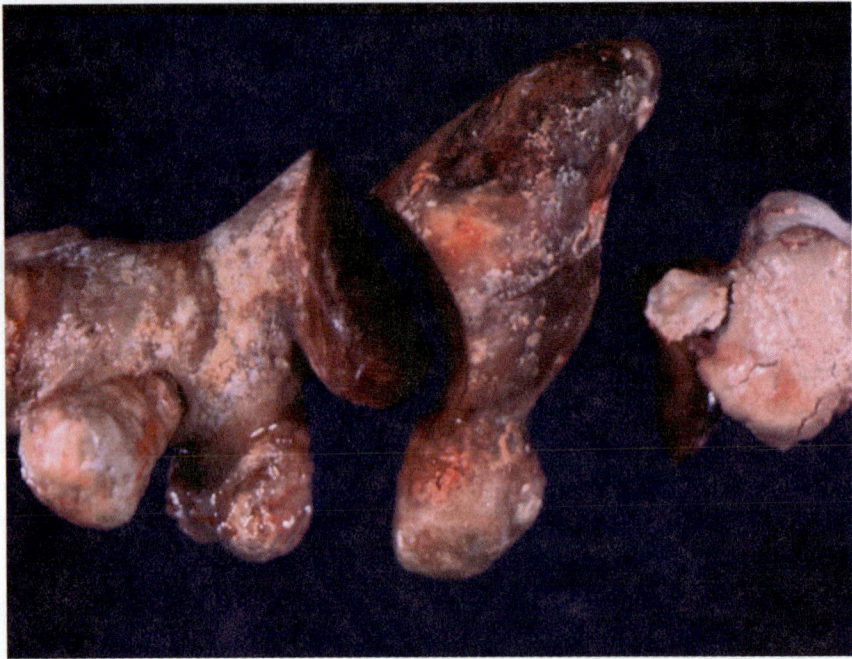

Figure 15-2. Struvite (Magnesium Ammonium Phosphate) Stone Forming Staghorn Calculi
© Katsumi M. Miyai, M.D., Ph.D.; Regents of the University of California. Used with permission.

- **Pathology.** Most stones are unilateral stones that are formed in the calyx, pelvis, and urinary bladder.
- **Clinical features.** Calcium stones are radiopaque and can be seen on x-ray. Renal colic may occur if small stones pass into the ureters. Stones may cause hematuria, urinary obstruction, and predispose to infection.
- **Treatment of stones** is with lithotripsy or endoscopic removal.

CHRONIC RENAL FAILURE

Chronic renal failure is the end stage of many different renal diseases. It is characterized pathologically by bilaterally shrunken kidneys. Clinically, it causes progressive irreversible azotemia, normocytic anemia, platelet dysfunction, renal osteodystrophy, and hypertension.

VASCULAR DISORDERS OF THE KIDNEY

Renal artery stenosis of any etiology causes decreased blood flow to the involved kidney, with resulting secondary hypertension that is often not responsive to antihypertensive medications. Treatment is usually surgical.

- Atheromatous plaque is the most common cause of renal artery stenosis.
- Dysplastic lesions ("fibromuscular dysplasia") are an important additional cause of renal artery stenosis.

Benign nephrosclerosis is caused by hypertension. The kidneys have a finely granular external surface and on microscopy show hyaline arteriolosclerosis, tubular atrophy, interstitial fibrosis, and glomerulosclerosis. Lab findings include mild proteinuria, hematuria, and azotemia.

Malignant (accelerated) hypertension can damage the kidney, causing fibrinoid necrosis of arterioles, glomerulitis, and hyperplastic arteriolosclerosis. Clinically, it causes cerebral edema, papilledema, retinal hemorrhage, intracerebral hemorrhage, and oliguric acute renal failure. The cortical surface shows pinpoint petechial hemorrhages ("flea-bitten" look).

Renal infarction is due to thrombi from the left side of the heart, atheroembolic disease, and vasculitis. It presents with sudden onset of flank pain and hematuria. Small infarcts may be asymptomatic.

Sickle cell anemia can cause medullary infarctions due to blockage of blood flow in the medullary vessels, which can result in asymptomatic hematuria, loss of urine concentrating ability, renal papillary necrosis, and pyelonephritis.

Diffuse cortical necrosis can cause anuria; the condition can occur with obstetric emergencies and disseminated intravascular coagulation.

TUMORS OF THE KIDNEY

Benign tumors of the kidney are as follows:

- **Cortical adenomas** are small, encapsulated cortical nodules measuring <3 cm; they are a common finding at autopsy. They may be composed of tubular or papillary structures. The papillary adenomas share the same chromosomal gains as papillary renal cell carcinoma.
- **Angiomyolipomas** are hamartomas composed of fat, smooth muscle, and blood vessels, common in patients with tuberous sclerosis.
- **Oncocytomas** are large, benign tumors that are resected to rule out renal cell carcinoma when they are found incidentally on imaging studies. They are brown on cut surface and have abundant pink cytoplasm on microscopy.
  Renal cell carcinoma (RCC) is most common, with males affected more than females.

  Risk factors include cigarette smoking, chronic analgesic use, asbestos exposure, chronic renal failure, acquired cystic disease, and von Hippel-Lindau disease (VHL tumor suppressor gene).

  In 10% of cases, the "classic" triad occurs:

- Hematuria
- Palpable mass
- Flank pain

A variety of paraneoplastic syndromes from ectopic hormone production can occur:

- Polycythemia (erythropoietin production)
- Hypertension (renin production)
- Cushing syndrome (corticosteroid synthesis)
- Hypercalcemia (PTH-like hormone)
- Feminization or masculinization (gonadotropin release)

Renal cell carcinoma may also cause secondary amyloidosis, a leukemoid reaction, or eosinophilia.

Gross examination typically demonstrates a large, solitary yellow mass found most commonly in the upper pole. Areas of necrosis and hemorrhage are commonly present. The tumor often invades the renal vein and may extend into the inferior vena cava and heart.

Wilms tumor (nephroblastoma) typically presents age 2-5 as a large abdominal mass.

- Pathologically, Wilms tumor causes a large, solitary tan mass. Microscopic examination reveals a tumor containing 3 elements: metanephric blastema, epithelial elements (immature glomeruli and tubules), and stroma.

Transitional cell carcinomas can involve the renal pelvis as well as the urinary bladder.

OBSTRUCTIVE DISORDERS OF THE URINARY SYSTEM

Hydronephrosis is a common complication of urinary tract obstruction. It is characterized by dilation of the ureter and renal pelvis. Specific causes include renal stones, retroperitoneal fibrosis, benign prostatic hyperplasia, and cervical cancer.

- In **unilateral hydronephrosis**, the kidney may enlarge to 20 cm. It may be found incidentally on physical exam. The parenchyma becomes compressed. If complete obstruction occurs suddenly, **necrosis of the renal papillae** may result.

- **Bilateral obstruction** that is complete presents as anuria; incomplete bilateral obstruction may present as polyuria.

URETERAL DISORDERS

Congenital anomalies include double ureters and congenital megaureter.

Ureteropelvic junction (UPJ) obstruction is the most common cause of hydronephrosis in infants and children. **Congenital UPJ obstruction** can also be identified in adults. It is often seen with other congenital anomalies. Treatment is surgical.

Ureteritis cystica describes chronic inflammation which causes formation of small mucosal cysts in the ureter. This condition can predispose for adenocarcinoma of the ureter.

Renal stones commonly lodge in the ureters.

Retroperitoneal fibrosis is usually an idiopathic condition causing severe fibrosis of the retroperitoneal area, which can entrap the ureters.

Transitional cell carcinoma is the most common ureteral carcinoma.

URINARY BLADDER PATHOLOGY

Congenital anomalies of the bladder. Exstrophy of the bladder is a developmental failure of the formation of the abdominal wall and bladder which leaves the bladder open at the body surface. Urachal cyst remnants may permit drainage of urine from a newborn's umbilicus, and may also be a cause of bladder adenocarcinoma.

Cystitis. The etiology of cystitis varies, with important causes including organisms, notably from fecal flora (*Escherichia coli, Proteus, Klebsiella, Enterobacter*); radiation cystitis (may follow radiation therapy); and chemotherapy agents such as cyclophosphamide (hemorrhagic cystitis).

Clinically, it affects females far more than males. Symptoms include frequency, urgency, dysuria, and suprapubic pain; systemic signs such as fever and malaise are uncommon. Predisposing factors include benign prostatic hypertrophy, bladder calculi, and cystocele.

Malakoplakia is a bladder inflammatory pattern associated with a defect in macrophage function. The cause is unknown.

Urinary bladder tumors are most commonly due to transitional cell carcinoma. There is an increasing incidence of urinary bladder tumors; males are affected more than females, and peak incidence is age 40-60. Risk factors include:

- Cigarette smoking and occupational exposure to azo dye production (transitional cell carcinoma) (both due to 2-naphthylamine)
- Chronic bladder infection with *Schistosoma haemotobium* (squamous cell carcinoma) (Africa including Egypt and the Middle East)

Bladder cancer usually presents with painless hematuria, but it may also cause dysuria, urgency, frequency, hydronephrosis, and pyelonephritis.

Prognosis of bladder cancer depends on the tumor grade and stage. There is a high incidence of recurrence.

Precursors of invasive transitional cell carcinoma can arise from a flat or papillary lesion.

- **Carcinoma in situ (CIS)** is a high-grade lesion with cytologic atypia in the full thickness of the epithelium. It is frequently multifocal. In 50-75% of untreated cases, it progresses to invasive cancer.
- Papillary precursors to invasive carcinoma include **papilloma ⇒ papillary urothelial neoplasia of low malignant potential ⇒ low-grade urothelial carcinoma ⇒ high-grade urothelial carcinoma.** Other bladder tumors include papillomas, adenocarcinoma, and embryonal rhabdomyosarcoma.

Miscellaneous bladder conditions

- **Acquired diverticuli** can complicate urinary tract outlet obstruction due to benign prostatic hyperplasia or other causes.
- **Cystocele** is the term used for prolapse of the bladder into the vagina. It is common in middle-aged to elderly women.
- **Cystitis cystica et glandularis** causes formation of small cysts and glands in the bladder mucosa related to chronic inflammation. It is associated with an increased risk of adenocarcinoma.

Gastrointestinal Tract Pathology 16

Learning Objectives

❏ Answer questions about esophagus, stomach, and small and large intestine pathology

❏ Solve problems concerning gastrointestinal familial syndromes and neoplasms

ESOPHAGUS

Congenital and Mechanical Disorders

Tracheoesophageal fistula may arise as a congenital connection between the esophagus and trachea that is often associated with esophageal atresia. It is often discovered soon after birth because of aspiration. In adults the condition can occur secondary to malignancy, trauma, or iatrogenic causes.

Esophageal webs are web-like protrusions of the esophageal mucosa into the lumen which typically present with dysphagia. Plummer-Vinson syndrome is a disease of middle-aged women characterized by esophageal webs, iron deficiency anemia, and increased risk of carcinoma. Schatzki rings are web-like narrowings at the gastroesophageal junction.

Achalasia is a failure of the lower esophageal sphincter (LES) to relax with swallowing. The etiology is unknown in most cases; in South America, achalasia may be caused by Chagas disease. Presentation is with progressive dysphagia. The esophagus is characteristically dilated proximal to the lower esophageal sphincter; barium swallow shows a "bird-beak" sign. Microscopically, there is a loss of ganglion cells in the myenteric plexus. Achalasia carries an increased risk for esophageal carcinoma.

Hematemesis and Esophageal Bleeding

Mallory-Weiss syndrome is esophageal bleeding due to linear lacerations at the gastroesophageal junction from severe prolonged vomiting; the most common cause is acute alcohol ingestion and/or chronic alcoholism. Esophageal rupture (Boerhaave syndrome) may result.

Esophageal varices are dilated submucosal veins in the lower third of the esophagus, usually secondary to portal hypertension. The most common cause is cirrhosis. Clinically, the presentation is asymptomatic, though there is massive hematemesis when the varices are ruptured. Complications include potentially fatal hemorrhage.

Esophagitis

Gastroesophageal reflux disease (reflux esophagitis) (GERD) is esophageal irritation and inflammation due to reflux of gastric secretions into the esophagus. Reflux typically presents with heartburn and regurgitation. Complications include bleeding, stricture, bronchospasm and asthma, and Barrett esophagus.

Barrett esophagus is a metaplasia of the squamous esophageal mucosa to a more protective columnar type (intestinal metaplasia). It occurs because of chronic exposure to gastric secretions, usually in the setting of GERD. The endoscopic appearance is of an irregular gastroesophageal junction with tongues of red granular mucosa extending up into the esophagus. Barrett has an increased risk for dysplasia and esophageal adenocarcinoma. The incidence of Barrett esophagus is increasing in the United States.

Esophageal Carcinoma

Squamous cell carcinoma (SCC) of the esophagus is the most common type of esophageal cancer in the world. It affects males more than females, and African Americans more than Caucasians; typical age is usually age >50. Risk factors include:

- Heavy smoking and alcohol use
- Achalasia
- Plummer-Vinson syndrome
- Tylosis
- Lye ingestion

In a Nutshell

Tylosis is an autosomal dominant syndrome. The phenotypic hallmarks are oral leukoplakia and hyperkeratosis of the palms and soles. Squamous cell carcinoma of the esophagus results in up to 95% of affected individuals.

The presentation of squamous cell carcinoma of the esophagus varies; it is often asymptomatic until late in the course. When symptoms do develop they may include progressive dysphagia, weight loss and anorexia, bleeding, hoarseness, and cough. Diagnosis is by endoscopy with biopsy. Treatment is surgery though the prognosis is poor.

Adenocarcinoma of the esophagus affects Caucasians more than African Americans. It arises in the distal esophagus. The progression from Barrett metaplasia to dysplasia and eventually to invasive carcinoma occurs due to the stepwise accumulation of genetic and epigenetic changes. The prognosis is poor.

In the United States, adenocarcinoma and squamous cell carcinoma of the esophagus occur with equal frequency.

STOMACH

Congenital Disorders

Pyloric stenosis is a congenital stenosis of the pylorus due to marked muscular hypertrophy of the pyloric sphincter, resulting in gastric outlet obstruction. It affects male infants more than females. It is associated with Turner and Edwards syndromes. Presentation is the onset of regurgitation and vomiting in week 2 of life; waves of peristalsis are visible on the abdomen and there is a palpable oval abdominal mass.

Congenital diaphragmatic hernia occurs when a congenital defect is present in the diaphragm, resulting in herniation of the abdominal organs into the thoracic cavity. The stomach is the most commonly herniated organ due to left-sided congenital diaphragmatic hernia. Congenital diaphragmatic hernia is often associated with intestinal malrotation. It may be complicated by significant lung hypoplasia.

Hypertrophic Gastropathy

Ménétrier disease is a rare disease of middle-aged men. It is caused by profound hyperplasia of surface mucous cells, accompanied by glandular atrophy. It is characterized by enlarged rugal folds in the body and fundus; clinically, patients experience decreased acid production, protein-losing enteropathy, and increased risk of gastric cancer.

Zollinger-Ellison syndrome. See discussion of gastrinoma in the Pancreas chapter.

Acute Inflammation and Stress Ulcers

Acute hemorrhagic gastritis causes acute inflammation, erosion, and hemorrhage of the gastric mucosa, secondary to a breakdown of the mucosal barrier and acid-induced injury. The etiology is diverse, with initiating agents including chronic aspirin or NSAID use, alcohol use, smoking, recent surgery, burns, ischemia, stress, uremia, and chemotherapy. Patients present with epigastric abdominal pain, or with gastric hemorrhage, hematemesis, and melena.

Gastric stress ulcers are multiple, small, round, superficial ulcers of the stomach and duodenum. Predisposing factors include:

- NSAID use
- Severe stress
- Sepsis
- Shock
- Severe burn or trauma
- Elevated intracranial pressure (Cushing ulcers)

ICU patients have a high incidence of gastric stress ulcer. These ulcers may be complicated by bleeding.

Chronic Gastritis

Chronic gastritis is chronic inflammation of the gastric mucosa, eventually leading to atrophy (chronic atrophic gastritis).

Fundic type chronic gastritis is an autoimmune atrophic gastritis that involves the body and the fundus. It is caused by autoantibodies directed against parietal cells and/or intrinsic factor. The result is loss of parietal cells, decreased acid secretion, increased serum gastrin (G-cell hyperplasia), and pernicious anemia (megaloblastic anemia due to lack of intrinsic factor and B12 malabsorption). Women are affected more than men.

Grossly, one sees a loss of rugal folds in the body and fundus. Microscopically, mucosal atrophy is seen with loss of glands and parietal cells, chronic lymphoplasmacytic inflammation, and intestinal metaplasia. Patients are at increased risk for gastric carcinoma.

Antral type chronic gastritis (also called *Helicobacter pylori* gastritis) is the most common form of chronic gastritis in the United States. The *H. pylori* organisms are curved, gram-negative rods which produce urease. The risk of infection increases with age. Infection is also associated with duodenal/gastric peptic ulcer, and gastric carcinoma with intestinal type histology.

Microscopically, *H. pylori* organisms are visible in the mucous layer of the surface epithelium. Other microscopic features include foci of acute inflammation, chronic inflammation with lymphoid follicles, and intestinal metaplasia.

Chronic Peptic Ulcer (Benign Ulcer)

Peptic ulcers are ulcers of the distal stomach and proximal duodenum caused by gastric secretions (hydrochloric acid and pepsin) and impaired mucosal defenses. Predisposing factors include the following:

- Chronic NSAID and aspirin use
- Steroid use
- Smoking
- *H. pylori* infection

Patients present with burning epigastric pain. Diagnosis is by endoscopy with or without biopsy. Treatment is acid suppression (H2 blocker, proton pump inhibitor, etc.) and eradication of *H. pylori*.

Complications of peptic ulcer include hemorrhage, iron deficiency anemia, penetration into adjacent organs, perforation (x-ray shows free air under the diaphragm), and pyloric obstruction.

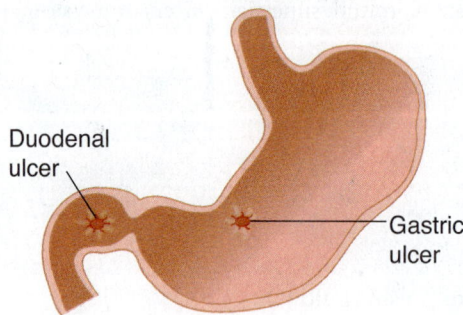

Duodenal peptic ulcers are more common than gastric peptic ulcers. Associations include the following:

- *H. pylori* (~100%)
- Increased gastric acid secretion
- Increased rate of gastric emptying
- Blood group O
- Multiple endocrine neoplasia (MEN) type I
- Zollinger-Ellison syndrome
- Cirrhosis
- Chronic obstructive pulmonary disease

Most duodenal peptic ulcers are located in the anterior wall of the proximal duodenum.

Gastric peptic ulcers are associated with *H. pylori* (75%). Most are located in the lesser curvature of the antrum. Grossly, they are small (<3 cm), sharply demarcated ('punched out'), solitary with round/oval shape, smooth borders, and radiating mucosal folds.

Gastric Carcinoma (Malignant Ulcer)

Gastric carcinoma is more common in Japan than in the United States, and has a decreasing incidence in the United States. Dietary factors can be risk factors:

- Smoked fish and meats
- Pickled vegetables
- Nitrosamines
- Benzpyrene
- Reduced intake of fruits and vegetables

Other risk factors include *H. pylori* infection, chronic atrophic gastritis, smoking, blood type A, bacterial overgrowth in the stomach, prior subtotal gastrectomy, and Ménétrier disease.

Gastric carcinoma is often (90%) asymptomatic until late in the course, when it can produce weight loss and anorexia. It can also present with epigastric abdominal pain mimicking a peptic ulcer, early satiety, and occult bleeding with iron deficiency anemia.

Most gastric carcinomas are located in the lesser curvature of the antrum. They are large (>3 cm) ulcers with heaped-up margins and a necrotic ulcer base. They may also occur as a flat or polypoid mass.

Gastric carcinoma may specifically metastasize to the left supraclavicular lymph node (Virchow sentinel node) and to the ovary (Krukenberg tumor).

Diagnosis is by endoscopy with biopsy.

GASTRIC LYMPHOMA

Marginal zone B-cell lymphoma and diffuse large B-cell lymphoma occur in the stomach.

SMALL AND LARGE INTESTINES

Mechanical Obstruction

Volvulus is a twisting of a segment of bowel on its vascular mesentery, causing intestinal obstruction and infarction. It is often associated with congenital abnormalities such as intestinal malrotation. Common locations include the sigmoid colon and small bowel; complications include infarction and peritonitis.

Intussusception is the telescoping of a proximal segment of the bowel into the distal segment. It is most common in infants and children. Children present with vomiting, abdominal pain, passage of blood per rectum, and lethargy; a sausage-shaped mass is often palpable in the right hypochondrium.

In adults, intussusception may be caused by a mass or tumor. The intussuscepted segment can become infarcted.

Incarcerated hernia is a segment of bowel that is imprisoned within a hernia; the condition can become complicated by intestinal obstruction and infarction.

Hirschsprung disease (or congenital aganglionic megacolon) is caused by congenital absence of ganglion cells in the rectum and sigmoid colon, resulting in intestinal obstruction. The condition affects males more than females, and can be associated with Down syndrome. Hirschsprung may present with delayed passage of meconium, or with constipation, abdominal distention, and vomiting.

Grossly, the affected segment is narrowed, and there is dilation proximal to the narrow segment (megacolon). Microscopically, there is an absence of ganglion cells in Auerbach and Meissner plexuses, and the diagnosis is established when rectal biopsy demonstrates the absence of ganglion cells.

Malabsorption Syndromes

Celiac sprue (or gluten-sensitive enteropathy and nontropical sprue) is caused by hypersensitivity to gluten (and gliadin), resulting in loss of small bowel villi and malabsorption. Microscopic exam demonstrates a loss of villi, with increased intraepithelial lymphocytes and increased plasma cells in the lamina propria.

Clinically, it often presents in childhood with malabsorption. Symptoms include abdominal distention, bloating, and flatulence, along with diarrhea, steatorrhea, and weight loss. Dermatitis herpetiformis may occur age >20. In adults, celiac presents between decades 4-7. Treatment is dietary restriction of gluten. There is an increased risk of gastrointestinal cancer.

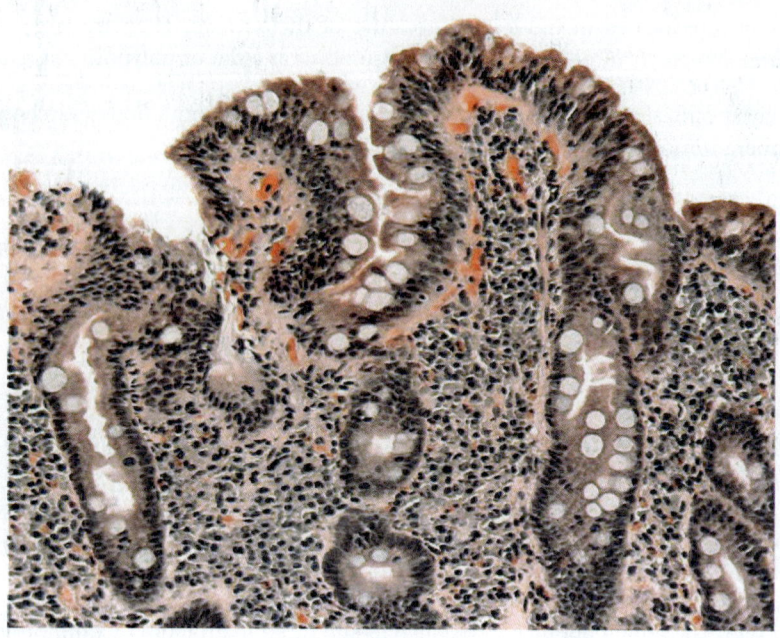

Figure 16-1. Celiac Disease

wikimedia.org.

Environmental enteropathy (previously known as **tropical sprue**) is a maladaptive disease of unknown etiology (infection and/or nutritional deficiency). If affects residents of low-income countries. Biopsy shows blunting of villi and a lymphocytic infiltrate.

Whipple disease is a rare infectious disease involving many organs, including small intestines, joints, lung, heart, liver, spleen, and central nervous system. It typically affects Caucasian males age 30-50.

The infecting organism is *Tropheryma whipplei*. Microscopically, the small bowel lamina propria is filled with macrophages stuffed with the PAS-positive, gram-positive, rod-shaped bacilli. Patients present with malabsorption, weight loss, and diarrhea. Treatment is antibiotics.

Inflammatory bowel disease (IBD). There are two categories of IBD:

- **Crohn's disease (CD)** (or regional enteritis)
- **Ulcerative colitis (UC)**

Colitis of indeterminate type describes cases that cannot be clearly classified.

Caucasians develop IBD more frequently than non-Caucasians. The incidence of IBD is increasing.

Age distribution varies with the disease:

- CD has a bimodal distribution with peaks at age 10–30 and 50–70
- UC peaks at age 20–30

Note

Damage to the ileal mucosa can cause deficiencies of vitamin B12 and folate.

IBD can present with episodes of bloody diarrhea or stools with mucus, crampy lower abdominal pain, or fever. CD may present with malabsorption or extraintestinal manifestations. It may mimic appendicitis. CD may cause perianal fistulas.

Diagnosis of IBD requires endoscopic biopsy and clinicopathologic correlation.

New studies indicate that risk of colorectal carcinoma (CRC) in CD and UC are equivalent for similar extent and duration of disease; the risk of CRC is not as high as previous studies suggested.

Table 16-1. Crohn's Disease Versus Ulcerative Colitis

	Crohn's Disease	Ulcerative Colitis
Most common site	Terminal ileum	Rectum
Distribution	Mouth to anus	Rectum → colon "back-wash" ileitis
Spread	Discontinuous/"skip"	Continuous
Gross features	• Focal aphthous ulcers with intervening normal mucosa • Linear fissures • Cobblestone appearance • Thickened bowel wall • "Creeping fat"	Extensive ulceration Pseudopolyps
Micro	Noncaseating granulomas	Crypt abscesses
Inflammation	Transmural	Limited to mucosa and submucosa
Complications	• Strictures • "String sign" on barium studies • Obstruction • Abscesses • Fistulas • Sinus tracts	Toxic megacolon
Genetic association		HLA-B27
Extraintestinal manifestations	Common (e.g., migratory polyarthritis, ankylosing spondylitis, primary sclerosing cholangitis, erythema nodosum, pyoderma gangrenosum, uveitis)	Common (e.g., migratory arthritis, ankylosing spondylitis, primary sclerosing cholangitis, erythema nodosum, pyoderma gangrenosum, uveitis)

Miscellaneous Conditions

Ischemic bowel disease is caused by decreased blood flow and ischemia of the bowel, secondary to atherosclerosis with thrombosis, thromboembolism, or reduced cardiac output from shock. It is most common in older individuals.

Typical presentation is with abdominal pain and bloody diarrhea. The disease distribution tends to involve watershed areas (e.g., splenic flexure), and affected areas typically show hemorrhagic infarction.

Hemorrhoids are tortuous, dilated anal submucosal veins caused by increased venous pressure. Risk factors include constipation and prolonged straining during bowel movements, pregnancy, and cirrhosis. Complications include painful thrombosis and streaks of bright red blood on hard stool.

Angiodysplasia is arteriovenous malformations of the intestines. It occurs in the cecum and right colon. Individuals age >55 are most commonly affected, presenting with multiple episodes of rectal bleeding.

Melanosis coli is common with laxative abuse; it causes black pigmentation of the colon due to the ingestion of the laxative pigment by macrophages in the mucosal and submucosa. It can mimic colitis or malignancy.

Pseudomembranous colitis (antibiotic-associated colitis) is an acute colitis characterized by the formation of inflammatory pseudomembranes in the intestines. It is usually caused by *Clostridium difficile* infection (often brought on by a course of broad-spectrum antibiotics, especially clindamycin and ampicillin), but it can be caused by ischemic bowel disease.

Gross examination shows yellow-tan mucosal membranes. Microscopic exam shows the pseudomembranes are composed of an adherent layer of acute inflammatory cells, mucus and necrotic debris overlying sites of colonic mucosal injury. Presentation is with diarrhea, fever, and abdominal cramps. Diagnosis is established with detection of *C. difficile* toxin in the stool. Treatment of clostriadial pseudomembranous colitis is vancomycin or metronidazole.

Appendicitis is most commonly caused by obstruction of the appendix by a fecalith. It often starts with periumbilical pain that subsequently localizes to the right lower quadrant. Nausea, vomiting, and fever may also be present. Lab studies show an elevated white blood cell count. A complication is appendiceal rupture leading to peritonitis. Grossly, a fibrinopurulent exudate may be seen on the appendiceal serosa; microscopically, neutrophils are present within the mucosa and muscular wall (muscularis propria) of the appendix.

Diverticula

Meckel diverticulum is a congenital small bowel diverticulum caused by persistance of a remnant of the vitelline (omphalomesenteric) duct (*see* Anatomy Lecture Notes).

Most Meckel diverticula are asymptomatic but they may contain rests of ectopic gastric mucosa and present with intestinal bleeding.

Colonic diverticulosis is an acquired outpouching of the bowel wall, characterized by herniation of the mucosa and submucosa through the muscularis propria (pseudodiverticulum). It is extremely common in the United States.

- Incidence increases with age
- Major risk factor is a low-fiber diet, which leads to increased intraluminal pressure
- Most common location is sigmoid colon

Many cases are asymptomatic and picked up on screening colonoscopy. When symptomatic, it can cause constipation alternating with diarrhea, left lower quadrant abdominal cramping and discomfort, occult bleeding and an iron deficiency anemia, or lower gastrointestinal tract hemorrhage. Complications include diverticulitis, fistulas, and perforation with accompanying peritonitis.

Polyps

Hamartomatous polyps include nonfamilial juvenile polyps and polyps associated with a familial (Peutz-Jeghers) syndrome. Nonsyndromic polyps do not have malignant potential.

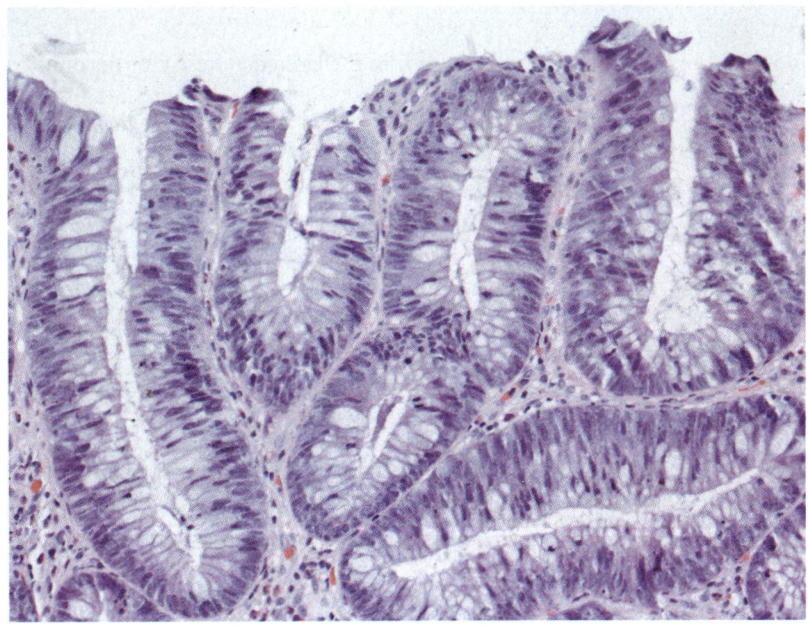

Figure 16-2. Tubular Adenoma
© Gregg Barré, M.D. Used with permission.

Hyperplastic polyps are the most common histologic type; they occur most often in the left colon and are usually <5 mm. Although previously considered not to have malignant potential, newer studies suggest they are part of a group of polyps with serrated histology and risk of progression to cancer. **Serrated polyps** occur more often in the right colon.

Tubular and villous adenomas have long been known to have malignant potential. Microscopically, they show cellular dysplasia and either pure tubular, pure villous or tubulovillous histology.

Familial Syndromes

Familial adenomatous polyposis (FAP), also called adenomatous polyposis coli (APC), is due to an autosomal dominant mutation of the *APC* gene on chromosome 5q21.

Affected individuals may develop **thousands of colonic adenomatous polyps**; the diagnosis is made with discovery of >100 adenomatous polyps on endoscopy. **Complications:** by age 40, virtually 100% will develop an invasive adenocarcinoma and increased risks for developing duodenal adenocarcinoma and adenocarcinoma of the papilla of Vater.

Gardner syndrome is an autosomal dominant variant of familial adenomatous polyposis characterized by numerous colonic adenomatous polyps, multiple osteomas, fibromatosis, and epidermal inclusion cysts.

Turcot syndrome is a rare variant of familial adenomatous polyposis characterized by numerous colonic adenomatous polyps and central nervous system tumors (gliomas).

Hereditary nonpolyposis colorectal cancer (HNPCC), or Lynch syndrome, is due to an autosomal dominant mutation of a DNA nucleotide mismatch repair gene that predisposes for colon cancer. It is associated with an increased risk of cancer at other sites, including the endometrium and the ovary.

Peutz-Jeghers syndrome is an autosomal dominant condition characterized by multiple hamartomatous polyps (primarily in the small intestine); melanin pigmentation of the oral mucosa; and increased risk of cancer at numerous sites including the lung, pancreas, breast, and uterus.

Neoplasia

Colonic adenocarcinoma is the third most common tumor in the United States, in terms of incidence and mortality. Risk factors include:

- Dietary factors (low fiber, low fruits/vegetables and high in red meat and animal fat)
- Colon polyps (isolated adenomatous polyps, hereditary polyposis syndromes)
- Other colon disease (Lynch syndrome, ulcerative colitis)

Diagnosis is established via endoscopy with biopsy.

Cancer genetics: Mutations of the *APC* gene cause activation of the Wnt pathway, leading β-catenin to translocate to the nucleus where it causes the overexpression of growth-promoting genes. DNA mismatch repair causes microsatellite instability, which is another genetic carcinogenesis pathway.

The pattern of spread in colonic adenocarcinoma includes lymphatic spread to mesenteric lymph nodes, with distant spread to liver, lungs, and bone. Staging is with the TNM system. Treatment can include surgical resection and chemotherapy (for metastatic disease); CEA levels can be used to monitor for disease recurrence.

In a Nutshell

TNM Staging of Colorectal Cancer

Stage I (T1-2N0M0): tumors that do not penetrate through mucosa (T1) or muscularis (T2)

Stage II (T3N0M0): tumors that have penetrated through the muscularis but have not spread to the lymph nodes

Stage III (TXN1M0): regional lymph node involvement

Stage IV (TXNXM1): metastasis to distant sites

Screening is recommended for the general population beginning age 50. Current guidelines suggest:

- Colonoscopy every 10 years or annual fecal occult blood test (FOBT), or
- Combination of FOBT (every 3 years) and sigmoidoscopy (every 5 years)

Carcinoid tumors are neuroendocrine tumors that often produce serotonin. Locations include the appendix (most common) and the terminal ileum. Metastasis to the liver may result in carcinoid heart disease.

Carcinoid syndrome is characterized by diarrhea, cutaneous flushing, bronchospasm and wheezing, and fibrosis. The diagnosis is substantiated by demonstrating elevated urinary 5-HIAA (5-hydroxyindoleacetic acid).

Gastrointestinal stromal tumor (GIST) is the most common sarcoma of the GI tract. Most cases have a *KIT* mutation. The peak incidence is in decade 7. Treatment is resection and a tyrosine-kinase inhibitor.

Note

Histologically, carcinoid tumors appear similar to other neuroendocrine tumors, with nests of small uniform cells.

Pancreatic Pathology 17

Learning Objectives

❏ Demonstrate understanding of congenital anomalies of the pancreas

❏ Use knowledge of inflammation of the pancreas or tumors of the pancreas to solve problems

CONGENITAL ANOMALIES OF THE PANCREAS

- **Pancreatic agenesis** is incompatible with life.
- **Pancreatic divisum** is a variant of pancreatic duct anatomy.
- **Annular pancreas** encircles the duodenum and presents as obstruction.
- **Ectopic pancreatic tissue** can hemorrhage, become inflamed, or give rise to a neuroendocrine tumor. These rests most often arise in the stomach, duodenum, or jejunum.

INFLAMMATION OF THE PANCREAS

Acute pancreatitis is acute inflammation caused by injury to the exocrine portion of the pancreas. The etiology is diverse:

- Gallstones
- Alcohol
- Hypercalcemia
- Drugs
- Shock
- Infections
- Trauma
- Scorpion stings

Pancreatic acinar cell injury results in activation of pancreatic enzymes and enzymatic destruction of the pancreatic parenchyma.

Symptoms include stabbing epigastric abdominal pain radiating to the back. Severe acute pancreatitis can also cause shock. Lab studies show elevated serum amylase and lipase. Complications include acute respiratory distress syndrome (ARDS), disseminated intravascular coagulation (DIC), pancreatic pseudocyst; pancreatic calcifications, and hypocalcemia. Severe cases have a 30% mortality rate.

- Gross pathologic examination shows focal hemorrhage and liquefication in the pancreas, accompanied by chalky, white-yellow fat necrosis of adjacent adipose tissue.
- Microscopically there is liquefactive necrosis of the pancreatic parenchyma with acute inflammation and enzymatic fat necrosis.
- Necrosis of blood vessels causes hemorrhage.

Chronic pancreatitis refers to irreversible changes in pancreatic function with accompanying chronic inflammation, atrophy, and fibrosis of the pancreas secondary to repeated bouts of pancreatitis. Manifestations include abdominal pain, pancreatic insufficiency and malabsorption, pancreatic calcifications, pseudocyst, and secondary diabetes mellitus (late complication).

It is common in middle-aged male alcoholics. Pathology shows grossly firm, white, and fibrotic pancreas. Microscopically there is extensive fibrosis with parenchymal atrophy and chronic inflammation.

Autoimmune pancreatitis can occur in association with IgG4-associated fibrosing disorders; this variant responds to steroid therapy.

PANCREATIC TUMORS

Pancreatic neuroendocrine tumors (islet cell tumors) are less common than exocrine tumors. Most are considered low grade malignancies. Some patients lack laboratory evidence of hormone overproduction. These tumors are not distinguishable from each other on the basis of gross appearance or histology.

- **Insulinoma (β-cell tumor)** (most common type of islet cell tumor)
  - Produces insulin
  - Can cause hypoglycemia, sweating, hunger, confusion, and insulin coma
  - Surgical excision is curative
- **Gastrinoma (G-cell tumor)**
  - Produces gastrin
  - Excess gastrin manifests as Zollinger-Ellison syndrome, which is characterized by thick gastric folds, elevated serum gastrin, gastric hyperacidity, and intractable peptic ulcers
  - Gastrinomas may arise outside the pancreas
  - May be associated with MEN I
- **Glucagonoma (α-cell tumor)**
  - Produces glucagon
  - Excess glucagon causes hyperglycemia (diabetes), anemia, and skin rash
- **Somatostatinoma (δ-cell tumor)**
  - Produces somatostatin
  - Excess somatostatin inhibits insulin secretion, leading to diabetes
  - Can also inhibit gastrin secretion (leading to hypochlorhydria) and cholecystokinin secretion (leading to gallstones and steatorrhea)
  - Prognosis is poor
- **VIPoma**
  - Produces vasoactive intestinal peptide (VIP)
  - Excess VIP causes WDHA syndrome: watery diarrhea, hypokalemia, and achlorhydria

Pancreatic carcinoma is the fifth most common cause of cancer death in the United States, and the incidence is rising.

- Most common ages 60-80
- Smoking is a risk factor
- Presents with only vague signs and symptoms until late in course
- When more definitive signs and symptoms develop, they can include abdominal pain, migratory thrombophlebitis, and obstructive jaundice

The tumor may occur in the head (60%), body (15%), and tail (5%). Microscopically, the adenocarcinoma arises from the duct epithelium. Tumor desmoplasia and perineural invasion are common. Tumor markers for pancreatic carcinoma include CEA and CA19-9, but they are not useful screening assays.

Treatment is surgical excision (Whipple procedure). The prognosis is very poor, with 5-year survival only ~5%.

Pancreatic cystic neoplasms: Serous neoplasms account for 25% of pancreatic cystic neoplasms; most are benign (cystadenomas) and the tumors carry a mutation of *VHL*.

Mucinous neoplasms: Mucinous cystic neoplasms are common in women and can harbor dysplasia or carcinoma.

Intraductal papillary mucinous neoplasms are common in men and tend to arise in the head of the pancreas; carcinoma may arise in the neoplasm.

Gallbladder and Biliary Tract Pathology

18

Learning Objectives

❏ Use knowledge of gallstones (cholelithiasis), inflammatory conditions of the gallbladder, and miscellaneous conditions to solve problems

❏ Explain information related to biliary tract cancer

GALLSTONES (CHOLELITHIASIS)

Gallstones are frequently asymptomatic but can cause biliary colic (right upper quadrant pain due to impacted stones). Diagnosis is by ultrasound; the majority of stones are not radiopaque. Complications include cholecystitis, choledocholithiasis (calculi within the biliary tract), biliary tract obstruction, pancreatitis, and cholangitis.

Note

Formation of cholesterol stones involves the precipitation of cholesterol from supersaturated bile.

Cholesterol stones are composed mostly of cholesterol monohydrate. The incidence increases with age. Risk factors include female gender, obesity, pregnancy, oral contraceptives, and hormone replacement therapy.

Pigmented bilirubinatestones are composed of calcium salts and unconjugated bilirubin. Risk factors are chronic hemolytic anemias, cirrhosis, bacterial infection, and parasites (*Ascaris* or *Clonorchis* [*Opisthorchis*] *sinensis*).

INFLAMMATORY CONDITIONS

Acute cholecystitis is an acute inflammation of the gallbladder, usually caused by cystic duct obstruction by gallstones. It can present with biliary colic, right upper quadrant tenderness on palpation, nausea and vomiting, low-grade fever, and leukocytosis. Complications include gangrene of the gallbladder, perforation and peritonitis, fistula formation and gallstone ileus (small bowel obstruction by a large gallstone). Acute acalculous cholecystitis is associated with surgery, trauma, and sepsis.

Chronic cholecystitis is ongoing chronic inflammation of the gallbladder, usually caused by gallstones. Well-developed examples show stromal and mural lymphocytic and plasmacytic infiltrates. Macrophages and granulomas may also be present. The wall is thickened.

Ascending cholangitis is a bacterial infection of the bile ducts ascending up to the liver, usually associated with obstruction of bile flow oftentimes from bile duct stones. It presents with biliary colic, jaundice, high fever, and chills. The infecting organisms are usually gram-negative enteric bacteria.

MISCELLANEOUS CONDITIONS

Cholesterolosis refers to an accumulation of cholesterol-laden macrophages within the mucosa of the gallbladder wall. Gross examination shows yellow speckling of the red-tan mucosa ("strawberry gallbladder"). Microscopic examination shows lipid-laden macrophages within the lamina propria.

Hydrops of the gallbladder (mucocele) occurs when chronic obstruction of the cystic duct leads to the resorption of the normal gallbladder contents and enlargement of the gallbladder by the production of large amounts of clear fluid (hydrops) or mucous secretions (mucocele).

BILIARY TRACT CANCER

Gallbladder cancer is frequently asymptomatic until late in the course. When the tumor does present, it may be with cholecystitis, enlarged palpable gallbladder, or biliary tract obstruction (uncommon). X-ray may show a calcified "porcelain gallbladder." Microscopically, the tissues show adenocarcinoma. The prognosis for gallbladder cancer is poor; 5-year survival rate is ~12%.

Bile duct cancer. Bile duct carcinoma is carcinoma of the **extrahepatic** bile ducts, while cholangiocarcinoma is carcinoma of the **intrahepatic** bile ducts. Klatskin tumor is a carcinoma of the bifurcation of the right and left hepatic bile ducts. Risk factors for bile duct cancer include *Clonorchis (Opisthorchis) sinensis* (liver fluke) in Asia and primary sclerosing cholangitis. Bile duct cancer typically presents with biliary tract obstruction. Microscopic examination shows adenocarcinoma arising from the bile duct epithelium. The prognosis is poor.

Adenocarcinoma of the ampulla of Vater may exhibit duodenal, biliary, or pancreatic epithelium. Patients present with painless jaundice. The 5-year survival rate is <50% in spite of resection.

Liver Pathology

Learning Objectives

❏ Solve problems concerning jaundice, cirrhosis, viral hepatitis, chemical hepatitis, amebic liver abscess, and alcoholic liver disease

❏ Differentiate metabolic liver disease from hemodynamic liver disease

❏ Solve problems concerning liver tumors

❏ Answer questions about dental-related hepatitis concepts

LIVER DYSFUNCTION

Dysfunction of the liver may be divided into 4 categories that may coexist:

- **Hepatic failure** occurs in the setting of hepatic necrosis secondary to acute liver failure, chronic liver disease, and hepatocyte dysfunction.
- **Portal hypertension** occurs in the setting of cirrhosis or increased portal venous blood flow.
- **Cholestasis** occurs in the setting of impaired bile flow due to hepatocyte dysfunction or biliary obstruction.
- **Cirrhosis** occurs in the setting of hepatocyte injury and is usually an irreversible nodular regeneration that is end stage.

JAUNDICE

Clinical jaundice occurs with bilirubin levels >2–3 mg/dL. The classic presentation is yellow skin (jaundice) and sclera (icterus). Causes of jaundice include overproduction of bilirubin, defective hepatic bilirubin uptake, defective conjugation, and defective excretion.

Table 19-1. Unconjugated Versus Conjugated Bilirubinemia

Unconjugated (Indirect) Bilirubinemia	Conjugated (Direct) Bilirubinemia
Increased RBC turnover (hemolytic anemias)	Biliary tract obstruction
Physiologic (newborn babies)	Biliary tract disease (PSC and PBC)
Hereditary (Gilbert and Crigler-Najjar syndromes)	Hereditary (Dubin-Johnson and Rotor syndromes)
	Liver disease (cirrhosis and hepatitis)

Increased red blood cell (RBC) turnover. RBCs are the major source of bilirubin. Jaundice related to overproduction of bilirubin can be seen in hemolytic anemia and ineffective erythropoiesis (thalassemia, megaloblastic anemia, etc.). Laboratory studies show increased unconjugated bilirubin. Chronic hemolytic anemia patients often develop pigmented bilirubinate gallstones. The most common cause of marked jaundice in the newborn is blood group incompatibility (most commonly ABO) between mother and child, causing **hemolytic disease of the newborn.**

Physiologic jaundice of the newborn is a transient unconjugated hyperbilirubinemia due to the immaturity of the liver. Risk factors include prematurity and hemolytic disease of the newborn (erythroblastosis fetalis). Physiologic jaundice of the newborn can be complicated by kernicterus; treatment is phototherapy. Jaundice also occurs in newborns who have infections.

Hereditary hyperbilirubinemias

When hyperbilirubinemia is prolonged in the newborn, a mutation affecting bilirubin conjugation enters the differential diagnosis.

- **Gilbert syndrome** is a common benign inherited disorder that causes unconjugated hyperbilirubinemia due to bilirubin UDP-glucuronosyltransferase (UGT) deficiency. Kernicterus rarely occurs.
- **Crigler-Najjar syndrome** causes unconjugated hyperbilirubinemia due to bilirubin glucuronosyltransferase (UGT) absence or deficiency.

Biliary tract obstruction may have multiple etiologies, including gallstones; tumors (pancreatic, gallbladder, and bile duct); stricture; and parasites (liver flukes—*Clonorchis [Opisthorchis] sinensis*). The presentation can include jaundice and icterus; pruritus due to increased plasma levels of bile acids; abdominal pain, fever, and chills; dark urine (bilirubinuria); and pale clay-colored stools. Lab studies show elevated conjugated bilirubin, elevated alkaline phosphatase, and elevated 5′-nucleotidase.

Primary biliary cirrhosis (PBC) is a chronic liver disease that is characterized by inflammation and granulomatous destruction of intrahepatic bile ducts. Females have 10 times the incidence of primary biliary cirrhosis compared to males; the peak incidence is age 40–50.

Presentation includes obstructive jaundice and pruritus; xanthomas, xanthelasmas, and elevated serum cholesterol; fatigue; and cirrhosis (late complication). Most patients have another autoimmune disease (scleroderma, rheumatoid arthritis or systemic lupus erythematosis).

Laboratory studies show elevated conjugated bilirubin, elevated alkaline phosphatase, and elevated 5′-nucleotidase. **Antimitochondrial autoantibodies** (AMA) are present in >90% of cases, which further supports an autoimmune basis. Microscopically, lymphocytic and granulomatous inflammation involves interlobular bile ducts.

Primary sclerosing cholangitis (PSC) is a chronic liver disease characterized by segmental inflammation and fibrosing destruction of intrahepatic and extrahepatic bile ducts. The exact etiologic mechanism is not known but growing evidence supports an immunologic basis.

The male to female ratio is 2:1; peak age 20–40. Most cases of PSC are associated with ulcerative colitis. The presentation is similar to PBC. Complications include biliary cirrhosis and cholangiocarcinoma.

Microscopically, there is periductal chronic inflammation with concentric fibrosis around bile ducts and segmental stenosis of bile ducts. Cholangiogram shows "beaded appearance" of bile ducts.

CIRRHOSIS

Cirrhosis is end-stage liver disease characterized by disruption of the liver architecture by bands of fibrosis which divide the liver into nodules of regenerating liver parenchyma.

Causes of cirrhosis include alcohol, viral hepatitis, biliary tract disease, hemochromatosis, cryptogenic/idiopathic, Wilson disease, and α-1-antitrypsin deficiency.

On gross Pathology, **micronodular** cirrhosis has nodules <3 mm, while **macronodular** cirrhosis has nodules >3 mm; mixed micronodular and macronodular cirrhosis can also occur. At the end stage, most diseases result in a mixed pattern, and the etiology may not be distinguished based on the appearance.

Cirrhosis has a multitude of **consequences**, including portal hypertension, ascites, splenomegaly/hypersplenism, esophageal varices, hemorrhoids, caput medusa, decreased detoxification, hepatic encephalopathy, spider angiomata, palmar erythema, gynecomastia, decreased synthetic function, hepatorenal syndrome and coagulopathy.

Clinical Correlate

Prothrombin time, not partial thromboplastin time, is used to assess the coagulopathy due to liver disease.

VIRAL HEPATITIS

Viral hepatitis can be asymptomatic or it can present with malaise and weakness, nausea and anorexia, jaundice, or dark urine. Lab studies show markedly elevated alanine aminotransferase (ALT) and aspartate aminotransferase (AST). Diagnosis is by serology.

Clinical Correlate

Non-hepatitis viruses which may infect the liver include:

- *Epstein-Barr virus* (EBV)–infectious mononucleosis
- *Cytomegalovirus* (CMV)
- Herpes
- Yellow fever

Acute viral hepatitis is viral hepatitis with signs and symptoms for <6 months. It can be caused by any of the hepatitis viruses.

Microscopically, the liver shows lobular disarray, hepatocyte swelling (balloon cells), apoptotic hepatocytes (Councilman bodies), lymphocytes in portal tracts and in the lobule, hepatocyte regeneration, and cholestasis.

Chronic viral hepatitis is viral hepatitis with signs and symptoms for >6 months. It can be caused by hepatitis viruses B, C, and D.

- Microscopically, **chronic persistent hepatitis** shows inflammation confined to portal tracts.
- **Chronic active hepatitis** shows inflammation spilling into the parenchyma, causing interface hepatitis (piecemeal necrosis of limiting plate).

Hepatitis B often has "ground glass" hepatocytes (due to cytoplasmic HBsAg).

Clinical Correlate

Hepatitis D requires hepatitis B to propagate

Table 19-2. The Hepatitis Viruses

Common Virus Name	Hepatitis A (HAV)	Hepatitis B (HBV)	Hepatitis C (HCV)	Hepatitis D (HDV)	Hepatitis E (HEV)
Common disease name	"Infectious"	"Serum"	"Post-transfusion" or "non-A, non-B"	"Delta"	"Enteric"
Virus	*Hepatovirus* nonenveloped capsid RNA	*Hepadnavirus* enveloped DNA	*Flavivirus* enveloped RNA	Defective enveloped circular RNA	*Hepevirus* nonenveloped capsid RNA
Transmission	Fecal-oral	Parenteral, sexual, perinatal	Parenteral, sexual	Parenteral, sexual	Fecal-oral
Severity	Mild	Occasionally severe	Usually subclinical	Co-infection with HBV occasionally severe; super-infection with HBV often severe	Normal patients: mild; pregnant patients: severe
Chronicity or carrier state	No	Yes	Yes (high)	Yes	No
Clinical diseases	Acute hepatitis	• Acute hepatitis • Chronic hepatitis • Cirrhosis • Hepatocellular carcinoma (HCC)	• Chronic hepatitis • Cirrhosis • HCC	• Acute hepatitis • Chronic hepatitis • Cirrhosis • HCC	• Acute hepatitis
Laboratory diagnosis	Symptoms and anti-HAV IgM	Symptoms and serum levels of HBsAg, HBeAg, and anti-HBc IgM	Symptoms and EIA for anti-HCV	Anti-HDV ELISA	Tests not routinely available
Prevention	Vaccine, hygiene	Vaccine		Hep B vaccine (indirectly)	Hygiene
Treatment	Supportive	Antivirals, interferons, transplant	Antivirals, interferons, transplant	See hepatitis B	Supportive

Table 19-3. Hepatitis B Terminology and Markers

Abbreviation	Name and Description
HBV	Hepatitis B virus, a hepadnavirus (enveloped, partially double-stranded DNA virus); Dane particle = infectious HBV
HBsAg	Antigen found on surface of HBV; also found on spheres and filaments in patient's blood: positive during acute disease; continued presence indicates carrier state
HBsAb	Antibody to HBsAg; provides immunity to hepatitis B
HBcAg	Antigen associated with core of HBV
HBcAb	Antibody to HBcAg; positive during window phase; IgM HBcAb is an indicator of recent disease
HBeAg	A second, different antigenic determinant on the HBV core; important indicator of transmissibility
HBeAb	Antibody to e antigen; indicates low transmissibility
Delta agent	Small RNA virus with HBsAg envelope; defective virus that replicates only in HBV-infected cells

Table 19-4. Hepatitis A Serology

Acute or recent infection	anti-HAV IgM
Prior infection or immunization	anti-HAV IgG

Table 19-5. Hepatitis B Serology

	HBsAg HBeAg* HBV-DNA	HBcAb IgM	HBcAb IgG	HBsAb IgG
Acute infection	+	+	−	−
Window period	−	+	−	−
Prior infection	−	−	+	+
Immunization	−	−	−	+
Chronic infection	+	−	+	−

*HBeAg—correlates with viral proliferation and infectivity

CHEMICAL (TOXIC) HEPATITIS

Although hepatitis is most often associated with viral disease (A, B, C, D, E), chemical non-viral hepatitis can occur. Common chemical causes can include:

Acetaminophen (Tylenol): Overdoses and/or acetaminophen taken concurrently with alcohol are often involved. Recent reactions to this condition have resulted in reductions of maximum daily recommended intake to 3,000 mg or less. Also of note is the contribution of combination over-the counter medications to raising the intake without the patient's knowledge. Many combination cold/flu medications combine acetaminophen with other ingredients.

Isoniazid (INH): Taken as a first line anti-tuberculosis drug or prophylaxis, it can result in chemical hepatitis.

Organic solvents, PCBs, and vinyl chloride can also cause toxic hepatitis.

AMEBIC LIVER ABSCESS

Amebic liver abscess is rare in the United States except in those who have traveled to/from tropical areas with poor sanitation. The causative organism is *Entamoeba histolytica*. The presentation, which may occur years after travel, includes RUQ pain, fever, and hepatic tenderness.

Detection of a space-occupying liver lesion with positive serology is diagnostic.

ALCOHOLIC LIVER DISEASE

Fatty change (steatosis) is reversible with abstinence. The gross appearance is of an enlarged, yellow, greasy liver. Microscopically, the liver initially shows centrilobular macrovesicular steatosis (reversible) that can eventually progress to fibrosis around the central vein (irreversible).

Alcoholic hepatitis is an acute illness that usually follows a heavy drinking binge. Some patients have no symptoms and others develop RUQ pain, hepatomegaly, jaundice, malaise, anorexia, or even fulminant liver failure.

Microscopically, the liver shows hepatocyte swelling (ballooning) and necrosis, Mallory bodies (cytokeratin intermediate filaments), neutrophils, fatty change, and eventual fibrosis around the central vein. The prognosis can be poor, since each episode has a 20% risk of death, and repeated episodes increase the risk of developing cirrhosis.

Alcoholic cirrhosis develops in 15% of alcoholics, and is typically a micronodular or Laennec cirrhosis.

METABOLIC LIVER DISEASE

Wilson disease (hepatolenticular degeneration) is a genetic disorder of copper metabolism resulting in the accumulation of toxic levels of copper in various organs. It affects the liver (fatty change, chronic hepatitis, and micronodular cirrhosis), cornea (Kayser-Fleischer rings [copper deposition in Descemet's membrane]), and brain (neurological and psychiatric manifestations, movement disorder).

The disease is autosomal recessive. Wilson disease presents in children or adolescents with liver disease.

Hemochromatosis is a disease of increased levels of iron, leading to tissue injury. **Hereditary (primary) hemochromatosis** is a recessive disorder of the *HFE* gene on chromosome 6p, which increases small intestine absorption of iron. **Secondary hemochromatosis** can follow transfusions for chronic anemias. Hemochromatosis affects 5 times as many males as females.

Hemochromatosis can cause micronodular cirrhosis and hepatocellular carcinoma (200 times the normal risk ratio); secondary diabetes mellitus; hyperpigmented skin ("bronzing"); congestive heart failure and cardiac arrhythmias; and hypogonadism. Diagnosis is established by demonstrating markedly elevated serum iron and ferritin or increased tissue iron levels (Prussian blue stain) on liver biopsy.

α-1-antitrypsin deficiency is an autosomal recessive disorder characterized by production of defective α-1-antitrypsin (α1-AT), which accumulates in hepatocytes and causes liver damage and low serum levels of α1-AT.

α-1-antitrypsin deficiency affects the liver (micronodular cirrhosis and an increased risk of hepatocellular carcinoma) and lungs (panacinar emphysema). Microscopically, PAS positive, eosinophilic cytoplasmic globules are found in hepatocytes.

Reye syndrome is a rare, potentially fatal disease that occurs in young children with viral illness (varicella or influenza) treated with aspirin. The disease mechanism is unknown; mitochondrial injury and dysfunction play an important role. Reye causes hepatic fatty change (microvesicular steatosis) and cerebral edema/encephalopathy. There is complete recovery in 75% of patients, but those that do not recover may experience permanent neurologic deficits. Coma and death may result. Treatment is supportive.

Nonalcoholic fatty liver disease is a disease of lipids accumulating in hepatocytes that is not associated with heavy alcohol use. It occurs equally in men and women, and is strongly associated with obesity, hyperinsulinemia, insulin resistance, and type 2 diabetes mellitus.

The pathogenesis involves lipid accumulation in hepatocytes that can progress to steatohepatitis (NASH—nonalcoholic steatohepatitis) and finally cirrhosis. Nonalcoholic fatty liver disease is a diagnosis of exclusion.

HEMODYNAMIC LIVER DISEASES

Budd-Chiari syndrome (hepatic vein thrombosis) refers to occlusion of the hepatic vein by a thrombus, often resulting in death. While a few cases are idiopathic, more often there is an underlying process predisposing for the thrombosis e.g., polycythemia vera, pregnancy, oral contraceptives, paroxysmal nocturnal hemoglobinuria, or hepatocellular carcinoma. It presents with abdominal pain, hepatomegaly, ascites, jaundice, splenomegaly, and in some cases, death.

The initial diagnostic test is ultrasonography. Microscopically, the liver shows centrilobular congestion and necrosis. In the chronic form, fibrosis develops.

Chronic passive congestion of the liver refers to a "backup of blood" into the liver, usually due to right-sided heart failure. Grossly, the liver characteristically has a nutmeg pattern of alternating dark (congested central areas) and light (portal tract areas) liver parenchyma. Microscopically, the liver shows centrilobular congestion.

Complications include centrilobular necrosis, which is an ischemic necrosis of centrilobular hepatocytes. Long-standing congestion can lead to centrilobular fibrosis, which can eventually become cardiac cirrhosis (sclerosis).

LIVER TUMORS

Hemangioma is the most common primary tumor of the liver, mostly affecting women. It is a benign vascular tumor that typically forms a subcapsular, red, spongy mass. It is often asymptomatic and detected incidentally on CT or MRI.

Hepatocellular adenoma (HCA) affects young women and is related to oral contraceptive use. Half of cases are asymptomatic. Symptoms include abdominal pain or spontaneous intraperitoneal hemorrhage.

Focal nodular hyperplasia is subcapsular lesion often discovered incidentally by the radiologist. Laboratory values are generally normal. It is a nodular proliferation in response to a vascular anomaly. There is a central, stellate scar.

Hepatocellular carcinoma (HCC) is the most common primary malignant tumor of the liver in adults. The incidence is higher in Asia and Japan than in the United States. Risk factors include cirrhosis, hepatitis B and C viruses, alcohol, aflatoxin B1.

HCC has a tendency for hematogenous spread and invasion of portal and hepatic veins. The tumor marker is α-fetoprotein (AFP).

Angiosarcoma is a rare, fatal tumor associated with exposure to vinyl chloride.

Hepatoblastoma is the most common hepatic malignancy in infants and children. Histology shows immature precursor cells.

Metastatic tumors are the most common tumors found within the liver. Common primary sites include the colon, breast, and lung. Metastatic tumors tend to occur as multiple well-circumscribed masses.

Central Nervous System Pathology

Learning Objectives

❑ Solve problems concerning infections across the blood brain barrier

❑ Answer questions about cerebrovascular disease, CNS trauma, and brain herniation

❑ Explain information related to demyelinating disorders

❑ Solve problems concerning degenerative and dementing disorders

❑ Describe CNS tumors

INFECTIONS

Meningitis is inflammation of the 2 inner meningeal layers, the pia and the arachnoid.

Acute aseptic (viral) meningitis is caused by leptomeningeal inflammation due to viruses (enterovirus most frequent); the inflammation produces a lymphocytic infiltration of leptomeninges and superficial cortex. Patients present with fever, signs of meningeal irritation, and depressed consciousness. Mortality is low. Viral meningitis carries a better prognosis than bacterial meningitis.

Acute viral meningitis is the most common neurologic symptom associated with primary HIV infection; it presents around the time of seroconversion with an acute confusional state. Symptoms resolve after one month with supportive care.

Acute purulent (bacterial) meningitis is a purulent leptomeningeal inflammation.

- *Streptococcus pneumoniae* is the most common cause of meningitis in infants, young children, and adults.
- Neonates are infected most frequently with group B streptococci but *Eschericia coli* causes a greater number of fatalities.
- *Neisseria meningitidis* is seen in teens and young adults and is often associated with a maculopapular rash.
- The incidence of *Listeria monocytogenes* increases after age 50. This pathogen also tends to infect people with poor cell-mediated immunity.

The leptomeninges are opaque on gross examination. Microscopic examination shows neutrophilic infiltration of the leptomeninges, extending variably to cortex. Diffuse cerebral edema carries a risk of fatal herniations. The classic triad of bacterial meningitis is fever, nuchal rigidity, and altered mental status.

Mycobacterial meningoencephalitis can be caused by *Mycobacterium tuberculosis* or atypical mycobacteria. It occurs in patients who have reactivation of latent infection and immunocompromised patients such as AIDS patients (*Mycobacterium avium-intracellulare*). Diagnosis requires microscopy/culture of large volumes of CSF. MRI is the imaging test of choice and shows basal meningeal enhancement and hydrocephalus. It usually involves the basal surface of the brain, and may cause characteristic tuberculomas within the brain and dura mater.

The **viral encephalitides** have common features of perivascular cuffs, microglial nodules, neuron loss, and neuronophagia. Clinical manifestations are variable, and can include mental status change, fever, and headache, often progressing to coma.

- Arthropod-borne forms can be due to St. Louis, Eastern and Western equine, and Venezuelan encephalitides.
- Herpes simplex type 1 produces a characteristic **hemorrhagic necrosis of temporal lobes**. Cowdry type A bodies are intranuclear inclusions seen in neurons and glial cells.
- **Rabies** has characteristic Negri bodies in the cytoplasm of hippocampal and Purkinje cells.
- **HIV encephalopathy** shows histopathology of microglial nodules and diagnostic multinucleated giant cells. Spinal involvement leads to vacuolar myelopathy, which is similar to vitamin B12 deficiency–associated subacute combined degeneration.
- **Progressive multifocal leukoencephalopathy (PML)** is caused by JC polyomavirus. It occurs in immuno-compromised patients and patients taking immunomodulatory therapies. Neurologic symptoms are varied and include impairment of cognition and motor function. Tissue sections show areas of demyelination and enlarged oligodendrocytes.

Fungal meningoencephalitides. *Candida*, *Aspergillus*, *Cryptococcus*, and *Mucor* species are the most frequent agents. *Aspergillus* and *Mucor* have a marked tropism for blood vessels, which leads to vasculitis, rupture of blood vessels, and hemorrhage. *Cryptococcus* causes diffuse meningoencephalitis, which leads to invasion of the brain through the Virchow-Robin space (a continuation of the subarachnoid space around blood vessels entering the neuropil) and soap bubble lesions.

Toxoplasmosis is caused by the protozoan parasite *Toxoplasma gondii*. It is common in AIDS patients, and the condition causes cerebral abscess with central necrosis and chronic inflammation. MRI/CT scan shows a characteristic ring-enhancing lesion.

Cerebral abscess can occur as a result of either hematogenous dissemination or direct spread from contiguous foci. **Systemic predisposing conditions** include acute bacterial endocarditis, cyanotic heart disease (right-to-left shunt), and chronic pulmonary abscesses. **Local predisposing conditions** include mastoiditis, paranasal sinusitis, acute otitis, open fracture, and previous neurosurgery. CT/MRI scan characteristically shows a ring-enhancing lesion. Clinical manifestations include signs of increased intracranial pressure (headache, vomiting, and papilledema). Focal neurological deficits vary depending on the site of lesion.

Subacute sclerosing panencephalitis is a rare complication of measles (rubeola) virus infection. Persistent immune-resistant measles virus infection causes slow-virus encephalitis. The typical scenario is a child who had measles age <2 and then 6-15 years later develops progressive mental deterioration with seizures.

Creutzfeldt-Jakob disease (CJD) is the most common human transmissible spongiform encephalopathy due to a prion (a protein with the capacity to be an infectious agent) that can change the conformation of normal prion protein(s). This can lead to rapidly progressive dementia, memory loss, personality changes, and hallucinations.

- The **prion protein** (PrP) is a 30-kD protein normally present in neurons. Its normal conformation is an α-helix: **PrP^c**. In disease states, PrP^c changes to a β-pleated sheet conformation: **PrP^{sc}**.
- PrP^{sc} is responsible for **cerebral pathologic changes**, characteristically resulting in spongiform change. This change is a fine vacuolization of the neuropil in the gray matter (especially cortex), which is due to large membrane-bound vacuoles within neuronal processes. There is an associated neuronal loss and astrogliosis. Kuru plaques are deposits of amyloid composed of altered PrP protein.
- About 85% of Creutzfeld-Jakob cases are sporadic, and 15% are familial. Affected patients are typically middle-aged to elderly patients who develop rapidly progressive dementia and memory loss with startle myoclonus or other involuntary movements.
- Variant Creutzfeldt-Jacob disease occurs in younger patients and results from exposure to bovine spongiform encephalopathy.

Table 20-1. Prion Diseases

Disease	Infectious Agent	Host	Comments
Kuru	Prion	Human	Subacute spongiform encephalopathy (SSE); Fore Tribe in New Guinea; consuming infected brains
Creutzfeldt-Jakob	Prion	Human	SSE Genetic predisposition
Gerstmann-Straussler	Prion	Human	SSE
Fatal familial insomnia	Prion	Human	SSE
Scrapie	Prion	Sheep	SSE—scraping their wool off on fences

HIV-associated neurocognitive disorder (HAND) presents as cognitive decline with behavioral changes and motor symptoms. Diagnosis is based on clinical features and the exclusion of other etiologies.

CEREBROVASCULAR DISEASE

Cerebrovascular disease is the third most frequent cause of death in industrialized countries, and it is the leading cause of serious disability in the United States. Risk factors are similar to coronary artery disease.

- **Global cerebral ischemia** (diffuse ischemic encephalopathy) is caused by a fall in blood flow to the brain, due to processes such as shock, cardiac arrest, and hypotensive episodes. While the entire brain can be damaged, some regions have selective vulnerability, including Purkinje neurons, hippocampus, CA1 (Sommer sector), and pyramidal neurons of cortex.

- **Transient ischemic attack** (TIA) is due to small platelet thrombi or atheroemboli and is characteristically reversible, with symptoms lasting less than 24 hours.

- **Stroke** can be due to infarction or hemorrhage.

- Infarction causes 85% of all stroke cases.

  ○ Can be due to **thrombotic occlusion** in the setting of atherosclerosis of the cerebral arteries; the thrombotic infarction is characteristically an anemic (white) infarct.

  ○ Can be due to **embolic occlusion**, most often due to thromboemboli from cardiac chambers and less frequently due to atheroemboli. Embolic infarction produces a hemorrhagic infarct. Small-vessel disease is a cause of small, lacunar infarcts or lacunae, and it is related to hypertension, resulting in hyaline arteriolosclerosis.

  ○ Atherosclerotic aneuryms are fusiform, involve the basilar artery, and present with infarction.

  ○ Clinical manifestations depend on the affected arterial distribution.
  Hemorrhage causes 15% of strokes.

- **Intracerebral (intraparenchymal) hemorrhage** causes severe headache, frequent nausea/vomiting, steady progression of symptoms over 15–20 minutes, and coma. It is most frequently due to hypertension, and in those instances, it most commonly involves the basal ganglia, cerebellum, pons, and centrum semiovale. Other causes include vascular malformations (especially arteriovenous malformations), cerebral amyloid angiopathy, neoplasms, vasculitides, abnormal hemostasis, hematological malignancies, infections, and diabetes mellitus.

- **Subarachnoid hemorrhage** is most frequently caused by ruptured berry aneurysm. Less frequent causes include extension of an intracerebral or subdural hematoma, vascular malformations, trauma, abnormal hemostasis, and tumors. Subarachnoid hemorrhage causes sudden headache ("worst headache of my life"), nuchal rigidity, neurological deficits on one side, and stupor.

  o **Berry aneurysms** are thin-walled saccular outpouchings, consisting of intima and adventitia only. They are the most frequent cause of subarachnoid hemorrhage. The most frequent sites are the anterior circle of Willis at branching points. Rupture is precipitated by a sudden increase in blood pressure; the prognosis after rupture is that one-third die, one-third recover, and one-third rebleed. The pathogenesis involves a congenital focal weakness of vessel media that is not identifiable at birth. Associated disorders include Marfan syndrome, Ehlers-Danlos type 4, and adult polycystic kidney disease. Hypertension and cigarette smoking predispose to formation.

CNS TRAUMA AND HERNIATIONS

Cranial Cavity and Brain

Concussion is mild traumatic brain injury with a transient loss of brain function. The trauma is commonly due to a change in the momentum of the head (impact against a rigid surface). Concussion causes loss of consciousness and reflexes, temporary respiratory arrest, and amnesia for the event. The pathogenesis is uncertain. Parenchymal injuries may or may not be evident at autopsy.

Contusions are bruises of the brain tissue. Common sites of injury include crests of orbital gyri in frontal and temporal poles, in addition to *coup* (site of injury) and *contrecoup* (site diametrically opposite) injuries. Coup and contrecoup develop when the head is mobile at the time of impact.

- **Acute contusion** is characterized by hemorrhage of brain tissue in a wedge-shaped area.
- **Subacute contusion** shows necrosis and liquefaction of brain.
- **Remote contusion** causes a depressed area of cortex with yellow discoloration ("*plaque jaune*").

Epidural hematoma (See Anatomy Lecture Notes.)

Subdural hematoma is caused by the rupture of bridging veins (from the cerebral convexities to the sagittal sinus); it is usually traumatic in older individuals. Predisposing conditions include brain atrophy (due simply to aging) and abnormal hemostatis. Symptoms include headache, drowsiness, focal neurological deficits, and sometimes dementia. It recurs frequently.

Diffuse axonal injury refers to damage to axons at nodes of Ranvier with impairment of axoplasmic flow. It causes coma after trauma without evidence of direct parenchymal injuries. There is a poor prognosis, related to duration of coma. The injury to the white matter is due to acceleration/deceleration forces with shearing of axons.

The histopathology shows axonal swellings appreciable in the white matter. It is diffuse, but with a predilection for the corpus callosum, periventricular white matter, and hippocampus, as well as cerebral and cerebellar peduncles.

Spinal cord injuries are usually traumatic, due to vertebral displacement. Symptomatology depends on the interruption of ascending and descending tracts.

- Lesions to thoracic segments or below cause paraplegia.
- Lesions to cervical segments cause tetraplegia.
- Lesions above C4 cause respiratory arrest due to paralysis of the diaphragm.

Chronic traumatic encephalopathy is a neurodegenerative disorder that occurs years or decades after a sports career with repetitive brain trauma. Neuropathological changes include neurofibrillary tangles, cerebellar atrophy and gliosis, hypopigmentation of the substantia nigra, and cavum septum pellucidum.

Cerebral Herniations

Subfalcine (cingulate gyrus) herniation occurs when the cingulate gyrus is displaced underneath the falx to the opposite side. Compression of the anterior cerebral artery can occur.

Transtentorial (uncal) herniation occurs when the uncus of the temporal lobe is displaced over the free edge of the tentorium. Clinical features include compression of the third nerve, ipsilateral pupillary dilatation, and infarction of the tissue supplied by the posterior cerebral artery. Advanced stages of transtentorial herniation can cause Duret hemorrhages within the central pons and midbrain.

Cerebellar tonsillar herniation occurs when there is displacement of cerebellar tonsils through the foramen magnum. Compression of the medulla may lead to cardiorespiratory arrest.

DEVELOPMENTAL ABNORMALITIES AND PERINATAL BRAIN INJURY

Neural tube defects are the most common developmental central nervous system abnormalities. They result from defective closure of the neural tube, and they tend to occur at the two extremities of the neuraxis. Folate deficiency is involved in the pathogenesis.

- **Anencephaly** is the absence of cranial vault. It is incompatible with life; babies die soon after birth.
- **Neural tube defects of the spinal cord** may take a variety of forms. Significant defects lead to paraplegia and urinary incontinence from birth.
  - ○ **Spina bifida occulta** is a bony defect of the vertebral arch.
  - ○ **Meningocele** is a bony defect with outpouching of meninges.
  - ○ **Meningomyelocele** is a defective formation of the bony arch with cystic outpouching of meninges, spinal cord, and spinal roots.
  - ○ **Myelocele** is a defective bony arch with complete exposure of the spinal cord.

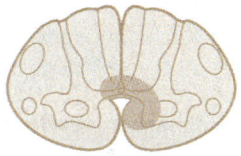

Syringomyelia

Syringomyelia is an ependymal-lined, CSF-filled channel parallel to and connected with the central canal in the spinal cord. (*Hydromyelia* means the central canal is dilated with CSF.) About 90% of cases are associated with Arnold-Chiari type 2; the remaining 10% are posttraumatic or associated with intraspinal tumors. *Syrinx* (the cyst) enlarges progressively and destroys the spinal parenchyma. Symptoms include paralysis and loss of sensory functions. (*See* Anatomy Lecture Notes.)

Perinatal brain injury is injury to the brain during prenatal or immediately postnatal period. This is the most common cause of cerebral palsy, and it occurs most frequently in premature babies.

Fetal alcohol syndrome is characterized by structural abnormalities (microcephaly, agenesis of the corpus callosum, cerebellar hypoplasia), functional impairments including learning disabilities, and neurological impairments including epilepsy.

Cerebellar Malformations

Cerebellar malformations have chromosomal, single-gene and complex inheritance.

- **Dandy-Walker malformation** is a non-communicating hydrocephalus with dilation of the fourth ventricle and hypoplasia of the cerebellar vermis.
- **Arnold-Chiari malformations**

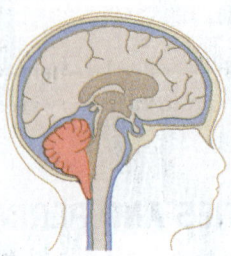

Arnold-Chiari Malformation

- ○ **Type 1** (common) is a downward displacement of cerebellar tonsils and the medulla through the foramen magnum. This lesion is mostly asymptomatic.
- ○ **Type 2** is due to a faulty craniospinal junction, resulting in a small posterior fossa, with abnormal development of the cerebellar vermis and medulla leading to downward displacement. It is mostly symptomatic because of compression of the fourth ventricle with obstructive hydrocephalus.
- ○ Other frequently related manifestations include syringomelia and lumbar meningomyelocele.

DEMYELINATING DISORDERS

Multiple sclerosis (MS) is a chronic relapsing-remitting disorder of probable autoimmune origin characterized by recurrent episodes of demyelination in the brain (including optic nerves) and spinal cord; it results in progressive neurological deficits.

- The overall prevalence of MS is 1/1,000, with higher prevalence in northern countries.
- Women have 2x the risk of men.

Genetic and environmental factors contribute to the pathogenesis. Environmental factors include viral infection, vitamin D deficiency, and smoking.

- **Acute lesions** on gross examination show well-circumscribed gray lesions (plaques), with bilateral distribution that is frequently periventricular. Histology shows chronic inflammation with phagocytosis of myelin by macrophages; axons are initially preserved.
- **Chronic lesions** have no inflammation, with axons showing remyelination. Remyelination is defective because myelin sheaths are thinner with shorter internodes.

During an acute attack, nerve conduction is entirely blocked, leading to acute neurological deficits. Chronic plaques are associated with slower nerve conduction, allowing for partial recovery. Recurrent attacks cause progressive neurological deterioration.

Clinical onset is typically in decades 3–4. About 85% of cases show a relapsing-remitting course; a minority of cases show primary progressive (slow deterioration) or progressive-relapsing (slow progression punctuated by acute exacerbations) course. Recovery from each episode of demyelination occurs in weeks or months.

Early symptoms include sensory problems, paresis, and visual dysfunction. As the disease progresses, other symptoms include fatigue, bladder dysfunction, spasticity and ataxia. Neuropsychological symptoms affect 40–60% of patients.

Diagnosis of MS requires the demonstration of the dissemination of disease in space and time. Clinical history, MRI, CSF studies and electrophysiological studies are important.

Central pontine myelinolysis (CPM) is a focal demyelination of the central area of the basis pontis. It probably derives from rapid correction of hyponatremia, and the condition is very often fatal. Patients at risk include the severely malnourished and alcoholics with liver disease.

DEGENERATIVE AND DEMENTING DISORDERS

Parkinson disease (PD) is a progressive neurodegenerative disease that involves genetic and environmental factors. The *SNCA* gene (alpha-synuclein) has been identified as a risk factor, and gene mutations and multiplications are associated with familial PD, but the majority of cases are sporadic. PD is due to loss of dopaminergic neurons in the substantia nigra, leading to tremor, rigidity, and akinesia.

- **Parkinson disease** is the idiopathic form.
- **Parkinson syndrome** is secondary to known injuries to the substantia nigra (e.g., infection, vascular condition, toxic insult).

  Parkinson disease is common, affecting 2% of the population. Clinical onset is typically in decades 5–8. Loss of dopaminergic neurons is still unexplained, though theories emphasize oxidative stress. Pesticides and meperidine have been associated with increased risk, while smoking and caffeine are protective.

On gross examination there is pallor of the substantia nigra. Histology shows loss of pigmented (dopaminergic) neurons in the substantia nigra. Residual neurons show Lewy bodies, which are intracytoplasmic round eosinophilic inclusions that contain α-synuclein. Electron microscopy shows filaments most likely of cytoskeletal origin. There is also a secondary degeneration of dopaminergic axons in the striatum.

Loss of the extrapyramidal nigrostriatal pathway leads to inhibition of movement of proximal muscles and disruption of fine regulation of distal muscles. Involvement of the amygdala, cingulate gyrus and higher cortical regions causes dementia and psychosis.

About 60% of patients experience dementia 12 years after diagnosis; 50% also experience depression and psychosis.

A clinical diagnosis is difficult to make early in disease because symptoms overlap with other conditions. Early symptoms include hyposmia, constipation, and fatigue. Key features are bradykinesia, rigidity, tremor and postural instability. Early in the disease course, a response to levodopa can help confirm the diagnosis.

Huntington disease (HD) is an autosomal dominant disorder. It is characterized pathologically by the degeneration of GABAergic neurons of the caudate nucleus, and clinically by involuntary movements, cognitive decline, and behavioral changes.

The pathophysiology is that loss of caudate nucleus GABAergic neurons removes inhibitory influences on extrapyramidal circuits, thus leading to chorea.

Clinical onset is typically in decades 3–5. The chorea is characterized by sudden, unexpected, and purposeless contractions of proximal muscles while awake. Psychiatric symptoms may predate motor symptoms. Disease progression leads to dependency and death.

Gross examination shows atrophy of the caudate nucleus with secondary ventricular dilatation. Histology shows loss of small neurons in the caudate nucleus followed by loss of the larger neurons.

A definitive diagnosis can be based on clinical symptoms with an affected parent. Otherwise, DNA determination is the gold standard.

Alzheimer disease (AD) causes 60% of all cases of dementia. It is the most common cause of dementia in people age >65.

- Incidence is 2% at age 65 and doubles every 5 years
- Risk factors include aging and significant head trauma
  - Aluminum is an epiphenomenon, not a risk factor
- Protective factors include high level of education and smoking

About 5–10% of AD cases are hereditary, early onset, and transmitted as an autosomal dominant trait.

AD is characterized by amyloid-β deposition, neurofibrillary tangle formation, and neuronal degeneration.

- **Abnormal proteins.** Aβ amyloid is a 42-residue peptide derived from a normal transmembrane protein, the amyloid precursor protein (APP). There is also an abnormal tau (a microtubule-associated protein).
- **Neuritic plaques** have a core of Aβ amyloid and are surrounded by abnormal neurites.
- **Neurofibrillary tangles** are intraneuronal aggregates of insoluble cytoskeletal elements, mainly composed of abnormally phosphorylated tau forming paired helical filaments.
- **Cerebral amyloid angiopathy** is accumulation of Aβ amyloid within the media of small and medium-size intracortical and leptomeningeal arteries; it may occur by itself and cause intracerebral hemorrhage.

  Affected areas are involved in learning and memory. Lesions involve the neocortex, hippocampus, and several subcortical nuclei including forebrain cholinergic nuclei (i.e., basal nucleus of Meynert). The earliest and most severely affected are the hippocampus and temporal lobe. Small numbers of neuritic plaques and neurofibrillary tangles also form in intellectually normal aging persons.

Macroscopic changes include atrophy of affected regions, producing brains that are smaller (atrophic), with thinner gyri and wider sulci. Hippocampi and temporal lobes are markedly atrophic.

Clinical manifestations have insidious onset, typically beginning in decades 7–8. They include progressive memory impairment, especially related to recent events; alterations in mood and behavior; progressive disorientation; and aphasia (loss of language skills) and apraxia (loss of learned motor skills). Within 5–10 years patients become mute and bedridden.

Lewy body dementia is a progressive brain disease associated with the formation of Lewy bodies in neurons involving neocortex and subcortical nuclei. The etiopathogenesis is obscure, with no known risk factors; it is the second leading cause of degenerative dementia in the elderly.

The histopathological hallmark is the Lewy body. Neuron loss accompanies Lewy body formation. Sites involved include the neocortex (especially the limbic system and cingulate gyrus), and subcortical nuclei, including basal nucleus of Meynert, amygdala, and substantia nigra.

The involvement of the neocortex and substantia nigra is responsible for cognitive deterioration and parkinsonism. Clinical manifestations include memory loss, parkinsonism, and visual hallucinations.

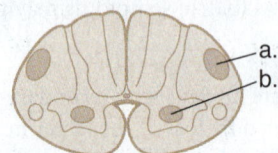

ALS
a. Primary lateral sclerosis
   (corticospinal tract)
b. Progressive spinal muscular
   atrophy (ventral horn)

Amyotrophic lateral sclerosis (ALS) is the most common adult-onset, progressive motor neuron disease.

The clinical diagnosis is supported by a biopsy of muscles. The etiopathogenesis is obscure; 5–10% of cases are hereditary, and a small number are caused by mutation of the gene encoding zinc-copper superoxide dismutase on chromosome 21.

- **Loss of upper motor neurons** produces hyperreflexia and spasticity. In some cases, involvement of cranial nerve nuclei also occurs.
- **Loss of lower motor neurons** produces weakness, atrophy, and fasciculations.

There is no cure for ALS. Ultimately, involvement of respiratory muscles will lead to death.

Friedreich ataxia is an autosomal recessive disorder which leads to degeneration of nerve tissue in the spinal cord, especially those sensory neurons connected to the cerebellum affecting muscle movement of the arms and legs. Onset is early childhood.

Mitochondrial iron builds up, leading to free radical damage and mitochondrial dysfunction.

Clinical manifestations include gait ataxia, dysarthria, hand clumsiness, loss of sense of position, impaired vibratory sensation, and loss of tendon reflexes. There is an increased incidence of heart disorders and diabetes. Patients become wheelchair-bound by age 5.

Wilson disease (*See* Liver Pathology chapter.)

Acute intermittent porphyria is an autosomal dominant defect in porphyrin metabolism with deficient uroporphyrinogen synthase. Both porphobilinogen and aminolevulinic acid are increased. Urine is initially colorless but on exposure to light turns dark red. Patients may develop recurrent severe abdominal pain, psychosis, neuropathy, and dementia.

Vitamin B12 deficiency causes megaloblastic anemia, demyelination of the spinal cord posterior columns and lateral corticospinal tracts (subacute combined degeneration of the spinal tract). It also causes dementia and peripheral neuropathy.

Alcohol abuse causes generalized cortical and cerebellar atrophy, as well as Wernicke-Korsakoff syndrome. The neurologic disease is usually related to thiamine deficiency. There can be hemorrhages in the mamillary bodies and the walls of the third and fourth ventricles. Neuronal loss and gliosis may be prominent.

- **Wernicke encephalopathy** has reversible confusion, ataxia, and nystagmus.
- **Korsakoff psychosis** is more severe and has irreversible anterograde and retrograde amnesia.
- **Central pontine myelinolysis** may cause death.

CNS TUMORS

CNS tumors account for 20% of all pediatric tumors. Most pediatric tumors mainly arise in the posterior fossa, while adult tumors arise in the supratentorial region. Factors determining prognosis and response to therapy include the following:

- Age
- Tumor location
- Grade
- Extent of surgical resection
- Molecular subgroupings

The World Health Organization (WHO) grading system assigns grades I–IV, with grade IV tumors the most aggressive.

Tumors of Neuroepithelial Tissue

Tumors of neuroepithelial tissue are categorized as **astrocytic** tumors, **oligodendroglial** tumors, **ependymal** tumors, and **embryonal** tumors (further broken down as **medulloblastoma** or **CNS primitive neuroectodermal tumor**).

Astrocytoma originates from astrocytes and exhibits fibrillary background, immunoreactivity for glial fibrillary acidic protein (GFAP), and diffuse (ill-demarcated) pattern of growth.

- **Glioblastoma** is the most common CNS primary malignancy in adults.
  - Histology shows necrosis and/or vascular proliferation in addition to features seen in anaplastic astrocytoma.

The prognosis of astrocytomas varies.

- Well-differentiated astrocytomas grow slowly; affect younger patients.
- Anaplastic astrocytomas and glioblastoma are aggressive; affect older patients; median survival for glioblastoma is 15 months.

Oligodendroglioma occurs more often in adults than in children. Its cortical location may cause seizures. Histologically, perinuclear halos are a fixation artifact that is not seen on frozen section. This tumor is slow-growing.

Ependymoma is typically located in the fourth ventricle in children, where it presents with obstructive hydrocephalus. In adults the spinal cord is the most common site. Pseudorosettes are a helpful diagnostic feature on microscopic study.

Embryonal (primitive) tumors are a group of small round cell tumors that occur predominantly in children. In the cerebellum, they are called medulloblastoma. Medulloblastoma is the most common malignant brain tumor in children.

Tumors of Cranial and Paraspinal Nerves

Schwannoma originates from Schwann cells of cranial or spinal nerves. The most frequent location is on CN 8 at the cerebellopontine angle (CPA). Schwannoma manifests characteristically with unilateral loss of hearing and tinnitus.

Tumors of the Meninges

Meningioma is a tumor that originates from meningothelial cells of the arachnoid. It is common in adults (women > men) and rare in children. It is a dura-based mass that can recur if the brain has been invaded, but invasion is unusual. It has varied clinical features but commonly presents with headache, seizures, and neurological deficits. Histology shows cellular whorls and psammoma bodies. Many patterns are seen; the syncytial pattern is common.

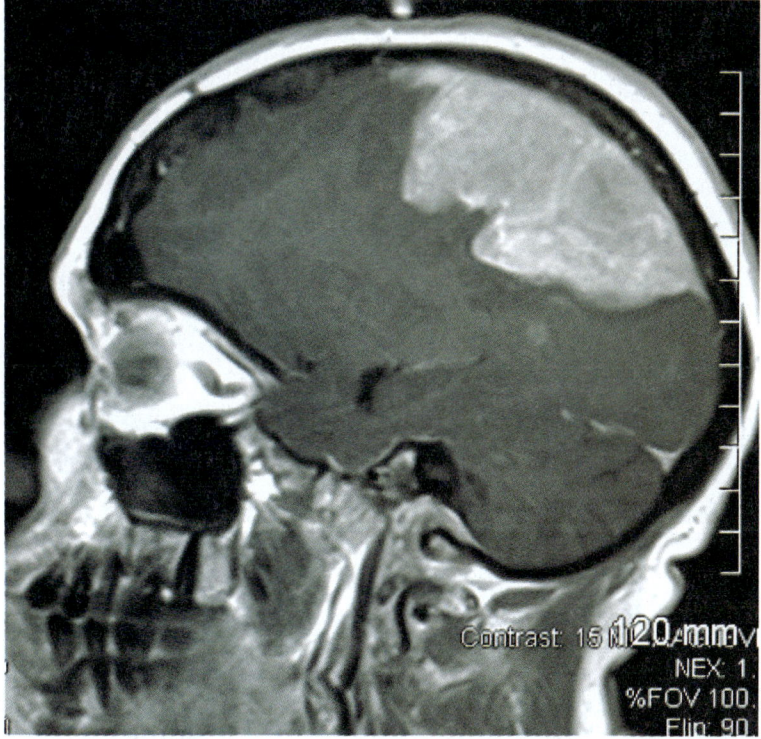

Figure 20-1. Large Meningioma Pushing into the Cerebral Cortex.
Note the thin dark shadow around the lesion which occurs because the
tumor is not actually invading the brain.

© Steven J. Golstein, University of Kentucky. Used with permission.

Tumors of the Sellar Region

Craniopharyngioma arises from rests of odontogenic epithelium within the suprasellar/diencephalic region. It most commonly affects children and young adults. The most common presenting symptoms are headache, hypopituitarism, and visual field disturbances.

- Contains deposits of calcium, evident on x-ray
- Histology shows squamous cells and resembles **ameloblastoma,** a tumor of ameloblasts.
- Is benign but tends to recur after resection

Other Neoplasms

- **Lymphomas** are the most common CNS tumors in the immunosuppressed. Primary CNS lymphomas may be multiple, unlike other histologic types.
- **Germ cell tumors** are more common in children than adults. The germinoma is the most common histologic type. It resembles the seminoma of the testis and the dysgerminoma of the ovary; the cells are large with a prominent nucleolus.

Metastatic Tumors

About 25–50% of all CNS tumors are metastatic tumors from sources outside the CNS. **Carcinomas** are the most common.

Hematopoetic Pathology–White Blood Cell Disorders & Lymphoid and Myeloid Neoplasms

Learning Objectives

❑ Explain information related to reactive changes in white blood cells

❑ Describe lymphoid, mature B-cell, peripheral T-cell, and natural killer cell neoplasms

❑ Solve problems concerning diseases of histiocytes and dendritic cells

❑ Demonstrate understanding of mast cell diseases

❑ Answer questions about diseases of the spleen and thymus

REACTIVE CHANGES IN WHITE BLOOD CELLS

Leukocytosis

Leukocytosis is characterized by an elevated white blood cell count. It has the following features:

- **Increased neutrophils** (neutrophilia)
  - Increased bone marrow production is seen with acute inflammation associated with pyogenic bacterial infection or tissue necrosis
  - Increased release from bone marrow storage pool may be caused by corticosteroids, stress, or endotoxin
  - Increased bands ("left shift") noted in peripheral circulation
  - Reactive changes include Döhle bodies (aggregates of rough endoplasmic reticulum), toxic granulations (prominent granules), and cytoplasmic vacuoles of neutrophils
- **Increased eosinophils** (eosinophilia) occurs with allergies and asthma (type I hypersensitivity reaction), parasites, drugs (especially in hospitals), and certain skin diseases and cancers (adenocarcinomas, Hodgkin disease).
- **Increased monocytes** (monocytosis) occurs with certain chronic diseases such as some collagen vascular diseases and inflammatory bowel disease, and with certain infections, especially TB.
- **Increased lymphocytes** (lymphocytosis) occurs with acute (viral) diseases and chronic inflammatory processes.
  - **Infectious mononucleosis**, an acute, self-limited disease, which usually resolves in 4–6 weeks, is an example of a viral disease that causes lymphocytosis. The most common cause is Epstein-Barr virus (a herpesvirus) though other viruses can cause it as well (heterophile-negative infectious mononucleosis is most likely due to cytomegalovirus).
    - Age groups include adolescents and young adults ("kissing disease").
    - The "classic triad" includes fever, sore throat with gray-white membrane on tonsils, and lymphadenitis involving the posterior auricular nodes. Another sign is hepatosplenomegaly.
    - Complications include hepatic dysfunction, splenic rupture, and rash if treated with ampicillin.
    - Diagnosis is often made based on symptoms. Lymphocytosis and a rising titer of EBV antibodies are suggestive of the infection. Atypical lymphocytes may be present in peripheral blood.
- **Increased basophils** are seen with chronic myeloproliferative disorders such as polycythemia vera.

Leukopenia

Leukopenia is characterized by a decreased white blood cell count. It has the following features:

- **Decreased neutrophils** can be due to decreased production (aplastic anemia, chemotherapy), increased destruction (infections, autoimmune disease such as systemic lupus erythematosus), and activation of neutrophil adhesion molecules on endothelium (as by endotoxins in septic shock).

- **Decreased eosinophils** are seen with increased cortisol, which causes sequestering of eosinophils in lymph nodes; examples include Cushing syndrome and exogenous corticosteroids.

- **Decreased lymphocytes** are seen with immunodeficiency syndromes such as HIV, DiGeorge syndrome (T-cell deficiency), and severe combined immunodeficiency (B- and T-cell deficiency); also seen secondary to immune destruction (systemic lupus erythematosus), corticosteroids, and radiation (lymphocytes are the most sensitive cells to radiation).

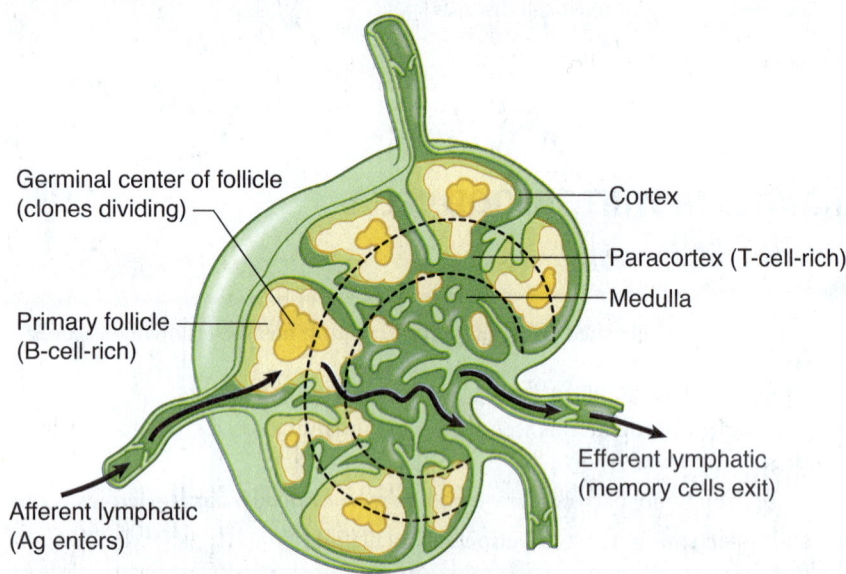

Figure 21-1. Lymph Node

Lymphadenopathy

Lymphadenopathy is lymph node enlargement due to reactive conditions or neoplasia.

- **Acute nonspecific lymphadenitis** produces tender enlargement of lymph nodes; focal involvement is seen with bacterial lymphadenitis. Microscopically, there may be neutrophils within the lymph node. Cat scratch fever (due to *Bartonella henselae*) causes stellate microabscesses. Generalized involvement of lymph nodes is seen with viral infections.

- **Chronic nonspecific lymphadenitis** causes nontender enlargement of lymph nodes. Follicular hyperplasia involves B lymphocytes and may be seen with rheumatoid arthritis, toxoplasmosis, and early HIV infections. Paracortical lymphoid hyperplasia involves T cells and may be seen with viruses, drugs (Dilantin), and systemic lupus erythematosus. Sinus histiocytosis involves macrophages and, in most cases, is nonspecific; an example is lymph nodes draining cancers.

- **Neoplasia** usually causes nontender enlargement of lymph nodes. The most common tumor to involve lymph nodes is metastatic cancer (e.g., breast, lung, malignant melanoma, stomach and colon carcinoma), which is initially seen under the lymph node capsule. Other important causes of lymphadenopathy are malignant lymphoma and infiltration by leukemias.

LYMPHOID NEOPLASMS

Lymphoid neoplasia is grouped according to the 2008 WHO classification as follows (note that B and T lymphoblastic lymphoma/leukemia is grouped by the WHO with myeloid neoplasia):

- Mature B-cell neoplasms
- Mature T-cell and NK-cell neoplasms
- Hodgkin lymphoma
- Histiocytic and dendritic cell neoplasms
- Posttransplantation lymphoproliferative disorders

MATURE B-CELL NEOPLASMS

Chronic lymphocytic leukemia (CLL) and **small lymphocytic lymphoma (SLL)** are very similar; they both represent an abnormal proliferation of B cells. Patients who present with **lymph node findings** are classified as having SLL. Patients who present with **blood findings** are classified as having CLL; 50% of CLL patients also have lymph node involvement.

- CLL is the most indolent of all of the leukemias.
- Mean age at time of diagnosis is age 60.
- The malignant cells are nonfunctional, so patients develop hypogammaglobulinemia, leading to an increased risk of infections.
- CLL is associated with warm autoimmune hemolytic anemia (AIHA) (10% of cases), which will cause spherocytes to be observed in peripheral blood.
- CLL rarely transforms into a worse disease such as prolymphocytic leukemia or large cell lymphoma (Richter syndrome).

CLL and SLL can be categorized by the markers present on the B cells:

- **B-chronic lymphocytic leukemia cells** (95% of cases) have B-cell markers, such as CD19 and CD20. One T-cell marker, CD5, is also present.
- **T-chronic lymphocytic leukemia cells** (5% of cases) have T-cell markers. The histology of affected lymph nodes reveals only a diffuse pattern (not nodular), but proliferation centers may also be present.
- Peripheral blood findings show increased numbers of normal-appearing lymphocytes. Numerous smudge cells ("parachute cells") are also present; the smudge cells result from the fact that the neoplastic lymphocytes are unusually fragile.
- Bone marrow shows numerous normal-appearing neoplastic lymphocytes.

Hairy cell leukemia is a rare B-cell neoplasm that causes indolent disease in middle-aged Caucasian men. There can be a "dry tap" with bone marrow aspiration. Lymphocytes have "hairlike" cytoplasmic projections.

Physical examination shows a markedly enlarged spleen (splenomegaly) due to infiltration of red pulp by malignant cells.

Follicular lymphoma is a well-differentiated B-cell lymphoma with follicular architecture. All follicular lymphomas are derived from B lymphocytes.

- Most common form of non-Hodgkin lymphoma in the United States
- Frequently presents with disseminated disease (more advanced stage)
- Prognosis is better than diffuse lymphoma, but it doesn't respond to therapy (unlike the more aggressive diffuse non-Hodgkin lymphomas)

Diffuse large B-cell lymphoma is a high grade large B-cell lymphoma with a diffuse growth pattern. It is an aggressive, rapidly proliferating tumor which may respond to therapy. Special subtypes include immunodeficiency-associated B-cell lymphomas (often infected with Epstein-Barr virus) and body-cavity large B-cell lymphomas (sometimes associated with human herpes virus [HHV]-8).

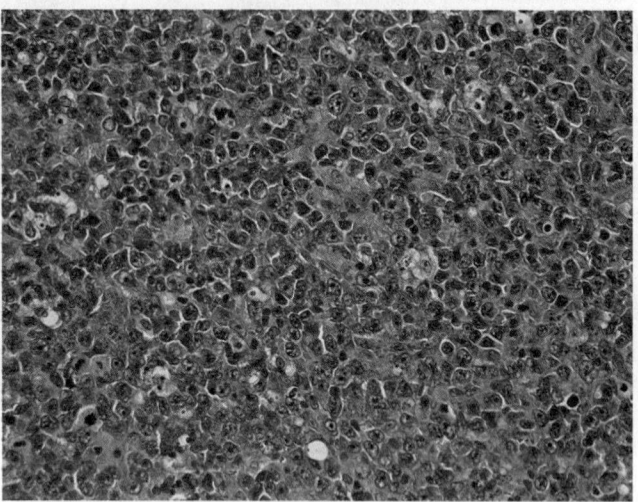

Figure 21-2. Diffuse Large B-Cell Lymphoma

© Bradley Gibson, M.D. Used with permission.

Small noncleaved lymphoma (Burkitt lymphoma) is a high grade B-cell lymphoma. It is composed of intermediate-sized lymphoid cells with a "starry sky" appearance due to numerous reactive tingible-body macrophages (phagocytosis of apoptotic tumor cells).

- **African type:** endemic form
  - Involvement of mandible or maxilla is characteristic; is associated with Epstein-Barr virus
- **American type:** nonendemic, sporadic form
  - Involvement of the abdomen (such as bowel, retroperitoneum, or ovaries); has a high incidence in AIDS patients

Both endemic and sporadic forms of Burkitt lymphoma are seen most often in children and young adults.

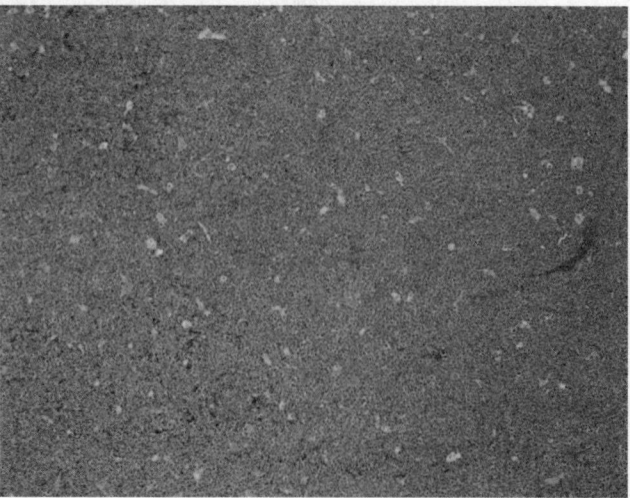

Figure 21-3. "Starry Sky" Appearance of Burkitt Lymphoma

© Bradley Gibson, M.D. Used with permission.

Mantle cell lymphoma (MCL) is a rare B-cell lymphoma in which the tumor cells arise from mantle zone B lymphocytes.

Marginal zone lymphoma (MALToma) is a diverse group of B-cell neoplasms that arise within lymph nodes, spleen, or extranodal tissue. It is associated with mucosa-associated lymphoid tissue (MALTomas). The lesion begins as a reactive polyclonal reaction and may be associated with previous autoimmune disorders or infectious disease (e.g., Sjögren disease, Hashimoto thyroiditis, *Helicobacter* gastritis). The lymphoma remains localized for long periods of time.

Multiple myeloma is a malignant neoplasm of plasma cells.

- Most common primary tumor arising in the bone marrow of adults
- Lab studies show increased serum protein with normal serum albumin; an M spike in serum electrophoresis is a monoclonal immunoglobulin spike—most commonly IgG (60%) and next most commonly IgA (20%)
- Bence Jones proteins are light chains that are small and can be filtered into urine.

Histologically, bone marrow shows increased plasma cells (>20% is characteristic). Peripheral blood may show rouleaux formation ("stack of coins"). Multiple lytic bone lesions are due to the osteoclastic activating factor. Lytic bone lesions cause hypercalcemia, bone pain, and increased risk of fracture.

Increased risk of infection is the most common cause of death. Other complications include renal disease (such as myeloma nephrosis) and primary amyloidosis (10% of patients) due to amyloid light (AL) chains.

Plasmacytoma is a solitary myeloma within bone or soft tissue.

- **Within bone**: precursor lesion that can later develop into myeloma
- **Outside bone** (extramedullary): usually found within upper respiratory tract

Monoclonal gammopathy of undetermined significance (MGUS) (an old name was benign monoclonal gammopathy). Serum M protein is found in 1–3% of asymptomatic individuals age >50; the incidence increases with increasing age. The annual risk of developing a plasma cell dyscrasia, usually multiple myeloma, is 1–2% per year. MGUS may also evolve into Waldenström macroglobulinemia, primary amyloidosis, B-cell lymphoma, or CLL.

Lymphoplasmacytic lymphoma (Waldenström macroglobulinemia) is a small lymphocytic lymphoma with plasmacytic differentiation. It is a cross between multiple myeloma and SLL.

Like myeloma, it has an M spike (IgM). Like SLL (and unlike myeloma), the neoplastic cells infiltrate many organs (e.g., lymph nodes, spleen, bone marrow). Also unlike multiple myeloma, there are no lytic bone lesions and there is no increase in serum calcium. Russell bodies (cytoplasmic immunoglobulin) and Dutcher bodies (intranuclear immunoglobulin) may be present.

- May have hyperviscosity syndrome, because IgM is a large pentamer
- Visual abnormalities may be due to vascular dilatations and hemorrhages in the retina
- Neurologic symptoms include headaches and confusion
- Bleeding and cryoglobulinemia can be due to abnormal globulins, which precipitate at low temperature and may cause Raynaud phenomenon

PERIPHERAL T-CELL AND NATURAL KILLER CELL NEOPLASMS

Peripheral T-cell lymphoma, unspecified is a "wastebasket" diagnostic category.

Adult T-cell leukemia/lymphoma (ATLL) is a malignant T-cell disorder (CD4-T cells) due to HTLV-1 infection. It is often seen in Japan and the Caribbean. Clinical symptoms include skin lesions, hypercalcemia, enlarged lymph nodes, heptomegaly, and splenomegaly. Microscopically, characteristic hyperlobated "4-leaf clover" lymphocytes can be found in the peripheral blood.

Mycosis fungoides is a malignant T-cell disorder (CD4+ cells) that has a better prognosis than ATLL. It can present with a generalized pruritic erythematous rash (no hypercalcemia), which develops as a sequence of skin changes:

inflammatory eczematous stage → plaque stage → tumor nodule stage

Microscopically, atypical PAS-positive lymphocytes are present in the epidermis (epidermotropism); aggregates of these cells are called Pautrier microabscesses. If there is erythroderma and cerebriform Sézary cells are present in peripheral blood, the condition is called **Sézary syndrome**.

HODGKIN LYMPHOMA

Hodgkin lymphoma has some characteristics that are different from non-Hodgkin lymphoma.

- May present similar to infection (with fever)
- Spread is contiguous to adjacent node groups
- No leukemic state
- Extranodal spread is uncommon

The malignant cells are the diagnostic **Reed-Sternberg cells**; these malignant cells are intermixed with reactive inflammatory cells. The Reed-Sternberg cell is a large malignant tumor cell that has a bilobed nucleus with a prominent large inclusion-like nucleolus in each lobe.

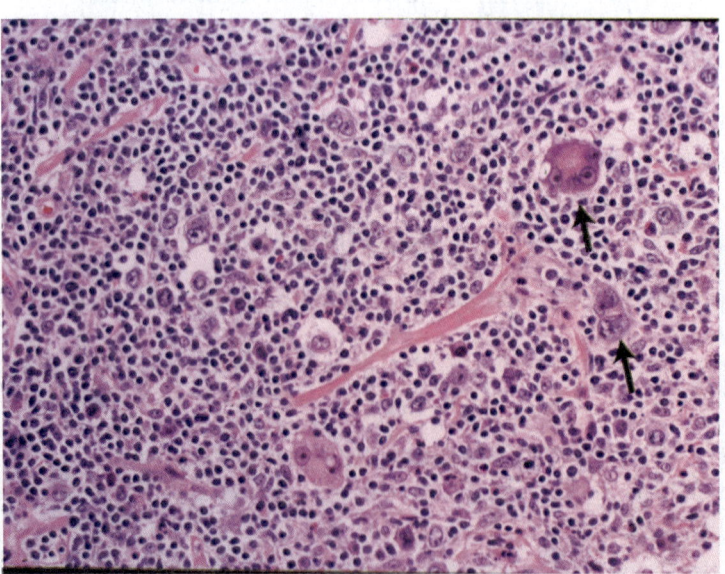

Figure 21-4. Reed-Sternberg Cells (arrows) of Hodgkin Lymphoma Appear as Large Binucleate Cells with Macronucleoli

© Katsumi M. Miyai, M.D., Ph.D.; Regents of the University of California. Used with permission.

Hodgkin lymphoma has a bimodal age group distribution (age late 20s and >50). Patients usually present with painless enlargement of lymph nodes.

Poor prognosis is directly proportional to the number of Reed-Sternberg cells present. Survivors of chemotherapy and radiotherapy have increased risk for secondary non-Hodgkin lymphoma or acute leukemia.

ACUTE LEUKEMIAS

In acute leukemias, the peripheral blood has decreased mature forms and increased immature forms called **blasts**, which have immature chromatin with nucleoli. The bone marrow has increased immature cells (blasts). Acute symptoms are secondary to marrow failure, which can produce decreased erythrocytes (causing anemia and fatigue), decreased leukocytes (permitting infections and fever), and decreased platelets (inducing bleeding).

B AND T LYMPHOBLASTIC LYMPHOMA/LEUKEMIA

Acute Lymphoblastic Leukemia (ALL)

- **Karyotypic abnormalities:** Most pre-B-cell tumors are hyperdiploid. Translocations are common in both B-ALL and T-ALL.
- **B-ALL** is more common in children; symptoms include fever, anemia, and bleeding
- **T-ALL** often presents as a mediastinal mass in an adolescent male

Lymphoblastic Lymphoma

Most cases of lymphoblastic lymphoma are T-cell neoplasms that are aggressive and rapidly progressive. Most patients are young males with a mediastinal mass (think thymus). The leukemic phase of lymphoblastic lymphoma is similar to T-ALL and some consider them the same entity.

Clinical Correlate

ALL is associated with infiltration of the CNS and testes (**sanctuary sites**). Thus, prophylactic radiation and/ or chemotherapy to the CNS is used because malignant cells in the brain are protected from chemotherapy by the blood–brain barrier.

MYELOID NEOPLASMS

Acute Myelogenous Leukemia

Acute myelogenous leukemia is a cancer of the myeloid line of blood cells. Median age at diagnosis is age 50. Symptoms include fatigue, unusual bleeding, and infections.

Lab findings: Myeloid blasts or promyelocytes represent at least 20% of the marrow cells. **Auer rods** (linear condensations of cytoplasmic granules) are characteristic of AML and are not found in normal myeloid precursors.

Myelodysplastic Syndromes (MDS)

MDS are classified according to the number of blasts in the marrow. Dysplastic changes include Pelger-Huët cells ("aviator glasses" nuclei), ring sideroblasts, nuclear budding, and "pawn ball" megakaryocytes. MDS are considered preleukemias, so patients are at increased risk for developing acute leukemia.

MDS mainly affect older adults (age 50–70); they also predispose to infection, hemorrhage and anemia. Transformation to AML is common.

Myeloproliferative Neoplasms (MPN)

MPN are clonal neoplastic proliferations of multipotent myeloid stem cells. The bone marrow is usually markedly hypercellular (hence the name *myeloproliferative*). All cell lines are increased in number (erythroid, myeloid, and megakaryocytes).

- **Chronic myelogenous leukemia (CML)** is a clonal proliferation of pluripotent granulocytic precursor stem cells.

  ○ CML has an insidious onset (i.e., chronic) and causes massive splenomegaly. Progression is typically slow (50% develop accelerated phase <5 years), unless blast crisis develops. In blast crisis, 70% of cases show myeloid blasts and 30% show lymphoid blasts.

  ○ Microscopically, the bone marrow is hypercellular, with all cell lines increased in number. Peripheral leukocytosis is present, including markedly increased neutrophils (and bands and metamyelocytes), as well as increased eosinophils and basophils (as in the other MPS).

- **Polycythemia vera** is a stem cell disorder with trilineage (erythroid, granulocytic, megakaryocytic) proliferation. It may develop into a "spent phase" with myelofibrosis. It causes an increased risk for acute leukemia. Phlebotomy is therapeutic.

  Polycythemia vera characteristically shows the following:

  ○ Increased erythroid precursors with increased red cell mass

  ○ Increased hematocrit

  ○ Increased blood viscosity, which can cause deep vein thrombosis and infarcts

  ○ Decreased erythropoietin, but erythrocytes have increased sensitivity to erythropoietin and overproliferate

  ○ Increased basophils. Histamine release from basophils can cause intense pruritus and gastric ulcer (bleeding may cause iron deficiency).

  ○ Increased eosinophils (like all of the MPS)

  ○ High cell turnover can cause hyperuricemia, resulting in gout. Other clinical characteristics include plethora (redness) and cyanosis (blue).

- **Essential thrombocythemia** is characterized by increased megakaryocytes (and other cell lines) in bone marrow. Peripheral blood smear shows increased platelets, some with abnormal shapes. There are also increased leukocytes. Clinical signs include excessive bleeding and occlusion of small vessels.

DISEASES OF HISTIOCYTES AND DENDRITIC CELLS

Langerhans histiocytosis is common in children. It can affect many sites, including skin, bone, CNS (diabetes insipidus), and lungs. Biopsy is required for diagnosis. The Langerhans cells are CD1a positive and on electron microscopy show cytoplasmic Birbeck granules (tennis racket–shaped organelles).

- Multisystem variant: Letterer-Siwe disease (marrow involvement can be fatal)
- Hand-Schuller-Christian triad is calvarial involvement, diabetes insipidus, and exophthalmos
- Unisystem variant: eosinophilic granuloma (most often found in bone)

DISEASES OF THE SPLEEN AND THYMUS

Splenomegaly (splenic enlargement) can be caused by multiple things:

- Vascular congestion (portal hypertension)
- Reactive hyperplasia of white pulp (autoimmune disorder, infectious mononucleosis, malaria)
- Infiltrative disease (metastatic non-Hodgkin lymphoma, primary amyloidosis, leukemia)
- Accumulated macrophages in red pulp (Gaucher, Niemann-Pick disease)
- Extravascular hemolysis
- Extramedullary hematopoiesis in splenic sinusoids

Hypersplenism will result in thrombocytopenia.

Splenic dysfunction will result in a loss of ability to remove damaged red cells, which leads to Howell-Jolly bodies in peripheral red blood cells. Splenectomized, asplenic, and hyposplenic individuals are at risk for infection (sepsis, peritonitis), particularly due to *Streptococcus*, *Haemophilus*, and *Salmonella*.

Thymomas are low-grade tumors of the thymic epithelium with many histologic patterns. Recent large case series have shown that tumor behavior does not always correlate with histopathological features.

True thymic hyperplasia is enlargement of a histologically normal thymus; it can occur as a complication of chemotherapy.

Thymic lymphoid hyperplasia shows germinal center hyperplasia.

Female Genital Pathology 22

Learning Objectives

❏ Demonstrate understanding of the pathology of the vulva, vagina, cervix, uterus, and ovary

❏ Solve problems concerning the placenta

VULVA

Infections

- **Human papillomavirus (HPV)** causes warty lesions (condylomata acuminata) and precursor dysplastic lesions of squamous cell carcinoma called vulvar intraepithelial neoplasia (VIN). Vulvar HPV is commonly subtype 6 and 11 and therefore has low oncogenic potential.
- **Herpes simplex virus (HSV)**. Most cases of vulvar herpes are caused by HSV-2. Painless vesicles progress to pustules and painful ulcers.
- **Syphilis** is a sexually transmitted disease caused by *Treponema pallidum*. The primary lesion is a chancre, a painless ulcer that does not scar after healing.
- **Molluscum contagiosum** is a viral disease caused by a DNA poxvirus. It presents as smooth papules and has characteristic cytoplasmic viral inclusions.
- **Bartholin gland abscess** is a polymicrobial infection requiring drainage or excision.

Tumors

- **Squamous cell carcinoma** is the most common malignancy of the vulva. The most common form occurs in women age >60. The less common form occurs in younger women with HPV serotypes 16 and 18.
- **Melanoma** can occur on the vulva, and must be differentiated from lentigo simplex which is more common.

VAGINA

- **Vaginal adenosis and clear cell adenocarcinoma** are rare conditions with increased risk in females exposed to diethylstilbestrol (DES) *in utero*.
- **Embryonal rhabdomyosarcoma** (sarcoma botryoides) affects infants and young children (age <5), in whom it can cause a polypoid, "grapelike," soft tissue mass that protrudes from the vagina. Microscopically, the mass is characterized by polypoid epithelial growth with an underlying immature (cambium) proliferation of spindle-shaped tumor cells with rare cross-striations. Tumor cells are positive for desmin.
- **Primary forms of vaginal squamous cell carcinoma** are usually related to HPV infection; secondary forms are more common and are usually due to extension from a cervical cancer. Treatment is radiotherapy.
- **Rhabdomyoma** is a benign skeletal muscle tumor that can involve the vagina. It occurs in middle-aged women.

- **Gartner duct cyst** is a cyst of the lateral wall of the vagina that is due to persistence of a mesonephric (Wolffian) duct remnant. Urinary tract abnormalities may exist.

- **Vaginitis/vaginosis:** All of the following conditions require vaginal swab for definitive diagnosis; molecular diagnostic tests may be indicated in certain situations.

   ◦ **Vulvovaginal candidiasis** can occur spontaneously or from antibiotic therapy; it is not usually sexually transmitted. Symptoms include discharge and pruritis. Yeast cells and pseudohyphae are seen on microscopy.

   ◦ **Bacterial vaginosis (BV)** is implicated in preterm labor and pelvic inflammatory disease. Some patients are asymptomatic. BV is a sexually transmitted bacterial infection of polymicrobial origin (although it used to be attributed only to *Gardnerella vaginalis*); recurrence rate is high after treatment with antibiotics. "Clue cells" are squamous cells coated with coccobacilli that may be seen microscopically in swab material.

   ◦ ***Trichomonis vaginalis*** is a sexually transmitted motile protozoan. Most infected people are asymptomatic. It can also cause cervicitis, but "strawberry cervix" is not a consistent diagnostic feature.

CERVIX

Pelvic inflammatory disease (PID) is an ascending infection (sexually transmitted disease) from the cervix to the endometrium, fallopian tubes, and pelvic cavity. The infecting organisms are most frequently nongonococcal organisms, including *Chlamydia*, *Mycoplasma hominis* and endogenous flora.

The distribution of disease includes the endometrium (endometritis), fallopian tubes (salpingitis), and pelvic cavity (peritonitis and pelvic abscesses). **Fitz-Hugh–Curtis syndrome** (perihepatitis) can occur, characterized by "violin-string" adhesions between the fallopian tube and liver capsule. Symptoms include the following:

- Vaginal discharge (cervicitis)
- Vaginal bleeding and midline abdominal pain (endometritis)
- Bilateral lower abdominal and pelvic pain (salpingitis)
- Abdominal tenderness and peritoneal signs (peritonitis)
- Pleuritic right upper quadrant pain (perihepatitis)

Clinical Correlate

Tubal ectopic pregnancies usually occur in the ampulla of the fallopian tube. Tubal rupture will cause severe, acute lower abdominal pain.

Complications of PID include tubo-ovarian abscess; tubal scarring (increasing risk of infertility and ectopic tubal pregnancies), and intestinal obstruction secondary to fibrous adhesions.

Table 22-1. Malignant Tumors of the Lower Female Genital Tract in the U.S.

Order of Incidence	Order of Greatest Mortality
1. Endometrial cancer	1. Ovarian cancer
2. Ovarian cancer	2. Endometrial cancer
3. Cervical cancer	3. Cervical cancer

Cervical carcinoma is most commonly squamous cell carcinoma but can also be adenocarcinoma or small cell neuroendocrine carcinoma. It is the third most common malignant tumor of the lower female genital tract in the United States, with peak incidence at ages 35–44. Risk factors include the following:

- Early age of first intercourse
- Multiple sexual partners
- Multiple pregnancies
- Oral contraceptive use
- Smoking
- STDs (including human papilloma virus)
- Immunosuppression

Human papilloma virus infection is the most important risk factor.

The precursor lesion is **cervical intraepithelial neoplasia (CIN)**, which is increasing in incidence and occurs commonly at the squamocolumnar junction (transformation zone). Cervical intraepithelial lesions show a progression of changes on histologic examination:

- Low grade SIL (squamous intraepithelial lesion)
- High grade SIL
- Carcinoma in situ
- Superficially invasive squamous cell carcinoma
- Invasive squamous cell carcinoma

Squamous cell carcinoma of the cervix may be asymptomatic or may present with postcoital vaginal bleeding, dyspareunia, and/or malodorous discharge. To establish the diagnosis, the Papanicolaou (**Pap**) test is useful for early detection, and colposcopy with biopsy for microscopic evaluation.

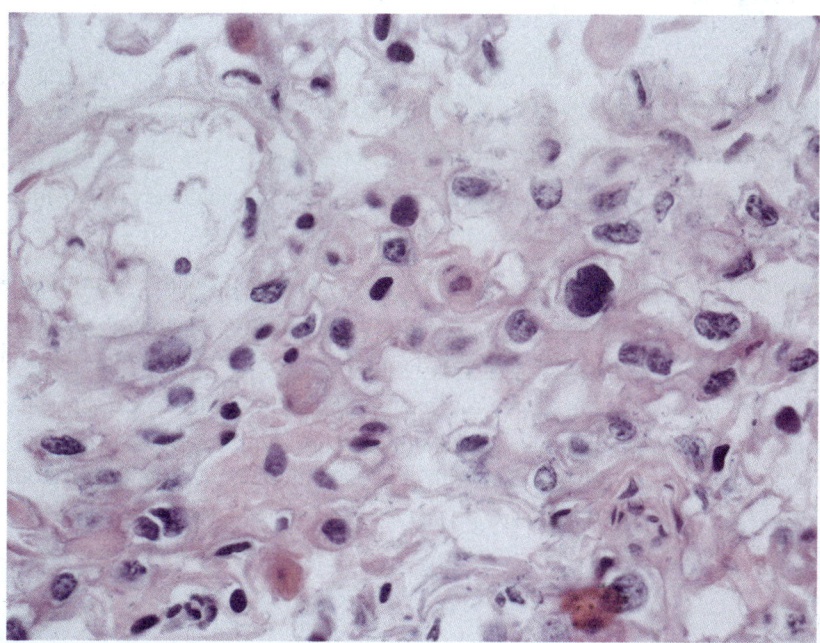

Figure 22-1. Cervix Biopsy Showing Squamous Cells with Nuclear Hyperchromasia and Perinuclear Vacuoles, Characteristic of HPV Cytopathic Effect

© Gregg Barré, M.D. Used with permission.

Acute cervicitis and chronic cervicitis are common and usually nonspecific inflammatory conditions.

- Acute cervicitis is often caused by *C. trachomatis*, *N. gonorrhoeae*, *T. vaginalis*, *Candida*, and herpes simplex type 2.
- A specific, severe form of chronic cervicitis (**follicular cervicitis**) can be caused by *C. trachomatis*; it can result in neonatal conjunctivitis and pneumonia in infants delivered vaginally through an infected cervix. **Cervical polyp** is a common non-neoplastic polyp that can be covered with columnar or stratified squamous epithelium.

UTERUS

Endometritis is inflammation of the endometrial lining in the uterus. It can be acute or chronic.

- **Acute endometritis** is an ascending infection from the cervix; it is associated with pregnancy and abortion.
- **Chronic endometritis** is associated with PID and intrauterine devices; plasma cells are seen in the endometrium.

Endometriosis is the presence of endometrial glands and stroma outside the uterus. It most commonly affects women of reproductive age. Common sites of involvement are the ovaries, ovarian and uterine ligaments, pouch of Douglas, serosa of bowel and urinary bladder, and peritoneal cavity. It can present with chronic pelvic pain, dysmenorrhea and dyspareunia, rectal pain and constipation, abnormal uterine bleeding, or infertility.

Grossly, endometriosis causes red-brown serosal nodules (an *endometrioma* is an ovarian "chocolate" (hemolyzed blood) cyst).

Leiomyoma (fibroid), the most common tumor of the female genital tract, is a benign, smooth muscle tumor of the myometrium. Leiomyomas have a high incidence in African Americans, though they are common across all populations. Their growth is estrogen-dependent.

Leiomyomas may present with menorrhagia, abdominal mass, pelvic/back pain, suprapubic discomfort, or infertility and spontaneous abortion.

Grossly, leiomyomas form well-circumscribed, rubbery, white-tan masses with a whorled, trabeculated appearance on cut section. Leiomyomas are commonly multiple, and may have subserosal, intramural, and submucosal location. The malignant variant is leiomyosarcoma.

Endometrial hyperplasia refers to a histological proliferation of endometrial glands with 2 important histopathologic categories:

- **Benign endometrial hyperplasia** shows uniform remodeling of glands with cyst formation.
- **Endometrial intraepithelial neoplasia** shows crowded architecture and cytologic alteration on biopsy.
  - Patients are at high risk for endometrial adenocarcinoma.
  - Treatment options include total hysterectomy or progestin therapy with biopsy surveillance.

Endometrial adenocarcinoma is the most common malignant tumor of the lower female genital tract. It most commonly affects postmenopausal women who present with abnormal uterine bleeding. Risk factors are mostly related to estrogen:

- Early menarche and late menopause
- Nulliparity
- Hypertension and diabetes
- Obesity
- Chronic anovulation
- Estrogen-producing ovarian tumors (granulosa cell tumors)

- ERT and tamoxifen
- Endometrial hyperplasia (complex atypical hyperplasia)
- Lynch syndrome (colorectal, endometrial, and ovarian cancers)

Endometrial adenocarcinoma typically forms a tan polypoid endometrial mass; invasion of myometrium is prognostically important.

Less common types of uterine malignancy include **leiomyosarcoma**, a malignant, smooth muscle tumor, and **carcinosarcoma**, which contains both malignant stromal cells and endometrial adenocarcinoma.

Adenomyosis is an invagination of the deeper layers of the endometrium into the myometrium, which causes menorrhagia and dysmenorrhea.

Anovulation can cause abnormal uterine bleeding, especially in women near menarche and menopause. Biopsy shows glandular and stromal breakdown in a background of proliferative phase endometrium.

OVARY

Polycystic ovarian disease (Stein-Leventhal syndrome) is an endocrine disorder of unknown etiology showing signs of androgen excess (clinical or biochemical), oligoovulation and/or anovulation, and polycystic ovaries.

Accurate diagnosis requires exclusion of other endocrine disorders that might affect reproduction. Patients are usually young women of reproductive age who present with oligomenorrhea or secondary amenorrhea, hirsutism, infertility, or obesity. Treatment is lifestyle change and hormone therapy.

Lab studies show elevated luteinizing hormone (LH), low follicle-stimulating hormone (FSH), and elevated testosterone. Gross examination is notable for bilaterally enlarged ovaries with multiple cysts; microscopic examination shows multiple cystic follicles.

Epithelial Ovarian Tumors

Epithelial ovarian tumors are the most common form of ovarian tumor. Risk factors include nulliparity, family history, and germline mutations.

Previously, epithelial tumors were characterized by histology into the categories cystadenoma (benign), borderline, and cystadenocarcinoma. Now, **serous tumors** are classified as **low grade** and **high grade** for prognostic significance.

- Low grade serous tumors are associated with *KRAS*, *BRAF*, or *ERB2* mutations.
- Most high grade serous tumors have *TP53* mutations.

Note
• The Pap test has reduced the incidence of cervical cancer in the United States.
• There is no screening test for ovarian cancer.

The most common malignant ovarian tumor is **serous cystadenocarcinoma**. Hereditary risk factors include *BRCA1* (breast and ovarian cancers) and Lynch syndrome.

Ovarian Germ Cell Tumors

- **Teratoma** (dermoid cyst)
  - Vast majority (>95%) of ovarian (but not testicular) teratomas are benign; commonly occurs in early reproductive years
  - Include elements from all three germ cell layers: ectoderm (skin, hair, adnexa, neural tissue), mesoderm (bone, cartilage), and endoderm (thyroid, bronchial tissue)
  - Complications include torsion, rupture, and malignant transformation
  - Can contain hair, teeth, and sebaceous material
  - The term *struma ovarii* is used when there is a preponderance of thyroid tissue
  - Immature teratoma is characterized by histologically immature tissue

- **Dysgerminoma**
  - Malignant; commonly occurs in children and young adults
  - Risk factors include Turner syndrome and disorders of sexual development
  - Gross and microscopic features are similar to seminomas

Ovarian Sex Cord–Stromal Tumors

- **Ovarian fibroma**
  - Most common stromal tumor; forms a firm, white mass
  - **Meigs syndrome** refers to the combination of fibroma, ascites, and pleural effusion.
- **Granulosa cell tumor**
  - Potentially malignant, **estrogen-producing** tumor
  - Presentation depends on age
  - Complications include endometrial hyperplasia and cancer
  - Tumor forms a yellow-white mass that microscopically shows polygonal tumor cells and formation of follicle-like structures (Call-Exner bodies)
- **Sertoli-Leydig cell tumor** (androblastoma) is an **androgen-producing tumor** that presents with virilization, usually in young women.

Primary sites for **metastatic tumor** to the ovary include breast cancer, colon cancer, endometrial cancer, and gastric "signet-ring cell" cancer (Krukenberg tumor).

Breast Pathology 23

Learning Objectives

❑ Explain information related to mastitis

❑ Demonstrate understanding of fibrocystic changes

❑ Solve problems concerning benign and malignant neoplasms

❑ Answer questions about gynecomastia

MASTITIS

Mastitis is an infection of the breast tissue.

Acute mastitis causes an area of erythema and firmness in the breast, commonly during lactation. The most common infecting organism is *S. aureus*. The breast is often biopsied to differentiate the condition from inflammatory carcinoma, another painful breast condition. Microscopically there is acute and chronic inflammation with abscess formation in some cases.

Fat necrosis is often related to trauma or prior surgery, and it may produce a palpable mass or a discrete lesion with calcifications on mammography. Microscopic changes include fat necrosis, chronic inflammation, hemosiderin deposits and fibrosis with calcification.

FIBROCYSTIC CHANGES

Fibrocystic changes (formerly called *fibrocystic disease*) are a group of very common, benign changes that can be classified as **proliferative** (having an increase in the glandular elements or epithelial cells) or **nonproliferative**. Because they carry varying degrees of risk for breast cancer, it is important to identify each type histologically.

Fibrocystic changes primarily affect women in their reproductive years. The changes most often involve the upper outer quadrant and may produce a palpable mass or nodularity.

- **Fibrosis** may mimic a tumor on clinical exam and U/S.
- **Cysts** can usually be diagnosed by U/S.
- **Apocrine metaplasia** is often seen in cyst walls.
- **Microcalcifications** occur in benign and malignant processes.
- **Ductal hyperplasia** is classified as usual or atypical on the basis of cytology and microlumen architecture; **atypical ductal hyperplasia** is differentiated from DCIS on the basis of microscopic extent.
- **Atypical lobular hyperplasia** is differentiated from LCIS histologically on the basis of the percentage of acini involved.
- **Sclerosing adenosis** is distinguished from carcinoma histologically by the preservation of the myoepithelial layer.

Table 23-1. Features That Distinguish Fibrocystic Change from Breast Cancer

Fibrocystic Change	Breast Cancer
Often bilateral	Often unilateral
May have multiple nodules	Usually single
Menstrual variation	No menstrual variation
May regress during pregnancy	Does not regress during pregnancy

BENIGN NEOPLASMS

Fibroadenoma is the most common benign breast tumor in women age <35. It causes a palpable, round, movable, rubbery mass, which on cross-section shows small, cleft-like spaces. Microscopically, the mass shows proliferation of benign stroma, ducts, and lobules.

Phyllodes tumor (cystosarcoma phyllodes) usually involves an older patient population (age 50s) and can be benign or malignant. Local recurrence is common but the incidence of metastasis is low. Microscopically, the mass shows increased stromal cellularity, clefts lined by epithelium, stromal overgrowth, and irregular margins.

Intraductal papilloma commonly presents as a bloody nipple discharge. Microscopically, papilloma causes benign papillary growth within lactiferous ducts or sinuses; the myoepithelial layer is preserved.

MALIGNANT NEOPLASMS

Carcinoma of the breast is the most common cancer in women and affects 1 in 9 women in the United States. It is also the second most common cause of cancer death. The incidence is increasing and is higher in the United States than in Japan. Many risk factors have been identified.

The incidence increases with the following factors:

- Age
- Unusually long/intense exposure to estrogens (long length of reproductive life, nulliparity, obesity, exogenous estrogens)
- Presence of proliferative fibrocystic changes, especially **atypical hyperplasia**
- First-degree relative with breast cancer

Hereditary influences are thought to be involved in 5-10% of breast cancers, with important genes as follows:

- *BRCA1* (error-free repair of DNA double-strand breaks) chromosome 17q21
- *BRCA2* (error-free repair of DNA double-strand breaks) chromosome 13q12.3
- *TP53* germline mutation (Li-Fraumeni syndrome)

Carcinoma in situ and risk of invasive carcinoma. About 35% of women with untreated DCIS will develop invasive cancer, usually in the same quadrant of the breast. About 35% of women with LCIS will develop invasive lobular or ductal carcinoma, in either breast.

Breast cancer is most common in the upper outer quadrant. Gross examination of a breast cancer typically shows a stellate, white-tan, gritty mass. Clinically, it can cause:

- Mammographic calcifications or architectural distortion
- Palpable solitary painless mass
- Nipple retraction or skin dimpling
- Fixation of breast tissue to the chest wall

Paget disease of the nipple is an intra-epidermal spread of tumor cells from an underlying ductal carcinoma in situ or invasive ductal carcinoma. The tumor cells often lie in lacunae, and there can be a dermal lymphocytic infiltrate.

Histologic variants of breast cancer are as follows:

- **Preinvasive lesions** include ductal carcinoma in situ (**DCIS**) and lobular carcinoma in situ (**LCIS**). Preservation of the myoepithelial cell layer distinguishes them from their invasive counterparts.
- **Invasive (infiltrating) ductal carcinoma** is the most common form (>80% of cases). Microscopically, it shows tumor cells forming ducts within a desmoplastic stroma.

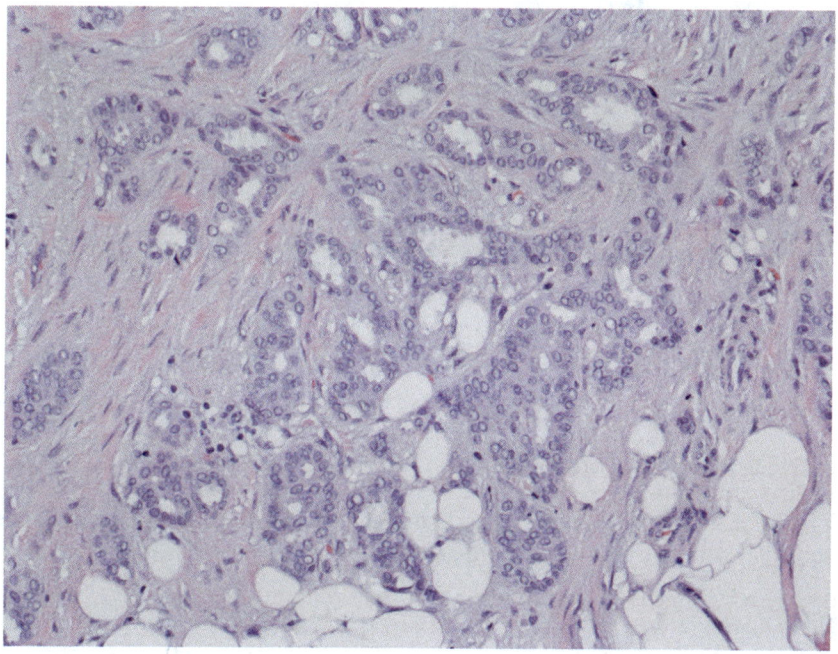

Figure 23-1. Invasive Ductal Carcinoma

© Gregg Barré, M.D. Used with permission.

- **Invasive (infiltrating) lobular carcinoma** (5–10% of cases) is characterized by small, bland tumor cells forming a single-file pattern.
- Multifocal and bilateral disease occurs commonly.
- **Mucinous (colloid) carcinoma** is characterized microscopically by clusters of bland tumor cells floating within pools of mucin. It has a better prognosis.
- **Tubular carcinoma** rarely metastasizes and has an excellent prognosis.
- **Medullary carcinoma is characterized microscopically by pleomorphic tumor cells forming syncytial** groups surrounded by a dense lymphocytic host response. It has a better prognosis.

- **Inflammatory carcinoma** is related to tumor invasion into the dermal lymphatics with resulting lymphatic edema; it presents with red, warm, edematous skin. The prognosis is poor.

  o The term *peau d'orange* is used when the thickened skin resembles an orange peel. This is caused by the accentuation of the attachments of the suspensory ligaments of Cooper to the dermis.

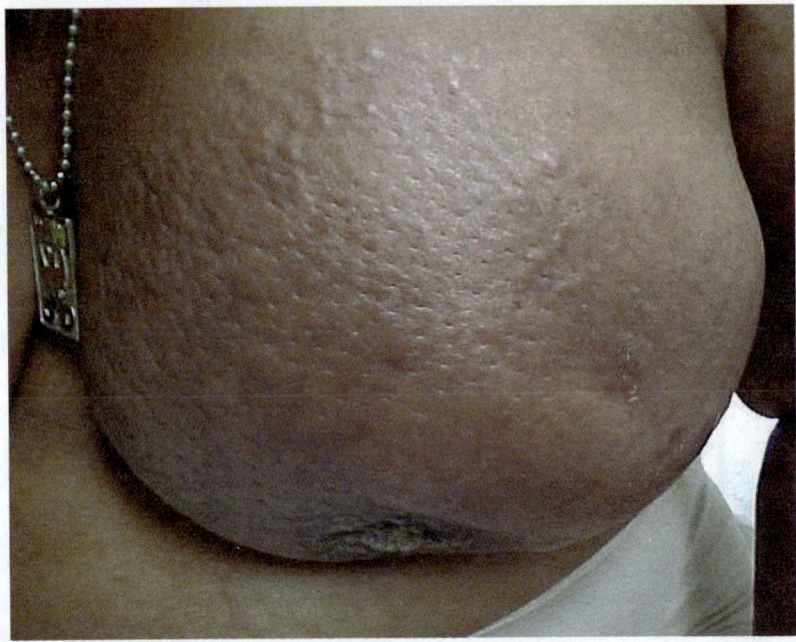

Figure 23-2. Advanced Breast Cancer with Peau d'Orange Skin Involvement

© Richard P. Usatine, M.D. Used with permission.

Mammary Paget disease (Paget disease of the nipple) is commonly associated with an underlying invasive or in situ ductal carcinoma. It may present with ulceration, oozing, crusting, and fissuring of the nipple and areola. Microscopic examination shows intraepidermal spread of tumor cells (Paget cells), with the cells occurring singly or in groups within the epidermis; there is often a clear halo surrounding the nucleus.

Although the majority of cancers in the breast are primaries, **cancer from other organs can spread to the breast.** Lung cancer may spread by contiguity or via the lymphatics.

GYNECOMASTIA

Gynecomastia is a unilateral or bilateral benign breast enlargement in a male. It is usually caused by an altered androgen-estrogen balance that favors estrogen effect. Microscopically, it is characterized by:

- Ductal epithelial hyperplasia
- Ductal elongation and branching
- Proliferation of periductal fibroblasts
- Increase in vascularity in the involved tissue

Male Pathology 24

Learning Objectives

❏ Explain information related to the pathology of the penis and testes

❏ Solve problems concerning testicular cancer

❏ Solve problems concerning prostate disease

PENIS

Malformations of the penis include epispadias and hypospadias. Both may be associated with undescended testes. **Epispadias** is a urethral opening on the dorsal surface of the penis, while **hypospadias** is a urethral opening on the ventral surface. Both have an increased risk of urinary tract infection and infertility.

Balanitis/balanoposthitis is inflammation of the glans penis, and the glans and foreskin, respectively. Causes include poor hygiene and lack of circumcision.

Peyronie disease is penile fibromatosis resulting in curvature of the penis during erection.

Condyloma acuminatum is a warty, cauliflower-like growth, with the causative agents most frequently being HPV serotypes 6 and 11.

Squamous cell carcinoma (SCC) is uncommon in the United States, and is often related to infection with HPV serotypes 16 and 18. There is an increased risk in uncircumcised males (multicentric carcinoma in situ).

Priapism is a persistent painful erection that can be caused by sickle cell anemia (causes blood sludging in penis), trauma, and drugs.

Erectile dysfunction (ED). Causes of impotence include psychological factors, decreased testosterone, vascular insufficiency (most common cause age >50), neurologic disease (multiple sclerosis, diabetic neuropathy, radical prostatectomy), some medications, hypothyroidism, prolactinoma, and penile disorders.

TESTES

Varicocele is a dilated pampiniform venous plexus and internal spermatic vein, usually on the left side. It may cause infertility. Clinically, it resembles a "bag of worms" superior to the testicle.

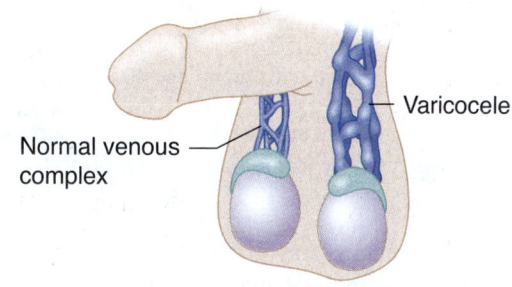

Figure 24-1. Varicocele

Hydrocele refers t`o fluid within the tunica vaginalis.

Spermatocele is an epididymal cyst containing sperm.

Epididymitis presents with fever and gradual onset of scrotal pain.

- Acute epididymitis that affects men age <35 is often caused by *N. gonorrhoeae* or *C. trachomatis*.
- Acute epididymitis that affects men age >35 is often caused by *E. coli* or *Pseudomonas*.
- Chronic epididymitis can be caused by TB.

Orchitis presents with sudden onset of testicular pain and fever. It is frequently viral, particularly due to the mumps virus.

Testicular torsion is twisting of the spermatic cord; may be associated with physical activity or trauma; and is a clinical emergency that can cause painful hemorrhagic infarction leading to gangrene.

Cryptorchidism is a failure of one or both testes to descend; the undescended testes are most commonly found in the inguinal canal. The undescended testes have an increased risk for developing seminoma.

Male infertility

- Decreased sperm count due to **primary testicular dysfunction** can be caused by Leydig cell dysfunction or seminiferous tubule dysfunction.
- Decreased sperm count due to **secondary hypogonadism** can be caused by pituitary and hypothalamic dysfunction.
- Inability of sperm to exit the body in sufficient numbers may be caused by **obstruction of the vas deferens** or **disordered ejaculation**.

TESTICULAR CANCER

Testicular cancer typically presents with a firm, painless testicular mass; nonseminomatous tumors may present with widespread metastasis. Caucasians have a higher incidence than African Americans.

Risk factors include:

- Cryptorchidism (3-5 times increased risk)
- Testicular dysgenesis (testicular feminization and Klinefelter syndrome)
- Positive family history

Clinically, testicular cancer typically shows an intratesticular mass. Serum tumor marker studies can be helpful in confirming the diagnosis.

Germ Cell Tumors

Germ cell tumors are usually hyperdiploid.

Seminoma is the most common germ cell tumor in adults, with mean age 40.

On gross examination the tumor has a pale tan, bulging cut surface. Microscopic exam shows sheets of monotonous cells (with clear cytoplasm and round nuclei) separated by fibrous septae. Lymphocytes, granulomas, and giant cells may be seen.

Embryonal carcinoma is more aggressive than seminoma and affects adults ages 20–40. It causes bulky masses with hemorrhage and necrosis. Microscopy shows large primitive cells.

Choriocarcinoma is a highly malignant tumor that often has widespread metastasis at the time of diagnosis; hematogenous spread to lungs and liver is particularly common. The often small tumor has extensive hemorrhage and necrosis. Microscopically, syncytiotrophoblasts and cytotrophoblasts are seen.

Yolk sac tumor (endodermal sinus tumor) is the most common germ cell tumor in children; in pediatric cases, the prognosis is good. In adults, the prognosis may depend on the other histologic types that are admixed. Microscopically, yolk sac tumors show numerous patterns. Schiller-Duval bodies are glomeruloid structures.

Teratoma often causes cystic masses which may contain cartilage and bone. Microscopically, mature teratoma usually contains ectodermal, endodermal, and mesodermal tissue in a haphazard arrangement. Immature elements contain embryonic tissue. Prepubertal cases are benign regardless of immature elements; teratomas in adults have malignant potential.

Mixed germ cell tumors. As many as 60% of germ cell tumors contain >1 component. When both teratoma and embryonal carcinoma are present, the name *teratocarcinoma* is used.

Sex Cord–Stromal Tumors

Sex cord–stromal tumors include Leydig cell and Sertoli cell tumors.

- **Leydig cell tumors** cause painless testicular masses, and have a bimodal distribution (prepubertal and age >50). They may produce androgens and estrogens.
    - In adults, the hormonal secretion can produce gynecomastia; in children, it can produce precocious puberty.
    - Benign tumors (90%) have an excellent prognosis; malignant tumors (10%) can be refractory to chemotherapy and radiation therapy.
    - Tumor cells have abundant pink cytoplasm.
- **Sertoli cell tumors** are rare and usually benign. Microscopically, they show tubule formation.

Other Tumors

- **Testicular lymphoma** is the most common testicular tumor in men >age 60. It is most commonly non-Hodgkin lymphoma, diffuse large cell type.
- **Scrotal squamous cell carcinoma** is associated with exposure to soot (chimney sweeps).

PROSTATE

Benign prostatic hyperplasia (BPH) (also called nodular hyperplasia; glandular and stromal hyperplasia) is extremely common. Androgens (dihydrotestosterone) play an important role in the pathogenesis, and the lesion is not premalignant. The incidence increases with age (age 60 is 70%; age 70 is 80%). BPH typically presents with the following:

- Decreased caliber and force of stream
- Trouble starting (hesitancy)/stopping the stream
- Postvoid dribbling
- Urinary retention
- Incontinence
- Urgency/frequency
- Nocturia/dysuria
- Possible elevation in prostate specific antigen (PSA) but usually <10 ng/mL

Complications include urinary tract infection, urinary bladder trabeculation and diverticula formation, and hydronephrosis and renal failure (rare).

Grossly, BPH causes an enlarged prostate with well-demarcated nodules in the transition and central (periurethral) zones, which often results in slit-like compression of the prostatic urethra. Microscopically, the lesion shows glandular and stromal hyperplasia resulting in the characteristic prostate enlargement.

Prostate adenocarcinoma is the most common cancer in men in the United States and the second most common cause of cancer death in men. The incidence increases with age, and the highest rate is in African Americans.

- Often clinically silent but may present with lower back pain secondary to metastasis
- Advanced localized disease may present with urinary tract obstruction or UTI (rare)
- Tumor can be detected with digital rectal exam (induration), serum PSA level, and transrectal U/S and biopsy
- Metastases most commonly involve obturator and pelvic lymph nodes
- Osteoblastic bone metastasis to lumbar spine can occur, and can be associated with elevated alkaline phosphatase
- The disease course can be monitored with PSA levels.

Pathologically, an ill-defined, firm, yellow mass commonly arises in the posterior aspect of the peripheral zone.

Prostatitis

- Acute prostatitis is usually caused by intraprostatic reflux of urinary tract pathogens.
- Chronic prostatitis may develop following recurrent acute prostatitis, and bacterial pathogens may not be detectable. Chronic nonbacterial prostatitis (**chronic pelvic pain syndrome**) is more common than bacterial prostatitis.
- Clinical findings can include fever (acute prostatitis), pain (lower back, perineal, or suprapubic), painful prostate on rectal exam, and dysuria (with possible hematuria).

Learning Objectives

❏ Demonstrate understanding of disease of the thyroid, parathyroid, adrenal, pituitary, and pineal gland

❏ Describe the relationship between the hypothalamus and pituitary gland

❏ Solve problems concerning multiple endocrine neoplasia syndromes

❏ Explain information related to diabetes mellitus

THYROID GLAND

Note: additional information can be found in Chapter 27 of Part 2: Physiology.

Multinodular goiter (nontoxic goiter) refers to an enlarged thyroid gland with multiple colloid nodules. Females are affected more often than males. It is frequently asymptomatic, and the patient is typically euthyroid, with normal T4, T3, and TSH. **Plummer syndrome** is the development of hyperthyroidism (toxic multinodular goiter) late in the course.

Microscopically, the tissue shows nodules of varying sizes composed of colloid follicles. Calcification, hemorrhage, cystic degeneration, and fibrosis can also be present.

Hyperthyroidism

The term *hyperthyroidism* is used when the mean metabolic rate of all cells is increased due to increased T4 or T3. Clinical features include tachycardia and palpitations; nervousness and diaphoresis; heat intolerance; weakness and tremors; diarrhea; and weight loss despite a good appetite. Lab studies show elevated free T4.

- In primary hyperthyroidism, TSH is decreased.
- In secondary and tertiary hyperthyroidism, TSH is elevated.

Graves disease is an autoimmune disease characterized by production of IgG autoantibodies to the TSH receptor. Females are affected more frequently than males, with peak age 20–40. Clinical features include hyperthyroidism, diffuse goiter, ophthalmopathy (exophthalmus), and dermopathy (pretibial myxedema). Microscopically, the thyroid has hyperplastic follicles with scalloped colloid.

Other causes of hyperthyroidism include toxic multinodular goiter, toxic adenoma (functioning adenoma producing thyroid hormone), and Hashimoto and subacute thyroiditis (transient hyperthyroidism).

Hypothyroidism

The term hypothyroidism is used when the mean metabolic rate of all cells is decreased due to decreased T4 or T3. Clinical features include fatigue and lethargy; sensitivity to cold temperatures; decreased cardiac output; myxedema (accumulation of proteoglycans and water); facial and periorbital edema; peripheral edema of the hands and feet; deep voice; macroglossia; constipation; and anovulatory cycles. Lab studies show decreased free T4.

- In primary hypothyroidism, TSH is elevated.
- In secondary and tertiary hypothyroidism, TSH is decreased.

Iatrogenic hypothyroidism is the most common cause of hypothyroidism in the United States, and is secondary to thyroidectomy or radioactive iodine treatment. Treatment is thyroid hormone replacement.

Congenital hypothyroidism (cretinism) in endemic regions is due to iodine deficiency during intrauterine and neonatal life, and in nonendemic regions is due to thyroid dysgenesis. Patients present with failure to thrive, stunted bone growth and dwarfism, spasticity and motor incoordination, and mental retardation. Goiter is seen in endemic cretinism.

Endemic goiter is due to dietary deficiency of iodine; it is uncommon in the United States.

Thyroiditis

Hashimoto thyroiditis is a chronic autoimmune disease characterized by immune destruction of the thyroid gland and hypothyroidism. It is the most common noniatrogenic/nonidiopathic cause of hypothyroidism in the United States; it most commonly causes painless goiter in females more than males, with peak age 40–65.

Hashimoto thyroiditis is the most common cause of hypothyroidism (due to destruction of thyroid tissue), though the initial inflammation may cause transient hyperthyroidism (hashitoxicosis). Hashimoto may be associated with other autoimmune diseases (SLE, rheumatoid arthritis, Sjögren syndrome, etc.), and it has an increased risk of non-Hodgkin B-cell lymphoma. Grossly, Hashimoto produces a pale, enlarged thyroid gland; microscopically, it shows lymphocytic inflammation with germinal centers and epithelial "Hürthle cell" changes.

Subacute thyroiditis (also called de Quervain thyroiditis and granulomatous thyroiditis) is the second most common form of thyroiditis; it affects females more than males, with peak age 30–50. Patients may complain of odynophagia (pain on swallowing).

- Typically preceded by a viral illness
- Produces a tender, firm, enlarged thyroid gland
- May be accompanied by transient hyperthyroidism

Microscopy shows granulomatous thyroiditis. The disease typically follows a self-limited course.

Riedel thyroiditis is a rare disease of unknown etiology, characterized by destruction of the thyroid gland by dense fibrosis and fibrosis of surrounding structures (trachea and esophagus). It affects females more than males, and most patients are middle-aged.

Microscopic exam shows dense fibrous replacement of the thyroid gland with chronic inflammation. Reidel thyroiditis is associated with retroperitoneal and mediastinal fibrosis.

Thyroid Neoplasia

Thyroglossal duct cyst presents as a midline neck mass in a young patient. Its epithelium varies with location (squamous/respiratory). It may become infected and painful. Treatment is surgical.

Adenomas: follicular adenoma is the most common. Clinically, adenomas are usually painless, solitary, encapsulated nodules that appear "cold" on thyroid scans. They may be functional and cause hyperthyroidism (toxic adenoma).

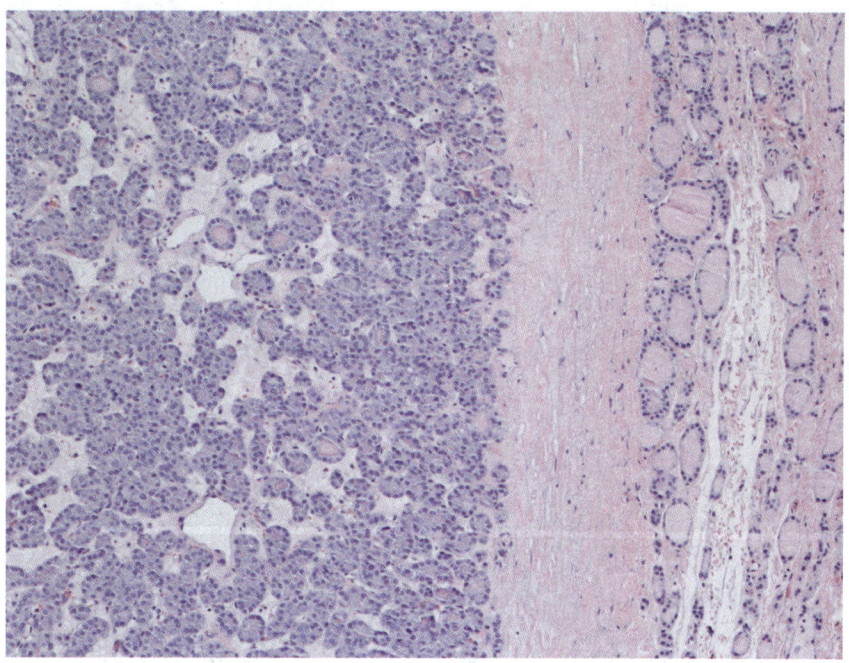

Figure 25-1. Follicular Adenoma *(left)*, Separated from Normal Thyroid
Parenchyma *(right)*, by the Capsule *(center)*

© Gregg Barré, M.D.Used with permission.

Papillary carcinoma accounts for 80% of malignant thyroid tumors. It affects females more than males, with peak age 20–50. Radiation exposure is a risk factor.

Microscopically, the tumor typically exhibits a papillary pattern. Occasional psammoma bodies may be seen. Characteristic nuclear features include clear "Orphan Annie eye" nuclei, nuclear grooves, and intranuclear cytoplasmic inclusions. Lymphatic spread to cervical nodes is common.

Follicular carcinoma accounts for 15% of malignant thyroid tumors. It affects females more than males, with peak age 40–60. Hematogenous metastasis to the bones or lungs is common. These cancers are microscopically distinguished from follicular adenoma by the presence of capsular invasion.

Medullary carcinoma accounts for 5% of malignant thyroid tumors. It arises from C cells (parafollicular cells) and secretes calcitonin. Microscopic exam shows nests of polygonal cells in an amyloid stroma.

Anaplastic carcinoma affects females more than males, with peak age >60. It can present with a firm, enlarging, and bulky mass, or with dyspnea and dysphagia. The tumor has a tendency for early widespread metastasis and invasion of the trachea and esophagus. Microscopically, the tumor is composed of undifferentiated, anaplastic, and pleomorphic cells. This very aggressive tumor is often rapidly fatal.

PARATHYROID GLANDS

Primary hyperparathyroidism can be caused by the following:

- Adenomas (80%);
- Parathyroid hyperplasia (15%)
  - Characterized by diffuse enlargement of all 4 glands; the enlarged glands are usually composed of chief cells
  - Parathyroid carcinoma is very rare
- Hyperparathyroidism can also occur as a paraneoplastic syndrome of lung and renal cell carcinomas.

The excess production of parathyroid hormone (PTH) leads to hypercalcemia, with lab studies showing elevated serum calcium and PTH.

In a Nutshell

Osteitis fibrosa cystica (von Recklinghausen disease) is seen when excessive parathyroid hormone (hyperparathyroidism) causes osteoclast activation and generalized bone resorption (causing possible bone pain, deformities, and fractures). It is common in primary hyperparathyroidism.

- Excess parathyroid hormone may be produced by parathyroid adenoma or parathyroid hyperplasia
- "Brown tumors" are masses produced by cystic enlargement of bones with areas of fibrosis and organized hemorrhage

---

Primary hyperparathyroidism is often asymptomatic, but may cause kidney stones, osteoporosis and osteitis fibrosa cystica, metastatic calcifications, or neurologic changes.

Secondary hyperparathyroidism is caused by any disease that results in hypocalcemia, leading to increased secretion of PTH by the parathyroid glands; it can result from chronic renal failure, vitamin D deficiency, or malabsorption.

Hypoparathyroidism can result from the surgical removal of glands during thyroidectomy, DiGeorge syndrome, or a hereditary autoimmune syndrome caused by mutations in the autoimmune regulator gene *AIRE*. Patients present with muscle spasm and tingling of toes and lips. The hypocalcemia may also cause psychiatric disturbances and cardiac conduction defects.

PITUITARY GLAND, HYPOTHALAMUS, AND PINEAL GLAND

Note: additional information can be found in Chapter 21 of Part 2: Physiology.

Pituitary adenomas are categorized as follows:

- **Microadenoma** if <1 cm
- **Macroadenoma** if >1 cm

Macroadenomas cause visual field defects.

- **Prolactinoma** is the most common type of pituitary adenoma. Lactotroph cells secrete prolactin, which results in hyperprolactinemia. Clinical features include galactorrhea, amenorrhea, and infertility, or decreased libido and impotence.
- **Nonfunctional adenoma** may produce hypopituitarism.
- **Growth-hormone–producing adenoma** is characterized by elevated growth hormone (GH) and elevated somatomedin C (insulin-like growth factor 1 [IGF-1]). It causes gigantism in children and acromegaly in adults.

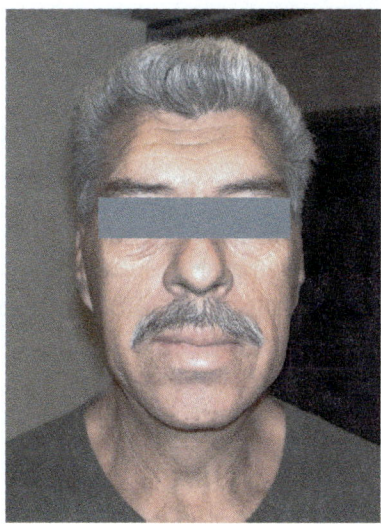

Figure 25-2. Coarse Facial Features and Protruding Jaw
Seen with Acromegaly

© Richard P. Usatine, M.D. Used with permission.

Sheehan syndrome is ischemic necrosis of the pituitary secondary to hypotension from postpartum hemorrhage resulting in panhypopituitarism.

Posterior pituitary syndromes include the following:

- **Diabetes insipidus**
  - ○ Central diabetes insipidus is caused by ADH deficiency, which results in hypotonic polyuria, polydipsia, hypernatremia, and dehydration. Causes include head trauma and tumors.
  - ○ Nephrogenic diabetes insipidus is caused by a lack of renal response to ADH.
- **Syndrome of inappropriate ADH secretion (SIADH)** is caused by excessive production of antidiuretic hormone (ADH), resulting in oliguria, water retention, hyponatremia, and cerebral edema. Causes include paraneoplastic syndrome and head trauma.
  Craniopharyngioma is a benign pituitary tumor derived from Rathke pouch remnants that is usually located above the sella turcica, but can extend downward to destroy the pituitary. It is the most common cause of hypopituitarism in children.

Hypothalamic disorders can cause a variety of problems:

- **Hypopituitarism** (including dwarfism) can be due to a lack of releasing hormones from the hypothalamus.
- **Central diabetes insipidus** is due to lack of ADH synthesis.
- **Precocious puberty** is usually due to a midline hamartoma in boys.
- The hypothalamus can also be affected in **hydrocephalus**.
- **Visual field changes** can complicate hypothalmic disorders.
- Masses can affect the hypothalamus, i.e., pituitary adenoma, craniopharyngioma, midline hamartoma, and Langerhans histiocytosis.
- Inflammatory processes can affect the hypothalamus, i.e., sarcoidosis and meningitis.
  Pineal diseases include dystrophic calcification (a useful landmark for radiologists) and rarely tumors, with most being germ cell tumors.

ADRENAL GLAND

Note: additional information can be found in Chapter 23 and 24 of Part 2: Physiology.

Cushing syndrome is characterized by increased levels of glucocorticoids. The most common cause is exogenous glucocorticoid administration.

Endogenous causes include:

- Cushing disease (hypersecretion of ACTH, usually due to a pituitary microadenoma)
- Secretion of ACTH from nonpituitary tumors (e.g., small cell lung cancer)
- ACTH-independent Cushing syndrome due to adrenal neoplasia

Clinical manifestations include hypertension, weight gain (truncal obesity, "buffalo hump" and moon facies), cutaneous striae, hirsutism and mental disturbances.

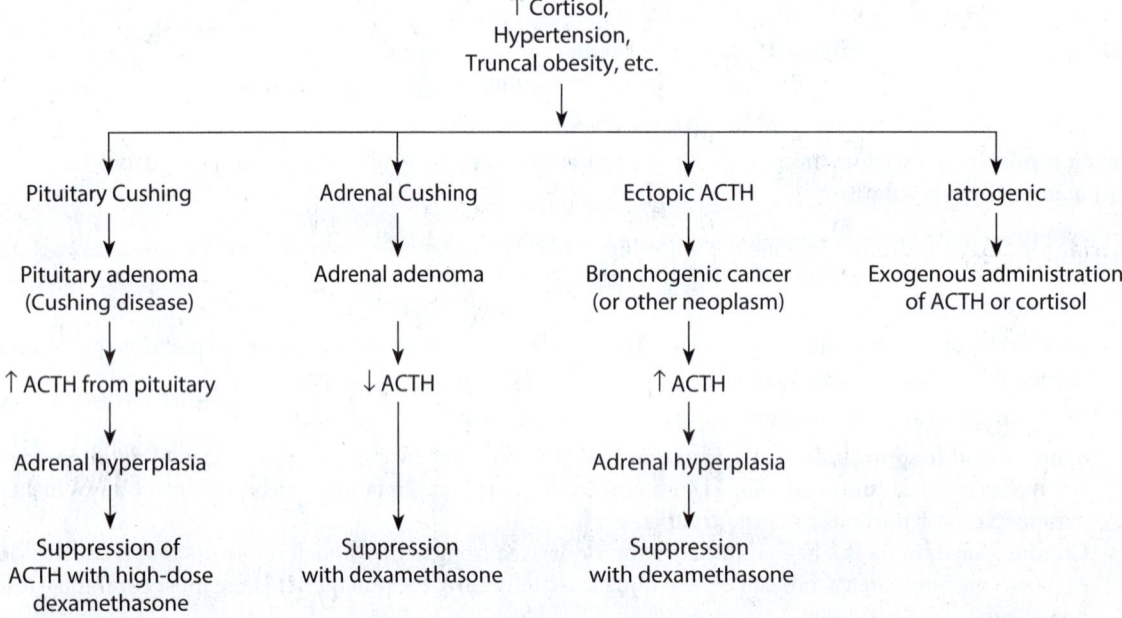

Figure 25-3. Cushing Syndrome and Its Effects

Hyperaldosteronism may cause hypertension and hypokalemia.

- **Primary** (decreased plasma renin)
  - Adrenocortical neoplasm: adenoma (Conn syndrome)
    - Circumscribed yellow nodule with vacuolated cells
    - Carcinoma: poorly demarcated lesion with cystic change and pleomorphic cells
  - Bilateral nodular hyperplasia of the adrenal
- **Secondary** (increased plasma renin) (e.g., renal artery stenosis)

Bridge to Embryology

The cells of the **adrenal medulla** are derived from neural crest cells.

The cells of the **adrenal cortex** are derived from mesoderm.

Adrenogenital syndromes are adrenal disorders characterized by excess production of androgens and virilization. They are caused either by adrenocortical adenoma/carcinoma, which produces androgens, or by congenital adrenal hyperplasia, a cluster of autosomal recessive enzyme defects (most common is 21-hydroxylase deficiency).

Waterhouse-Friderichsen syndrome (acute adrenal insufficiency) is a potentially fatal, bilateral hemorrhagic infarction of the adrenal glands associated with sepsis, often due to a *N. meningitidis* infection in children. It is clinically characterized by disseminated intravascular coagulation (DIC), acute respiratory distress syndrome, hypotension and shock, and acute adrenal insufficiency.

Addison's disease (chronic adrenocortical insufficiency) is caused by destruction of the adrenal cortex, leading to a deficiency of glucocorticoids, mineralocorticoids, and androgens. The most common cause is autoimmune adrenalitis, though adrenal involvement by TB or metastatic cancer are other possible causes. Patients present with gradual onset of weakness, skin hyperpigmentation, hypotension, hypoglycemia, poor response to stress, and loss of libido. Treatment is steroid replacement.

Secondary adrenocortical insufficiency may be caused by disorders of the hypothalamus or pituitary (cancer or infection, for example). Since ACTH levels are low, hyperpigmentation does not occur.

Pheochromocytoma ("dark/dusky-colored tumor") is an uncommon benign tumor of the adrenal medulla, which produces catecholamines (norepinephrine and epinephrine). It can present with sustained or episodic hypertension and associated severe headache, tachycardia, palpitations, diaphoresis, and anxiety.

Urinary vanillylmandelic acid (VMA) and catecholamines are elevated. Microscopically, the tumor shows nests of cells (Zellballen) with abundant cytoplasm.

MULTIPLE ENDOCRINE NEOPLASIA SYNDROMES

Multiple endocrine neoplasia (MEN) syndromes are autosomal dominant conditions with incomplete penetrance that are characterized by hyperplasia and tumors of endocrine glands occurring at a young age.

- **MEN 1** (Werner syndrome) features tumors of the pituitary gland, parathyroids, and pancreas.
- Associated with peptic ulcers and Zollinger-Ellison syndrome
- **MEN 2A** (Sipple syndrome) features medullary carcinoma of the thyroid, pheochromocytoma, and parathyroid hyperplasia or adenoma.
- **MEN 2B** features medullary carcinoma of the thyroid, pheochromocytoma, and mucocutaneous neuromas.

DIABETES MELLITUS

Note: additional information can be found in Chapter 25 of Part 2: Physiology.

Diabetes mellitus (DM) is a chronic systemic disease characterized by insulin deficiency or peripheral resistance, resulting in hyperglycemia and nonenzymatic glycosylation of proteins. Diagnosis is established by demonstrating **either** of the following:

- Fasting glucose >126 mg/dL on at least two separate occasions
- Positive glucose tolerance test

A glycated hemoglobin (HbA1c) assay is used for certain patient populations. The diagnostic cutoff is 6.5%.

Type 1 diabetes (T1D) represents 10% of cases of diabetes.

- Affects children and adolescents, usually age <20
- Risk factors include Northern European ancestry and specific HLA types
- Pathogenesis is a lack of insulin due to autoimmune destruction of β cells (type IV hypersensitivity reaction)
- Patients are absolutely dependent on insulin to prevent ketoacidosis and coma
- Thought to be caused by autoimmune reaction triggered by an infection (Coxsackie B virus) in a genetically susceptible individual

T1D can present with polydipsia, polyuria, and polyphagia; dehydration and electrolyte imbalance; metabolic ketoacidosis; and coma and potentially death. Microscopically, lymphocytic inflammation involves the islets of Langerhans (insulitis), leading to loss of β cells and fibrosis of the islets. Treatment is insulin.

Type 2 diabetes (T2D) represents 90% of cases.

- Affects obese individuals, both children and adults
- Approximately 10 million people in the United States are affected (half are undiagnosed), and incidence increases with age
- Risk factors include obesity, increasing age, and genetic predisposition
- Pathogenesis involves relatively reduced insulin secretion; *peripheral insulin resistance* is the term used for reduced tissue sensitivity to insulin due to decreased numbers of insulin receptors on the cell membranes.

T2D is often asymptomatic, but it can present with either polydipsia, polyuria, and polyphagia, or with hyperosmolar nonketotic diabetic coma. Microscopically, the changes are nonspecific, and can include focal atrophy and amyloid deposition in islets (hyalinization). Treatment is diet/weight loss, oral antidiabetic drugs, and insulin as needed (more common in long-standing cases).

Vascular pathology. Diabetes is a major risk factor for atherosclerosis and its complications, including myocardial infarction (most common cause of death), stroke (CVA), and peripheral vascular disease. The vascular disease can lead to atrophy of skin and loss of hair of the lower extremities, claudication, nonhealing ulcers, and gangrene of lower extremities.

Diabetic effects on oral tissue include more rapid progression of periodontal disease, loss of attachment, and alveolar bone loss. Research shows a two-way relationship of HbA1c and periodontal disease. Elevated HbA1c results in worsened periodontal condition, while improvements to periodontal condition can lower HbA1c.

In dental treatment, uncontrolled diabetics require antibiotics more regularly for periodontic treatment and oral surgery. Uncontrolled diabetes is also a contraindication for implants.

Diabetic nephropathy includes glomerular lesions, arteriolosclerosis, and pyelonephritis (*see* Renal chapter).

Diabetic retinopathy. Nonproliferative retinopathy is characterized by microaneurysms, retinal hemorrhages, and retinal exudates. Proliferative retinopathy is characterized by neovascularization and fibrosis. Diabetics also have an increased incidence of cataracts and glaucoma.

Diabetic neuropathy can cause peripheral neuropathy, neurogenic bladder, and sexual impotence.

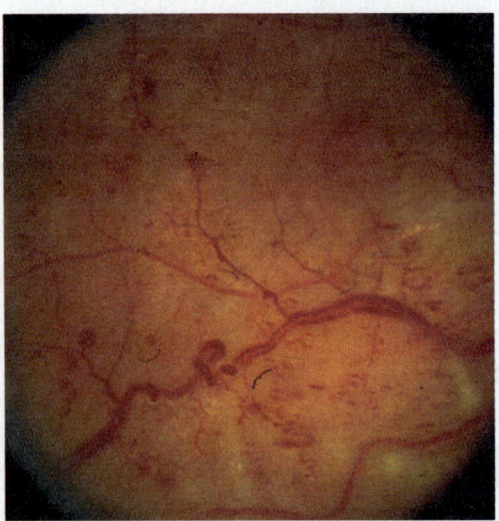

Figure 25-4. Diabetic Retinopathy with Hemorrhages, Venous Beading, and Looping of Vessels

© Richard P. Usatine, M.D. / Paul D. Comeau, M.D. Used with permission.

Bone Pathology 26

Learning Objectives

❏ Describe normal bone

❏ Explain information related to hereditary bone disorders

❏ Answer questions about Paget disease

❏ Differentiate osteoporosis, osteomalacia, and rickets

❏ Solve problems concerning osteomyelitis, benign tumors of bone, and malignant tumors of bone

NORMAL BONE

Normal bone is composed of organic matrix and inorganic matrix.

- The **organic matrix** includes cells, type I collagen (90% of bone protein), osteocalcin, glycoproteins, and proteoglycans.
- The **inorganic matrix** includes calcium hydroxyapatite $Ca_{10}(PO_4)_6(OH)_2$, magnesium, potassium, chloride, sodium, and fluoride.

There are three cell types.

- **Osteoblasts** are responsible for the production of osteoid (unmineralized bone); they contain high amounts of alkaline phosphatase, have receptors for parathyroid hormone (PTH), and modulate osteoclast function.
- **Osteocytes** are responsible for bone maintenance; they are osteoblasts that have become incorporated in the matrix.
- **Osteoclasts** are responsible for bone resorption; they contain high amounts of acid phosphatase and collagenase, and resorb bone within Howship's lacunae.

Bone remodeling occurs throughout life and is necessary to maintain healthy bones. Bone resorption by osteoclasts is tightly balanced with bone formation by osteoblasts.

Important hormones involved in bone physiology include parathyroid hormone (PTH), calcitonin, vitamin D, estrogen, thyroid hormone, cortisol, and growth hormone.

Formation of bones is as follows:

- **Intramembranous bone** occurs as direct bone formation without a "cartilage model." Intramembranous bones include flat bones such as the flat bones of the skull (frontal, parietal, flat portions of the temporal and occipital, most of the maxilla and the mandible, except for the condyle), clavicle, vertebrae, wrist, and ankle bones.
- **Endochondral bone** is indirect bone formation from a "cartilage model" at the epiphyseal growth plates; this type of bone formation occurs in long bones such as the femur, humerus, tibia, fibula, etc. In the head and neck, the sphenoid, ethmoid, and non-flat parts of the occipital and temporal bones are endochondral. The condyle (only) of the mandible is endochondral.

HEREDITARY BONE DISORDERS

Achondroplasia is the most common form of inherited dwarfism. It is caused by an autosomal dominant mutation which inhibits cartilage synthesis at the epiphyseal growth plate, resulting in decreased enchondral bone formation and premature ossification of the growth plates.

- Long bones are short and thick, leading to dwarfism with short extremities.
- Cranial and vertebral bones are spared, leading to relatively large head and trunk.
- Intelligence, life span, and reproductive ability are normal.

Osteogenesis imperfecta (OI) ("brittle bone disease") is a hereditary defect leading to abnormal synthesis of type I collagen.

- Patients have generalized osteopenia (brittle bones), resulting in recurrent fractures and skeletal deformity
- Abnormally thin sclera with blue hue is common
- Laxity of joint ligaments leads to hypermobility
- Involvement of inner and middle ear bones produces deafness
- Occasional dentinogenesis imperfecta, characterized by small, fragile, and discolored teeth due to a deficiency of dentin
- Dermis may be abnormally thin, and skin is susceptible to easy bruising
- Treatment is supportive

Osteopetrosis (or marble bone disease) is a hereditary defect leading to decreased osteoclast function, with resulting decreased resorption and thick sclerotic bones. X-ray shows symmetrical generalized osteosclerosis. Long bones may have broadened metaphyses, causing an "Erlenmeyer flask"-shaped deformity. Treatment is hematopoietic stem cell transplantation.

- **Autosomal recessive** type (**malignant**):
  - Affects infants and children (causes multiple fractures and early death due to anemia, infection, and hemorrhage)
- **Autosomal dominant** type (**benign**):
  - Affects adults (causes fractures, mild anemia, and cranial nerve impingement)

Pathology shows increased bone density and thickening of bone cortex. Myelophthisic anemia may result from marrow crowding. Cranial nerve compression due to narrowing of cranial foramina may result in blindness, deafness, and facial nerve palsies. Hydrocephalus may develop due to obstruction of CSF.

PAGET DISEASE

Paget disease (osteitis deformans) is a localized disorder of bone remodeling, resulting in excessive bone resorption followed by disorganized bone replacement, producing thickened but weak bone that is susceptible to deformity and fracture. There is an association with paramyxovirus.

- Seen in those age >40
- Common in those of European ancestry
- Common sites of involvement include the skull, pelvis, femur, and vertebrae
- Majority of cases are polyostotic and mild

Paget disease develops in three stages:

- **Osteolytic stage** (osteoclastic activity predominates)
- **Mixed osteolytic-osteoblastic stage**
- **Osteosclerotic stage** (osteoblastic activity predominates in this "burnout stage")

Paget disease can cause bone pain and deformity, fractures, and warmth of the overlying skin due to bone hypervascularity. X-rays show bone enlargement with lytic and sclerotic areas. Lab studies show highly elevated serum alkaline phosphatase and increased levels of urinary hydroxyproline. Complications include arteriovenous shunts within marrow, which may result in high-output cardiac failure and an increased incidence of osteosarcoma and other sarcomas.

Microscopically, there is a haphazard arrangement of cement lines, creating a "mosaic pattern" of lamellar bone. Involved bones are thick but weak and fracture easily. Skull involvement leads to increased head size and foraminal narrowing that can impinge on cranial nerves, often leading to deafness. Involvement of facial bones may produce a lion-like facies.

OSTEOPOROSIS

Osteoporosis is decreased bone mass (osteopenia), resulting in thin, fragile bones susceptible to fracture. It is the most common bone disorder in the United States. It most commonly occurs in postmenopausal Caucasian women and the elderly.

Note

In osteoporosis, bone is formed normally but in decreased amounts.

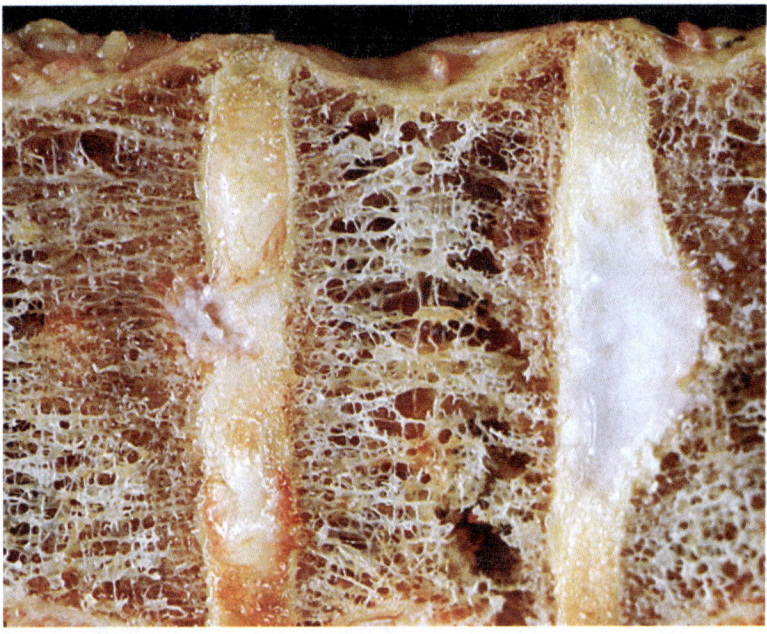

Figure 26-1. Marked Thinning of Bony Trabeculae in Osteoporosis
© Katsumi M. Miyai, M.D., Ph.D.; Regents of the University of California. Used with permission.

Primary causes of osteoporosis include the following:

- Estrogen deficiency (postmenopausal, Turner syndrome)
- Genetic factors (low density of original bone)
- Lack of exercise
- Old age
- Nutritional factors

Secondary causes include immobilization, endocrinopathies (e.g., Cushing disease, thyrotoxicosis), malnutrition (e.g., deficiencies of calcium, vitamins C and D, protein), corticosteroids, smoking/alcohol consumption, genetic disease (e.g., Gaucher disease).

- Patients may experience bone pain and fractures; weight-bearing bones are predisposed to fractures.
- Common fracture sites include vertebrae (compression fracture); femoral neck (hip fracture); and distal radius (Colles fracture).
- Kyphosis and loss of height may result.
- X-rays show generalized radiolucency of bone (osteopenia).

Dual-energy X-ray absorptiometry (DEXA) can measure bone mineral density to predict fracture risk. Lab studies may show normal serum calcium, phosphorus, and alkaline phosphatase, but the diagnosis is not based on labs. Microscopically, the bone has thinned cortical and trabecular bone.

Treatment can include estrogen replacement therapy (controversial; not recommended currently); weight-bearing exercise; calcium and vitamin D; bisphosphonate (alendronate); and calcitonin.

OSTEOMALACIA AND RICKETS

Osteomalacia and **rickets** are both characterized by decreased mineralization of newly formed bone. They are usually caused by deficiency or abnormal metabolism of vitamin D. Specific causes include dietary deficiency of vitamin D, intestinal malabsorption, lack of sunlight, and renal and liver disease. Treatment is vitamin D and calcium supplementation.

Osteomalacia (adults) is due to impaired mineralization of the osteoid matrix resulting in thin, fragile bones susceptible to fracture. The patient may present clinically with bone pain or fractures (vertebrae, hips, and wrist). X-rays show transverse lucencies called Looser zones. Lab studies show low serum calcium, low serum phosphorus, and high alkaline phosphatase.

Rickets (children) occurs in children prior to closure of the epiphyses. Both remodeled bone and bone formed at the epiphyseal growth plate are undermineralized. Enchondral bone formation is affected, leading to skeletal deformities. Skull deformities include craniotabes (softening, seen in early infancy) and frontal bossing (hardening, later in childhood). The "rachitic rosary" is a deformity of the chest wall as a result of an overgrowth of cartilage at the costochondral junction. Pectus carinatum, lumbar lordosis, bowing of the legs, and fractures also occur.

Note

Rickets and osteomalacia are disorders of osteoid mineralization; osteoid is produced in normal amounts but is not calcified properly.

OSTEOMYELITIS

Pyogenic osteomyelitis is bone inflammation due to bacterial infection. The most common route of infection is **hematogenous spread** (leading to seeding of bone after bacteremia); this type of spread often affects the metaphysis. Other routes of spread include direct inoculation (e.g., trauma) and spread from an adjacent site of infection (e.g., prosthetic joint).

The most common infecting organism is *S. aureus*; other important pathogens include *E. coli*, streptococci, gonococci, *H. influenzae*, *Salmonella* (common in sickle cell disease), and *Pseudomonas* (common in IV drug abusers and diabetics).

Clinically, osteomyelitis is characterized by fever and leukocytosis; and localized pain, erythema, and swelling. X-ray studies may be normal for up to t weeks, and then initially show periosteal elevation followed by a possible lytic focus with surrounding sclerosis. MRI and nuclear medicine studies are more sensitive and specific.

Microscopic examination shows suppurative inflammation. Vascular insufficiency can lead to ischemic necrosis of bone; a sequestrum is an area of necrotic bone, while an involucrum is the new bone formation that surrounds the sequestrum. The diagnosis is established with blood cultures or with bone biopsy and culture.

Complications include fracture, intraosseous (Brodie) abscess, secondary amyloidosis, sinus tract formation, squamous cell carcinoma of the skin at the site of a persistent draining sinus tract, and, rarely, osteogenic sarcoma.

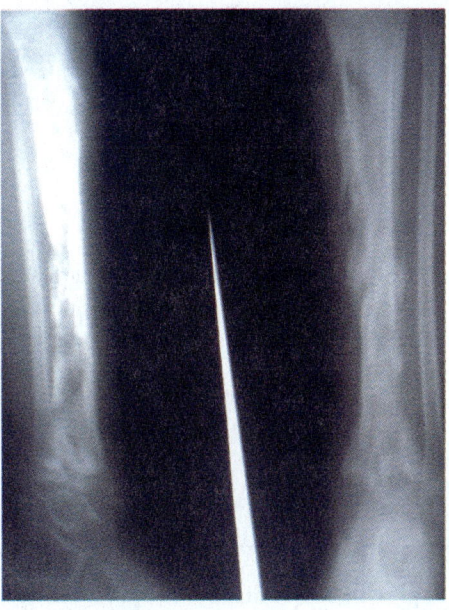

Figure 26-2. Tibial Radiolucencies Representing Osteomyelitis.
Source: commons.wikimedia.org

Tuberculous osteomyelitis is seen in 1% of cases of TB. It presents with pain or tenderness, fever, night sweats, and weight loss. Biopsy shows caseating granulomas with extensive destruction of the bones. Common sites of involvement include thoracic and lumbar vertebrae ("Pott disease"). Complications include vertebral compression fracture, psoas abscesses, and secondary amyloidosis.

MISCELLANEOUS BONE DISORDERS

Avascular necrosis (or aseptic necrosis and osteonecrosis) is the term used for ischemic necrosis of bone and bone marrow. Causes include trauma and/or fracture (most common); idiopathic; steroid use; sickle cell anemia; Gaucher disease; and caisson disease. Avascular necrosis can be complicated by osteoarthritis and fractures.

Osteitis fibrosa cystica (or von Recklinghausen disease of bone) is seen when excessive parathyroid hormone (hyperparathyroidism) causes osteoclast activation and generalized bone resorption, resulting in possible bone pain, bone deformities, and fractures.

- Seen commonly in primary hyperparathyroidism
- Excess parathyroid hormone may be produced by parathyroid adenoma or parathyroid hyperplasia
- Can be resolved if hyperparathyroidism is treated

Microscopic exam shows excess bone resorption with increased number of osteoclasts, fibrous replacement of marrow, and cystic spaces in trabecular bone (dissecting osteitis). "Brown tumors" are brown bone masses produced by cystic enlargement of bones with areas of fibrosis and organized hemorrhage.

Hypertrophic osteoarthropathy presents with painful swelling of wrists, fingers, ankles, knees, or elbows.

- Seen in the setting of bronchogenic carcinoma (a paraneoplastic syndrome), chronic lung diseases, cyanotic congenital heart disease, and inflammatory bowel disease
- Can regress if underlying disease is treated

Pathologically, the ends of long bones show periosteal new bone formation, which can produce digital clubbing and often arthritis of adjacent joints.

Osgood-Schlatter disease is a common cause of knee pain in adolescents. It develops when stress from the quadriceps during rapid growth causes inflammation of the proximal tibial apophysis at the insertion of the patellar tendon. Permanent changes to the knees (knobby knees) may develop. The lesion is not usually biopsied.

Fibrous dysplasia presents with painful swelling, deformity, or pathologic fracture of involved bone (typically ribs, femur, or cranial bones), usually in children and young adults. Gene mutations cause osteoblasts to produce fibrous tissue (microscopically, irregularly scattered trabelculae) rather than bone.

BENIGN TUMORS OF BONE

Osteoma is a benign neoplasm that frequently involves the skull and facial bones. Osteoma can be associated with Gardner syndrome. Malignant transformation doesn't occur.

Osteoid osteoma is a benign, painful growth of the diaphysis of a long bone, often the tibia or femur. Males are affected more than females, with peak age 5–25. Pain tends to be worse at night and relieved by aspirin. X-rays show central radiolucency surrounded by a sclerotic rim. Microscopically, ostoblasts line randomly connected trabeculae.

Osteoblastoma is similar to an osteoid osteoma but larger (>2 cm) and often involves vertebrae.

Osteochondroma (exostosis) is a benign bony metaphyseal growth capped with cartilage, which originates from epiphyseal growth plate. It typically presents in adolescent males who have firm, solitary growths at the ends of long bones. It may be asymptomatic, cause pain, produce deformity, or undergo malignant transformation (rare). *Osteochondromatosis* (multiple hereditary exostoses) produces multiple, often symmetric, osteochondromas.

Enchondroma is a benign cartilaginous growth within the medullary cavity of bone, usually involving the hands and feet. It is typically solitary, asymptomatic, and requires no treatment.

Giant cell tumor of bone ("osteoclastoma") is a benign neoplasm containing multinucleated giant cells admixed with stromal cells. It is uncommon but occurs more often in females than in males, with peak age 20–50. Clinically, the tumor produces a bulky mass with pain and fractures. X-rays show an expanding lytic lesion surrounded by a thin rim of bone, with a possible "soap bubble" appearance. In spite of being considered benign, approximately 2% will metastasize to the lungs.

Grossly, the tumor causes a red-brown mass with cystic degeneration that often involves the epiphyses of long bones, usually around the knee (distal femur and proximal tibia). Microscopically, multiple osteoclast-like giant cells are distributed within a background of mononuclear stromal cells.

MALIGNANT TUMORS OF BONE

Osteosarcoma (osteogenic sarcoma) is the most common primary malignant tumor of bone. It occurs more frequently in males than in females, with most cases in teenage years (ages 10–25). Patients with familial retinoblastoma have a high risk.

Osteosarcoma presents with localized pain and swelling. The classic x-ray findings are Codman triangle (periosteal elevation), "sun burst" pattern, and bone destruction. Hematogenous metastasis to the lungs is common. **Secondary osteosarcoma** is seen in the elderly; these highly aggressive tumors are associated with Paget disease, irradiation, and chronic osteomyelitis.

Grossly, osteosarcoma often involves the metaphyses of long bones, usually around the knee (distal femur and proximal tibia). It produces a large, firm, white-tan mass with necrosis and hemorrhage. Microscopically, anaplastic cells producing osteoid and bone are seen.

Chondrosarcoma is a malignant tumor of chondroblasts which may arise *de novo* or secondary to a preexisting enchondroma, exostosis, or Paget disease. Males are affected more frequently than females, with peak ages 30–60. It presents with enlarging mass with pain and swelling, and it typically involves the pelvic bones, spine, and shoulder girdle. Microscopically, there is cartilaginous matrix production. Radiographs show osteolytic destruction and "popcorn" calcification.

Ewing sarcoma is a malignant neoplasm of undifferentiated cells arising within the marrow cavity. Males are affected slightly more often than females, with most cases in teenage years (ages 5–20).

Clinically, patients present with pain, swelling, and tenderness. X-ray studies show concentric "onion-skin" layering of new periosteal bone with soft tissue extension. Treatment is chemotherapy, surgery, and/or radiation; the 5-year survival rate is 75%.

Grossly, Ewing sarcoma often affects the diaphyses of long bones, with the most common sites being the femur, pelvis, and tibia. The tumor characteristically produces a white-tan mass with necrosis and hemorrhage. Microscopically, Ewing sarcoma is characterized by sheets of undifferentiated small, round, blue cells resembling lymphocytes, which may form Homer Wright pseudorosettes. The tumor cells erode through the cortex and periosteum and invade surrounding tissues.

Metastasis to bone is much more common than primary bone tumor. Common primary sites include prostate (often osteoblastic), breast, lung, thyroid, and kidney.

Joint Pathology 27

Learning Objectives

❏ Solve problems concerning osteoarthritis, rheumatoid arthritis, and seronegative spondyloarthropathies

❏ Describe arthritis related to crystal deposition, infectious arthritis, and neuropathic arthropathy (Charcot joint)

Table 27-1. Osteoarthritis vs RA

Osteoarthritis	RA
"Wear and tear"	Systemic autoimmune disease
	(+) Rheumatoid factor
	(+) Rheumatoid nodules
Degeneration of articular cartilage	Synovial proliferation
Knees and hands (DIP) in women; hips in men	Hands (PIP) and feet
Asymmetrical	Symmetrical and migratory

OSTEOARTHRITIS

Osteoarthritis (OA) (degenerative joint disease) is joint degeneration with loss of articular cartilage, with no to minimal inflammation. It is the most common form of arthritis. Risk increases with age; OA affects at least 1 joint in 80% of people age >70.

Clinically, there is an insidious onset of joint stiffness; deep, aching joint pain, which worsens with repetitive motion; decreased range of motion; crepitus; and joint effusions and swelling. Osteophytes may cause nerve compression. X-ray studies show narrowing of the joint space due to loss of cartilage; osteosclerosis and bone cysts; and osteophytes (osteophytic lipping).

The pathogenesis involves both biomechanical factors (aging or wear and tear of articular cartilage) and biochemical factors (chondrocyte injury and abnormal collagen activity). Predisposing factors include obesity, previous joint injury, ochronosis, diabetes, and hemarthrosis.

OA affects weight-bearing joints (knees, hips, and spine), often with asymmetrical involvement.

- There is degeneration and loss of articular cartilage with eburnation (exposed bone becomes polished) and subchondral bone sclerosis.
- The changes may include subchondral bone cysts, loose bodies (joint mice), which are free-floating fragments of cartilage and bone, and osteophytes (bone spurs), which are reactive bony outgrowths.
- **Heberden nodes** are osteophytes at the distal interphalangeal (DIP) joints, while **Bouchard nodes** are osteophytes at the proximal interphalangeal (PIP) joints.

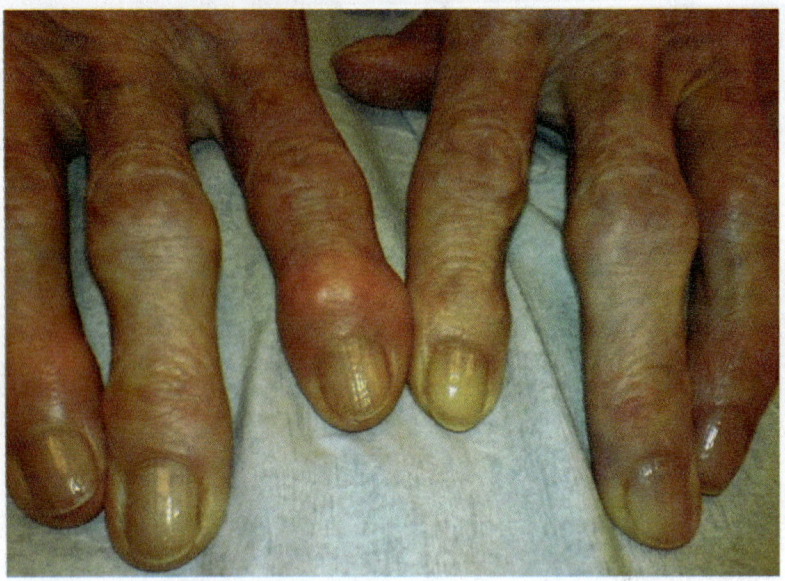

Figure 27-1. Heberden (Distal Interphalangeal Joint) and Bouchard (Proximal Interphalangeal Joint) Nodes in Patient with Osteoarthritis

© commons.wikimedia.org.

RHEUMATOID ARTHRITIS

Rheumatoid arthritis (RA) is a systemic, chronic, inflammatory disease characterized by progressive arthritis, production of rheumatoid factor, and extra-articular manifestations. It affects females 4x more than men, with highest incidence at ages 20–50. Some cases have a genetic predisposition.

RA is thought to be caused by an autoimmune reaction triggered by an infectious agent in a genetically susceptible individual.

RA most commonly affects the hand, wrist, knee, and ankle joints, and the involvement tends to be symmetrical. There is often morning stiffness which improves with activity.

- There is typically fusiform swelling, redness, and warmth of the proximal interphalangeal (PIP) joint.
- X-ray studies show juxta-articular osteoporosis and bone erosions; joint effusion may also be present.
- RA causes a diffuse proliferative synovitis, pannus formation (proliferation of the synovium and granulation tissue over the articular cartilage of the joint), fibrous and bony ankylosis (joint fusion), and joint deformities. Joint deformities can include:
  - Radial deviation of the wrist and ulnar deviation of the fingers
  - Swan neck deformity (hyperextension of PIP joint and flexion of DIP joint
  - Boutonniere deformity (flexion of PIP and extension of DIP joints)
- Baker cysts (synovial cysts in the popliteal fossa) may be present.

Lab studies show elevated sedimentation rate and hypergammaglobulinemia. Rheumatoid factor (RF) is an autoantibody (usually IgM) against the Fc fragment of IgG; it is present in 80% of cases. RF may circulate and form immune complexes, and titer of RF correlates with the severity of the arthritis and prognosis.

- Extra-articular manifestations may be prominent. Systemic symptoms include low-grade fever, malaise, fatigue, lymphadenopathy, and weakness. Arteries may show acute necrotizing vasculitis due to circulating antigen-antibody complexes.

- Rheumatoid nodules, subcutaneous skin nodules, are present in 25% of cases. They are usually found on extensor surfaces of the forearms and elbows, but can also be found in the heart valves, lung, pleura, pericardium, and spleen. They are composed of central fibrinoid necrosis surrounded by epithelioid macrophages, lymphocytes, and granulation tissue.

- **Sjögren syndrome** may be present in 15%. In **Felty syndrome**, RA accompanies splenomegaly and neutropenia. In **Caplan syndrome**, RA is associated with pneumoconiosis.

- Secondary amyloidosis may also complicate RA.

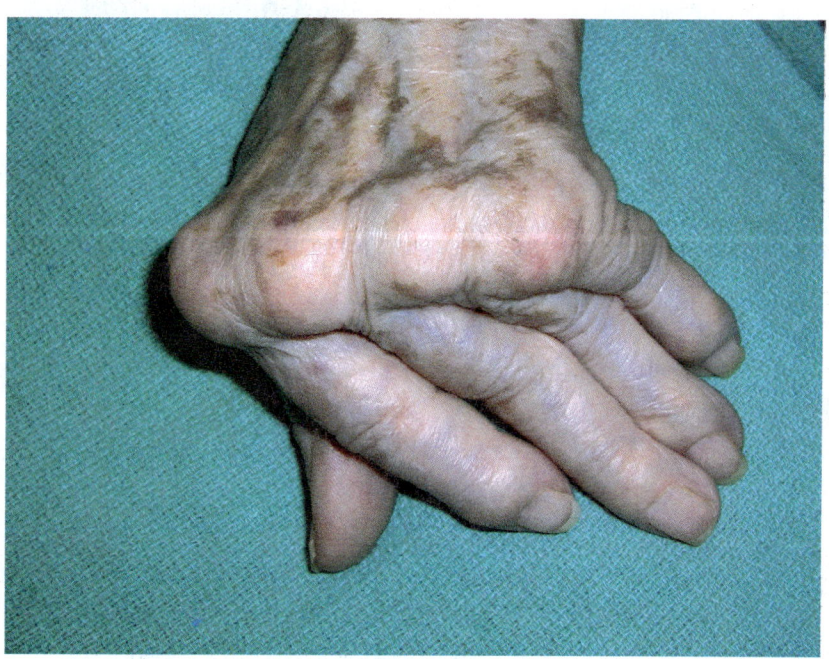

Figure 27-2. Ulnar Deviation at the Metacarpophalangeal Joints
in Advanced Rheumatoid Arthritis

© Richard P. Usatine, M.D. Used with permission.

SERONEGATIVE SPONDYLOARTHROPATHIES

Seronegative spondyloarthropathies are a group of disorders characterized by the following:

- Rheumatoid factor seronegativity
- Involvement of the sacroiliac joints
- Association with HLA-B27

Ankylosing spondylitis occurs predominantly in young men with HLA-B27 (90% of cases); usually involves the sacroiliac joints and spine; and may be associated with inflammatory bowel disease.

Clinical Correlate
Complete fusion of the spine can occur in ankylosing spondylitis and can cause complete rigidity of the spine. The resulting condition is known as bamboo spine, which can be seen on X-ray.

Reactive arthritis is characterized by a classic triad of conjunctivitis, urethritis, and arthritis. The arthritis affects the ankles and knees. It affects males more than females, with onset age 20s–30s. Onset often follows a venereal disease or bacillary dysentery.

Enteropathic arthritis occurs in 10–20% of patients with inflammatory bowel disease.

Psoriatic arthritis affects 5–10% of patients with psoriasis; is often a mild and slowly progressive arthritis, with pathology similar to RA.

ARTHRITIS RELATED TO CRYSTAL DEPOSITION

In **gout**, hyperuricemia and the deposition of monosodium urate crystals in joints will result in recurrent bouts of acute arthritis. The hyperuricemia can be caused by overproduction or underexcretion of uric acid.

- **Primary gout** (90%) is idiopathic, affects males more than females, and is typically seen in older men.
- **Secondary gout** (10%) is seen with excessive cell breakdown (chemotherapy), decreased renal excretion (drugs), and Lesch-Nyhan syndrome.

Bridge to Biochemistry
Uric acid is the end product of purine metabolism.

Gout affects the great toe (podagra, characterized by an exquisitely painful, inflamed big toe), ankle, heel, and wrist.

Joint aspiration shows birefringent, needle-shaped uric acid crystals and numerous neutrophils. **Tophi** are deposits of crystals surrounded by inflammation. Skin ulceration and destruction of adjacent joints may occur. Complications include joint destruction and deformity, uric acid renal calculi, and renal failure.

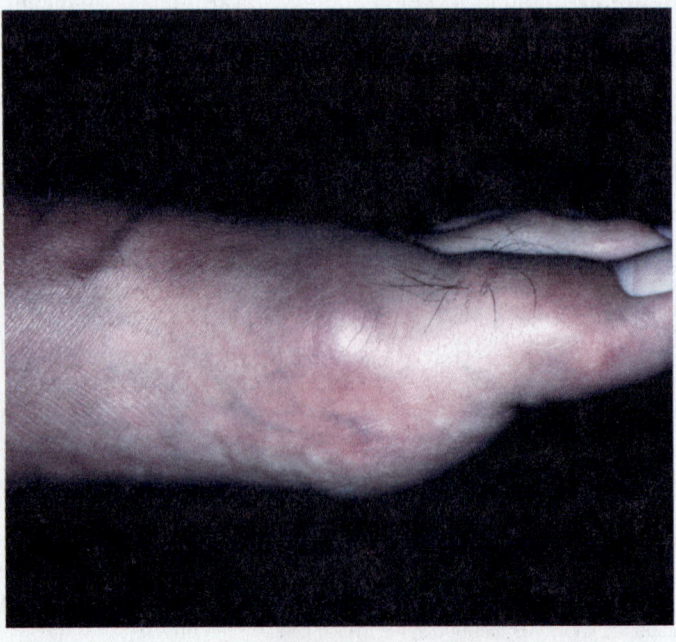

Figure 27-3. Gout
© Richard P. Usatine, M.D. Used with permission.

Pseudogout (chondrocalcinosis) is deposition of calcium pyrophosphate crystals in joints, leading to inflammation. Affected patients are usually age >50. The knee joint is most commonly involved. Aspiration of the joint demonstrates positively birefringent (weak), rhomboid-shaped crystals. Pseudogout is associated with many metabolic diseases (e.g., diabetes, hypothyroidism, ochronosis), and it may mimic OA or RA.

INFECTIOUS ARTHRITIS

Suppurative arthritis may result from seeding of the joint during bacteremia. Other routes include spread from an adjacent site of infection and direct inoculation. Infecting organisms include gonococci, *Staphylococcus*, *Streptococcus*, *H. influenzae*, and gram-negative bacilli.

Suppurative arthritis causes a tender, painful, swollen, and erythematous joint. Large joints (knee, hip, shoulder) are most often infected, and the arthritis is usually monoarticular. Joint aspiration shows cloudy synovial fluid that clots readily and has a high neutrophil count. Gram stain and culture are positive in 50–70% of cases.

Lyme disease is caused by the spirochete *Borrelia burgdorferi*. The disease is arthropod-borne, spread by deer ticks (*Ixodes dammini*). Symptoms are skin rash (erythema chronicum migrans), and migratory arthritis involving the knees, shoulders, and elbows. The histology of the arthritic joint is similar to RA. Lyme disease can also have CNS and cardiac involvement. Serologic tests may remain negative until infection has been present for several weeks.

NEUROPATHIC ARTHROPATHY (CHARCOT JOINT)

Charcot joint refers to joint damage secondary to impaired joint innervation (neuropathy), leading to an inability to sense pain. The damage also leads to destruction of joint surfaces, debris in joints, deformity, and dislocations.

Different **underlying neurologic diseases** tend to affect different joints.

- Diabetes mellitus (most common cause) tends to damage the tarsometatarsal joint in the midfoot.
- Syringomyelia (cavity in spinal cord) tends to damage the shoulder, elbow, and wrist joints.
- Tabes dorsalis (neurosyphilis) tends to damage the hip, knee, and ankle joints.

Skeletal Muscle and Peripheral Nerve Pathology

28

Learning Objectives

❏ Demonstrate understanding of inflammatory myopathies and neuropathies

❏ Describe the mechanism of action of myasthenic syndromes

❏ Explain information related to muscular dystrophy

❏ Solve problems concerning soft tissue and peripheral nerve tumors

Type I (red) skeletal muscle is used in postural weight bearing. It produces a slow twitch as a result of aerobic metabolism of fatty acids.

Type II (white) skeletal muscle is used for purposeful movement. It produces a fast twitch as a result of anaerobic glycolysis of glycogen.

Table 28-1. Type I (Slow-Twitch) Versus Type II (Fast-Twitch) Muscles

	Type I	Type II
Twitch rate	Slow twitch	Fast twitch
Function	Postural weight bearing	Purposeful movement
	Sustained tension	Short, quick bursts
Metabolism	Aerobic (Krebs cycle)	Anaerobic (glycolysis)
Energy source	Fatty acids	Glycogen
Mitochondria	Many	Few
Color	Red	White
Fatigue	Slow fatigue	Rapid fatigue

INFLAMMATORY MYOPATHIES

Polymyositis is an autoimmune disease seen in adults. It presents with bilateral proximal muscle weakness. Microscopic exam demonstrates endomysial lymphocytic inflammation (mostly cytotoxic T8) and skeletal muscle fiber degeneration and regeneration. Patients respond to immunosuppression.

Dermatomyositis is a connective tissue disorder involving inflammation of skeletal muscle and skin. It can affect both children and adults. It presents with bilateral proximal muscle weakness, skin rash of the upper eyelids, and periorbital edema. Microscopic exam demonstrates perimysial and vascular lymphocytic inflammation, perifascicular fiber atrophy, and skeletal muscle fiber degeneration and regeneration. Adult patients are at increased risk of lung, colon, breast, and gynecologic cancers.

Inclusion body myositis affects adults age >50, causing slowly progressive, asymmetrical, distal muscle weakness. Light microscopy demonstrates autophagic vacuoles and inclusion bodies in addition to inflammation and necrosis.

MYASTHENIC SYNDROMES

Myasthenia gravis is an autoimmune disease characterized by autoantibodies against the acetylcholine (ACh) receptor of the neuromuscular junction, resulting in muscular weakness predominantly affecting the facial muscles. Females are affected more frequently than males.

- Extraocular muscle weakness may lead to ptosis and diplopia; the weakness worsens with repeated contractions.
- Respiratory muscle involvement may lead to death.
- There is an association with thymic hyperplasia and thymomas.

Lambert-Eaton myasthenic syndrome frequently arises before a diagnosis of cancer is made, often in cases of small cell lung cancer. Patients report dry mouth and proximal muscle weakness. Autoantibodies are directed against presynaptic calcium channels of the neuromuscular junction.

MUSCULAR DYSTROPHY

Duchenne muscular dystrophy is a recessive X-linked form of muscular dystrophy leading to rapid progression of muscle degeneration. It is the most common and severe form of muscular dystrophy. The affected gene is the dystrophin gene on the X chromosome (Xp21); dystrophin protein is an important muscle structural protein, and mutation results in a virtual absence of the dystrophin protein.

Affected boys are normal at birth but have onset of symptoms by age 5. Clinical features include:

- Progressive muscular weakness
- Calf pseudohypertrophy
- Proximal weakness of shoulder and pelvic girdles
- Possible heart failure and arrhythmias
- Respiratory insufficiency and pulmonary infections as a result of decreased mucociliary clearance

Lab studies show elevated serum creatine kinase. Muscle biopsy shows muscle fibers of various sizes; necrosis, degeneration, and regeneration of fibers; fibrosis; and fatty infiltration. Immunostains show decreased dystrophin protein. Diagnosis can also be confirmed with genetic testing.

Becker muscular dystrophy is a recessive X-linked inherited disorder leading to slowly progressive muscle weakness of the legs and pelvis.

- Less severe than Duchenne
- Not as common as Duchenne
- Has a later onset than Duchenne, with variable progression
- Mutation produces an altered dystrophin protein
- Cardiac involvement is rare, and patients can have relatively normal lifespan

INFLAMMATORY NEUROPATHY

Guillain-Barré syndrome is an autoimmune disease leading to the destruction of Schwann cells and peripheral nerve demyelination. Clinically, it is preceded by a viral illness. Muscular weakness occurs with an ascending paralysis, accompanied by loss of deep tendon reflexes. Diagnosis can be established with nerve conduction studies; lumbar puncture shows elevated protein.

Microscopic examination demonstrates inflammation and demyelination of peripheral nerves and spinal nerve roots, resulting in muscular weakness. Guillain-Barré syndrome is fatal in 5% of cases because of respiratory paralysis.

SOFT TISSUE AND PERIPHERAL NERVE TUMORS

Lipoma is a benign adipose tissue tumor that most often arises in subcutaneous tissue of trunk, neck, or proximal extremities. It is the most common benign soft tissue tumor. The tumor is usually more of a cosmetic problem than a medical one. Microscopically, it is composed of mature fat cells but can contain other mesenchymal elements.

Liposarcoma is a malignant adipose tissue tumor that most often arises in the thigh or retroperitoneum. It is the most common adult sarcoma. It is distinguished from lipoma by the presence of **lipoblasts**. Grossly, it tends to be larger than lipoma, and the cut surface shows fibrous bands. Microscopically, well-differentiated liposarcoma consists of mature fat with varying numbers of hyperchromatic spindle cells and multivacuolated lipoblasts. Metastases are rare but retroperitoneal tumors tend to recur.

Dermatofibroma is a benign dermal spindle cell proliferation that most often arises in the extremities. A small, red nodule is seen, which is tender and mobile on examination.

Fibromatosis is a non-neoplastic proliferative connective tissue disorder that can histologically resemble a sarcoma. Fibrous tissue infiltrates muscle or other tissue, and may cause a mass lesion. The cut surface is trabeculated. Microscopically, bundles of fibroblasts and collagen are seen.

- **Superficial fibromatoses** arise from fascia or aponeuroses. Palmar fibromatosis is the most common type. Penile fibromatosis is known as Peyronie's disease.
- **Deep fibromatoses** (desmoids) occur in extraabdominal sites (children) and abdominal wall and extraabdominal sites (adults). Abdominal desmoids often occur in women within a year of pregnancy. They may also follow surgery or trauma. Intraabdominal fibromatosis is commonly associated with Gardner syndrome (*see* Gastrointestinal Tract Pathology).

Fibrosarcoma is a malignant fibrous tumor, commonly seen on the thigh and upper limb. It may arise spontaneously or after therapeutic/accidental irradiation. Microscopically, there are uniform spindle cells with a "herringbone" pattern. Metastases are hematogenous, often to the lung.

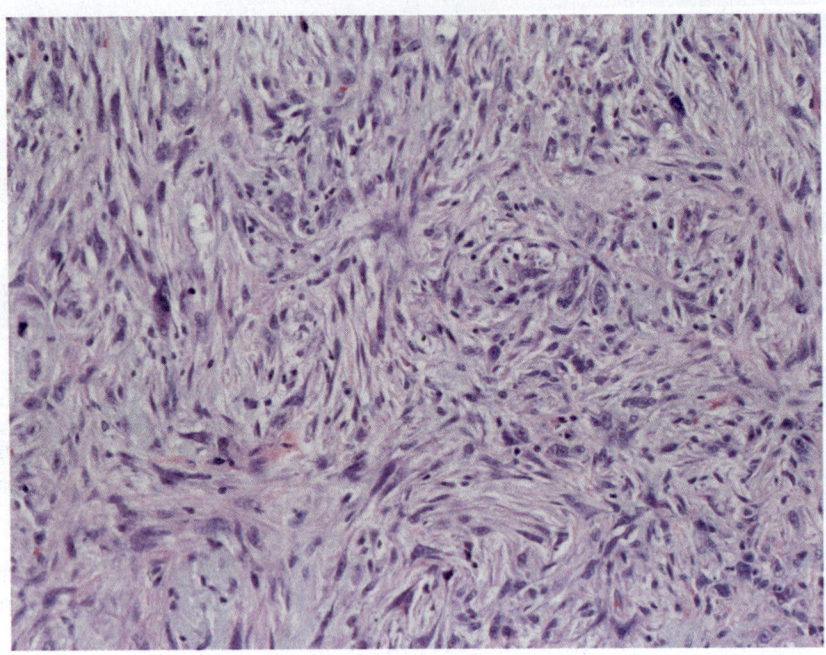

Figure 28-1. Fibrosarcoma
© Gregg Barré, M.D. Used with permission.

Undifferentiated pleomorphic sarcoma (previously known as malignant fibrous histiocytoma) is a large multilobulated tumor seen in the extremities and retroperitoneum of older adults. Microscopically, they may have a storiform (cartwheel-like) pattern. They recur and metastasize.

Rhabdomyoma (*See* Female Genital and Cardiac Pathology.)

Embryonal rhabdomyosarcoma (*See* Female Genital Pathology.)

Leiomyoma is a benign smooth muscle tumor most often seen in the uterus (*see* Female Genital Pathology) and gastrointestinal tract. Less often it is seen in skin, and only rarely in deep soft tissue.

Leiomyosarcoma of soft tissue is less common than its counterpart in the gastrointestinal tract and uterus (*see* Female Genital Pathology). In soft tissue, it usually arises in the retroperitoneum of older women.

Grossly, the tumor is fleshy and white with hemorrhage and necrosis. Microscopically, the tumor nuclei are blunt ended ("cigar-shaped"). Longitudinal striations can be seen with Masson trichrome staining. The tumor is highly aggressive in the retroperitoneum, where complete resection may not be possible.

Synovial sarcoma occurs in young adults. The knee is a common location. The gross appearance is variable but calcification is common. Microscopically, tumors may be biphasic (epithelial and spindle cells) or monophasic (spindle cell or epithelial).

Benign peripheral nerve sheath tumors

- **Schwannoma** is an encapsulated nerve sheath tumor with alternating Antoni A and B areas (*see* Central Nervous System Pathology).
- **Neurofibroma** is nonencapsulated and may have a solitary, diffuse, or plexiform pattern. Microscopically, neoplastic cells are interspersed among wavy, loose or dense collagen bundles.

Malignant peripheral nerve sheath tumor may arise from neurofibromas or *de novo* in a peripheral nerve. It typically occurs in young adults in major nerve trunks (sciatic nerve, brachial plexus, and sacral plexus). Microscopically, it resembles fibrosarcoma. Recurrence and distant metastases are common.

Dental Anatomy

General Characteristics

Learning Objectives

❏ Describe the general characteristics and anatomy of teeth

❏ Understand basic anatomical terms applied to tooth structure

❏ Understand structure and relationship of tooth tissue types

DEFINITIONS

General

Maxilla: Stationary, upper jaw

Mandible: Moveable, lower jaw

Arch trait: Characteristics of the teeth of one arch vs. the other (3 roots in a maxillary molar vs. 2 in a mandibular molar)

Type trait: Differences between the arch components of each tooth class that make them easily identifiable (difference between mandibular central incisor and mandibular lateral incisor)

Class trait: Characteristic of major tooth type (incisor vs. molar) based on overall structure and function (tearing, grinding)

Set trait: Characteristic that identifies what dentition the tooth belongs to (deciduous or permanent)

Types of Teeth

Deciduous:

- Primary teeth
- 20 teeth
- Must be exfoliated

Exfoliation:

- Process of shedding or losing deciduous teeth

Permanent:

- Adult dentition
- 32 teeth
- Usually erupt between 6–18 years

Succedaneous:

Take the place of the exfoliated primary teeth (note: molars are not succedaneous). For example, the first premolar is the succedaneous tooth for the first primary molar.

Mixed dentition:

Containing a combination of both primary and permanent teeth

ANATOMY OF A TOOTH

Crown

- Surface portion that erupts through the gingiva
- Composed of enamel, dentin, and pulp

Root

- Anchoring portion of the tooth
- Composed of cementum, dentin, and pulp

Clinical crown

- Portion visible in the oral cavity

Anatomic crown

- Begins at cementoenamel junction
- Anatomic crown is covered by enamel

Gingiva

- Soft tissue surrounding crown and boundary between clinical crown and root

Alveolus

- Bony socket anchoring tooth

Cervical line

- Boundary between anatomic crown and root (at cementoenamel junction)

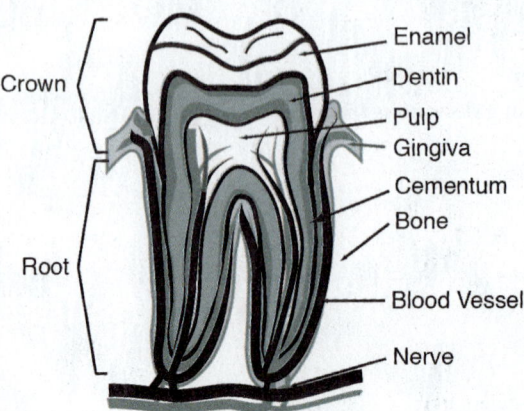

Figure 1-1. General tooth anatomy and terminology

Root Structure (Most common, with exceptions)

Single-rooted teeth: all anteriors, maxillary second premolar, mandibular first and second premolars (general rule with exceptions)

Double-rooted teeth (Bifurcation): maxillary first premolar, mandibular molars

Triple-rooted teeth (Trifurcation): maxillary molars

Root trunk: common part of the tooth root before the root separates*

Cervical line: boundary between the enamel of the anatomical crown and the cementum of the anatomical root (cementoenamel junction)

*Note that the root form of 3rd molars of both arches is highly variable.

Each root usually has one root canal, except:**

- Maxillary:
  - second premolar (occasionally 2)
  - molars (mesiobuccal root can have 2, especially in maxillary first molar)

- Mandibular
  - central (occasionally 2)
  - lateral (occasionally 2)
  - canine (occasionally 2)
  - first premolar (occasionally 2)
  - second premolar (occasionally 2)
  - molars (mesial root usually has 2 canals; distal may have 1 or 2)

**Note that there are many exceptions to rules about roots.

Pulp Cavity

Pulp chambers and **pulp canals** make up the pulp cavity.

The **pulp chamber** is generally in the coronal portion of the tooth. It is a singular chamber in all teeth and extends into the root trunk, generally 1–2 mm below the cervical line. The chamber outline follows the basic outline of the tooth.

Pulp horns are projections of the pulp chamber into the major cusps of the teeth. They are also found in mammelons of the maxillary incisors when teeth are young.

Table 1-1. Tooth Tissue Types

	Composition	Characteristics	Function	Location	Strength
Enamel	96–98% inorganic material (mineral)	Hard, translucent Cannot repair itself Complete at time of eruption	Protects biting surface of tooth	Covers anatomic crown	Hardest substance in body
Cementum	50% organic 50% inorganic	2 types: cellular, acellular Blood supply through the cementum (nourishment from outside tooth)	Provides anchoring mechanism to tooth (periodontal ligament between cementum and alveolar bone)	Covers surface of anatomic root	Less dense than enamel
Dentin	22% organic* 65% inorganic* 13% water* Composed of tubules (extension of nerve tissue from pulp protrudes into these tubules)	Makes up bulk of tooth **2 types:** primary (produced during development) and secondary (formed to protect the pulp)	Provides elasticity to tooth	Beneath the enamel and cementum	Softer and less brittle than enamel
Pulp	Nerves, blood vessels, lymph	Formative (will produce dentin throughout life) Contains odontoblasts to produce dentin	Provides nutrients to tooth Sensory (pain from heat, cold, decay, etc.)	Innermost portion of the tooth	Soft tissue

*Values vary in some texts; % inorganic depends on whether water is included in total

TOOTH DEVELOPMENT

A. **Background:** The first sign of tooth development occurs at about 6 weeks of embryonic life. The embryo is now 11 mm long. There is a thickening of the oral epithelium. This thickening forms a band that runs along the outline of the future dental arches. This band or thickening is continuous around each arch and is called the dental lamina.

At certain points along the dental lamina, there are further bulb-like thickenings corresponding roughly to the location of the 20 maxillary and mandibular deciduous teeth. These bulb-like thickenings are referred to as **tooth buds.**

A tooth bud consists of three parts:

1. Enamel organ: derivative of oral ectoderm. It produces tooth enamel.
2. Dental papilla: derivative of mesenchyme. It produces pulp and dentin.
3. Dental sac: derivative of mesenchyme. It produces cementum and the periodontal ligament.

Note

Enamel is an ectodermal derivative. Dentin is a mesodermal (mesenchymal) derivative.

B. The **stages of tooth development** are named according to the shape of the epithelial part of the tooth and are: the **bud, cap,** and **bell stages.**

1. **Bud stage:** This is the stage already mentioned, where there are ovoid swellings at 10 different points on each arch corresponding to the positions of the deciduous teeth.

2. **Cap stage:** The bud stage proliferates and expands; however, it does not expand everywhere equally. The result is a shallow invagination on the deep surface of the bud.

   The following are seen during the cap stage:

   a. **Outer and inner enamel epithelium:**
      i   Outer enamel epithelium = cuboidal cells on periphery of cap stage
      ii Inner enamel epithelium = tall cells on concavity of cap

   b. **Stellate reticulum:** Cells that lie between the inner enamel epithelium and outer enamel epithelium begin to separate by an increase in intercellular fluid and arrange themselves into a network. This network is called the stellate reticulum.

   c. **Enamel knot:** Densely packed cells in center of enamel organ

   d. **Dental papilla:** As the epithelium of the enamel organ proliferates, the mesenchyme, partially enclosed by the invaginated portion of the inner enamel epithelium, proliferates. This mesenchyme further condenses to form the dental papilla.

      The dental papilla is the formative organ of the dentin and primordium of the pulp.

   e. **Dental sac:** As the enamel organ and dental papilla are developing, there also occurs a condensation of the mesenchyme surrounding these two structures. Gradually, there appears a dense, fibrous layer referred to as the dental sac.

      The dental sac derivatives are cementum and the PDL.

3. **Bell stage:** As the invagination of the epithelium develops further and deepens, the enamel organ develops a bell-shaped appearance.

   The following are seen during the bell stage:

   a. **Inner enamel epithelium:** Cells of the inner enamel epithelium will differentiate into ameloblasts.

   b. **Stratum intermedium:** Several layers of squamous cells between the inner enamel epithelium and the stellate reticulum. Their function is not clear but they seem to be essential if enamel is to be formed.

   c. **Stellate reticulum:** This looks the same as in the cap stage but has expanded more.

   d. **Outer enamel epithelium:** These cells eventually flatten to low cuboidal cells.

   e. **Dental lamina:** All teeth except for the permanent molars; there is a proliferation of the dental lamina to give rise to the enamel organs of the permanent teeth.

f. **Dental papilla:** Cells close to the inner enamel epithelium within the dental papillae differentiate into odontoblasts. The odontoblasts will lay down the dentin.

g. **Dental sac:** The dental sac now shows a circular arrangement of its fibers and resembles a capsular structure. When the root develops, fibers of the dental sac will differentiate into the periodontal fibers that will become embedded in cementum and alveolar bone.

h. **Vestibular lamina:** There occurs an epithelial thickening, labial and buccal, to the dental lamina. This is the vestibular lamina. It will hollow and form the oral vestibule between the alveolar portion of the jaws and the lips and cheeks.

The sequence is as follows:

i. Cells of the inner enamel epithelium differentiate into ameloblasts (morphogenic stage).

ii. Some protein factor is transported from the ameloblasts across the basement membrane into the dental papilla (organizing stage).

iii. Cells of the dental papilla differentiate into odontoblasts under the influence of this inducing factor.

iv. The odontoblasts begin to lay down predentin.

v. Through a reciprocal factor transported across the basement membrane, the ameloblasts can now lay down their initial enamelin, which will later mineralize to form enamel (formative stage).

C. **Root formation:** The development of the roots begins after enamel and dentin formation has reached the future CEJ (cementoenamel junction). The enamel organ plays a crucial role in root formation. The enamel organ forms the **epithelial root sheath of Hertwig**. The components of this root sheath are fused inner and outer enamel epithelium only. There is no stratum intermedium or stellate reticulum present. The root sheath molds the shape of the roots and initiates dentin formation.

When the cells of the root sheath have induced the differentiation of connective tissue cells into odontoblasts and the first layer of dentin has been laid down, the root sheath loses its continuity and begins to degenerate. It does not disappear altogether, however, and remnants of the root sheath of Hertwig are called the **Malassez rests**. These rests may form granulomas in pathologic processes, or they form cementicles if they become calcified. The Malassez rests will only be found in the PDL.

Cementum is a derivative of the dental sac, which is a derivative of mesechyme. It is formed when cells of the primitive periodontal connective tissue come into contact with the dentin after the root sheath of Hertwig has broken up. These cells, similar to fibroblasts, differentiate into cementoblasts and begin to lay down **cementoid**, which subsequently mineralizes to form cementum. Some of the cells in the apical third of the root structure become entrapped in their own secretions. This region of mature cementum will contain cells within it and will hence be referred to as cellular cementum. The occlusal two thirds of the root structure usually possess acellular cementum.

TOOTH COMPONENTS: ENAMEL, DENTIN, CEMENTUM, AND PULP

A. **Enamel:** hardest structure of the body; an ectodermal derivative; laid down first as "enamelin" by the ameloblasts

1. **Color:** yellow white to grayish white

2. **Chemical composition:** It is 96% inorganic (main constituent = hydroxyapatite), 1% organic, 3% water.

The enamel forms a protection over the entire surface of the crown. It is well adapted to bear up under masticatory stresses. Enamel is a brittle structure, as well as being very hard. Enamel has been shown to be slightly permeable, and this permeability decreases as one gets older.

Note

Dentin is much more "bone-like" histologically than is enamel.

The enamel consists of thin **rods or prisms** that stand upright on the surface of the dentin. After a wavy course, they reach the enamel surface and are perpendicular to the enamel surface at every point on the crown. Every rod runs through the entire thickness of the enamel layer. The enamel rods or prisms and the "interprismatic" substance have been shown to be composed of apatite crystals and a bit of organic material. The more or less regular change in the direction of the enamel rods is responsible for the appearance of Hunter-Schreger bands or the lines of Schreger.

In a cross-section of the crown, the enamel shows concentric lines, which are brown in transmitted light and colorless in reflected light. In the longitudinal section, they run obliquely inward from the surface and toward the root. These are the **lines of Retzius** or **incremental lines of Retzius.** They illustrate the incremental pattern of enamel, i.e., the successive apposition of layers of enamel during formation of the crown. The incremental lines of Retzius have been compared with the growth rings of a tree.

Other enamel structures with which to be familiar are:

a. **Perikymata:** These are transverse, wave-like grooves thought to be external manifestations of the striae (lines) of Retzius. They are continuous around the tooth and lie parallel to each other and to the CEJ.

b. **Enamel spindles:** Some dentinal tubules penetrate a short distance into the enamel and end blindly. These spindle-shaped odontoblastic processes are called enamel spindles.

c. **Tomes processes:** The surfaces of the ameloblasts facing the developing enamel are not smooth. There is an interdigitation of the cells and the enamel rods they produce. This interdigitation is due to the fact that the long axes of the ameloblasts are not parallel to the long axes of the rods. The projections of ameloblasts into the enamel matrix are referred to as **Tomes processes**.

Local disturbances of the enamel during development cause the enamel lamellae and tufts.

d. **Enamel lamellae:** Thin structures of organic material (very little mineral content) extending from the surface of the enamel toward and sometimes into the dentin. These usually develop in areas of tension between enamel prisms.

e. **Enamel tufts:** These extend from the dentinoenamel junction (DEJ) into the enamel for one fifth to one third of its thickness. The tuft shape, however, is an optical illusion due to the projection onto one plane of fibers lying in different planes. Tufts are basically hypocalcified enamel rods and interprismatic substance.

3. **Age changes in enamel:**

a. Attrition or wear of occlusal surfaces and proximal contact points due to mastication

b. Flattening of perikymata and disappearance of the rod ends

c. Eventual disappearance of the perikymata

d. Decreased permeability of enamel

e. Teeth become darker and more resistant to decay.

Remember that enamel development occurs in two phases:

i. Matrix formation

ii. Maturation

If there are developmental disturbances in matrix formation, enamel hypoplasia will result, i.e., a defect in enamel itself.

If there are developmental disturbances in maturation, or if maturation is lacking or not complete, enamel will be hypocalcified, i.e., a deficiency in the mineral content of the enamel.

B. **Dentin:** mesodermal derivative from dental papilla; laid down first as predentin by odontoblasts; harder than compact bone, although it resembles bone in its structure, chemical nature, and development

1. **Color:** yellowish to semitransparent in fresh condition

2. **Chemical composition:** roughly 70% inorganic material; 30% organic material and water (note some variations in this number from source to source)

Unlike enamel, which is very hard and brittle, dentin is subject to slight deformation and is somewhat elastic. It is harder than compact bone, yet softer than enamel. In ground sections of dentin, the dentin has a radially striated appearance. This is due to the presence of **dentinal tubules**. The course of the dentinal tubules is somewhat curved and resembles an "S" shape. They start at right angles from the pulp surface and then follow their "S"-shaped course.

Remember: The tubules are farther apart in the peripheral layers of dentin (near the enamel and cementum). The dentinal tubules house the odontoblastic processes (Tomes fibers). You should be familiar with the following terms:

a. **Peritubular dentin:** The zone of dentin immediately surrounding the odontoblastic process. This stains darker in a histologic preparation. It is thought that this dentin is more mineralized than is the intertubular dentin.

b. **Intertubular dentin:** The main bulk of dentin is composed of intertubular dentin. Even though it is fairly mineralized, greater than half of its volume is taken up by organic matrix. (The matrix of dentin is basically collagenous fibers enveloped in an amorphous ground substance.)

c. **Incremental lines of von Ebner:** Seen as fine lines that in cross-section run at right angles to the dentinal tubules. They correspond to the lines of Retzius in enamel and represent the incremental apposition of the dentin layers. Also known as **imbrication lines**.

d. **Contour lines of Owen:** Sometimes, the incremental lines mentioned above are accentuated due to disturbances in the mineralization process. These lines are known as the contour lines of Owen. An exaggerated incremental line or contour line of Owen due to the trauma of birth is known as the **neonatal line**.

e. **Interglobular dentin:** You may remember that the odontoblasts first produce a matrix material known as predentin, which will subsequently mineralize. (The first sign of predentin formation is the laying down of a fan-like arrangement of collagen fibers known as Korff fibers.) This mineralization begins in small, globular areas that normally fuse to form a uniformly calcified dentin layer. If fusion of these globular areas does not take place, there will be hypomineralized or unmineralized regions between the globules referred to as interglobular dentin.

Note: Interglobular dentin is found mainly in the crown near the dentino-enamel junction (DEJ). This does not interfere with the course of the dentinal tubules.

f. **Tomes granular layer:** Minute areas of interglobular dentin in the dentin subjacent to cementum.

Dentin is sensitive to touch, to cold, and to acid-containing foods. Only occasional nerve fibers penetrate the dentin and extend for short distances. These are small unmyelinated nerve fibers that are in close contact with the odontoblastic process.

3. **Age and functional changes in dentin:** Remember that the dentin houses the odontoblastic processes and is certainly a vital tissue. The effects of aging or pathologic processes are seen by deposition of new layers of dentin (reparative dentin) and by alteration of the original dentin (sclerotic dentin).

a. **Secondary dentin:** Remember that dentin deposition may continue throughout life. The dentin formed in later life is separated from that previously formed by a darkly stained line. The tubules of this secondary dentin are more wavy but less numerous than the original dentin. They are also naturally found closer to the pulp tissues.

b. **Reparative dentin:** Remember that dentin is a vital tissue. If by excess wear, erosion, caries, operative procedures, etc., the odontoblastic processes are cut or damaged, the damaged odontoblast may degenerate or it may continue to form hard dentin as a protection from further injury. If the odontoblast degenerates, it may be replaced by an undifferentiated cell from the pulp, which will produce new dentin. The dentin that these odontoblasts lay down is reparative dentin. The tubules of this dentin are twisted and fewer of them exist.

Note

The pulp is living tissue and can produce new dentin through stimulation of odontoblasts at any age.

---

c. **Sclerotic dentin:** Seen in the teeth of elderly people. This dentin is **transparent** and results from calcium salts being deposited in or around degenerating odontoblastic processes. The calcium salts may even obliterate the tubules.

C. **Cementum:** a mesodermal derivative; derives from dental sac; laid down first as cementoid by cementoblasts, most "bone-like" of dental tissue

1. **Color:** light yellow, lacks luster that enamel possesses

2. **Chemical composition:** It is 60–65% inorganic (mainly hydroxyapatite) and 35–40% organic material and water.

3. There are two types of cementum:

a. **Acellular cementum:** occlusal two thirds of root structure. Consists of calcified intercellular substance and embedded Sharpey fibers. Cementoblasts line its structure.

b. **Cellular cementum:** found in apical third of root. The cells included in cellular cementum are cementocytes. They lie in spaces called lacunae. The cell body has long processes ("**canaliculi**") extending from it. These processes may branch and anastomose with neighboring cells. There are no Haversian systems in cementum, however.

Note

The compact bone containing Sharpey fibers is often termed "bundle bone."

---

c. **Secondary cementum:** Due to severe trauma or pathologic processes, cementum may reabsorb. If it does, cells of the PDL differentiate into cementoblasts and lay down secondary cementum. Secondary cementum can be reabsorbed more easily. Secondary cementum resembles cellular cementum in some ways.

Remember: Cellular cementum, secondary cementum, and bone are similar in that they contain cells in lacunae, have canaliculi that extend primarily toward the nutritional source, and can be reabsorbed. Cementum, however, reabsorbs less than bone.

4. **Function of cementum:**

    a. Anchors tooth to the bony socket by attachment of fibers (Sharpey fibers; PDL fibers)

    b. Compensates by means of its growth for loss of tooth substance due to occlusal wear

    c. Contributes, via growth, to the continuous occlusomesial eruption of the teeth

    Remember that cementum is not reabsorbed under normal conditions, whereas bone is reabsorbed constantly with the apposition of new bone. Both cementum and bone reabsorb on the pressure side (side to which tooth is moved) and are laid down on the tension side (side from which tooth is moved away) of tooth movement. To repeat, cementum is more resistant to reabsorption than is bone.

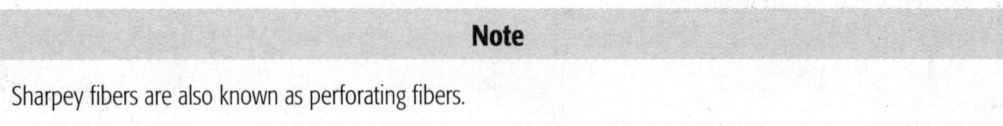

Note

Sharpey fibers are also known as perforating fibers.

5. **Hypercementosis:** This is an abnormal thickening of cementum. This is seen occasionally in connection with chronic periapical inflammation. A thickening of cementum is also observed on teeth that are not in function (hypofunction).

D. **Pulp:** of mesodermal origin; derives from dental papilla. The pulp contains most of the cellular and fibrous elements that are present in loose connective tissue.

The primary function of the pulp is the production of dentin.

1. The pulp has the following functions:

    a. **Nutritive:** Pulp provides nourishment to dentin via the odontoblasts and processes.

    b. **Sensory:** Nerves of pulp contain both sensory and GVE (general visceral efferent or sympathetic) fibers. The sensory fibers of the pulp mediate the sensation of pain only. Sympathetics go to the smooth muscle of the pulpal blood vessels.

Note

Due to the type of sensory nerve fibers in the pulp, cold, heat, chemicals, and touch sensation are all interpreted as pain.

    c. **Defensive:** It was noted that cells of the pulp could, if provoked, differentiate into odontoblasts and produce reparative dentin. The pulp can also respond to injury by an inflammatory process.

    Remember that the pulp is a nonexpandable tissue. The walls of the pulp chamber are made of rigid dentin. If there is severe inflammation and there is enough edema and exudative fluid, the pulp may "strangle" its own blood vessels and necrose. This is an example of where the protective wall around the pulp can be seen as a disadvantage.

2. In the **embryonic pulp**, the fibers are argyrophilic. There are no mature collagenous fibers. As the development of the tooth germ progresses, the pulp becomes increasingly vascular and fibroblasts differentiate from the primitive mesenchymal cells.

3. In **adult pulp**, one sees cells, fibroblasts, and an intercellular substance. This intercellular substance consists of collagenous and argyrophilic fibers and ground substance. **There are no elastic fibers in the pulp.** There

are defense cells (histiocytes) in the pulp, and remember that the odontoblasts are a part of the dental pulp. There are numerous capillary and nerve plexi found in the pulp.

4. **Blood and lymph vessels:** Pulp is extremely vascular. The vessels enter the pulp through the apical foramen. The vessels of the pulp communicate with the vessels of the PDL via accessory canals. Lymph vessels are also found in the pulp.

5. **Nerves:** Usually nerve bundles follow blood vessels. Most nerve fibers entering the pulp are myelinated. They mediate pain. The unmyelinated fibers belong to the sympathetic nervous system and regulate the lumen size of the blood vessels.

   Remember that the pulp cannot differentiate between heat, touch, cold, pressure, or chemicals. **The result is pain only.**

6. Age changes within the pulp. **Pulpstones** (denticles) seem to be normal structures seen frequently in the adult pulp. Classified as true denticles, false denticles, or diffuse calcifications. **True denticles** show real dentin structure with tubules, etc. **False denticles** do not show the structure of dentin. They only show concentric layers of calcified tissue. **Diffuse calcifications** can be large and are very amorphous calcifications usually associated with collagen fiber bundles or blood vessels. Pulpstones may also be classified as **free** (surrounded by pulp tissue completely), **attached** (fused to dentin), or **embedded** (surrounded entirely by dentin).

Table 1-2. General Characteristics of Tooth Classes (Permanent teeth)

Class	Number per Quadrant	Characteristics	Function	Position
Incisors (I)	2	Front teeth, single rooted Straight incisal edge	Cutting, aesthetics, phonetics, biting	Central—closest to midline Lateral—2nd position from midline
Canines (C)	1	Canine prominence of tooth seen at corner of mouth Long rooted	Cutting, shearing, tearing	3rd position from midline
Premolars (PM)	2	Single roots, except for maxillary first premolar (2 roots)	Mastication	4th and 5th position from midline
Molars (M)	3	Grinding, chewing 4 cusps or more Wide masticating surface	Mastication	6th, 7th, and 8th position from midline

ANATOMIC DIVISIONS AND ORIENTATIONS (PERMANENT TEETH)

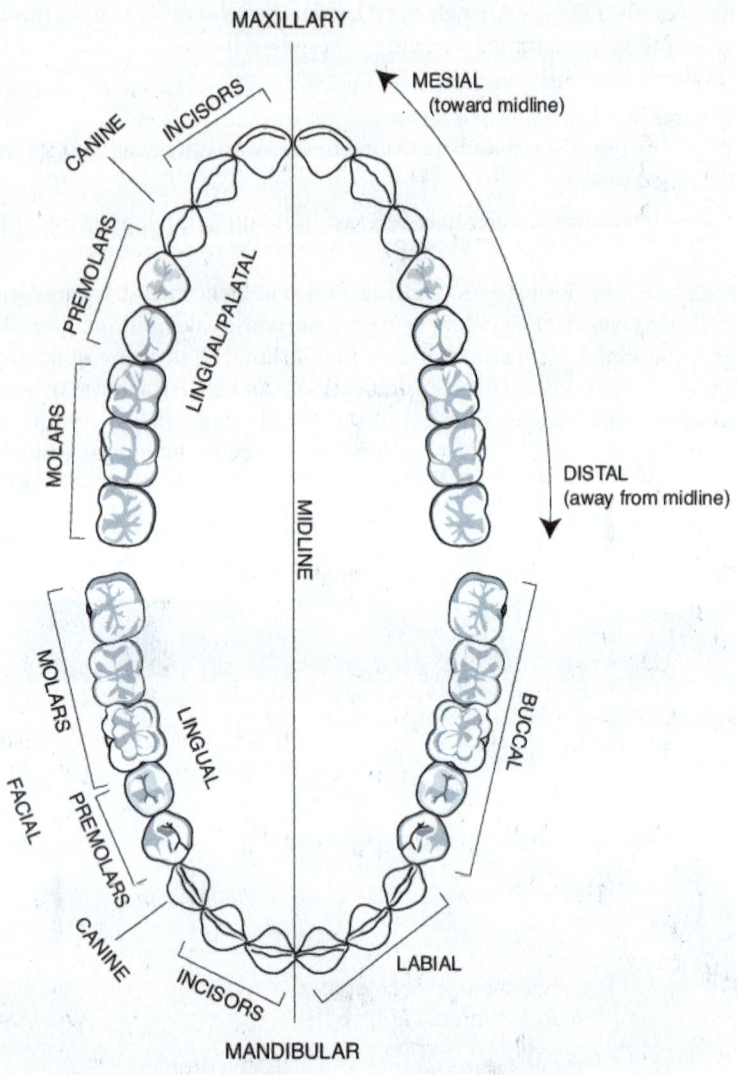

Figure 1-2. Tooth types and orientation for permanent dentition

Surfaces

Occlusal: biting surface of posterior teeth

Incisal: biting surface of anterior teeth

Gingival/Cervical: area near gingiva

Contact area: area that contacts an adjacent tooth on the proximal surface of the tooth

Definitions

Mesial: closer to midline

Distal: away from midline

Proximal: area between two teeth (for example: mesial or distal)

Lingual: surface facing the tongue (also **palatal** in maxilla)

Facial: outer surface facing toward cheek

Labial: surface facing cheek in anterior teeth

Buccal: surface facing cheek in posterior teeth

Note

Facial, labial, and buccal are often used interchangeably.

Anterior teeth: incisors and canines

Posterior teeth: premolars and molars

Anatomic Thirds

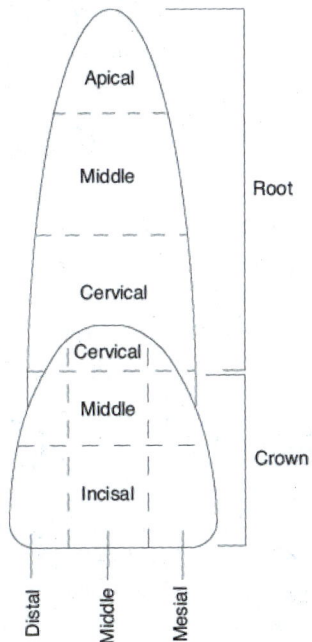

Figure 1-3. Anatomic regions (thirds) of tooth crown and root

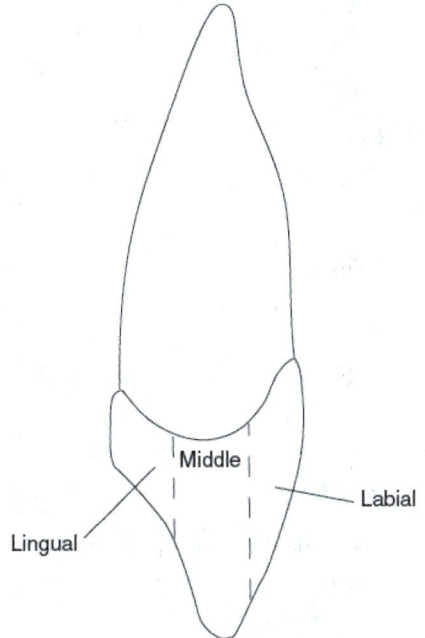

Figure 1-4. Proximal view of crown anatomic thirds (anterior tooth)

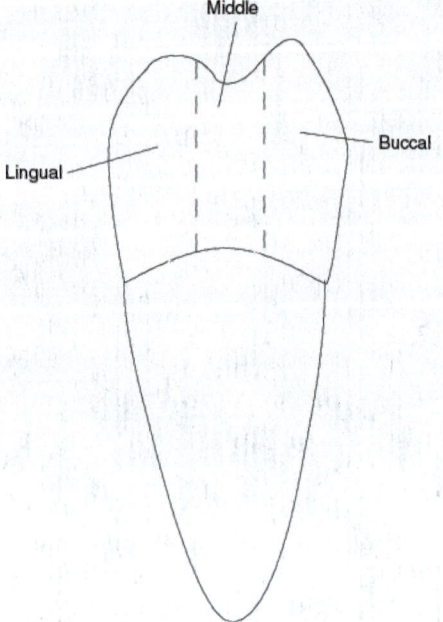

Figure 1-5. Proximal view of crown anatomic thirds (premolar)

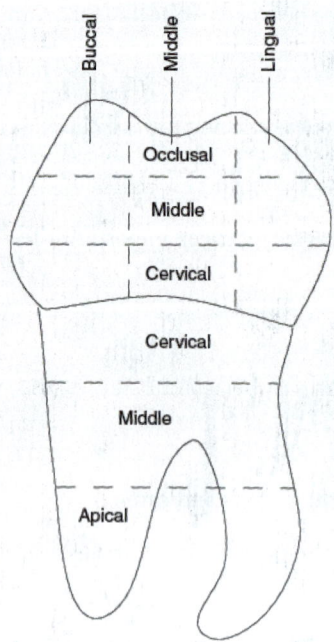

Figure 1-6. Proximal view of crown and root anatomic thirds (molar tooth)

Nomenclature

Shorthand

Permanent Dentition

Universal System

Teeth are numbered from 1–32 starting with the permanent maxillary right third molar, i.e., perm/max/right/central incisor = #8.

Note
Although other numbering systems exist, the universal system will be used on Dental Boards questions.

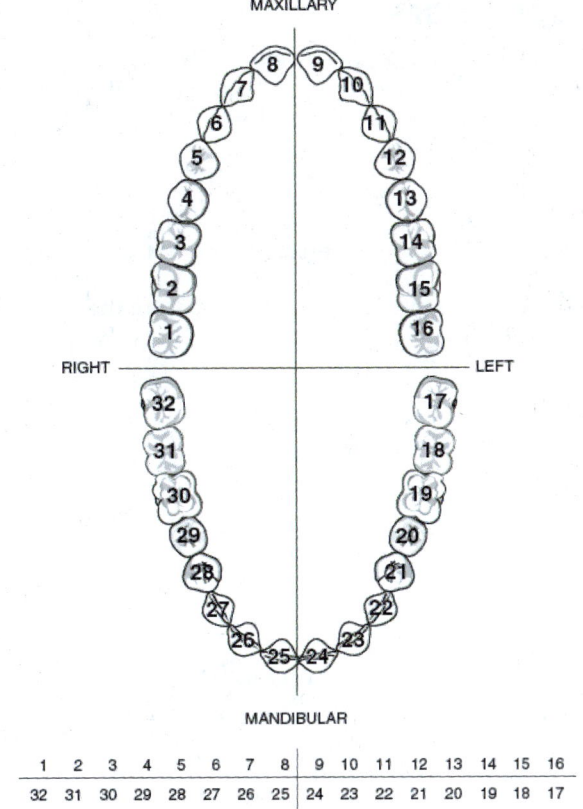

Figure 1-7. Permanent dentition universal numbering system

Primary Dentition

Universal System

Teeth are numbered from A–T starting with the primary maxillary right second molar, i.e., prim/max/right/central incisor = E.

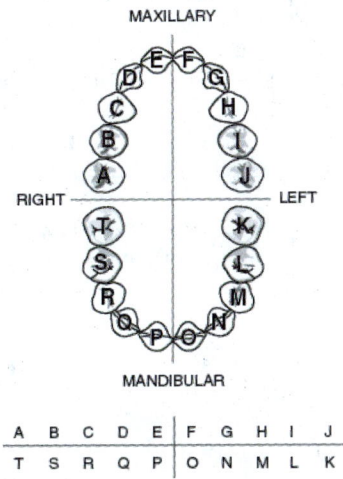

Figure 1-8. Primary dentition universal numbering system

Development of Cusps and Lobes

Tooth germs (or tooth buds) are small groupings of cells that develop during the eighth week of embryonic development. **Calcification**, the hardening of tooth tissues by the deposition of minerals found within, begins at the fourth to fifth month of fetal life. Calcification begins in permanent teeth just after birth.

Lobes

All anterior teeth develop from **four major growth centers** called **lobes**, i.e., **mammelons** and **cingula**.

The posterior teeth develop from four to five lobes. Cusps develop from the lobes, and the coalescence of lobes is marked by developmental grooves.

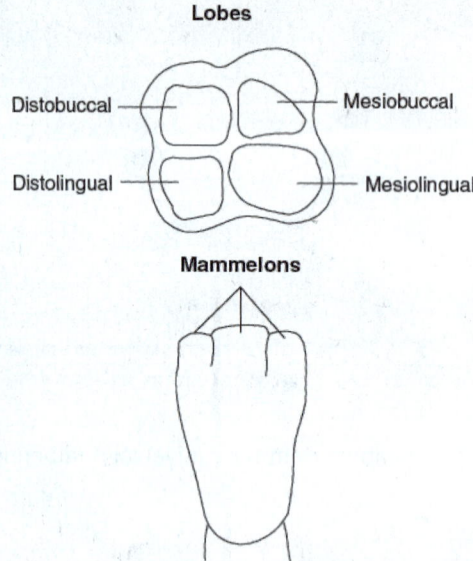

Figure 1-9. Mammelons of a permanent incisor

The lobes of a tooth act as the major centers of the formation of enamel. In the fully developed tooth, these lobes give rise to the formation of **cusps, mammelons, and cingula**. The coalescence of the lobes is marked by the formation of developmental depressions (anterior teeth) and developmental grooves (posterior teeth).

Anterior teeth (incisors and canines) have three facial lobes: distolabial, middlelabial, mesiolabial, and one lingual lobe, cingulum.

Premolars have four lobes: distobuccal, middlebuccal, mesiobuccal, and one lingual lobe, (lingual cusp).

Molars have **four lobes:** distolingual, distobuccal, mesiolingual, and mesiobuccal. The maxillary first molar may have a fifth lobe, the cusp of Carabelli (a small fifth cusp), and the mandibular first molar has a fifth lobe (distal cusp).

Dental Terminology

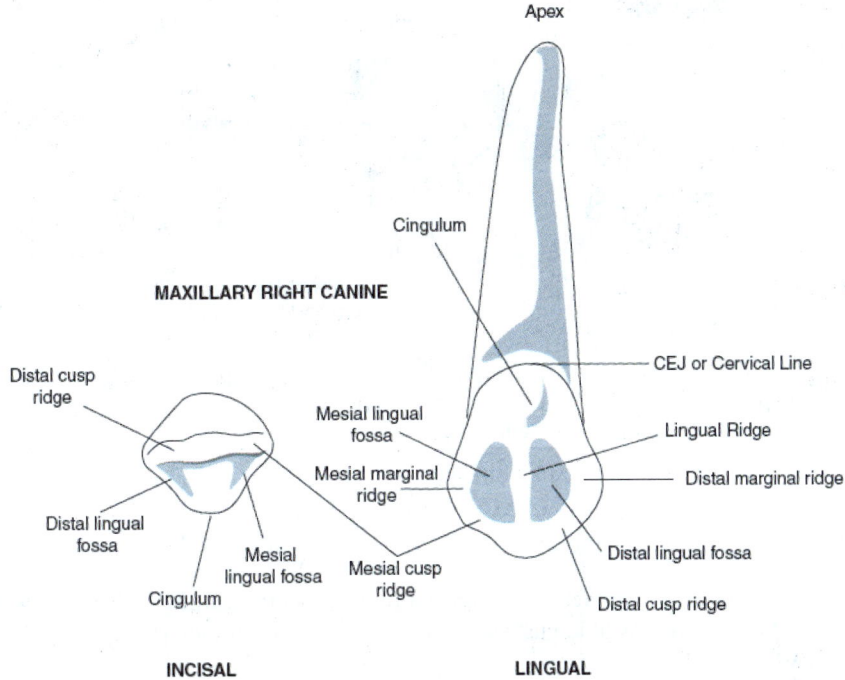

Figure 1-10. Anatomical features of a canine

Fossa: irregular rounded depression on surface of crown

Lingual fossa: broad shallow depression on lingual surface of anterior teeth

Central fossa: deep depression in central portion of anterior or posterior teeth

Triangular fossa: triangular fossa located in the marginal ridges of the posterior teeth

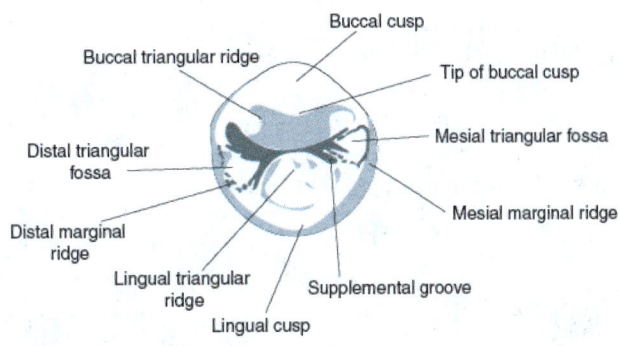

MAXILLARY RIGHT SECOND PREMOLAR

Cusp: elevation on the crown portion of tooth; forms the bulk of the occlusal surface

Cingulum: rounded eminence or bulge on lingual side of anterior teeth

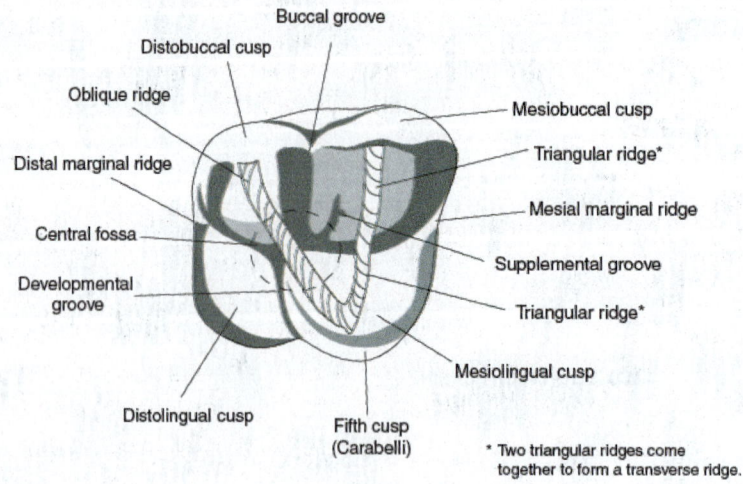

Buccal groove
Distobuccal cusp
Oblique ridge
Distal marginal ridge
Central fossa
Developmental groove
Mesiobuccal cusp
Triangular ridge*
Mesial marginal ridge
Supplemental groove
Triangular ridge*
Mesiolingual cusp
Distolingual cusp
Fifth cusp (Carabelli)

* Two triangular ridges come together to form a transverse ridge.

▨▨▨ represents triangle formed by the major ridges of the maxillary first molar.

MAXILLARY RIGHT FIRST MOLAR

Ridge: any linear elevation on surface of tooth; named according to location

Marginal ridge: rounded borders of enamel; form mesial and distal margins of occlusal surfaces of premolars and molars; form mesial and distal margins of lingual surfaces of incisors and canines

Triangular ridge: prominent elevation, triangular in cross-section

Transverse ridge: union of two triangular ridges crossing the occlusal surface of posterior tooth

Incisal ridge: found on newly erupted anterior teeth (mammelons)

Oblique ridge (maxillary molars only): transverse ridge that runs from distal buccal to mesial lingual cusp

Table 1-3. Maxillary Versus Mandibular Teeth

	Maxillary	Mandibular
Anterior	Wider, less symmetrical crown	Long, narrow symmetric crown
Molars	Wider in a faciolingual direction 3 roots—2 facial, 1 lingual (palatal) [MB, ML, P]	Wider in a mesiodistal direction 2 roots—1 mesial, 1 distal
Premolars	First premolar has 2 roots; others are single roots	All single roots
Posteriors	More centered in a faciolingual direction	Somewhat lingually placed
Occlusal tables	Centered over root trunk	Somewhat lingually placed
Buccal cusps	Displaced from midline in faciolingual direction; height of contour low	Buccal cusp more toward middle of tooth in the faciolingual direction
Lingual cusps	Displaced from midline in faciolingual direction	Lingual almost in line with lingual profile of root
Occlusal view	Equal amounts of buccal and lingual surfaces seen	More buccal (up to 1/3) than lingual surface seen
Contours	Buccal height of contour is low; lingual height of contour relatively high on crown	Buccal height of contour very low, near cervical

Fundamental Geometric Shapes of Crowns

Table 1-4. Axial Views

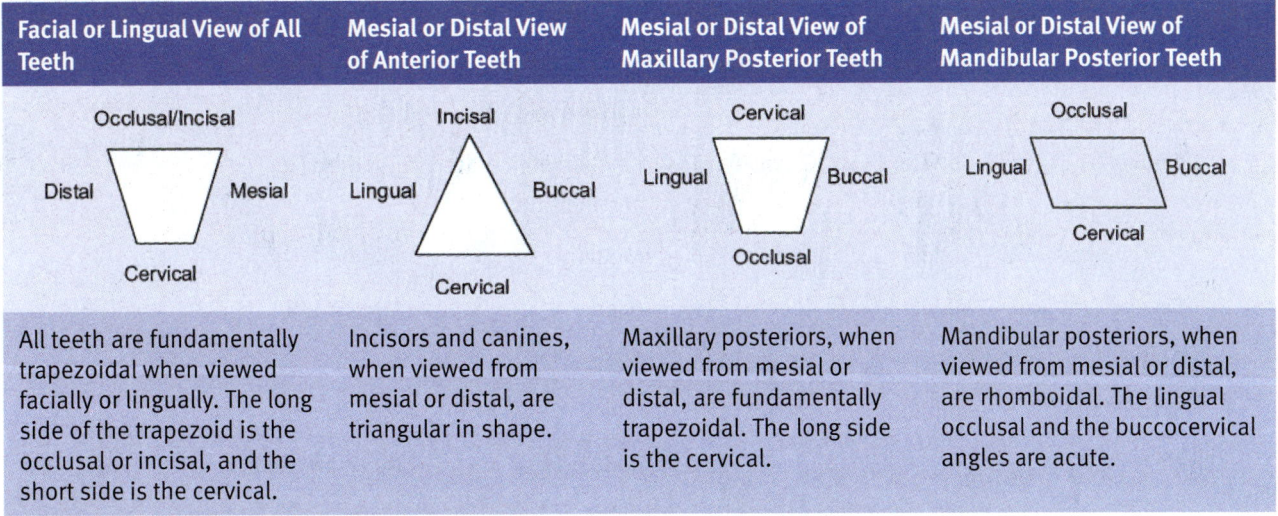

Facial or Lingual View of All Teeth	Mesial or Distal View of Anterior Teeth	Mesial or Distal View of Maxillary Posterior Teeth	Mesial or Distal View of Mandibular Posterior Teeth
All teeth are fundamentally trapezoidal when viewed facially or lingually. The long side of the trapezoid is the occlusal or incisal, and the short side is the cervical.	Incisors and canines, when viewed from mesial or distal, are triangular in shape.	Maxillary posteriors, when viewed from mesial or distal, are fundamentally trapezoidal. The long side is the cervical.	Mandibular posteriors, when viewed from mesial or distal, are rhomboidal. The lingual occlusal and the buccocervical angles are acute.

Note that all teeth are wider buccolingually than mesiodistally, except maxillary incisors and mandibular molars.

Heights of Contours and Contacts

The **height of contour, or the crest of curvature,** is the greatest elevation of the tooth. The contact areas are also considered the location of the height of contour on the proximal surfaces.

Knowing the heights of contour helps to understand contact relationships.

- Generally, the **mesial height of contour** is more incisal or occlusal than is the distal, except for the mandibular central incisor, premolars, and possibly molars.
- The **lingual height of contour** of the mandibular posteriors is much more occlusal than that of the maxillary posteriors.
- The **facial height of contour** of the maxillary posteriors is generally more occlusal than that of the mandibular posteriors.
- The **facial and lingual heights of contour** generally have a convexity of approximately 0.5 mm, except for the lingual of the mandibular posteriors, where it may measure up to 1 mm.

Table 1-5. Maxillary Heights of Contours/Contacts

	Lingual	Facial	Mesial Contact	Distal Contact
Central incisor	Cervical 1/3	Cervical 1/3	Incisal 1/3	Junction of middle and incisal 1/3
Lateral incisor	Cervical 1/3	Cervical 1/3	Junction of middle and incisal 1/3	Middle 1/3
Canine	Cervical 1/3	Cervical 1/3	Junction of middle and incisal 1/3	Middle 1/3
First premolar	Middle 1/3	Cervical 1/3	Middle 1/3	Middle 1/3
Second premolar	Middle 1/3	Cervical 1/3	Middle 1/3	Middle 1/3
First molar	Middle 1/3	Cervical 1/3	Middle 1/3	Middle 1/3
Second molar	Middle 1/3	Cervical 1/3	Middle 1/3	Middle 1/3
Third molar	Middle 1/3	Cervical 1/3	Middle 1/3	No distal contact

Table 1-6. Mandibular Heights of Contours/Contacts

	Lingual	Facial	Mesial Contact	Distal Contact
Central incisor	Cervical 1/3	Cervical 1/3	Incisal 1/3	Incisal 1/3
Lateral incisor	Cervical 1/3	Cervical 1/3	Incisal 1/3	Incisal 1/3
Canine	Cervical 1/3	Cervical 1/3	Incisal 1/3	Middle 1/3
First premolar	Junction of cervical and middle 1/3	Cervical 1/3	Middle 1/3	Middle 1/3
Second premolar	Middle 1/3	Cervical 1/3	Junction of middle and occlusal 1/3	Junction of middle and occlusal 1/3
First molar	Middle 1/3	Cervical 1/3	Junction of middle and occlusal 1/3	Middle 1/3
Second molar	Middle 1/3	Cervical 1/3	Middle 1/3	Middle 1/3
Third molar	Middle 1/3	Cervical 1/3	Middle 1/3	No distal contact

Contact Areas

Contact areas are influenced by the **size**, **form**, and **alignment** of the teeth. They are located at the **widest portion of a tooth** and correspond to the height of the contour. They function to:

- Stabilize the arch
- Prevent food impaction
- Protect the interproximal gingival tissue

Interproximal caries typically form immediately apical to the contact area.

Contact areas are described by **two coordinates: incisocervical** (occlusocervical) and **faciolingual.**

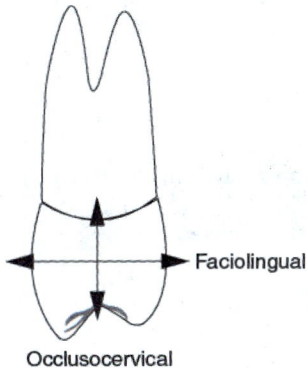

Incisocervical or occlusocervical contact

- At the mesial and distal heights of contour
- Mesial contact area is generally more occlusal or incisal than the distal (except for mandibular central incisors, premolars, possibly molars.

Faciolingual contact

- Anterior teeth contact centered faciolingually
- Posterior teeth contact placement may be more facial in the buccal third.

Junctions

DEJ (Dentinoenamel)

Dentin meeting enamel

Found only in crown

CEJ (Cementoenamel)

Between cementum and enamel; border of anatomic crown

Mesial curvature of CEJ greater than on distal of same tooth

Curvature becomes less distinct as you move toward posterior

Molar's CEJ relatively straight

Greatest mesial CEJ curvature of all teeth on maxillary central incisor (~3.5 mm; mesial surface)

CDJ (Cementodentinal)

Cementum meets dentin

Found only in root

Line angle—where two surfaces come together to form a line, e.g., mesiolabial, distolabial

Point angle—where three surfaces come together to form a point; takes name of surfaces involved, i.e., mesiolingual/occlusal, mesiobuccal/occlusal

Embrasures

Definition

Gap between two adjacent teeth, as teeth curve away from contact area

Form is dependent upon size, shape, and form of teeth

Four embrasures per contact area: lingual, facial, incisal/occlusal, gingival

Functions

Act as spillways for food from occlusal surfaces

Make teeth more self-cleansing

Characteristics

Maxillary anteriors

Lingual is greater than facial

Mandibular anteriors

Facial is greater than lingual

Posteriors

Lingual is generally greater than the facial (except maxillary molars)

Incisals

Incisal/occlusal is smaller than the gingival

Incisal may be missing between the mandibular central incisors because of high placement of mesial contact areas. This is the smallest incisal/occlusal embrasure found in the mouth.

Adult Dentition 2

Learning Objectives

❏ Describe general characteristics of maxillary and mandibular teeth

❏ Answer questions concerning specific anatomical details of individual teeth

❏ Recognize specific exceptions and variations to normal tooth anatomy

GENERAL

Incisors are involved with all of the main dental functions: **mastication, aesthetics, and phonetics.**

There are **8** permanent incisors (2 per quadrant). The central incisors are at the midline with the lateral incisors distal to the centrals.

Incisors are the **first succedaneous teeth to erupt.**

All incisors except the mandibular central have rounder distoincisal angles than mesioincisal angles (mandibular central is symmetric).

Smallest tooth—mandibular central incisor

Bilaterally symmetric—mandibular central incisor

Most distinct lingual anatomy—maxillary lateral incisor

Incisal edge not perpendicular to labiolingual bisecting line—mandibular lateral incisor ("twisted" on its axis)

Incisors

Maxillary	Mandibular
Larger	Smaller
Wider mesiodistal diameter (arch trait)	Wider labiolingual diameter
More distinct lingual anatomy	Less distinct lingual anatomy
May have lingual pits	Does not have lingual pits
Incisal edge is centered labiolingually	Incisal edge is lingual to labiolingual midpoint
Heights of contour more toward middle/incisal	Heights of contour more incisal
Lingual embrasure is greater than facial	Facial embrasure is greater than lingual
Contacts more cervically located	Contacts near incisal edge
More rounded distoincisal angles	Labial surface is straighter and flatter

Table 2-1. Summary of Lateral Versus Central Maxillary Incisors

	Maxillary Central Incisor	**Maxillary Lateral Incisor**
Crown	Not as rounded as lateral	Characterized by roundness; slightly more round on mesioincisal (distinctly so on distoincisal angles)
Root Cross-Section	Round	Ovoid
Other Features	Distinct lingual anatomy	More distinct lingual anatomy
	Distinct mammelons on incisal edge	Mammelons may be present only on newly erupted tooth
		Highly variable crown (peg laterals, etc.)
		May have distinct lingual pit

Table 2-2. Summary of Lateral Versus Central Mandibular Incisors

Mandibular Central Incisor	**Mandibular Lateral Incisor**
Smallest tooth	Not as small as central
Bilaterally symmetric	Not symmetric
Mirror mesial and distal axial surfaces	Distoincisal angle more round
Incisal edge perpendicular to a labiolingual bisecting line	Incisal edge not perpendicular to a labiolingual bisecting line ("twisted" on its axis)

Maxillary Central Incisor

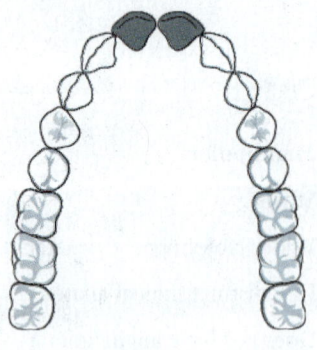

Position (tooth #)		
	Right	**Left**
Universal	8	9

Width: Wider mesiodistally than labiolingually

Root: Conical in shape-round in cross section

Angle: Distoincisal angle more rounded than mesioincisal

Developmental Data

First evidence of calcification: 3–4 months after birth

Enamel completed: 4–5 years

Eruption: 7–8 years

Root completed: 10 years

Number of roots: 1

Number of pulp horns: 3

Developmental lobes: 4

Table 2-3. Maxillary Right Central Incisor

Labial	Lingual	Mesial	Distal	Incisal
Surface convex in both directions	Slightly more narrow than labial	Triangular (wedge-shaped)	Similar to mesial	Triangular
Developmental depressions, lobulated appearance	Trapezoid	Apex of root toward labial	Wedge-shaped, more rounded	Incisal edge centered, straight, three mammelons
Mammelons at time of eruption	Lingual fossa scoop-like	Crest of curvature in cervical third	Less cervical line curvature	Cingulum toward distal
Trapezoid	Tendency for lingual fossa and cingulum to have central pit	Greatest cervical line curvature		Cross section at the cervical line is roundish
Incisal outline straight	Distinct mesial and distal marginal ridges and lingual fossa	Contour relatively straight		
Root cone-shaped				
Imbrication lines (faint curved lines parallel to CEJ)				

Variations on the Central Incisor (some may also be found on other teeth)

- Microdontia
- Macrodontia
- Hypercementosis—excessive amount of cementum
- Gemination (split)—

    Partial (1 pulp, 1 large tooth)

    Complete (results in twin teeth)

- Fusion—two teeth fused together along cementum; each tooth has own pulp
- Dilaceration—sharp angle of the root of tooth
- Plexion—sharp bend
- Extra incisor—supernumerary (accessory tooth between two maxillary central incisors called **mesiodens**)

Maxillary Lateral Incisor

The maxillary lateral incisor is the **most variable** of teeth, ranging from absent to peg-shaped to normal incisor shape. Its lingual surface can be flat, bulbous, or deeply pitted. It is characterized also by the **roundness of its disto-incisal and mesioincisal angles** and is the incisor **most likely to need a lingual restoration**.

The lateral incisors complement the central incisors. They are **smaller** in dimension, **except in root length**, and the **features** of the **lateral** are more **prominent**.

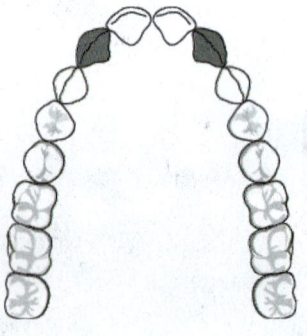

Position (tooth #)		
	Right	**Left**
Universal	7	10

Width: Wider mesiodistally than labiolingually

Root: Conical in shape

Angle: Distoincisal angle more rounded than the mesioincisal

Variations on the Lateral Incisor

- Missing altogether—partial anodontia
- Incomplete development of mesial and distal lobe—"peg lateral"
- Lingual surface—deep pit, dens en dente

Developmental Data

First evidence of calcification: 1 year

Enamel completed: 4–5 years

Eruption: 8–9 years

Root completed: 11 years

Number of roots: 1

Number of pulp horns: 1–3

Developmental lobes: 4

Table 2-4. Maxillary Right Lateral Incisor

Labial	Lingual	Mesial	Distal	Incisal
Surface has more curvature than central	Smaller than central	Crest of curvature in cervical third	Cervical line not as deep as in mesial	More ovoid in shape
Distal outline more rounded	Distinct anatomy: **mesial and distal marginal ridges, cingulum, lingual fossa, central pit**	Cervical line deeper than on distal		Mesiolabial and distolabial line angle more rounded
Root surface length greater in proportion to crown than in central	Incisal edge well developed			Evidence of lobes seen
	Lingual fossa more concave			
	Tendency to have lingual pit			
	Cingulum appears more prominent			
	Surface may be lobulated and slightly convex			

Mandibular Central Incisor

The mandibular central incisor is the **narrowest** and **most symmetric** of all teeth. **Mesial and distal profiles mirror each other.**

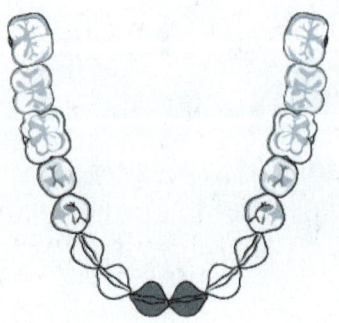

Position (tooth #)		
	Right	**Left**
Universal	25	24

Width: Narrowest of all teeth

Root: Ovoid on cross section;

wider labiolingually than mesiodistally;

symmetry

Angles: Mesioincisal and distoincisal angles very sharp

Developmental Data

First evidence of calcification: 3–4 months after birth

Enamel completed: 4–5 years

Eruption: 6–7 years

Root completed: 9 years

Number of roots: 1

Number of pulp horns: 1–3

Developmental lobes: 4

Table 2-5. Mandibular Right Central Incisor

Labial	Lingual	Mesial	Distal	Incisal
Root relatively long and straight	Indistinct lingual anatomy	Roots are wide faciolingually with depressions on both sides	Distal surface of crown and root very similar to mesial view	Symmetry between mesial and distal
Cervical line more rounded than on lingual	Root relatively long and straight	Incisal edge on or lingual to root axis	Distal contact area more toward cervical than mesial contact	Incisal edge toward lingual
Smooth surfaces (no marginal ridge)	Small cingulum			
Almost perfectly symmetrical crown	Almost perfectly symmetrical crown			

Mandibular Lateral Incisor

Mandibular lateral incisors are similar to mandibular centrals, except for the following:

- Lingual anatomy is indistinct.
- Mesial contour is straight with a height of contour at incisal edge.
- Incisal edge is **lingual to the labiolingual midpoint of the crown,** but the edge itself is not at right angles to a line bisecting the crown. However, it does follow arch curvature, making the distal end more lingually placed. The incisal edge appears to be rotated on the root.
- The root itself is very ovoid, being wider labiolingually than mesiodistally and may have mesial and distal depressions.

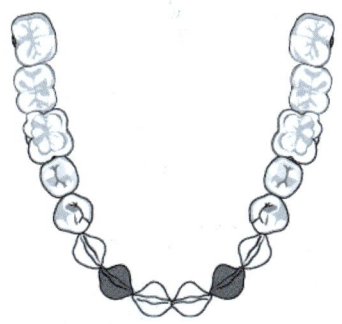

Position (tooth #)		
	Right	**Left**
Universal	26	23

- **Width:** Wider mesiodistally than central incisor

Developmental Data

First evidence of calcification: 3–4 months after birth

Enamel completed: 4–5 years

Eruption: 7–8 years

Root completed: 10 years

Number of roots: 1

Number of pulp horns: 1–3

Developmental lobes: 4

Table 2-6. Mandibular Right Lateral Incisor

Labial	Lingual	Mesial	Distal	Incisal
Asymmetric crown	Anatomy indistinct Cingulum distal to the long axis of tooth	Greater height of curvature of the CEJ From mesial, more of the lingual is visible (distal tilt)	Distal portion of incisal edge has a lingual turn	Incisal edge not straight mesiodistally and curves toward lingual on distal edge Cingulum is slightly toward distal Marginal ridge longer on mesial than distal side

Canines

There is only **one canine per quadrant** in the human. They are the only teeth with a **single cusp**. The canines are the **longest** and **most stable teeth** in the adult permanent dentition and have an **oversized root**.

Maxillary	Mandibular
Wider mesiodistally	Narrower mesiodistally
Distinct lingual anatomy (lingual cingulum)	Less distinct anatomy on lingual (cingulum less pronounced)
Contact point more cervical	Contact areas and heights of contour higher; contact points more incisal

Maxillary	Mandibular
Anomalies rare (may have tubercle between cusp tip and lingual ridge); very stable	One anomaly is a bifurcated root
Longest tooth in mouth (total length)	Anatomic crown longer
Incisal edge centered labiolingually	Incisal edge lingual to the labiolingual midpoint
Buccal tip centered in the long axis of the tooth	Cusp tip distally displaced
Wider mesiodistally	Narrower mesiodistally
Longer total length	Shorter total length
Crown generally in line with root and is shorter, fatter	Longer, slimmer crown that appears distally bent
Incisal edge in labiolingual midpoint	Incisal edge lingual to labiolingual midpoint
Prominent distal and mesial marginal ridge	Less prominent marginal ridges
Lingual ridge from cusp to cingulum	Less prominent lingual ridge
Labial surface has prominent middle lobe running from cusp tip to cervical line	
Buccal surface marked by three-lobed appearance	

Maxillary Canine

The maxillary canine is pointed and the **longest tooth in the mouth.**

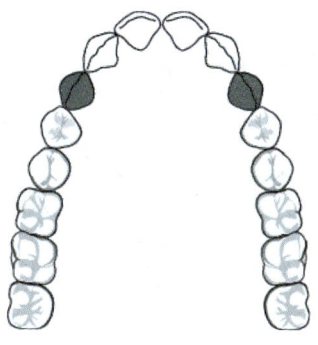

Position (tooth #)		
	Right	**Left**
Universal	6	11

Developmental Data

First evidence of calcification: 4–5 months after birth

Enamel completed: 6–7 years

Eruption: 11 to 12 years

Root completed: 14 to 15 years

Number of roots: 1

Number of pulp horns: 1–3

Developmental lobes: 4

Table 2-7. Maxillary Right Canine

Labial	Lingual	Mesial	Distal	Incisal
				D ◇ M
Root is long and tapers evenly Mesial ridge longer than distal Mesial incisal angle sharp One cusp tip	Outline similar to facial Pronounced cingulum Marginal ridges Lingual fossae (mesial and distal) Possible lingual pit	Root is straight (wider labial lingually than mesial distally) Mesial cervical line more curved than distal	Distal contour is very bulbous or convex	Cusp tip is facial and mesial in placement Cingulum is slightly distal Pulp cavity centered in root Root is wider faciolingually than mesiodistally

Mandibular Canine

The mandibular canine is also a long, pointed tooth in which the total length is less than the maxillary canine, but the crown is longer. It has a **trilobed buccal surface**.

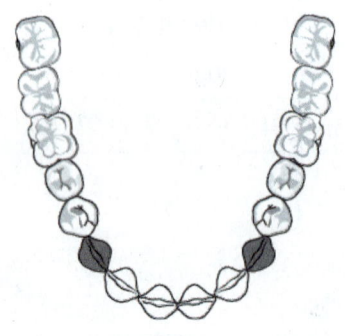

Position (tooth #)		
	Right	**Left**
Universal	27	22

Developmental Data

First evidence of calcification: 4–5 months after birth

Enamel completed: 6–7 years

Eruption: 9–10 years

Root completed: 12–14 years

Number of roots: 1

Number of pulp horns: 1–3

Developmental lobes: 4

Table 2-8. Manibular Right Canine

Labial	Lingual	Mesial	Distal	Incisal
Mesial cusp ridge is shorter than distal	Anatomy is less distinct than maxillary canine. Lingual pit is rare	Profile straight. Possible root concavity. Mesial cervical line more curved than distal	Similar to mesial view	Crown is distally inclined with cusp tip slightly distally displaced. Incisal edge is lingual to labiolingual midpoint. Cingulum is distally positioned. More symmetric than maxillary canine

Anomalies

One anomaly associated with the mandibular canine is a bifurcated root.

Premolars

General

There are two premolars per quadrant. The buccal cusp is more predominant than the lingual, and each premolar has **two cusps**. Premolars are also known as bicuspsids.

Maxillary and mandibular premolars are **approximately the same size mesiodistally and in total length**.

Know the premolars well. A surprisingly large number of dental anatomy questions involve these teeth.

Maxillary	Mandibular
Greater faciolingual diameter	Smaller faciolingual diameter
More distinct lingual cusps	Less distinct lingual cusps
Occlusal table centered faciolingually	Occlusal table lingually displaced
Two roots (buccal and lingual) in maxillary first	Both premolars with one root
Buccal surface is straighter from height of contour to cusp tip	Buccal surface more convex
Prominent mesial root concavities, especially maxillary first	Rounder roots on cross-section

Table 2-9. Comparison of Developmental Data of Premolars

	Maxillary First	Maxillary Second	Mandibular First	Mandibular Second
First evidence of calcification	1½–1¾ years	1–2½ years	1¾–2 years	2¼–2½ years
Enamel completed	5–6 years	6–7 years	5–6 years	6–7 years
Eruption	10–11 years	10–12 years	10–12 years	11–12 years
Root completed	12–13 years	12–14 years	12–13 years	13–14 years
Number of lobes	4	4	4	4–5
Number of roots	2	1	1	1

Table 2-10. Comparison of the Premolars

	Maxillary First	Maxillary Second	Mandibular First	Mandibular Second
Root	2 roots	1 root	1 root Relatively round and conical	1 root Roundest and most conical root on cross section
Cusps	Distally displaced buccal cusp and mesially displaced lingual cusp	Buccal and lingual cusps equal and centered mesiodistally	Large buccal cusp dominates Canine-like in appearance	**2 to 3 cusps** If 3, 2 are lingual, with mesiolingual larger than distolingual "Y" occlusal pattern for 3 cusps; "H" occlusal pattern for 2 cusps
Occlusal table	Trapezoidal	Rectangular	**Lingually inclined**	Square-shaped Less inclined than first premolar
Occlusal outlines	Hexagonal	Ovoid	Diamond	Square
Grooves	Mesial intraradicular groove Mesial marginal developmental groove	Short central groove Numerous supplemental grooves	**Mesiolingual developmental groove**	Lingual groove with 2 lingual cusps (3-cusp type)

	Maxillary First	Maxillary Second	Mandibular First	Mandibular Second
Ridges	Lingual convergence Buccal cusp ridge inclines toward mesiolingual (twisted appearance)	Little lingual convergence	**Transverse ridge** Well-developed buccal ridge Mesial ridge less distinct than distal marginal ridge Lingual convergence	Little lingual convergence
Other distinguishing features	"Broad-shouldered" Prominent mesial concavity Prominent buccal lobes	"Narrow shouldered" Less prominent mesial axial concavity than maxillary first	Most resembles **canine** **Lingual cusp that resembles a cingulum** Transitional tooth Greatest discrepancy in size of buccal and lingual cusps and width (buccal dominant) Mesial/distal fossae with pits Prominent mesial bulge Sloping occlusal table	Central pit Equal buccal and lingual surfaces

Maxillary First Premolar

The maxillary first premolar has a **prominent buccal ridge**, and its buccal surface is wider than the lingual surface. It is the **only premolar that has two roots** (one buccal and one lingual) and **two cusps**.

The maxillary first premolar and its **intraradicular groove** is important to know for the **NBDE Part I**. Root planing of the mesial side and adapting a matrix band on the mesial side can both be difficult because of this groove.

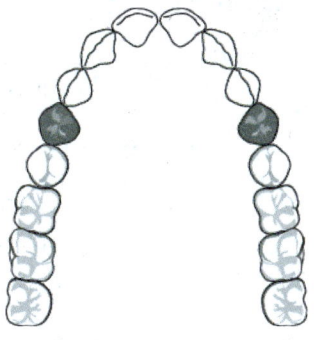

Position (tooth #)		
	Right	**Left**
Universal	5	12

Table 2-11. Maxillary Right First Premolar

Buccal	Lingual	Mesial	Distal	Occlusal
				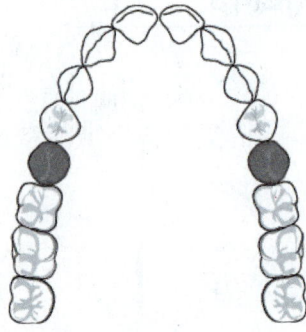
Rounded, long cusp Prominent buccal ridge running axially and bordered by depressions that give the surface a 3-lobed appearance Buccal surface wider than lingual surface ("broad-shouldered")	Lingual cusp smaller Lingual cusp slightly mesial to midpoint and smaller than buccal cusp Surface rounded	Marked mesial concavity runs onto mesial root surface (**mesial interradicular groove**) **Mesial marginal developmental groove** (extension of central groove) interrupts mesial marginal ridge and progresses down mesial surface	Buccal cusp distally placed and larger than lingual cusp Also has developmental depression	**Hexagonal crown profile** (mesial and distal surfaces converge toward lingual) **Trapezoidal occlusal table** 2 cusps that are well defined: buccal is larger, and lingual is shifted mesially

Variants and Anomalies

- Single root (rare)
- Occasionally 3 rooted (rare)

Maxillary Second Premolar

The maxillary second premolar is a **"narrow-shouldered"** tooth from the buccal and is **slightly smaller** than the first premolar. It has **indistinct lobes**; a slight mesial concavity or even convexity may be seen on the mesial surface. **The mesial marginal ridge is not interrupted by a groove. Cusps** are more **equal in height and length**, and the **tips are centered** on the tooth in a mesiodistal direction.

Position (tooth #)		
	Right	**Left**
Universal	4	13

Table 2-12. Maxillary Right Second Premolar

Buccal	Lingual	Mesial	Distal	Occlusal
				D M
Indistinct lobes	Lingual cusp almost as big as buccal cusp	Surface round	Surface round	**Ovoid to round** shape
Buccal cusp is **shorter and rounde**r than first premolar	Lingual cusp tip shifted mesially	Mesial marginal ridge is **not** interrupted by groove		**Rectangular** occlusal table
				Little lingual convergence

Variants and Anomalies

More variability than in first maxillary premolar

Mandibular First Premolar

The mandibular first premolar may be viewed as a **transitional tooth, resembling a canine**. Its buccal cusp is much larger than is the lingual cusp, which may resemble a cingulum. It is the **only posterior tooth with a lingually inclined occlusal table.**

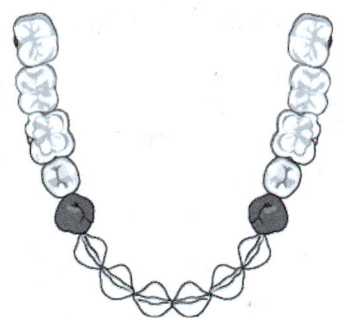

Position (tooth #)		
	Right	Left
Universal	28	21

Table 2-13. Mandibular Right First Premolar

Buccal	Lingual	Mesial	Distal	Occlusal
Outline is almost bilaterally symmetrical	**Smallest and indistinct cusp of all premolars**	Prominent mesial bulge	Very large buccal cusp tip centered over root tip	**Diamond shaped,** with convergence to the lingual
Large pointed buccal cusp	Lingual cusp may resemble a cingulum	Very large buccal cusp tip centered over root tip	Reduced lingual cusp	Marginal ridges well developed
Well-developed buccal ridge	**Mesiolingual developmental groove** produces slight concavity at about the mesiolingual line angle	Reduced lingual cusp	Mesial/distal fossae with pits	Mesial and distal fossae with pits
		Mesial/distal fossae with pits	Marginal ridges well developed	Mesiolingual developmental groove
		Marginal ridges well developed		

Variants and Anomalies

- Grooved or bifurcated roots
- Crown and root may be variable

Mandibular Second Premolar

The mandibular second premolar is generally larger than the mandibular first premolar. It is distinguished by its **two variations of the lingual cusp.** If the mandibular second premolar has three cusps (more common) instead of two, the two appear on the lingual view and the mesiolingual is much larger than the distolingual. The mesiolingual cusp is also separated by a lingual groove extending from the central pit.

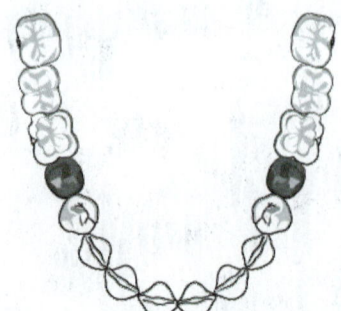

Position (tooth #)		
	Right	Left
Universal	29	20

Chapter 2 • Adult Dentition

Table 2-14. Mandibular Right Second Premolar

Buccal	Lingual	Mesial	Distal	Occlusal

Buccal	Lingual	Mesial	Distal	Occlusal
Buccal width nearly equal with lingual; buccal cusp size more equal with lingual cusp size	Lingual width nearly equal with buccal; lingual cusp size more equal with buccal cusp size If 3 cusps, 2 are lingual, with mesiolingual larger than distolingual Mesiolingual and distolingual cusp separated by lingual groove extending from central pit Little occlusal surface seen from the lingual In the single lingual cusp variant, its tip is shifted mesially	Buccal cusp is slightly shorter than first mandibular premolar Buccal cusp slightly longer than lingual cusp		Square in outline Central pit Variant groove patterns: • Y (3 cusps with central pit) • H (2 cusps with single developmental groove crossing transverse ridge from mesial to distal)

Variants and Anomalies

- One or two lingual cusps
- Missing altogether

Molars

General

The molar is derived from *mola*, Latin for "millstone." The main function of molars is to grind food, thus explaining their **large occlusal surfaces**. The most complicated of the adult human dentition, they can have from **three to five cusps** and **two to three roots**.

Questions on NBDE part I concerning molar anatomy will usually focus more on the first molar. This is because of increasing variation in the second and third molars.

Maxillary Molar (First)

3 roots

4 pulp horns

4 cusps (and extra variable Carabelli cusp (trait)

Buccal cusps unequal

Lingual cusps unequal; cusp of Carabelli mostly present

Oblique ridge diagonal

Occlusal table centered labiolingually

Equal amounts of buccal and lingual surfaces may be seen from occlusal

Lingual height of contour in middle third just above junction of middle and cervical thirds

Wider faciolingually than mesiodistally

Distolingual groove

Mandibular Molar (First)

2 roots

2 pulp horns

5 cusps

Buccal cusps equal

Lingual cusps equal; cusp of Carabelli absent

Oblique ridge not found

Occlusal table lingually placed

More buccal surface than lingual surface may be seen from occlusal

Lingual height of contour in middle third just below the junction of the middle and occlusal thirds

Wider mesiodistally than faciolingually

Buccal pit

Table 2-15. Developmental Data

	Maxillary			Mandibular		
	First	Second	Third	First	Second	Third
First evidence of calcification	Birth	2 ½ years	7–9 years	Birth	2½–3 years	8–10 years
Enamel completed	3–4 years	7–8 years	12–16 years	2½–3 years	7–8 years	12–16 years
Eruption	6 years	12–13 years	17–21 years	6–7 years	11–13 years	17–21 years
Root completed	9–10 years	14–16 years	18–25 years	9–10 years	14–15 years	18–25 years
Number of lobes	5	4	4	5	4	4
Number of roots	3	3	3 (may be fused into 1; highly variable)	2	2	2 (may be fused into 1; may be 3; highly variable)

Table 2-16. Comparison of the Maxillary Molars

	Maxillary First	Maxillary Second	Maxillary Third
Root	**3 roots** (2 buccal, 1 lingual) Buccal roots look like "pliers handles"; distobuccal smallest Large lingual palatal root longest, "banana shaped" (almost straight) and centered between buccal roots 30% have fourth canal found in mesiobuccal root	**3 roots** (2 buccal, 1 lingual) Buccal roots distally inclined Roots are within crown profiles when seen from all angles	**3 roots** (2 buccal, 1 lingual) Often short Very distally inclined Tend to fuse (lingual to buccal)
Cusps	**4 major** (2 buccal, 2 lingual) **Fifth** minor cusp: **Carabelli** ML and MB cusps very large DB cusp large; DL cusp smaller 4 pulp horns (1 per major cusp)	**4 major** No Carabelli trait ML and MB cusps smaller than first DB cusp smaller; DL cusp even smaller (may be missing) 4 pulp horns (1 per major cusp)	**Usually 3** No Carabelli trait ML and MB cusps smaller than second DB cusp much smaller; DL cusp usually missing
Occlusal outlines	Rhomboidal	Rhomboidal or heart-shaped	Heart-shaped or triangular
Grooves	Lingual groove separates lingual cusps Buccal groove runs between buccal cusps Distal groove extends from central pit distolingually toward oblique ridge	Usually a short buccal groove; no buccal pit Similar to first molar	Variable pattern
Ridges	Oblique ridge most prominent, connects distobuccal cusp to mesiolingual cusp Mesial marginal ridge longer and more distinct than distal marginal ridge	Oblique ridge from distobuccal to mesiolingual Similar to first molar	Oblique ridges may be missing Variable pattern
Other distinguishing features	Looks like two premolars stuck together Distal and central fossa Distal triangular fossa contains distal pit Cusp size: Mesiolingual > mesiobuccal > distobuccal > distolingual	More exaggerated difference in cusp size: mesiolingual > mesiobuccal > distobuccal > distolingual	More variable morphology than any other tooth May be the most often congenitally missing

Table 2-17. Comparison of the Mandibular Molars

	Mandibular First	Mandibular Second	Mandibular Third
Root (for more details, see individual tooth)	2 roots Rounded apex Mesial root largest Roots less distally inclined than in second molar	2 roots More distinctly distally inclined Pointed apex Proximal root concavities not usually seen	2 roots Extremely distally inclined Short, often fused
Cusps	5 cusps	4 cusps	4 cusps (highly variable)
Occlusal outlines	Pentagonal	Rectangular	Ovoid
Grooves	2 buccal grooves (MB and DB) Mesial and distal marginal grooves	Single buccal groove No marginal grooves	Single buccal groove No marginal grooves
Ridges	Two transverse ridges, no oblique ridge	Two transverse ridges, no oblique ridge	Two transverse ridges, no oblique ridge
Other distinguishing features	Prone to misshapen enamel defect: mulberry molar Largest of the mandibular teeth	Most symmetric of the molars No distal cusp	Often has variable morphology May be the most often congenitally missing Common tooth to have enamel pearls

Maxillary First Molar

The **Carabelli trait** is the most distinguishing feature of the maxillary first molar, and is highly variable, from being a full cusp to being barely visible. It is found attached to ML cusp when present.

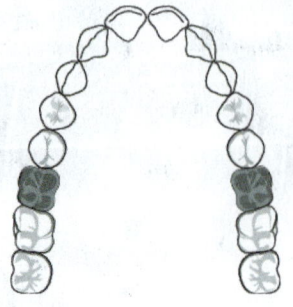

Position (tooth #)		
	Right	**Left**
Universal	3	14

Table 2-18. Maxillary Right First Molar

Buccal	Lingual	Mesial	Distal	Occlusal

Larger mesiobuccal cusp

Cervical line straight

Mesiobuccal and distobuccal dominate

Buccal developmental groove

Roots: Buccal roots joined in common root trunk (extends 2.5–3.5 mm from cervical line)

Root trunk may have deep developmental groove

All roots can be seen from buccal view, with lingual root in between

Lingual surface convex throughout

Lingual developmental groove (extension of distolingual groove)

Larger mesiolingual cusp sometimes has Carabelli trait

Root: Lingual is largest root (greatest diameter in mesiodistal direction)

Massive root trunk

Vertical depression on its lingual surface extending from cervical line

Mesiobuccal has a mesial contour; distobuccal has distal contour

Flat to concave surface

Cusp of Carabelli seen

Roots: From mesial view, only mesiobuccal and lingual roots seen (distobuccal blocked by mesiobuccal)

Convex surface throughout, except for concave-to-flat area immediately above distobuccal root

Distal marginal ridge shorter than mesial

Rhomboid shape

Angles: Mesiobuccal and distolingual **acute**; distobuccal and mesiolingual **obtuse**

4 major cusps

Cusp of Carabelli on mesiolingual cusp

Lingual groove separates lingual cusps

Oblique ridge (mesiolingual to distobuccal cusps)

Major fossae: distal and central

Minor fossa: mesial triangular, distal triangular

Distal pit

Largest crown of all maxillary molars

Maxillary Second Molar

The maxillary second molar is very similar to the first molar, with the following exceptions: *1)* **the distobuccal cusp is relatively smaller and the distolingual cusp is smaller or absent,** *2)* **the absence of the cusp of Carabelli,** *3)* the mesiobuccal and distolingual angles are more acute, whereas the mesiolingual and distobuccal angles are more obtuse, and *4)* there are **more supplemental grooves** on the occlusal surface.

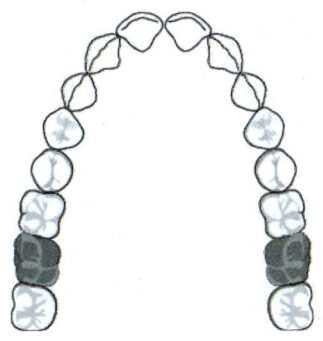

	Position (tooth #)	
	Right	**Left**
Universal	2	15

Table 2-19. Maxillary Second Right Molar

Buccal	Lingual	Mesial	Distal	Occlusal

D · M

| Crown is shorter occlusocervically and is narrower mesiodistally

Distobuccal cusp is smaller

Root: Mesiobuccal and distobuccal root are inclined distally and are more parallel and usually the same length | Distolingual cusp smaller

No Carabelli cusp

Root: Lingual root may be distally inclined (no "pliers handles") | Crown is shorter than first molar

Roots confine themselves to width of crown | | **Rhomboidal** (large distolingual cusp) or **heart-shaped** (smaller distolingual cusp)

Distobuccal cusp smaller and less defined than first molar

Oblique ridge less dominant

Differences in cusp size more exaggerated than on first molar

Distolingual cusp smaller to absent |

Variants and Anomalies

- Distolingual cusp absent
- Occlusal shape rhomboidal or heart-shaped
- Fused root

Maxillary Third Molar

The maxillary third molar, as well as the maxillary lateral incisor, is known for **extreme variability of form.** Pointed, peg-like maxillary third molars are not uncommon. The sometimes fused, pointed roots can make extraction of these teeth easier than expected.

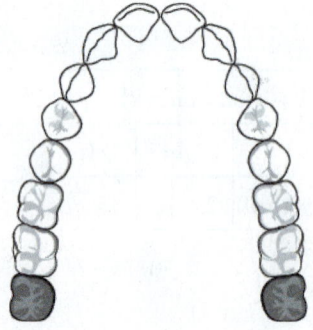

Position (tooth #)		
	Right	**Left**
Universal	1	16

Table 2-20. Maxillary Third Right Molar

Buccal	Lingual	Mesial	Distal	Occlusal
Distobuccal cusp smaller than mesiobuccal (sometimes missing) **Roots:** Buccal roots most often fused	Distolingual cusp often absent (mostly one large lingual cusp) **Root:** Lingual root often fused to buccal cusps	Crown outline rounded, bulbous	**No contact point** on distal surface Crown outline also rounded, bulbous	**Heart-shaped or triangular** Oblique ridge may be small or missing Smallest crown of the maxillary molars Mesiolingual cusp is largest; distobuccal is smallest (or distolingual, if present)

Variants and Anomalies

- Impaction common
- Many cusps and grooves possible
- Distobuccal cusp small
- Distolingual cusp missing

Mandibular First Molar

The mandibular first molar has a **distinctive pentagonal ("home plate") occlusal outline**, and two buccal and one lingual groove form the pattern distinctive to this tooth. The **buccal half is divided into three cusps, and the lingual is divided into two.**

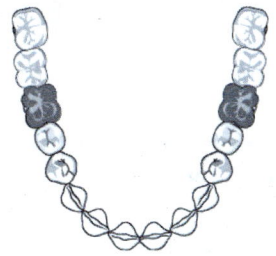

Position (tooth #)		
	Right	**Left**
Universal	30	19

Table 2-21. Mandibular Right First Molar

Buccal	Lingual	Mesial	Distal	Occlusal

(Tooth illustrations: Buccal, Lingual, Mesial, Distal, and Occlusal views with M and D labels)

Buccal	Lingual	Mesial	Distal	Occlusal
3 cusps seen	3 cusps seen	Rhomboid (tilted lingually)	3 cusps seen (distobuccal, distal, distolingual)	**Pentagonal** ("home plate") shape
2 developmental grooves (mesiobuccal and distobuccal)	Developmental groove separates 2 lingual cusps	Lingual surface straighter than convex buccal surface	Tooth tapers toward distal	**5** functional cusps
Mesiobuccal groove ends in **buccal pit** on buccal surface	Prominent cervical ridge height	Mesial marginal groove notches mesial marginal ridge	Distal marginal ridge notched by distal marginal groove	**3 fossae, each with pit:** central, mesial, and distal
Trapezoidal shape (wider at occlusal)	**Roots:** 2 visible	Buccal cervical ridge	**Root:** Curves distally; blunt, distal smaller than mesial; may have shallow proximal root concavity; joined with mesial at common root trunk	Buccal outline divided into 3 (mesiobuccal and distobuccal grooves)
Distal outline more rounded		**Root:** Mesial root is the broadest root in the arch in a buccolingual direction; curves distally; distinct proximal root concavity on mesial surface; blunt; joined with distal at common root trunk		Lingual outline divided into 2 (lingual groove)
Mesiobuccal cusp widest; distobuccal smallest				Distal marginal ridge smaller than mesial marginal ridge (both ridges cut through by developmental grooves)
Roots: 2 clearly seen; distal root is less curved than mesial				

Variants and Anomalies

- Distal cusp absent
- Occasionally 2 mesial roots
- Sixth cusp rare

Mandibular Second Molar

The mandibular second molar is similar to the first molar except that it is *1)* smaller, *2)* the **distal cusp is missing**, *3)* the lingual and buccal surfaces are similar in length, *4)* there is **only one buccal groove**; *5)* the crown is also shorter, and *6)* there are **no developmental grooves interrupting the marginal ridges.** Finally, *7)* roots are more distally inclined than the first molar and have a more pointed apex.

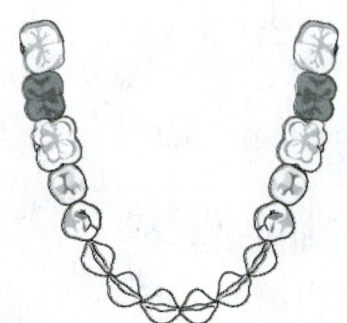

Position (tooth #)		
	Right	**Left**
Universal	31	18

Table 2-22. Mandibular Second Right Molar

Buccal	Lingual	Mesial	Distal	Occlusal
Buccal groove separates mesiobuccal from disto-buccal cusps Trapezoidal shape No distal cusp (4 cusps) **Roots:** Closer together than first mandibular molar and are distally inclined	Trapezoidal shape Lingual groove **Roots:** Closer together than first mandibular molar and are distally inclined	Looks similar to first molar Cusps of equal height	Cusps of equal height Distal marginal ridge helps form profile Cervical line flat	**Rectangular** 4 cusps 3 grooves (buccal, lingual, central) 3 fossae, each with pit (central, medial, distal) Two transverse ridges

Variants and Anomalies

- 2 root canals for each root
- Five cusps (rare)

Mandibular Third Molar

Third molars vary in shape and **do not have a standard form**. They are usually smaller than the second molar.

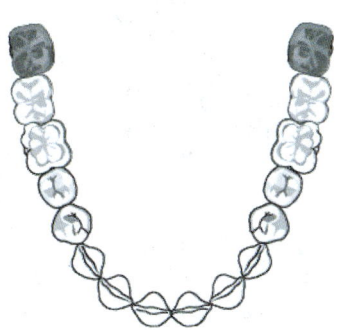

Position (tooth #)		
	Right	**Left**
Universal	32	17

Table 2-23. Mandibular Third Right Molar

Buccal	Lingual	Mesial	Distal	Occlusal
Crown short and bulbous		Resembles first and second molars, but shorter crown		**Ovoid to round**
Roots: distally inclined; poorly developed				4–5 cusps
				May have indistinct grooves

Variants and Anomalies

- Most commonly missing permanent teeth
- Often under- or oversized
- Supernumerary (fourth molars)
- May be partially erupted (susceptible to periodontal infections)
- Occlusal surface may be crenulated (numerous grooves)
- Often fail to erupt

Primary Dentition

Learning Objectives

❏ List general characteristics of primary teeth

❏ Answer questions concerning development, calcification, eruption, and shedding of primary teeth

❏ Describe specific characteristics of individual primary teeth

GENERAL

In addition to performing the normal chewing function, the deciduous dentition (also called "primary" or "baby" teeth) helps permanent teeth develop proper alignment, spacing, and occlusion. As stated in the first few pages of the General Characteristics section, there are 20 primary teeth (10 maxillary and 10 mandibular).

MAXILLARY

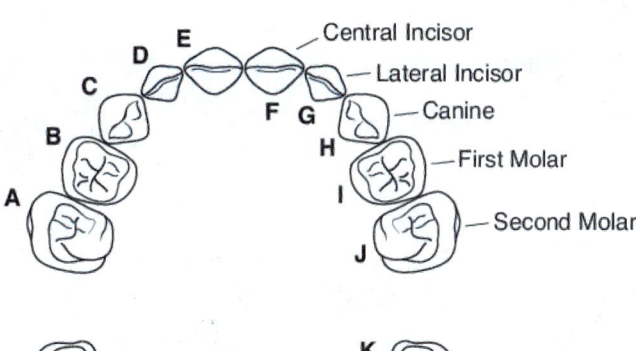

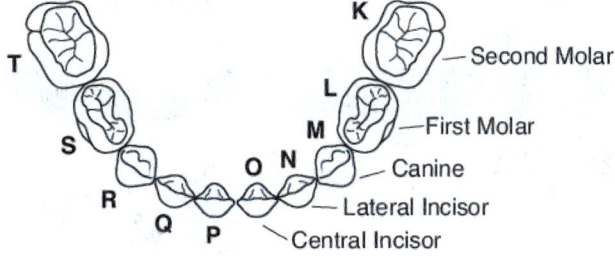

MANDIBULAR

Figure 3-1. Deciduous Teeth

Table 3-1. Eruption and shedding of primary teeth

Maxillary	Eruption* (months)	Shedding (years)
Central incisor	8–12	6–7
Lateral incisor	9–13	7–8
Canine (cuspid)	16–22	10–12
First molar	13–19	9–11
Second molar	25–33	10–12
Mandibular		
Central incisor	6–10	6–7
Lateral incisor	10–16	7–8
Canine (cuspid)	17–23	9–12
First molar	14–18	9–11
Second molar	23–31	10–12

*Note that teeth tend to erupt in pairs.

Also, eruption and shedding patterns are seen earlier in girls.

Table 3-2. Calcification and root formation of primary teeth

Maxillary	Calcification (weeks in utero)	Root Formation Complete (months)
Central incisor	14	10
Lateral incisor	16	11
Canine (cuspid)	17	19
First molar	15	16
Second molar	19	26
Mandibular		
Central incisor	14	8
Lateral incisor	16	13
Canine (cuspid)	17	20
First molar	15½	16
Second molar	18	27

Primary Teeth Characteristics as Differing from Permanent Teeth

In general, the primary teeth are **smaller and whiter** than permanent teeth and generally resemble the teeth that replace them, **except for the first molars**, which resemble nothing in the permanent dentition. **Primary molars** are replaced by **permanent premolars**. Crown-to-root ratios are generally less than those of permanent teeth (crowns are relatively smaller). Pulps are relatively larger.

Development of Primary Teeth

- Development begins at 6 weeks in utero
- Calcification begins at approximately 14 weeks in utero (approx 4–6 months)
- By the age of 3, apices are completely formed

Table 3-3. Comparison of primary and permanent teeth–general characteristics

Features	Comparison with Permanent Teeth
Crowns	Crown-to-root ratio is smaller Shorter and fatter Rounded
Roots	Marked bowing and flaring Molars: long and slender with little or no trunk Incisors and canines: longer and slender
Enamel	Whiter
Surfaces	Lingual and facial cervical bulges Facial and lingual surfaces are flatter No mammelons on anterior teeth
Arch	More circular
Ridges	Cervical ridges more prominent

Anterior Teeth

The primary incisors and canines resemble the permanent ones, **except for traits listed in the following table.** A notable characteristic of the anteriors is **cervical constricture**.

Table 3-4. Characteristics of primary anterior teeth

Tooth	Position (Right/Left)	Replaced by	Differences from Permanent Replacement
Maxillary primary central incisor*	E/F	Maxillary permanent central incisor	Smooth labial surface No mammelons Cingulum may be prominent Cervical constricture: facial and lingual cervical bulges Height of crown smaller than mesiodistal diameter
Maxillary primary lateral incisor*	D/G	Maxillary permanent lateral incisor	Labial surface smoother than permanent No mammelons Cervical constricture
Maxillary primary canine*	C/H	Maxillary permanent canine	Diamond-shaped crown from facial Labial surface smoother Prominent cingulum (cusped appearance) Mesial and distal contacts are at same level Longer mesial incisal slope than distal incisal slope Height of crown less than mesiodistal diameter
Mandibular primary central incisor	P/O	Mandibular permanent central incisor	Labial surface smooth, unmarked, flat Prominent cingulum on lingual Often, developmental groove or depression on distal of root Cervical contricture
Mandibular primary lateral incisor	Q/N	Mandibular permanent lateral incisor	Prominent cingulum on lingual Cervical constricture
Mandibular primary canine	R/M	Mandibular permanent canine	Arrow-shaped from facial Smooth labial surface Longer distal incisal ridge than mesial incisal ridge

*These teeth are most damaged by baby bottle tooth decay (BBTD) or early childhood caries (ECC).

Posterior Teeth

The primary first molar resembles nothing in the adult dentition. In general, **upper molars** have **3 roots**, whereas the **lower molars** have only **2**. First molars are also distinguished by a bulge on the buccal surface (cervical bulge).

Table 3-5. Characteristics of primary posterior teeth

Tooth	Position	Replaced by	Traits
Maxillary primary first molar	B/I	Maxillary permanent first premolar	Resembles nothing in permanent dentition
			Two-cusped (mesiobuccal and mesiolingual with small distobuccal cusp area)
			Nodule resembling small cusp may be present on mesial ridge of the mesiobuccal cusp
			Occlusal table outline is rectangular with deep prominent **buccal developmental groove** (terminates in central pit)
			Frequently, **oblique ridge** from mesiolingual cusp to distobuccal cusp area
			Heights of contour low and prominent
			Three roots very divergent (room for developing premolar), without trunk root; looks like "elephant charging" when viewed from lingual and inverted
Maxillary primary secondary molar	A/J	Maxillary permanent Second premolar	Closely resembles maxillary permanent first molar (see "Isomorphy" below) (4 cusps, Carabelli trait), except:
			• Squatter and more bulbous
			• More prominent cervical bulges
			• Very little root trunk
Mandibular primary first molar	S/L	Mandibular permanent first premolar	Resembles nothing in permanent dentition
			Looks more like a molar than maxillary primary first molar
			4 cusps (2 buccal, 2 lingual); mesiobuccal and mesiolingual largest
			Transverse ridge between mesiobuccal and mesiolingual (largest) cusps
			Mesial/distal profiles: highly convex
			Occlusal **outline rhomboidal** because of buccal cervical ridge
			Occlusal **table rectangular**
			Buccal profile: **low, prominent buccal cervical ridge** (unique; gives "pregnant" appearance)
			Deep buccal groove, shallow lingual groove; may have mesial marginal groove
			2 roots: mesial larger
			Central pit radiating a central groove (goes to mesial pit and buccal and lingual grooves)
Mandibular primary second molar	T/K	Mandibular permanent second premolar	Closely resembles mandibular permanent second molar (see "Isomorphy" below), except:
			• 2 roots more divergent and without root trunk
			• Cervical bulges
			• All 3 buccal cusps equal in size

Isomorphy of Primary Second and Permanent First Molars

In summary, there is a remarkable resemblance between the maxillary and mandibular second primary molars and their first permanent molar counterparts, even down to the smallest details.

Summary of Some Important Primary Teeth Characteristics

This information about primary teeth is important to know for the NBDE Part I exam:

- The mandibular first primary molar has the most unique buccal cervical bulge or ridge.
- The mandibular first primary molar has a prominent transverse ridge.
- The mandibular first and maxillary first primary molars resemble nothing in permanent dentition. (The maxillary first primary molar somewhat resembles a premolar.)
- The mandibular second and maxillary second primary molars resemble the mandibular first and maxillary first permanent molars, respectively.

Learning Objectives

- ❏ Describe basic properties of occlusion
- ❏ Understand relationship of tooth anatomy to occlusion
- ❏ Answer questions concerning specific tooth to tooth occlusal relationships

Occlusion is the general contact relationship between the occlusal surfaces of the maxillary and mandibular arches and individual teeth.

Arch-to-Arch Relationships

When the two arches come together, each tooth opposes two teeth in the opposite arch, with the exception of the **mandibular central incisor** and **the maxillary third molar**, each of which only opposes one tooth. Knowing the general relationships described below is critical when answering most occlusion questions.

The Maxillary Arch

Each tooth in the maxillary arch opposes two teeth in the mandibular arch—its counterpart in the mandibular arch, plus the tooth distal to its counterpart, except the maxillary third molar.

Example

The first maxillary premolar opposes the first mandibular premolar and second mandibular premolar.

The Mandibular Arch

Each tooth in the mandibular arch opposes two teeth in the maxillary arch—its counterpart in the maxillary arch, plus the tooth mesial to its counterpart, except the mandibular central incisor.

Example

The first mandibular molar opposes the first maxillary molar (its counterpart), plus the second maxillary premolar (tooth mesial to its counterpart).

Note: The tip of the maxillary canine is placed in the labial embrasure.

The arch form of the maxilla is larger compared with the mandible, providing an overlapping of the maxillary teeth over the mandibular teeth. The **horizontal overlap** is referred to as **overjet,** and the **vertical overlap** is referred to as **overbite.** This overhanging provides a protective feature during opening and closing movements of the jaws. Soft tissues are displaced during the act of closure until the teeth have come together in occlusal contact. Therefore, the cheeks, lips, and tongue are less likely to be caught and injured during mandibular movements.

Concepts and Definitions

The numbers in the first column of the table correspond with the figure.

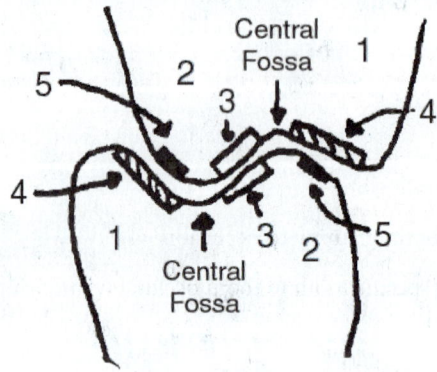

Figure 4-1. Occlusal surfaces

Table 4-1. Occlusal cusps, surfaces, and contacts

	Area	Definition	Examples
1	**Guiding cusp**	Cusp of tooth **not in contact in occlusion** but **outside** occluding area Opposing embrasures or grooves in the opposing dentition	Buccal cusps of maxillary posteriors and lingual cusps of mandibular posteriors
2	**Supporting (holding) cusp**	Cusp of tooth that **contacts the opposing arch on marginal ridges or central fossa area** Responsible for **supporting the forces of occlusion**	Buccal cusps of mandibular posteriors and lingual cusps of maxillary posteriors
3	**Occlusal slope**	Inclines of slopes of holding cusps	Buccal inclines of lingual cusps of maxillary posteriors and lingual inclines of buccal cusps of mandibular posteriors
4	**Guiding incline**	Inclines or slopes of the guiding cusps from the guiding cusp tip toward the center of tooth	Lingual inclines of buccal cusps of maxillary posteriors and buccal inclines of lingual cusps of mandibular posteriors
5	**Functional outer aspect (FOA)**	The outside 1–2 mm of supporting cusp Makes contact with guiding inclines of guiding cusps of opposing dentition when in occlusion	1–2 mm wide strip from buccal cusp tips of mandibular posteriors on buccal surface, and 1–2 mm wide strip from lingual cusp tips of maxillary posteriors on lingual surface

Posterior Teeth in General

The **buccal cusps of the mandibular posteriors** and **the lingual cusps of the maxillary posteriors** are the holding, supporting, or occluding cusps, and they contact marginal ridges and central fossae in the opposing arch.

The **buccal cusps of the maxillary posteriors** and the **lingual cusps of the mandibular posteriors** are the guiding cusps and oppose the embrasures and grooves of the opposing dentition.

Therefore, on each posterior tooth, we should expect **3 areas of contact** during occlusion:

1. The FOA of the holding cusp contacting the guiding incline(s) of the guiding cusp in the opposing dentition
2. The occlusal slope of the holding cusp contacting the occlusal slope of the opposing holding cusp
3. The guiding incline(s) of the guiding cusp contacting the FOA of the holding cusp of the opposing dentition

Summary of Occlusal Contacts

Table 4-2. Tooth Contacts in a Class I Normal Occlusion*

Maxillary Teeth	Mandibular Occlusal Contact	Mandibular Teeth	Maxillary Occlusal Contact
Central incisor	Central and lateral	Central incisor	Maxillary central incisor
Lateral incisor	Lateral incisor and canine	Lateral incisor	Central and lateral incisors
Canine	Canine and first premolar	Canine	Lateral incisor and canine
First premolar	First and second premolars	First premolar	Canine and first premolar
Second premolar	Second premolar and first molars	Second premolar	First and second premolar
First molar	First and second molars	First molar	Second premolar and first molar
Second molar	Second and third molars	Second molar	First and second molar
Third molar	Third molar	Third molar	Second and third molar

*The mandibular central incisor is the only anterior tooth that occludes with only one tooth. The maxillary third molar is the only posterior tooth that occludes with only one tooth.

GENERAL RULE OF MAXILLARY POSTERIOR HOLDING CUSPS

The holding cusps of the maxillary posteriors occlude on the distal marginal ridge of its counterpart in the mandibular arch plus the mesial marginal ridge of the tooth distal to its counterpart, with the exception of the **mesiolingual cusps** of the molars, which occlude in the central fossae of their counterpart molars in the mandibular arch.

1. **First maxillary premolar** (lingual cusp): contacts the distal marginal ridge (DMR) of the first mandibular premolar plus the mesial marginal ridge (MMR) of the second mandibular premolar.
2. **Second maxillary premolar** (lingual cusp): contacts DMR of the second mandibular premolar plus the MMR of the first mandibular molar.

3. **First maxillary molar:** (lingual cusps)

   a. **Mesiolingual cusp:** occludes in the central fossa of the first mandibular molar.

   b. **Distolingual cusp:** occludes in the DMR of the first mandibular molar plus the MMR of the second mandibular molar.

4. **Second maxillary molar:** (lingual cusps):

   a. **Mesiolingual cusp:** occludes in the central fossa of the second mandibular molar.

   b. **Distolingual cusp:** occludes on the DMR of the second mandibular molar plus the MMR of the third mandibular molar.

5. **Third maxillary molar:** (lingual cusps):

   a. **Mesiolingual cusp:** occludes in the central fossa of the third mandibular molar.

   b. **Distolingual cusp:** is usually missing.

GENERAL RULE OF MANDIBULAR POSTERIOR HOLDING CUSPS

These holding cusps occlude on the mesial marginal ridge of their counterpart in the maxillary arch plus the distal marginal ridges of the tooth mesial to its counterpart, with the exception of the **distobuccal cusp** of the molars, which occludes in the central fossa of the counterpart molar in the maxillary arch and **distal cusp of the mandibular first molar**, which occludes in the **distal triangular fossa of the maxillary first molar** and the buccal cusp of the mandibular first premolar, which only contacts the MMR of the maxillary first premolar.

1. **First mandibular premolar** (buccal cusps): contacts the MMR of the first maxillary premolar and is slightly out of contact with the DMR of the maxillary canine.

2. **Second mandibular premolar** (buccal cusps): contacts the DMR of the first maxillary premolar plus the MMR of the second maxillary premolar.

3. **First mandibular molar** (buccal cusps):

   a. Mesiobuccal cusp: contacts the DMR of the second maxillary premolar plus the MMR of the maxillary first molar.

   b. Distobuccal cusp: contacts the central fossae of the first maxillary molar.

   c. Distal cusp: occludes in the distal triangular fossa of the first maxillary molar.

4. **Second mandibular molar** (buccal cusps):

   a. Mesiobuccal cusp: occludes on the DMR of the maxillary first molar plus the MMR of the maxillary second molar.

   b. Distobuccal cusp: occludes in the central fossa of the second maxillary molar.

5. **Third mandibular molar** (buccal cusps):

   a. Mesiobuccal cusp: occludes on the DMR of the maxillary second molar plus the MMR of the maxillary third molar.

   b. Distobuccal cusp: occludes in the central fossa of the third maxillary molar.

GENERAL RULE OF MAXILLARY GUIDING CUSPS

The buccal cusps of the maxillary posterior teeth oppose the facial embrasure between its counterpart in the mandibular dentition and the tooth distal except for the mesiobuccal cusps of the molars, which oppose the buccal groove of its counterpart mandibular molar and the distobuccal cusp of the maxillary first molar, which opposes the distobuccal groove of the mandibular first molar.

1. **Maxillary first premolar** (buccal cusp): opposes the facial embrasure between the mandibular first premolar and the mandibular second premolar.

2. **Maxillary second premolar** (buccal cusp): opposes the facial embrasure between the mandibular second premolar and the mandibular first molar.

3. **Maxillary first molar** (buccal cusps):

   a. Mesiobuccal cusp: opposes the mesiobuccal groove of the first mandibular molar.

   b. Distobuccal cusp: opposes the distobuccal groove of the first mandibular molar.

4. **Maxillary second molar:**

   a. Mesiobuccal cusp: opposes the buccal groove of the second mandibular molar.

   b. Distobuccal cusp: opposes the facial embrasure between the second mandibular molar and third mandibular molar.

5. **Maxillary third molar:** Mesiobuccal cusp opposes the buccal groove of the third mandibular molar.

GENERAL RULE OF MANDIBULAR GUIDING CUSPS

A. The lingual cusps of the mandibular posterior teeth oppose the lingual embrasure between its counterpart in the maxillary dentition and the tooth mesial to it except the distolingual cusps of the molars, which oppose the lingual grooves of their maxillary counterpart molar.

B. **Anterior teeth** do not occlude or touch in normal occlusion. The maxillary anteriors overlap the mandibular anteriors. This in essence places the labioincisal angle of the mandibular incisors in opposition to the upper (incisal) lingual aspect of the maxillary incisors (i.e., the mesial and distal marginal ridge and lingual fossa). This makes the upper lingual surface of the maxillary incisors like a guiding slope and the labioincisal angle and incisal 1–2 mm of the labial surface of the mandibular incisors in essence a FOA.

   1. **First mandibular premolar** (lingual cusp): Very small cusp not really acting as guiding cusp will oppose the lingual embrasure between the maxillary canine and maxillary first premolar.

   2. **Second mandibular premolar** (lingual cusp): opposes the lingual embrasure between the maxillary first premolar and maxillary second premolar.

   3. **First mandibular molar:**

      a. **Mesiolingual cusp:** opposes the lingual embrasure between the maxillary second premolar and the maxillary first molar.

      b. **Distolingual cusp:** opposes the lingual groove of the maxillary first molar.

   4. **Second mandibular molar:**

      a. **Mesiolingual cusp:** opposes the lingual embrasure between the maxillary first and maxillary second molars.

      b. **Distolingual cusp:** opposes the lingual groove of the maxillary second molar.

   5. **Third mandibular molar**

      a. **Mesiolingual cusp:** opposes the lingual embrasure between the maxillary second and the maxillary third molars.

SUMMARY OF OPPOSITION

A. **Mandibular central incisor:** The labioincisal angle opposes the mesial marginal ridge of the maxillary central incisor, as well as the maxillary central's lingual fossa.

B. **Mandibular lateral incisor:** The labioincisal angle opposes the distal marginal ridge of the maxillary central and the mesial marginal ridge of the maxillary lateral, as well as the lingual fossa.

C. **Mandibular canine:** The cusp tip is located in the lingual embrasure between the maxillary canine and the maxillary lateral incisor.

D. **Maxillary central incisor:** Overlaps (vertically and horizontally) the mandibular central and lateral incisors, and its lingual surface is in opposition to them.

E. **Maxillary lateral incisor:** Overlaps the mandibular lateral and canine, and the lingual surface may be considered in opposition to them.

F. **Maxillary canine:** Cusp tip is located in the facial embrasure between the mandibular canine and first premolar.

Tooth Guidance in Mandibular Movements

Canine guided—The maxillary and mandibular canine contact during working side mandibular movement, causing all posterior teeth to disocclude.

Group function—The maxillary canine and buccal cusps of the posterior teeth contact during working side mandibular movement, causing the disocclusion of the posterior teeth on the nonworking side.

Anterior guidance—Contact between the lingual surface of the maxillary teeth and the facial surfaces of the mandibular teeth during protrusive movement of the mandible disocclude all the posterior teeth.

Arch (Angle) Classifications

Detailed information on Angle classification is not needed until the NBDE Part II. Know the classes described here.

Class I

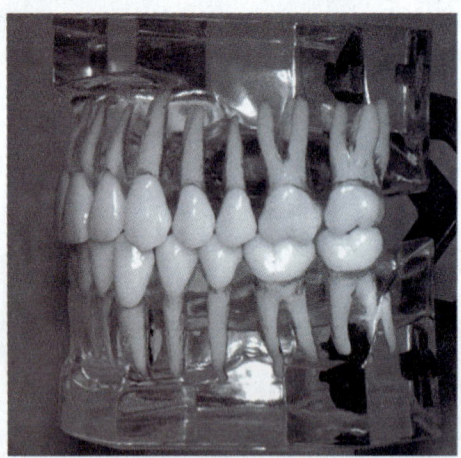

In reality, the class I type of occlusion described by Angle is a **malocclusion**. Even though it has a normal cusp-groove relationship, there may be anterior crowding. Normal occlusion is not classified by Angle's system. The mesiobuccal cusp of the first maxillary molar is **opposite** the mesiobuccal groove of the mandibular first molar. The maxillary canine is **in the labial embrasure** between the mandibular canine and the mandibular first premolar. Class I occlusion is often called neutroclusion.

Class II

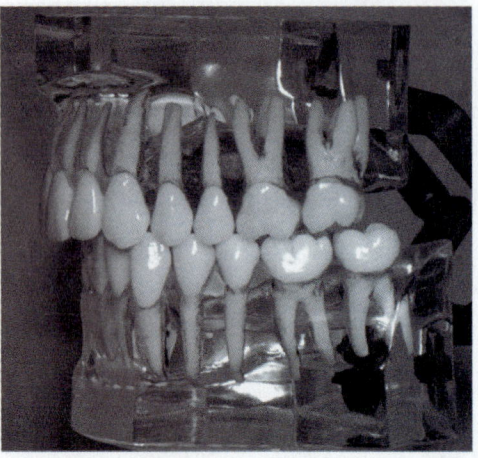

In class II occlusion, the mandible is small or **micrognathic**. The mesiobuccal cusp of the first maxillary molar is **anterior** to the mesiobuccal groove of the mandibular first molar. The maxillary canine is **anterior** to the **labial embrasure** of the mandibular canine and the mandibular first premolar (often called **distoclusion**). The lower teeth are abnormally distal to the upper teeth.

Class III

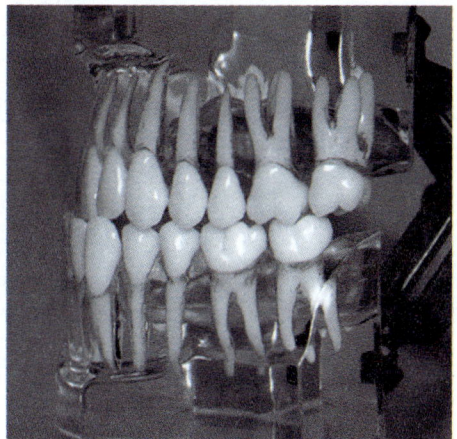

In class III occlusion, the mandible is large or **prognathic**. The mesiobuccal cusp of the first maxillary molar is **posterior** to the mesiobuccal groove of the mandibular first molar. The maxillary canine is **posterior** to the labial embrasure of the mandibular canine and the mandibular first premolar (often called **mesioclusion**). The lower teeth are mesial to the upper teeth.

Curves

Curve of Spee

The anterior−posterior relation of the teeth viewed from the lateral, i.e., from the side.

- The **maxillary** arch is **convex**.
- The **mandibular** arch is **concave**.

Curve of Wilson

The tilting of the mandibular posteriors lingually when the arches are viewed from the front (the maxillary posteriors tilt facially or buccally).

- The **maxillary** arch is **convex**.
- The **mandibular** arch is **concave.**

Table 4-3. Root Angulation

Roots	Angles
Mandibular	Anterior teeth angled distally
	Posterior teeth angled facially
Maxillary	Anterior teeth angled distally
	Posterior teeth angled lingually, except distobuccal root of first maxillary molar (inclined buccally)

Masticatory Muscle Function

Closing (elevating the mandible): Masseter, medial pterygoid, temporalis

Opening (depressing the mandible): Lateral pterygoid, mylohyoid, digastric, geniohyoid

Protruding: Lateral pterygoid

Lateral motion: Lateral pterygoid

- **Right lateral pterygoid:** moves the mandible to the **left**
- **Left lateral pterygoid:** moves the mandible to the **right**

Retruding: Temporalis, especially the posterior fibers. Mylohyoid, digastric, and geniohyoid are sometimes considered to be secondary retruders.

Temporomandibular Joint (TMJ)

The temporomandibular joint is both a **ginglymoarthrodial** joint (**hinge and gliding**) and a**diarthrosis** joint (**capable of free movement**). It is located between the mandibular (glenoid) fossa of the temporal bone and the condylar head of the mandible.

The **mandibular condyle** is an oblong process wider mediolaterally than anteroposteriorly with a rounded posterior aspect and concave anterior aspect (**fovea pterygoidea**). Its articulating surface, the **superior anterior aspect**, is slightly convex. The condyle, as well as the articular tubercle, is covered by a rather thick layer of fibrous avascular tissue (fibrous connective tissue). The **articular eminence** is located anterior to the rather thin-boned articular fossa of the temporal bone.

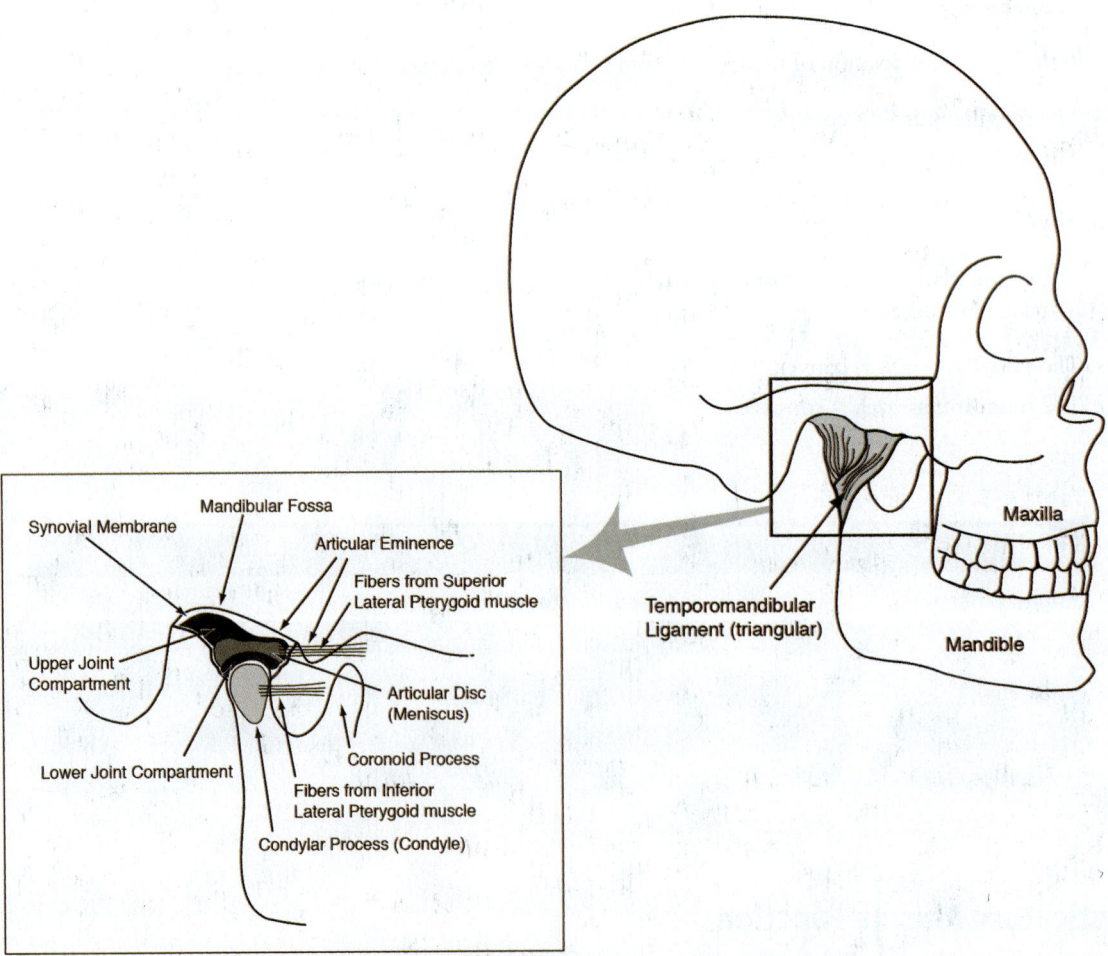

Figure 4-2. Structure of temporomandibular joint

Table 4-4. Detailed structure and histology of the TMJ

Bone	Condyle	**Cancellous (spongy)** bone covered by a thin layer of compact bone
		Marrow is red, except in older persons, where it may be replaced by fatty marrow
	Glenoid (mandibular) fossa	Roof of fossa consists of thin layer of compact bone
	Articular eminence	Consists of spongy bone covered with a thin layer of compact bone
Joint components	**Articular disc**	Dense, fibrous connective tissue with a few elastic fibers
		Center is very dense connective tissue; no blood vessels; thinner and avascular in center; more vascular in posterior and periphery
	Articular space	Divided into two compartments: • Lower—between condyle and disc (hinge movement, rotation) • Upper—between disc and temporal bone (sliding movement, translation)
Ligaments	**Temporomandibular (Lateral)**	Consists of two short, fibrous bands attached to: *(1)* the lateral surface of zygomatic arch and to the tubercle on its inferior border superiorly, and *(2)* the lateral surface and posterior border of the neck of the mandible inferiorly.
	Lateral ligament	Provides strong reinforcement of anterior lateral wall of capsule and helps prevent excess lateral and posterior displacement of mandible
	Sphenomandibular	Thin band attached to spine of sphenoid bone and descends to the lingula of the mandible, near the foramen; gives support to mandible and helps limit the maximum opening of the jaw
	Stylomandibular	Extends from near the apex of the styloid process of temporal bone to the angle and posterior border of the ramus of the mandible; relaxed when the mouth is closed and when in extreme protrusion becomes tense
	Capsular ligament (fibrous capsule)	Surrounds entire joint; composed of fibrous tissue reinforced by accessory ligaments; restricts movement of mandibular condyle on wide opening

Functional Contacting Movements

Working Side

When the mandible is moved to the left or right, it is the side to which the mandible is moved. (i.e.: When the mandible moves right, the right side is the working side.)

Non-Working Side (Balancing Side)

When the mandible is moved to the left or right, it is the side away from which the mandible moves. (i.e: When the mandible moves right, the left side is the balancing side.)

Table 4-5. Standard condylar movements with associated condylar positioning

	Movement of the Mandible	Working Side Condyle	Non-Working Side Condyle
Protrusive	Mandible moves directly forward	Both condyles move simultaneously **forward and downward** along the articular eminence	
Lateral	Mandible moves to right or left without moving forward	Condyle **rotates**	Condyle moves f**orward and downward**
Lateral protrusive	Combination of lateral and protrusive movements	Condyle **rotates** and moves **forward and down**	Condyle moves **anteriorly, downward, and medially**
Retrusive	Mandible moves directly backward	Both condyles move **upward and back** into mandibular fossa	

Mandibular Contacting Movement

When interpreting mandibular contacting movement, remember that the **maxillary teeth** are stationary and the **mandible** moves. If given a diagram of the maxillary arch with mandibular cusp pathways shown, the movement indicated would be the true movement of the mandible. If a diagram of mandibular teeth was shown, and maxillary cusps were illustrated, the movement of the maxillary cusps would be opposite the movement of the mandible.

The balancing side or nonworking side should not contact during the lateral contacting movements because of the mandibular condyles moving downward on the articular eminence.

The figures below illustrate contacting movement.

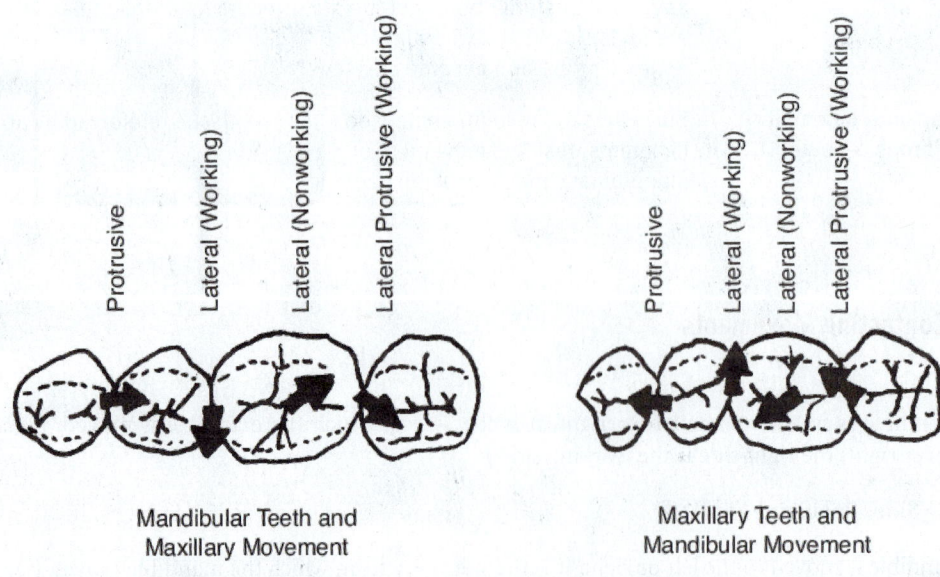

Mandibular Teeth and Maxillary Movement

Maxillary Teeth and Mandibular Movement

Figure 4-3. Relative movements of mandible and maxilla

Note that diagram on **right** is **actual** movement, diagram on **left** is **relative** movement. Arrows in diagrams are all opposite.

Recording Mandibular Movements

Expect at least one question on the Posselt envelope of motion. Remember that the outline is the extreme position of all movements. The mandible can take any position within this outline.

Posselt Envelope of Motion

The **Posselt envelope of motion** defines the border movements of the mandible. To arrive at this diagram, one could place a tracer in the mandible between the two central incisors and record the position of the tracer when the mandible moves. The tracing records the **anterior–posterior** and **inferior–superior** positions. Remember that this is a recording of mandibular motion **viewed from the lateral**.

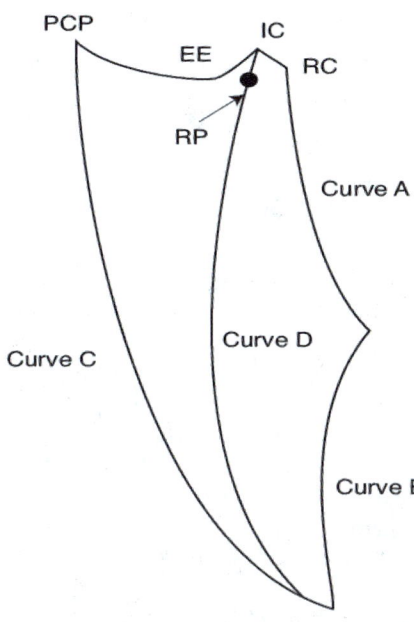

Intercuspal (IC) Position

The **intercuspal** (IC) position is the **highest position of the mandible** and is seen when the teeth are in maximum intercuspation. Also known as **centric occlusion**.

Retruded Contract (RC) Position

Retruded contact (RC) is the most retruded position of the mandible (retruded contacting position, centric relation). In 90% of the population, the IC (or centric occlusion) is approximately 1.25 mm anterior to the **centric relation,** and in the other 10%, IC corresponds to RC. When going to this RC position, the mandible must move downward and posteriorly from its height in the intercuspal position. This is because of the holding cusps of the mandibular teeth sliding on the mesial inclines of maxillary cusps located posterior to them.

Opening Movements

The **mandibular condyles** are capable of two types of **opening** movement when in retruded contacting position:

- **Pure rotational movement** (curve A in figure)—The rotatory movement accounts for the first 20 or so millimeters of mandibular opening, and then ligaments become taut. For further opening, the ligaments must be loosened, and this is achieved by the mandibular condyles moving down the articular eminence.
- **Translational movement** (curve B in figure)—The mandible opens further (translational movement) to its maximal opening (40–50 mm separation of the anterior teeth).

The line that connects the position of maximal opening to protruded contact position (curve C in figure) is the **protrusive opening path.** This line describes the curve made if the mandible were placed as far forward as possible and then opened as far as possible.

Curve D represents normal chewing movement.

Protruded Contact Position (PCP)

The protruded contact position (PCP) describes the most protruded or anterior position of the mandible. If the jaw is in this position, the incisors would not be in an edge-to-edge relationship, but instead the mandibular incisors would be more anterior than the maxillary incisors.

Edge to Edge (EE)

From PCP, remaining in tooth contact, the mandible is pulled backward until the incisors are edge to edge (**position EE, or "edge to edge"**). The mandible must move down so that the incisors can come edge to edge.

Moving from EE to IC, the mandibular cusps slide up the distal inclines of the maxillary cusps anterior to them. Curve D illustrates the mandibular path when opening to the position of maximum opening. This curve is not pure rotatory motion, but rather rotatory and **translational movement.** It is not a border movement because it occurs within the envelope of motion.

Normal Rest Position (RP)

Point RP is the normal position of the mandible. At rest, the teeth are not contacting. This position is also known as the **postural position** or **physiologic rest position**. The distance from RP to IC is called **freeway space.** That is, it represents the space between the teeth when the mandible is in the postural position (2–3 mm).

Rest position is determined primarily by musculature.

Frontal View

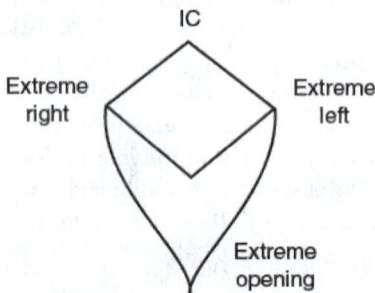

This figure represents the same movement as above, but here, in the lateral contacting positions, the mandible is opened to its maximum.

The **chewing stroke,** or **masticatory stroke,** when seen from the anterior on the lateral, is well within the borders of the mandibular movement. It is described as a pear- or tear-shaped movement. When chewing, the chewing is usually unilateral, favoring a particular side. This accounts for the displacement towards one side of the inferior portion of this movement.

Horizontal View (view from above or below)

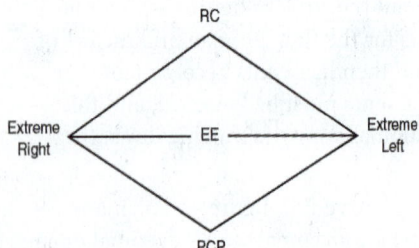

This diamond-shaped figure is a tracing of the mandible when starting in the RC position and then moving to the extreme right (right lateral contacting position), then moving to PCP (protruded contact position), then to the extreme left (left lateral contacting position), and finally back again to RC.

Oral Mucosa, Soft Tissue, Bone and Musculature

5

Learning Objectives

❏ Understand the histology of mucosa, bone, salivary glands, and other oral tissue

❏ Describe the process of mastication and swallowing

❏ Answer questions concerning non-tooth oral structures

The oral cavity is lined throughout with **oral epithelium(stratified, squamous epithelium)** and the underlying **lamina propria (connective tissue layer)**. Under the oral mucosa is the submucosa, which also differs from place to place, depending on the function of the particular area.

The surface epithelium may be categorized as **keratinized** or **non-keratinized**. A full keratinized potential does not present in mucosal cells under normal conditions, except in the masticatory mucosa. Mastication mucosa is found in the hard palate, gingiva, and dorsum of the tongue.

In **non-keratinized** oral epithelium, the outer two layers are termed the **intermediate** and **superficial** layers.

Table 5-1. Layers of Oral Epithelium

Layer	Characteristics
Stratum basal layer (stratum germinativum)	Single layer of cuboidal to low columnar cells Basal layer provides new cells for the other epithelial layers Found in both keratinized and non-keratinized epithelium Mitosis or cell division occurs at this level
Stratum spinosum (prickle cell layer)	A multilayer of polyhedral-like cells bound together by means of numerous desmosomal junctions Found in both keratinized and non-keratinized epithelium Toward the surface, these cells flatten and widen considerably **No further changes occur in the non-keratinizing epithelium**
Stratum granulosum*	Flattened polygonal cells filled with basophilic keratohyalin granules This layer is found in keratinized epithelium **only.**
Stratum corneum*	Flat cells filled with keratin This layer is found in keratinized epithelium **only.**

*In non-keratinized epithelium, the stratum granulosum and stratum coneum are not present, and the two outer layers are termed "intermediate" and "superficial" layers.

The **lamina propria** is a dense layer of connective tissue. Its papillae indent the epithelium and carry both blood vessels and nerves. Between the connective tissue papillae are the epithelial rete pegs.

Note that the epithelial layer down **not** have blood vessels.

Three types of stratified squamous epithelium are found in the oral cavity.

Table 5-2. Types of Stratified Squamous Epithelium

Type	Location	Characteristics	Appearance
Non-keratinized (nonmasticatory)	Buccal mucosa Cheeks Floor of the mouth Lips Soft palate Ventral surface of the tongue Alveolar mucosa	Basal cell, prickle cell, intermediate and outer most (superficial) non-keratinized layers	It appears as a soft, moist surface
Orthokeratinized (masticatory–stratum corneum cells lose their nuclei)	Gingiva (70-80%) Dorsum of the tongue Hard palate	Basal cell, prickle cell, granular layers. Stratum corneum cells are anuclear	Coral-pink in color and highly vascular
Parakeratinized – stratum corneum cells retain their nuclei	Gingiva (20-30%) Dorsum of the tongue	Basal cell, prickle cell, granular layers. Stratum corneum cells with nuclei.	Associated with lingual papillae of the tongue Taste buds present in this tissue

---

Note

In orthokeratinized epithelium, stratum corneum cells do **not** have a nucleus. In parakeratinized cells, they retain their nucleus.

Periodontium: Gingival Unit

The **gingival unit** consists of the **free gingiva, attached gingiva**, and **alveolar mucosa.** The gingival unit has a lining epithelium of either **masticatory mucosa**, which is thick keratinized epithelium with a dense collagenous connective tissue corium, or **lining mucosa**, which is thin, non-keratinized epithelium with loose connective tissue corium containing elastic, and sometimes muscle, fibers.

Masticatory mucosa is found in the free and the attached gingiva, hard palate, and dorsum of the tongue, and lining mucosa is found elsewhere in the oral cavity.

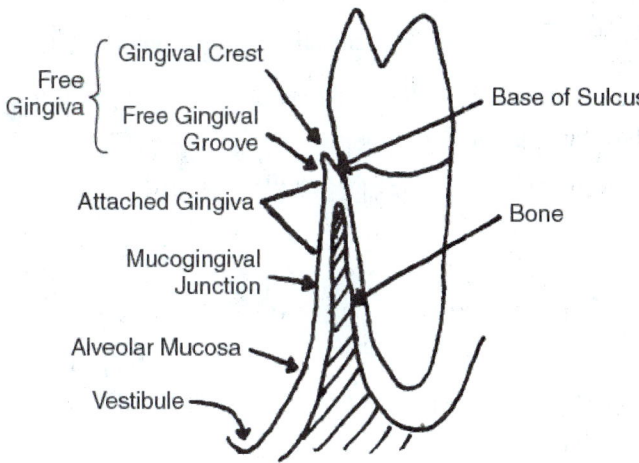

Free Gingiva: Gingiva located above the base of the gingival sulcus

Gingival Sulcus: Area between free gingiva and tooth surface

Free Gingival Groove: Indented line separating free gingiva from attached gingiva

Attached Gingiva: Gingiva below the free gingival groove and above the mucogingival junction

Alveolar Mucosa: Below the mucogingival junction

Attachment Apparatus

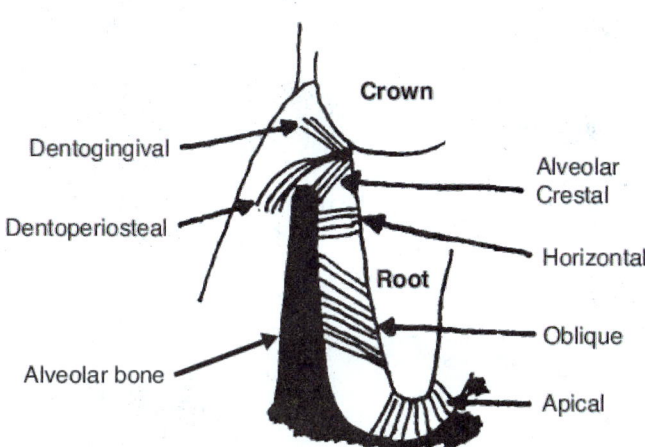

The attachment apparatus consists of the cementum, periodontal ligament, and alveolar bone. The periodontal ligament surrounds the tooth and connects to the bone, acting like a hammock. The attachment apparatus provides proprioceptive information to stimuli like pressure and pain. The bone and cementum can be resorbed when under controlled pressure, allowing for orthodontic movement of the teeth.

Principal Fiber Group

The principal fiber group comprises collagen fibers, which **do not attach to alveolar bone**.

- **Dentogingival:** Runs from the cementum into the free gingiva
- **Dentoperiosteal:** Runs from the cementum apically, over the alveolar crest of the bone, into the periosteum of the attached gingiva
- **Transseptal:** Runs from the cementum of one tooth, over the alveolar crest bone, to the cementum of an adjacent tooth
- **Circular:** Not attached to cementum; runs in the free gingiva around the tooth in a circular manner

Periodontal Fiber Group

The periodontal fiber group comprises collagen fibers, which **run from cementum to alveolar bone**.

- **Alveolar crestal:** Runs from supra-alveolar cementum down to the alveolar crest
- **Horizontal:** Runs from the cementum directly across to the alveolar bone
- **Oblique:** Largest group of fibers; runs from the cementum, from the root to the bone, in a diagonal coronal direction
- **Apical:** Runs from apex of root to alveolar bone in base of alveolus

The Periodontal Ligament (PDL)

The periodontal ligament (PDL) is the connective tissue that surrounds the root of the tooth and attaches the root of the tooth to the bony alveolus.

Functions

- **Formative:** cementoblasts, fibroblasts, and osteoblasts are derived from cells in the PDL
- **Supportive:** maintains the tooth in its position
- **Sensory:** extremely good innervation in PDL
- **Nutritive:** extremely good blood supply in the PDL

Blood supply

1. Periosteal blood supply from alveolar bone (**major source**)
2. Arteries of gingiva, which anastomose with the PDL (**minor source**)
3. Arteries of the periapical area, which arise from the vessels entering the pulp (**minor source**)

Nerve supply

- Nerves follow path of blood vessels
- Free nerve endings are receptors for pain and proprioceptive stimuli*

Lymphatics

- Follow path of blood vessels
- Flow of lymph is from ligament toward and into alveolar bone

    *Note: The proprioceptive information regulates the masticatory musculature and protects the tooth from sudden overload due to severe masticatory stresses.

Damage to the PDL

In Loss of Function

1. The PDL narrows.
2. The regular arrangement of fibers is lost.
3. The PDL becomes a thin membrane with irregularly arranged fibers.
4. Cementum may become thickened.

In Occlusal Trauma

1. Alveolar bone is reabsorbed.
2. PDL is widened.
3. Tooth becomes loose.
4. When source of trauma removed, repair usually occurs.

THE AVEOLAR PROCESS

The alveolar process is that part of the mandible and maxilla that forms and supports the sockets of the teeth. There is no anatomic boundary between the body of the maxilla or mandible and their respective alveolar processes.

There are two parts of the alveolar process:

1. **Alveolar bone proper:** consists of thin lamellar bone that surrounds the root of the tooth and gives attachment to the principal fibers of the PDL
2. **Supporting alveolar bone:** surrounds the alveolar bone proper and gives support to the socket

The supporting alveolar bone is divided into two parts:

1. **Cortical plates:** compact bone. These form the outer and inner plates of the alveolar processes.
2. **Spongy bone:** fills in the area between the cortical plates.

    Remember that the marrow spaces of the alveolar process may contain **hematopoetic marrow**, but they are usually found to contain **fatty marrow**. Hematopoetic marrow may be found in the adult in the condylar process, the angle of the mandible, the maxillary tuberosity, and in other areas.

SWALLOWING (DEGLUTITION)

The act of swallowing (deglutition) is generally broken down into three phases:

1. **Voluntary (oral)**
2. **Pharyngeal**
3. **Esophageal**

VOLUNTARY STAGE

A. After the bolus is prepared by mastication for swallowing to be initiated, the **oral cavity** must be sealed. This is normally done by closing the lips.

B. The mandible is stabilized by contraction of the masseter, internal (medial) pterygoid, and temporal muscles. This sometimes results in tooth contact, but not always. One of the few times that teeth would normally come together occurs during this process.

C. The **nasal cavity** is sealed by raising the soft palate.

D. The bolus on the tongue is carried to the posterior area of the oral cavity by raising the posterior part of the tongue. The bolus then slides into the oral pharynx, and the involuntary or reflex stages of swallowing take place (i.e., the pharyngeal and esophageal).

    Note: Tongue thrusting, a habit that may be developed to seal the oral cavity if the lips are unable to accomplish this necessary step in deglutition, may cause abnormal tongue pressure on the maxillary anteriors, causing an anterior open bite.

E. Teeth normally only contact during swallowing, and this contact is not necessary for swallowing.

MUSCLES OF MASTICATION

Four muscles are considered to be the primary muscles of mastication. Three others (to be listed later) also insert on the mandible and produce motion of the mandible.

A. The **temporalis** fibers arise from beneath the fascia overlying the lateral side of the temporal bone as well as sections of the frontal, occipital and sphenoid bones. They pass below the zygomatic arch and insert on the coronoid process of the mandible. Anterior and middle sections **elevate** the mandible, whereas posterior sections **retract** it.

B. The **masseter** arises from the zygomatic arch (medial and lateral sections) and inserts in periosteum of the lateral side of the angle of the mandible. It **elevates** the mandible.

C. The **medial pterygoid** arises from the medial surface of the pterygoid plate, the pyramidal process of the palatine bone, and the tubercle of the maxilla. It inserts in the medial side of the periosteum of the angle of the mandible. It **elevates** the mandible.

D. One head of the **lateral pterygoid** arises from the infratemporal surface of the sphenoid bone and inserts into the temporomandibular joint capsule and disc (superior head). The other head arises from the lateral surface of the pterygoid plate and inserts on the condyle of the mandible (inferior head). The lateral pterygoids **protrude**, **depress** (open), and **move the mandible from side to side**. Both lateral pterygoids acting together **protrude** the mandible or depress (open) the mandible, whereas one acting alone moves the mandible forward and laterally to the **opposite** side (*left* lateral pterygoid contraction moves the mandible to the *right*).

> ### Note
>
> Expect a number of questions in Dental Anatomy and Anatomic Sciences concerning the four major muscles of mastication.

The **masseteric sling consists** of the **medial pterygoid** (medially) and **masseter** (laterally). It supports the mandible and provides powerful closing (elevating) action.

Note: All four muscles are innervated by the **mandibular division of the trigeminal nerve** (CN V3). Also innervated by CN V3 are the mylohyoid, tensor tympani, tensor veli palatini, and the *anterior* diagastric.

The lateral surface of the medial pterygoid contacts the parotid gland, inferior alveolar artery, lingual nerve, inferior alveolar nerve, and chorda tympani nerve, which all run alongside it.

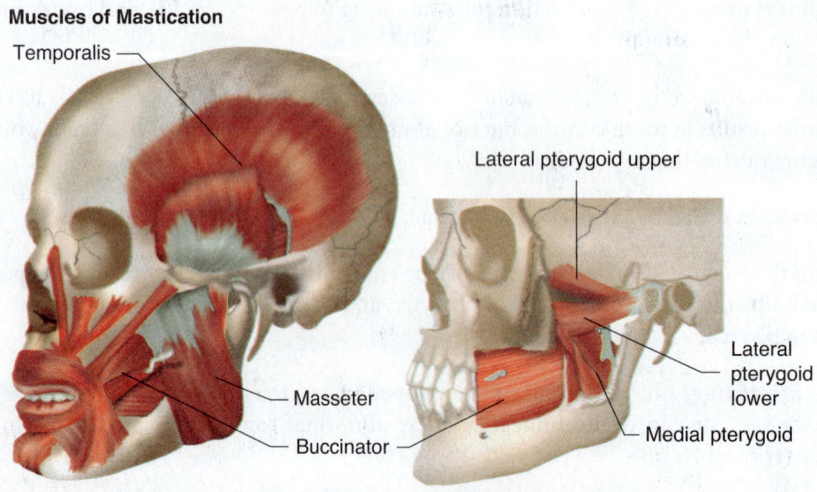

Muscles of Mastication

Temporalis

Lateral pterygoid upper

Lateral pterygoid lower

Masseter

Medial pterygoid

Buccinator

Figure 5-1. Mastication Muscle

E. The **digastric** has two sections: the anterior belly, which arises from the trochlea (hyoid sling) of the hyoid bone and inserts into the digastric fossa of the mandible, and the posterior belly, which arises from the mastoid process and passes through the trochlea of the hyoid bone. The anterior section is innervated by the mylohyoid branch of the mandibular nerve (CN V3). The posterior section is innervated by the digastric branch of the facial nerve (CN VII). It can depress (open) and retract the mandible.

Note

The major jaw opener (depressor) is the lateral pterygoid. The diagastric, mylohyoid, and geniohyoid are often called "accessory depressors."

F. The **mylohyoid** arises from both sides of the mandible, on the mylohyoid line. The two sections meet in a midline fibrous raphe, which connects to the hyoid bone. The mylohyoid forms a sling under the floor of the mouth. The mylohyoid is innervated by the **mylohyoid branch of the mandibular nerve** (V3). It can **depress** (open) the **mandible**.

G. The **geniohyoid** arises from the hyoid bone and inserts into the midline of the mandible (genio = chin). It is innervated by **fibers of C1 carried by the hypoglossal nerve** (XII). It can help **retract and depress** the mandible.

H. **Pharyngeal constrictor muscles:**

1. **Superior:** attaches to pterygomandibular raphe (with buccinator), pharyngeal raphe, and basioccipital bone

2. **Middle:** attaches to pharyngeal raphe, hyoid bone, and stylohyoid ligament

3. **Inferior:** attaches to pharyngeal raphe, thyroid cartilage, and cricoid cartilage

   All pharyngeal constrictors are innervated by CN X (vagus).

I. **Other pharyngeal muscles:**

1. Palatopharyngeus

2. Salpingopharyngeus

3. Both are innervated by CN X (vagus).

4. Stylopharyngeus is innervated by CN IX.

J. **Other innervations:**

1. **Facial expression:** (including buccinator) CN VII (facial)

2. **Digastric:** anterior—CN V3; posterior—CN VII

3. **Tensor veli palatini:** CN V3

4. **Levator palatini:** CN X (vagus)

5. **Sternocleidomastoid:** CN XI (accessory)

6. **Trapezius:** CN XI (accessory)

Note

All pharyngeal muscles are innervated by CN X except stylopharyngeus, which is innervated by CN IX (glossopharyngeal). It is the only muscle innervated by CN IX.

REVIEW OF MASTICATORY MUSCLE FUNCTIONS

A. **Closing (elevating):** masseter, medial pterygoid, temporalis (anterior and middle fibers)

B. **Opening (depressing):** lateral pterygoid, mylohyoid, digastric, geniohyoid

C. **Protruding:** lateral pterygoid

D. **Lateral motion:** lateral pterygoid. Right lateral pterygoid moves the mandible *left*. Left lateral pterygoid moves the mandible *right*.

E. *Cut* a lateral pterygoid, and mandible will move *toward* side of injury.

F. **Retruding:** temporalis, especially posterior fibers (minor retruders = geniohyoid, digastric)

INNERVATIONS OF IMPORTANT ORAL STRUCTURES

A. **Tongue:** The sensory (nontaste) innervation of the anterior two thirds of the tongue is by the **lingual branch of the mandibular nerve** (CN V3). The taste sensation of the anterior two thirds is by the **chorda tympani of the facial nerve**(CN VII) (except for the vallate papillae). Taste to the posterior one third of the tongue *and* the vallate papillae *and* general sensation to the posterior third is provided by the **lingual branch of the glossopharyngeal nerve**(CN IX). Some taste sensation to the posterior region of the valleculae is provided by the **superior laryngeal nerve of the vagus nerve**(CN X). Motor innervation to the entire tongue is provided by the **hypoglossal nerve**(CN XII).

B. **Teeth:** Lower molar and premolar teeth are innervated by branches of the **inferior alveolar nerve of the mandibular nerve** (CN V3). Lower incisors are innervated by the **incisal branches** of the same nerve. In the maxilla, there is overlap of innervation, but generally the third through first molars receive innervation from the **posterior superior alveolar nerve of the maxillary nerve** (CN V2). The first molar and premolars receive innervation from the **middle superior alveolar nerve of the maxillary nerve**. Canines and incisors are innervated by the **anterior superior alveolar nerve of the maxillary nerve**.

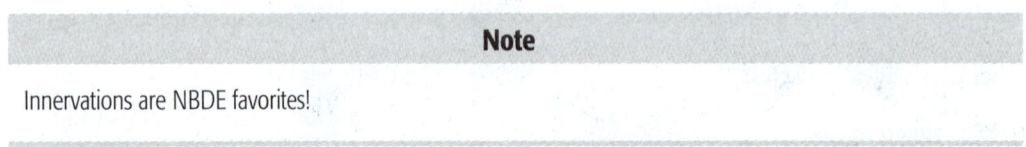

Note
Innervations are NBDE favorites!

C. **Supporting tissue:** On the lower arch, lingual gingiva and supporting tissues are innervated by the **lingual nerve of the mandibular nerve** (CN V3). Buccal surfaces in the molar region are innervated by branches of the **inferior alveolar nerve**, as well as by branches of the **buccal nerve**. Those supporting tissues in the buccal areas anterior to the molars are innervated by branches of the **mental nerve**.

On the upper arch, the buccal supporting tissues are innervated by the **anterior, middle, and posterior superior alveolar nerves**, whereas those areas on the lingual (palatal) side are innervated by the **greater palatine nerve**, except in the incisal area, where they are innervated by the **nasopalatine nerve**.

Table 5-3. Innervation of the Teeth and Supporting Structures

Teeth	Type	Innervation
	Lower molar and premolar	Inferior alveolar nerve of the mandibular nerve **(CN V3)**
	Lower incisors	Inferior alveolar nerve of the mandibular nerve **(CN V3)** incisal branch
	Maxillary third through first molar (except MO of first molar)	Posterior superior alveolar nerve of the maxillary nerve **(CN V2)**
	Mesial buccal root of the maxillary first molar and the maxillary premolars	Middle superior nerve of the maxillary nerve
	Maxillary canines and incisors	Anterior superior alveolar nerve of the maxillary nerve
Supporting Tissues	**Tissue**	**Innervation**
Mandibular	Lingual gingiva and supporting tissue	Lingual nerve of the mandibular nerve **(CN V3)**
	Buccal molar region	Inferior alveolar nerve and the buccal nerve (long buccal nerve)
	Anterior to molars	Mental nerve
Maxillary	Buccal tissues	Anterior, middle, and posterior superior alveolar nerve
	Posterior lingual (palatal)	Greater palatine nerve
	Anterior lingual (palatal)	Nasopalatine nerve

Note: The trigeminal nerve CN V supports both the dental (teeth) and the periodontal tissues. The maxillary nerve (CN V2) innervates the maxillary structures. The mandibular nerve (CN V3) innervates the mandibular structures.

SALIVARY GLANDS

A. **Specific Glands**

Saliva </ix>contains water, sodium, potassium, calcium, chloride bicarbonate, other mineral salts, immunoglobulins (especially secretory IgA), amylase, and mucopolysaccharides. It serves to lubricate, aid swallowing, digest starch to maltose, buffer acids, and cleanse the teeth and other oral structures.

1. **Parotid:** This is the **largest** of the salivary glands and contains **serous** (watery, nonmucous type) acini (secretory units). It has the highest level of **amylase** of any salivary gland. It produces approximately 30% of the total salivary volume. The parotid duct (**Stensen duct**) opens into the oral cavity near the upper second molars. Innervation to the gland is as follows: Secretomotor nerve fibers originate in the **glossopharyngeal nerve** (CN IX), pass in the **tympanic branch**, the **lesser petrosal nerve**, and synapse in the **otic ganglion**. Postganglionic fibers reach the gland in the **auriculotemporal nerve**. Sympathetic fibers reach the gland by traveling with the external carotid artery.

> **Note**
>
> Injections of anesthetic near the parotid can diffuse through the gland to the nearby facial nerve (CN VII).

2. **Sublingual:** The **smallest** of the three major glands, with the **lowest amylase content** and the **highest mucus content**. It empties through 10 to 20 ducts in the floor of the mouth (Plica sublingualis). Some of its secretion pushes through the Bartholin's duct to connect to the Wharton duct below. It is innervated by preganglionic fibers from the **chorda tympani** of the **facial nerve** (CN VII). They synapse in the **submandibular ganglion**, and postganglionic fibers travel directly to the gland. Sympathetic fibers reach the gland by traveling with the facial artery.

> **Note**
>
> Most texts describe the sublingual as almost (but not entirely) completely mucous.

3. **Submandibular:** Intermediate between the parotid and sublingual in size (about half the size of the parotid) and composition (**mixed serous and mucous**). The sublingual duct (**Wharton duct**) opens into the floor of the mouth on the sublingual papilla. Its innervation is the **same as that of the sublingual**. The submandibular produces the highest volume of saliva.

4. **Note:** Be aware of the following minor salivary glands:

von Ebner (of tongue)—serous	Palatine—mucous
Anterior lingual (Blandin or Nuhn)—mixed	Buccal—mixed
Labial— mixed	Glossopalatine—mucous

B. **Structure**

1. In mixed glands, mucous cells are nearer the duct opening, and serous cells are further back. Serous cells in mixed glands are often in "demilunes" or crescents surrounding the mucous cells. Their secretions pass by the enclosed mucous cells through "secretory capillaries" or "canaliculi."
2. Myoepithelial cells (basket cells) are presumed to help force out secretions through contractile action. They are located between secretory cells and the basal lamina.

C. **Ducts**

1. **Intercalated:** located closer to salivary production, structural ducts of cuboidal epithelium
2. **Striated:** Located farther toward duct. Striated ducts modify salivary concentrations. The striated appearance is due to mitochondria in rows. These mitochondria provide energy needed for active transport of ions. Striated duct cells are generally columnar epithelium.

D. **General histology: Gland types**

1. **Holocrine:** Entire cell becomes secretion (e.g., sebaceous).
2. **Apocrine:** Apex (only) of cell becomes secretion (e.g., lipid part of milk secretion).
3. **Merocrine:** (Most common) secretion through membrane by exocytosis. Cell cytoplasm itself is not lost as part of the secretion.
4. **Simple glands:** One secretory section is attached to one duct.
5. **Compound:** branched, with many secretory sections converging, eventually into one duct

DEVELOPMENT AND GROWTH OF UPPER AND LOWER JAWS

A. **Background:** Bones of the skull develop either by endochondral ossification replacing the cartilage or by **intramembranous ossification** in the mesenchyme (primitive connective tissue).

1. The **endochondral bones** are:

   a. The bones at the base of the skull

      i. Ethmoid bone

      ii. Inferior concha

      iii. Body, lesser wings, basal part of greater wings, and lateral plate of the pterygoid process of the sphenoid bone; petrosal part of temporal bone; basilar, lateral, and some of the squamous portion of the occipital bone condyle (**only**) of the mandible.

2. The **intramembranous bones** are:

   b. Frontal bones

   c. Parietal bones

   d. Squamous and tympanic parts of temporal bone

   e. Parts of the greater wings and medial plate of the pterygoid process of the sphenoid bone

   e. Upper part of the squamous portion of the occipital bone

   Remember: All the bones of the upper face develop by intramembranous ossification. The mandible develops as **intramembranous bone** lateral to the cartilage of the mandibular arch (Meckel cartilage), except for the condyle, which is endochondral.

B. **The maxilla:** The human maxilla is a derivative of two bones: the maxilla proper and the premaxilla. The premaxilla carries the maxillary incisor teeth and forms the anterior portion of the hard palate. The maxilla is primarily intramembranous.

   The upper jaw grows downward and forward due to appositional growth at the sutures of the maxillae and palatine bones.

C. **The mandible:** Remember that the mandible, as well as the maxilla, is a derivative of branchial arch I. The mandible is first seen in the sixth week of embryonic life as a thin plate of bone lateral to Meckel's cartilage. The mandible, except the condyle, develops by intramembranous ossification. Right through fetal life, the mandible is a paired bone. Right and left mandibles are joined in the midline by fibrocartilage in the mandibular symphysis. At the end of year 1, the fibrocartilage ossifies and the mandible becomes one bone.

   The lower jaw grows downward and forward due to appositional growth at the posterior border of the ramus of the mandible.

The Tongue

Table 5-4. Papillae Types

Papillae Type	Vascular/Nonvascular	Taste Buds?	Location
Filiform	Nonvascular	No	Rows, anterior to middle, keratinized
Fungiform	Vascular	Yes	Anterior only–non-keratinized
Circumvallate (vallate)	Vascular	Yes	10 to 12 only, V-shaped row near anterior/posterior border–non-keratinized
Foliate	Nonvascular	No	Lateral border of the tongue–non-keratinized

Foramen Caecum

Remnant of thyroglossal duct; located at the apex of the "V" formed by the circumvallate papillae.

Other Taste Buds

Additional taste buds can be found on the posterolateral palate, epiglottis, and the pharynx.

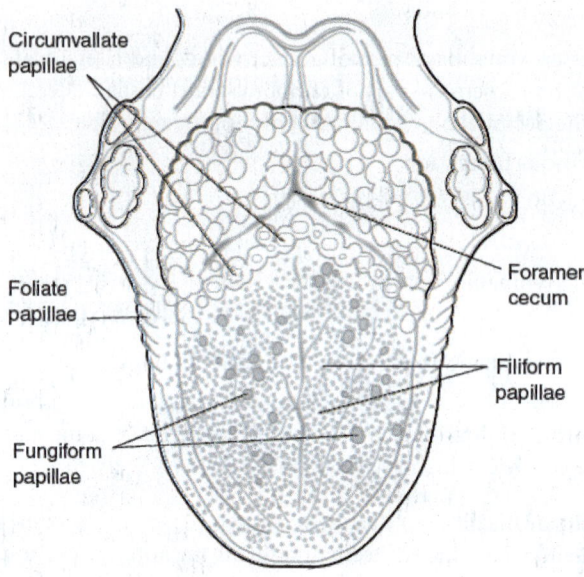

Figure 5-2. Tongue histology and papillae

Table 5-5. Innervation of the Tongue

Tongue	Function	Innervation
Anterior 2/3	Sensory, nontaste	Lingual branch of the mandibular nerve **(CN V)**
Anterior 2/3	Taste	Chorda tympani of the facial nerve **(CN VII)**
Posterior 1/3	Taste, general sensory	Lingual branch of the glossopharyngeal nerve **(CN IX)**
Most posterior tongue (base, root)	Taste, general sensory	Vagus nerve **(CN X)**
Entire tongue	Motor innervation	Hypoglossal nerve **(CN XII)** for intrinsic and extrinsic tongue muscles except palatoglossus **(CN X)**

Tongue Development

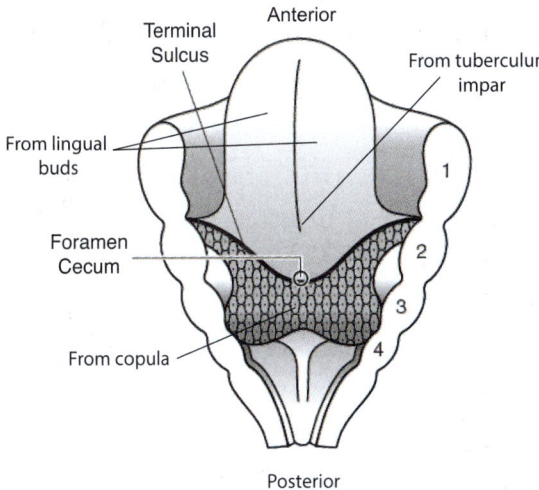

Development of the tongue

Branchial arches 1–4

Lingual buds (bilateral swellings, lateral)

Tuberculum impar (central)

Copula

Branchial arch and associated cranial nerve*

Arch 1—CN V

Arch 2—CN VII

Arch 3—CN IX

Arch 4—CN X

*Note that the order of innervation of the branchial arches is the same as the anterior to posterior innervation of the formed tongue.

Index